Emergency
Care and Transportation of the Sick and Injured

Real-life emergencies go beyond the curriculum, and so does the Seventh Edition of the Orange Book.

This book is part of an integrated training program that combines comprehensive medical content with exciting new features, design and technology to better support instructors and to help prepare students for the field.

The Seventh Edition contains significantly increased coverage of:

- **NEW** Patient Assessment and Ongoing Assessment
- **NEW** Anatomy and Physiology
- **NEW** Stroke and Seizure and Neurologic Emergencies
- **NEW** Medical Conditions with chapters on:
  - Acute Abdomen
  - Behavioral Emergencies
- **NEW** Specific Trauma Injuries with chapters on:
  - Kinematics of Trauma
  - Abdomen and Genitalia Injuries
  - Eye Injuries
  - Face and Throat Injuries
  - Chest Injuries
- **NEW** Pediatrics with chapters on:
  - Pediatric Airway and Resuscitation
  - Pediatric Assessment and Medical Emergencies
  - Pediatric Trauma
- **NEW** Geriatrics with a chapter on Geriatric Assessment and Transfer

This preview guides you through all of the new features and innovative enhancements designed to better meet the needs of today's EMT students and tomorrow's EMS providers.

162

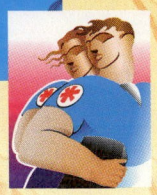

you are the emt

Rescue 6 please respond to the Altwood Apartments at 126th and Lexington for a man having shortness of breath. He is in Building C, apartment 9. Be advised that Engine 7 is already en route.

Calls for "breathing problems" are dispatched routinely every day. In fact, this is the most common reason people call 9-1-1. This chapter will prepare you to respond to many types of respiratory problems that you will encounter as an EMT-B and will help you to answer the following questions:

1. What type of respiratory emergencies should I expect to see as an EMT-B?

2. What is my role in caring for patients with this type of emergency?

NEW

you are the emt

Each chapter opens with a scenario. "you are the emt" captures students' attention and prepares them for important concepts presented in the chapter.

NEW

vital vocabulary

"vital vocabulary" highlights terms that students must know in the field. A comprehensive list of definitions is included in the "prep kit" at the end of the chapter. Pronunciations of terms are available at www.emtb.com so that students can listen to the proper pronunciation of difficult terms.

NEW

web links

"web links" directs students to the best EMS sites on the Internet. Web links reinforce and expand on important information from the chapters.

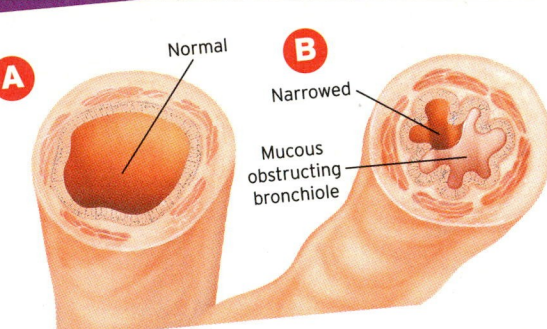

A Normal   **B** Narrowed

Mucous obstructing bronchiole

FIGURE 12-10 Acute spasms in the bronchioles cause asthma. **A:** Cross section of a normal bronchiole. **B:** The bronchiole in spasm; a mucus plug has formed and partially obstructed the bronchiole.

ruptures, often during coughing. A patient with a spontaneous pneumothorax becomes dyspneic (short of breath) and can complain of <u>pleuritic chest pain</u>, a sharp, stabbing pain on one side that is worse during breathing or with certain movement of the chest wall. By listening to the chest with the stethoscope, you can sometimes tell that breath sounds are absent or decreased on the affected side. However, altered breath sounds are very difficult to detect in a patient with severe emphysema. Spontaneous pneumothorax may be the cause of sudden dyspnea in a patient with underlying emphysema.

Asthma and Allergic Reactions

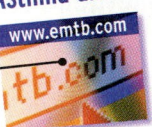

<u>Asthma</u> is an acute spasm of the smaller air passages called bronchioles, associated with excessive mucus production and sometimes with spasm of the bronchiolar muscles (Figure 12-10). It is a common but serious disease, affecting about 6 million Americans and killing some 4,000 to 5,000 Americans each year. Asthma produces a characteristic wheezing as patients attempt to exhale through partially obstructed air passages. These same air passages open easily during inspiration. In other words, when patients inhale, breathing appears relatively normal; the wheezing is heard only when they exhale. This wheezing may be so

---

substance that causes the reaction ever, there is no identifiable subst triggers the body's immune system be considered an allergen. An al tain foods or some other allergen asthma attack. Between attacks normally. In its most severe for can produce anaphylaxis and e This, in turn, may cause resp severe enough to result in co attacks may also be caused by exercise, or respiratory infectio

Most patients with asthma symptoms and know when Typically, they will have appr with them or at home. You what these patients tell you what they need.

Asthma and anaphylactic not have asthma may still ha The same allergens that may cause anaphylaxis, a reacti swelling and dilation of blo which may lower blood pre laxis may be associated wit asthmalike condition. The a breathing problems can pr in breathing to total airwa few minutes. Most anaph 30 minutes of exposure anything from eating certa injection. For some patie they had such a reaction t may not know what cause tion. In other cases, the p but not be aware of exp rine is the treatment o tamines are also usefu should guide appropria

Hay fever. A much m problem is hay fever. T tion to pollen. In so pollen is present in fever is almost a univ

preview

caring for kids

Asthma is a common childhood illness. When assessing a pediatric patient, look for retraction of the skin above the sternum and between the ribs. Retractions are typically easier to see in children than in adults. Cyanosis is a late finding in children. Keep in mind that a cough may not be a symptom of a cold; it could signal pneumonia or asthma. Even if you do not hear much wheezing, the presence of a cough can indicate that some degree of reactive airway disease, or a frank asthma attack may be taking place.

The emergency care of a child with shortness of breath is the same as it is for an adult, including the use of supplemental oxygen. However, many small children will not tolerate (or may refuse to wear) a face mask. Rather than fighting with the child, hold the oxygen mask in front of the child's face or ask the parent to hold the mask (Figure 12-16). Many children with asthma also will have prescribed hand-held metered-dose inhalers. Use these inhalers just as you would with an adult.

caring for kids

"caring for kids" is a feature dedicated to pediatrics and puts the special needs of pediatric patients into the context of the chapter.

caring for the elderly

"caring for the elderly" focuses on geriatric considerations and puts the special needs of geriatric patients into the context of the chapter.

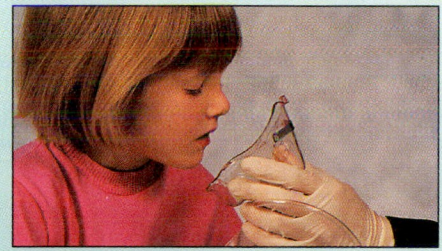

FIGURE 12-16 Because children may refuse to wear an oxygen mask, you may have to hold the mask in front of the child's face. If the child still refuses, enlist the parents' help.

caring for the elderly

As we get older, normal aging processes alter the respiratory system and our ability to exchange oxygen and carbon dioxide. If the patient is a smoker, the disease processes of emphysema or chronic bronchitis can hasten or worsen these changes.

Several changes occur as we age. The chest wall, including the muscles and ribs, become less resilient. Additionally, the bronchi and bronchioles lose their muscle mass or tone, and the air sacs (alveoli) become stiffer and less able to recoil (relax and empty) in exhaling. If the chest wall, including muscles and ribs, is weaker or less flexible, the chest cavity cannot expand as easily, and the total amount of air that is allowed into the lungs will be reduced. With decreased recoil of the lungs, alveoli can become distended with air trapped inside. If you are required to ventilate, the (nonbreathing)

The geriatric patient is at an increased risk of pneumonia or a worsening of asthma or COPD if the airways have lost muscle mass or tone. Secretions might not be expelled from the airways, allowing pneumonia to develop.

The result of normal changes with aging is a reduction of the total amount of air the lungs can hold, air becoming trapped in overstretched alveoli, and increased resistance to air flow into and out of the lungs. Ultimately, all these changes cause a decreased oxygen/carbon dioxide exchange in the respiratory system with reduced oxygen delivery to the cells. Be sure to consider changes in aging that affect the respiratory system and provide adequate ventilation and oxygenation according to the patient's needs. The [geriatric] patient may need ventilatory support for [conditi]ons that, in the younger adult, are easily [accomm]odated by the respiratory system.

SKILL EMT-B DRILL

Stabilizing a Suspected Neck Injury

Figure 20-13

skill drills

"skill drills" provide a step-by-step, visual summary of the most important skills and procedures for easy reference.

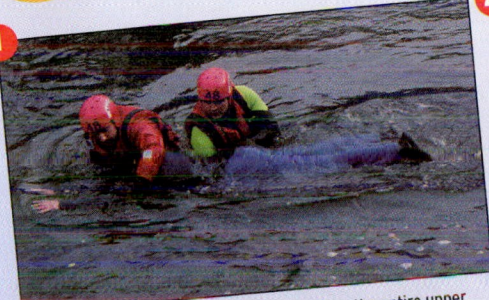

1 Turn the patient to a supine position by rotating the entire upper half of the body as a single unit.

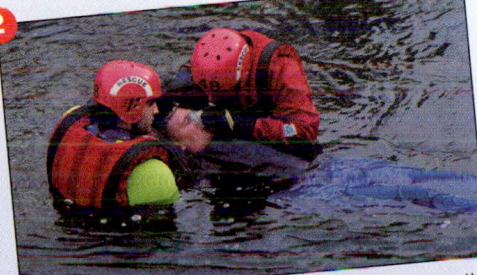

2 As soon as the patient is turned, begin artificial ventilation using the mouth-to-mouth method or a pocket mask.

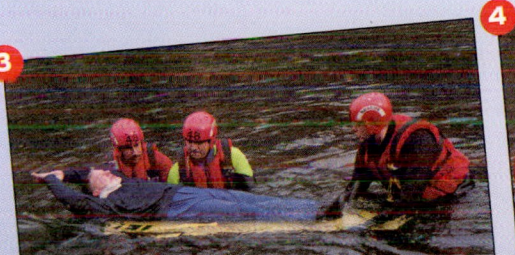

3

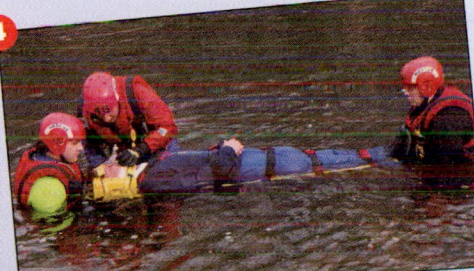

4

preview

NEW

Patient Assessment Flowchart
A flowchart provides a quick, visual reference for the patient assessment process.

The chapter is divided into 6 sections. The Patient Assessment Flowchart is repeated at the beginning of every section to show students "at a glance" where they are in the patient assessment process.

Each section of the flowchart is color-coded and numbered for easy reference.

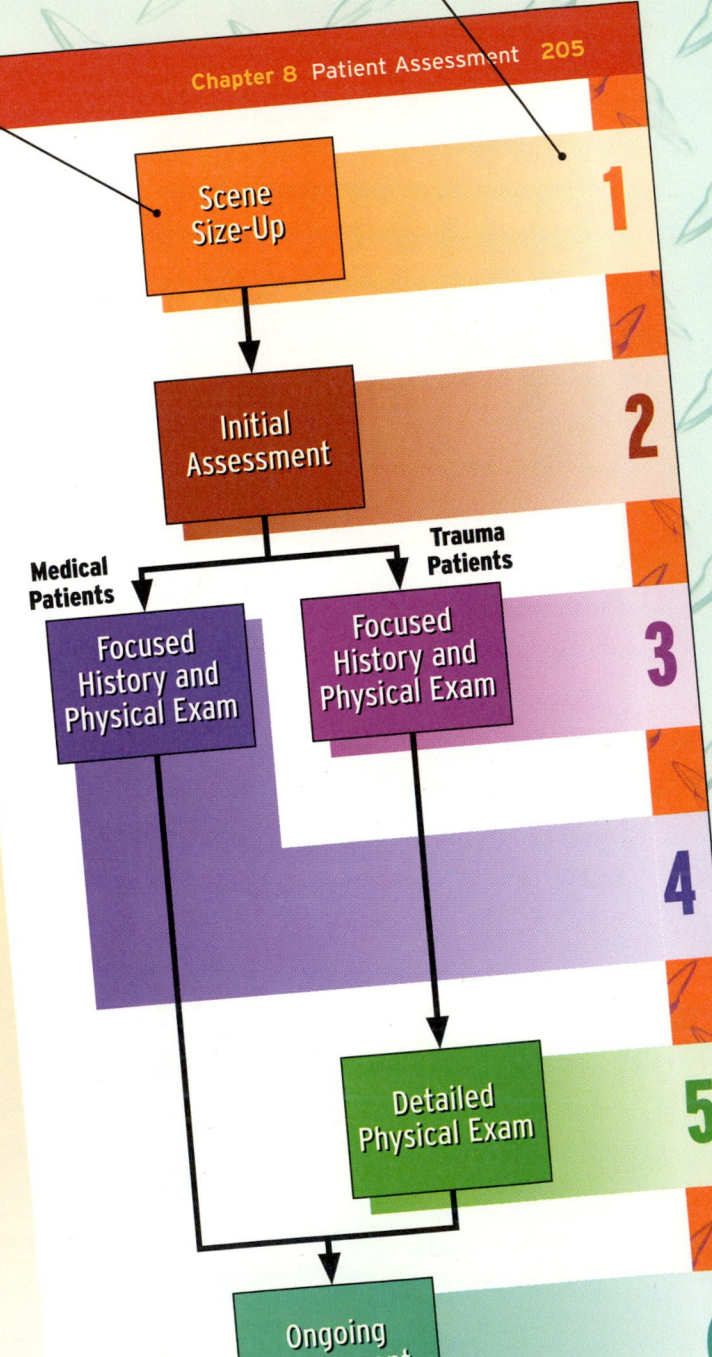

Chapter 8 Patient Assessment **205**

PATIENT ASSESSMENT FLOWCHART

Scene Size-Up

1 Scene Size-Up

2 Initial Assessment

Medical Patients — Focused History and Physical Exam

Trauma Patients — Focused History and Physical Exam

3

4

5 Detailed Physical Exam

6 Ongoing Assessment

An outline provides an overview of each section of the patient assessment process, which follows the DOT National Standard EMT-B Curriculum.

NEW

prep kit

End-of-chapter activities reinforce important concepts and improve student comprehension. The activities are expanded upon in the student workbook. Additional instructor support and answers to all activities are contained in the Instructor's Resource Kit for a truly integrated teaching and learning system.

NEW

ready for review

"ready for review" thoroughly summarizes the chapter.

---

180 Medical Emergencies Section 4

prep kit

ready for review

Dyspnea is a common complaint that may be caused by numerous medical problems, including infections of the upper or lower airways, acute pulmonary edema, chronic obstructive pulmonary disease, spontaneous pneumothorax, asthma or allergic reactions, pleural effusions, mechanical obstruction of the airway, pulmonary embolism, and hyperventilation. Each of these lung disorders interferes in one way or another with the exchange of oxygen and carbon dioxide that takes place during respiration. This interference may be in the form of damage to the alveoli, separation of the alveoli from the pulmonary vessels by fluid or infection, obstruction of the air passages, or air or excess fluid in the pleural space. Patients with longstanding lung diseases often have chronically high levels of blood carbon dioxide; in some cases, giving too much oxygen to these patients may depress or stop respirations. However, judicious use of oxygen is always an important priority in patients with dyspnea.

Signs and symptoms of breathing difficulty include unusual breath sounds, including wheezing, stridor, rales, and rhonchi; nasal flaring; pursed lip breathing; cyanosis; inability to talk; use of accessory muscles to breathe; and sitting in the tripod position, which allows the diaphragm the most room to function.

In treating dyspnea, it is important to reassure the patient and provide supplemental oxygen. Remember to maintain the patient in a position that is comfortable for breathing, usually sitting upright. If the patient is not breathing, use a BVM device to assist breathing. If the patient is breathing with great difficulty, apply oxygen through a nonrebreathing face mask with the oxygen flow set at 10 to 15 L/min. Next, perform a focused history and physical exam, including vital signs. If the patient has a prescribed inhaler or epinephrine injector, consult medical control to assist with its use. Then transport the patient to the hospital, monitoring his or her condition on the way. Talking with the patient is a good way to monitor a breathing problem.

Remember, a patient who is breathing rapidly may be getting insufficient oxygen as a result of respiratory distress from a variety of problems, including pneumonia or a pulmonary embolism; trying to "blow off" more carbon dioxide to compensate for acidosis caused by a poison, a severe infection, or a high level of blood glucose; or having a stress reaction. In every case, prompt recognition of the problem, giving oxygen, and prompt transport are essential.

prep kit

vital vocabulary

allergen A substance that causes an allergic reaction.

asthma A disease of the lungs in which muscle spasm in the small air passageways and the production of large amounts of mucus result in airway obstruction.

bronchitis Irritation of the major lung passageways, from either infectious disease or irritants such as smoke.

carbon dioxide retention A condition characterized by a chronically high blood level of carbon dioxide in which the respiratory center no longer responds to high blood levels of carbon dioxide.

chronic obstructive pulmonary disease (COPD) A slow process of dilation and disruption of the airways and alveoli, caused by chronic bronchial obstruction.

common cold Usually associated with swollen nasal mucous membranes and the production of fluid from the sinuses and nose.

croup An infectious disease of the upper respiratory system that may cause partial airway obstruction and is characterized by a barking cough; usually seen in children.

diphtheria An infectious disease in which a membrane lining the pharynx is formed that can severely obstruct passage of air into the larynx.

dyspnea Shortness of breath or difficulty breathing.

embolus A blood clot or other substance that has formed in a blood vessel or in the heart that breaks off and travels to another blood vessel, where it causes blockage.

emphysema A disease of the lungs in which there is extreme dilation and eventual destruction of pulmonary alveoli with poor exchange of oxygen and carbon dioxide; it is one form of chronic obstructive pulmonary disease (COPD).

www.emtb.com

epiglottitis An infectious disease in which the epiglottis becomes inflamed and enlarged and may cause upper airway obstruction.

hyperventilation A lowering of blood carbon dioxide levels, usually through rapid or deep breathing.

hypoxia A condition in which the body's cells and tissues do not have enough oxygen.

pleural effusion A collection of fluid between the lung and chest wall that may compress the lung.

pleuritic chest pain Sharp, stabbing pain in the chest that is worsened by a deep breath; often caused by inflammation or irritation of the pleura.

pneumonia An infectious disease of the lung that damages and destroys lung tissue.

pneumothorax A partial or complete accumulation of air in the pleural space.

pulmonary edema A buildup of fluid in the lungs, usually as a result of congestive heart failure.

pulmonary embolism The condition in which a blood clot breaks off from a large vein and travels to the blood vessels of the lung, causing obstruction of blood flow.

rales Crackling, rattling breath sounds signaling fluid in the air spaces of the lungs.

rhonchi Coarse breath sounds heard in patients with chronic mucus in the airways.

stridor A harsh, high-pitched inspiratory sound, such as the sound often heard in acute laryngeal (upper airway) obstruction.

wheeze A high-pitched, whistling breath sound, characteristically heard on expiration in patients with asthma or COPD.

NEW

vital vocabulary

"vital vocabulary" pronunciations are available at www.emtb.com. Your students can listen to the proper pronunciation of difficult terms.

preview

NEW

assessment in action

"assessment in action" promotes critical thinking and provides you with discussion points to use in class.

assessment in action

You receive a call for assistance from a local bookseller specializing in old and antique books. When you arrive, you find one of the customers, a 38-year-old man, seated in a hunched-over position in one of the back aisles. You notice immediately that the patient seems to be breathing very fast. As you begin to ask him questions, you find that he can speak only in short, three- and four-word bursts. He manages to tell you that he had been looking at old books for the last hour when his chest started to tighten up, possibly from the dust. The patient also tells you that he uses a Ventolin inhaler, but he left it in his car. The patient says that he smokes about two packs of cigarettes a week. Your partner obtains baseline vital signs. The patient has a blood pressure of 152/90 mm Hg, a regular pulse of 122 beats/min, and shallow respirations of 34 breaths/min.

1. Which of the following steps would be **LEAST** helpful in assessing this patient's respiratory status?
   A. Assessing the depth of the breaths
   B. Evaluating the use of accessory muscles
   C. Counting the number of breaths in a minute
   D. Compressing the rib cage for injuries or deformity

2. Another customer offers to let the patient use her inhaler when he states that he thinks he needs an inhaler. The most appropriate course of action would be to:
   A. thank the other customer and state that the patient needs his own inhaler.
   B. check for breath sounds, then let the patient use the other customer's inhaler.
   C. observe the patient as the other customer helps the patient use her inhaler.
   D. obtain another set of vital signs, then let the patient use the other customer's inhaler.

3. Which of the following statements about administering medication via an inhaler is **FALSE**?
   A. The medication in the inhaler does not expire.
   B. The inhaler should be shaken vigorously before each use.
   C. The inhaler should be used at room temperature or warmer.
   D. The medication in the inhaler relaxes the muscles that surround the bronchioles.

4. The patient finds an almost-empty inhaler in his briefcase and uses it. Which of the following would **NOT** be considered a side effect of using his inhaler?
   A. Nervousness
   B. Symptom relief
   C. Increased pulse
   D. Tremors or shaking

5. Which of the following facts from the patient's history is **LEAST** important as you assess the patient and plan his care?
   A. The patient is a 38-year-old man.
   B. The patient uses Ventolin to treat his asthma.
   C. The patient smokes two packs of cigarettes a week.
   D. The patient is currently taking antibiotics for a sinus infection.

prep kit 12

points to ponder

Objectives 1-2.5, 1-2.6

You are returning from lunch when you hear the dispatch of another unit to a drowning at an apartment complex about half a block away from where you are. You "jump" the call and turn into the complex. You arrive at the pool as the rescuers hand out an 18-month-old child. The child is cyanotic and unresponsive. You find a pulse but no breathing. Your partner has a child about that same age and is shaken by this call. Just before transport, the child "crashes," losing its pulse also. Even with the best care you could provide, the child does not make it. Now you are back out on duty, your partner is barely functioning, and when you close your eyes, you can see the child and the look on your partner's face as you took control of the scene. There are about six hours left in your shift.

- Would you stay on duty? What would you do to help your partner? What would you do to help yourself?

online outlook

The term "chronic obstructive pulmonary disease" (COPD) comprises emphysema and chronic bronchitis. The number of lives that are claimed by chronic lung disease has increased sharply. In 1979, it accounted for about 50,000 deaths. In 1982, the number rose to 59,000, and by 1992, the number of deaths reached 86,974. To learn more about COPD, complete Exercise 12 at the www.emtb.com.

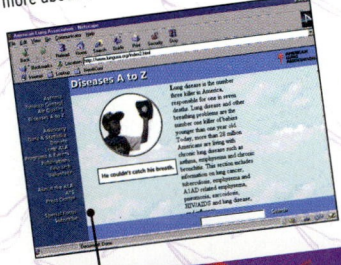

NEW

points to ponder

"points to ponder" tackle cultural, social, ethical, and legal issues that directly relate to curriculum objectives.

NEW

online outlook

"online outlook" guides exploration of the World Wide Web. In addition, activities reinforce and expand on important information from the chapter.

preview

registry review

A practice exam based on the blueprint for the National Registry Exam will help your students to better prepare for tests.

appendix b

...ear-old patient should ...epth and rate of:

A. ½" to 1", at a rate of 140/min.
B. 1" to 1½", at a rate of 100/min.
C. 1" to 2", at a rate of 60 to 80/min.
D. ¾" to 2", at a rate of 100 to 120/min.

12. A local celebrity has severe injuries as a result of an automobile-truck accident. The highway is closed by law enforcement officials, but the media is allowed to cover the story. A reporter approaches you and asks the condition of the patient. You should:

A. ignore the reporter.
B. answer the reporter's questions as best you can.
C. tell the reporter the patient will be fine to pro-tect his privacy.
D. explain that you cannot comment and that the reporter should contact the hospital.

13. Gastric distention during artificial ventilation is considered dangerous because it can:

A. stimulate hyperventilation.
B. result in bacterial pneumonia.
C. cause the patient to vomit during CPR.
D. increase lung volume by elevating the diaphragm.

14. The best way to estimate a ...

17. In most instances, cardiac arrest in infants and children results from:

A. electrocution.
B. respiratory arrest.
C. severe head trauma.
D. severe hypothermia.

18. In which of the following situations has expressed consent been given?

A. A 5-year-old child who says, "Make me better"
B. An unconscious 26-year-old woman who has a bleeding head wound
C. A 35-year-old man who has a slight concussion but holds his bleeding arm out for bandaging
D. An 86-year-old man who stares blankly at his bleeding leg and says, "What happened to me?"

19. Which of the following signs is seen in respiratory depression?

A. Rapid, shallow respirations
B. Deep, labored, noisy respirations
C. Strong airflow at the nose and mouth
D. Little or no movement of the chest and abdomen

20. If an injured patient needs to be moved, ...
in immediate dang... ...

online outlook is as easy as 1...2...3

1 Go to www.emtb.com and select online outlook

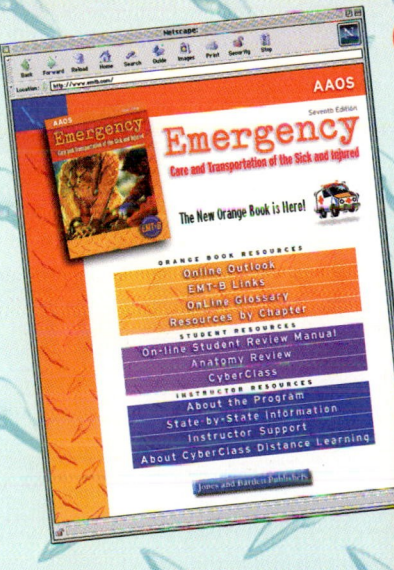

2 Link to Chapter 12 online outlook

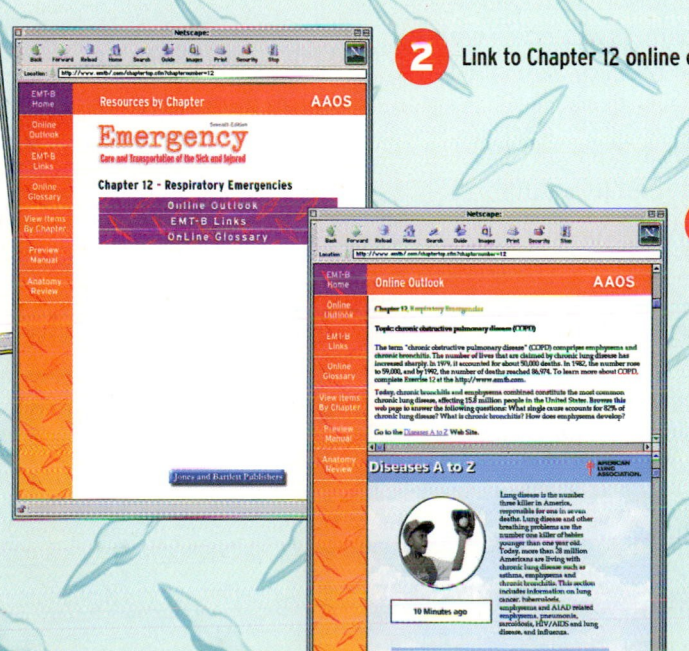

3 A brief recap of a topic is presented again on the web site. The student is then asked to complete activities using the links provided.

Links to outside web sites provide up-to-date information. Links will be changed as new information is uncovered, or if links are broken.

Instructor Resources:

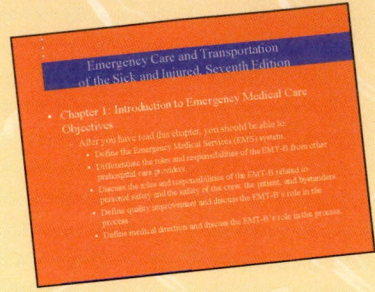

Instructor's CD-ROM and PowerPoint Presentation

We have made it easier for you with:

NEW

- Lesson plans laid out in a customizable PowerPoint presentation
- Online Outlook and www.emtb.com screen captures show students interesting Internet sites
- Images from the text to incorporate into class lectures
- Video clips

ISBN: 0-7637-0929-8

Instructor's Resource Kit

The **Instructor's Resource Kit** has been designed to be your quick-reference guide. The IRK practically plans each class for you.

It is a series of self-contained booklets, one for each section of the text, and includes:

- Detailed lesson plans for both curriculum objectives and enhancement materials with sample lectures, lesson quizzes, and suggested readings
- Teaching tips and ideas to enhance your presentation, cuts down on prep time
- Activities and games to enhance classroom learning

ISBN: 0-7637-0936-0

Monthly Newsletter

Instructors who adopt *Emergency Care and Transportation of the Sick and Injured, Seventh Edition* will be connected to EMS educators worldwide, via a free monthly e-mail newsletter. You will benefit from shared teaching tips, classroom experiences, and strategies.

NEW ## Instructor's Video Set

10 compelling videos that capture real-life scenes from the street. Each video has been enriched with thought-provoking questions to stimulate classroom discussion and encourage critical thinking. (Set includes: Patient Assessment, Lifting and Moving, Geriatrics, Pediatrics (2), Trauma, Communications, The EMS Call The Well-Being of the EMS Provider, and Airway.)

ISBN: 0-7637-1025-3

Videos are also sold separately.

Instructor's Test Bank

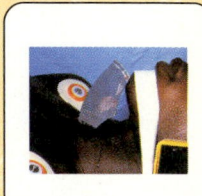

Created exclusively by EMS educators, this new test bank follows the cognitive objectives of the EMT-B National Standard Curriculum.

- Over 1,500 multiple-choice questions
- Each question has been correlated to the appropriate cognitive objective in the EMT-B National Standard Curriculum and page in the text
- The Test Bank is available in two formats; print and instructor customizable electronic versions

ISBN: PRINT 0-7637-0931-X
IBM 0-7637-0933-6

Instructor's Slide Set

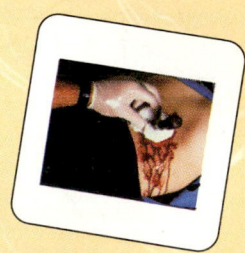

1,200 informative slides emphasize key points and stimulate discussion with realistic examples for EMT training.

ISBN: 0-7637-0934-4

Trauma Slide Set

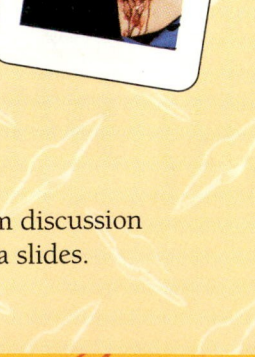

Bring the "real world" to your classroom discussion with approximately 100 real-life trauma slides.

ISBN: 0-7637-0656-6

Student Resources:

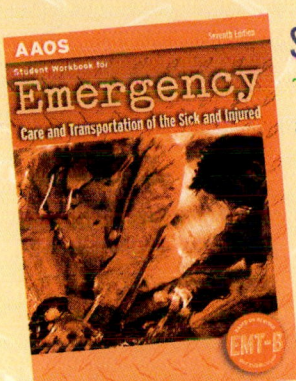

Student Workbook

The self-correcting workbook's additional review questions focus on curriculum objectives, basic concepts, and principles, as they appear in the Seventh Edition.

ISBN: 0-7637-0804-6

Student CD-ROM

This CD-ROM covers key EMT-B topics, and has been developed to challenge students' mastery through scenario-based learning, and full motion video clips.

ISBN: 0-7637-0928-X

NEW

EMT-B Student Review Manual, 3rd Edition

The review manual provides students with an easy and convenient way to test their knowledge. The **Student Review Manual** corresponds directly to the Seventh Edition. The following features are included for each chapter:

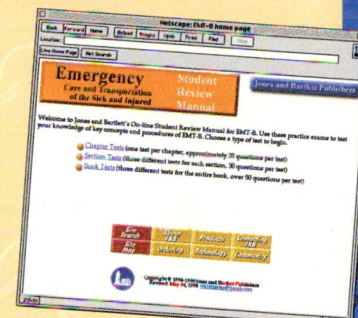

- 20-40 multiple choice questions
- Brief explanations for those questions answered incorrectly
- A page-by-page correlation of the question/answer to the text

NEW

The Student Review Manual is also available on-line at www.emtb.com, with approximately 650 images and an automated grading feature.

ISBN: Text—0-7637-1026-1
      Disk—0-7637-1043-1
      Text & Disk—0-7637-1042-3

Internet Resources

NEW

www.emtb.com

www.emtb.com has been specifically developed to complement the Seventh Edition, and is regularly updated.

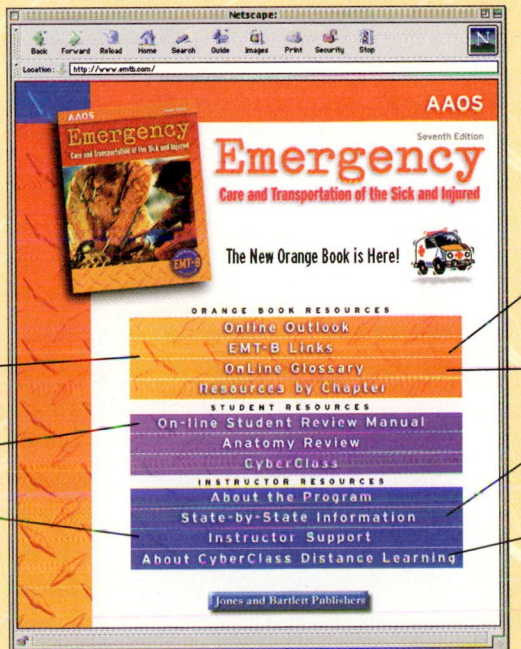

Offers value-added activities and links to the best EMS sites on the Internet.

Quizzes on the material found in the text.

Provides teaching tips, strategies, and other instructor support.

Reinforces and expands on topics discussed within the chapter.

Defines key terms and includes images and pronunciations.

State-specific information as related to EMT-B.

This is an invaluable class-management and communication tool for you and your students. An ideal way for students to catch up on lectures when they miss a class.

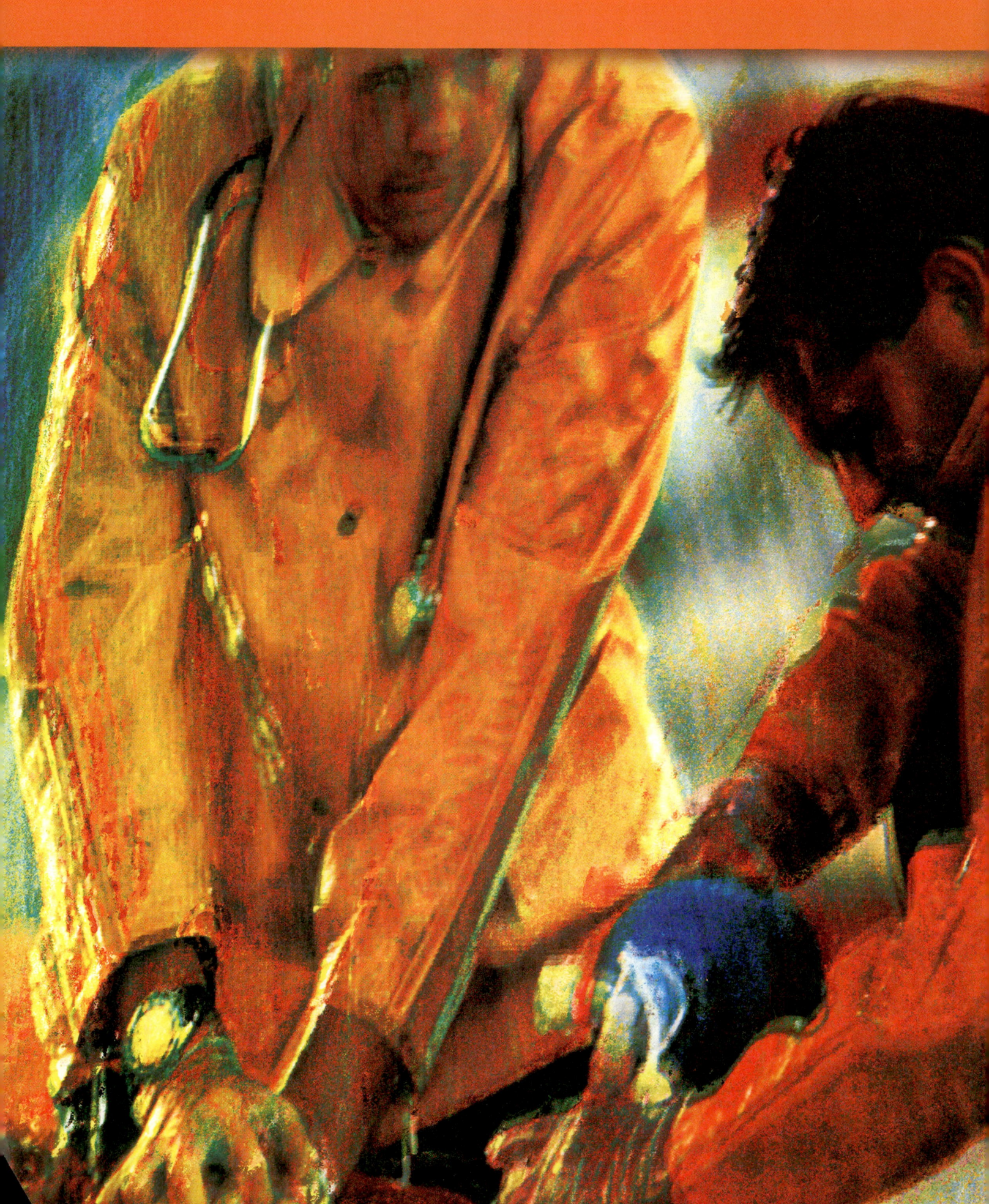

Seventh Edition

Emergency
Care and Transportation of the Sick and Injured

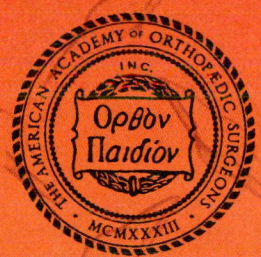

American Academy of Orthopaedic Surgeons

Editors:

Bruce D. Browner, MD, FAAOS

Lenworth M. Jacobs, MD, MPH, FACS

Andrew N. Pollak, MD, EMT-P, FAAOS

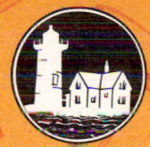

JONES AND BARTLETT PUBLISHERS

Sudbury, Massachusetts

BOSTON   TORONTO   LONDON   SINGAPORE

Jones and Bartlett Publishers

40 Tall Pine Drive
Sudbury, MA 01776
978-443-5000
www.emtb.com
www.jbpub.com

Jones and Bartlett Publishers Canada
P.O. Box 19020
Toronto, ON M5S 1X1
CANADA

Jones and Bartlett Publishers International
Barb House, Barb Mews
London W6 7PA
UK

Production Credits
Chief Executive Officer: Clayton Jones
Executive Vice President, Publisher: Tom Walker
Vice President, Senior Managing Editor: Judith H. Hauck
Vice President of Sales: Tom Manning
Emergency Care Editor: Tracy Murphy Foss
Production Director: Anne Spencer
Senior Production Editor: Cynthia Knowles Maciel
Marketing Director: Rich Pirozzi
Marketing Manager: Kimberly Brophy
Interactive Technology Director: Mike Campbell
Manufacturing Director: Therese Bräuer
Manufacturing Buyer: Kristen Guevara
Design and Composition: Studio Montage
Cover Photograph: © Bruce Ayres, Tony Stone Images
Color Separation: Eastern Rainbow
Printing and Binding: Banta Company

This textbook is intended solely as a guide to the appropriate procedures to be employed when rendering emergency care to the sick and injured. It is not intended as a statement of the standards of care required in any particular situation, because circumstances and the patient's physical condition can vary widely from one emergency to another. Nor is it intended that this textbook shall in any way advise emergency personnel concerning legal authority to perform the activities or procedures discussed. Such local determinations should be made only with the aid of legal counsel.

Notice: The patients described in "you are the emt" and "assessment in action" throughout this text are fictitious.

Library of Congress Cataloging-in-Publication Data

Emergency care and transportation of the sick and injured. — 7th ed. / [edited by] Bruce Browner, Lenworth Jacobs.
    p.   cm.
    Includes index.
    ISBN 0-7637-0796-1
    1. Medical emergencies. 2. Transport of sick and wounded. I. Browner, Bruce D. II. Jacobs, Lenworth M. III. American Academy of Orthopaedic Surgeons.
    [DNLM: 1. Emergency Medical Services. 2. Emergency Treatment. 3. Transportation of Patients. WX 215 E509 1998]
    RC86.7.A43 1998
    616.025—21
    DNLM/dc21   98-20963
    for Library of Congress   CIP
ISBN 0-7637-0796-1 (soft cover)
ISBN 0-7637-1044-X (hard cover)

Additional credits appear on page 959 which constitutes a continuation of the copyright page.

Printed in the United States of America
02 01 00 99   10 9 8 7 6 5 4 3 2

Brief Contents

Contents

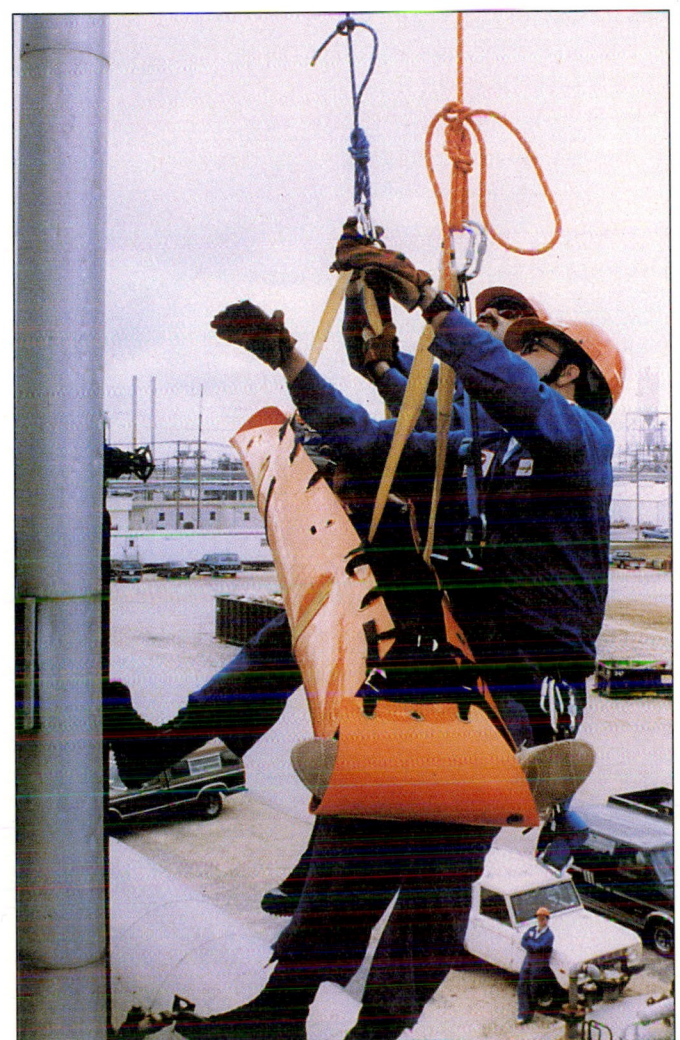

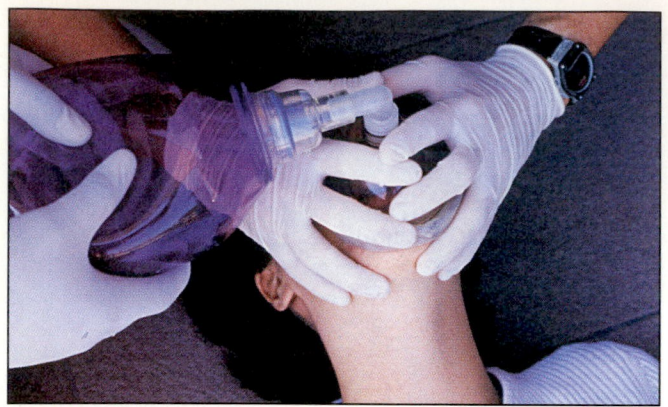

Section 2
Airway

Section 3
Patient Assessment

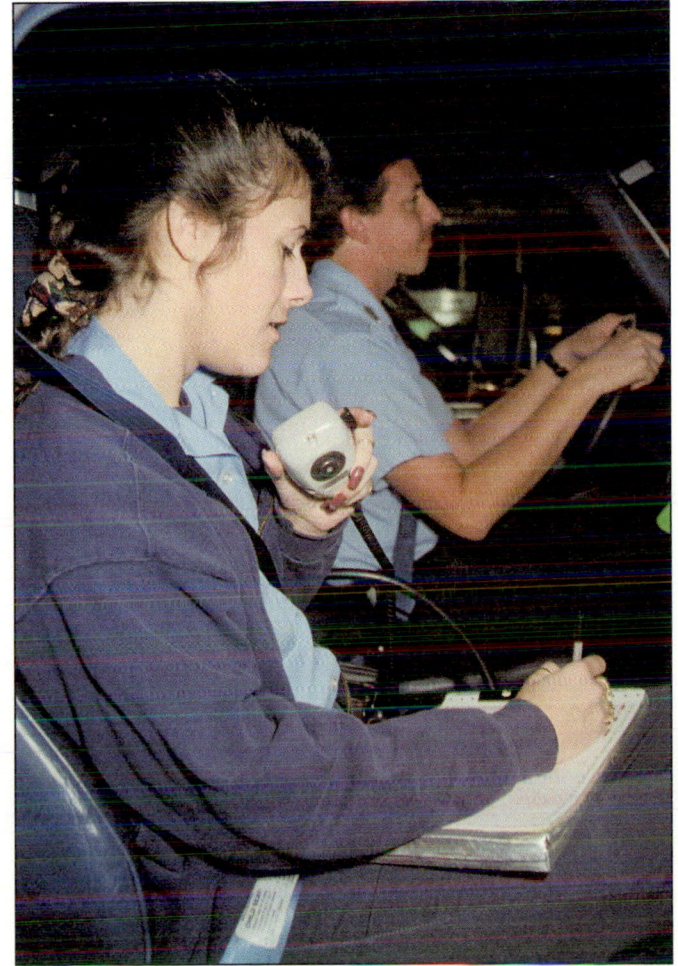

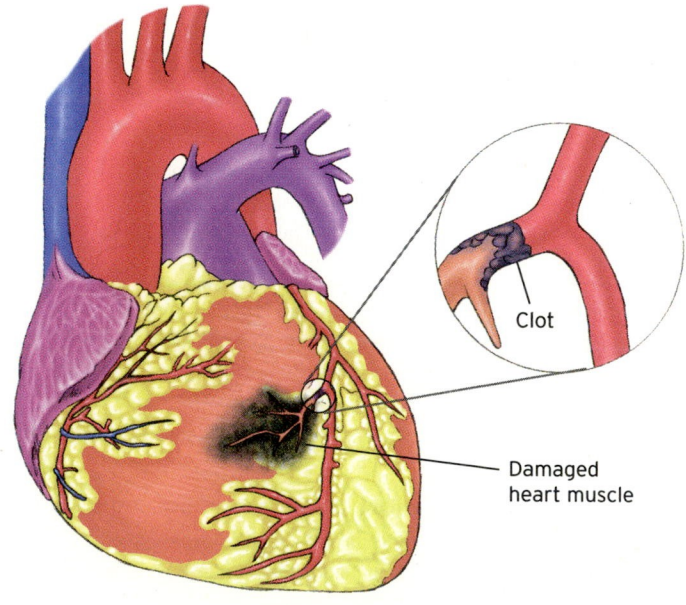

Clot

Damaged
heart muscle

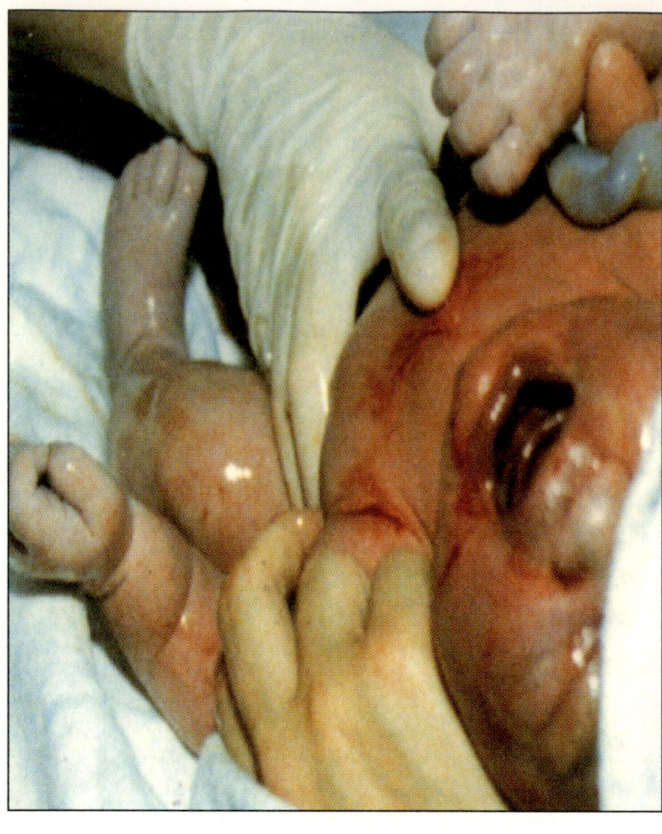

Section 5
Trauma

Cardiac muscle

Skeletal muscle

Smooth muscle

Section 6
Infants and Children

Section 7
Operations

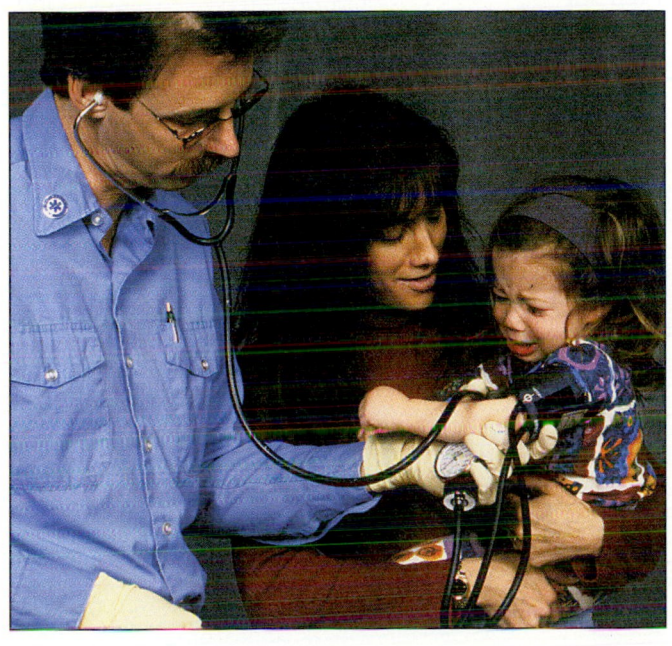

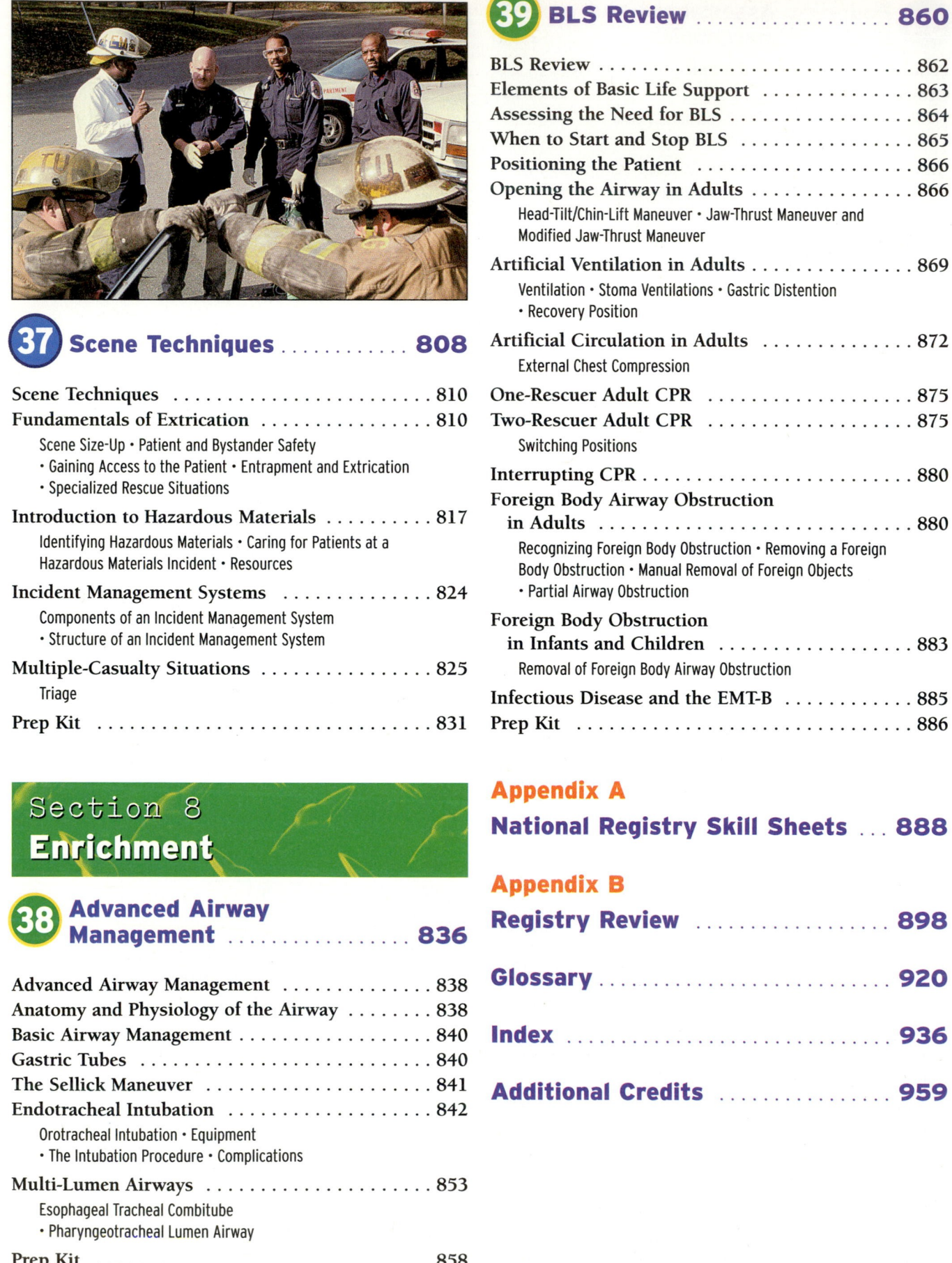

EMT-B Skill Drills

Acknowledgments

Editors

Bruce D. Browner, MD, FAAOS

Dr. Browner is a senior member of the orthopaedic trauma community in the United States. He has been active at both the national and international levels in clinical program and technology development, education, research, and health policy. Prior to his orthopaedic residency, he completed a fellowship at the Shock Trauma Research Unit at Albany Medical College. Upon completion of his training, he spent four years on the faculty of the Maryland Shock Trauma Center. He subsequently spent ten years at the University of Texas Medical School in Houston and Hermann Hospital where he served as Director of the Division of Orthopaedic Surgery and Chief of the Orthopaedic Service. Six years ago, he assumed his current position in Connecticut. Dr. Browner has served on the Board of Directors, and the Committees on Injuries, Health Care Finance, and International Affairs of the American Academy of Orthopaedic Surgeons. He is currently Chairman of the Advisory Council for Orthopaedic Surgery, member of the Board of Governors and a senior member of the Committee on Trauma of the American College of Surgeons. He has also been appointed the Founding Chairman of Trauma Committee by Societe International de Chirurgie Orthopedique et de Traumatologie (S.I.C.O.T.). Dr. Browner was a founding member and past President of the Orthopaedic Trauma Association. He is the senior editor of *Skeletal Trauma,* the leading textbook on fractures and dislocations in the world.

Gray-Gossling Professor and Chairman
Department of Orthopaedic Surgery
University of Connecticut
* Health Center*
Farmington, CT
Director of Orthopaedic Department
Hartford Hospital
Hartford, CT

Lenworth M. Jacobs, MD, MPH, FACS

Dr. Jacobs has been actively involved in EMS and EMS education for many years. In 1976, he served as Associate Director of Emergency Medical Services for the Department of Health and Hospitals in Boston and from 1977 to 1983 as Director of EMS and Director of the Paramedic Training Program. Since 1985, he has been Director of the LIFE STAR Helicopter Program at Hartford Hospital. He served as Division Chief of Emergency Medicine and is currently Chairman of the Department of Traumatology and Emergency Medicine at the University of Connecticut School of Medicine. Dr. Jacobs has served on numerous boards as an EMS consultant and policy maker at the local, regional, and national levels. His current responsibilities include being Chairman of the Connecticut Chapter of the American College of Surgeons Committee on Trauma, Vice President of the American Association for the Surgery of Trauma, and a member of the Emergency Medical Services Advisory Board at the Connecticut Committee on Trauma of the American College of Surgeons. He is an Affiliate Faculty Member of the American Heart Association and a member of the National Advanced Trauma Life Support Faculty of the American College of Surgeons.

Professor and Chairman
Department of Traumatology and
* Emergency Medicine*
Professor of Surgery
University of Connecticut
* School of Medicine*
Director, EMS/Trauma Program
Hartford Hospital
Hartford, CT

Andrew N. Pollak, MD, EMT-P, FAAOS

Dr. Pollak began his EMS career in 1980 as a junior volunteer firefighter and first responder. He remained active in EMS through college and medical school. During his career he has served as an EMS provider at the EMT-A, EMT-P and physician levels having worked as a flight physician with a hospital-based aeromedical ambulance service. He is currently a faculty member at the University of Maryland School of Medicine and Attending Orthopaedic Surgeon at the R Adams Cowley Shock Trauma Center in Baltimore, Maryland. He remains active in EMS as an educator, administrator, and a participant in a hospital-based rapid response field unit—the Shock Trauma Go Team.

Assistant Professor of Surgery
Attending Orthopaedic Traumatologist
University of Maryland School of Medicine
R Adams Cowley Shock Trauma Center
Baltimore, MD

Editorial Board

Kevin S. Brame, MA
Chief Training Officer
Orange County Fire Authority
Orange, CA

Bruce D. Browner, MD
Gray-Gossling Professor and Chair
Department of Orthopaedic Surgery
University of Connecticut
  Health Center
Farmington, CT
Director of Orthopaedic Department
Hartford Hospital
Hartford, CT

Alasdair K.T. Conn, MD
Chief of Emergency Services
Emergency Services
Massachusetts General Hospital
Boston, MA

Alice Dalton (Twink), RN, MS
EMS Education Coordinator
Omaha Fire Department
Omaha, NE

Lenworth M. Jacobs, MD, MPH, FACS
Professor and Chairman
Department of Traumatology and
  Emergency Medicine
Professor of Surgery
University of Connecticut
  School of Medicine
Director, EMS/Trauma Program
Hartford Hospital
Hartford, CT

Richard L. Judd, PhD, EMSI
President and Professor of
  Emergency Medical Sciences
Central Connecticut State University
New Britain, CT

Paul E. Pepe, MD, MPH, FACEP, FCCM
Professor of Surgery, Emergency
  Medicine and Public Health
Allegheny University of the
  Health Sciences
Pittsburgh, PA

Andrew N. Pollak, MD, EMT-P, FAAOS
Assistant Professor of Surgery
Attending Orthopaedic
  Traumatologist
University of Maryland
  School of Medicine
R Adams Cowley Shock
  Trauma Center
Baltimore, MD

James S. Seidel, MD, PhD
Chief, General and Emergency
  Pediatrics
Professor of Pediatrics
Department of Emergency Medicine
Harbor-UCLA Medical Center
Torrance, CA

Mike Smith, MICP
Vice President
Emergency Medical Training
  Associates, Inc.
Olympia, WA

J.J. Tepas III, MD
Professor of Surgery
Chairman, Department of Surgery
University of Florida Health Science
  Center -Jacksonville
Jacksonville, FL

Contributors

Scott S. Bourn, RN, MSN, EMT-P
Clinical Instructor
Director, Emergency Health Services
Beth-El College of Nursing and
  Health Sciences University of
  Colorado
Colorado Springs, CO

Stephen M. Belkoff, PhD, EMT-B
Director and Assistant Professor
Orthopaedic Biomechanics
  Laboratory
Orthopaedic Surgery and
  Mechanical Engineering
University of Maryland
Baltimore, MD

Kenneth J. Bouvier, NREMT-I
EMS Education
New Orleans, LA

Andrew R. Burgess, MD
Director, Division of Orthopaedic
  Surgery
University of Maryland School
  of Medicine
Chief, Section of Orthopaedic
  Traumatology
R Adams Cowley Shock Trauma
  Center
Orthopaedics
Baltimore, MD

Alexander M. Butman, BA, DSc, REMT-P
Executive Director
Emergency Training Institute
Fairlawn, OH

Jack P. Campbell, MD
Associate Professor
EMS Medical Director
Emergency Department
Truman Medical Center-West
Kansas City, MO

Eduardo E. Castro, MD
Director of Prehospital Medicine
Department of Emergency Medicine
Massachusetts General Hospital
Boston, MA

Contributors—cont'd.

John "Chip" Coleman, SSgt, USAF, NREMT-P
USAF School of Healthcare Sciences
Sheppard AFB, TX

Alice Dalton (Twink), RN, MS
EMS Education Coordinator
Omaha Fire Department
Omaha, NE

Suzanne Goodrich, RN, MSN
Prehospital Care Coordinator
UCI Medical Center
Orange, CA

Cressy Goodwin, MPH
Emergency Medical Services
    Coordinator
Department of Traumatology
    and Emergency Medicine
Hartford Hospital
Hartford, CT

Carol Gupton, BSEMS, NREMT-P
EMS Faculty
Training Division
Omaha Fire Department
Omaha, NE

Fred Harchelroad, MD, FAAEM, FACMT
Associate Professor
Department of Emergency Medicine
Allegheny University of the Health
    Sciences
Pittsburgh, PA

Deborah Parkman Henderson, PhD, RN
Assistant Professor
UCLA School of Medicine
Department of Pediatrics
Harbor-UCLA Medical Center
Torrance, CA

L. Scott Levin, MD
Associate Professor
Division of Orthopaedic Surgery
Duke University Center
Durham, NC

Hilary C. Onyiuke, MD
Assistant Professor
Neurosurgery
Hartford Hospital
Hartford, CT

Craig B. Ordway, MD
Assistant Professor of
    Orthopedic Surgery
State University of New York
Stony Brook, NY

Edward L. Pesanti, MD
Professor of Medicine
Assistant Professor of
    Orthopaedic Surgery
University of Connecticut
    Health Center
Farmington, CT

Jonathan Politis, BA, NREMT-P
Director, Town of Colonie
Department of Emergency
    Medical Services
Latham, NY

Andrew N. Pollak, MD
Assistant Professor of Surgery
Attending Orthopaedic
    Traumatologist
University of Maryland
    School of Medicine
R Adams Cowley Shock
    Trauma Center
Baltimore, MD

Pamela Poore, RN
Clinical Supervisor
Little Company of Mary
Emergency Department
Torrance, CA

Linda Quan, MD
Chief, Emergency Services
Children's Hospital Regional
    Medical Center
Seattle, WA

Vincent M. Santoro, MD
Chief, Orthopaedic Trauma Service
Department of Orthopedics
Hartford Hospital
Hartford, CT

Michael R. Sayre, MD
Assistant Professor
Department of Emergency Medicine
University of Cincinnati
Cincinnati, OH

James S. Seidel, MD, PhD
Chief, General and
    Emergency Pediatrics
Professor of Pediatrics
Department of Emergency Medicine
Harbor-UCLA Medical Center
Torrance, CA

Mike Smith, MICP
Vice President
Emergency Medical Training
    Associates, Inc.
Olympia, WA

Samuel J. Stratton, MD
Medical Director, Los Angeles
    County EMS Agency
Associate Professor
Department of Emergency Medicine
Harbor-UCLA Medical Center
Torrance, CA

Vincent P. Tamariz, MD
Fellow, Pediatric Emergency
    Medicine
Department of Emergency Medicine
Harbor-UCLA Medical Center
Torrance, CA

Stephen H. Thomas, MD
Associate Director of Prehospital
    Medicine
Department of Emergency Medicine
Massachusetts General Hospital
Boston, MA

John M. Watson, MD
Trauma/Critical Care Fellow
Department of EMS/Trauma
Hartford Hospital
Hartford, CT

Brian S. Zachariah, MD
Chief, EMS Section
Division of Emergency Medicine
University of Texas, Southwestern
Dallas, TX

Reviewers

Barbara Aehlert, RN, BSPA
President
Southwest EMS Education
Glendale, AZ

Ken Beers, MS
Program Coordinator
Public Safety Training Center
Monroe Community College
Rochester, NY

Greg P. Carlson, NREMT-P
EMS Teaching Specialist
EMS
Wisconsin Indianhead
    Technical College
New Richmond, WI

Les Chatelain
Health Promotion and Education
    Department
University of Utah
Salt Lake City, UT

Paul Coffey
Massachusetts Department of Public
    Health
OEMS
Basic EMT Training Coordinator
Boston, MA

Holly Frost Davis, BS, NREMT-P
EMS Faculty
Emergency Medical
    Services Technology
Northern Virginia
    Community College
Annandale, VA

Kim Dickerson, EMT-P, RN
EMS Coordinator
Emergency Medical Services
    Technology
Edison Community College
Fort Myers, FL

Richard Ellis, NREMT-P, AAS
USAF EMT Program Manager
United States Air Force Base
Sheppard AFB, TX

Ned Fowler, MA Ed., EMT-P
Chairman
Emergency Medical
    Science Department
Asheville-Buncombe Technical
    Community College
Asheville, NC

Larry G. Gosdin, RN, BA, EMT-P
Director
Emergency Medical
    Services Program
Gadsden, AL

Donald Graesser, PhD
Assistant Director - EMT Coordinator
Bergen County EMS
    Training Center
Paramus, NJ

Jack T. Grandey, NREMT-P
Operations Director
Wilderness EMS Institute
Pittsburgh, PA

Jaime S. Greene, BA, EMT-B
EMT Program Director
Adult, Vocational, and
    Community Education
School District of
    Palm Beach County
West Palm Beach, FL

Barbara L. Klingensmith, BA, MS, NREMT-P
Director, Public Services
Edison Community College
Fort Myers, FL

Rebecca Layman, EMT-B
EMS Coordinator
R Adams Cowley Shock
    Trauma Center
Baltimore, MD

Scott A. McConnell, BA, EMT-P
Chairman, EMS Technology Program
Lima Technical College
Lima, OH

Jeff McDonald
Coordinator
Emergency Medical
    Technology Program
Tarrant County Junior College
Fort Worth, TX

Michael G. Miller, RN, NREMT-P
EMS Coordinator
Department of Emergency Medicine
West Suburban Hospital
    Medical Center
Oak Park, IL

Anthony J. Misner, EMT-P, BA
Emergency Services Coordinator
Emergency Services Programs
Yosemite Community
    Education Center
Oakhurst, CA

Robert G. Nixon, BA, EMT-P
President
Lifecare Medical Training
Walnut Creek, CA

John Rinard, BBA, EMT-P
Faculty
EMS Program
Texas Tech University Health Science
    Center
Lubbock, TX

Fredrick H. (Ted) Rogers, NREMT-P
Lead Instructor, EMT Program
St. Petersburg Junior College
St. Petersburg, FL

Jose V. Salazar, MPH, NREMT-P
President
Jose Salazar & Associates
Sterling, VA

Dave Schottke, RN, REMT-P, MPH
Washington, D.C.

Sandra Stinson, RN, NREMT-P, I/C
EMS Program Director
EMS Education
Southwest Mississippi Regional Medical
    Center
McComb, MS

Donna Tidwell, BS, RN, EMT-P
Director, EMT-Paramedic Program
Columbia State
    Community College
Columbia, TN

Denise Tiedeman
Instructor/Coordinator
Tidewater Community College
Virginia Beach, VA

John Todaro, REMT-P, RN
EMS Training Coordinator
Seminole County Department
    of Public Safety
Sanford, FL

Ed Travers, RN, CEN, EMT-P
Assistant Professor and Director of EMT
    and Paramedic Education
Massachusetts Bay Community College
Boston, MA

Technical and Photographic Consultants

Abbott Ambulance, Inc.
American Heart Association
American Lung Association
Anderson Ambulance Service
Anne Arundel County EMS/Fire/Rescue
BCI International
Baltimore City Fire Department
Baltimore County Fire Department
Brimfield Township Fire Department
Catherine Emery Design and Photography
Center Laboratories
Chicago Fire Department
Cowenton Volunteer Fire Department
Deaton Specialty Hospital & Home
Dolton Fire Department
Downers Grove Fire Department
Emergency Products and Research
Franklin Park Medical Department
Gibbons/McClincy
Hinsdale Fire Department
Kingsville Volunteer Fire Department
Lemont Fire Department
Leon Valley Fire Department

Maryland Express Care
Maryland Institute for Emergency Medical Services Systems
Maryland State Police - Aviation Division
Mayo Clinic
New Lenox Fire Department
Oak Lawn Fire Department
Prince George's County Fire and EMS Department
Prospect Heights Fire District
R Adams Cowley Shock Trauma Center
Riverside Department of Fire, Rescue & Emergency Services
Rollin Schnieder
Rosemont Department of Public Safety
San Antonio Fire Department
Sheridan Catheter Corp.
St. Petersberg Fire Department
Stickney Fire Department
Texas Department of Health, Bureau of Emergency Management
University of Texas at Galveston
WesTech

I am grateful to my co-editors for their support during this project. Lenworth Jacobs, MD, MPH, provided a broad perspective and philosophic guidance from his many years of involvement with pre-hospital care, flight service operations, emergency medicine and trauma surgery. Andrew Pollak, MD, used his formal training and previous working background as an EMT-P to supplement his current experience as an orthopaedic trauma surgeon. He and David Stanley from the Academy Publications Department were tireless in their efforts to review and revise all of the photographs and illustrations. The new illustration program is outstanding.

The other members of the Editorial Board, Alasdair Conn, MD, Alice "Twink" Dalton, BSN, NRPM, Richard Judd, PhD, Paul Pepe, MD, MPH, James Seidel, PhD, MD, Mike Smith, MICP, and J.J. Tepas III, MD, approached their work with true devotion, demonstrating a rare mixture of extensive field experience and expertise as teachers.

No one worked harder or with more dedication on this project than Lynne Shindoll, our Managing Editor, who integrated the activity of all contributors throughout the project and attended to every detail with a consistently high level of professionalism.

It was a great privilege to serve as the lead editor of this exceptional team. I will always be greatful for their energetic collaboration and impressed with their extraordinary dedication.

Dr. Bruce Browner

Preparing to be an EMT-B

Richard L. Judd, PhD, EMSI

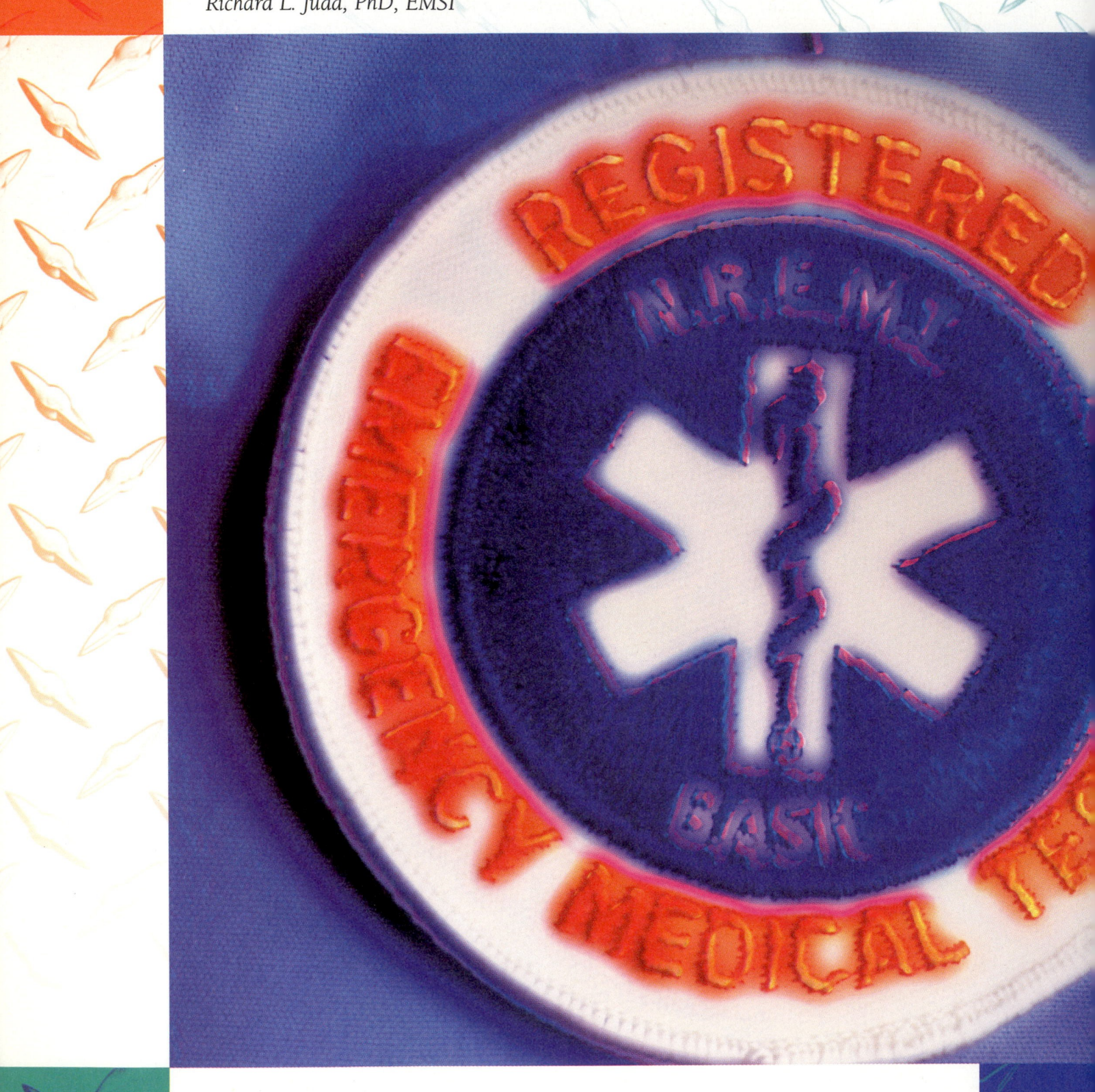

Introduction to Emergency Medical Care

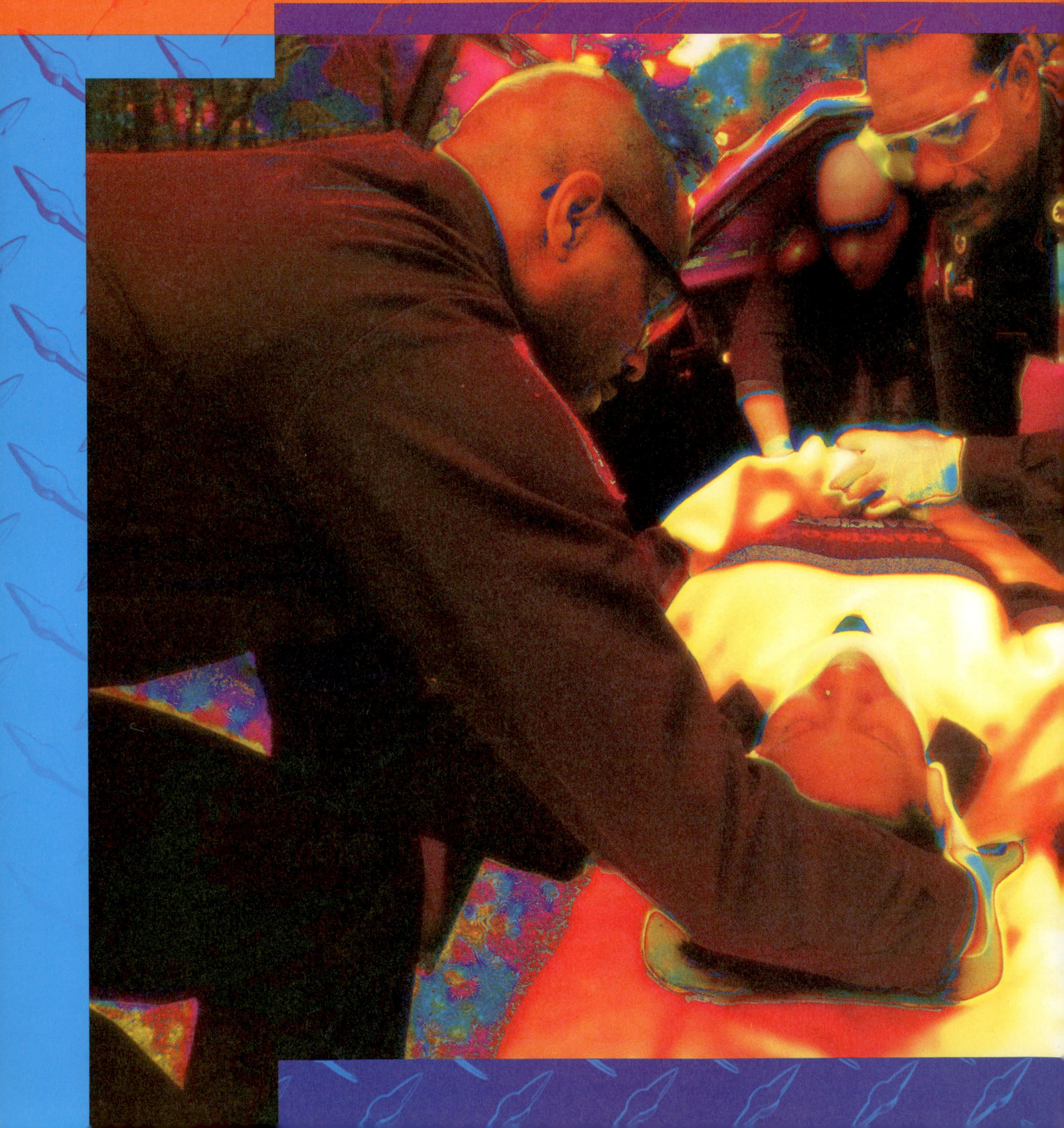

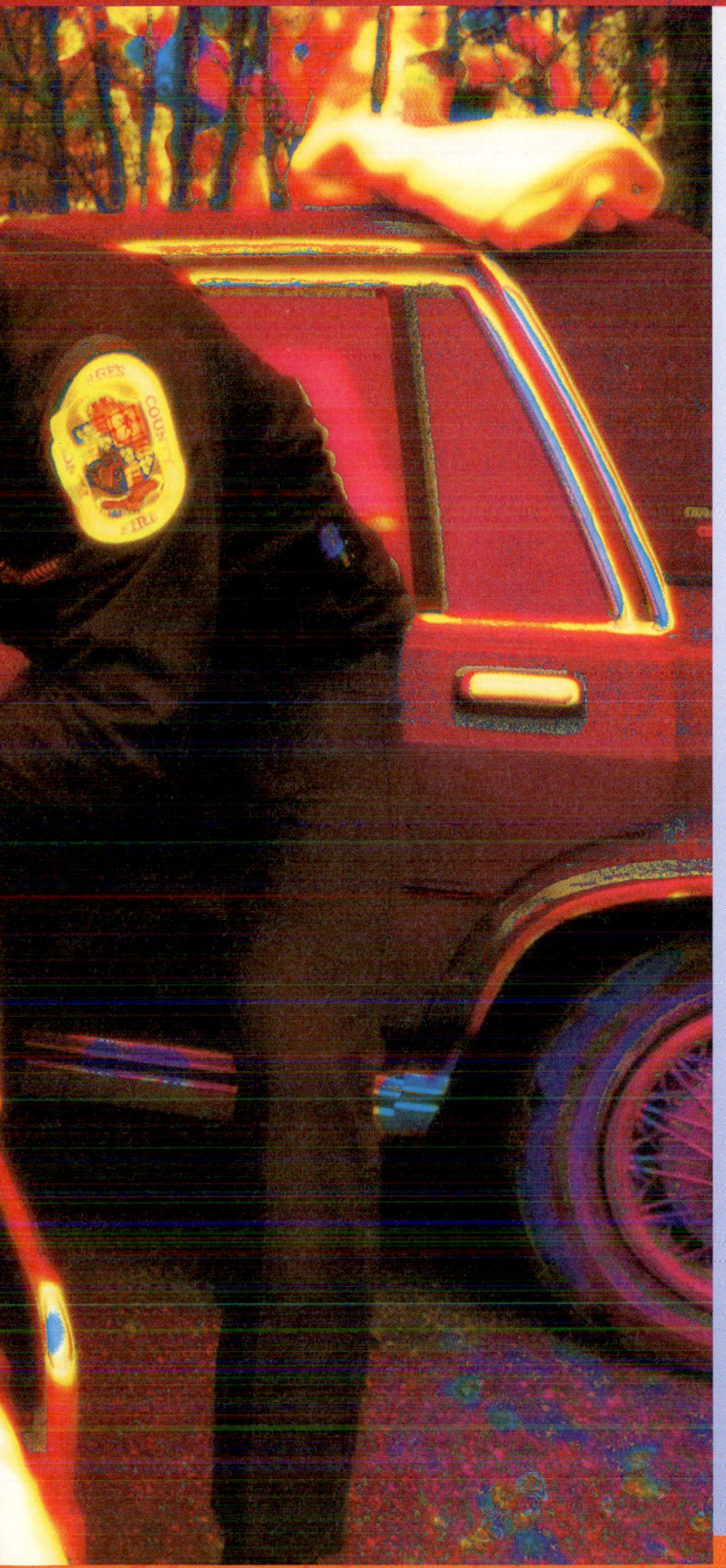

objectives

Cognitive

1. Define Emergency Medical Services (EMS) systems.

2. Differentiate the roles and responsibilities of the EMT-B from other prehospital care providers.

3. Describe the roles and responsibilities related to personal safety.

4. Discuss the roles and responsibilities of the EMT-B towards the safety of the crew, the patient, and bystanders.

5. Define quality improvement and discuss the EMT-B's role in the process.

6. Define medical direction and discuss the EMT-B's role in the process.

7. State the specific statutes and regulations in your state regarding the EMS system.

Affective

8. Assess areas of personal attitude and conduct of the EMT-B.

9. Characterize the various methods used to access the EMS system in your community.

Psychomotor

None

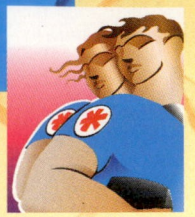

At some point in your life, an ambulance probably raced by and you wondered where it was going. Now that you have enrolled in an EMT-Basic course, you will find out exactly where those ambulances go and what kind of situations EMTs encounter daily.

This chapter will help to introduce you to the exciting profession of EMS. It will also help you to answer the following questions:

1. What is an emergency? How do emergency calls meet the expectations of EMS providers?
2. Where do EMTs and the EMS system fit into the continuum of patient care for both medical and traumatic events?

Introduction to Emergency Medical Care

This book has been designed to serve as the text and primary resource for the emergency medical technician basic (EMT-Basic) course. This chapter describes the content and objectives of the EMT-Basic course. It also discusses what will be expected of you during the course and what other requirements you will have to meet to be licensed or certified as an EMT-Basic in most states. The differences between basic first aid training, a Department of Transportation (DOT) First Responder training course, and the training for the EMT-Basic, EMT-Intermediate, and EMT-Paramedic are described.

Emergency medical services (EMS) is a system. The key components of this system and how they influence and affect the EMT-Basic and his or her delivery of emergency care are carefully discussed. Next, the administration, medical direction, quality control, and regulation of EMS services are presented. The chapter ends with a detailed discussion of the roles and responsibilities of the EMT-Basic as a healthcare professional.

Course Description

You are about to enter an exciting field. **Emergency medical services (EMS)** consists of a team of healthcare professionals who, in each area or jurisdiction, are responsible for and provide prehospital emergency care and transportation to the sick and injured (Figure 1-1). Each emergency medical service is part of a local or regional EMS system that provides the many varied prehospital and hospital components required for the delivery of proper emergency medical care. The standards for prehospital emergency care and the individuals who provide it are governed by the laws in each state and are typically regulated by a state office of EMS (OEMS).

The individuals who provide the emergency care in the field are trained and, except for licensed physicians, must be state-licensed or certified **emergency medical technicians (EMT)**. EMTs are categorized into three training and licensure levels: EMT-Basic, EMT-Intermediate, and EMT-Paramedic. An **EMT-Basic** (EMT-B) has training in basic emergency care skills, including automated defibrillation, use of definitive airway adjuncts, and assisting patients with certain medications. An **EMT-Intermediate** (EMT-I) has advanced training in specific aspects of

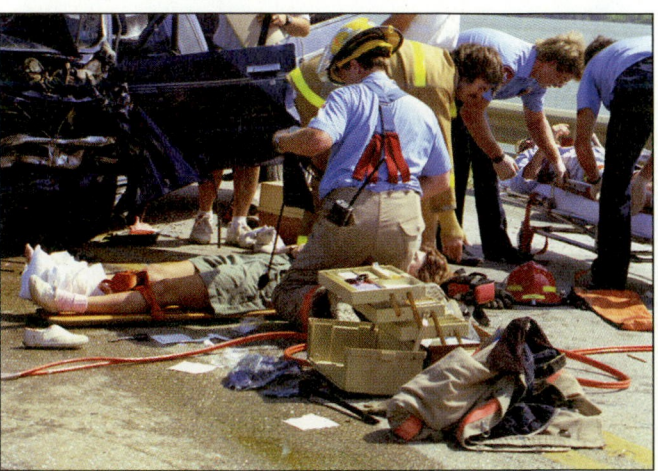

FIGURE 1-1 As an EMT-B, you will be part of a larger team that responds to a variety of calls and provides a wide range of prehospital emergency care.

advanced life support, such as intravenous (IV) therapy. An **EMT-Paramedic** (EMT-P) has extensive training in advanced life support, including IV therapy, pharmacology, cardiac monitoring, and other advanced assessment and treatment skills.

Although the specific training and licensure requirements vary from one state to another, the training that is required in almost every state follows or exceeds the guidelines that are recommended in the current U.S. DOT National Standard Curriculum for each EMT level.

After successfully completing the BLS/CPR course for healthcare providers and meeting the other prerequisites, you are ready to take the EMT-B course. Like any introductory course, the EMT-B course covers a great deal of information and introduces many skills. Everything you learn in the course will be important to your ability to provide high-quality emergency care once you are licensed and ready to practice. In addition, the knowledge, understanding, and skills that you acquire in the EMT-B course will serve as the foundation for the additional knowledge and training that you will receive in future years.

This textbook covers the material and skills that are identified in the U.S. DOT 1994 EMT-Basic National Standard Curriculum and in the 1994 National EMS Education and Practice Blueprint. In addition to the required core content, it includes additional information that will help you to understand and apply the material and skills that are included in the EMT-B level. Your instructor will furnish you with reading assignments. It is important that you complete the assigned reading *before* each class.

In class, the instructor will review the key parts of the reading assignment and clarify and expand on them.

TABLE 1-1	Study Tips for Using This Textbook

- **Do each assignment** diligently and carefully.
- **Read the textbook** like a textbook, not like a newspaper, magazine, or novel.
- **Read each chapter** several times and underline key points. Take notes!
- **Ask your instructor** to clarify any questions you note in your reading or in class.
- **Take additional notes** when the assigned material is expanded upon in class.
- **Remember:** The only absurd question is the one that a student has and fails to ask.

He or she will also answer any questions that you have and will clarify any points that you or others found confusing (Figure 1-2). Unless you have carefully read the assignment and made notes before coming to class, you will not fully understand or benefit from the classroom presentation and discussions. You will also need to take additional notes during class (Table 1-1).

The EMT-B course will include four types of learning activities:

1. **Reading assignments** from the textbook and presentations and discussions held in class will provide you with the necessary knowledge base.

2. **Step-by-step demonstrations** will teach you hands-on skills that you then need to practice repeatedly in supervised small group workshops.

3. **Summary skills sheets** will help you to memorize the sequence of steps in complex skills that contain a large number of steps or variations so that you can perform the skill with no errors or omissions.

4. **Case presentations and scenarios** used in class will help you learn how to apply the knowledge and skills acquired in class in situations like those you will find in the field.

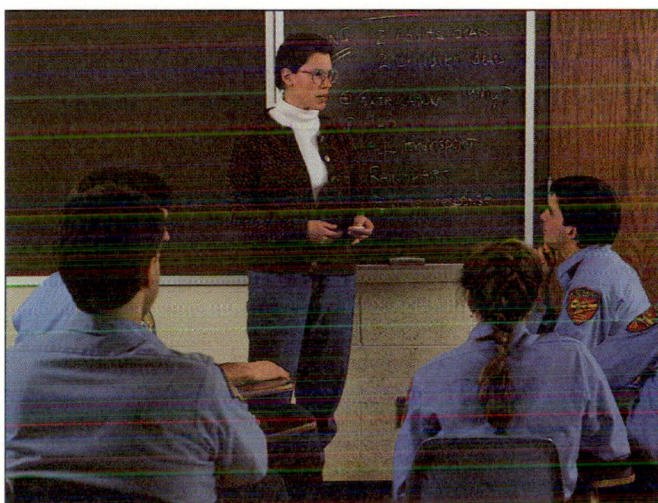

FIGURE 1-2 In the classroom, you will learn both cognitive and practical skills to prepare you for many types of calls.

Everything you learn in the EMT-B course will be important to your ability to provide high-quality emergency care.

EMT-B Training Focus and Requirements

EMT-B training is divided into three main categories. The first and most important category focuses on the care of life-threatening or potentially life-threatening conditions. To deal with these, you will learn how to do the following:

- Size up the scene and situation

- Ensure that the scene is safe

- Perform an initial assessment of the patient

- Obtain a history of this episode and a pertinent past medical history

- Identify life-threatening injuries/conditions

- Establish and maintain an open airway

- Provide adequate ventilation

- Manage conditions that prevent proper ventilation

- Provide high-flow supplemental oxygen

- Perform cardiopulmonary resuscitation (CPR)

- Perform automated or semiautomated external defibrillation (AED)

- Control external bleeding

- Recognize and treat shock

- Care for cases of poisoning

- Care for patients in an acute life-threatening medical emergency

- Assist patients in taking certain emergency medications that they carry and that their physician has prescribed for an acute episode

- Identify and rapidly package (positioning, covering, and securing a patient for transport) patients for whom the rapid initiation of transport is important

> As an EMT-B, you will be joining a long tradition of people who have provided emergency medical care to their fellow human beings.

The second category of training covers conditions that, although not life threatening, are key components of emergency care or are necessary to prevent further harm before the patient is moved. You will learn to do the following:

- Identify patients for whom spinal precautions should be taken and immobilize them properly

- Dress and bandage wounds

- Splint injured extremities

- Care for burns

- Deliver a baby

- Assess and care for a newborn infant

- Manage patients with behavioral/psychological problems

- Cope with the psychological stresses on patients, families, your fellow EMT-Bs, and yourself.

The third category covers important issues that are related to your ability to provide emergency care. You will develop the following related skills:

- Understanding the role and responsibilities of the EMT-B

- Following your service's protocols and direct medical directions

- Understanding ethical and medicolegal problems

- Learning emergency vehicle and defensive driving

- Using equipment carried on the ambulance

- Checking and stocking the ambulance

- Communicating with patients and others at the scene

- Using the radio and communicating with the dispatcher

- Giving a precise patient radio report and obtaining direct medical direction

- Giving a full verbal report when transferring the patient's care at the hospital

- Preparing proper documentation and completing the written run report

- Working with other responders at an accident scene

- Cooperating with operations at special rescue, mass-casualty, and hazardous materials incidents

Certification Requirements

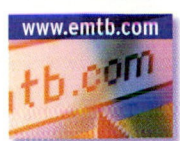 To be recognized and perform as an EMT-B, you must meet certain training and other requirements. The specific requirements differ from state to state. You should ask your instructor or contact your state EMS office to find out about the requirements in your state. Generally, the criteria will include the following:

- High school diploma or equivalent
- Proof of immunization against certain communicable diseases
- Valid driver's license
- Successful completion of a recognized healthcare provider's BLS/CPR course
- Successful completion of a state-approved EMT-Basic course
- Successful completion of a state-recognized written certification examination
- Successful completion of a state-recognized practical certification examination
- Demonstrating that you can meet the mental and physical criteria necessary to be able to safely and properly perform all the tasks and functions described in the defined role of an EMT-B
- Compliance with other state and local provisions

Many states require substantiation that no criminal and/or mental history exist in the potential licensure or certification of an EMT-B.

The **Americans with Disabilities Act (ADA)** of 1990 protects individuals who have a disability from being denied access to programs and services that are provided by state or local governments and prohibits employers from failing to provide full and equal employment to the disabled. To obtain further information about the ADA and employment as an EMT-B, you should contact your state EMS office.

In most states, individuals who have a history of a health problem that could make their performance of an EMT-B's tasks dangerous to themselves or others, have been convicted of driving while under the influence of drugs or alcohol, or have been convicted of certain felonies may be denied certification as an EMT-B.

Overview of the Emergency Medical Services System

History of EMS

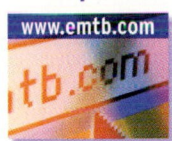 As an EMT-B, you will be joining a long tradition of people who have provided emergency medical care to their fellow human beings. With the early use of motor vehicles in warfare, volunteer ambulance squads were organized and went overseas to provide care for the wounded in World War I. In World War II, the military trained special corpsmen to provide care in the field and bring the casualties to aid stations staffed by nurses and physicians. In the Korean conflict, this evolved to the field medic and rapid helicopter evacuation to nearby Mobile Army Surgical Hospital (MASH) units, where immediate surgical intervention was provided. Many advances in the immediate care of trauma patients resulted from the casualty experiences in the Korean and Vietnam conflicts.

Unfortunately, emergency care of the injured and ill at home had not progressed to a similar level. As late as the early 1960s, emergency ambulance service and care across the United States varied widely. In some places, it was provided by well-trained advanced first aid squads that had well-equipped modern ambulances. In a few urban areas, it was provided by hospital-based ambulance services that were staffed with interns and early forms of medics. In many places, the only emergency care and ambulance service was provided by the local funeral home using a Cadillac-type hearse that could be converted to carry a cot and serve as an ambulance. In other places, the police or fire department used a station wagon that carried a cot and a first aid kit. In most cases, both of these were staffed by a driver and an attendant who had some basic first aid training. In the few areas where a commercial ambulance was available to transport the ill, it was usually similarly staffed and served primarily as a means to transport the patient to the hospital.

Many communities had no formal provision for prehospital emergency care or transportation. Accident victims were given basic first aid by police or fire personnel at the scene and were transported to the hospital in a police or fire officer's car. Customarily, patients with an acute illness were transported to the hospital by a relative or neighbor and were met by their family physician or an on-call hospital physician, who assessed them and then summoned any specialists and operating room staff that were needed. Except in large urban centers, most hospitals did not have the staffed emergency departments to which we are accustomed today.

EMS as we know it today had its origins in 1966 with the publication of *Accidental Death and Disability: The Neglected Disease of Modern Society*. This report, prepared jointly by the Committees on Trauma and Shock of the National Academy of Sciences/National Research Council, revealed to the public and Congress serious inadequacy of prehospital emergency care and transportation in many areas. A number of key items were recommended in the report, some of which follow:

- Development of national courses of instruction for prehospital emergency care and transportation by fire, police, rescue, and ambulance personnel

- Development of nationally accepted textbooks and training aids for these courses

- Development of federal guidelines for the design of ambulances and the equipment they carry

- Development and adoption of general policies and regulations pertaining to ambulance services and qualification and supervision of ambulance personnel in each state

- Adoption by each municipality (or district or county) of means to supply the necessary proper prehospital emergency care and transport within its jurisdiction

- Establishment of hospital emergency departments with staffing by physicians, nurses, and other personnel who are trained in resuscitation and the immediate care of the seriously injured and ill

As a result, Congress mandated that two federal agencies address these issues. The National Highway Traffic Safety Administration (NHTSA) of the Department of Transportation, through the Highway Safety Act of 1966, and the Department of Health and Human Services (HHS), through the Emergency Medical Act of 1973, created funding sources and programs to develop improved systems of prehospital emergency care.

In the early 1970s, DOT developed and published the first National Standard Curriculum to serve as the guideline for the training of EMTs. To support the EMT course, the American Academy of Orthopaedic Surgeons prepared and published the first EMT textbook—the first edition of *Emergency Care and Transportation of the Sick and Injured*—in 1971. Through the 1970s, following the recommended guidelines, each state developed the necessary legislation, and the EMS system was developed throughout the United States. During the same period, emergency medicine became a recognized medical specialty, and the fully staffed emergency departments that we know today became the accepted standard of care.

In the late 1970s and early 1980s, DOT developed a recommended National Standard Curriculum for the training of paramedics and identified a part of the course to serve as additional training for the EMT to allow advancement to the EMT-Intermediate level.

By 1980, EMS had been established throughout the nation. The system was based on the following two key changes:

- The introduction of legislation that made it the responsibility of each municipality, township, or county to provide proper prehospital emergency care and transportation within its boundaries

- The establishment of recognized and regulated standards for the training of ambulance personnel and equipment required on each ambulance

These changes ensured that, regardless of where an individual became hurt or acutely ill, he or she would receive timely, proper emergency care and transport to the hospital. During the 1980s, many areas enhanced the EMT National Standard Curriculum by adding EMTs with higher levels of training who could provide key components of **advanced life support (ALS)** care (advanced lifesaving procedures). The availability of paramedics (EMT-P) and ALS on calls that require or benefit from advanced care has grown steadily in recent years. In addition, with the evolution in training and new technology available, the EMT-B and EMT-I can now perform a number of important advanced skills in the field that were formerly reserved for the EMT-P.

The way EMS systems work may differ depending on the geographic area and population served. Regardless of the area, however, NHTSA is available to evaluate EMS systems, based on the following 10 criteria in their Technical Assistance Program Assessment Standards:

1. Regulation and policy

2. Resource management

3. Human resources and training

4. Transportation equipment and system

5. Medical and support facilities

6. Communications system

7. Public information and education

8. Medical direction

9. Trauma system and development

10. Evaluation

Levels of Training

Public Basic Life Support and Immediate Aid

With the development of EMS and increased awareness of the need for immediate emergency care, millions of laypeople have been trained in CPR/basic life support (BLS). In addition to CPR, many individuals have taken short basic first aid courses that include control of bleeding and other simple skills that may be required to provide immediate essential care. These courses are designed to train individuals so that those in the workplace, teachers, coaches, babysitters, and the like, can provide the necessary critical care in the minutes before EMTs or other responders arrive at the scene.

In addition, many individuals, such as those who regularly accompany groups on camping trips or are in other situations in which the arrival of EMS may be delayed because of remote location, are trained in advanced first aid. This course includes basic life support and the essential additional care and packaging that may be necessary until the help of rescuers and EMTs can be obtained at a remote location.

First Responders

Because the presence of a person who is trained and able to initiate basic life support and other urgent care cannot be ensured, the EMS system includes immediate care by first responders, such as law enforcement officers, fire fighters, park rangers, ski patrollers, or other organized rescuers who often arrive at the scene before the ambulance and EMTs (Figure 1-3). DOT has established a First Responder Curriculum and course outline to provide these individuals with the training necessary to initiate immediate care and then assist the EMTs on their arrival. The course focuses on providing immediate basic life support and urgent care with limited equipment. It also familiarizes the student with the additional procedures, equipment, and packaging that EMTs may use and with which the first responder may be called upon to assist.

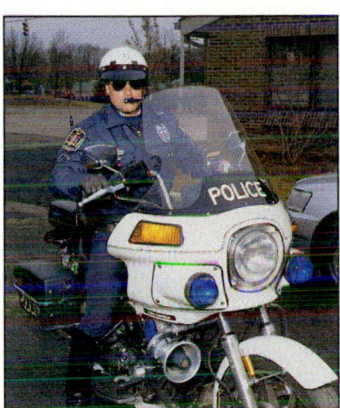

FIGURE 1-3 First responders, such as law enforcement officers, are trained to provide immediate basic life support until EMTs arrive on the scene.

Just as it is essential for the first responder to do enough for the patient, it is also essential for the first responder not to try to do too much. One of the most serious dangers to patients is improper removal from a vehicle or accident scene. Permanent paralysis and other injuries have been caused by these well-intentioned but potentially dangerous actions.

First responders should be trained by using the DOT First Responder Curriculum, which includes training in cardiopulmonary resuscitation (CPR). First responders can provide BLS before the ambulance arrives by assessing the injury or illness, providing air to the lungs and blood to the brain, and controlling bleeding, all of which can be done with little or no equipment.

EMT-Basic

The EMT-B course requires approximately 110 hours (more in some states) and includes the essential knowledge and skills required to provide basic emergency care in the field. The course serves as the foundation on which additional knowledge and skills are built in advanced EMT training. On arrival at the scene, you and the other EMTs who have responded with the ambulance should assume responsibility for the assessment and care of the patient, followed by proper packaging and transport of the patient to the emergency department. With the publication and adoption of the U.S. DOT 1994 EMT-Basic National Standard Curriculum, three ALS skills have been added to this level. These skills include automated defibrillation, use of a definitive airway adjunct, and assisting patients with the use of certain previously prescribed medications, such as nitroglycerin, epinephrine, or a metered-dose inhaler (Figure 1-4).

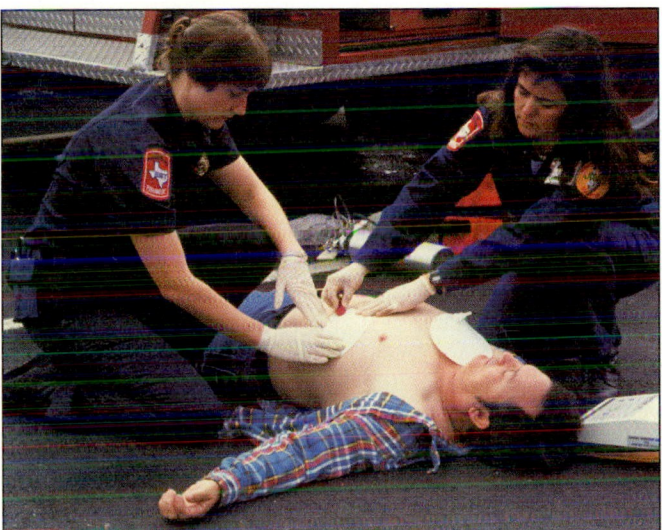

FIGURE 1-4 EMT-Bs are trained to perform automated defibrillation.

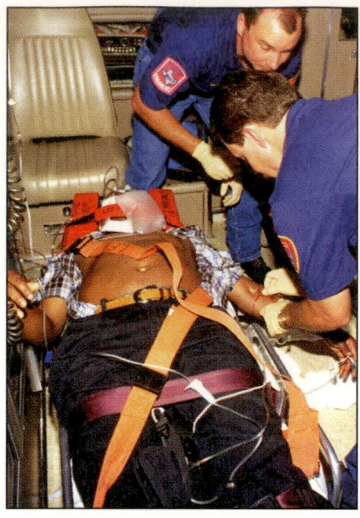

FIGURE 1-5 Advanced training covers a wide range of ALS skills, including IV therapy.

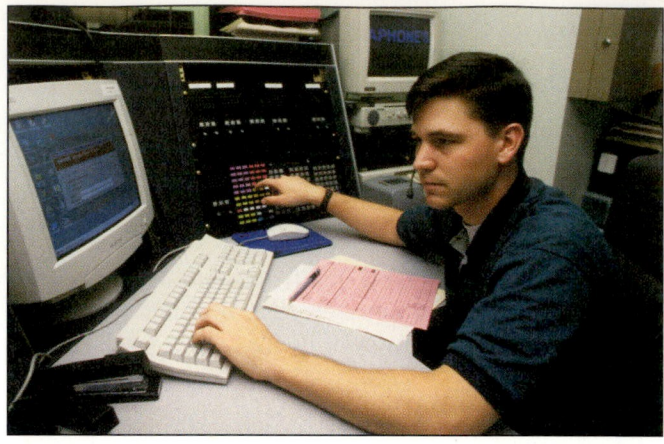

FIGURE 1-6 Trained dispatchers obtain information about the call and then send responders to the scene as needed.

EMT-Intermediate

The EMT-Intermediate (EMT-I) course and training are designed to add increased knowledge and additional skills in specific aspects of ALS to individuals who have been trained and have experience in providing emergency care as an EMT-B. These additional skills include IV therapy, interpretation of cardiac rhythms and defibrillation, orotracheal intubation, and, in some states, the knowledge and skills necessary to administer certain prescribed drugs.

EMT-Paramedic

The EMT-Paramedic (EMT-P) has completed an extensive course of training that significantly increases knowledge and mastery of basic skills and covers a wide range of ALS skills (Figure 1-5). These skills include the following:

- ECG monitoring and interpretation of cardiac rhythms
- Advanced cardiac life support (ACLS) protocols and skills
- Manual defibrillation and external cardiac pacing
- Various techniques for orotracheal and nasotracheal intubation
- Performing a cricothyroidostomy and percutaneous transtracheal ventilation
- Decompressing a tension pneumothorax
- IV therapy
- Advanced pharmacology
- Drug calculations
- Techniques necessary to administer emergency medications orally, by injection, and by IV

Components of the EMS System

Access

Easy access to help needed in an emergency is essential. In most of the country, an emergency communications center that dispatches fire, police, rescue, and EMS units can be reached by dialing 9-1-1. At the communication center, trained dispatchers obtain the necessary information from the caller and, following dispatch protocols, dispatch the ambulance crew and other equipment and responders that may be needed (Figure 1-6).

In an enhanced 9-1-1 system, the address of the phone from which the call is made is displayed on a screen. The connection is frozen until the dispatcher releases it so that if the caller is unable to speak, his or her location remains displayed. Most emergency communications centers also include special equipment so that individuals with speech or hearing disabilities can communicate with the dispatcher via a keyboard and printed messages. In some areas, rather than 9-1-1, a different special published emergency number may be used to call for EMS. Training the public in how to summon an EMS unit is an important part of the public education responsibility of each service.

In many municipalities, EMS is a part of the fire department. In others, it is a part of the police department or is an independent public safety service. In some areas, a contractor may provide either the basic EMS or ALS service. In some areas, ALS is provided by paramedics who are based at a hospital or who may cover a number of towns in a region.

Administration and Policy

Each EMS service operates in a designated **primary service area (PSA)** in which it is responsible for the provision of prehospital emergency care and the transportation of the sick and injured to the hospital.

EMS services are usually administered by a senior EMS official. Daily operations and overall direction of the service is provided by an appointed chief executive officer and several other officers who serve under him or her. When the EMS service is a part of a fire or police department, the department chief will usually delegate the responsibility for directing EMS to an assistant chief or other officer whose sole responsibility is to manage the EMS activities of the department. To provide clear guidelines, most services have written operating procedures and policies. When you join a service, you will be expected to learn and follow them.

The chief executive of the service is in charge of both the necessary administrative tasks (e.g., scheduling, personnel, budgets, purchasing, vehicle maintenance) and the daily operations of the ambulances and crews. Except for medical matters, he or she operates as the chief (similar to a fire chief or police chief) of EMS for the service and the PSA that it covers.

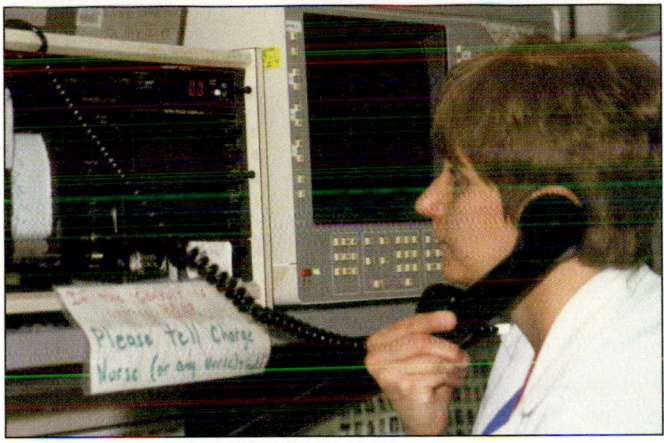

FIGURE 1-7 On-line or direct medical control is provided by a physician.

Medical Direction and Control

Each EMS system has a physician **medical director** who authorizes the EMTs in the service to provide medical care in the field. The appropriate care for each injury, condition, or illness that you will encounter in the field is determined by the medical director and is described in a set of written standing orders, or protocols. **Medical control** is either off-line (indirect) or on-line (direct), as authorized by the medical director. Standing orders are known as indirect medical direction. Each EMT must know and follow the protocols prescribed by his or her medical director.

The service's protocols will also identify a medical control hospital or center at which an EMS physician designated by the service's medical director can be reached by radio or phone for medical control during a call (Figure 1-7). This is called direct medical control. On each call, once the squad has initiated any immediate urgent care and gives its radio report, the on-line medical control physician will either confirm or modify the proposed treatment plan and will prescribe any additional special orders that the EMT-Bs are to follow for that patient. The point at which the EMT-Bs should give their radio report and obtain on-line medical direction varies from place to place.

The medical director provides the ongoing working liaison between the medical community, hospitals, and the EMTs in the service. If treatment problems arise or different procedures should be considered, these are referred to the medical director for his or her decision

and action. To ensure that the proper training standards are met, the medical director determines and approves the continuing education and training that are required of each EMT in the service and approves any that individuals obtain elsewhere.

Quality Control and Improvement

The medical director is responsible for maintaining **quality control**, ensuring that all staff members who are involved in caring for patients meet appropriate medical care standards on each call. To provide the necessary quality control, the medical director and other involved staff review each written patient run report that EMTs complete and the impressions noted by the physician who received the patient in the emergency department.

Continuous quality improvement (CQI) is a circular system of continuous internal and external reviews and audits of all aspects of an EMS call. To provide CQI, periodic run review meetings are held in which all those who are involved in patient care review the run reports and then discuss any areas of care that appear to need change or improvement. Areas that are done well are also discussed. If a problem appears to be repeated by a single EMT or crew, the medical director will discuss the details with the individuals involved and, if necessary, assign remedial training or some other development activity. The medical director is also responsible for ensuring that appropriate continuing education and training are available.

Information and skills in emergency medical care change constantly. You need refresher training or continuing education as new modalities of care, equipment, and understanding of critical illnesses and trauma develop. Equally, when you have not used a particular procedure or skill for some time, skill decay occurs. Therefore, your medical director might establish a CQI

> Each EMS system has a physician medical director who authorizes the EMTs in the service to provide medical care in the field.

process to correct the deficit. For example, an emergency department physician noted that despite their assessments, many EMT-Bs were missing a high number of closed long bone fractures, resulting in poor prehospital care. A subsequent audit of calls led to a review and retraining session for assessment and care of fractures. This same issue is involved in BLS/CPR or any other type of skill that you do not use often. Ensuring that your skills and knowledge are current is one of the ongoing commitments of being an EMT.

Other Physician Input

EMS is an extension of the emergency medical care provided in the emergency department by physicians and the other specialists who provide definitive care in the hospital. Besides the direction that the medical director and direct on-line medical control physicians provide, your training and practices are based on input from many specialty professional associations at the national, state, and local levels.

As an EMT-B, you are part of the professional continuum of care provided to patients who often have life-threatening conditions. Physicians are at the top of the professional continuum pyramid. Many physician experts from the specialties of emergency medicine, traumatology, orthopaedics, cardiology, anesthesiology, radiology, and other medical disciplines participate in the ongoing work of EMS. The efforts of these groups—often through professional associations such as the American Academy of Orthopaedic Surgeons, the American College of Emergency Physicians, the American College of Surgeons —include research, the establishment of standards for quality assurance, continuing education, and publications. These efforts and other beneficial work assist EMS in the day-to-day work of EMTs.

Regulation

Although each EMS system, medical director, and training program has vast latitude, their training, protocols, and practices must conform with the EMS legislation, rules, regulations, and guidelines adopted by each respective state. The state OEMS is responsible for authorizing, auditing, and regulating all EMS services, training institu-

tions, courses, instructors, and providers within the state. In most states, the state EMS office obtains input from an advisory committee made up of representatives of the services, service medical directors, medical associations, hospitals, training programs, instructors' associations, EMT associations, and the public in that state.

Equipment

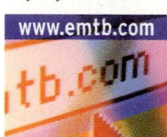

As an EMT-B, you will use a wide range of different emergency equipment. During the EMT-B course, you will be introduced to, and learn how to use, a variety of the different appliances and devices that you may need to use on a call. You will also learn when the use of each is indicated and when it is contraindicated because it will not be of benefit or may cause harm. Although the use of different models and brands of a given device will follow the same generic principles and methods, some variation and peculiarities exist from one model to another. When you join a service, you should check each key piece of equipment before going on duty to ensure that it is in its assigned place, that it is working properly, and that you are familiar with the specific model carried on your ambulance.

The Ambulance

Each EMT-B may be called upon to drive the ambulance (Figure 1-8). Therefore, you must familiarize yourself with the roads in your PSA or sector. Before going on duty, you should check all the equipment and supplies that the ambulance carries and make sure that it is fully fueled, that it has sufficient oil and other key fluids, and that the tires are in good condition and properly inflated. You should also test each of the driver's controls and each built-in unit and control in the patient compartment. If you have not driven the specific ambulance before, it is a good idea to take it out and become familiar with it before you respond to a call. Maintenance and safe driving of the ambulance are discussed in detail in Chapter 36.

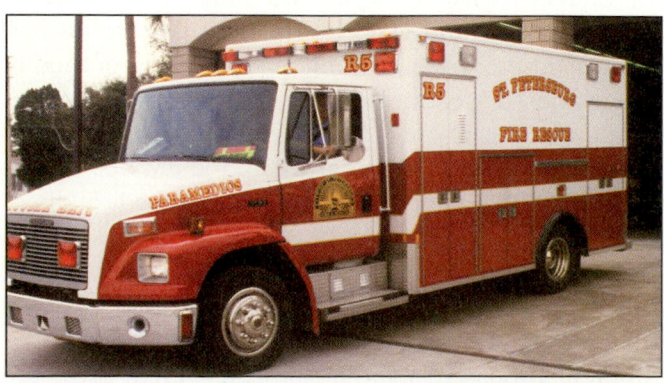

FIGURE 1-8 You may be called upon to drive the ambulance.

Transport to Specialty Centers

In addition to hospital emergency departments, many EMS systems include specialty centers that focus on specific types of care (e.g., trauma, burns, poison, or psychiatric conditions) or specific types of patients (e.g., children). Specialty centers require in-house staffs of surgeons and other specialists; other facilities must page operating teams, surgeons, or other specialists from outside the hospital. Typically, only a few hospitals in a region are designated as specialty centers. Transport time to a specialty center may be slightly longer than that to an emergency department, but patients will receive definitive care more quickly at a specialty center. You must know the location of the centers in your area and when, according to your protocol, you must transport the patient directly to one. Sometimes, air medical transport will be necessary. Local, regional, and state protocols will guide your decision in these instances.

Working with Hospital Staff

You should become familiar with the hospital by observing hospital equipment and how it is used, the functions of staff members, and the policies and procedures in all emergency areas of the hospital. You will also learn about advances in emergency care and how to interact with hospital personnel (Figure 1-9). This experience will help you to understand how your care influences the patient's recovery and will emphasize the importance and benefits of proper prehospital care. It will also show you the consequences of delay, inadequate care, or poor judgment.

Physician, nurses, and other medical professionals are not likely be in the field with you to provide personal, on-the-spot instructions. However, you may consult with appropriate medical staff over the radio through established medical control procedures.

In the emergency department, hospital staff may train you by showing you assessment and treatment techniques on actual patients. A physician or nurse may serve as an instructor for medical subjects in your training program. Through these experiences, you will become more comfortable using medical terms, interpreting patient signs and symptoms, and developing patient management skills.

Hospital staff are usually willing to help you improve your skills and efficiency throughout your career. Some physicians and nurses may have completed the EMT curriculum as part of their formal medical training. The best patient care occurs when all emergency care providers have a close rapport. This allows you and hospital staff the opportunity to discuss mutual problems and to benefit from each other's experiences.

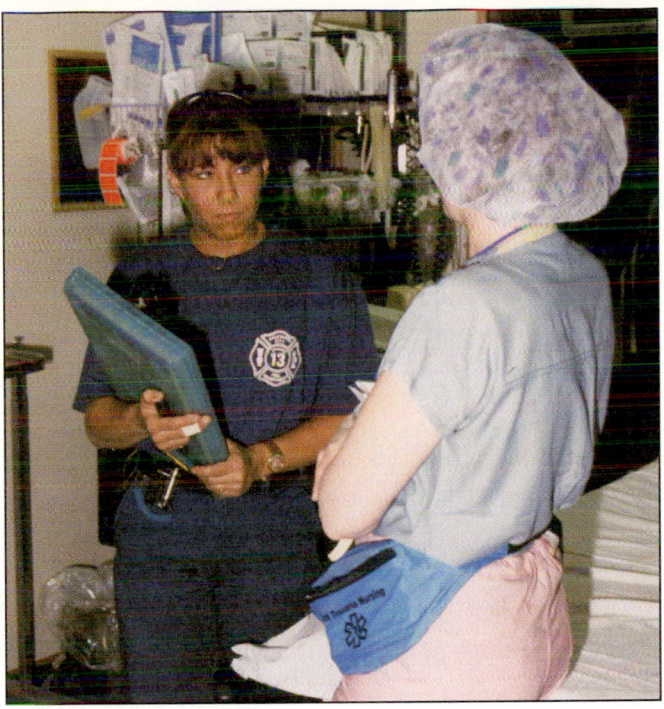

FIGURE 1-9 As an EMT-B, you will interact with hospital staff.

Working with Public Safety Agencies

Some public safety workers have EMS training. As an EMT-B, you must become familiar with all the roles and responsibilities of these agencies. Personnel from certain agencies are better prepared than you to perform certain functions. For example, employees of a utility company are better equipped to control downed power lines than you or your partner. Law enforcement personnel are better able to handle violent scenes and traffic control, while you and your partner are better able to provide emergency medical care. If you work together and recognize that each person has special talent and a job to do at the scene, effective scene and patient management will result. Remember that the best, most efficient patient care is achieved through cooperation among agencies.

Training

Your training will be conducted by many knowledgeable EMS educators. In most states, the instructors who are responsible for coordinating and teaching the EMT-B course and continuing education courses are approved and certified by the state EMS. To be certified, an instructor must have extensive medical and educational training, and teach for a designated period while being observed and supervised by an experienced instructor.

Most ALS training is provided in either a college or hospital setting. In most states, educational programs that provide ALS training must be approved by the state and have their own medical director. In these courses, many of the lectures and small group sessions will be presented by the medical director or other physicians and nurses. In clinical sessions in which supervised practice is obtained in the emergency department or other in-hospital settings, students are also supervised directly by physicians and other medical staff.

The quality of care that you will provide depends on your ability and the quality of your training. Therefore, your instructor and the many others who developed and participated in your training program are key members of the emergency care team.

Providing a Coordinated Continuum of Care

The emergency care of patients occurs in three progressive phases:

1. **The first phase** consists of patient assessment, initial prehospital care, proper packaging, and safe transport to the hospital.

2. **In the second phase,** the patient receives continued assessment and stabilization in the hospital emergency department.

3. **In the third phase,** the patient receives the necessary specialized definitive care.

These three phases must be provided in a coordinated continuum of care to maximize survival and reduce suffering and lasting adverse effects. The EMS system is designed to produce such a coordinated effort among the local EMS services, emergency department staff, and the medical staff who provide definitive care.

Roles and Responsibilities of the EMT-B

As an EMT-B, you will be the first healthcare professional to assess and treat the patient; as such, you have certain roles and responsibilities (Table 1-2). Often, patient outcomes are determined by the care that you provide in the field and your identification of patients who need prompt transport.

Professional Attributes

As an EMT-B, whether paid or volunteer, you are a healthcare professional. Part of your responsibility is to make sure that patient care is given a high priority without endangering your own safety or the safety of others.

TABLE 1-2   Roles and Responsibilities of the EMT-B

- Locating and safely driving to the scene
- Sizing up the scene and situation
- Ensuring your own safety and the safety of your fellow EMT-Bs, the patient, and others at the scene
- Rapidly assessing the patient's gross neurologic, respiratory, and circulatory status
- Providing any essential immediate intervention
- Performing a thorough, accurate patient assessment
- Obtaining an expanded SAMPLE history
- Reaching a clinical impression and providing prompt, efficient, prioritized patient care based on your assessment
- Communicating effectively with the patient and advising him or her of any procedures you will perform
- Properly interacting and communicating with fire, rescue, and law enforcement responders at the scene
- Identifying patients who require rapid packaging, and initiating transport without delay

- Identifying patients who do not need emergency care and will benefit from further detailed assessment and care before they are moved and transported
- Properly packaging the patient
- Safely lifting and moving the patient to the ambulance and loading the patient into it
- Providing safe, appropriate transport to the hospital emergency department or other ordered facility
- Giving the necessary radio report to the medical control center or receiving hospital emergency department
- Providing any additional assessment or treatment while en route
- Monitoring the patient and checking vital signs while en route
- Documenting all findings and care on the run report
- Unloading the patient safely and, after giving a proper verbal report, transferring the patient's care to the emergency department staff
- Safeguarding the patient's rights

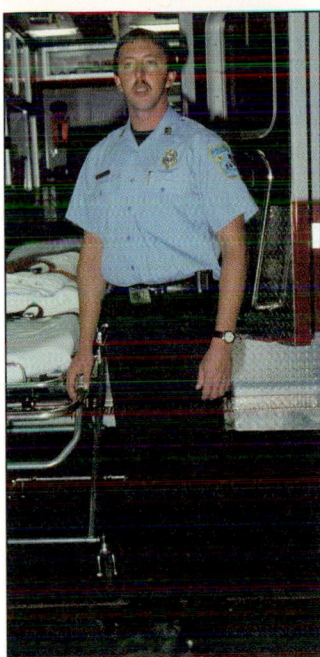

FIGURE 1-10 A professional appearance and manner help to build confidence and ease patient anxiety.

Another part of the responsibility to yourself, other EMTs, the patient, and other healthcare professionals is to maintain a professional appearance and manner at all times. Your attitude and behavior must reflect that you are knowledgeable and sincerely dedicated to serving anyone who is injured or in an acute medical emergency.

As a professional, you must take pride in your appearance, grooming, and hygiene (Figure 1-10). A professional appearance and manner help to build confidence and ease the patient's anxiety. You will be expected to perform under pressure with composure and self-confidence. Patients and families who are under stress need to be treated with understanding, respect, and compassion.

Most patients will treat you with respect and appreciation, but some will not. Some patients are uncooperative, demanding, unpleasant, ungrateful, and verbally abusive. You must be nonjudgmental and overcome your instincts to react poorly to such behavior. Remember that when individuals are hurt, ill, under stress, frightened, despondent, under the influence of alcohol or drugs, or feel threatened, they will often react with inappropriate behavior, even toward those who are trying to help and care for them. *Every patient, regardless of his or her attitude, is entitled to compassion, respect, and the best care that you can provide.*

Most individuals in this country can obtain proper routine medical care when they are ill and are surrounded by relatives and friends who will help to take care of them. However, when you are called to a home for a medical problem that is clearly not an emergency, remember that for some individuals, calling an ambulance and being transported to the emergency department for an illness are the only way to obtain medical care.

As a new EMT-B, you will be given a lot of advice and training from the more experienced EMT-Bs with whom you serve. Some may voice a callous disregard for some types of patients. You should not be influenced by the unprofessional attitude of these individuals, regardless of how experienced or skilled they appear.

As a healthcare professional and an extension of physician care, you are bound by patient confidentiality. You should not discuss your findings or any disclosures made by the patient with anyone but those who are treating the patient or, as required by law, the police or other social agencies. When discussing a call with others, you should be careful to avoid any information that might disclose the name or identity of patients you have treated. Be careful not to gossip about calls and patients with others, even in your own home.

Continuing Education

Once you no longer have the structured learning environment that is provided in a course, you must assume the responsibility for directing your own study and learning. As an EMT-B, you will be required to attend a certain number of hours of continuing education each year to maintain, update, and expand your knowledge and skills. In many services, the required hours are provided by the training officer and medical director. In addition, most EMS education programs and hospitals offer a number of regular continuing education opportunities in each region. You may also attend state and national EMS conferences to help keep you up-to-date about local, state, and national issues affecting EMS. Whether you take advantage of these opportunities depends on you. Whether you decide to remain an EMT-B or achieve a higher level of training and certification, the key to being a good EMT and providing high-quality care is your commitment to continual learning and ever increasing knowledge and skills.

EMTs possess special knowledge and skills that are directed to the care of patients in emergency situations. The authority that is delegated to you to care for patients is a very special one. Maintaining your knowledge and skills is a substantial responsibility. Knowledge and skills that are learned in any profession decay and weaken when they are not used on a continual basis. Consider BLS/CPR. If you have not used these skills since your original training, it is likely that you will perform CPR in a way that is less than desirable. Continuing education and refresher courses are one way by which you can maintain your skills and knowledge.

Every patient, regardless of his or her attitude, is entitled to compassion, respect, and the best care that you can provide.

prep kit

ready for review

EMS is the system that provides the emergency medical care that is needed by people who have been injured or have an acute medical emergency. When the dispatcher at the 9-1-1 emergency communications center receives a call for emergency care, he or she dispatches to the scene the designated EMS ambulance squad and any fire, rescue, or police units that may be needed. The EMS ambulance is staffed by EMTs who have been trained to the EMT-Basic, EMT-Intermediate, or EMT-Paramedic level according to recommended national standards and have been certified/licensed by the state. After the EMTs size up the scene and assess the patient, they provide the emergency care that is indicated by their findings and ordered by their medical director in the service's standing order protocols or the physician who is providing on-line medical direction. The EMTs then package the patient and provide transport to the nearby hospital or designated specialized care facility (eg, trauma center, pediatric hospital) for further evaluation and stabilization in the emergency department and, after admission, definitive surgical or medical care.

The EMT-B course that you are now taking will present the information and skills that you will need to pass the required examinations for licensure and start as an EMT-B in the field. This course will provide you with the training that you need to function as an EMT-B and will serve as the essential foundation upon which you can advance your training and expertise.

The following are the essential keys to being a good EMT-B:

- Compassion and motivation to reduce suffering, pain, and death in those who are injured or acutely ill
- Desire to provide each patient with the best possible care
- Commitment to obtain the knowledge and skills that this requires
- The drive to continually increase your knowledge, skills, and ability

Once you have successfully completed this course and have been certified as an EMT-B, you will enter the next key phase of your training. When you join an EMS service, your first task will be to learn the medical protocols and operating procedures of the squad. You will also have to learn where each piece of equipment is kept on the ambulance and become familiar with how the specific models that you will be using operate. From your experience and the guidance provided by your crew chief and the other experienced EMT-Bs you work with, you will gain increased mastery of the skills that you learned in the course and learn how to apply your knowledge and skills in the diverse situations that are actually encountered in the field.

Once you have completed the course, you must assume responsibility for directing your own study through continuing education provided by your service's training officer and medical director and through other opportunities available to you. Your commitment to continuing learning is the key to being a good EMT.

vital vocabulary

www.emtb.com

advanced life support (ALS) Advanced lifesaving procedures, some of which are now being provided by the EMT-B.

Americans with Disabilities Act (ADA) Comprehensive legislation that is designed to protect individuals with disabilities against discrimination.

continuous quality improvement (CQI) A system of internal and external reviews and audits of all aspects of an EMS system.

emergency medical services (EMS) A multidisciplinary system that represents the combined efforts of several professionals and agencies to provide prehospital emergency care to the sick and injured.

emergency medical technician (EMT) An EMS professional who is trained and licensed by the state to provide emergency medical care in the field.

EMT-Basic An EMT who has training in basic emergency care skills, including automated defibrillation, use of a definitive airway adjunct, and assisting patients with certain medications.

EMT-Intermediate An EMT who has advanced training in specific aspects of advanced life support, such as intravenous therapy.

EMT-Paramedic An EMT who has extensive training in advanced life support, including intravenous therapy, pharmacology, cardiac monitoring, and other advanced assessment and treatment skills.

first responder The first trained individual, such as a police officer, fire fighter, or other rescuer, to arrive at the scene of an emergency to provide initial medical assistance.

medical control Physician instructions that are given directly by radio (on-line/direct) or indirectly by protocol/guidelines (off-line/indirect), as authorized by the medical director.

medical director The physician who authorizes or delegates the authority to perform medical care in the field.

primary service area (PSA) The area in which the EMS service is responsible for the provision of prehospital emergency care and transportation to the hospital.

quality control The responsibility of the medical director to ensure that the appropriate medical care standards are met by EMT-Bs on each call.

assessment in action

You are on your way to becoming an EMT-Basic, the backbone of the EMS system. In this course, you will learn new terms, theories, and techniques. These fundamental concepts and principles serve as the very foundation of patient care skills.

To help you develop critical thinking skills, expanded scenarios called Assessment in Action appear at the end of each chapter.

These scenarios are followed by discussion and multiple-choice questions that are designed to stimulate discussion with your classmates or your instructor. These discussions, along with the rest of your course work, will help you to develop the skills that you need to become a successful EMT-B.

1. Which of the following is **NOT** considered one of the roles and responsibilities of an EMT-B?
   A. Ensuring your own safety during an emergency response
   B. Treating only patients who are able to pay for your services
   C. Providing safe transport of patients in your care to the hospital
   D. Providing quality patient care based on your assessment findings

2. What aspect of EMS is most likely to contribute to reducing permanent injury and disability to the general population?
   A. Health care insurance for all Americans
   B. Rapid access to EMS using 9-1-1 systems
   C. Increased Medicare reimbursement for hospitals
   D. Smaller, faster, and more fuel-efficient ambulances

3. Which of the following is **NOT** an attribute of a professional EMT-B?
   A. Having total recall of local EMS protocols
   B. Meeting continuing education requirements
   C. Maintaining a neat, clean personal appearance
   D. Placing personal needs before the patient's needs

4. Continuous quality improvement in EMS is best described as:
   A. a local concept with little practical importance except to attorneys and legislators.
   B. a government mandate that ensures that each state receives the same amount of tax-based funding.
   C. an ongoing system of audits and reviews that ensures that the public receives the highest standard of patient care.
   D. a philosophy that suggests that only young, healthy individuals be employed in EMS to reduce on-the-job injuries.

5. The medical director of an EMS provider agency is **NOT** responsible for:
   A. reviewing run reports to ensure compliance with protocols.
   B. developing and implementing protocols or standing orders.
   C. providing on-line medical direction during emergency calls.
   D. deciding which patients will be reimbursed for insurance claims.

prep kit 1

points to ponder

Objectives 1-1.2, 1-1.8

You are a volunteer for a rural ambulance agency and are dispatched to a two-car automobile accident about 12 miles out of town. There are six reported victims, at least two of whom are in bad shape. When you arrive, there are two people on scene who identify themselves as first responders, and they begin telling you what they have been doing. Shortly after your arrival, a car stops, and an EMT from a fire department in another city gets out and assumes control of the scene. It is quickly determined that the EMT is an EMT-B with less than a year of experience.

- Describe how you would deal both with the first responders and with the other EMT. What is the primary goal at the scene of any emergency?

online outlook

The National Highway Traffic Safety Administration's (NHTSA) mission is to save lives, prevent injuries, and reduce traffic-related health care and other economic costs. Learn more about the NHTSA's involvement in EMS by completing Exercise 1 at www.emtb.com.

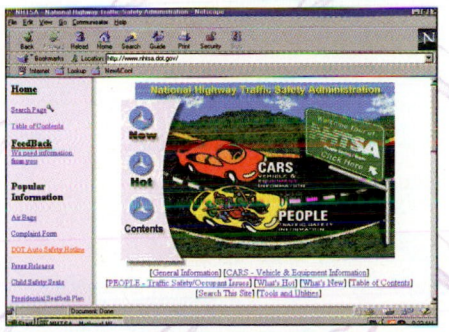

The Well-Being
of the EMT-B

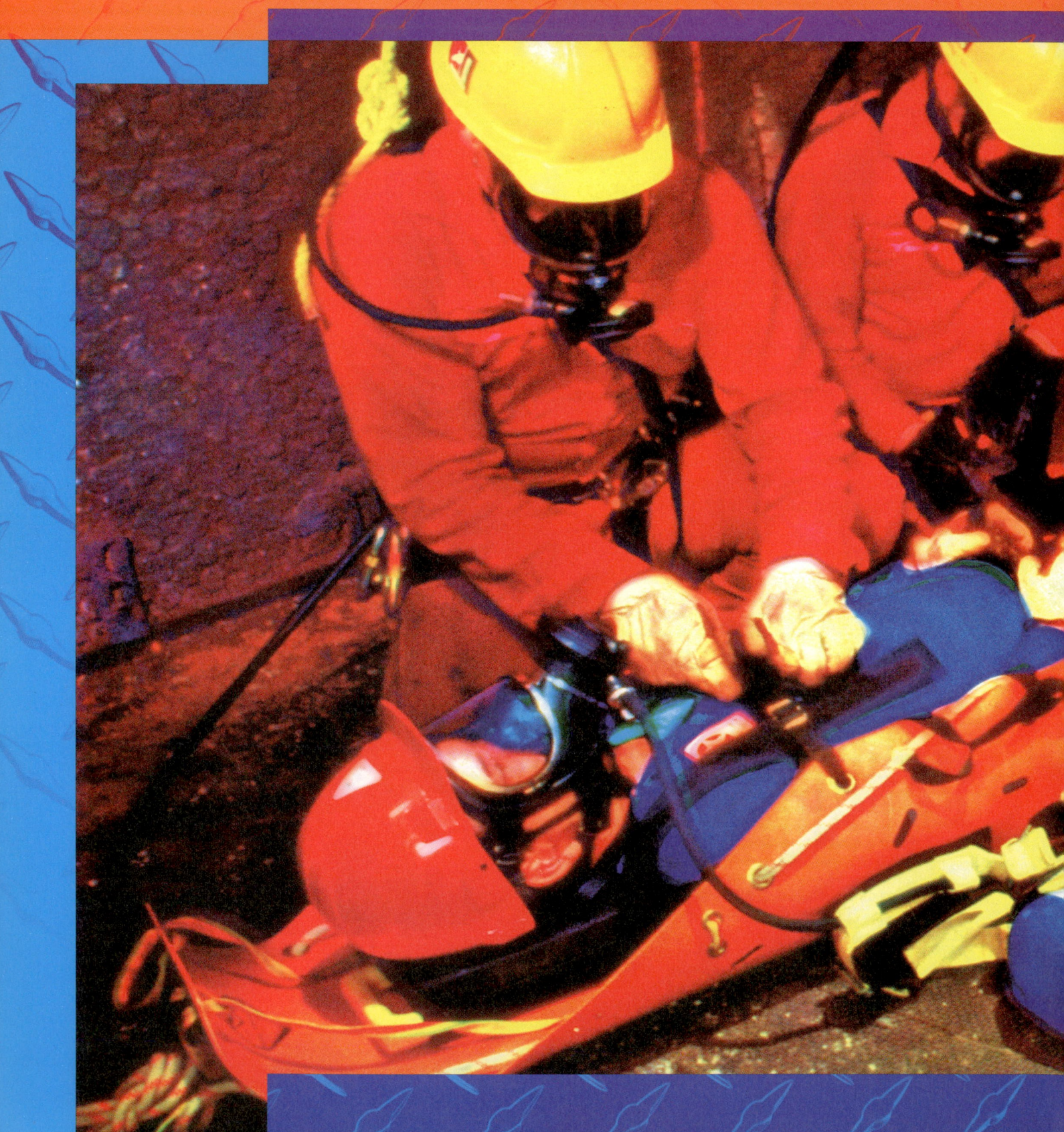

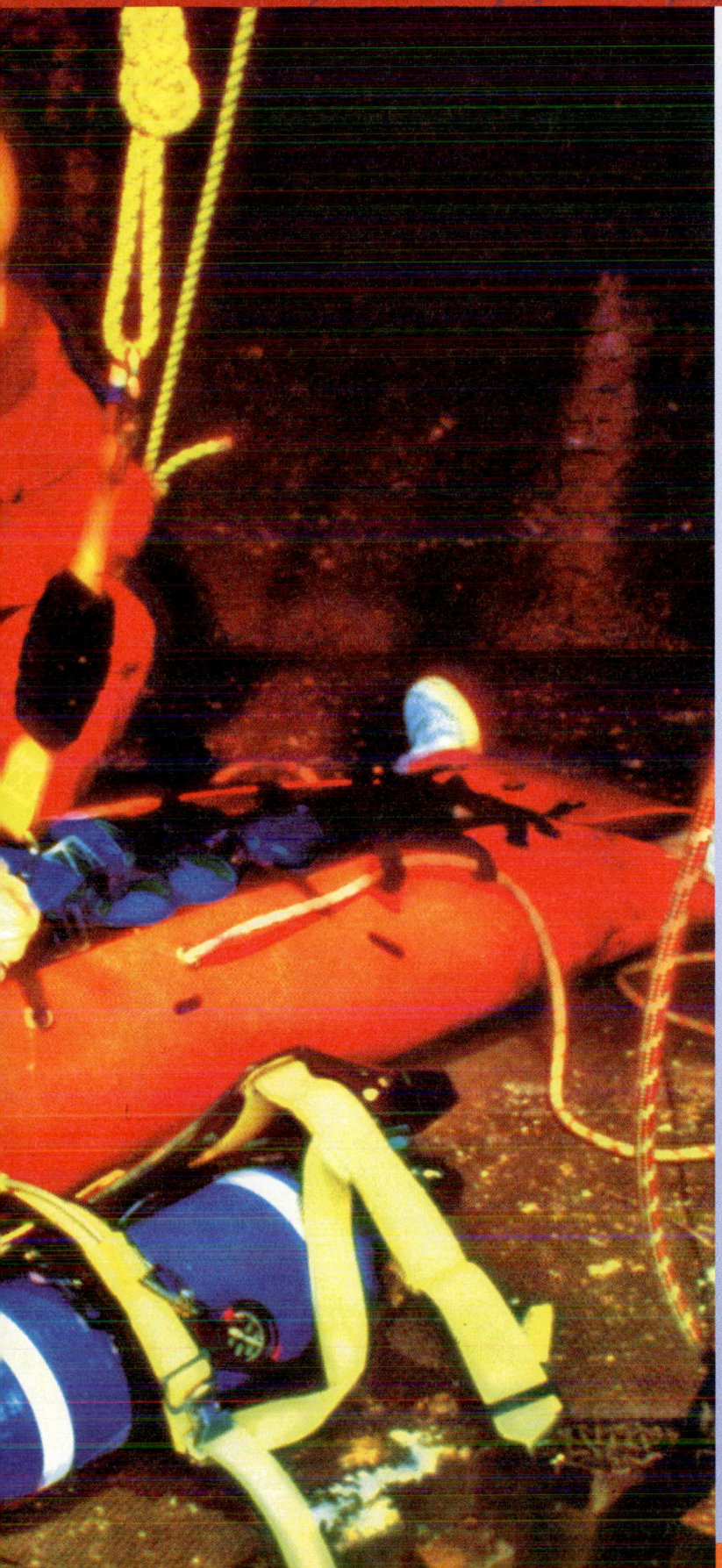

objectives

Cognitive

1. List possible emotional reactions that the EMT-B may experience when faced with trauma, illness, death, and dying.

2. Discuss the possible reactions that a family member may exhibit when confronted with death and dying.

3. State the steps in the EMT-B's approach to the family confronted with death and dying.

4. State the possible reactions that the family of the EMT-B may exhibit due to their outside involvement in EMS.

5. Recognize the signs and symptoms of critical incident stress.

6. State possible steps that the EMT-B may take to help reduce/alleviate stress.

7. Explain the need to determine scene safety.

8. Discuss the importance of body substance isolation (BSI).

9. Describe the steps the EMT-B should take for personal protection from airborne and bloodborne pathogens.

10. List the personal protective equipment necessary for each of the following situations:
    - Hazardous materials
    - Rescue operations
    - Violent scenes
    - Crime scenes
    - Exposure to bloodborne pathogens
    - Exposure to airborne pathogens

Affective

11. Explain the rationale for serving as an advocate for the use of appropriate protective equipment.

Psychomotor

12. Given a scenario with potential infectious exposure, the EMT-B will use appropriate personal protective equipment. At the completion of the scenario, the EMT-B will properly remove and discard the protective garments.

13. Given the above scenario, the EMT-B will complete disinfection/cleaning and all reporting documentation.

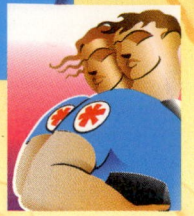

you are the emt

Squad 7 please respond to a home at 251 Redondo Circle for emergency assistance of a patient with terminal cancer.

A patient with a terminal illness might wish to die at home, and the family might call for help when death is imminent. Death is a part of life and will be part of your experience as an EMT-B. This chapter will help you to understand how to cope with difficult situations and emphasize the importance of your personal well-being. It will also help you to answer the following questions:

1. What are the warning signs of stress? When should you seek professional assistance for yourself or your co-workers?
2. What can you do to reduce some of the risks associated with being an EMT-B?

The Well-Being of the EMT-B

There is an ancient proverb, "Physician, heal thyself." As providers of health care, doctors need to look after themselves—in all respects—so that they can minister to others. An ill physician is in no position to render care as he or she was trained to do. That dictum applies to all healthcare providers and goes well beyond just physical factors. In caring for the critically ill and injured, there are many factors and situations that can interfere with the EMT-B's ability to treat the patient.

The personal health, safety, and well-being of all EMT-Bs are vital to an EMS operation. As a part of your training, you will learn how to recognize possible hazards and protect yourself from them. These hazards vary greatly, ranging from personal neglect to environmental and human-made threats to your health and safety. You will also learn about the mental and physical stress that you must cope with as a result of caring for the sick and injured. Death and dying challenge you to deal with the realities of human weaknesses and the emotions of the survivors.

It is important to remain calm to perform effectively when you are confronted with horrifying events, life-threatening illness, or injury. A special kind of self-control is needed to respond efficiently and effectively to the suffering of others. This self-control is developed through the following:

- Proper training
- Ongoing experience in dealing with all types of physical and mental distress
- A dedication to serve humanity

Emotional Aspects of Emergency Care

At times, even the most experienced healthcare providers have difficulty overcoming personal reactions and proceeding without hesitation. Patients need to be removed from life-threatening situations. Life support measures need to be given to patients who are severely injured. You may also be called upon to recover human remains from highway accidents, aircraft disasters, or explosions (Figure 2-1). In all of these situations, you must be calm and act responsibly as a member of the emergency medical care team. You must also realize that even though

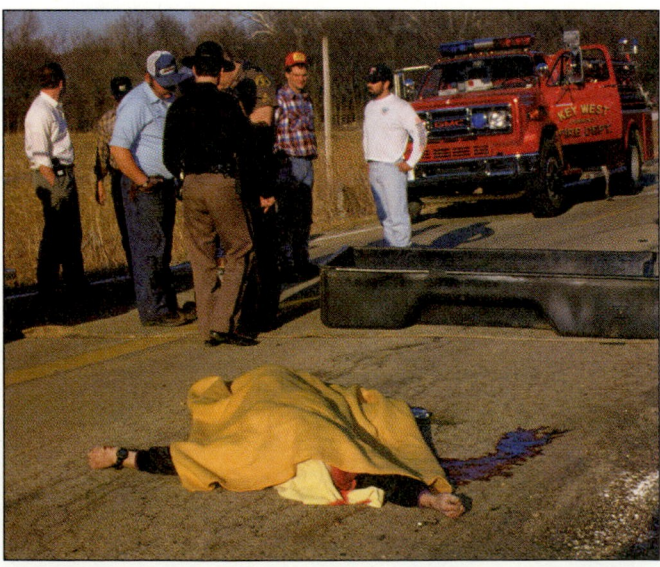

FIGURE 2-1 As an EMT-B, you will be called upon to recover human remains from disaster scenes, such as highway accidents, airline crashes, or explosions.

your personal emotions must be kept under control, these are normal feelings. Every EMT-B who must deal with such situations has these feelings. The struggle to remain calm in the face of horrible circumstances contributes to the emotional stress of the job.

Death and Dying

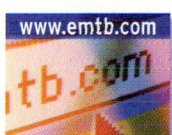

Today, life expectancy has dramatically increased; nearly two-thirds of all deaths occur among those age 65 and older. Sixty percent of all deaths today are attributed to heart disease. From the age of 1 to the age of 34, trauma is the leading cause of death. Death today is likely to occur either quite suddenly or after a prolonged terminal illness. The environment of death has changed since our nation's earlier days; it no longer occurs in the home setting. The setting of death is somewhere else—in the hospital, a hospice, or a convalescent home, at the workplace, or on the highway. For this reason, we are less familiar with death than our ancestors were. We tend to deny death in America. Illness can be much more drawn-out and much more removed from daily life. Life support systems and impersonal care remove the whole experience of death from most people's awareness. The mobility of families also makes it less likely that there will be extended family support when death does occur.

Death was once both an expected and accepted fact in earlier American history. Life expectancy was brief (compared to today's), mortality rates (the ratio of number of deaths to a given population size) were high, and childbirth was hazardous, often resulting in the death of both the mother and the baby. Hardships of the times, both natural and human-made, were great. Children and adults died from disease, injuries, and the traumas of war. Most people had experienced the death of someone close to them. There were no funeral homes; mourning occurred at home in the family setting. The presence of the dead body was a natural event.

No matter what the frequency of response to emergency calls, death is something that every EMT-B will sometime face. For some of you, it may be infrequent. Others, in urban settings, may see death many times in responding to motor vehicle crashes, drug overdoses, suicides, or homicides. Some EMT firefighters may have to deal with the mass-casualty incident of an airplane crash or a hazardous materials accident. In all these cases, coming to grips with your thoughts, understandings, and adjustment to death is not only important personally, but also a function of delivering emergency medical care.

Physical Signs of Death

Determination of the cause of death is the medical responsibility of a physician. There are both definitive and presumptive signs of death. In many states, death is defined as the absence of circulatory and respiratory function. Many states have also adopted "brain death" provisions; these provisions refer to irreversible cessation of all functions of the brain and brain stem. Questions often arise as to whether to begin basic life support. In the absence of physician orders such as do not resuscitate (DNR), the general rule is: If the body is still warm and intact, initiate emergency medical care. An exception to this rule is cold temperature (hypothermia) emergencies. Hypothermia is a general cooling of the body in which the internal body temperature becomes abnormally low: 95°F (35°C). It is considered a serious condition and is often fatal. At 86°F (30°C), the brain can survive without perfusion for about 10 minutes. When the core temperature drops to 82.4°F (28°C), the patient is in grave danger; however, individuals have survived a hypothermia accident with a temperature of 64.4°F (18°C). In cases of hypothermia, the patient should not be considered dead until the patient is warm and dead.

Presumptive Signs of Death. Most medicolegal authorities will consider the presumptive signs of death that are listed in Table 2-1 adequate, particularly when they follow a severe trauma or occur at the end stages of long-term illness such as cancer or other prolonged diseases. These signs would not be adequate in cases of sudden death due to hypothermia, acute poisoning, or cardiac arrest. Usually, in these cases, some combination of the signs is needed to declare death, not just one of them alone.

TABLE 2-1   Presumptive Signs of Death
• Unresponsiveness to painful stimuli
• Lack of a pulse or heartbeat
• Absence of breath sounds
• No deep tendon or corneal reflexes
• Absence of eye movement
• No systolic blood pressure
• Dependent lividity: blood settling to the lowest point of the body, causing discoloration of skin
• Profound cyanosis
• Lowered or decreased body temperature

Definitive Signs of Death. Definitive or conclusive signs of death that are obvious and clear to even non-medical persons include the following:

- Obvious mortal damage, such as a body in parts (decapitation)

- Rigor mortis, the stiffening of body muscles caused by chemical changes within muscle tissue. It develops first in the face and jaw, gradually extending downward until the body is in full rigor. The rate is affected by the body's ability to lose heat to its surroundings. A thin body loses heat faster than a fat body. A body on a tile floor loses heat faster than a body wrapped up in a blanket in a bed. Rigor mortis occurs sometime between 2 to 12 hours after death.

- Putrefaction (decomposition of body tissues). Depending on temperature conditions, this occurs sometime between 40 to 96 hours after death.

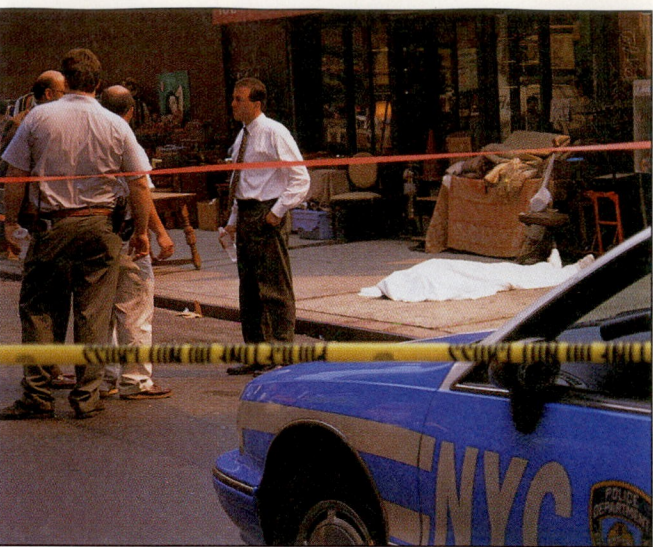

FIGURE 2-2 When trauma is a factor or the death involves a suspected criminal situation, the medical examiner is required.

Medical Examiner Cases

Involvement of the medical examiner, or the coroner in some states, depends on the nature and scene of the death. In most states, when trauma is a factor or the death involves suspected criminal or unusual situations such as hanging or poisoning, the medical examiner is required (Figure 2-2). When the medical examiner or coroner assumes responsibility of the scene, that responsibility supersedes all others at the scene, including the family's. The following are considered medical examiner's cases:

- When the person is dead on arrival (DOA)
- Death without previous medical care or when the physician is unable to state the cause of death
- Suicide (self-destruction)
- Violent death
- Poisoning, known or suspected
- Death resulting from accidents, direct or indirect
- Suspicion of a criminal act

If emergency medical care has been initiated, keep thorough notes of what was done or found. These records may be important during a subsequent investigation.

The Grieving Process

The death of a human being is one of the most difficult events for another human being to accept. If the survivor is a relative or close friend of the deceased, it is even more difficult. Emotional responses to the loss of a loved one or friend are appropriate and should be expected. In fact, it is expected that you will feel emotional about the death of a patient. Feelings and emotions are part of the grieving process. All of us experience these feelings after a stressful situation that causes us personal pain. The stages of grieving are as follows:

1. **Denial.** Refusal to accept diagnosis or care, unrealistic demands for miracles, or persistent failure to understand why there is no improvement.

2. **Anger, hostility.** Projection of bad news onto the environment and commonly in all directions, at times almost at random. The person lashes out. Someone must be blamed, and those who are responsible must be punished. This is usually an ugly phase.

3. **Bargaining.** An attempt to secure a prize for good behavior or promise to change lifestyle. "I promise to be a 'perfect patient' if only I can live until 'x' event."

4. **Depression.** Open expression of grief, internalized anger, hopelessness, the desire to die. It rarely involves suicidal threats, complete withdrawal, or giving up long before the illness seems terminal. The patient is usually silent.

5. **Acceptance.** The simple "yes." Acceptance grows out of a person's conviction that all has been done and the person is ready to die.

Even though the event (death) has not yet happened, the patient knows that it will happen. The patient has no control over this process. The patient will die whether or not he or she is ready to die. Furthermore, being ready to die does not mean that the patient will be happy about dying. You may encounter situations in which the patient is close to death, and you may have to help the patient with this process.

TABLE 2-2	Responding to Grief
Don't Say...	**Try Instead...**
Give it time. Things will get better.	I'm sorry.
You should not question God's will.	It is okay to be angry.
You have to get on with your life.	It must be hard to accept.
You have to keep on going.	That must be painful for you.
You can always have another child.	Tell me how you are feeling.
You're not the only one who suffers.	Let's spend some time together.
The living must go on.	If you want to cry, it's okay.
I know how you feel.	People really cared for…

What Can the EMT-B Do?

Do helpful things, and make simple suggestions. Ask whether there is anything that you can do that will be of help, such as calling a relative or religious advisor. Provide gentle and caring support. Reinforcing the reality of the situation is important. This can be accomplished by merely saying to a grieving person, "I am so sorry for your loss; this is very sad." It is not important that you have a well-rehearsed script, for it is not likely that your exact words or consolations will be remembered. Being yourself and sincere is important.

Some statements tend to be trite, and some suggest a kind of silver lining behind the clouds. Although they may be intended to make the person feel better about a situation, they also can be viewed as an attempt to diminish the person's grief. The grieving person needs to grieve. Statements like these can also indicate our inability to comprehend the profound sadness of grief because we have not experienced that kind of loss.

Attempts to take grief away too quickly are not good. If you do not know how the person really feels, you should not say so. People may be offended by responses that give advice or explanations about the death (Table 2-2). Statements such as "Oh, you shouldn't feel that way" are judgmental. If you judge what the grieving person is feeling, it is likely that he or she will stop talking with you. There is no reason why grieving people should not feel what they are feeling.

Statements and comments that suggest action on your part are generally helpful. These statements imply a sense of understanding; they focus on the grieving person's feelings. It is not necessary to go into an extensive discussion. All you need to do is be sincere and say, "I am so sorry. I just want you to know that I am thinking about you." What people really appreciate is somebody who will listen to them. Simply ask, "Would you like to talk about how or what you are now feeling?" Then accept the response.

Dealing with the Patient and Family Members

There is no right or wrong way to grieve. Each person will experience grief and respond to it in his or her own way. Family members may express rage, anger, and despair. Many people will be rational and cooperative. Their concerns will usually be relieved by your calm, efficient manner. Your actions and words, even a simple touch, can communicate caring. While you must treat all patients with respect and dignity, use special care with dying patients and their families. Be concerned about their privacy and their wishes, and let them know that you take their concerns seriously. However, it is best to be honest with patients and their families; do not give them false hope.

Initial Care of the Dying, Critically Ill, or Injured Patient

Individuals who are in the process of dying as a result of trauma, an acute medical emergency, or a terminal disease will feel threatened. That threat may be related to their concern about survival. These concerns may involve feelings of helplessness, disability, pain, and separation. They are related to the individual's sense of self and understanding of death (Table 2-3).

TABLE 2-3	Major Concerns of the Dying, Critically Ill, or Injured Patient

- Anger and hostility
- Anxiety
- Dependency
- Depression
- Guilt
- Mental health problems
- Pain and fear
- Receiving unrelated bad news

Anxiety. Anxiety is a response to the anticipation of danger. The source of the anxiety is often unknown; but in the case of seriously injured or ill patients, the source is usually recognizable. What may increase the anxiety are the unknowns of the current situation. Patients may ask the following:

- What will happen to me?
- What are you doing?
- Will I make it?
- What will my disabilities be?

Patients who are anxious may exhibit the following signs and symptoms:

- Upset
- Sweaty and cool (diaphoretic)
- Rapid breathing (hyperventilating)
- Fast pulse (tachycardic)
- Restless
- Tense
- Fearful
- Shaky (tremulous)

For the anxious patient, time seems to be extended; seconds seem like minutes, and minutes seem like hours.

Pain and fear. Pain and fear are very closely interrelated. Pain often is associated with illness or trauma. Fear is generally thought of in relation to the oncoming pain and the outcome of the damage. It is often helpful to encourage patients to express their pains and fears, since expression of them begins the process of adjustment to the pain and acceptance of the emergency medical care that may be necessary. Some individuals have difficulty in openly admitting their fear. The fear may be expressed as bad dreams, withdrawal, tension, restlessness, "butterflies" in the stomach, or nervousness. In some cases, it may be expressed as anger.

Anger and hostility. Anger may be expressed by very demanding and complaining behavior. Often, this may be related to the fear and anxiety of the emergency medical care that is being given. Sometimes, the fear is so acute that the patient may want to express anger toward you or others but is unable to do so because of the dependency factor. If you find that you are the target of the patient's anger, make sure that you are safe, but do not take the anger or insults personally. Be tolerant, and do not become defensive.

The anger may also be expressed physically, and you may be the target of the displaced aggression. If the patient or a relative becomes so emotionally upset that you are physically assaulted or you believe that this could happen, back out of the situation. Such hostility must be contained. If emergency medical care is not possible under these circumstances, law enforcement intervention is required.

Depression. Almost all dying patients feel some degree of depression because of internalized anger and other factors. Some patients may have many dissatisfactions and regrets about their lives; others may be wrapped up in concerns about financial, legal, social, or family problems. The patient should be encouraged to express his or her feelings. Assisting the patient and his or her family in resolving unsettled matters may decrease feelings of depression.

Dependency. When emergency medical care is given to any individual, a sense of dependency develops. Individuals who are placed in this position often feel helpless and may become resentful. The resentfulness may arouse feelings of inferiority, shame, or weakness.

Guilt. Many patients who are dying, or families of those patients, may feel quite guilty over what has happened to them. Most of the time, no one can explain these feelings, and the magnitude of the guilt may be very great. Sometimes, feelings of guilt can result in delay in seeking emergency medical care.

Mental health problems. Mental health problems such as disorientation, confusion, or delusions may develop in the dying patient. In these instances, the patient may display behavior that departs from normal patterns of thinking, feeling, or acting. Common characteristics of such behavior may include the following:

- Loss of contact with reality
- Distortion of perception
- Regressive behavior and attitudes
- Diminished control of basic impulses and desires
- Abnormal mental content, including delusions and hallucinations

In some long-term situations, generalized personality deterioration may occur.

Receiving unrelated bad news. A patient who is in critical condition or is dying may not want to hear of unrelated bad news, such as the death of someone close to them. Such news may depress the patient or cause the patient to give up hope.

Caring for Critically Ill and Injured Patients

Patients need to know who you are and what you are doing. Let the patient know that you are attending to his or her immediate needs and that these are your primary

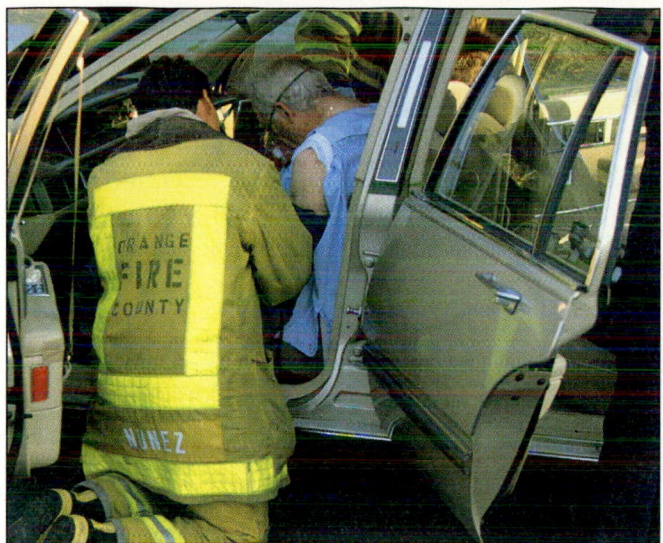

FIGURE 2-3 Let the patient know immediately that you are there to help.

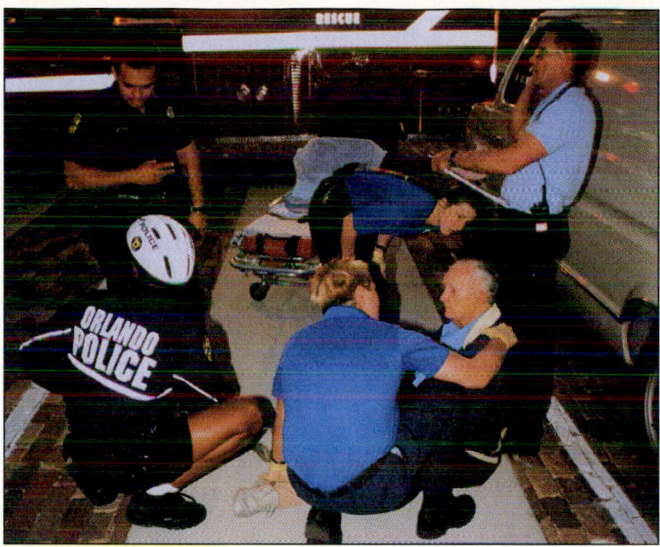

FIGURE 2-4 The aura of an emergency situation can be confusing and frightening to the patient. Make sure you explain to the patient what has happened.

concerns at this moment (Figure 2-3). As soon as possible, explain to the patient what is going on. Confusion, anxiety, and other feelings of helplessness will be decreased if you keep the patient informed at the scene.

Avoid Sad and Grim Comments

EMT-Bs, other safety personnel, family, and bystanders must avoid grim comments about a patient's condition. Remarks such as "This is a bad one" or "The leg is badly damaged, and I think he will lose it" are inappropriate. These remarks may depress the patient and compromise possible recovery outcomes. This is especially true for the patient who may be able to hear but not to respond.

Orient the Patient

You should expect a patient to be disoriented in an emergency situation. The aura of the emergency situation—lights, sirens, smells, and unknown personnel—is intense. The impact and effect of injuries or acute illness may cause the patient to be confused or unsettled. It is important to orient the patient to his or her surroundings (Figure 2-4). Use brief, concise statements such as "Mr. Smith, you have had an accident, and I am now splinting your arm. I am John Foxworth of the New Britain EMS; I will be caring for you."

Be Honest

In approaching any patient, you must decide how much each patient is able to understand and accept. You should be honest without additionally shocking the patient or giving information that is unnecessary or that may not be understood. Simply explain what you are

doing, and allow the patient to be part of the care being given; this can relieve feelings of helplessness as well as some of the fear.

Acknowledge the Seriousness of the Condition

There may be occasions when a patient may refuse emergency medical care and insist that you do nothing or leave him or her alone. In these cases, it is important to impress on the patient the seriousness of the condition without causing undue alarm. Saying, "Everything will be OK," when it is obvious that it is not, is not being truthful. Generally, seriously ill or injured patients know that they are in trouble. If the patient absolutely refuses emergency medical care, document this in your report. If possible, have the patient or other competent person sign a refusal of care form.

Allow for Hope

In trauma and acute medical conditions, patients may ask whether they are going to die. You may feel at a loss for words. You may also know, on the basis of past experience or in view of the seriousness of the present situation, that the prognosis is poor. But it is not up to you to tell the patient that he or she is dying. Statements such as "I don't know if you are going to die; let's fight this one out together" or "I am not going to give up on you, so do not give up on yourself" are helpful. These statements transmit a sense of trust and hope, and they let the patient know that you are doing everything possible to save his or her life. If there is the slightest chance of hope remaining, you want that message transmitted in your attitude and in the statements you make to the patient.

Locate and Notify Family Members

Many patients will be concerned and ask you to notify their family or others close to them. The patient may or may not be able to assist you in doing this. You should see to it that an appropriate and responsible person makes an effort to locate the desired persons. Assuring the patient that someone is going to do this may be a significant part of the patient's care.

Injured and Critically Ill Children

Injured and critically ill children who have life-threatening conditions should be cared for as any patient would be, insofar as ABCD and immediate life threats are concerned. Due regard should be given to the variations in height, weight, and size in providing emergency medical care. Because of the increased excitement and extraordinary nature of the emergency scene for a child, it is important that a relative or responsible adult accompany the child, to relieve anxiety and assist in care as appropriate.

Dealing with the Death of a Child

The death of a child is a tragic and dreaded event. It is not unusual to think about the fact that the dead or dying child has a lot more to do and should have many more years to live. In our society, we assume that only old people are supposed to die. Children die less frequently now than they did in earlier times, so most people are unprepared for what they will feel when a child dies. You may think about your own children and those whom you know: nephews, nieces, grandchildren, and children of close friends. And you may think, "Why should this child, who is only 5 years old, die?"

Answering the difficult questions of your own mortality will be of help when dealing with the death of a child. But, still, the death of a child will not be an easy subject to talk about. This will be especially so for the family. And as an EMT-B involved in a call that involves the death of a child, you will also likely experience stress.

One of your responsibilities may be to help the family through the initial period after the death. As an EMT-B, until more definitive and professional help can be available, you may be in the best position to help the family begin to cope with their loss. How a family initially deals with the death of a child will affect its stability and endurance. You can help a family through its initial period of grief and alert the family to the follow-up counseling and support services that are available.

Helping the Family

If the child is dead, acknowledging the fact of the death is important. This should be done in a private place, even if that is inside an ambulance. Often, the parents cannot believe that the death is real, even if they have been preparing for it, as in the case of a terminal illness such as leukemia. Reactions vary, but shock, disbelief, and denial are common. Some parents show little emotion at the initial news.

If it is possible, find a place where the mother and father can hold the child. This is important in the parent's grieving process; it helps to lessen the sense of disbelief and makes the death real. Even if the parents do not ask to see the child, you should tell them that they may. Your decision in permitting the parents to see the child may need some discretion. For example, in the case of a traumatic death in which there is significant disfigurement, that decision might have to be delayed. The delay may involve having support services available or contacting the family physician or others who can help the parents through this difficult situation. This may involve preparing the parents for what they will see and the changes brought on by rigor mortis, asphyxiation, and so forth.

Sometimes, you do not need to say much. In fact, silence can sometimes be more comforting than words. You can express your own sorrow. Do not overload grieving parents with a lot of information; at this point, they cannot handle it. Nonverbal communication, such as holding a hand or grasping a shoulder, may also be valuable. Let the family's actions be your guide about what is appropriate. It is important that parents be encouraged to talk about their feelings.

Stressful Situations

Many situations, such as mass-casualty scenes, serious automobile accidents, excavation cave-ins, house fires, infant and child trauma, amputations, infant/child/spousal/elderly abuse, and death of a coworker or other public safety personnel, will be stressful for everyone involved. During these situations, you must exercise extreme care in both your words and your actions. Be careful to present a professional demeanor in words and actions at the scene. Words that do not seem important, or that are said jokingly, may hurt someone. Conversations at the scene must be professional. You should not say, "Everything will be all right," or "There is nothing to worry about." A person who is trapped in a wrecked car, hurting from head to foot and worrying about a loved one, knows that all is not well. What will reassure the patient is your calm and caring approach to the emergency situation. Briefly explain your plan of action to assist the patient in the crisis. Inform the patient that you need his or her help and the assistance of family members or bystanders to carry out the plan of action.

How a patient reacts to injury or illness may be influenced by certain personality traits. Some patients may become highly emotional over what may seem to be a minor problem. Others may show little or no emotion, even after serious injury or illness. Many other factors influence how a patient reacts to the stress of an EMS incident. Among these factors are the following:

- Socioeconomic background
- Fear of medical personnel
- Alcohol or substance abuse
- History of chronic disease
- Mental disorders
- Reaction to medication
- Age
- Nutritional status
- Feelings of guilt

You are not expected to always know why a patient is having an unusual emotional response. However, you can quickly and calmly assess the actions of the patient, family members, and bystanders. This assessment will help you to gain the confidence and cooperation of everyone at the scene. In addition, you should use a professional tone of voice and show courtesy, along with sincere concern and efficient action. These simple considerations will go far to relieve worry, fear, and insecurity. Calm reassurance will inspire confidence and cooperation. Compassion is important, but you must be careful. Your professional judgment takes priority over compassion. For example, suppose a screaming child with no obvious life-threatening injuries is covered with another patient's blood. This frightened child appeals to your compassion and thus gets your attention. In the meantime, an unconscious, nonbreathing adult nearby could die from lack of care.

Patients must be given the opportunity to express their fears and concerns. You can easily relieve many of these concerns at the scene. Usually, patients are concerned about the safety or well-being of others who are involved in the accident and about the damage or loss of personal property. Your responses must be discreet and diplomatic, giving reassurance when appropriate. If a loved one has been killed or critically injured, you should wait, if possible, until clergy or emergency department staff can give the patient the news. They can then provide the psychologic support the patient may need.

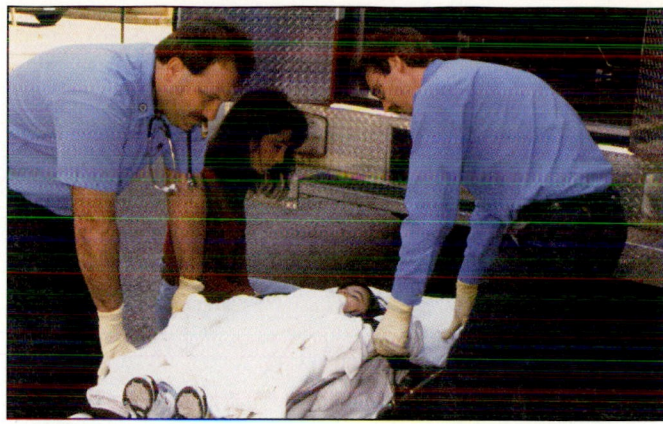

FIGURE 2-5 Children may be frightened when separated from family members. Parents should go with their children during transport.

Some patients, especially children and the elderly, may be terrified or feel rejected when separated from family members by the uniformed EMS provider team. Other patients may not want family members to share their stress, see their injury, or witness their pain. It is usually best if parents go with their children and relatives accompany elderly patients (Figure 2-5).

Religious customs or needs of the patient must also be respected. Some people will cling to religious medals or charms, especially if any attempt is made to remove them. Others will express a strong desire for religious counsel, baptism, or last rites if death is near. You must try to accommodate these requests. Some people have religious convictions that strongly oppose the use of drugs, blood, and blood products. If you obtain such information, it is imperative that you report it to the next level of care.

In the event of a death, you must handle the body with respect and dignity. It must be exposed as little as possible. Learn your local regulations and protocols about moving the body or changing its position, especially if you are at a possible crime scene. Even in these situations, cardiopulmonary resuscitation (CPR) and appropriate treatment must be given unless there are obvious signs of death.

Uncertain Situations

There will be times when you are unsure whether a true medical emergency exists. If you are unsure, contact medical control about the need to transport. If you cannot reach medical control, it is always best to transport the patient. For both ethical and medicolegal reasons, a physician must examine all patients who are transported and judge the degree of medical need.

You must also realize that the most minor symptoms may be early signs of severe illness or injury. Symptoms of many illnesses can be similar to those of substance abuse, hysteria, or other conditions. You must accept the patient's complaints and provide appropriate care until you are able to transfer care of the patient to a higher level (e.g., paramedic, nurse, or physician). Your local protocols will direct your actions in these uncertain situations. When in doubt, err on the side of caution, and acquire the patient's consent and transport to the medical facility.

Stress Warning Signs and the Work Environment

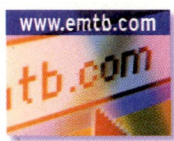 EMS is a high-stress job. Understanding the causes of stress and knowing how to deal with them is critical to one's job performance, health, and interpersonal relationships. To prevent stress from affecting your life negatively, you need to understand what stress is, its physiologic effects, what you can do to minimize these effects, and how to deal with stress on an emotional level.

Stress is the impact of stressors on your physical and mental well-being. Stressors include emotional, physical, and environmental situations or conditions that may cause a variety of physiologic, physical, and psychologic responses. The body's response to stress begins with an alarm response, followed by a stage of reaction and resistance, and then recovery or, if the stress is prolonged, exhaustion. This three-stage response is referred to as the general adaptation syndrome.

The physiologic responses involve the interaction of the endocrine and nervous systems, resulting in chemical and physical responses. This is commonly known as the *fight-or-flight response*. Positive stress, such as exercise, as well as negative forms of stress, such as shift work, long hours, or the frustration of losing a patient, all have the same physiologic manifestations. These include the following:

- Increased respirations and heart rate
- Increased blood pressure
- Dilated venous vessels near the skin surface (causes cool, clammy skin)
- Dilated pupils
- Tensed muscles
- Increased blood glucose levels
- Perspiration
- Decreased blood flow to the gastrointestinal tract

Stress may also have physical symptoms such as fatigue, changes in appetite, gastrointestinal problems, or headaches. Stress may cause insomnia or hypersomnia, irritability, inability to concentrate, and hyperactivity or underactivity. Additionally, stress may manifest itself in psychologic reactions such as fear, dull or nonresponsive behavior, depression, oversensitivity, anger, irritability, and frustration. Often, today's fast-paced lifestyles compound these effects by not allowing a person to rest and recover after periods of stress. Prolonged or excessive stress has been proven to be a strong contributor to heart disease, hypertension, cancer, alcoholism, and depression.

Many people are subject to cumulative stress, whereby insignificant stressors accumulate to a larger stress-related problem. In the emergency services environment (EMS, police, firefighters), stressors may also be sudden and more severe. Some events are unusually stressful or emotional, even by emergency services standards. These acute severe stressors result in what is referred to as critical incident stress. Events that can trigger critical incident stress include the following:

- Mass-casualty incidents
- Serious injury or traumatic death of a child
- Crash with injuries, caused by an emergency services provider while responding to or from a call
- Death or serious injury of a coworker in the line of duty

Posttraumatic stress disorder (PTSD) may develop after a person has experienced a psychologically distressing event. It is characterized by re-experiencing the event and overresponding to stimuli that recall the event. PTSD is sometimes referred to as "Vietnam veteran's disease" because of its classification as a mental disorder following the Vietnam conflict. Stressful events in EMS are sometimes psychologically overwhelming. Some of the symptoms include depression, startle reactions, flashback phenomena, and dissociative episodes (e.g., amnesia of the event).

An emergency services provider need not suffer through the emotional aftermath of these difficult situations. A process called **critical incident stress management (CISM)**, was developed to address this need. This process confronts the responses to critical incidents and defuses them, directing the emergency services personnel toward physical and emotional equilibrium. CISM can occur formally, as a debriefing for those who were on scene. A trained CISM team of peers and mental health professionals may facilitate this (Figure 2-6). Additionally, CISM can occur at an ongoing scene in the following circumstances:

- When personnel are assessed for signs and symptoms of distress while resting
- Before re-entering the scene
- During a scene demobilization in which personnel are educated about the signs of critical incident stress and given a buffer period to collect themselves before leaving

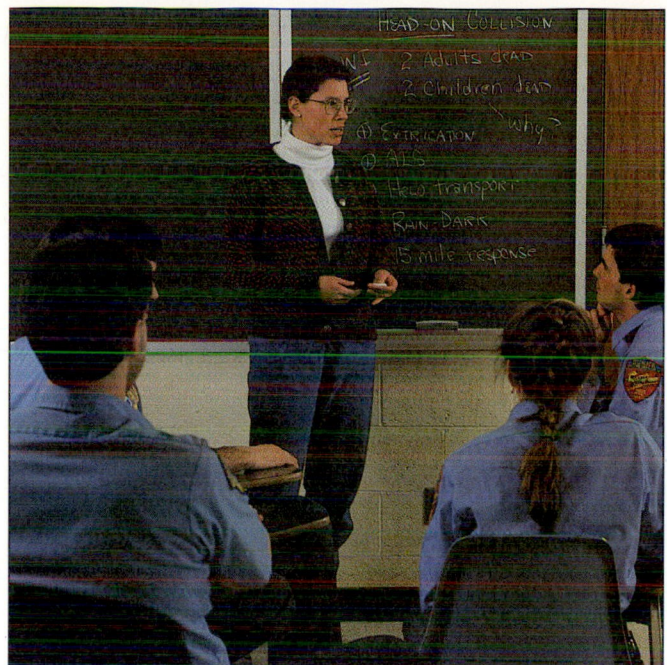

FIGURE 2-6 Critical incident stress management plays an important role in helping providers to relieve stress.

The most common form of CISM is peer diffusing, when a group informally discusses events that they experienced together.

Stress and Nutrition

Anyone can respond to a sudden physical stress for a short time. If stress is prolonged, especially if physical action is not a permitted response, the body can quickly be drained of its reserves. This can leave it depleted of key nutrients, weakened, and more susceptible to illness.

Your body's three sources of fuel—carbohydrates, fat, and protein—are consumed in increased quantities during stress, particularly if physical activity is involved. The quickest source of energy is glucose, taken from stored glycogen in the liver. However, this supply will last less than a day. Protein, drawn primarily from muscle, is a long-term source of glucose. Tissues can use fat for energy. The body also conserves water during periods of stress. To do so, it retains sodium by exchanging and losing potassium from the kidneys. Other nutrients that are susceptible to depletion are the vitamins and minerals that are not stored by the body in substantial quantities. These include such water-soluble B and C vitamins and most minerals.

As EMS providers, we do not have control of what stressors we will face on any given day. Consequently, stress in one form or another is an unavoidable part of our lives. As one would study for a test, dress properly for a day of snow skiing, or train for a sporting event, we should physically prepare our bodies for stress. Physical conditioning and proper nutrition are the two variables over which we have absolute control. Muscles will grow and retain protein only with sufficient activity. Bones will not passively accumulate calcium. In response to the physical stress of exercise, bones store calcium and become denser and stronger. Regular, well-balanced meals are essential to provide the nutrients that are necessary to keep your body fueled (Figure 2-7). Vitamin-mineral preparations that provide a balanced mix of all the nutrients may be necessary to supplement a less than perfectly balanced diet.

Stress Management

There are many methods of handling stress. Some are positive and healthy; others are harmful or destructive. Americans consume more than 20 tons of aspirin per day, and doctors prescribe muscle relaxers, tranquilizers, and

FIGURE 2-7 A healthy diet is illustrated by the USDA food guide pyramid.

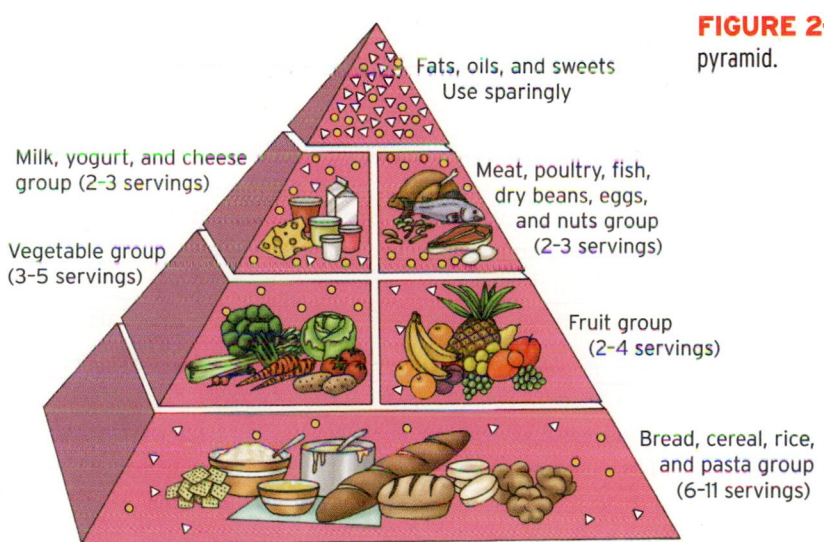

Fats, oils, and sweets
Use sparingly

Milk, yogurt, and cheese group (2-3 servings)

Meat, poultry, fish, dry beans, eggs, and nuts group (2-3 servings)

Vegetable group (3-5 servings)

Fruit group (2-4 servings)

Bread, cereal, rice, and pasta group (6-11 servings)

KEY
▣ Fat (naturally occurring and added)
▽ Sugar (added)
These symbols show fat and added sugars in foods.

TABLE 2-4   Strategies to Manage Stress

Change or eliminate stressors.

Change partners to avoid a negative or hostile personality.

Change work hours.

Cut back on overtime.

Change your attitude about the stressor.

Stop wasting your energy complaining or worrying about things that you cannot change, such as:

- Skid row alcoholics
- Abused children
- Nursing home transfers
- Cleaning contaminated EMS units

Try to adopt a more relaxed, philosophical outlook.

Expand your social support system apart from your co-workers.

Sustain friends and interests outside emergency services.

Minimize the physical response to stress by employing various techniques, including:

- A deep breath to settle an anger response
- Periodic stretching
- Slow, deep breathing
- Regular physical exercise
- Progressive muscle relaxation

sedatives more than 90 million times per year to patients in the United States. Although these medicines have legitimate uses, they do nothing to combat the stress that may cause the medical problems described previously.

The term "stress management" refers to the tactics that have been shown to alleviate or eliminate stress reactions. These may involve changing a few habits, changing your attitude, and perseverance (Table 2-4).

A clue to the management of stress comes from the fact that it is not the event itself but the individual's reaction to it that determines how much it will strain the body's resources. Remember that stress is defined as anything that you perceive as a threat to your equilibrium. Stress is an undeniable and unavoidable part of our everyday life. By understanding how it affects you physiologically, physically, and psychologically, you can more successfully manage it.

Supporting patients in emergency situations is difficult. It is stressful for them but also for you. You are vulnerable to all the stresses that go with your profession. It is critical that you recognize the signs of stress so that it does not interfere with your work or life away from work, including your family life. The signs and symptoms of chronic stress may not be obvious at first. Rather, they may be subtle and not present all the time (Table 2-5).

The following sections provide some suggestions for how to cope better with stress. Some of them may be useful in helping you to prevent problems from developing. Others may help you to solve problems, should they develop.

Lifestyle changes. Your well-being is of primary importance to effective EMS operations. The effectiveness and efficiency with which you do your job depend

TABLE 2-5   Warning Signs of Stress

Irritability toward co-workers, family, and friends

Inability to concentrate

Difficulty sleeping and nightmares

Anxiety

Indecisiveness

Guilt

Loss of appetite

Loss of interest in sexual activities

Isolation

Loss of interest in work

Increased use of alcohol

on your ability to stay in shape and avoid the risk of personal injury. Burnout is a condition of chronic fatigue and frustration that results from mounting stress over time. To avoid burnout, you need to be in good physical and mental health. Be aware of the potential hazards in rescue and emergency medical care. You must also learn how to avoid or prevent personal injury or illness.

Nutrition. To perform efficiently, you must eat nutritious food. Food is the fuel that makes the body run. The physical exertion and stress that are a part of your job require a high energy output. If you do not have a ready source of fuel, your performance may be less than

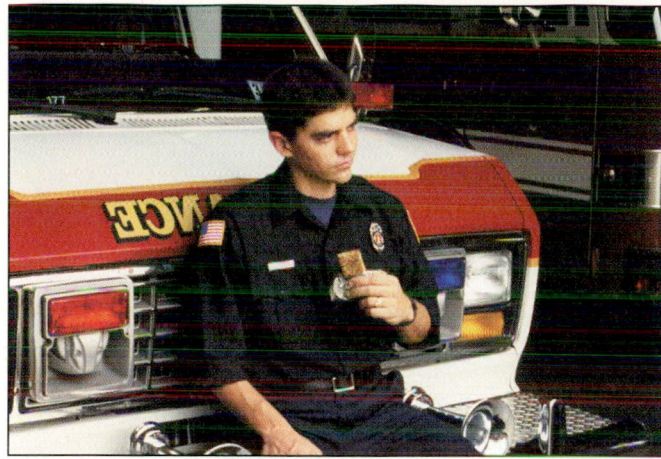

FIGURE 2-8 Carry a supply of high-energy food with you so that you can maintain your energy levels.

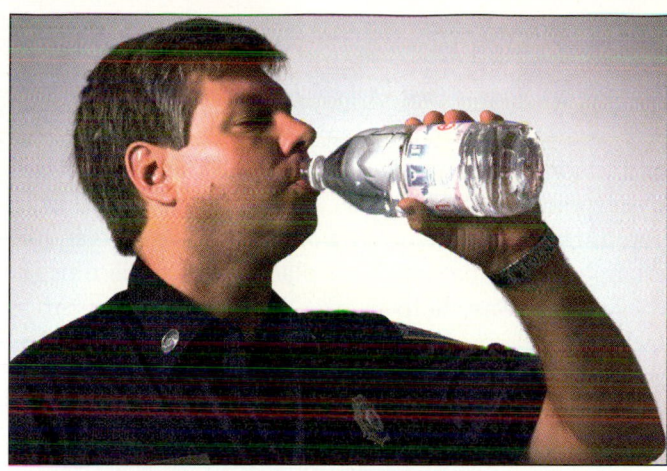

FIGURE 2-9 Maintain an adequate fluid intake by drinking plenty of water or other nonalcoholic, caffeine-free fluid.

satisfactory. This can be dangerous for you, your partner, and your patient. Therefore, it is important for you to learn about and follow the rules of good nutrition.

Candy and soft drinks contain sugar. These foods are quickly absorbed and converted to fuel by the body. But simple sugars also stimulate the body's production of insulin, which reduces blood glucose levels. For some people, eating a lot of sugar can actually result in lower energy levels.

Complex carbohydrates rank next to simple sugars in their ability to produce energy. Complex carbohydrates such as pasta, rice, and vegetables are among the safest, most reliable sources for long-term energy production. However, some carbohydrates take hours to be converted into usable body fuel.

Fats are also easily converted to energy, but eating too much fat can lead to obesity, cardiac disease, and other long-term health problems. The proteins in meat, fish, chicken, beans, and cheese take several hours to convert to energy.

Carry an individual supply of high-energy food to help you maintain your energy levels (Figure 2-8). Try eating several small meals throughout the day to keep your energy resources at constant high levels. Remember, however, that overeating may reduce your physical and mental performance. After a large meal, the blood that is needed for the digestive process is not available for other activities.

You must also make sure that you maintain an adequate fluid intake (Figure 2-9). Hydration is important for proper functioning. Fluids can be easily replenished by drinking any nonalcoholic, noncaffeinated fluid. Water is generally the best fluid available. The body absorbs it faster than any other fluid. Avoid fluids that contain high levels of sugar. These can actually slow the rate of fluid absorption by the body. They can also cause

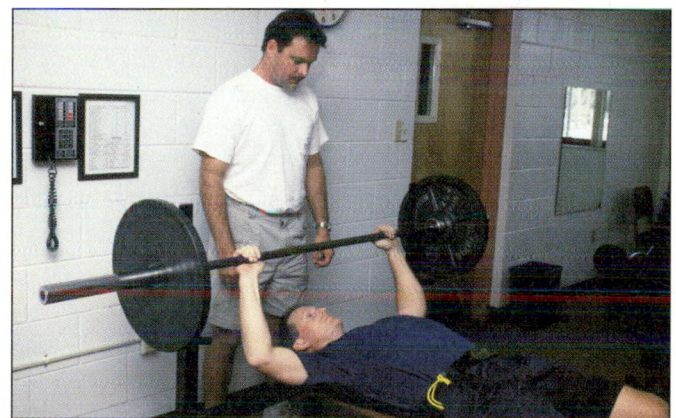

FIGURE 2-10 A regular program of exercise will increase strength and endurance.

abdominal discomfort. One indication of adequate hydration is frequent urination. Infrequent urination or urine that has a deep yellow color indicates dehydration.

Exercise and relaxation. A regular program of exercise will enhance the benefits of maintaining good nutrition and adequate hydration. When you are in good physical condition, you can handle job stress more easily. A regular program of exercise will increase your strength and endurance (Figure 2-10). You may wish to practice relaxation techniques, meditation, and visual imagery.

Balancing work, family, and health. As an EMT-B, you will often be called to assist the sick and injured any time of the day or night. Unfortunately, there is no rhyme or reason to the timing of illness and injury. Volunteer EMT-Bs may often be called away from family or friends during social activities. Shift workers may be required to be apart from loved ones for long periods of time. You should never let the job interfere excessively with your own needs. Find a balance between work and family; you owe it to yourself and to them. It is important to make sure that you have the time that you need to relax with family and friends.

It is also important to realize that coworkers, family, and friends often may not understand the stress caused by responding to EMS calls. As a result of a "bad call," you might not feel like going out to a movie or attending a family event that has been planned for some time. In these situations, help from a Critical Incident Stress Debriefing team or information sessions conducted by the EMS unit's employee assistance program may assist you in resolving these problems.

When possible, rotate your schedule to give yourself time off. If your EMS system allows you to move from station to station, rotate to reduce or vary your call volume. Take vacations to provide for your good health so that you will be able to respond the next time you are needed. If at any point you feel that the stress of work is more than you can handle, seek help. You may want to discuss your stress informally with your family or coworkers. Help from more experienced team members can be invaluable. You may also wish to get help from peer counselors or other professionals. Seeking this help does not make you weak in the eyes of others. Rather, it shows that you are in control of your life.

Critical Incident Stress Debriefing (CISD)

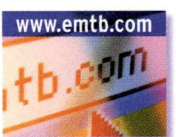

You may be called to a situation so horrible that you find it difficult to respond as you were trained. You may have an immediate or delayed negative response to the incident. Do not be ashamed of such feelings; almost all responders have had the same reaction at one time or another. If you feel overwhelmed, step back and call for help. Sometimes, simply knowing that help is on the way can help you to overcome your fear or anxiety and enable you to respond to the situation. Remember that if you have these feelings from time to time, your partner and other members of the team may have them, too. Keep an eye on other members of your team. See that they are under control and act appropriately during a major disaster.

After a stressful run or a disaster, there may be an emotional letdown. This letdown is often overlooked. However, it may be more important to deal with than the initial contact response. Critical Incident Stress Debriefing is a way to deal with this emotional letdown phase. A critical incident is any event that causes anxiety and mental stress to emergency workers. **Critical incident stress debriefing (CISD)** is a program in which severely stressful job-related incidents are discussed. These discussions are conducted in strict confidence

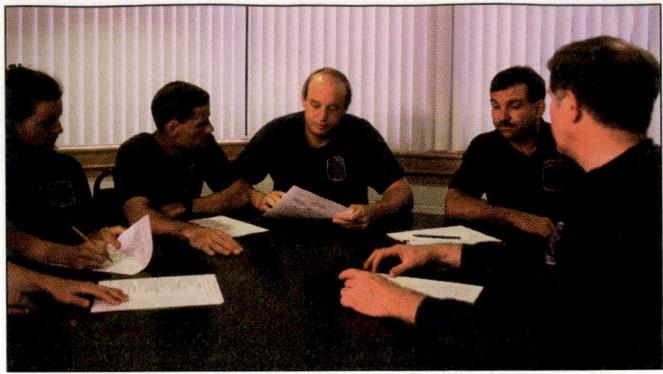

FIGURE 2-11 CISD sessions are conducted in strict confidence with other emergency workers who are trained in CISD.

with other emergency workers who are trained in CISD (Figure 2-11). The purpose of CISD is to relieve personal and group anxieties and stress. Never be ashamed to report your feelings, because such a debriefing can be vital to your emotional well-being. It should not be dismissed as trivial or nonessential.

CISD teams consist of peer counselors and mental health professionals who help you to deal with critical incident stress. Usually, CISD meetings are held within 24 to 72 hours of a major incident. CISD meetings may also have to be repeated at a later time. A CISD meeting is not an investigation or an interrogation. It is an opportunity to discuss your feelings, fears, and reactions to the event. All information that is discussed in the meeting should remain confidential. The CISD leaders and mental health professionals will help you by listening and then offering suggestions on how to overcome the stress. CISD is designed to accelerate the normal recovery process following a critical incident. These meetings are helpful to all rescuers who are involved in an incident, whether or not they think they were stressed. A CISD meeting provides a means to quickly vent feelings in a nonthreatening atmosphere.

CISD programs are located throughout the United States. CISD teams usually can be located by calling telephone directory assistance in your area and asking for CISD. The International Critical Incident Stress Foundation, Inc., has an emergency access number: (410) 313-2473. For general information, call (410) 750-9600, or contact the foundation by e-mail at icisf@erols.com.

A comprehensive CISM system includes the following 10 components:

- Preincident stress education
- On-scene peer support
- One-on-one support
- Disaster support services
- Defusings

- CISD
- Follow-up services
- Spouse and family support
- Community outreach programs
- Other health and welfare programs, such as wellness

Workplace Issues

As our society continues to grow more and more culturally diverse, some groups that may have been satisfied in the past to accept and participate in American cultural traditions may seek instead to assert, preserve, and nurture their differences. As our society grows more culturally diverse, so do EMS workplaces. There will be challenges as these changes continue to occur. With the greater involvement of people of different backgrounds, EMS has the opportunity to serve people with more sensitivity to cultural variances.

Cultural Diversity on the Job

Each individual is different, and you should communicate with coworkers and patients in a way that is sensitive to everyone's needs (Figure 2-12). Look at cultural diversity as a resource, and make the most of the differences among people in EMS, thus allowing them to provide optimum patient care. As the public safety workplace becomes more culturally diverse, changes may occur that could be considered disruptive. It is possible to build the strength of your workgroup through the use of diversity.

For many years, EMS and public safety have been dominated by white males, though to a lesser extent than police and fire departments because of the tradi-

tional involvement of female nurses in EMS. This trend continues to decline; more women and minorities are working in public safety. The proactive EMT-B understands the benefits of using cultural diversity to improve patient care and expects to work alongside workers with different backgrounds and to accept their differences.

As an arm of public safety, EMS has not been around for as long as law enforcement and fire departments. Therefore, there may be less resistance to cultural diversity in EMS than in the other areas of public safety. Depending on your work experience, you may or may not have worked with people of varying backgrounds, attitudes, beliefs, and values.

Compared with traditional workplaces, EMS might seem like chaos. People who work in an office or manufacturing facility can reasonably expect to go to work every day, see the same people, and perform basically the same tasks. In EMS and public safety work, you are exposed to people in crisis. This exposure brings out the traits and qualities that your partners and coworkers use to manage their stress. Coworkers in traditional workplaces may not be willing to show this side of themselves to others. Debriefing after the call will help in this process.

Cultural diversity in EMS allows EMT-Bs to enjoy the benefits of accentuating the skills of a broad range of people. When you accept coworkers as individuals, the need to fit them into rigid roles is eliminated. To be more sensitive to cultural diversity issues, you must first be aware of your own cultural background. Ask yourself, "What are my own issues relative to race, color, religion, and ethnicity?" Since culture is not restricted to different nationalities, you should also consider age, handicap, gender, sexual orientation, marital status, work experience, and education.

In sports, you play to your team's strengths. For example, in football, offensive lines have a fast side and a strong side, and they run plays toward either side depending on the situation. As part of an effective EMS team, you can make it part of your team culture to play to your group's strengths. This may be difficult to do; but once you begin the process, the benefits in terms of improved patient care are immeasurable.

Your Effectiveness as an EMT-B

To be an effective EMT-B, you need to discover the diverse cultural needs of your coworkers, as well as those of your patients and their families. Although it is unrealistic to expect EMT-Bs to become cross-cultural experts with knowledge about all ethnicities, you should learn how to relate effectively.

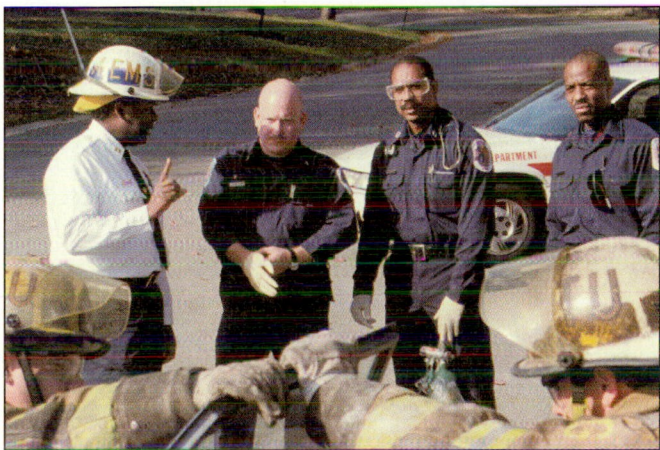

FIGURE 2-12 Communicate with coworkers in a way that is sensitive and respectful of individual differences.

Teamwork is essential in public safety and EMS. In order to work effectively as a team, you need to communicate to deal with cultural diversity issues.

As a healthcare professional, you should try to be a role model for new EMT-Bs by showing them the value of diversity. If you are working with a coworker or patient from a particular cultural group, be careful about any opinion you may have formed about that group. Do not assume that there is a language barrier, and do not appear patronizing by saying, "Some of my best friends are..." There are legitimate differences in how various cultures respond to stress. For example, you should be prepared to accept that people of different cultures might respond differently to the death of a loved one.

When working with patients or calling the hospital on the radio, other EMT-Bs may be sensitive to how you treat patients from their cultural group. Therefore, when referring to patients, you should use the appropriate terminology. Avoid using terms such as "cripple," "deformed," "deaf," "dumb," "crazy," and "retard" when referring to patients. Instead, use the term "disabled," and describe the specific disability.

You might want to consider taking multilingual training classes. This will not only be useful in communicating with your coworkers; it will also help to improve communication with your patients and sensitize you to the cultural richness of the people who are using the language.

Even the perception of discrimination can weaken morale and motivation and negatively affect the goal of EMS. Therefore, to achieve the benefits of cultural diversity in the EMS workplace, EMT-Bs must understand how to communicate effectively with coworkers from various backgrounds.

Avoiding Sexual Harassment

The number of sexual harassment lawsuits skyrocketed in the 1990s because of increased media attention to the problem. Furthermore, guilty verdicts encouraged others to bring suit concerning conduct that once would have gone unchallenged.

Sexual harassment is any unwelcome sexual advance, unwelcome requests for sexual favors, or other unwelcome verbal or physical conduct of a sexual nature when submitting is a condition of employment, submitting or rejecting is a basis for an employment decision, or such conduct substantially interferes with performance and/or creates a hostile or offensive work environment.

Supreme Court Justice Clarence Thomas's confirmation hearings brought sexual harassment to the nation's attention. These hearings raised our awareness of sexual harassment, how it occurs, its impact on victims, and why victims might not report the behavior. The Tailhook incident that resulted in the resignations of two top U.S. Navy officers also helped to increase our awareness.

There are two types of sexual harassment: quid pro quo (the harasser requests sexual favors in exchange for something else, such a promotion) and hostile work environment (jokes, touching, leering requests for a date, talking about body parts). Seventy percent of sexual harassment today is considered hostile work environment. Remember, it does not matter what the intent or who the harasser was. What matters are the other person's perception and what impact that behavior had on that person. For many years, it was not uncommon to walk into a fire station and see sexually suggestive posters, calendars, or cartoons and to hear sexual jokes or comments. This situation is changing because more women are working in EMS and public safety and because of high-profile events such as the ones mentioned above.

Because EMT-Bs and other public safety professionals depend on each other for their safety, it is especially important to try to develop nonadversarial relationships with coworkers. Some EMS facilities and fire stations make arrangements for different bunkrooms for men and women. If this is not the case at your facility, you should discuss this with your supervisor and talk openly with coworkers of the opposite gender to allow for their privacy.

If you are concerned about a particular behavior, it may be helpful to ask yourself these questions: "Would I do or say this in front of my spouse, significant other, or parents?" "Would I want my family members to be exposed to this behavior?" "Would I want my behavior videotaped and shown on the evening news?"

If you have been harassed, you should report it to your supervisor immediately and keep notes of what happened and what was said. You should confront the harasser if you feel comfortable doing so; however, this may not be for everyone. If you are asked for a date, say, "I'm not interested." If remarks or touching offends you, say, "Please don't say/do that to me; it offends me."

Substance Abuse

In the past, part of the fire service ritual was to go back to the fire station after the fire, clean and maintain the equipment, and discuss the call. At some locations, having a few beers was not uncommon. EMS today is very different from the ambulance service in which one of your parents may have participated years ago.

Drug and alcohol use in the workplace causes an increase in accidents and tension among workers, but most important, it can lead to poor treatment decisions. EMS personnel who abuse substances such as alcohol or marijuana are more likely to have problems with their work habits. They may be absent from work more often than other workers. If the abuse has occurred within hours before the start of their shift, their ability to render emergency medical care may be lessened because of mental or physical impairment. Since public safety workers depend so much on coworkers for their own safety, it is even more important that ways be found to manage this problem.

As an EMT-B, you will witness firsthand the tremendous effects of violence, trauma, and disease. Beyond CISD, members of the public safety community have a way of covering for each other. It is important to understand that the problem behavior will usually get worse before it gets better. Unfortunately, the stereotypical image of the alcoholic or addict lying in the gutter in an urban part of town often blinds EMS personnel to the existence of a coworker's drug or alcohol problem. Not all people with a substance abuse problem fit the stereotype.

As a member of the EMS team, you are responsible for responding to the community's emergency medical needs. Hazards in the EMS workplace are great. If you or one of the members of your team has a drug or alcohol problem, this risk increases. Furthermore, drug use that occurs off the job does not necessarily decrease the risk. Because of the tremendous risk potential, it is critical that EMT-Bs seek help or find a way to confront their partner or coworker even though there will be great pressure to allow the behavior to continue. Addicts and alcoholics develop great skill at covering their behavior; you might even decide not to bother your coworker because you feel that he or she has caught too many tough calls lately and needs to blow off some steam. Do not let this happen. You have to find a way to confront someone who has a substance abuse problem. Because of the tremendous hazard to patients, the public, and EMT-Bs, you have a legitimate right to confront coworkers with drug and alcohol problems.

When confronting a coworker with a potential drug or alcohol problem, make it clear to the worker that if the problem is personal, it is the worker's responsibility to take care of it. You have the power to assist this person. In many workplaces, coworkers are often in a position to notice a change in a coworker's behavior or attitude before a supervisor does. This is even more the case in EMS because of the close relationship that develops between people who work in the ambulance for so many hours and share rooms, meals, and social interaction while waiting for the next call. This may allow you to help someone before his or her job performance is negatively affected.

> One of the fundamental tools of the EMT-B is communication.

To help reduce the potential for drug and alcohol use in the EMS workplace, EMT-Bs can learn about drugs and alcohol. Beyond following company policy, EMT-Bs can agree among themselves what constitutes unacceptable behavior. The best time to confront these issues is usually after a call. Management sets the tone on these issues, but senior EMT-Bs can also emphasize to new EMT-Bs that drug abuse will not be tolerated.

In a manufacturing or office environment, supervisors refer employees with problems to employee assistance programs (EAPs). EMS operations might not lend themselves easily to EAPs. Operations may be geographically spread out with minimal supervision and irregular work hours. Calls may range from a relatively simple 5-minute call to complex mass-casualty incidents that last several hours. Your partners may change regularly. And since you depend so much on each other for your safety, there will be pressure not to rock the boat. You are not "turning someone in." You may be saving his or her life. Your coworker may be a great EMT-B, but if this person has unresolved substance abuse issues, the risk to fellow EMT-Bs and patients is just too great. If a substance abuse-related accident occurs during a call, it may dramatically increase the workload for other emergency responders when they respond to assist you. Early intervention is the best bet to ensure a safe, alcohol- and drug-free workplace.

Scene Safety and Personal Protection

The personal safety of all those involved in an emergency situation is very important. In fact, it is so important that the steps you take to preserve personal safety must become automatic. A second accident at the scene or an injury to you or your partner creates more problems, delays emergency medical care for patients, increases the burden on the other EMT-Bs, and may result in unnecessary death.

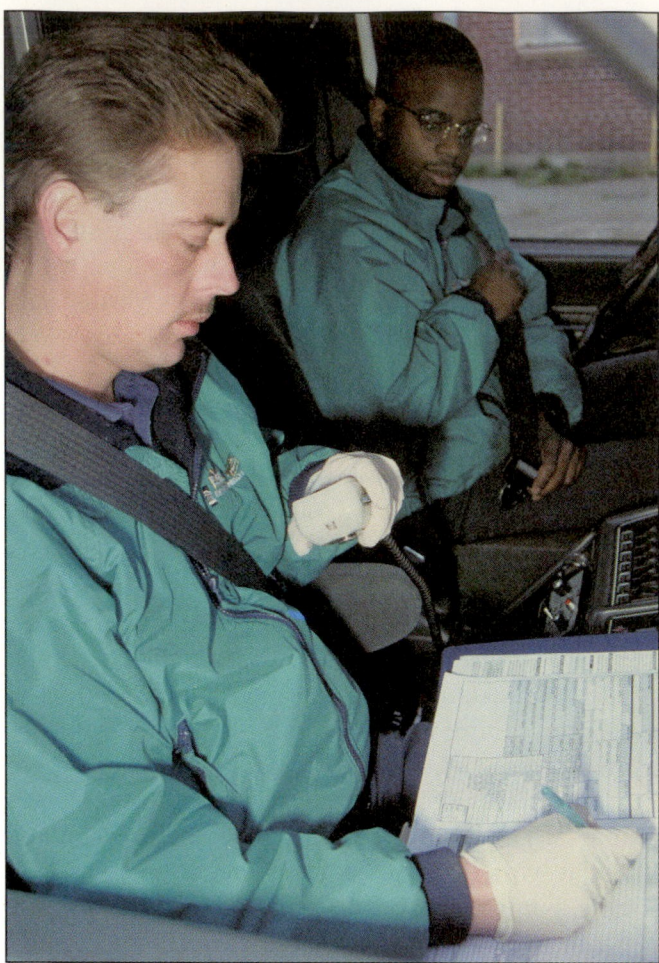

FIGURE 2-13 Wear seat belts and shoulder harnesses en route to the scene.

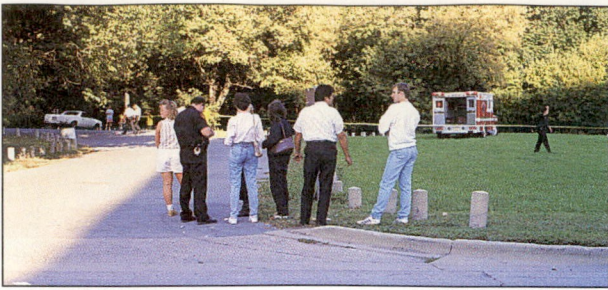

FIGURE 2-14 Make sure the accident scene is well marked to prevent a second accident that may damage the ambulance or result in injury to you, your partner, or the patient.

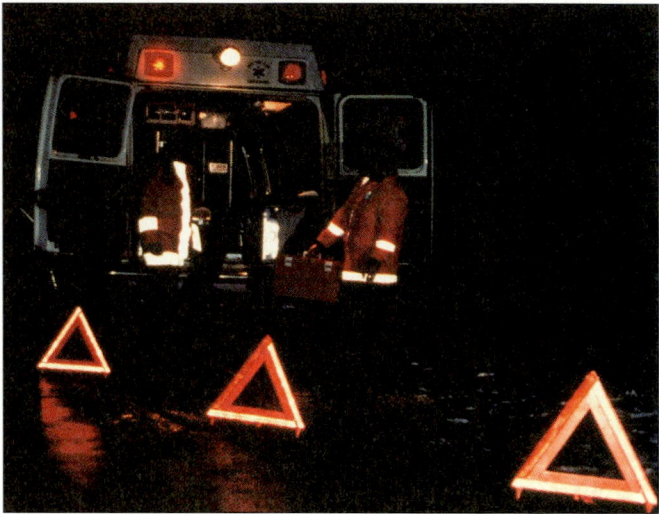

FIGURE 2-15 Wear reflective emblems or clothing to help make you more visible at night and improve your safety in the dark.

You should begin protecting yourself as soon as you are dispatched. Before you leave for the scene, begin preparing yourself both mentally and physically. Make sure you wear seat belts and shoulder harnesses en route to the scene. Wear seat belts and shoulder harnesses at all times unless patient care makes it impossible (Figure 2-13). Many EMS units have mandatory seat belt policies for the driver at all times, for all EMT-Bs during transit to the scene, and for anyone who is riding with a patient.

Protecting yourself at the scene is also very important. A second accident may damage the ambulance and may result in additional injury to you, your partner, or the patient. The scene must be well marked (Figure 2-14). If law enforcement has not already done so, you should make sure that proper warning devices are placed at a sufficient distance from the scene. This will alert motorists coming from both directions that an accident has occurred. You should park the ambulance at a safe but convenient distance from the scene. Before

attempting to access patients who are trapped in a vehicle, check the vehicle's stability. Then take any necessary measures to secure it. Do not rock or push on a vehicle to find out whether it will move. This can overturn the vehicle or send it crashing into a ditch.

When working at night, you must have plenty of light. Poor lighting increases the risk of further injury to both you and the patient. It also results in poor emergency medical care. Proper lighting is included in the equipment requirements for ambulances. Reflective emblems or clothing helps to make you more visible at night and decrease your risk of injury (Figure 2-15).

Body Substance Isolation

You should always follow body substance isolation techniques to protect yourself and your patient. **Body substance isolation (BSI)** is an infection control concept and practice that is designed to approach all body fluids as being potentially infectious. Modes of transmission include the following:

- Blood or fluid splash
- Surface contamination
- Needlestick exposure
- Oral contamination due to lack of or improper handwashing

Handwashing. Handwashing is perhaps one of the simplest yet most effective ways to control disease transmission. You should always wash your hands before and after contact with a patient, regardless of whether you wear gloves. You should wash your hands before performing a procedure, after glove removal, and between patients. If no running water is available, you may use waterless handwashing substitutes (Figure 2-16). If you use a waterless substitute in the field, make sure that you wash your hands once you arrive at the hospital. The proper procedure for handwashing is as follows:

1. Use soap and water.
2. Rub your hands together for at least 10 to 15 seconds to work up a lather.
3. Rinse your hands, and dry them with a paper towel.
4. Use the paper towel to turn off the faucet.

Gloves and eye protection. Gloves and eye protection are the minimum standard for all patient care if there is any possibility for exposure to blood or body fluids. Both vinyl and latex gloves provide adequate protection. Your department may prefer one type of glove over the other, or you may choose yourself. You may wish to select a particular type of glove for a particular patient care task. Wear double gloves if there is massive bleeding. You may also wear double gloves if you will be exposed to large volumes of other body fluids. Be sure to change gloves as you move from patient to patient. For cleaning and disinfecting the unit, you should use heavy-duty utility gloves (Figure 2-17). *You should never use lightweight latex or vinyl gloves for cleaning.*

Eye protection is important in case blood splatters into your eye (Figure 2-18). If this is a possibility, wearing goggles is your best protection. However, you need not wear goggles if you wear prescription glasses. Prescription glasses are acceptable as eye protection, but you must add removable side shields when on duty.

Mask and cover gowns. Occasionally, you may need to wear a mask and gown. A mask and gown provide protection from extensive blood splatter. Gowns may be worn in situations such as field delivery of a baby or major trauma. However, wearing a gown may not be practical in many situations. In fact, in some instances,

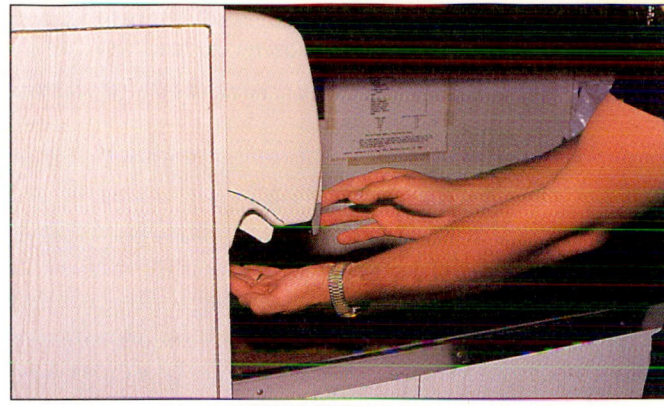

FIGURE 2-16 Use a waterless handwashing solution if there is no running water available. Be sure to wash your hands with soap once you arrive at the hospital.

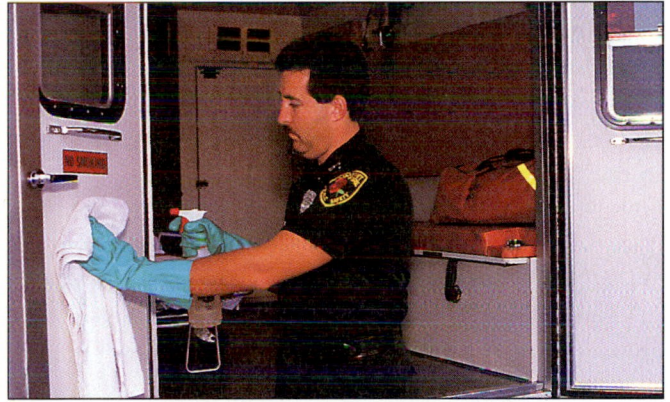

FIGURE 2-17 Use heavy-duty utility gloves to clean the unit. You should never use lightweight or vinyl gloves for cleaning.

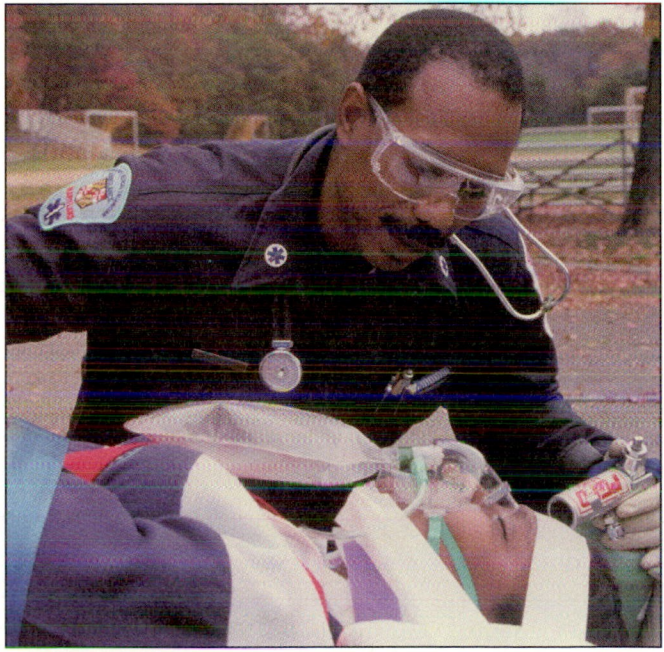

FIGURE 2-18 Wear eye protection to prevent blood splatter into your eyes.

a gown may pose a risk for injury. Your department will likely have a policy regarding gowns. Be sure you know your local policy. There are times when a change of uniform is preferred because trying to clean off contaminants is difficult and sometimes impossible without professional cleaning and disinfection or disposing of the uniform entirely.

The use of a mask is becoming a very complex issue in prehospital care. Many EMS systems have protocols that determine the type of mask that should be used in specific situations. If blood splatter is a real possibility, you should wear a standard surgical mask. If you suspect that a patient has an airborne disease, you should place a surgical mask on the patient. If you suspect that the patient has tuberculosis, you should place a surgical mask on the patient. In addition, you should wear a High-Efficiency Particulate Air (HEPA) respirator (Figure 2-19). You should not place a HEPA respirator on a patient.

Remember that the outside surfaces of these items are considered contaminated after they have been exposed to the patient. You must make sure that gloves, masks, gowns, and all other items that have been exposed to infectious processes or blood are properly disposed of according to local guidelines. If you are stuck by a needle, get blood in your eye, or have any body fluid contact with the patient, immediately report this incident to your supervisor.

The Occupational Safety and Health Administration (OSHA) develops and publishes guidelines concerning safety in the workplace. It is also responsible for enforcing these guidelines. OSHA requires all EMT-Bs to be trained in the handling of blood-borne pathogens and in approaching the patient who has a communicable or infectious disease. Training must also be provided for issues including blood and body fluid precautions, respiratory precautions, secretion precautions, and contamination precautions.

Hazards

In the course of your career, you will be exposed to many hazards. Some situations will be dangerous. Some will be life threatening. In these cases, you must be protected with the proper hazardous material suit and self-contained breathing apparatus (SCBA), as needed, or you must avoid the hazard completely.

Hazardous materials. Your safety is the most important consideration at a hazardous materials incident. Upon your arrival, you should first try to read labels and identification numbers. All hazardous materials should be marked with safety placards, though this is not

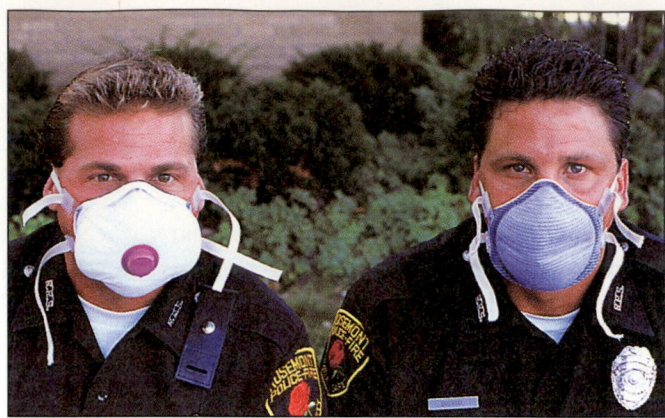

FIGURE 2-19 Wear a HEPA respirator if you treat a patient whom you suspect has tuberculosis. HEPA respirators may be reusable (left) or disposable (right).

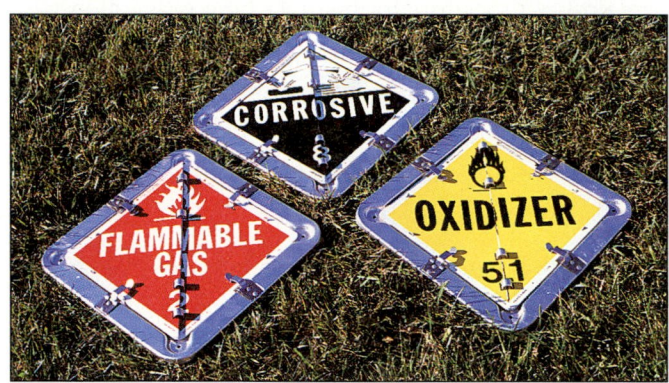

FIGURE 2-20 Hazardous materials safety placards are marked with colored diamond-shaped labels.

always done. These placards are marked with colored diamond-shaped labels (Figure 2-20). Although it is important for you to obtain information from the placards, you should never approach any object marked with a placard. It is useful to carry binoculars in the ambulance so that you can read the placards from a safe distance. A specially trained and equipped hazardous materials team will be called to handle disposal of materials and removal of patients. You should not begin caring for patients until they have been moved away from the scene or the scene is safe for you to enter.

The DOT's *Hazardous Materials: The Emergency Response Guidebook* is an important resource (Figure 2-21). It lists most hazardous materials and the proper procedures for scene control and emergency care of patients. Several similar resources are available. Some state and local government agencies may also have information about the hazardous materials in their areas. A copy of the *Guidebook* and other information relevant to your area should be available in your unit or at the dispatch center. Thus, you should be able to begin proper

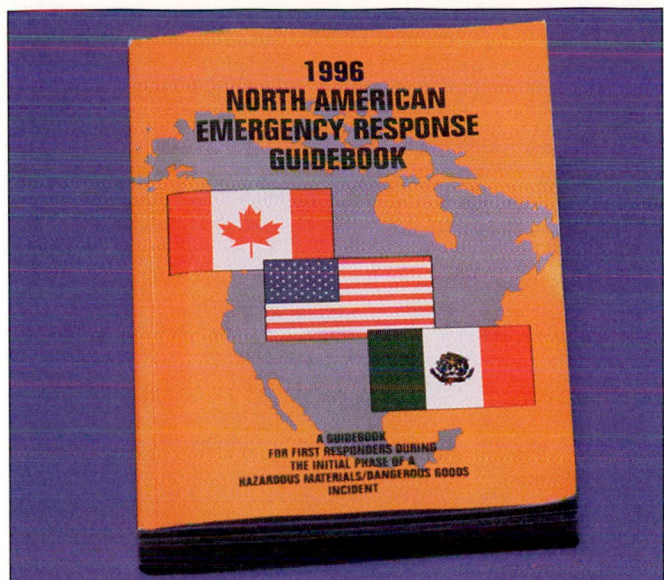

FIGURE 2-21 The DOT's *Emergency Response Guidebook* lists many hazardous materials and the proper procedures for scene control and emergency care of patients.

emergency management as soon as the hazardous material is identified. Again, do not go into an area and risk exposure to yourself. Do not enter the area unless you are absolutely sure that no hazardous spill has occurred.

Hazardous materials are classified according to toxicity levels, which dictate the level of protection required. The toxicity levels—0, 1, 2, 3, 4—measure the risk the substance poses to an individual. The higher the number, the greater is the toxicity and the greater is the protection needed (Table 2-6). It is important to remember that you are at great risk in hazardous materials situations. Do not enter the scene if a HazMat team is en route. If your area does not have such a team and you must enter, make sure you are wearing the proper protective gear.

Electricity. Electrical shock can be produced by human-made sources (power lines) or natural sources (lightning). No matter what the source, you must evaluate the risk to you and to the patient before you begin patient care.

The amount of current that is involved greatly affects the level of risk for injury. Your local power company can help you by providing training to evaluate the risks in electrical emergencies. Its staff can also teach you how to deal with power lines once the risks have been established. *You should not touch downed power lines.* Dealing with power lines is beyond the scope of EMT-B training. However, you should mark off a danger zone around the downed lines.

Energized, or "live" power lines, especially high-voltage lines, behave in unpredictable ways. You need in-depth training to be able to handle the equipment that is used in an electrical emergency. The equipment also has specific storage needs and requires careful cleaning. Dirt or other contaminants can make this equipment useless or dangerous.

At the scene of a motor vehicle crash, above-ground and below-grade power lines may become hazards. Disrupted overhead wires are usually a visible hazard. You must be careful even if you do not see sparks coming from the lines. Visible sparks are not always present in charged wires. The area around downed power lines is always a danger zone. This danger zone extends well beyond the immediate accident scene.

Use the utility poles as landmarks for establishing the perimeter of the danger zone. The danger zone must be a restricted area. Only emergency personnel, equipment, and vehicles are allowed inside this area.

If you must enter this type of situation, be sure to wear the proper protective equipment according to the type of incident. You should always wear a helmet with chin strap and face shield. The shell of the helmet should be made of a certified electrical nonconductor. The chin strap should not stretch. In fact, it should fasten securely so that the helmet stays in place if you are knocked down or a power line hits your head. You should also be able to

TABLE 2-6	Toxicity Levels of Hazardous Materials	
Level	**Hazard**	**Protection Needed**
0	Little to no hazard	None
1	Slightly hazardous	SCBA only
2	Slightly hazardous	SCBA only
3	Extremely hazardous	Full protection, with no exposed skin
4	Minimal exposure causes death	Special HazMat gear

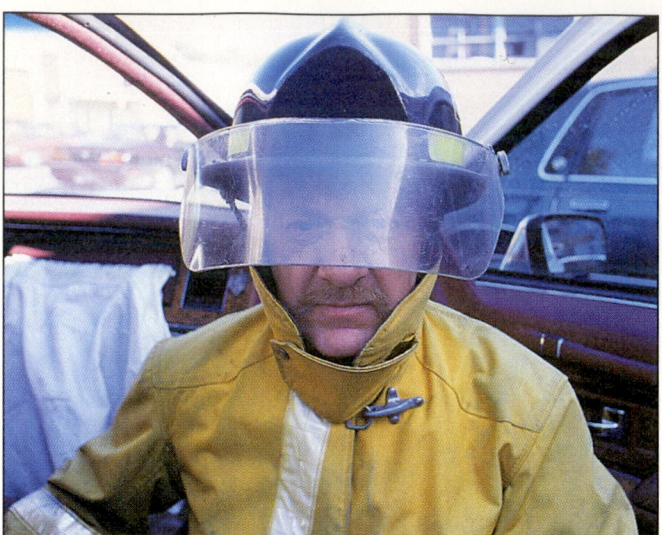

FIGURE 2-22 Wear a helmet made of a certified electrical nonconductor material, making sure that the chin strap is fastened securely and the face shield is locked.

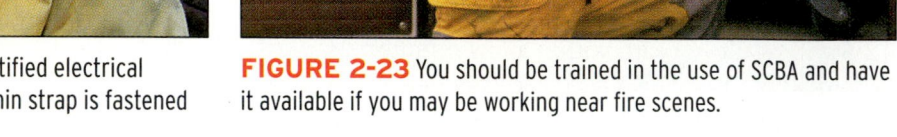

FIGURE 2-23 You should be trained in the use of SCBA and have it available if you may be working near fire scenes.

lock the face shield on the helmet. This will protect your face and eyes from power lines and flying sparks.

Turnout gear or a bunker jacket provides minimal protection from electrical shock. But it does protect you from heat, fire, possible flashover, and flying sparks. The front opening of the jacket should be fastened, and the jacket should be worn with the collar up and closed in front to protect your neck and upper chest (Figure 2-22). Proper fit is important so that you can move freely.

Lightning is a complex natural phenomenon. You are unwise to think that "lightning never strikes in the same place twice." If the right conditions remain, a repeat strike in the same area can occur.

Lightning is a threat in two ways: through a direct hit and through ground current. After the lightning bolt strikes, the current drains along the earth, following the most conductive pathway. To avoid being injured by a ground current, stay away from drainage ditches, moist areas, small depressions, and wet ropes. If you are involved in a rescue operation, you may need to delay it until the storm has passed. Recognize the warning signs just before a lightning strike. As your surroundings become charged, you may feel a slight tingling sensation on your skin, or your hair may even stand on end. In this situation, a strike may be imminent. Move immediately to the lowest possible area.

If you are caught in an open area, try to make yourself the smallest possible target for a direct hit or for ground current. To keep from being hit by the initial strike, stay away from projections from the ground, such as a single tree. Drop all equipment, particularly metal objects that project above your body. Avoid fences and other metal objects. These can transmit cur-

rent from the initial strike over a long distance. Position yourself in a low crouch. This position exposes only your feet to the ground current. If you sit, both your feet and your buttocks are exposed. Place an object made of nonconductive material, such as a blanket, under your feet. Get inside a car or your unit, if possible, as vehicles will protect you from lightning.

Fire

You will often be called to the scene of a fire. Therefore, you should understand some basic information about fire, if you do not know it already. There are five common hazards in a fire:

1. Smoke
2. Oxygen deficiency
3. High ambient temperatures
4. Toxic gases
5. Building collapse

Smoke is made up of particles of tar and carbon. These particles irritate the respiratory system on contact. Most smoke particles are trapped in the upper respiratory system, but many smaller particles enter the lungs. Some smoke particles not only irritate the airway, but also may be deadly. You must be trained in the use of appropriate airway protection, such as an SCBA or a disposable short-term device, and have it available at all fire scenes (Figure 2-23).

Fire consumes oxygen. Particularly in a closed space, such as a room, fire may consume most of the available oxygen. This will make breathing difficult for anyone in that space. The high ambient temperatures in a fire can result in thermal burns and damage to the respiratory system. Breathing air that is heated above 120°F (49°C) can damage the respiratory system.

A typical building fire emits a number of toxic gases, including carbon monoxide and carbon dioxide. Carbon monoxide is a colorless, odorless gas that is responsible for more fire deaths each year than any other by-product of combustion. Carbon monoxide combines with the hemoglobin in your red blood cells about 200 times more rapidly than oxygen does. It blocks the ability of the hemoglobin to transport oxygen to your body tissues. Carbon dioxide is also a colorless, odorless gas. Exposure causes increased respirations, dizziness, and sweating. Breathing concentrations of carbon dioxide above 10% to 12% will result in death within a few minutes.

During and after a fire, there is always a possibility that all or part of the burned structure will collapse. Often, there are no warning signs. Therefore, you should never run into a burning building. Your hasty entry into a burning structure may result in serious injury and possibly death. Once inside the burning building, you are subject to an uncontrolled, hostile environment. Fires are not selective about their victims. You must be extremely cautious whenever you are near a burning structure or one in which a fire has just been put out. Trained firefighters will be at the scene. Follow their instructions at the scene of any fire.

Fuel and fuel systems of vehicles that have been involved in accidents are also a hazard. Although vehicle fires rarely happen, any fuel may ignite under the right conditions. If you see or smell a known fuel leak, or if people are trapped in the vehicle, you must coordinate appropriate fire protection.

Make sure that you are properly protected if there is or has been a fire in the vehicle. Wear appropriate respiratory protection and thermal protection, as the smoke from a vehicle fire contains many toxic by-products. The use of full protective gear at an accident scene can reduce your risk of injury. Avoid using oxygen in or near a vehicle that is smoking, smoldering, or leaking fuel.

Protective Clothing

Wearing protective clothing and other appropriate gear is critical to your personal safety. Become familiar with the protective equipment that is available to you. Then you will know what clothing and gear are needed for the job. You will also be able to adapt or change items as the situation and environment change. Remember that pro-

tective clothing and gear are safe only when they are in good condition. It is your responsibility to inspect your clothing and gear. Learn to recognize how wear and tear can make your equipment unsafe. Be sure to inspect equipment before you use it, even if you must do so at the scene.

Clothing that is worn for rescue must be appropriate for the activity and the environmental conditions in which the activity will take place. For example, bunker gear that is worn for firefighting is usually too restrictive for working in a confined space. In every situation involving blood and/or other body fluids, be sure to follow BSI techniques. You must protect yourself and the patient by wearing gloves and eye protection, along with increasingly more protective clothing as needed.

Cold Weather Clothing

When dressing for cold weather, you should wear several layers of clothing. Multiple layers provide much better protection than a single thick cover. You have more flexibility to control your body temperature by adding or removing a layer. Cold weather protection should consist of at least three layers:

1. **A thin inner layer** (sometimes called the transport layer) next to your skin. This layer pulls moisture away from your skin, keeping you dry and warm. Underwear made of polypropylene or polyester material works well.

2. **A thermal middle layer** of bulkier material for insulation. Wool has been the material of choice for warmth, but newer materials, such as polyester pile, are also commonly used.

3. **An outer layer** that will resist chilling winds and wet conditions, such as rain, sleet, or snow. The two top layers should have zippers to allow you to vent some body heat if you become too warm.

When choosing clothing to protect yourself from the weather, pay attention to the type of material used. Cotton should be avoided in cold, wet environments. Cotton tends to absorb moisture, causing chilling from wetness. For example, if you wear cotton trousers and walk through wet grass, the cotton soaks up the moisture from the grass. This will chill you in cold weather. However, cotton is appropriate in warm, dry weather because it absorbs moisture and pulls heat away from the body.

As an outer layer in cold weather, you might consider plastic-coated nylon, as it provides good waterproof protection. However, it can also hold in body heat and perspiration, which makes you wet both inside and out.

Newer, less airtight materials allow perspiration and some heat to escape while the material retains its water resistance. Avoid flammable or meltable synthetic material anytime there is any possibility of fire.

Turnout Gear

Turnout or bunker gear is a fire service term for protective clothing, designed for use in structural firefighting environments (Figure 2-24). Turnout gear provides head-to-toe protection. It uses different layers of fabric or other material to provide protection from the heat of fire, to reduce trauma from impact or cuts, and to keep water away from the body. Like most protective clothing, turnout gear adds weight and reduces range of motion to some degree.

The exterior fabrics provide increased protection from cuts and abrasions. They also act as a barrier to high external temperatures. In cold weather, an insulated thermal inner layer of material that helps to retain body heat is recommended.

Gloves

You must wear latex or vinyl gloves any time you may be exposed to blood or other body fluids. In many EMS rescue operations, you must also protect your hands and wrists from injury. Firefighting gloves will provide the best protection from heat, cold, and cuts (Figure 2-25). Yet these gloves reduce manual dexterity. In addition, firefighting gloves will not protect you from electrical hazards. In rescue situations, you must be able to use your hands freely to operate rescue tools, provide patient care, and perform other duties. You may wear puncture-proof leather gloves, with latex gloves underneath. This combination will allow you free use of your hands with added protection from blood and body fluids. Remember that latex or vinyl gloves are considered medical waste and must be disposed of properly. Leather gloves must be treated as contaminated material until they can be properly decontaminated.

Helmets

You should wear a helmet any time you are working in a fall zone. A fall zone is an area where you are likely to encounter falling objects. The helmet should provide top and side impact protection. It should also have a secure chin strap (Figure 2-26). Objects will often fall one after another. If the strap is not secure, the first falling object may knock off your helmet. This leaves your head unprotected as the remaining objects fall.

Construction-type helmets are not well suited for rescue situations. They offer minimal impact protection

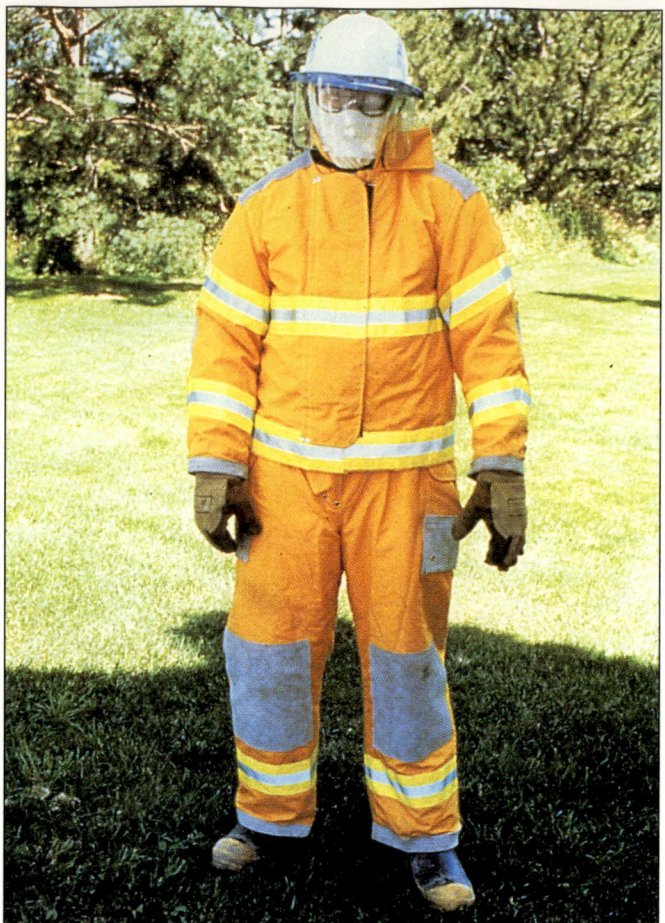

FIGURE 2-24 Turnout or bunker gear provides complete head-to-toe protection.

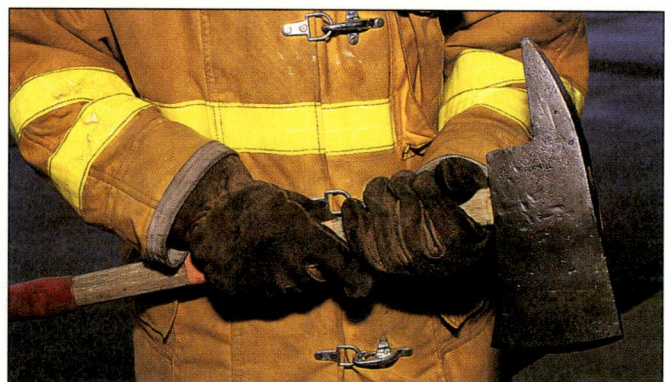

FIGURE 2-25 Firefighting gloves protect your hands and wrists from heat, cold, and injury.

and have inadequate chin straps. Modern fire helmets offer impact protection. However, the projecting brim at the back of the neck may get in your way in a rescue situation. In cold weather, you can lose a good bit of body heat if you are not wearing a hat or helmet. An insulated hat made from wool or a synthetic material can be pulled down over the face and the base of the skull to reduce heat loss in extremely cold weather.

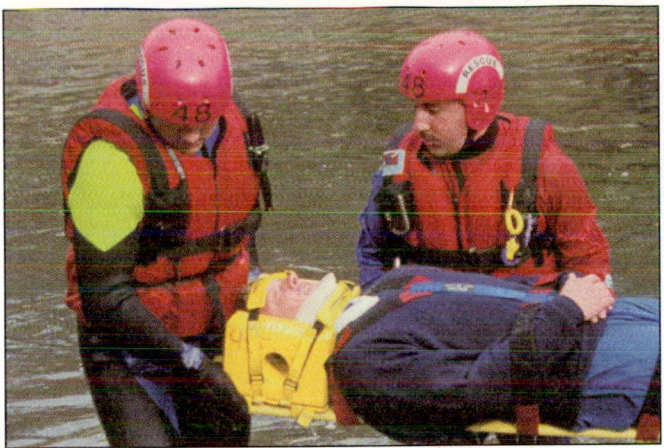

FIGURE 2-26 A helmet with side impact protection and a chin strap will not dislodge if struck by an object.

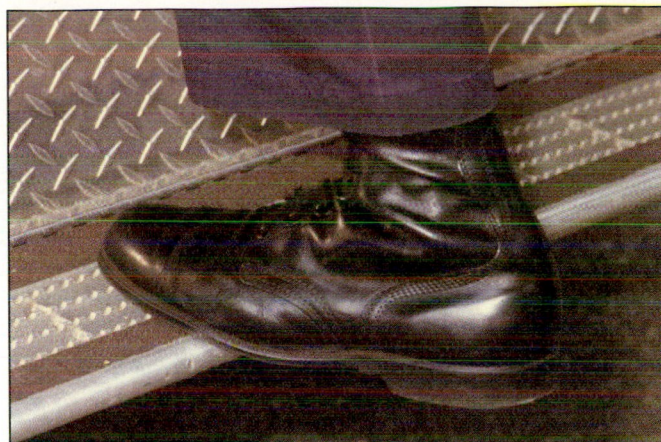

FIGURE 2-27 Boots should cover and protect your ankles, keeping out stones, debris, and snow.

Boots

Boots should protect your feet. They should be water resistant, fit well, and be flexible so that you can walk long distances comfortably. If you will be working outdoors, you should choose boots that cover and protect your ankles, keeping out stones, debris, and snow (Figure 2-27). In cold weather, your boots must also protect you from the cold. Leather is one of the best materials for boots. However, other materials, such as Gore-Tex water-repellent fabric, are also very good. The soles of your boots must provide traction. Lug-type soles may grip well in snow, but they become very slippery when caked with mud.

The fit of boots and shoes is extremely important, because a minor annoyance can develop into a disabling injury. You may develop painful blisters if your feet slip around inside your boots. However, make sure you have enough room to wiggle your toes.

Boots should be puncture resistant, protect the toes, and provide foot support. It may be difficult to obtain a good fit with firefighting boots; shoe inserts or sock layering may be needed for a comfortable fit. Make sure the tops of your boots are sealed off to keep rain, snow, glass, or other materials from getting into your boots.

Socks will keep your feet warm and provide some cushioning for you as you walk. In cold weather, two pairs of socks are generally preferable to one thick pair. A thin sock next to the foot helps to wick perspiration away to a thicker, outer sock. This tends to keep your feet warmer, drier, and generally more comfortable. When you purchase new shoes or boots, keep these points in mind.

Eye Protection

The human eye is very fragile, and permanent loss of sight can occur from very minor injuries. You need to protect your eyes from blood and other body fluids, foreign objects, plants, insects, and debris from extrication. You may wear eyeglasses with side shields during routine patient care. However, when tools are being used during extrication, you must wear a face shield and goggles. In these instances, prescription eyeglasses do not provide adequate protection. In snow or white sand, particularly at higher altitudes, you must protect your eyes from ultraviolet exposure. Specially designed glasses or goggles can provide this. In addition, your eye protection must be adaptable to the weather and the physical demands of the task. It is critical that you have clear vision at all times.

Ear Protection

Exposure to loud noises for long periods of time can cause permanent hearing loss. Certain equipment, such as helicopters, some extrication tools, and sirens, produces high levels of noise. Wearing soft foam industrial-type earplugs usually provides adequate protection.

Skin Protection

Your skin needs protection against sunburn while you are working outdoors. Long-term exposure to the sun increases the possibility of skin cancer. It might be considered simply an annoyance, but sunburn is a type of thermal burn. In reflective areas such as sand, water, and snow, your risk of sunburn increases. Protect your skin by applying a sunscreen with a minimum rating of SPF 15. It may also be necessary to wear masks and gowns when treating certain patients. Wearing them will protect both you and the patient. Remember that masks and gowns are considered medical waste and must be disposed of properly.

Violent Situations

The safety of you and your team is of primary concern. Civil disturbances, domestic disputes, and crime scenes, especially those involving gangs, can create many hazards for EMS personnel. Large gatherings of hostile or potentially hostile people are also dangerous. Several agencies will respond to large civil disturbances. In these instances, it is important for you to know who is in command and will be issuing orders (Figure 2-28). However, you and your partner may be on your own when a group of people seems to grow larger and become increasingly hostile. In these cases, you should call law enforcement immediately if they are not already at the scene. You may need to wait for law enforcement to arrive before you can treat the patient.

Remember that you and your partner must be protected from the dangers at the scene before you can provide patient care. Law enforcement must make sure the scene is safe before you and your partner enter. A crime scene often poses potential problems for EMS personnel. If the perpetrator is still somewhere on the scene, this person could reappear and threaten you and your partner or attempt to further injure the patient you are treating. Bystanders who are trying to be helpful may interfere with your emergency medical care. Family members may be very distraught and not understand what you are doing when you attempt to splint an injured extremity and the patient cries out that what you are doing hurts. Be sure that you have adequate assistance from the appropriate public safety agency in these cases.

Sometimes EMT-Bs will be at a scene where a dangerous situation is underway, such as a hostage situation or riot. In these instances, it may be necessary for EMS personnel to be protected from projectiles such as bullets, bottles, and rocks. Law enforcement personnel will ordinarily provide for concealment or cover of personnel who are involved in the response to the incident. **Cover** and concealment involve the tactical use of an impenetrable barrier for protection. EMT-Bs should not be placed in a position that will endanger their lives or safety during such incidents.

In some areas, EMS personnel wear body armor (bulletproof vests) if a scene has the potential to become violent. Several types of body armor are available. They range from extremely lightweight and flexible to heavy and bulky. The lighter vests do not stop large-caliber bullets. However, they offer more flexibility and are preferred by most law enforcement personnel. Lighter vests are commonly worn under a uniform shirt or jacket. The larger, heavier vests are worn on the outside of your uniform. Remember that your personal safety is of the utmost importance. You must thoroughly understand the risks of each environment you enter.

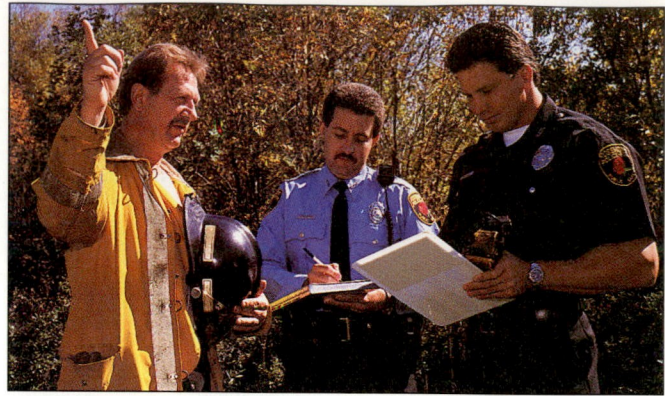

FIGURE 2-28 Several agencies may respond to large disturbances. It is important for you to know who is in command and will be issuing orders.

Whenever you are in doubt about your safety, do not put yourself at risk. Never enter an unstable environment, such as a shooting, a brawl, a hostage situation, or a riot. Therefore, as part of your scene size-up, evaluate the scene for the potential for violence. If it is a possibility, call for additional help. Failure to do so may put you and your partner at serious risk. Rely on the advice of law enforcement personnel as they have more experience and expertise in handling these situations.

It is also important for you to remember that if you believe that an event is a crime scene, you must attempt to maintain the chain of evidence. Briefly, make sure that you do not disturb the scene unless it is absolutely necessary in caring for the patient.

Behavioral Emergencies

Consider these questions as you evaluate the patient in terms of a behavioral or psychiatric emergency that may lead to violent patient reaction:

- How does this patient relate to you?
- Are your questions answered appropriately?
- Is the patient withdrawn or detached?
- Is the patient hostile or friendly? Overly friendly?
- Does the patient understand why you are there?
- How is the patient dressed? Is the dress appropriate for the time of the year and occasion? Are the clothes clean? Dirty?
- Are the patient's movements coordinated or jerky and awkward? Is there hyperactivity? What kind?
- Are the patient's movements purposeful, for example, in putting his or her clothes on? Are the actions aimless, such as sitting and rocking back and forth in a chair?
- Has the patient harmed herself or himself? Is there damage to the surroundings?

- Does the patient present as physically rigid, or is there waxy flexibility?
- Does the patient appear relaxed, stiff, or guarded?
- What are the patient's facial expressions? Are they bland or flat, or are they expressive? Does the patient show joy, fear, or anger to appropriate stimuli? If so, to what degree?
- Are the patient's vocabulary and expressions what you would expect under the circumstances? Are they related to the patient's social and educational background?

It might not be possible for you to gather all of the information that these questions suggest. Sometimes, a patient who is experiencing a behavioral emergency will not respond at all. In those cases, the patient's facial expressions, pulse and respirations, tears, sweating, and blushing may be significant indicators of his or her emotional state.

The following principal determinants of violence, though not intended to be the only ones specifically looked for, are of value for the EMT-B:

- **Past history.** Has this patient previously exhibited hostile, overly aggressive, or violent behavior? This information should be solicited by EMS personnel at the scene or requested from law enforcement personnel, family, previous EMS records, or hospital information.
- **Posture.** How is this person sitting or standing? Does the patient appear to be tense, rigid, or sitting on the edge of the bed, chair, or wherever he or she is positioned? The observation of increased tension by physical posture is often a warning signal for hostility.
- **Vocal activity.** What is the nature of the speech the patient is using? Loud, obscene, erratic, and bizarre speech patterns usually indicate emotional distress. The patient who is conversing in quiet, ordered speech is not as likely to strike out against others as is the patient who is yelling and screaming.
- **Physical activity.** Perhaps one of the most demonstrative factors to look for is the motor activity of a person who is undergoing a behavioral crisis. The patient who is pacing, cannot sit still, or is displaying protection of his or her boundaries of personal space needs careful watching. Agitation is a prognostic sign to be observed with great care and scrutiny.

Other factors to take into consideration for potential violence include the following:

- Poor impulse control
- The behavior triad of truancy, fighting, and uncontrollable temper
- Socioeconomic status, instability of family structure, inability to keep a steady job
- Tattoos, such as those with gang identification or statements like "born to kill" or "born to lose"
- Substance abuse
- Functional disorder (If the patient says that he or she is hearing voices that say to kill, believe it!)
- Depression, which accounts for 20% of violent attacks

Immunizations

As an EMT-B, you are at risk for acquiring an infectious or communicable disease. Using basic protective measures can minimize this risk. You are responsible for protecting yourself.

Prevention begins by maintaining your personal health. Annual health examinations should be required for all EMS personnel. A history of all your childhood infectious diseases should be recorded and kept on file. Childhood infectious diseases include chickenpox, mumps, measles, and whooping cough. If you have not had one of these diseases, you must be immunized.

The Centers for Disease Control and Prevention and OSHA have developed requirements for protection from blood-borne pathogens such as hepatitis B and human immunodeficiency viruses. An immunization program should be in place in your EMS system. Immunizations should be kept up to date and recorded in your file. Recommended immunizations include the following:

- Tetanus-diphtheria boosters
- Measles vaccine
- Rubella (German measles) vaccine
- Mumps vaccine
- Influenza vaccine (yearly)
- Hepatitis B vaccine

You should also have a skin test for tuberculosis before you begin working as an EMT-B. The purpose of the test is to identify anyone who has been exposed to tuberculosis in the past. Testing should be repeated every year.

If you know that you will be transporting a patient who has a communicable disease, you have a definite advantage. This is when your health record will be valuable. If you have already had the disease or been vaccinated, you are not at risk. However, you will not always know whether a patient has a communicable disease. Therefore, you should always follow BSI techniques if there is the possibility of exposure to blood or other body fluids.

prep kit

ready for review

EMT-Bs will encounter death, dying patients, and the families and friends of those who have died. Death will be no stranger in the work of emergency medical services. Therefore, coming to grips with death and dying and understanding the concerns of the dying patient, assisting a family following the death of loved one, and dealing with one's own feelings are both personally and professionally important.

When signs of stress such as fatigue, anxiety, anger, feelings of hopelessness, worthlessness, or guilt, and other such indicators manifest themselves, behavioral problems can develop. Recognizing the signs of stress is important for all EMT-Bs. CISD efforts, among other programs of support, are important in identifying potentially serious mental health problems, such as posttraumatic stress disorder, that can result from dealing with the overwhelming stress that sometimes develops in critical situations, such as the death of patients. Posttraumatic stress disorder is a syndrome with onset following a traumatic, usually life-threatening event.

As an EMT-B, you will arrive at scenes where potential danger to yourself is easily apparent, such as a motor vehicle crash where gasoline is leaking. As is mentioned in this chapter, every patient encounter should be considered to be potentially dangerous to you. One of the dangers is the potentially violent patient. Communicable diseases also pose a risk to you. Therefore, it is essential that you take all available precautions to minimize exposure and risk.

vital vocabulary

www.emtb.com

body substance isolation (BSI) An infection control concept and practice that assumes that all body fluids are potentially infectious.

burnout A condition of chronic fatigue and frustration that results from mounting stress over time.

cover The tactical use of an impenetrable barrier to conceal EMS personnel and protect them from projectiles (eg, bullets, bottles, rocks).

Critical Incident Stress Debriefing (CISD)
A confidential group discussion of a highly traumatic incident that usually occurs within 24 to 72 hours of the incident.

Critical Incident Stress Management (CISM)
A process that confronts the responses to critical incidents and defuses them, directing the emergency services personnel toward physical and emotional equilibrium.

Occupational Safety and Health Administration (OSHA) The federal regulatory compliance agency that develops, publishes, and enforces guidelines concerning safety in the workplace.

Posttraumatic Stress Disorder (PTSD) A delayed stress reaction to a prior incident. This delayed reaction is the result of one or more unresolved issues concerning the incident that may have been alleviated with the use of critical incident stress management.

prep kit 2

assessment in action

You and your partner are dispatched to an "unknown emergency" at a small apartment complex in town. When you arrive about 4 minutes later, you see that law enforcement is already there, trying to manage the 6 or 7 neighbors who have gathered outside a first-floor apartment. You enter the apartment to find a 31-year-old woman lying on the sofa and pills from a half-dozen bottles scattered on the carpet. From the doorway, the patient appears to be dead, but you approach her and perform an initial assessment. Her skin is cool to the touch, and as you suspected, rigor mortis appears to have occurred. Suddenly, the patient's mother enters and begins to yell at you, demanding to know why it took you so long to respond. The mother then threatens to sue you and your partner.

1. The patient's mother appears to be in what stage of coping with her daughter's unexpected death?
   A. Denial
   B. Anger
   C. Bargaining
   D. Acceptance

2. The most appropriate way to respond to the mother is to:
   A. ignore her.
   B. become defensive.
   C. be tolerant and empathetic.
   D. take the comments personally.

3. The patient's boyfriend arrives on the scene and says, "If only we hadn't had a fight last night, things would have been different." The patient's boyfriend is in what stage of coping with her death?
   A. Denial
   B. Anger
   C. Bargaining
   D. Acceptance

4. Approximately a month later, you continue to have dreams about the call. To help cope with this problem, you should:
   A. ignore the dreams.
   B. resign from the squad.
   C. seek professional help.
   D. drink and unwind with your friends.

5. Critical Incident Stress Management (CISM) is a forum that allows you and other participants to:
   A. discuss fears, feelings, and reactions to the incident.
   B. talk about your feelings 5 to 10 days after an incident.
   C. share information that would otherwise be considered confidential.
   D. provide the medical director with facts and details to critique the incident.

points to ponder

Objectives 1-2.2, 1-2.3

It is 7:30 A.M., and you are dispatched to the scene of an unconscious male. Upon arrival, you find a 54-year-old man who apparently died in his sleep during the night. It is obvious that the man has been dead for much of the night. His teenage children and wife are in the room when you enter. A quick check of pulse and breathing confirm that the man is both apneic and pulseless. When you tell the family that there is nothing you can do, they begin yelling at you to do something, and they become a little abusive.

- Explain how you would deal with this situation, including how you would tell the family that the man is beyond your help and how you would deal with their aggressive behavior.

online outlook

As a part of training you will begin to recognize and protect yourself from possible hazards. Nevertheless, injury and death to EMTs sometimes occur. Visit the National EMS Memorial Service Web Site and complete exercise 2 at www.emtb.com.

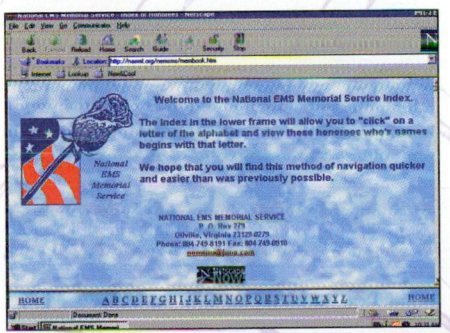

prep kit 2

Medical, Legal, and Ethical Issues

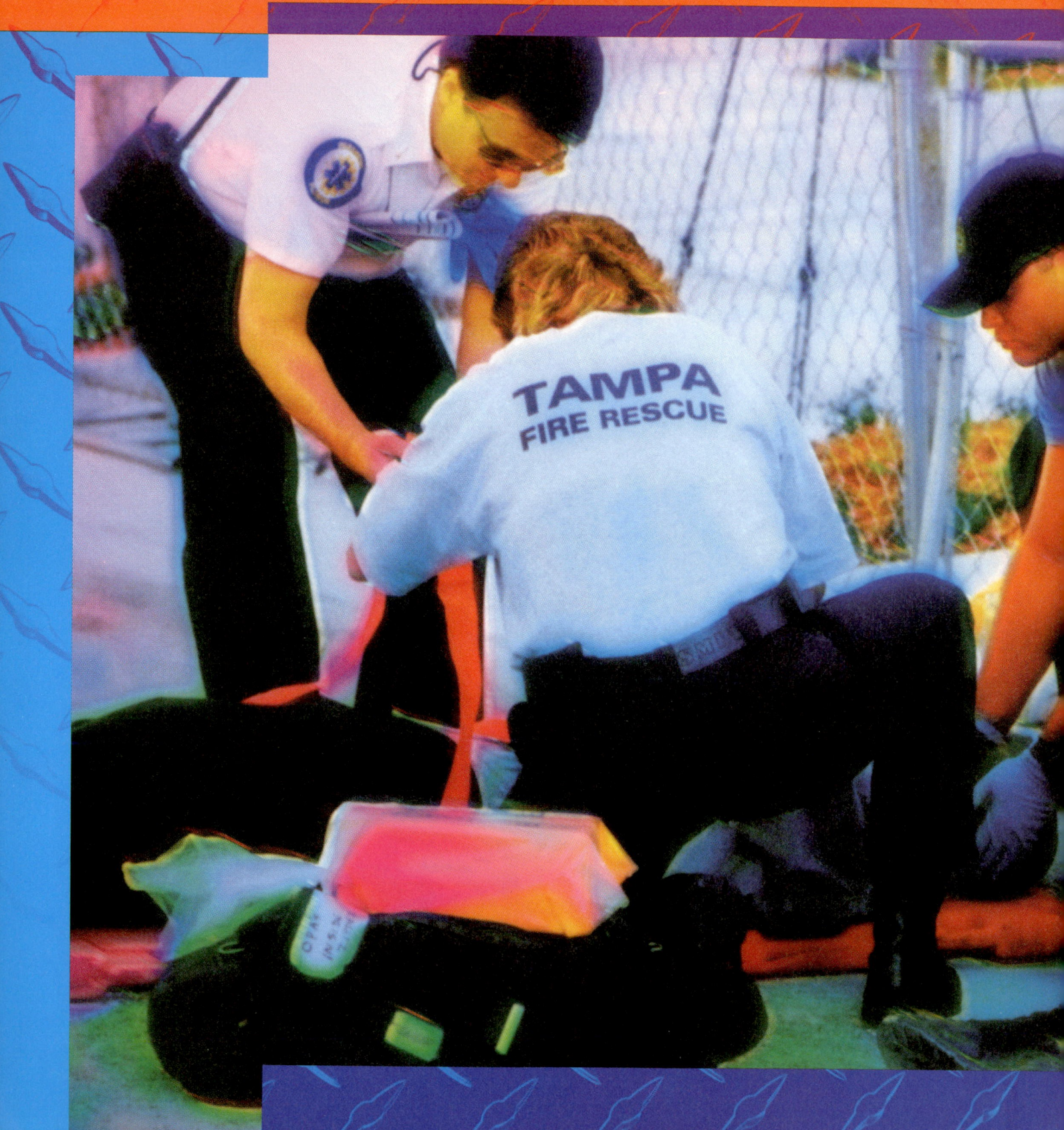

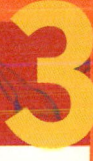
objectives

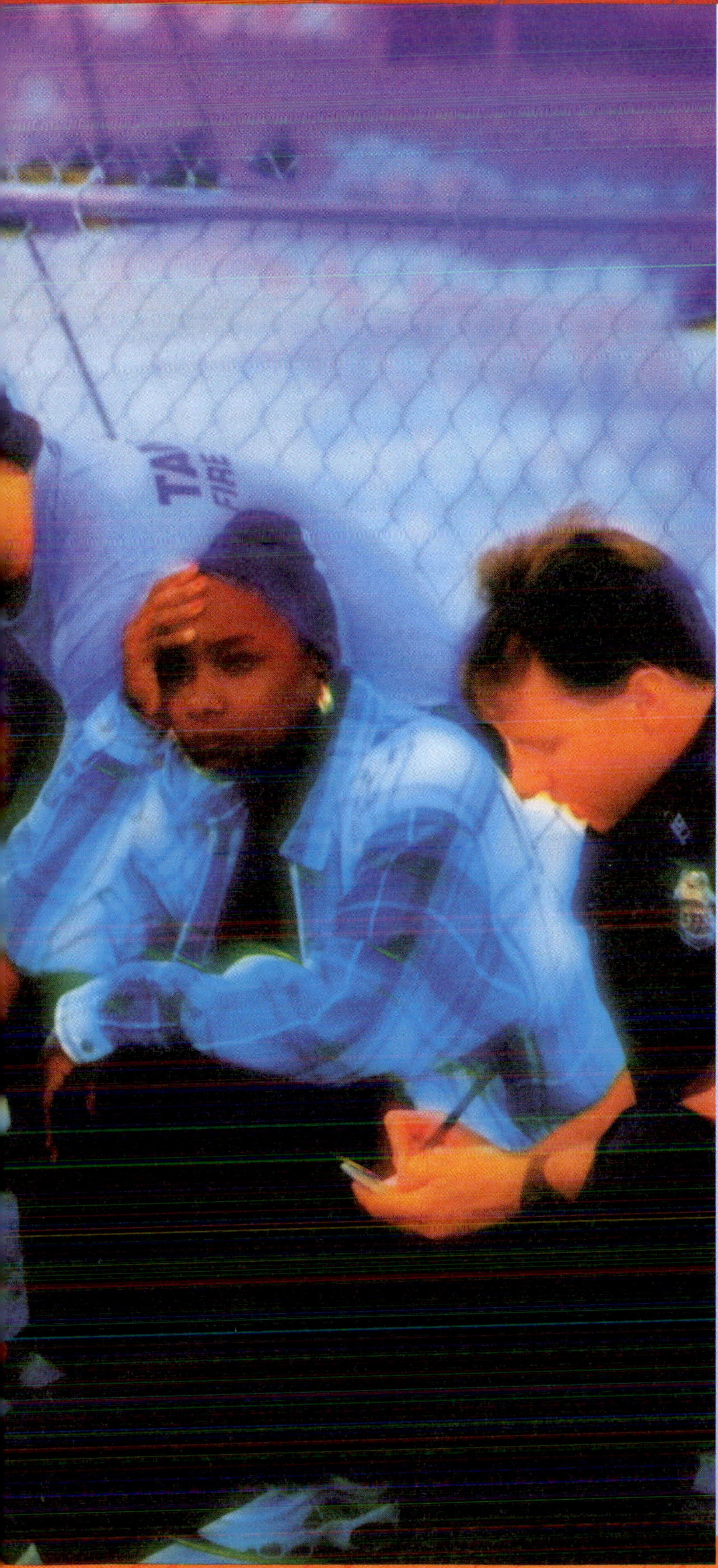

Cognitive

1. Define the EMT-B scope of practice.

2. Discuss the importance of do not resuscitate (DNR) [advance directives] and local or state provisions regarding EMS application.

3. Define consent and discuss the methods of obtaining consent.

4. Differentiate between expressed and implied consent.

5. Explain the role of consent of minors in providing care.

6. Discuss the implications for the EMT-B in patient refusal of transport.

7. Discuss the issues of abandonment, negligence, and battery and their implications to the EMT-B.

8. State the conditions necessary for the EMT-B to have a duty to act.

9. Explain the importance, necessity, and legality of patient confidentiality.

10. Discuss the considerations of the EMT-B in issues of organ retrieval.

11. Differentiate the actions that an EMT-B should take to assist in the preservation of a crime scene.

12. State the conditions that require an EMT-B to notify local law enforcement officials.

Affective

13. Explain the role of EMS and the EMT-B regarding patients with DNR orders.

14. Explain the rationale for the needs, benefits, and usage of advance directives.

15. Explain the rationale for the concept of varying degrees of DNR.

Psychomotor

None

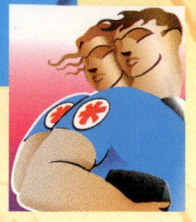

you are the emt

You are midway through your shift when the doorbell rings at your quarters. The man standing at the door hands you a subpoena ordering you to report to the district attorney's office to give a deposition for a lawsuit that was recently filed.

As much as every EMS provider would like to avoid this situation, it is part of the job. This chapter will explain the legal concepts that are most commonly encountered in prehospital medicine. It will also help you to answer the following questions:

1. What is your best defense when legal action is being taken against you?
2. What can you do to avoid being sued successfully?

Medical, Legal, and Ethical Issues

A basic principle of emergency care is to do no further harm. Any healthcare provider who acts in good faith and according to an appropriate standard of care usually avoids legal exposure. Providing emergency medical care in an organized system is a recent phenomenon. **Emergency medical care**, or immediate care or treatment, is often provided by an EMT, who may be the first link in the chain of prehospital care. As the scope and nature of emergency medical care becomes more complex and widely available, litigation involving participants in EMS systems will no doubt increase. Providing competent emergency medical care that conforms with the standard of care taught to you will help you to avoid both civil and criminal actions. Consider the following situations:

- You are transporting a patient, and while the gurney is being loaded into the ambulance, your partner slips, the gurney crashes to the ground, and the patient is injured.
- You are about to begin treating a child, and the father commands you to stop.

What should you do? Even when emergency medical care is properly rendered, there are times when you may be sued by a patient who seeks to obtain relief, often in the form of a monetary award, for pain and suffering. Or administrative action, such as suspension of your state license or EMT-B certificate, may be brought against you for failure to abide by the regulations of your state EMS agency. For this reason, you must understand the various legal aspects of emergency medical care.

You must also consider ethical issues. As an EMT-B, should you stop and treat patients who were involved in an automobile crash while you are en route to another emergency call? Should you begin CPR on a patient who, according to the family, has terminal cancer? Should patient information be released to a patient's attorney on the telephone?

Scope of Practice

The scope of practice, which is most commonly defined by state law, outlines the care you are able to provide for the patient. Your medical director further defines the scope of practice by developing protocols and standing orders. The medical director gives you the legal authorization to provide patient care through telephone or radio communication (on-line) or standing orders and protocols (off-line) (Figure 3-1).

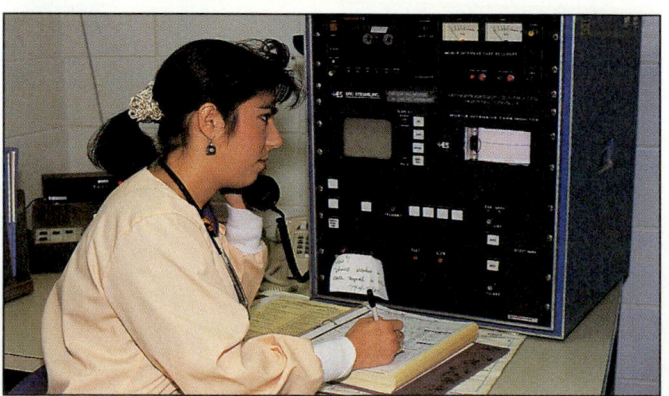

FIGURE 3-1 On-line medical direction is often communicated via radio.

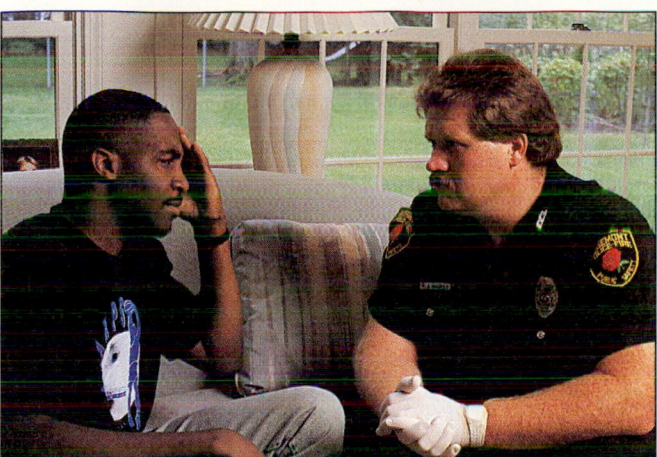

FIGURE 3-2 Act or behave toward others in a way that shows your concern about their safety and welfare, especially when your behavior or activities can cause others injury or harm.

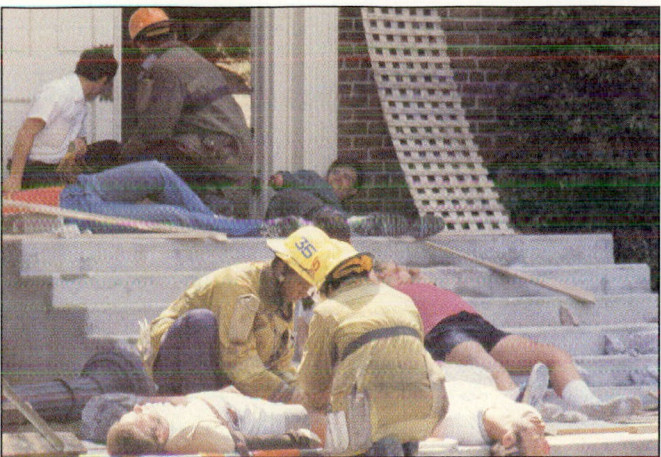

FIGURE 3-3 An emergency is a serious situation that arises suddenly, threatens the life or welfare of one or more individuals, and requires immediate intervention.

You and other EMS personnel have a responsibility to provide proper, consistent patient care and to report problems, such as possible liability or exposure to airborne or bloodborne pathogens or infectious disease, to your medical director immediately.

Standards of Care

The law requires you to act or behave toward other individuals in a certain, definable way, regardless of the activity involved. Under given circumstances, you have a duty either to act or not. Generally speaking, you must be concerned about the safety and welfare of others when your behavior or activities have the potential for causing others injury or harm (Figure 3-2). The manner in which you must act or behave is called a <u>standard of care</u>.

Standard of care is established in many ways, among them local custom, statutes, ordinances, administrative regulations, and case law. In addition, professional or institutional standards have a bearing on determining the adequacy of your conduct.

Standards Imposed by Local Custom

The standard of care is how a reasonably prudent person with similar training and experience would act under similar circumstances, with similar equipment, and in the same place. For example, the conduct of an EMT-B who is employed by an ambulance service is to be judged in comparison with the expected conduct of other EMT-Bs from comparable ambulance services. These standards are often based on locally accepted protocols.

As an EMT-B, you will not be held to the same standard of care as physicians or other more highly trained individuals would. In addition, your conduct must be judged in the light of the given emergency situation, taking into consideration the following factors:

- General confusion at the scene of the emergency
- The needs of other patients
- The type of equipment available

In this context, an <u>emergency</u> is a serious situation, such as injury or illness, that arises suddenly, threatens the life or welfare of a person or group of people, and requires immediate intervention (Figure 3-3).

The prevailing custom of the community is an important element in determining the standard of emergency care required.

Standards Imposed by Law

In addition to local customs, standards of emergency medical care may be imposed by statutes, ordinances, administrative regulation, or case law. In many jurisdictions, violating one of these standards is said to create *presumptive negligence*. Therefore, you must become familiar with the particular legal standards that may exist in your state. In many states, this may take the form of treatment protocols published by a state agency.

Professional or Institutional Standards

In addition to standards imposed by law, professional or institutional standards may be admitted as evidence in determining the adequacy of an EMT's conduct. Professional standards include recommendations published by organizations and societies that are involved in emergency medical care. Institutional standards include specific rules and procedures of the EMS service, ambulance service, or organization to which you are attached.

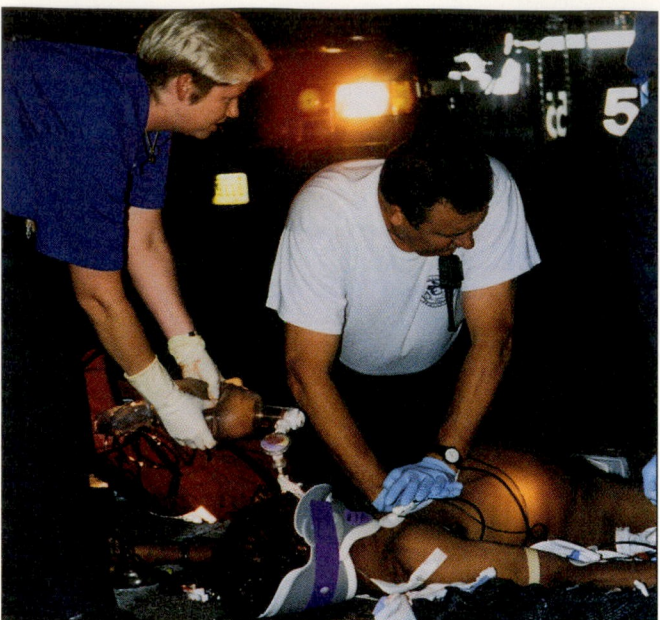

FIGURE 3-4 Many standards of care are imposed on you, such as those for performing BLS and CPR.

Two words of caution: First, you must be familiar with the standards of your organization. Second, if you are involved in formulating standards for a particular agency, they should be reasonable and realistic so that they do not impose an unreasonable burden on EMTs. Providing the best emergency medical care should be every EMT's goal, but it is not realistic to have institutional standards that *demand* the best care.

Many standards of care may be imposed on you. State health department regulations usually govern the scope and level of training. Court decisions have resulted in case law defining standards of care. Professional standards are also imposed, such as the American Heart Association's standard for BLS and CPR (Figure 3-4).

Ordinary care is a minimum standard of care. In general, it is expected that anyone who offers assistance will exercise reasonable care and act prudently. If you act reasonably, according to the accepted standard, the risk of civil suit is small. If you apply the standard practices you have been trained to use, you can likely avoid liability. For example, various organizations have defined standards for performing CPR. If you deviate from these standards, you may be liable for civil and possibly criminal prosecution. In addition, state regulatory agencies that oversee EMS operations can sanction EMS personnel for deviating from the standard of care.

Standards Imposed by States

Medical Practices Act. EMS personnel are exempt from the licensure requirements of the Medical Practices Act in most states because an EMT-B is regarded as a non-

medical professional. The practice of medicine is defined as the diagnosis and treatment of disease or illness. EMT-Bs and others in the prehospital care chain assess the need for life support and begin care. Therefore, the standard of care must be maintained within the scope of your state's provisions and licensing requirements.

Certification. Some states provide certification or licensure of individuals who perform emergency medical care. <u>Certification</u> is the process by which an individual, institution, or program is evaluated and recognized as meeting certain predetermined standards to ensure safe and ethical patient care. Once certified, you are obliged to conform to the standards that are generally recognized nationally by various registry groups and provide an important link in nationwide EMS. To be protected, you must ensure that your certification or licensure remains current; skill levels must be kept up to date.

Some organizations have recently changed their concept of certification. The American Heart Association, for example, now acknowledges only one's successful completion of a BLS/CPR course. Certification has specific legal meaning and is generally restricted to licensing agencies.

Duty to Act

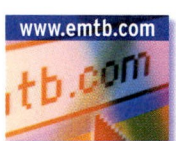

<u>Duty to act</u> is an individual's responsibility to provide patient care. Responsibility comes from either statute or function. A bystander is under no obligation to assist a stranger in distress; there is no duty to act. There may be a duty to act in certain instances, including the following:

- You are charged with emergency medical response.
- Your service or department's policy states that you must assist in any emergency.

Once your ambulance responds to a call or treatment is begun, you have a legal duty to act. If you are off duty and come upon an accident, you are not legally obligated to stop and assist patients. However, you do have a moral and ethical duty to act because of your special training and expertise.

Negligence

<u>Negligence</u> is the failure to provide the same care that a person with similar training would provide. It is deviation from the accepted standard of care that may result in further injury to the patient. Determination of negligence is based on the following four factors:

1. **Duty.** It is the EMT-B's responsibility to act reasonably. Conduct is measured by standards of care based on training. How would a person with similar training act under the same circumstances?

2. **Breach of duty.** There is a breach of duty when the EMT-B does not act within an expected and reasonable standard of care.

3. **Damages.** There are damages when a patient is physically or psychologically harmed in some noticeable way.

4. **Cause.** There must be a reasonable cause and effect. An example is dropping the patient during lifting, causing a fracture of the patient's leg. If a person has a duty and abuses it, causing harm to another individual, the EMT-B and/or the agency may be sued for negligence.

All four elements must be present for the legal doctrine of negligence to apply.

Abandonment

Abandonment is the unilateral termination of care by the EMT-B without the patient's consent and without making any provisions for continuing care by a medical professional with skills at the same or a higher level. For the EMT-B, once care is started, you have assumed a duty that must not stop until an equally competent person assumes responsibility. Not performing that duty exposes the patient to harm and is a basis for a negligence suit. Abandonment is legally and ethically a serious matter than can result in both civil and criminal actions against an EMT.

For example, suppose you arrive at the scene of a single-car accident and begin care of two injured patients. A passerby tells you of a two-car accident farther down the road in which five people are injured. You turn care of the two injured patients from the first accident over to the passerby and leave to go to the other accident. Abandonment has occurred because you did not turn care of the patients over to a person with the same or a higher level of skill than yours. Consider the following questions when you are faced with making a decision such as this one:

- What problems may develop from your actions?
- Are you neglecting your duty to the patients in the first accident?
- What is the passerby's level of training?
- Are you abandoning the patient if you leave the scene?
- Are you violating a standard of care?
- Are you acting prudently?

Consent

Under most circumstances, consent is required from every conscious, mentally competent adult before care can be started. A person receiving care must give permission, or **consent**, for treatment. If a person is in control of his or her actions, even though injured, and refuses care, you may not assist. In fact, doing so may be grounds for both criminal and civil action such as unlawful battery. Consent can be actual or implied and can involve the care of a minor or a mind-altered patient.

Expressed Consent

Expressed consent (or actual consent) is the type of consent in which the patient expressly authorizes you to provide care or transport. It must be **informed consent**, which means that the patient has been told of the potential risks, benefits, and alternatives to treatment and has given consent to treatment. The legal basis for this doctrine rests on the assumption that the patient has a right to determine what is to be done with his or her body. The patient must be of legal age and able to make a rational decision.

A patient might agree to certain emergency medical care but not to other care. For example, a patient might agree to be removed from a car but refuse further care. An injured person might agree to emergency care at home but refuse to be transported to a medical facility. Informed consent is valid if given orally; however, it may be difficult to prove. Having the patient sign a consent form does not eliminate your responsibility to tell that patient what is involved.

Implied Consent

When a person is unconscious and unable to give consent or when a serious threat to life exists, the law assumes that the patient would consent to care and transport to a medical facility (Figure 3-5). This is called **implied consent**. Implied consent is limited to true emergency situations and is appropriate when the patient is unconscious, delusional, unresponsive as a result of drugs or alcohol use, or otherwise physically unable to give expressed consent. However, many things may be unclear about what represents a "serious threat to life." Legal action would likely revolve around that question. This becomes a medicolegal judgment, which should be supported by the EMT-B's best efforts to obtain consent. **Medicolegal** is a term that relates to medical jurisprudence (law) or forensic medicine. In most instances, the law allows the spouse, a close relative, or next of kin to give consent for an injured person who is unable to give consent. Refusal of your intention to

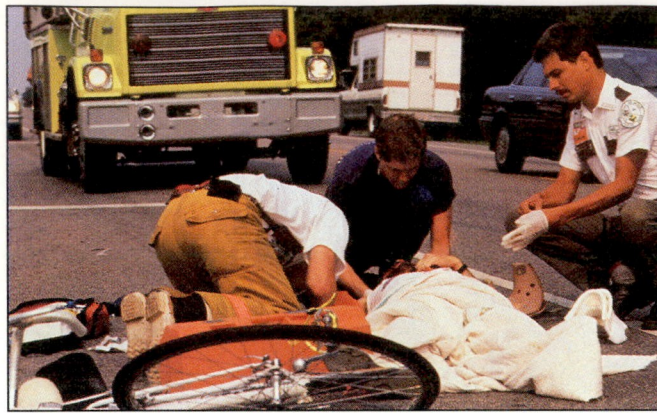

FIGURE 3-5 When a serious threat to life exists and the patient is unconscious or otherwise unable to give consent, the law assumes that the patient would give implied consent or consent to care and transport to the hospital.

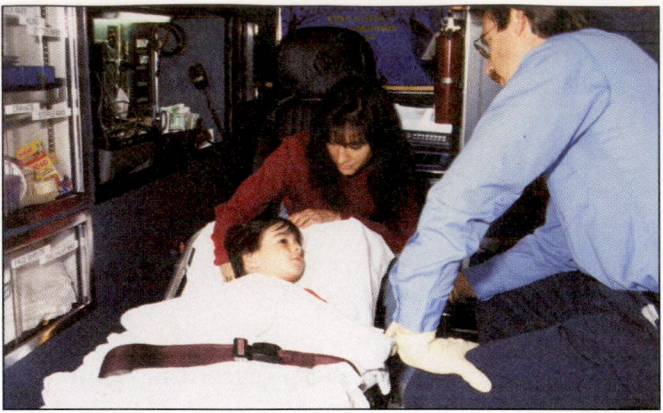

FIGURE 3-6 The law requires that a parent or legal guardian give consent for treatment or transport of a minor.

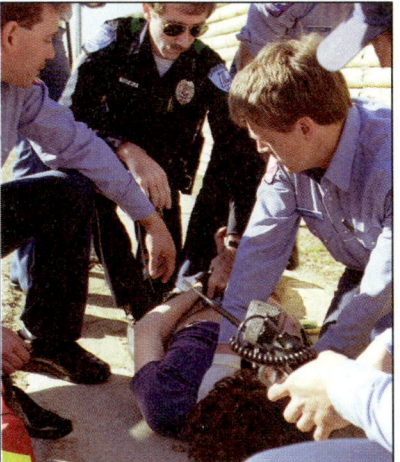

FIGURE 3-7 Be sure that you know the local laws about forcible restraint of a patient. In most states, only a law enforcement officer has the authority to restrain a patient.

render emergency care also may be implied. For example, a patient's action in pulling his or her arm from your splint may be an indication of refusal of consent.

Minors and Consent

Because a minor might not have the wisdom, maturity, or judgment to give valid consent, the law requires that a parent or legal guardian give consent for treatment or transport (Figure 3-6). However, in some states, a minor can give valid consent to receive medical care, depending on the minor's age and maturity. Many states also allow emancipated, married, or pregnant minors to be treated as adults for the purposes of consenting to medical treatment. You should obtain consent from a parent or legal guardian whenever possible; however, if a true emergency exists and the parent or legal guardian is not available, the consent to treat the minor is implied, just as with an adult. You must never withhold lifesaving care.

Mentally Incompetent Adults

Assisting patients who are mentally ill, in behavioral (psychological) crisis, under the influence of drugs or alcohol, or developmentally delayed is complicated. An adult patient who is mentally incompetent is not able to give informed consent. From a legal perspective, this situation is similar to those involving minors. Consent for emergency care should be obtained from someone who is legally responsible, such as a guardian or conservator. In many cases, however, such permission will not be readily obtainable. Many states have protective custody statutes allowing such a person to be taken, under law enforcement authority, to a medical facility. Know the provisions in your area. Remember that when a true emergency exists, you can assume that implied consent applies.

Forcible Restraint

Forcible restraint means confining an individual from being able to take any mental or physical action. Forcible restraint of a mentally disturbed individual may be required before emergency care can be rendered. If you believe that a patient will injure himself, herself, or others, you can legally restrain the patient. However, you must consult medical control for authorization to restrain or contact law enforcement personnel who have authority to restrain the patient. In most states, only a law enforcement officer may forcibly restrain an individual (Figure 3-7). You should be clearly informed about local laws. Restraint without authority exposes you to both litigation and possible personal danger. Restraint may be used only in circumstances of risk to yourself or others.

Your service should have clearly defined protocols to deal with situations involving restraint. After restraints are applied, they must not be removed en route even if the patient promises to behave.

Remember that if the patient is conscious and the situation is not urgent, consent is required. Adults who appear to be in control of their senses cannot be forced to submit to either care or transportation.

Assault and Battery

Assault is defined as unlawfully placing a person in fear of immediate bodily harm without the person's consent. Battery is unlawfully touching a person; this includes providing emergency care without consent. Serious legal problems may arise in situations in which a patient has not given consent for treatment. Battery could be considered if you apply a splint to a suspected fracture of the lower leg or use an Epi-Pen on a patient without the patient's consent. The patient may have grounds to sue you for assault, battery, or both. To protect yourself from these charges, make sure that you obtain expressed consent or that the situation allows for implied consent. Consult your medical director if you have questions or doubt about a specific situation.

The Right to Refuse Treatment

Mentally competent adults have the right to refuse treatment or withdraw from treatment at any time. However, these patients present you with a dilemma. Should you provide care against their will and risk being accused of battery? Should you leave them alone? If you leave patients alone, you risk being accused of negligence or abandonment if their condition becomes worse.

If a patient refuses treatment or transport, you must make sure that he or she understands, or is informed about, the potential risks, benefits, treatments, and alternatives to treatment. You must also fully inform the patient about the consequences of refusing treatment and encourage the patient to ask questions. Remember that competent adults who refuse specific kinds of treatment for religious reasons generally have a legal right to do so.

When a patient refuses treatment, you must assess whether the patient's mental condition is impaired. If the patient refusing treatment is delusional or confused, you cannot assume that the refusal is an informed refusal. When in doubt, it is always best to proceed with treatment. This is the best course of action because providing treatment is a much more defensible position than failing to treat a patient. Failure to treat a patient is considered abandonment.

You may also be faced with a situation in which a parent refuses to permit treatment of an ill or injured child. In this situation, you must consider the emotional impact of the emergency on the parent's judgment. In this and virtually all cases of refusal, you can usually resolve the situation with patience and calm persuasion. You may also need the help of others, such as law enforcement officials.

There will be times when you are not able to persuade the patient, guardian, conservator, or parent of a minor or mentally incompetent patient to proceed with treatment. In this case, you must obtain the signature of the individual who is refusing treatment on an official release form that acknowledges refusal. You must be sure to document any assessment findings and emergency care that you provided. You must also obtain a signature from a witness to the refusal. You should then keep the refusal with the run report and the medical incident report. In addition to the release form itself, you should write a note about the refusal on the medical incident report and the run report as well. If the patient refuses to sign the release form, the best you can do is inform your medical director and thoroughly document the situation and the refusal. You should never make an independent decision not to transport. Report to medical control, and/or follow your local protocols with regard to this situation. Make sure your department keeps a copy of the documentation for future reference.

Good Samaritan Laws and Immunity

Most states have adopted Good Samaritan laws, which are based on the common law principle that when you reasonably help another person, you should not be liable for errors and omissions that are made in giving good faith emergency care. However, Good Samaritan laws do not protect you from a lawsuit. Only a few statutory provisions provide immunity from a lawsuit, and those usually are reserved for governments. Good Samaritan laws provide an affirmative defense if you are sued for rendering care, but they do not protect you from liability or for failure to provide proper care, nor do they pertain to acts outside the scope of care. These laws do not protect anyone from wanton, gross, or willful negligence (eg, the failure to exercise due care).

Another group of laws grants immunity from liability to official emergency medical care providers, such as EMT-Bs. These laws, which vary from state to state, do not provide immunity when injury or damage is caused by gross negligence or willful conduct.

Most states have also adopted specific laws granting special privileges to EMS personnel, authorizing them to perform certain medical procedures. Many states also grant partial immunity to EMTs and physicians and nurses who give emergency instructions to EMS personnel via radio or other forms of communication. Consult your medical director for more information about the laws in your area.

Advance Directives

Occasionally, you and your partner may respond to a call in which a patient is dying from an illness. When you arrive at the scene, you may find that family members present do not want you to try to resuscitate the patient. Without written documentation from a physician, such as an advance directive or a do not resuscitate (DNR) order, this type of request places you in a very difficult position. An **advance directive** is a written document that specifies medical treatment for a competent patient, should he or she become unable to make decisions. In this situation, a **competent** patient is able to make rational decisions about his or her well-being. An advance directive is also commonly called a living will. DNR orders give you permission *not* to attempt resuscitation. Generally speaking, to be valid, **DNR orders** must meet the following requirements:

- Clearly state the patient's medical problem(s)

- Be signed by the patient or legal guardian

- Be signed by one or more physicians

- Be dated in the preceding 12 months

However, even in the presence of such a DNR order, you are still obligated to provide supportive measures (oxygen, pain relief, and comfort) whenever possible. Each ambulance service, in consultation with its medical director and legal counsel, must develop a protocol to follow in these circumstances.

Because of terminal nursing home placement and hospice and home health programs, you may be faced with this situation often. Specific guidelines vary from state to state, but the following four statements may be considered general guidelines:

1. **Patients have the right to refuse treatment,** including resuscitative efforts, provided that they are able to communicate their wishes.

2. **A written order from a physician is required** for DNR orders to be valid in a health care facility.

3. **You should periodically review** state and local protocols and legislation regarding advanced directives.

4. **When you are in doubt** or the written orders are not present, resuscitate.

Ethical Responsibilities

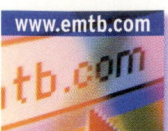

In addition to legal duties, you have certain ethical responsibilities to the public. Ethics are related to moral action, conduct, motive, or character. From an EMS standpoint, ethics are related to what the profession of emergency medical service providers deems right or fitting. Treating a patient ethically means doing so in a manner that conforms to professional standards of conduct. One ethical principle might be caring for all patients with a sense of excellence (Figure 3-8). Excellence in patient care and the quality of patient care, for example, may become guiding moral principles in seeking certain attributes and skills in the EMS work that you do.

You must meet your legal responsibilities and, at the same time, make the physical and emotional needs of the patient a priority. Patient needs vary, depending on the situation. You must practice and maintain your skills to the point of mastery. In other words, you must strive to be at your best at all times.

From time to time, you should review your performance. Assess your techniques, your response times, patient outcomes, and communication. Think about ways in which you can improve your performance. Through hands-on experience and critical review, you can maintain and improve your skills. Another way to maintain your skills is by taking continuing education classes and refresher programs.

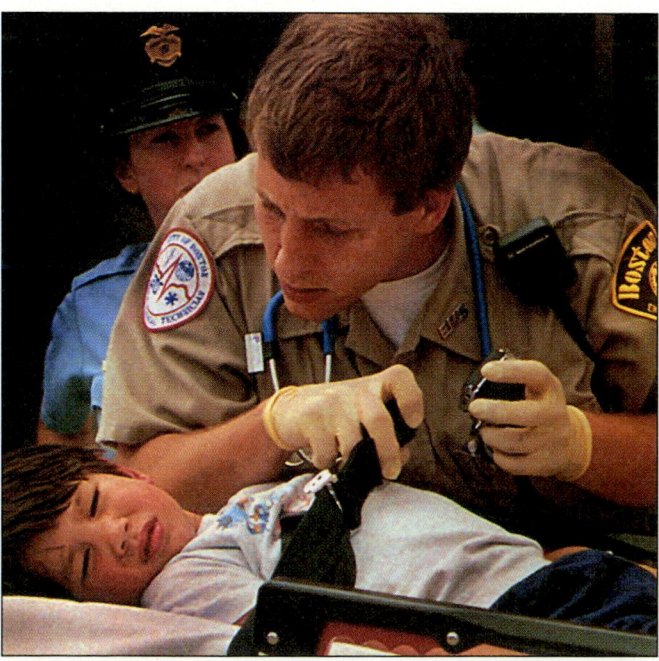

FIGURE 3-8 Care for all patients with a sense of excellence so that it becomes a guiding moral principle in the EMS work that you do.

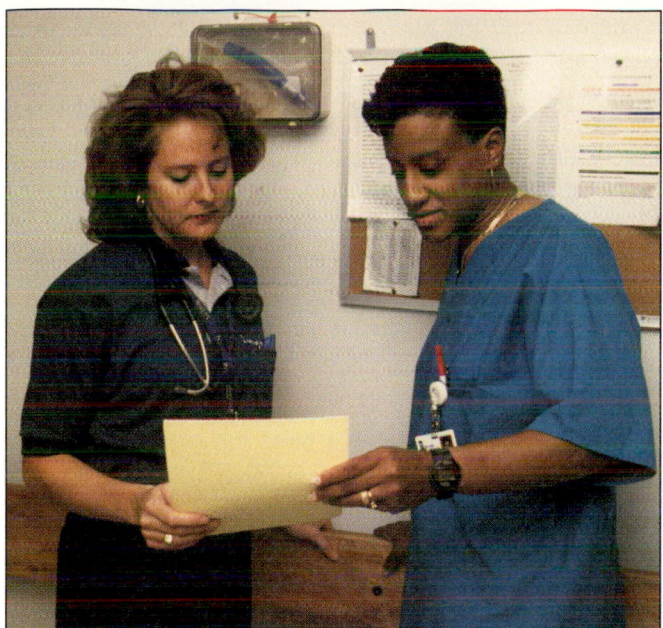

FIGURE 3-9 Provide a complete account of the event, along with details of patient care and professional duties.

Another ethical responsibility is honest reporting. Absolute honesty in reporting is essential. You must provide a complete account of the events and the details of all patient care and professional duties. Accurate records are also important for quality improvement activities (Figure 3-9).

Confidentiality

Communication between you and the patient is considered confidential and generally cannot be disclosed without permission from the patient or a court order. Confidential information includes the patient history, assessment findings, and treatment provided. You cannot disclose information regarding a patient's diagnosis, treatment, or mental or physical condition without consent; if you do, you may find yourself liable for breach of confidentiality.

In certain situations, you may release confidential information to designated individuals. In most states, records may be released when a legal subpoena is presented or the patient signs a written release. The patient must be mentally competent and fully understand the nature of the release.

Another means for disclosing information is with an automatic release, which does not require a written form. This type of release allows you to share information with other health care providers so that they may continue the patient's care.

In many states, you do not need a written release to report information about cases of rape or abuse to proper authorities. Third-party payment billing forms may also be completed without written consent.

Records and Reports

Society, through its government, has formulated a policy to protect individuals with health regulations and statutes. Because certain individuals are in a position to observe and gather information about diseases, injuries, and emergency events, an obligation to compile such information and report it to certain agencies may be imposed. Even if there is no such requirement, you should compile a complete and accurate record of all incidents in which you come into contact with sick or injured patients. Most medical and legal experts believe that a complete and accurate record of an emergency medical incident is an important safeguard against legal complications. The absence of a record or a substantially incomplete record may mean that you have to testify about the events, your findings, and your actions relying on memory alone, which can prove to be wholly inadequate and embarrassing in the face of aggressive cross-examination.

The courts consider the following two rules of thumb regarding reports and records:

- **If an action or procedure** is not recorded on the written report, it was not performed.
- **An incomplete or untidy report** is evidence of incomplete or inexpert emergency medical care.

You can avoid both of these potentially dangerous presumptions by compiling and maintaining accurate reports and records of all events and patients.

Special Reporting Requirements

Abuse of Children, the Elderly, and Others

All states and the District of Columbia have enacted laws to protect abused children, and some have added other protected groups such as the elderly and "at-risk" adults. Most states have a reporting obligation for certain individuals, ranging from physicians to any person. You must be aware of the requirements of law in your state. Such statutes frequently grant immunity from liability for libel, slander, or defamation of character to the individual who is obligated to report, even if the reports are subsequently shown to be unfounded, as long as the reports are made in good faith.

Injury During the Commission of a Felony

Many states have laws requiring the reporting of any injury that is likely to have occurred during the commission of a crime, such as gunshot wounds, knife wounds, or poisonings. Again, you must be familiar with the legal requirements of your state.

Drug-Related Injuries

In some instances, drug-related injuries must be reported. These requirements may affect the EMT-B. However, it should be stressed that the U.S. Supreme Court has held that drug addiction, in contrast to drug possession or sale, is an illness and not a crime. Hence, an injury as a result of a drug overdose may not be within the definition of an injury resulting from a crime.

Some states, by statute, specifically establish confidentiality and excuse certain specified individuals from reporting drug cases, either to a government agency or to a minor's parents, if, in the opinion of those individuals, withholding reporting is necessary for the proper treatment of the patient. Once again, you must be familiar with the legal requirements of your state.

Childbirth

Many states require that anyone who attends at a live birth in any place other than a licensed medical facility report the birth. As before, you must be familiar with state requirements.

Other Reporting Requirements

Other reporting requirements may include attempted suicides, dog bites, certain communicable diseases, assaults, and rapes.

Most EMS agencies require that all exposures to infectious diseases be reported. You may be asked to transport certain patients in restraints, which must also be reported. Each of these situations can present significant legal problems. You should learn your local protocols regarding these situations.

Scene of a Crime

If there is evidence at an emergency scene that a crime may have been committed, you must notify the dispatcher immediately so that law enforcement authorities can be informed. Such circumstances should not stop you from providing necessary emergency medical care to the patient; however, your safety is a priority, so you must ensure that the scene is safe to enter. At times, you may have to transport the patient to the hospital before the authorities arrive. While emergency medical care is being provided, you must be careful not to disturb the scene of the crime any more than absolutely necessary. Notes and drawings should be made of the position of the patient and of the presence and position of any weapon or other objects that may be valuable to the investigating officers. If possible, do not cut through holes in clothing from weapon or gunshot wounds. You should confer periodically with local authorities and be aware of their wishes as to any actions you should take at the scene of the crime. It is best if these guidelines can be established by protocol.

The Deceased

In most states, EMTs do not have the authority to pronounce a patient dead. If there is any chance that life exists or that the patient can be resuscitated, you must make every effort to save the patient at the scene and during transport. However, at times death is obvious, such as in the following circumstances:

- Rigor mortis (stiffening of the body) has set in.
- Mortal injury, such as decapitation, consumption of the body by fire, or a massive head injury with parts missing, has occurred.
- Dependent lividity (discoloration of the body as a result of pooling of the blood) is present (Figure 3-10).
- The body is decomposed.

In such instances, there is no urgent reason to move the body. The only immediate action that is required of you is to cover the body and prevent its disturbance. Local rules and protocols from the medical examiner or coroner will determine your ultimate action in these instances.

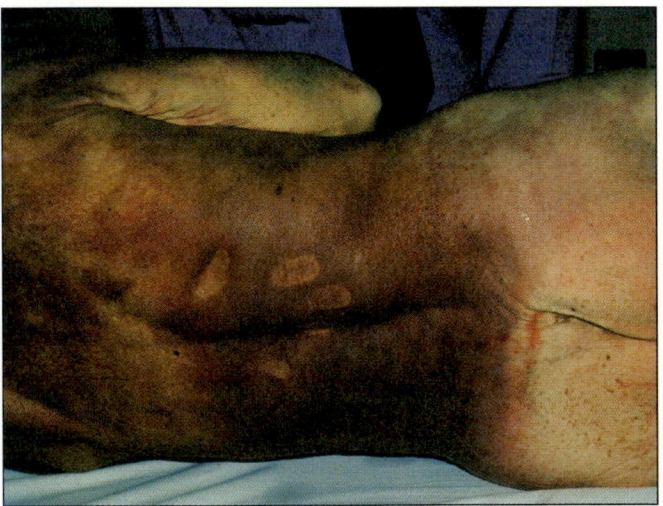

FIGURE 3-10 Dependent lividity is an obvious sign of death caused by discoloration of the body from pooling of the blood to the lower parts of the body.

Special Situations

Organ Donors

You may be called to a scene involving a potential organ donor. An individual who has expressed a wish to donate organs is a potential organ donor. Consent to organ donation must be voluntary and knowing. Consent is evidenced by either a donor card or a driver's license indicating that the individual wishes to be a donor (Figure 3-11). You must inform medical control immediately if you are faced with this situation.

You should treat a potential organ donor in the same way that you would any other patient needing treatment. The fact that a patient is a possible donor does not mean that you should not use all means necessary to keep that patient alive. Organs that are often donated, such as a kidney, heart, or liver, need oxygen at all times; you must give the possible donor oxygen, or the organs will be damaged and become useless.

Remember that your priority is to save the patient's life. If it seems that saving the patient's life is not possible, you must still provide the necessary care to make sure that the organs remain viable. This generally means providing adequate ventilation until you arrive at the hospital.

You may encounter potential organ donor situations at a multiple-casualty incident. The potential organ donor should be triaged with other patients and assigned a cat-

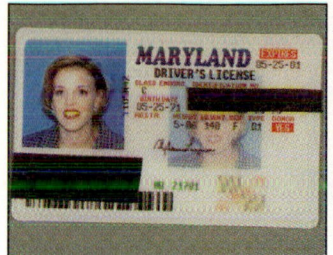 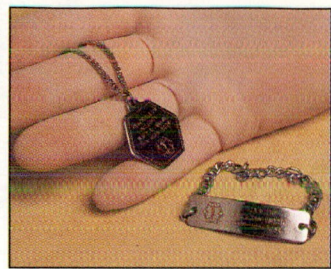

FIGURE 3-11 The patient may be carrying a donor card or driver's license indicating that he or she may wish to be an organ donor.

FIGURE 3-12 The patient may be carrying a medical identification card or wearing a bracelet or necklace that may indicate a serious medical condition.

egory; the potential organ donor may have to have a lower priority than other less severely injured patients.

Be sure to learn what the specific protocols are in your area regarding these situations.

Medical Identification Insignia

Many patients will carry important medical identification and information, often in the form of a bracelet, necklace, or card that will identify whether the patient has allergies, diabetes, epilepsy or some other serious condition (Figure 3-12). This information is helpful to you and can change the way you treat the patient. If you fail to take this information into account, you may harm the patient.

prep kit

ready for review

A basic principle of emergency care is to do no harm to the patient. As the scope of emergency medical care becomes more complex and widely available, litigation involving participants in emergency medical services will increase.

The scope of practice outlines the care you are able to provide to the patient and is most commonly defined by law; the medical director further defines the scope of practice. The standard of care is the manner in which you must act or behave when treating sick or injured patients. Some standards are imposed by local custom, some by the law, and some by institutions such as the American Heart Association.

A duty to act is the responsibility of an individual to provide patient care. If you are off duty or out of your jurisdiction, you may not have a legal duty to act; however, you do have a moral and ethical duty to act because of your training and expertise.

Negligence is the failure to provide the same care that a person of similar training would provide. Determination of negligence is based on the presence of four elements: duty, breach of duty, damages, and cause.

Abandonment is the termination of care without the patient's consent and without making provisions for the transfer of care to a medical professional with skills at the same or a higher level than yours. Abandonment is legally and ethically a very serious act.

You must receive consent from a patient before beginning care. A conscious adult patient who can make a rational decision will be able to give you expressed consent. Expressed consent must also be informed consent. When a patient is unconscious and unable to give consent, the law assumes implied consent. You should try to obtain consent from a parent or guardian of a minor whenever possible. You should never withhold lifesaving care.

(Continued)

prep kit

ready for review—cont'd.

Assault is defined as unlawfully placing a person in fear of immediate harm without the person's consent. Battery is unlawfully touching a person; this includes providing emergency care without the patient's consent. To protect yourself from these charges, be sure to obtain expressed consent whenever possible.

Mentally competent patients have the right to refuse treatment. In these instances, be sure to have the patient sign a refusal form, and make sure your department keeps a copy of the documentation for future reference.

Many states have adopted Good Samaritan laws and other laws that provide immunity to EMS personnel, provided that injury to the patient was not the result of gross negligence or willful conduct on the part of the EMT-B.

An advance directive is a written document that specifies medical treatment in case a mentally competent patient becomes unable to make decisions. DNR orders give you permission to not attempt resuscitation in the event of cardiac arrest. Your ambulance service, in consultation with the medical director and legal counsel, should have in place protocols to follow when you are faced with an advance directive or DNR orders.

Communication between you and the patient is confidential and should not be disclosed without permission from the patient or a court order.

Records and reports are an important part of the emergency care process. Make sure that you compile a complete and accurate record of each incident in which you come into contact with sick or injured patients. You may need to testify some day and will need the written information to effectively relate what happened. The courts consider an action or procedure that was not recorded on the written report as not having been performed, and an incomplete or untidy report is considered evidence of incomplete or inexpert medical care.

You should know what the special reporting requirements are involving abuse of children, the elderly, and others; injuries related to crimes; drug-related injuries; and childbirth. You should also know what to do when you are at the scene of a crime, when your patient is obviously dead, or when you are called to the scene and a potential organ donor is injured. Be sure to note whether patients are carrying some type of medical identification information. If you fail to take this information into account, you may cause harm to the patient.

prep kit

3

vital vocabulary

www.emtb.com

abandonment Unilateral termination of care by the EMT-B without the patient's consent and without making provision for transferring care to another medical professional with skills at the same level or higher.

advance directive Written documentation that specifies medical treatment for a competent patient should the patient become unable to make decisions; also called a living will.

assault Unlawfully placing a patient in fear of bodily harm.

battery Touching a patient or providing emergency care without consent.

certification A process in which a person, an institution, or a program is evaluated and recognized as meeting certain predetermined standards to provide safe and ethical care.

competent Able to make rational decisions about personal well-being.

consent Granting permission to another to render care.

DNR orders Written documentation giving permission to medical personnel not to attempt resuscitation in the event of cardiac arrest.

duty to act A medicolegal term relating to certain personnel who either by statute or by function have a responsibility to provide care.

emergency A serious situation, such as injury or illness, that threatens the life or welfare of a person or group of people and requires immediate intervention.

emergency medical care Immediate care or treatment; the EMT-B is often the first link in the chain of prehospital care.

expressed consent A type of consent in which a patient gives express authorization for provision of care or transport.

forcible restraint The process of confining an individual from being able to take any mental or physical action.

Good Samaritan laws Statutory provisions enacted by many states to protect citizens from civil and criminal liability for errors and omissions in giving good faith emergency medical care, unless there is wanton, gross, or willful negligence.

implied consent Type of consent in which a patient who is unable to give consent is given treatment under the legal assumption that he or she would want treatment.

informed consent Permission for treatment given by a competent patient after the potential risks, benefits, and alternatives to treatment have been explained.

medicolegal A term relating to medical jurisprudence (law) or forensic medicine.

negligence Failure to provide the same care that a person with similar training would provide. Also defined as a deviation from accepted standards of care.

standard of care Written, accepted levels of emergency care expected by reason of training and profession; written by legal or professional organizations so that patients are not exposed to unreasonable risk or harm.

assessment in action

No sooner does dispatch clear you for dinner when it comes back on the air to send you to a "woman down" out at a farm in the county. About 10 minutes later, you pull up in front of a small farmhouse. A couple of pushes on the doorbell followed by several hard knocks on the door produce no response. You try again, but you still get no reply, so you decide to find out whether the door is open. It is, so you tentatively enter and shout, "Is anybody home?" You see an elderly woman lying in the middle of the floor. Her bluish appearance immediately suggests cardiac arrest. Your partner is bending over to assess her level of consciousness and to open her airway when a huge, angry young man strides into the room and announces, "You touch my mom, and I'll kill you!"

1. If you were to choose to ignore the son's threat of harm, under what type of consent could you treat the patient and attempt resuscitation?
   A. Undue
   B. Informed
   C. Referred
   D. Implied

2. What term is used to describe the document in which a patient has declared his or her decision to refuse resuscitative efforts?
   A. Plea bargain
   B. Cardiac sign-off
   C. Advance directive
   D. EMS declaration

3. Suppose that this patient had been conscious, alert, and oriented and had refused care. If you ignored her wishes and treated her anyway, you could be charged with:
   A. battery.
   B. slander.
   C. ignorance.
   D. restitution.

4. Suppose this patient had only been asleep and, upon awakening, was alert and oriented to person, place, and time. Once awakened, she stated that she did not wish to go to the hospital. The most appropriate course of action would be to:
   A. ask her sign a patient refusal form and then leave.
   B. threaten legal action against her if she chooses not to go.
   C. secure her to the gurney and then transport her to the hospital.
   D. call law enforcement so that they could place her under arrest.

5. Which of the following statements regarding duty to act is true?
   A. All certified EMT-Bs are bound by a duty to act 24 hours a day, 7 days a week.
   B. Some form of contractual or legal obligation to act must exist.
   C. Only EMT-Bs who work for full-time services have a duty to act.
   D. Duty to act is a personal choice, so EMT-Bs can treat whom they wish.

prep kit 3

points to ponder

You and your partner are greeted at the door of a house by a middle-aged woman and are directed into a bedroom where an elderly woman lies, unresponsive, in the bed. Her pulse is very weak and irregular, and her breathing is coming in gasps. While you are assessing her, you hear her husband telling your partner that she is in the terminal stage of cancer and he does not want any resuscitation efforts made. He has handed your partner some papers that he says are "Do Not Resuscitate Orders." The woman who let you in immediately interrupts, saying that she is the daughter and that the children want their mother to have "every possible chance to live" and so you must treat her as needed.

- Explain how you would handle this situation. If the two sides cannot agree quickly, whose wishes would you follow?

online outlook

When you arrive at the scene of a terminally ill patient, you may find that family members present do not want you to try to resuscitate the patient. This places you in a very difficult situation. Learn more about this by completing Exercise 3 at www.emtb.com.

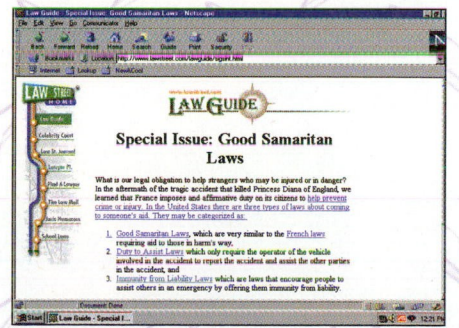

The Human Body

objectives

Cognitive

1. Identify and locate on the body the following topographic terms: medial, lateral, proximal, distal, superior, inferior, anterior, posterior, midline, right and left, midclavicular, bilateral, and midaxillary.

2. Describe the anatomy and function of the following major body systems: respiratory, circulatory, musculoskeletal, nervous, and endocrine.

Affective

None

Psychomotor

None

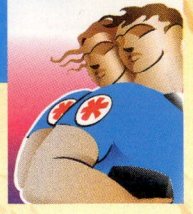

you are the emt

After stopping at headquarters to pick up some supplies, you and your partner look at the bulletin board for any new course listings. You see a notice for an anatomy and physiology course to be given next month in the cadaver laboratory. "A total waste of time," says your partner as he heads out to the unit. You think that he couldn't be more wrong.

This chapter introduces important material about the basic structure and design of the human body. It will also help you to answer the following questions:

1. Why is a working knowledge of anatomy and physiology important as they relate to the pathophysiology of illness and injury?

2. How does each body system work alone? How does each work with other body systems?

The Human Body

A working knowledge of human anatomy is important for you as an EMT-B. Even though you will not make diagnoses, you can help hospital personnel by communicating information using the correct medical terms. All EMT-Bs must be familiar with the language of topographic anatomy. By using the proper medical terms, you will be able to communicate correct information with the least possible confusion.

Using topographic anatomy is actually like using a road map. The terms that are introduced in this chapter will help you to identify the topographic (ie, on the surface) landmarks of the body. These landmarks are used as guides to locate the internal structures that lie under them. These terms also refer to the names of the major regions of the body and the way in which the locations of these regions are described in relation to one another.

Topographic Anatomy

The surface of the body has many definite visible features that serve as guides or landmarks to the structures that lie beneath them. You must be able to identify the superficial landmarks of the body—its **topographic anatomy**—to perform an accurate assessment. Understanding the terminology is also important so that you can describe patient findings correctly to your team, ALS personnel, and hospital personnel.

Learning the terms that are introduced in this chapter will make your job as an EMT-B easier, since you will be able to correctly identify structures as you complete and report your assessment findings. Hospital personnel will use these terms to ask you questions about a patient. Therefore, you must learn what these terms mean and how to use them.

The terms that are used to describe the topographic anatomy are applied to the body when it is in the **anatomic position**. This is a position of reference in which the patient stands facing you, arms at the side, with the palms of the hands forward.

The Planes of the Body

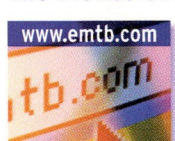
www.emtb.com

The anatomic planes of the body are imaginary straight lines that divide the body (Table 4-1). These planes help you to identify the location of internal structures and understand the relationships between and among the organs in the abdominal cavity.

TABLE 4-1	Anatomic Planes of the Body
Term	**Definition**
Anterior	Front
Posterior	Back
Midline	Line drawn through nose and umbilicus
Midclavicular	In the middle of the clavicle, parallel to the midline
Midaxillary	In the middle of the armpit, parallel to the midline

Anterior and posterior. <u>Anterior</u> refers to the front surface of the body, the side facing you. <u>Posterior</u> refers to the back surface of the patient, or the side away from you.

Midline. An imaginary vertical line drawn from the middle of the forehead through the nose and the umbilicus (navel) to the floor is called the <u>midline</u> of the body. This imaginary line divides the body into two halves that are mirror images. The nose, chin, umbilicus (navel), and spine are examples of midline structures.

Midclavicular line. The <u>midclavicular line</u> is an imaginary line drawn vertically through the middle portion of the clavicle and parallel to the midline. For example, the nipples of the breasts are in the midclavicular line on either side of the body.

Midaxillary line. The <u>midaxillary line</u> is an imaginary vertical line drawn through the middle of the axilla (armpit). This line is also in the middle of the anterior and posterior surfaces of the body.

Directional Terms

In this section, terms that indicate direction are introduced. These terms indicate distance and direction from the midline (Figure 4-1, Table 4-2).

Right and left. The terms "right" and "left" refer to the patient's right and left sides, not to your right and left sides.

Superior and inferior. The <u>superior</u> part of the body, or any body part, is the portion nearer to the head. The part nearer to the feet is the <u>inferior</u> portion. These terms are also used to describe the relationship of one structure to another. For example, the nose is superior to the mouth and inferior to the forehead.

Lateral and medial. Parts of the body that lie away from the midline are called <u>lateral</u> (outer) structures. The parts that lie toward the midline are called <u>medial</u> (inner) structures. For example, the knee has medial (inner) and lateral (outer) aspects.

Proximal and distal. The terms "proximal" and "distal" are used to describe the relationship of any two structures on an extremity. <u>Proximal</u> describes structures that are closer to the trunk. <u>Distal</u> describes structures that are farther from the trunk or nearer to the free end of the extremity. For example, the elbow is distal to the shoulder and proximal to the wrist and hand.

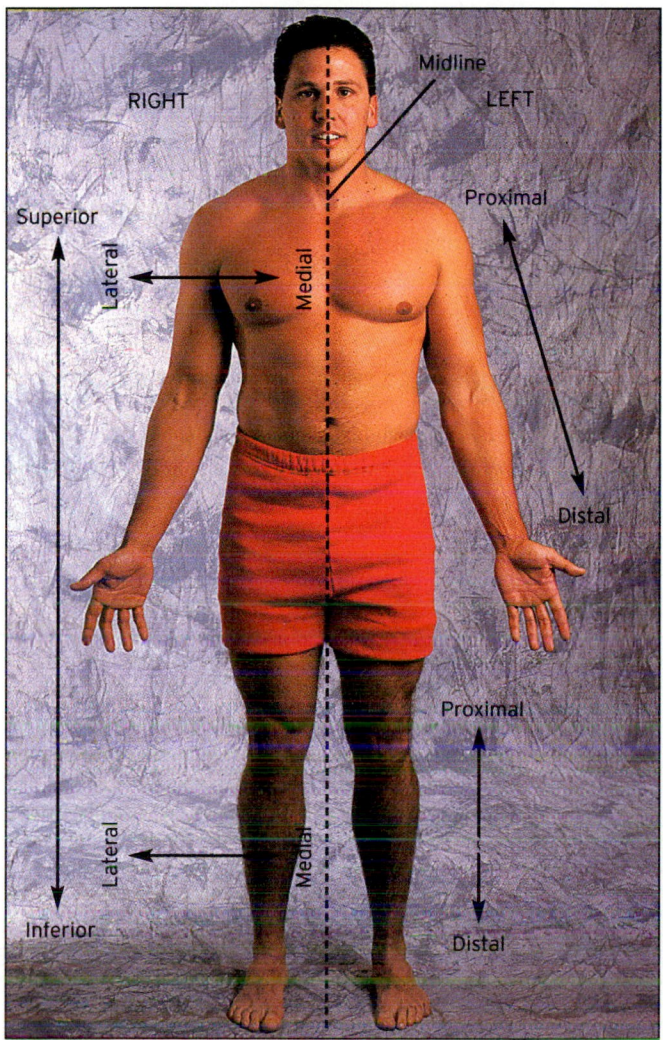

FIGURE 4-1 Directional terms indicate distance and direction from the midline.

TABLE 4-2	Directional Terms
Term	**Definition**
Right	The patient's right
Left	The patient's left
Lateral	Farther from midline
Medial	Closer to midline
Superior	Closer to the head, higher
Inferior	Farther from the head, lower
Proximal	Closer to the midline (in an extremity, closer to the trunk)
Distal	Farther from the midline (in an extremity, closer to the free end)
Dorsal	Toward the spine
Ventral	Toward the abdomen
Palmar	The front region of the hand
Plantar	The bottom of the foot

Superficial and deep. <u>Superficial</u> means closer to or on the skin. <u>Deep</u> means further inside the body and away from the skin.

Ventral and dorsal. <u>Ventral</u> refers to the anterior surface of the body. <u>Dorsal</u> refers to the posterior surface of the body, including the back of the hand.

Palmar and plantar. The front region of the hand is referred to as the palm or <u>palmar</u> surface. The bottom of the foot is referred to as the <u>plantar</u> surface.

Apex. The <u>apex (plural: apices)</u> is the tip or the topmost portion of a structure. For example, the tips of the shoulders are the apices of the shoulder. The most superior portions of the lungs are the apices of the lungs.

Other directional terms. Many structures of the body occur bilaterally. A <u>bilateral</u> structure is a body part that appears on both sides of the midline. For example the eyes, ears, hands, and feet are bilateral structures. This is also true for structures inside the body, such as the lungs and kidneys. Structures that appear on only one side of the body are said to occur unilaterally. For example, the spleen is on the left side of the body only, and the liver is on the right side.

As part of the assessment process, you will palpate the abdomen and report your findings. Therefore, it is important that you be able to describe the exact location of areas of the abdomen. The way to describe the sections of the abdominal cavity is by <u>quadrants</u>. Imagine two lines intersecting at the umbilicus dividing the abdomen into four equal areas (Figure 4-2). These are referred to as the right upper quadrant (RUQ), left upper quadrant (LUQ), right lower quadrant (RLQ), and left lower quadrant (LLQ). Remember that here, too, right and left refer to the patient's right and left, not yours.

It is important to learn all of these terms and concepts so that you can describe the location of any injury

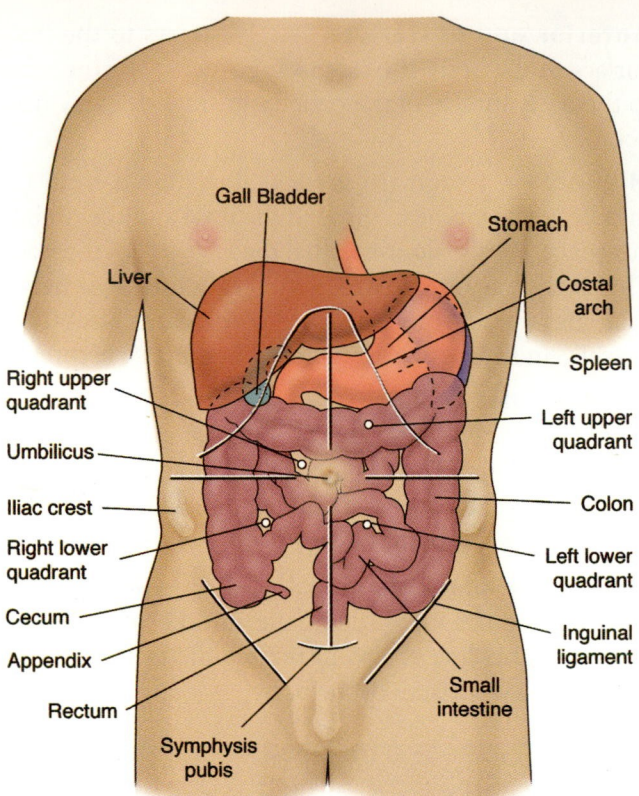

FIGURE 4-2 The abdomen is divided into four quadrants

or assessment findings. When you use these terms properly, any other medical personnel who care for the patient will know immediately where to look and what to expect.

Anatomic Positions

You will use these terms to describe the position of the patient as you find him or her or as you are to eventually transport the patient to the emergency department (Figure 4-3).

Prone and supine. These terms describe the position of the body. The body is in the <u>prone position</u> when lying face down; the body is in the <u>supine position</u> when lying face up.

Fowler's position. A patient who is sitting up with the knees bent is in <u>Fowler's position</u>.

Trendelenburg's position. In <u>Trendelenburg's position</u>, the body is supine with the head lower than the feet.

Shock position. In the <u>shock position</u>, or modified Trendelenburg's position, the head and torso (trunk) are supine, and the lower extremities are elevated 8" to 12". This helps to increase blood flow to the brain.

> The surface of the body has many definite visible features that serve as guides or landmarks to the structures that lie beneath them.

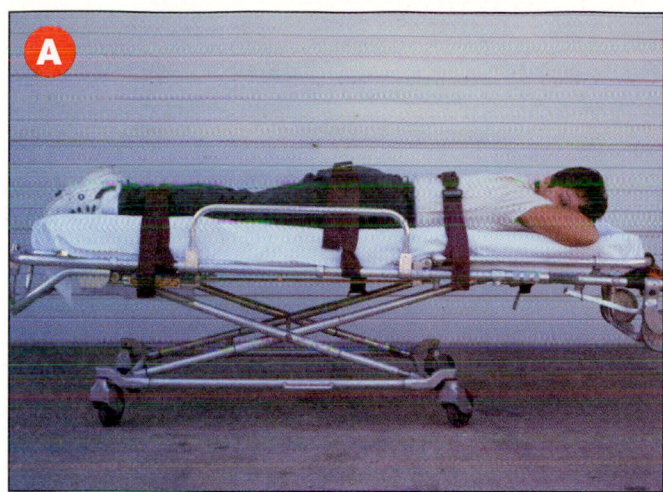

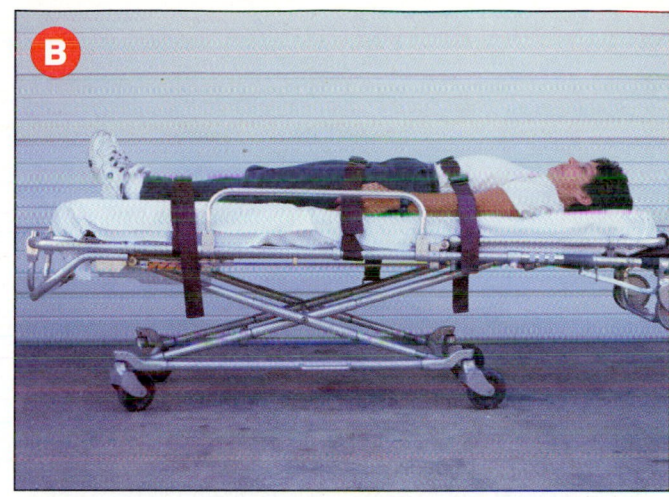

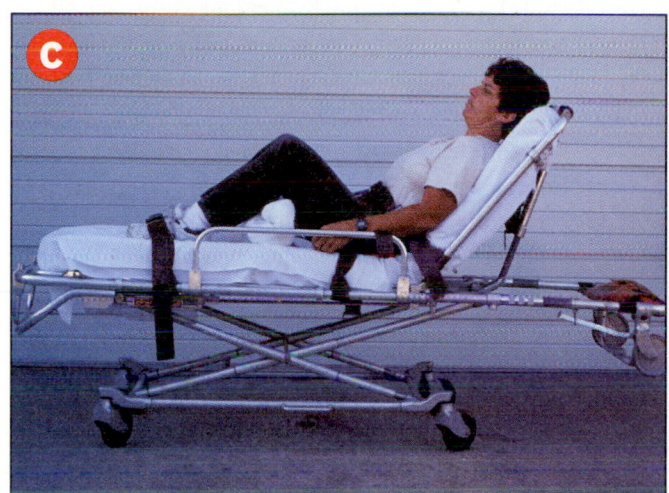

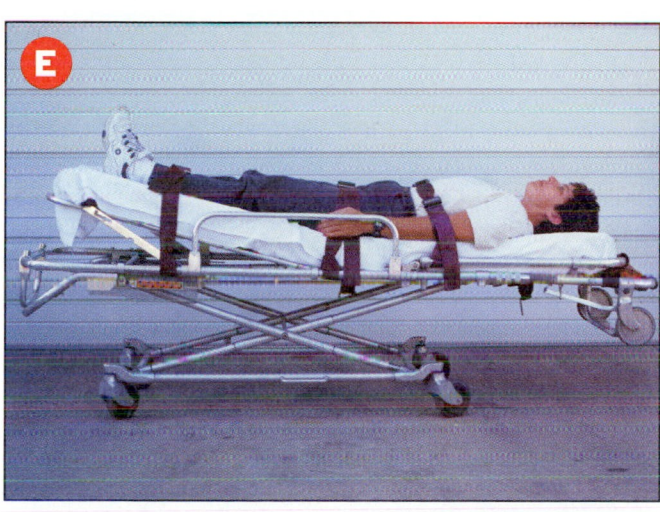

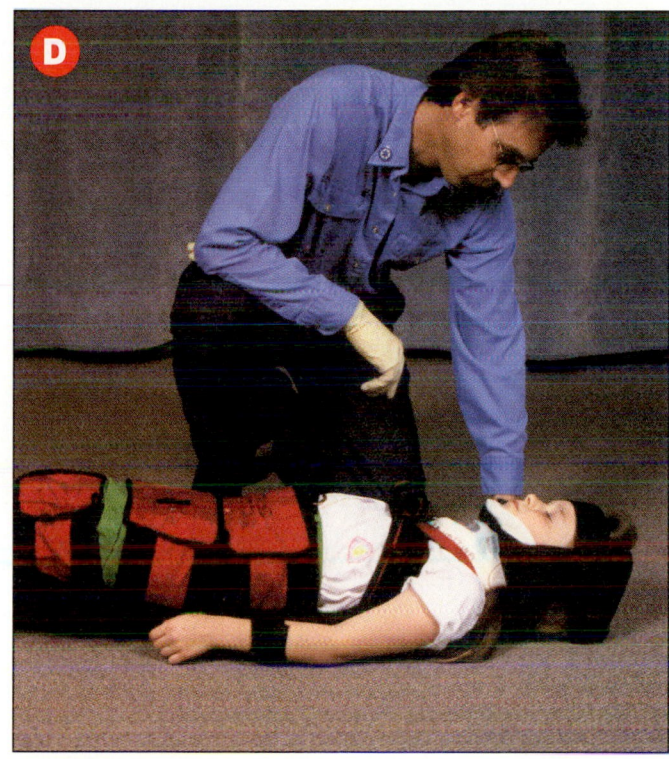

FIGURE 4-3
A: Prone.
B: Supine.
C: Fowler's position.
D: Trendelenburg's position.
E: Shock position (modified Trendelenburg's position).

The Skeletal System

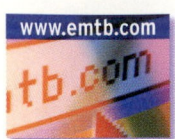

The skeleton gives us our recognizable human form and protects our vital internal organs (Figure 4-4). The brain lies within the skull. The heart, lungs, and great vessels are protected by the thorax, which is part of the torso. Much of the liver and spleen is protected by the lower ribs. The spinal cord is contained within and protected by a bony spinal canal formed by the vertebrae.

The 206 bones of the skeleton provide a framework for the attachment of muscles. The skeleton is also designed to allow motion of the body. Bones come into contact with one another at joints where, with the help of muscles, the body is able to bend and move.

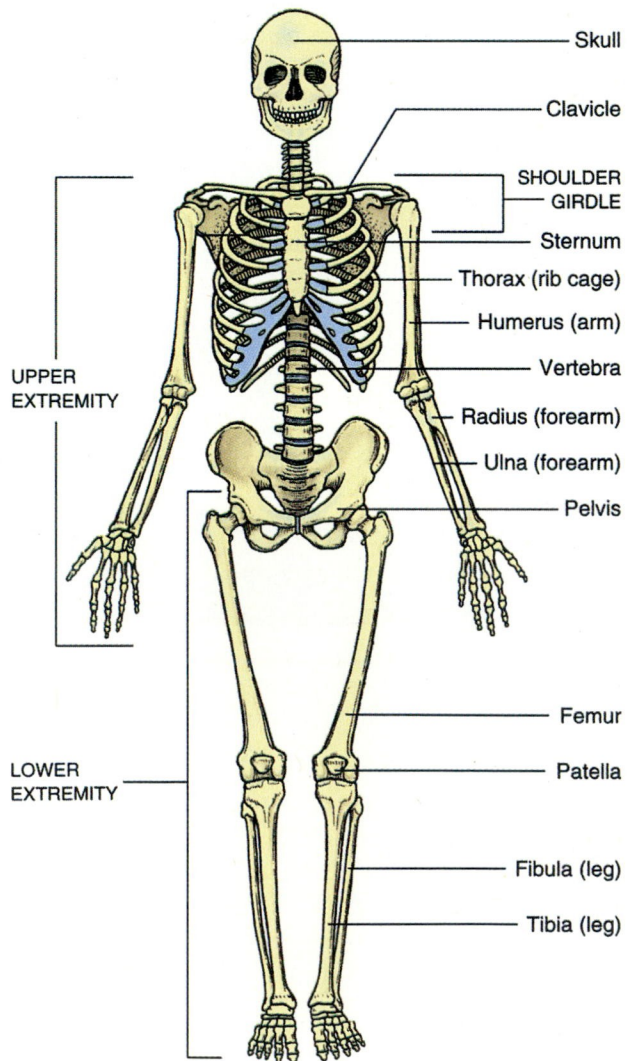

FIGURE 4-4 The 206 bones of the skeleton give us our form, protect our vital organs, and allow us to move.

The Skull

The skull has two major parts: the cranium and the face (Figure 4-5). The cranium is composed of a number of thick bones that fuse together to form a shell that holds and protects the brain. The brain connects to the spinal cord through a large opening at the base of the skull (the foramen magnum). The spinal cord is composed of virtually all the nerves that carry messages between the brain and the rest of the body.

The most posterior portion of the cranium is called the occiput. On each side of the cranium, the lateral portions are called the temples or temporal regions. Between the temporal regions and the occiput lie the parietal regions. The forehead is called the frontal region. Just anterior to the ear, in the temporal region, you can feel the pulse of the superficial temporal artery. The thick skin covering the cranium and usually bearing hair is called the scalp.

The face is composed of the eyes, ears, nose, mouth, and cheeks. Six bones—the nasal bone, the two maxillae (upper jawbones), the two zygomas (cheek bones), and the mandible (lower jawbone)—are the major bones of the face.

The orbit (eye socket) is made up of two facial bones: the maxilla and the zygoma. The orbit also includes the frontal bone of the cranium. Together, these bones form a solid bony rim that protrudes around the eye to protect it. If you look at the face from the side, you can see that the eyeball sits back within the orbit. The nasal bone is very short, because most of the nose is made of flexible cartilage. In fact, only the proximal one third of the nose, the bridge, is formed by bone. Unlike the nose, the exposed portion of the ear is made up entirely of cartilage that is covered by skin. The visible part of the ear is called the pinna. The earlobes are the fleshy parts at the bottom of each ear. About 1″ posterior to the external opening of the ear is a prominent bony mass at the base of the skull called the mastoid process.

The maxilla contains the upper teeth and forms the hard palate (roof of the mouth). The mandible is the only movable facial bone that has a joint (temporomandibular joint). This joint meets with the cranium just in front of each ear.

> The spinal cord is composed of virtually all the nerves that carry messages between the brain and the rest of the body.

FIGURE 4-5 The skull has two major parts: the cranium and the face.

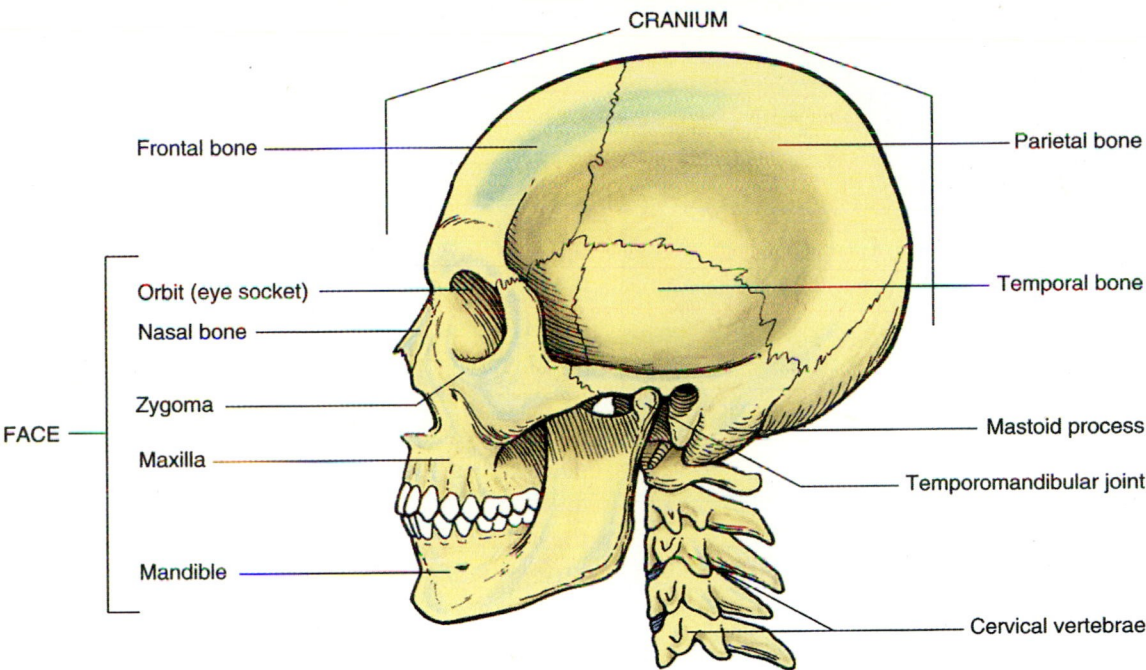

CRANIUM

Frontal bone

Parietal bone

Orbit (eye socket)

Temporal bone

Nasal bone

FACE

Zygoma

Mastoid process

Maxilla

Temporomandibular joint

Mandible

Cervical vertebrae

The Neck

The neck contains many important structures. It is supported by the cervical spine, or the first seven vertebrae in the spinal column (C1 through C7). The spinal cord exits from the foramen magnum and lies within the spinal canal formed by the vertebrae. The upper part of the esophagus and the <u>trachea</u> (windpipe) lie deep in the midline of the neck. The carotid arteries may be found on either side of the trachea, along with the jugular veins and several nerves.

Several useful landmarks can be palpated and seen in the neck (Figure 4-6). The most obvious is the firm prominence in the center of the anterior surface commonly known as the <u>Adam's apple</u>. Specifically, this prominence is the upper part of the larynx, the <u>thyroid cartilage</u>. It is more prominent in men than in women. The other portion of the larynx is the <u>cricoid cartilage</u>, a firm ridge of cartilage inferior to the thyroid cartilage, which is somewhat more difficult to palpate. Between the thyroid cartilage and the cricoid cartilage in the midline of the neck is a soft depression, the <u>cricothyroid membrane</u>. This is a thin sheet of connective tissue (<u>fascia</u>) that joins the two cartilages. The cricothyroid membrane is covered at this point only by skin.

Inferior to the larynx, several additional firm ridges are palpable in the anterior midline. These ridges are the cartilage rings of the trachea. The trachea connects the larynx with the main air passages of the lungs (the

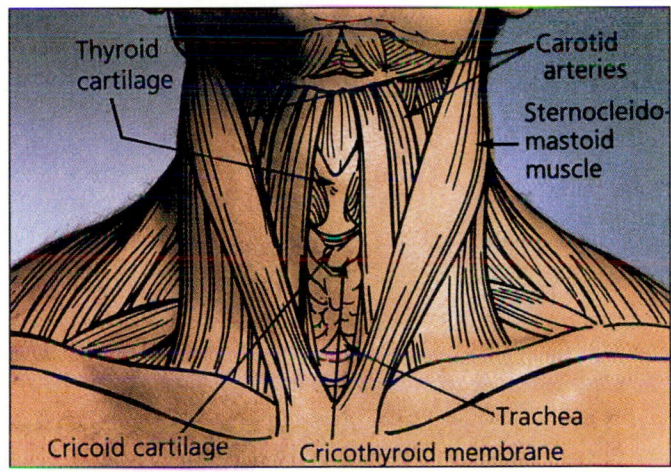

Thyroid cartilage

Carotid arteries

Sternocleido-mastoid muscle

Cricoid cartilage

Trachea

Cricothyroid membrane

FIGURE 4-6 The principal structures of the neck include the trachea, along with many blood vessels, muscles, and nerves.

bronchi). On either side of the lower larynx and the upper trachea lies the thyroid gland. Unless it is enlarged, this gland is usually not palpable.

Pulsations of the carotid arteries are easily palpable in a groove 0.4″ to 0.8″ lateral to the larynx. Lying immediately adjacent to these arteries, but not palpable, are the internal jugular veins and several important nerves. Lateral to these vessels and nerves lie the <u>sternocleido-mastoid muscles</u>. These muscles originate from the mastoid process of the cranium and insert into the medial border of each collarbone and the <u>sternum</u> (breastbone) at the base of the neck.

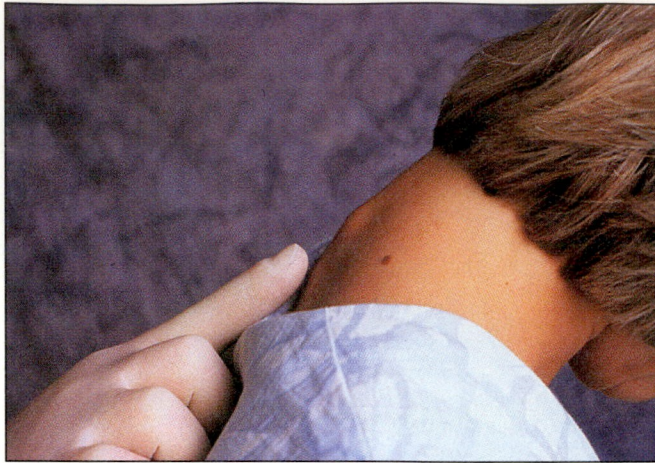

FIGURE 4-7 The most prominent of the cervical vertebrae is the spine of C7.

A series of bony prominences lie posteriorly, in the midline of the neck. They are the spines of the cervical vertebrae. The lower cervical spines are more prominent than the upper ones, and they are more easily palpable when the neck is flexed. At the base of the neck posteriorly, the most prominent spine is the seventh cervical vertebra (Figure 4-7).

The Spinal Column

The spinal column is the central supporting structure of the body and is composed of 33 bones, each called a vertebra. The vertebrae are named according to the section of the spine in which they lie and are numbered from top to bottom (Figure 4-8). From the top down, the spine is divided into five sections:

- **Cervical spine**. The first seven vertebrae (C1 through C7) form the cervical spine. The skull rests on the first cervical vertebra (the atlas) and articulates with it.

- **Thoracic spine**. The next 12 vertebrae make up the thoracic spine. One pair of ribs is attached to each of the thoracic vertebrae.

- **Lumbar spine**. The next five vertebrae form the lumbar or dorsal spine.

- **Sacrum**. The five sacral vertebrae are fused together to form one bone called the sacrum. The sacrum is joined to the iliac bones of the pelvis with strong ligaments at the sacroiliac joints to form the pelvis.

- **Coccyx**. The last three or four vertebrae form the coccyx or tailbone.

The **spinal cord** is an extension of the brain, composed of virtually all the nerves that carry messages between the brain and the rest of the body. It exits through a large hole in the base of the skull called the foramen magnum and is contained within and protected by the vertebrae of the spinal column. The spinal column is virtually surrounded by muscles. However, the posterior spinous process of each vertebra can be felt as it lies just under the skin in the midline of the back. The most prominent and most easily palpable spinous process is that of the seventh cervical vertebra at the base of the neck.

The anterior part of each vertebra consists of a round, solid block of bone called the body. The posterior part of each vertebra forms a bony arch. This series of arches from one vertebra to the next forms a tunnel that runs

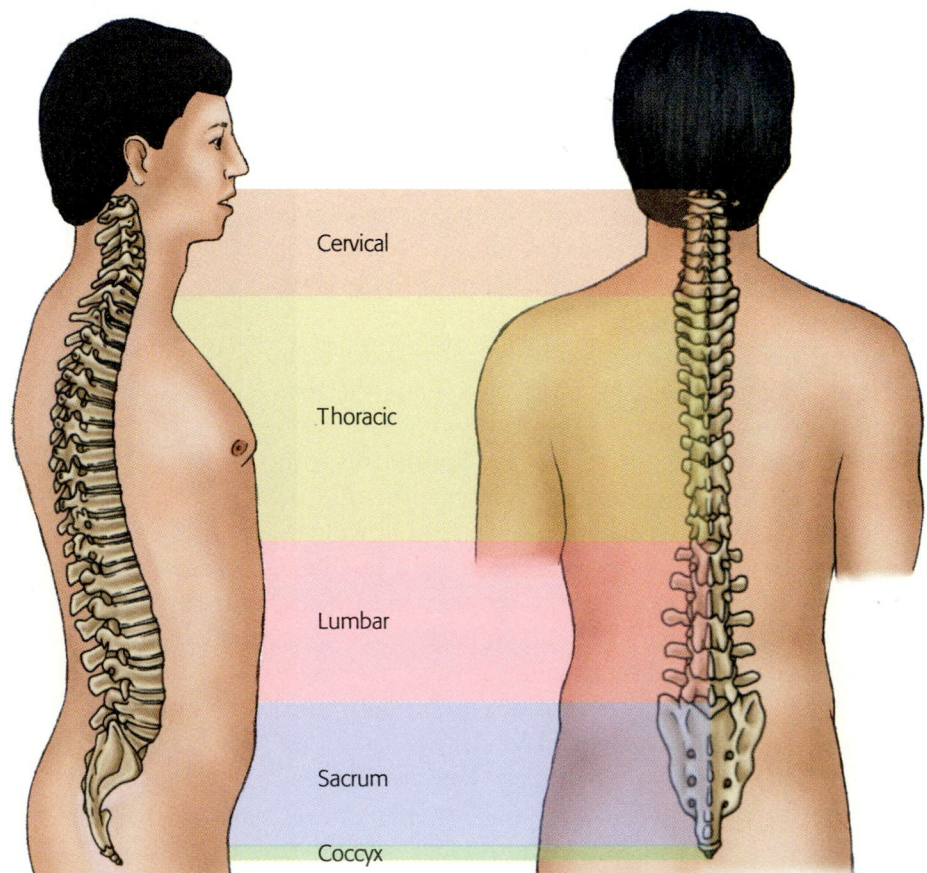

Cervical

Thoracic

Lumbar

Sacrum

Coccyx

FIGURE 4-8 The spinal column is composed of 33 bones divided into five sections.

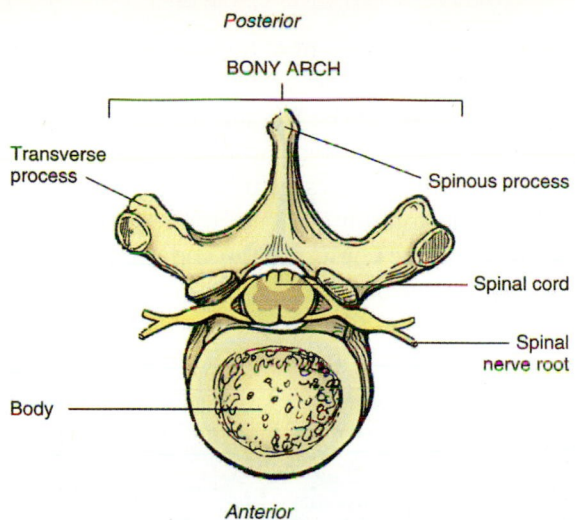

FIGURE 4-9 The bones of the spinal column encase and protect the spinal cord.

the length of the spine called the spinal canal. The bones of the spinal canal encase and protect the spinal cord (Figure 4-9). Nerves branch from the spinal cord and exit from the spinal canal between each two vertebrae to form the motor and sensory nerves of the body.

The vertebrae are connected by ligaments, and between each two vertebrae is a cushion called the intervertebral disk. These ligaments and disks allow some motion so that the trunk can bend forward and back.

However, they also limit motion of the vertebrae so that the spinal cord will not be injured. An injury to the spine may damage part of the spinal cord and its nerves that may not be protected by the vertebrae. Therefore, until the injury is stabilized, you must use extreme caution in caring for the patient to prevent injury to the spinal cord.

The Thorax

The thorax (chest) is the cavity that contains the heart, lungs, esophagus, and great vessels (the aorta and two venae cavae) (Figure 4-10). It is formed by the 12 thoracic vertebrae (T1 through T12) and their 12 pairs of ribs. The clavicle (collarbone) overlies its superior boundaries in front and articulates with the scapula (shoulder blade), which lies in the muscular tissue of the thoracic wall posteriorly. The inferior boundary of the thorax is the diaphragm, which separates the thorax from the abdomen.

Anterior aspects. The dimensions of the thorax are defined by the thoracic cage (bony rib cage) and its attachments. Anteriorly, in the midline of the chest is the sternum. The superior border of the sternum forms the easily palpable jugular notch. The sternum has three components: the manubrium, the body, and the xiphoid

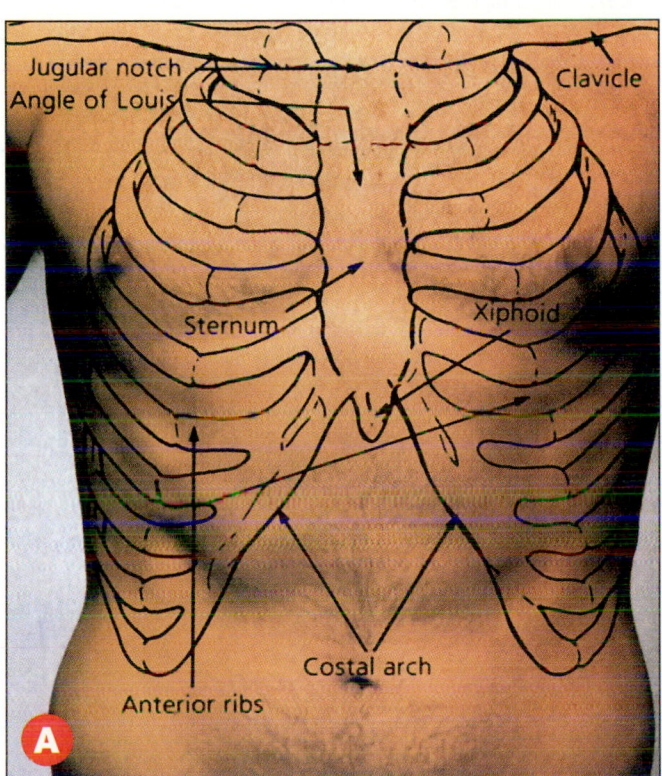

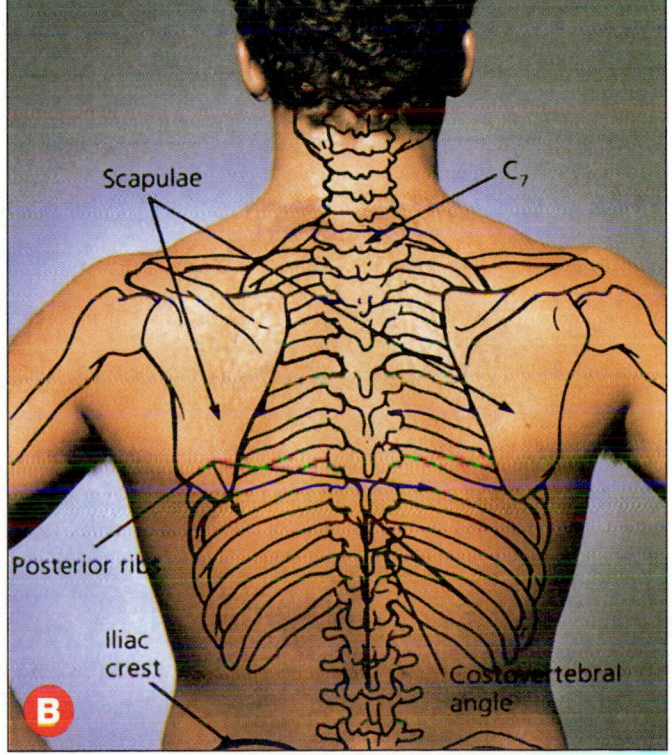

FIGURE 4-10 A: The anterior aspect of the thorax includes the following bony landmarks: the clavicle, the sternum, the xiphoid process, the angle of Louis, and the anterior ribs. **B:** The posterior aspect of the thorax includes the following bony landmarks: the scapulae, the thoracic vertebrae, and the posterior ribs.

process. The upper quarter of the sternum is called the **manubrium**. The body comprises the rest of the sternum except for a narrow, cartilaginous tip inferiorly, which is called the **xiphoid process**. The junction of the manubrium and the body forms a very prominent ridge on the sternum, called the angle of Louis. The **angle of Louis** lies at the level where the second rib is attached to the sternum; it provides a constant and reliable bony landmark on the anterior chest wall.

In the midline of the upper back, the spines of the 12 thoracic vertebrae can be palpated. Twelve ribs on each side form small joints with their respective thoracic vertebrae and extend around to the front to create the walls of the thoracic cage. The upper five ribs connect to the sternum through a short bridge of cartilage. The sixth through tenth ribs insert into the costal arch. The **costal arch** is a bridge of cartilage that connects the ends of the sixth through tenth ribs with the lower portion of the sternum. The eleventh and twelfth ribs are called **floating ribs**, because they do not attach to the sternum through the costal arch. The costal arch is easily palpable and represents the boundary between the lower border of the thorax and the upper border of the abdomen.

Posterior aspects. On the posterior chest wall, the scapulae overlie the thoracic wall and are surrounded by large muscles. When the patient is standing or sitting erect, the two scapulae should lie at approximately the same level, with their inferior tips at about the level of the seventh thoracic vertebra. In the lower part of the thorax on each side, an angle called the **costovertebral angle** is formed by the junction of the spine and the tenth rib. The kidneys lie deep to (beneath) the back muscles in the costovertebral angle.

Diaphragm. The **diaphragm** is a muscular dome that forms the inferior boundary of the thorax, separating the chest from the abdominal cavity (Figure 4-11). Anteriorly, it attaches to the costal arch; posteriorly, it attaches to the **lumbar vertebrae**. The diaphragm cannot be seen or palpated.

Organs and vascular structures. Within the thoracic cage, the largest structures are the heart and lungs (Figure 4-12). The heart lies immediately under the sternum. It extends from the second to the sixth ribs anteriorly and from the fifth to the eighth thoracic vertebrae posteriorly. The inferior border of the heart extends into the left side of the chest. Diseased hearts may be larger or smaller. The major blood vessels that travel to and from the heart also lie in the chest cavity. On the right side of the spinal column, the superior and inferior venae cavae carry blood to the heart.

Just beneath the manubrium of the sternum, the arch of the aorta and the pulmonary artery exit the heart. The arch of the aorta passes to the left and lies along the left side of the spinal column as it descends into the abdomen. The esophagus lies behind the great vessels and directly on the anterior aspect of the spinal column as it passes through the chest into the abdominal cavity.

All space within the chest that is not occupied by the heart, great vessels, and esophagus is occupied by the

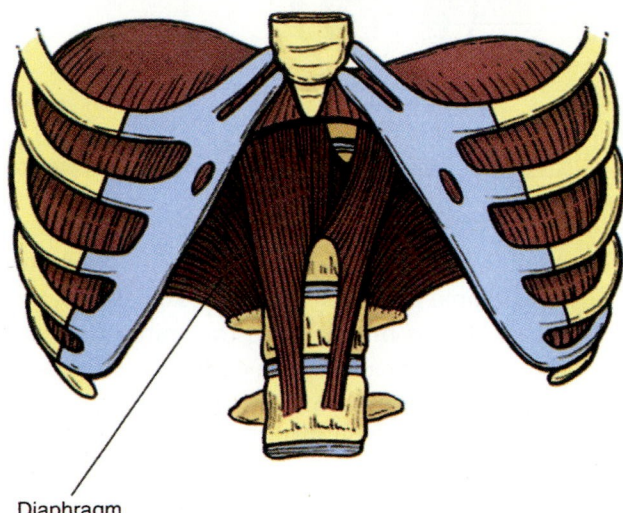

Diaphragm

FIGURE 4-11 The diaphragm forms the undersurface of the thorax, separating the chest from the abdominal cavity.

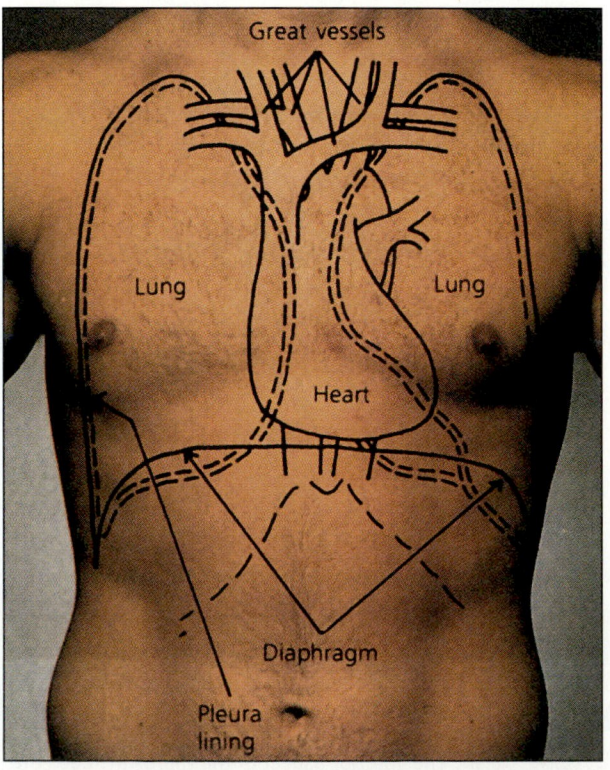

FIGURE 4-12 The anterior aspect of the thorax shows the relative positions of the principal organs beneath the surface.

lungs. Anteriorly, the lungs extend down to the surface of the diaphragm at the level of the xiphoid process. Posteriorly, the lungs extend farther inferiorly to the surface of the diaphragm at the level of the twelfth thoracic vertebra.

Anatomic landmarks. The major palpable landmarks in the chest are obviously the ribs. Most of them can be easily felt except for the first, which is hidden under and behind the clavicle. Both clavicles and the sternum can be easily palpated. The jugular notch is the top portion of the sternum. The angle of Louis is readily palpable in the upper portion of the sternum at the level of the space between the second and third ribs (the second intercostal space). Inferiorly, the costal arch is readily palpable on both sides of the anterior chest wall. In the midline, the tip of the xiphoid process is a tender and easily palpated landmark.

The Abdomen

The **abdomen** is the second major body cavity; it contains the major organs of digestion and excretion. The diaphragm separates the thorax from the abdomen. Anteriorly and posteriorly, thick muscular abdominal walls create the boundaries of this space. Inferiorly, the abdomen is separated from the pelvis by an imaginary plane that extends from the symphysis pubis through the sacrum (Figure 4-13). Many organs lie in both the abdomen and the pelvis, depending on the posture of the patient.

The simplest and most common method of describing the portions of the abdomen is by quadrants. In this system, the abdomen is divided into four equal parts by two imaginary lines that intersect at right angles at the umbilicus. On the anterior abdominal wall, the quadrants that are thus formed are right upper, right lower, left upper, and left lower (Figure 4-14). The terms "right quadrant" and "left quadrant" refer to the patient's right and left as you face them, not to your right and left sides. Pain or injury in a given quadrant usually arises from or involves the organs that lie in that quadrant. This simple means of designation will allow you to identify injured or diseased organs that require emergency attention.

Organs and vascular structures. In the right upper quadrant (RUQ), the major organs are the liver, the gallbladder, and a portion of the colon. Most of the liver lies in this quadrant, almost entirely under the protection of the eighth to twelfth ribs. The liver fills the entire anteroposterior depth of the abdomen in this quadrant. Therefore, injuries in this area are frequently associated with injuries of the liver.

In the left upper quadrant (LUQ), the principal organs are the stomach, the spleen, and a portion of the colon. The spleen is almost entirely under the protection of the left rib cage, whereas the stomach may sag well down into the left lower quadrant when full. The spleen lies in the lateral and posterior portion of this quadrant, under the diaphragm and immediately in

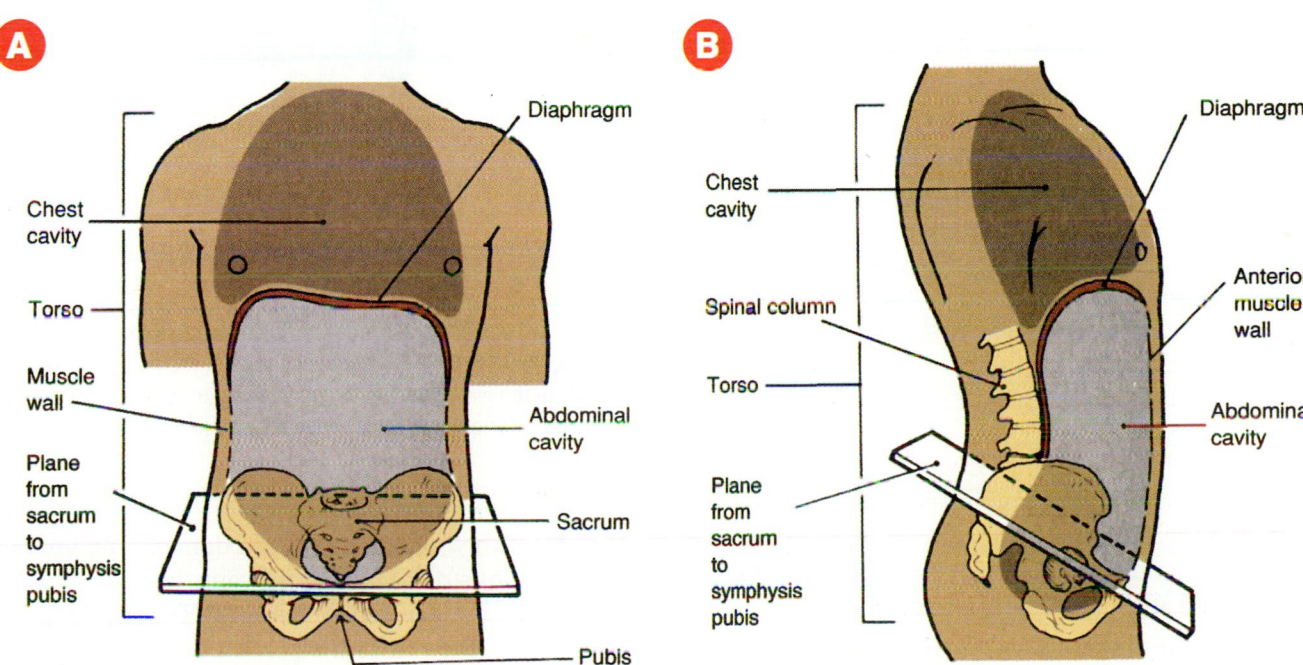

FIGURE 4-13 The boundaries of the abdomen are the anterior and posterior abdominal cavity walls, the diaphragm, and an imaginary plane from the symphysis pubis to the sacrum.

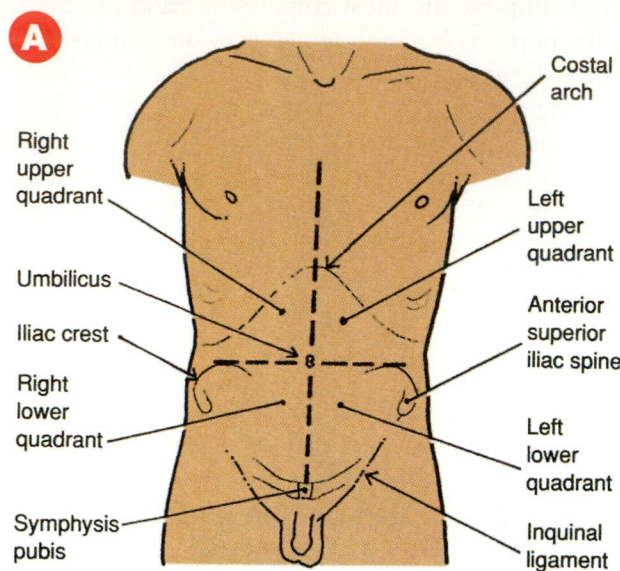

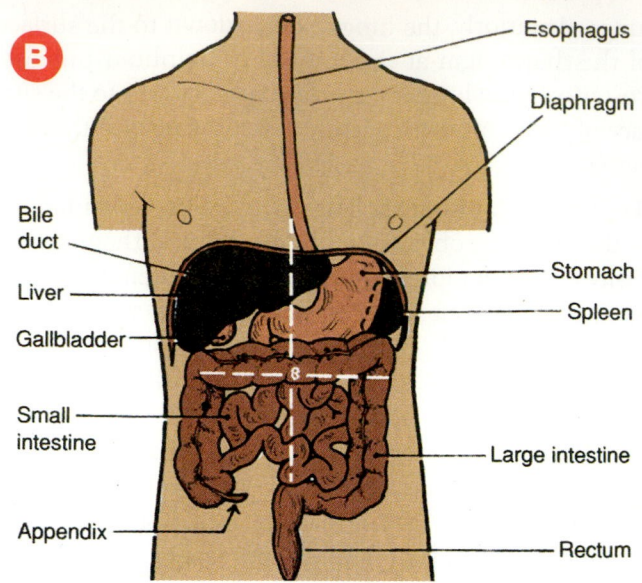

FIGURE 4-14 A: In the abdomen, quadrants are the easiest system for identifying areas. Major bony landmarks are also shown. **B:** Many of the organs in the abdomen lie in more than one quadrant.

front of the ninth to eleventh ribs. The spleen is frequently injured, especially when these ribs are fractured.

The right lower quadrant (RLQ) contains two portions of the large intestine: the <u>cecum</u> and the ascending colon. The <u>appendix</u> is a small tubular structure that is attached to the lower border of the cecum. Appendicitis is the most frequent cause of tenderness and pain in this region. In the left lower quadrant (LLQ) lie the descending and the sigmoid portions of the colon.

Several organs lie in more than one quadrant. The small intestine, for instance, occupies the central part of the abdomen around the umbilicus, and parts of it lie in all four quadrants. The pancreas lies just behind the abdominal cavity on the posterior abdominal wall in both upper quadrants. The large intestine also traverses the abdomen, beginning in the RLQ and ending in the LLQ as it passes through all four quadrants. The urinary bladder lies just behind the pubic symphysis in the middle of the abdomen and therefore lies in both lower quadrants and also in the pelvis.

The kidneys are called <u>retroperitoneal</u> organs because they lie behind the abdominal cavity (Figure 4-15). They are above the level of the umbilicus, extending from the eleventh rib to the third lumbar vertebra on each side. They are approximately 5″ long and lie just anterior to the costovertebral angle.

Anatomic landmarks. The chief landmarks in the abdomen are the costal arch, the umbilicus, the anterior superior iliac spines, the iliac crest, and the pubic symphysis. The costal arch, as was noted earlier, is the fused

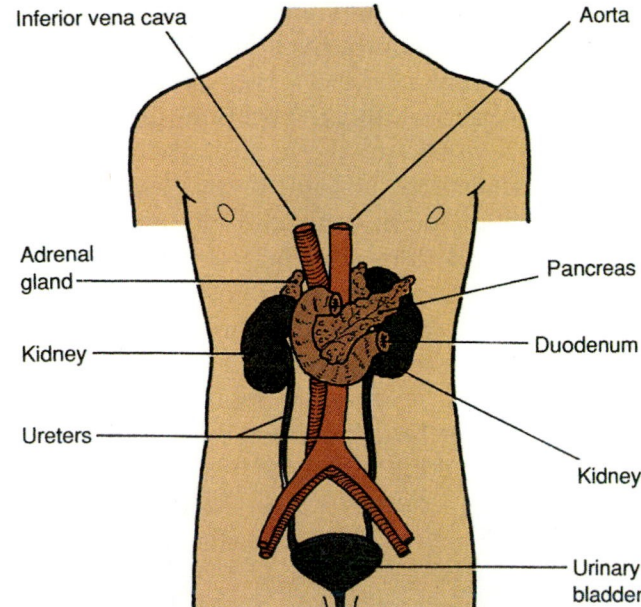

FIGURE 4-15 The major organs of the retroperitoneal space lie behind the abdominal cavity, above the level of the umbilicus, and extend from the eleventh rib to the third lumbar vertebra. Note that the bladder, inferior vena cava, and aorta also lie in this plane.

cartilages of the sixth through the tenth ribs. It forms the superior arching boundary of the abdomen. The umbilicus, a constant structure, is in the same horizontal plane as the fourth lumbar vertebra and the superior edge of the iliac crest, the rim of the pelvic bone. The <u>anterior superior iliac spines</u> are the hard bony prominences at the front on each side of the lower abdomen just below the plane of the umbilicus. In the midline in the lowermost portion of the abdomen is another hard bony prominence, the pubic symphysis. Between the lateral edge of the pubic symphysis and the anterior superior spine on each side you can palpate the tough **inguinal ligament**, which stretches between these two structures. Below the ligament lie the femoral vessels.

Posteriorly, you do not usually refer to abdominal quadrants. The posterior portion of the iliac crest can be palpated, as can the spines of the five lumbar vertebrae (Ll through L5) in the midline.

The Pelvis

The pelvis is a closed bony ring that consists of three bones: the sacrum and the two pelvic bones (Figure 4-16). Much like the skull, each pelvic bone is formed by the fusion of three separate bones. These three bones are called the **ilium**, the **ischium**, and the **pubis**. These bones meet at three joints: the two posterior sacroiliac joints and the anterior midline symphysis pubis. All three joints allow very little motion, as they are firmly held together by strong ligaments. On the lateral side of each pelvic bone—where the three component bones join—is the socket for the hip joint. This depression, in which the femoral head fits very snugly, is called the **acetabulum**

The pelvic cavity is bounded superiorly by an imaginary plane that runs from the symphysis pubis to the top of the sacrum. Its lateral walls are formed by the inner borders of the pelvic bone, and its inferior boundary is the pelvic outlet, a layer of muscles with openings for the gastrointestinal tract (the rectum), the female reproductive system (the vagina), and the urinary tract (the urethra). In addition, the pelvis contains the final portions of the gastrointestinal tract (the rectosigmoid colon), the female reproductive organs, and the urinary bladder.

Anterior aspects. The prominent anterior bony landmarks of the pelvis are the symphysis pubis in the midline and the anterior superior iliac spines. The inguinal ligament attaches to these two bony prominences and can be palpated in a thin person. Just distal to the midpoint of the inguinal ligament, the femoral artery can be palpated as it enters the thigh. From the anterior superior iliac spine, the ilium extends laterally and posteriorly to form the rim of the pelvis. This bony ridge is called the **iliac crest**, or wings of the pelvis.

Posterior aspects. Posteriorly, the pelvis appears flat, and in the middle third, the firm bony sacrum can be palpated. Just lateral to the sacrum on either side is a joint with the iliac portion of the pelvic bone (the sacroiliac joint). In the sitting position, a bony prominence is easily felt below the middle of each buttock. These prominences are the ischial tuberosities. The sciatic nerve, which is the major nerve to the lower extremity, lies just lateral to the tuberosity as it enters the thigh.

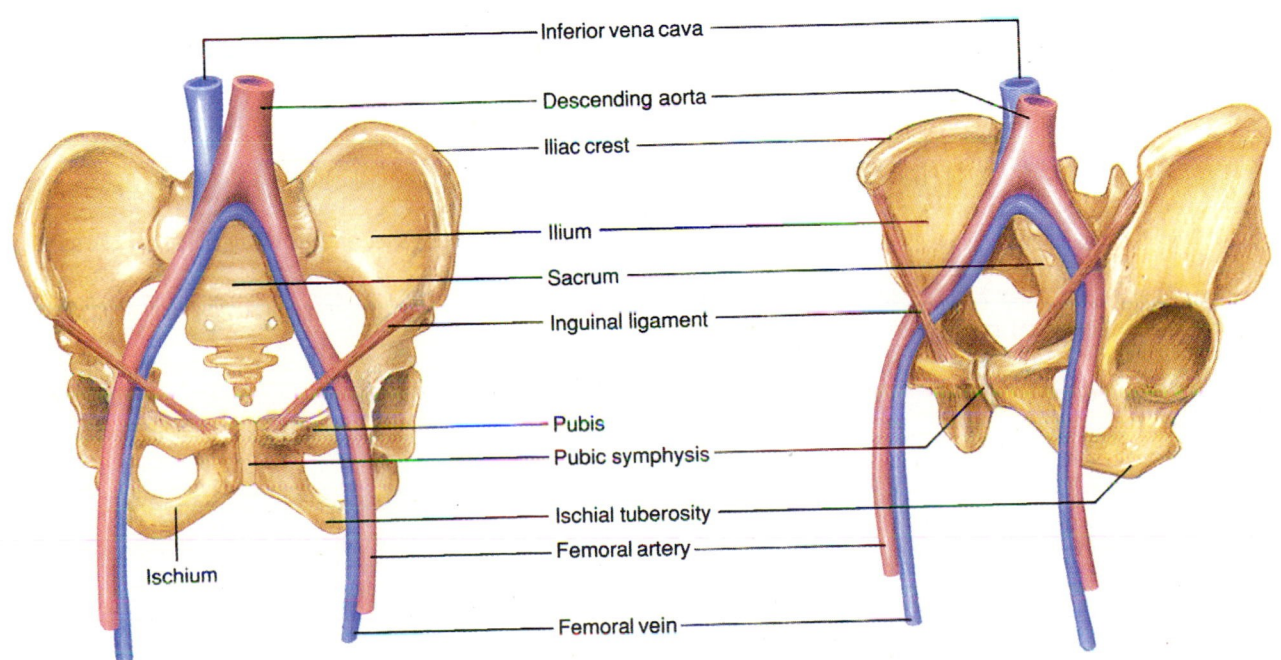

Inferior vena cava

Descending aorta

Iliac crest

Ilium

Sacrum

Inguinal ligament

Pubis

Pubic symphysis

Ischial tuberosity

Femoral artery

Ischium

Femoral vein

FIGURE 4-16 The pelvis is a closed bony ring that consists of the sacrum and two pelvic bones.

The Lower Extremity

The main parts of the lower extremity are the thigh, the leg, and the foot (Figure 4-17). Three joints connect the parts of the lower extremity: the hip, the knee, and the ankle. The joint between the thigh and pelvis is called the hip. The joint between the thigh and the leg is the knee. The joint between the leg and the foot is the ankle.

Thigh. On the proximal lateral side of the thigh, just below the hip joint, is a bony prominence called the greater trochanter. This prominence is sometimes called the "hip bone." During patient assessment, you should always compare the position of the greater trochanter with that on the opposite side as a guide to injury or deformity of the hip.

The femur (thigh bone) is the longest and one of the strongest bones in the body. The femoral head (at the top of the femur) forms the hip joint with the acetabulum of the pelvis. This ball-and-socket joint allows for flexion, extension, and motion toward (adduction) and away (abduction) from the midline. It also allows for internal and external rotation of the entire lower extremity. The shaft of the femur is surrounded by large muscles (the quadriceps in front and the hamstrings in back). Just above the knee, the medial and lateral femoral condyles can be palpated.

Knee. Between the thigh and the leg is the largest joint in the body: the knee. The knee is essentially a hinge joint, allowing only flexion and extension between the distal femur and the proximal tibia. Adduction, abduction, and rotation of the knee are resisted by complex ligaments that are quite susceptible to injury. Anterior to the knee is a specialized bone called the patella (kneecap). It lies within the tendon of the quadriceps muscle and protects the front of the knee from injury.

Leg. The leg lies between the knee and the ankle joint (Figure 4-18) and is composed of the tibia and the fibula. The tibia (shin bone) is the larger bone and lies in the front of the leg. You can palpate the entire length of the tibia on the anterior surface of the leg just under the skin. The fibula lies on the lateral side of the leg. You can palpate the head of the fibula on the lateral aspect of the knee joint. Its distal end forms the lateral malleolus of the ankle joint.

Ankle and foot. The ankle is a hinge joint that allows flexion and extension of the foot on the leg (Figure 4-19). The end of the tibia forms the medial malleolus, and the end of the fibula forms the lateral malleolus. These two bony prominences form the socket of the ankle joint. Both are surface landmarks of the ankle joint and are easily palpated. The foot contains seven tarsal bones.

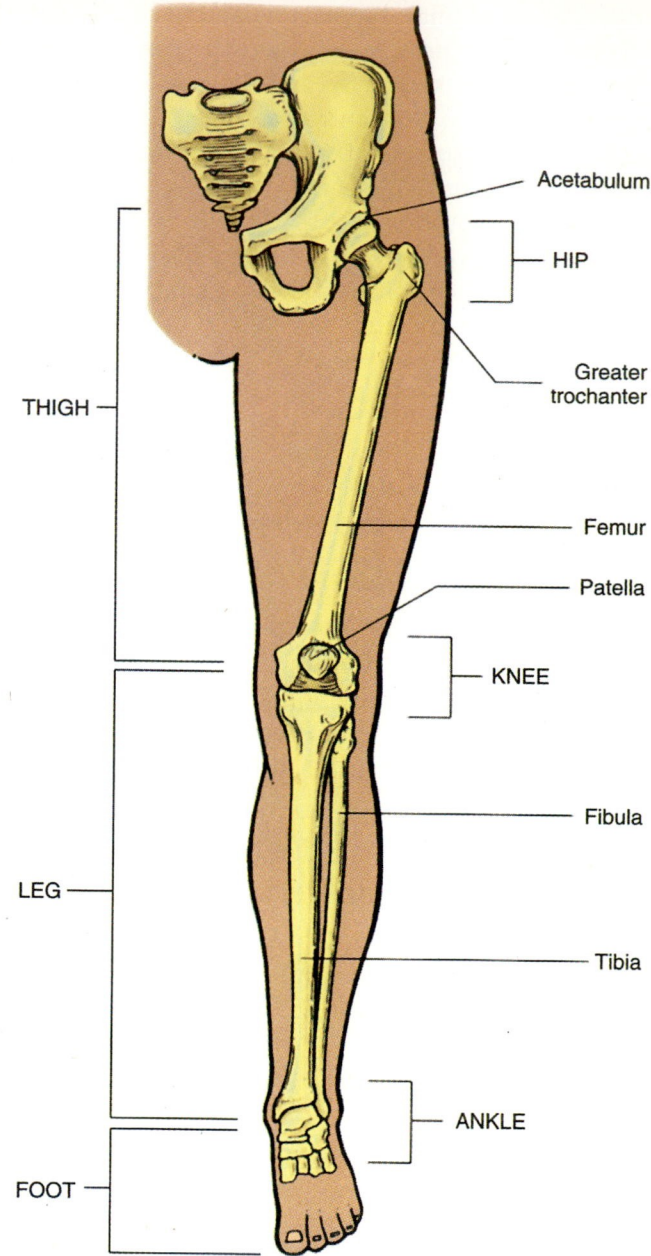

FIGURE 4-17 The principal parts of the lower extremity include the thigh, leg, and foot.

The talus is one of the largest; the calcaneus, which forms the prominence of the heel, is the other large tarsal bone. The Achilles tendon inserts into the back of the calcaneus. Five metatarsal bones form the substance of the foot. The five toes are formed by 14 phalanges—two in the great toe and three in each of the smaller toes.

The Upper Extremity

The upper extremity extends from the shoulder girdle to the fingertips and is composed of the arm, elbow, forearm, wrist, hand, and fingers. The arm extends from the shoulder to the elbow.

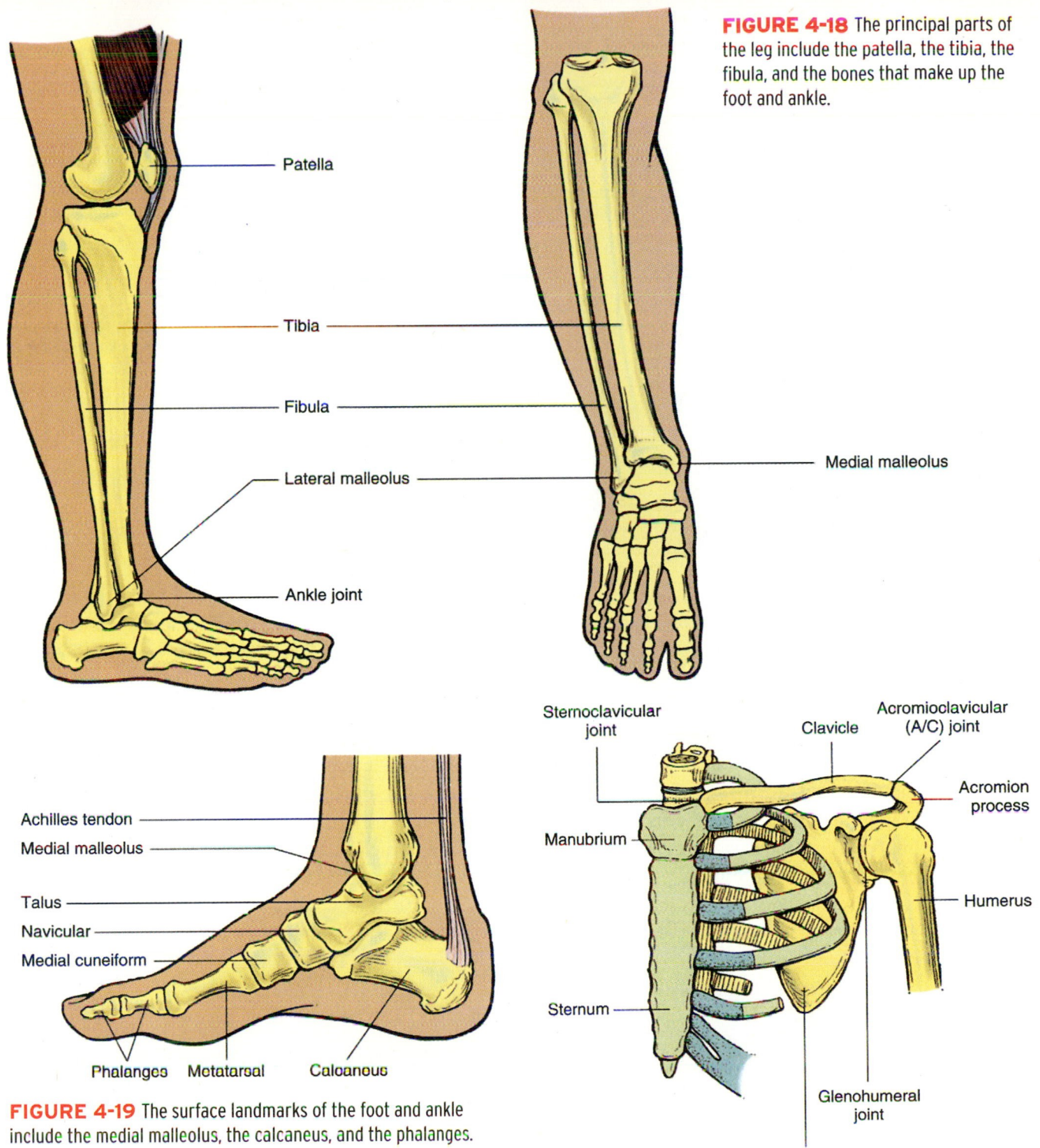

FIGURE 4-18 The principal parts of the leg include the patella, the tibia, the fibula, and the bones that make up the foot and ankle.

Patella

Tibia

Fibula

Lateral malleolus

Ankle joint

Medial malleolus

Achilles tendon

Medial malleolus

Talus

Navicular

Medial cuneiform

Phalanges   Metatarsal   Calcaneus

FIGURE 4-19 The surface landmarks of the foot and ankle include the medial malleolus, the calcaneus, and the phalanges.

Sternoclavicular joint

Acromioclavicular (A/C) joint

Clavicle

Acromion process

Manubrium

Humerus

Sternum

Glenohumeral joint

Scapula

FIGURE 4-20 The bones of the shoulder girdle include the clavicle, the scapula, and the humerus.

Shoulder girdle. The proximal portion of the upper extremity is called the <u>shoulder girdle</u> and consists of three bones: the clavicle, the scapula, and the humerus (Figure 4-20). The shoulder girdle is where the upper extremity attaches to the trunk. The upper extremity can move through a wide range of motion, allowing the hand to be placed in almost any position. This motion occurs at three joints within the shoulder girdle: the sternoclavicular joint, the acromioclavicular (A/C) joint, and the glenohumeral joint. Only slight motion occurs normally at the sternoclavicular and acromioclavicular (A/C) joints. The ball-and-socket arrangement of the glenohumeral joint allows great freedom of motion in almost any direction.

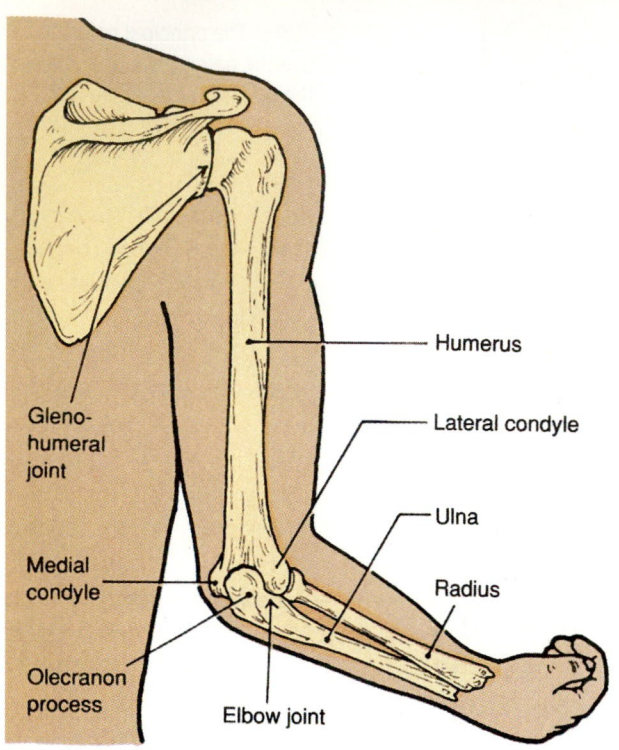

FIGURE 4-21 The principal bones in the arm and forearm include the humerus, the radius, and the ulna

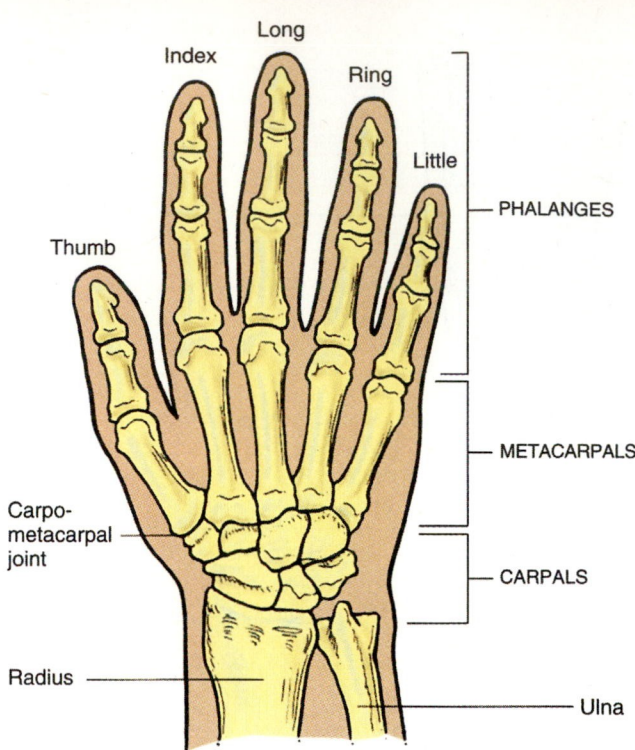

FIGURE 4-22 The principal bones in the wrist and hand include the carpals, the metacarpals, and the phalanges.

The clavicle is a long, slender bone that lies just under the skin and provides support for the upper extremity. The clavicle is palpable though its entire length from the sternum to its attachment to the scapula. Its medial end is attached by very strong ligaments to the manubrium of the sternum to form the sternoclavicular joint. Its lateral end forms a joint with the acromion process of the scapula to create the A/C joint.

The scapula is a large, flat, triangular bone that overlies the posterior wall of the thorax and is surrounded by large muscles. Because of these muscles, only small parts of this bone are palpable. The scapula has two specially named regions that form joints with the clavicle and the humerus. The acromion process in the front forms part of the A/C joint. The glenoid fossa joins with the humeral head to form the glenohumeral joint. The spine and medial border of the scapula can be seen and palpated posteriorly. The acromion process forms the rounded edge of the shoulder girdle. You can feel this if you slowly move your finger along the clavicle and across the A/C joint.

Arm. The supporting bone of the arm is the **humerus**. Its long, straight shaft serves as an effective lever for heavy lifting. As in the thigh, there are few bony landmarks in the arm because it is covered by large muscles: the **biceps** in the front and the **triceps** in the back. The

head of the humerus is covered by muscles that form the rounded prominence of the shoulder girdle laterally. The distal end articulates with both the radius and ulna at the elbow joint (Figure 4-21).

The humerus joins with the radius and ulna to form the elbow, which is a relatively simple hinge joint. You can easily see and feel three prominences on the back of the elbow: the medial and lateral condyles of the humerus and the olecranon process of the ulna.

Forearm. The forearm is composed of the radius and the ulna. The **ulna** is larger in the proximal forearm, and the **radius** is larger in the distal forearm. The olecranon process of the ulna forms most of the elbow joint. The entire ulnar shaft from the tip of the olecranon process distally can be palpated, because it lies just under the skin on the back of the forearm. The radius is covered by muscles and cannot be palpated except in the lower third of the forearm, where it enlarges to form a major portion of the wrist joint. The radius rotates about the ulna, which allows the palm of the hand to turn up or down. At the wrist, the ends of the radius and ulna (the styloid processes) lie directly under the skin and can be easily palpated. The radial styloid is slightly longer than the ulnar styloid. The radius lies on the lateral, or thumb, side of the forearm, and the ulna is on the medial or little finger side.

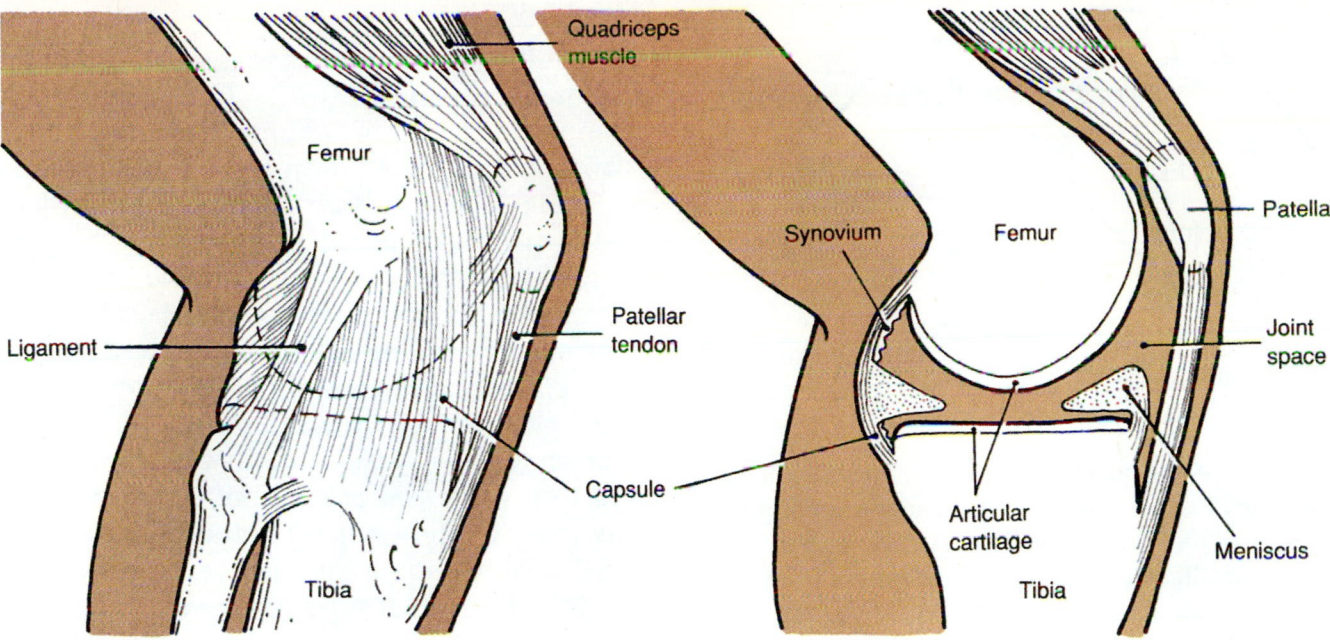

FIGURE 4-23 A joint consists of bone ends, the fibrous joint capsule, and ligaments. The degree to which a joint can move is determined by how the ligaments hold the bone ends and by the configuration of the bones themselves.

Wrist and hand. The wrist is a modified ball-and-socket joint formed by the ends of the radius and ulna and several small wrist bones (Figure 4-22). There are eight bones in the wrist, called carpal bones. Extending from the carpal bones are five metacarpals, which serve as a base for each of the five fingers or digits. The carpometacarpal joint (thumb joint) is a modified ball-and-socket joint that allows the thumb to rotate as well as to flex and extend. The other joints in the hand are simple hinge joints. In the thumb, there are two bones beyond the metacarpal: the proximal and distal phalanges. The remaining four digits of the hand are named in order: the index, middle, ring, and little finger. Each of these contains three phalanges.

Joints

Wherever two bones come in contact, a joint (articulation) is formed. A joint consists of the ends of the bones that make up the joint and the surrounding connecting and supporting tissue (Figure 4-23). Most joints in the body are named by combining the names of the two bones that form that joint. For example, the sternoclavicular joint is the articulation between the sternum and the clavicle. Most joints allow motion—for example, the knee, hip, or elbow—whereas some bones fuse with one another at joints to form a solid, immobile, bony structure. For instance, the skull is composed of several bones that fuse as a child grows. An infant, whose skull bones are not yet fused, has fontanels (soft spots) between the bones. The fontanels close as the bones fuse together when the infant's skull reaches the adult size. Some joints have slight, limited motion in which the bone ends are held together by fibrous tissue. Such a joint is called a symphysis.

The bone ends of a joint are held together by a fibrous sac joint capsule. At certain points around the circumference of the joint, the capsule is lax and thin so that motion can occur. In other areas, it is quite thick and resists stretching or bending. These bands of tough, thick tissue are called ligaments. A joint such as the sacroiliac joint that is virtually surrounded by tough, thick ligaments will have little motion, whereas a joint such as the shoulder, with few ligaments, will be free to move in almost any direction (and will, as a result, be more prone to dislocation).

The degree of freedom of motion of a joint is determined by the extent to which the ligaments hold the bone ends together and also by the configuration of the bone ends themselves. The hip joint is a **ball-and-socket joint**, which allows rotation as well as bending (Figure 4-24). The finger joints and the knee are **hinge joints**, with motion

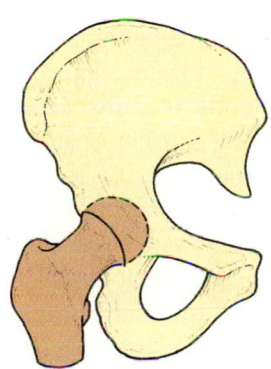

FIGURE 4-24 The hip is a typical ball-and-socket joint.

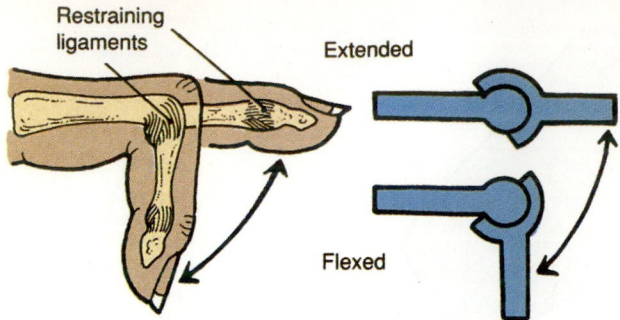

FIGURE 4-25 The finger joints are hinge joints, which allow motion in only one plane.

restricted to one plane (Figure 4-25). They can only **flex** (bend) and **extend** (straighten). Rotation is not possible because of the shape of the joint surfaces and the strong restraining ligaments on both sides of the joint. Thus, although the amount of motion varies from joint to joint, all joints have a definite limit beyond which motion cannot occur. When a joint is forced beyond this limit, damage to some structure must occur. Either the bones that form the joint will break, or the supporting capsule and ligaments will be disrupted.

The Musculoskeletal System

The human body is a well-designed system whose form, upright posture, and movement are provided by the **musculoskeletal** system. As its combination form suggests, the term musculoskeletal refers to the bones and voluntary muscles of the body. The musculoskeletal system also protects the vital internal organs of the body. Muscles are a form of tissue that allows body movement. Although there are more than 600 muscles in the musculoskeletal system, they are generally divided into three types: skeletal, smooth, and cardiac (Figure 4-26).

Skeletal Muscle

Skeletal muscle, so named because it attaches to the bones of the skeleton, forms the major muscle mass of the body. It is also called **voluntary muscle**, because all skeletal muscle is under direct voluntary control of the brain and can be stimulated to contract or relax at will. Skeletal muscle is also called **striated muscle**, because when viewed under the microscope, it has characteristic stripes (striations). All body movement results from skeletal muscle contraction or relaxation. Usually, a specific motion is the result of several muscles contracting and relaxing simultaneously.

All skeletal muscles are supplied with arteries, veins, and nerves (Figure 4-27). Arterial blood brings oxygen

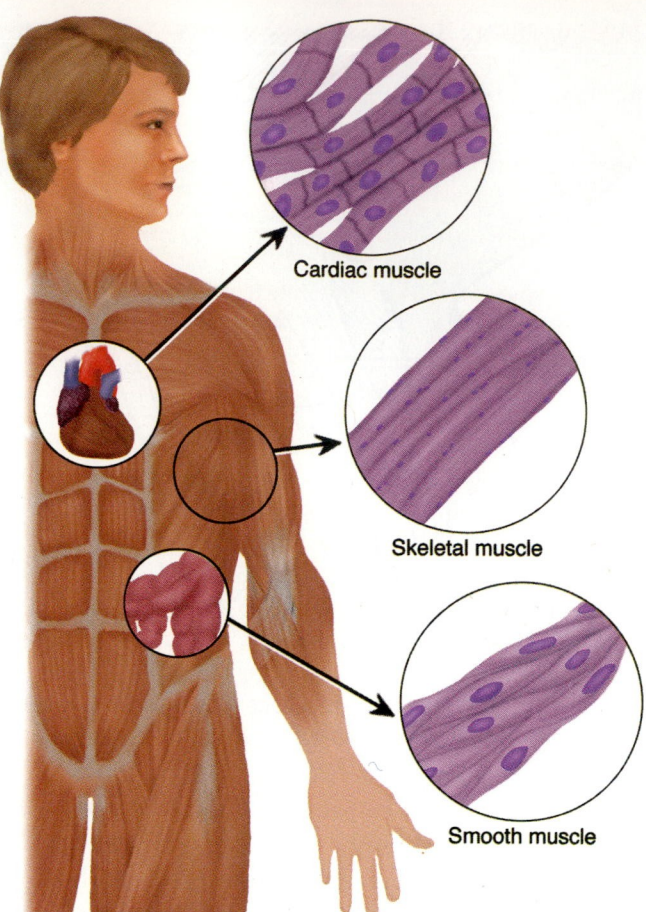

FIGURE 4-26 The three types of muscles are skeletal, smooth, and cardiac.

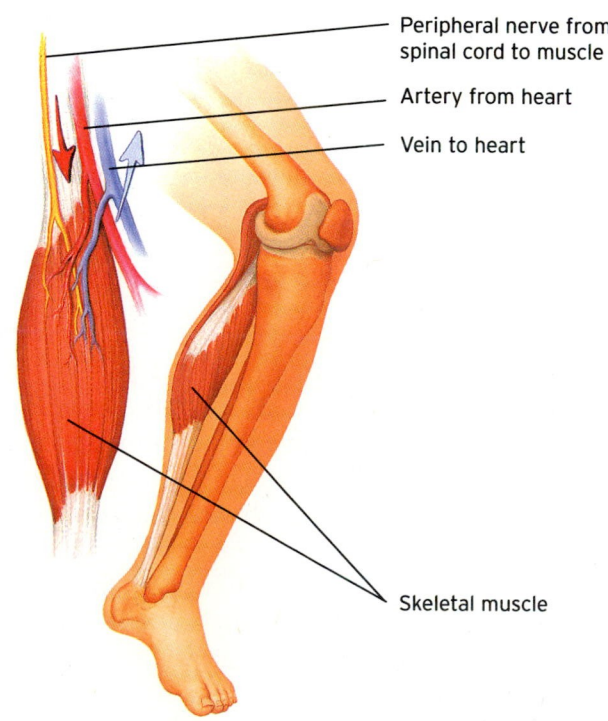

FIGURE 4-27 All skeletal muscles are supplied by arteries, veins, and nerves.

and nutrients to the muscle, and the veins carry away the waste products of muscular contraction (carbon dioxide and water). Muscles cannot function without this ongoing supply of oxygen and nutrients and removal of waste products. Muscle cramps result when insufficient oxygen or food is carried to the muscle or when acidic waste products accumulate and are not carried away.

Skeletal muscle is under the direct control of the nervous system and responds to a command from the brain to move a specific body part. Specific nerves pass directly from the brain to the spinal cord. There, they connect with other nerves that exit from the spinal cord and pass to each skeletal muscle. Electrical impulses are carried from the cells in the brain and spinal cord along the peripheral nerves to each muscle, signaling it to contract. When this normal nerve supply is lost through injury to the brain, spinal cord, or peripheral nerves, the voluntary control of the muscle is lost, and the muscle becomes paralyzed.

Most skeletal muscles attach directly to bone by tough, ropelike cords of fibrous tissue called tendons, which continue the fascia that covers all skeletal muscles. The fascia is much like the skin of a sausage in that it encases the muscle tissue. At either end of the muscle, the fascia extends beyond the muscle to attach to a bone. This musculotendinous unit crosses a joint and is responsible for the motion of that joint. The proximal point of attachment of the musculotendinous unit is its origin, and the distal bony attachment is called the insertion of the muscle. When a muscle contracts, a line of force is created between the origin and the insertion, which pulls the points of origin and insertion closer together (Figure 4-28). This motion occurs at the joint between the two bones.

Smooth Muscle

Smooth muscle carries out much of the automatic work of the body; therefore, it is also called **involuntary muscle**. Smooth muscle is found in the walls of most tubular structures of the body, such as the gastrointestinal tract, the urinary system, the blood vessels, and the bronchi of the lungs. Contraction and relaxation of smooth muscle propel or control the flow of the contents of these structures along their course. For example, the rhythmic contraction and relaxation of the smooth muscles of the wall of the intestine propel ingested food through it, and smooth muscle in the walls of a blood vessel can alter the diameter of the vessel to control the amount of blood flowing through it (Figure 4-29).

Smooth muscle responds only to primitive stimuli such as stretching, heat, or the need to relieve waste. An individual cannot exert any voluntary control over this type of muscle.

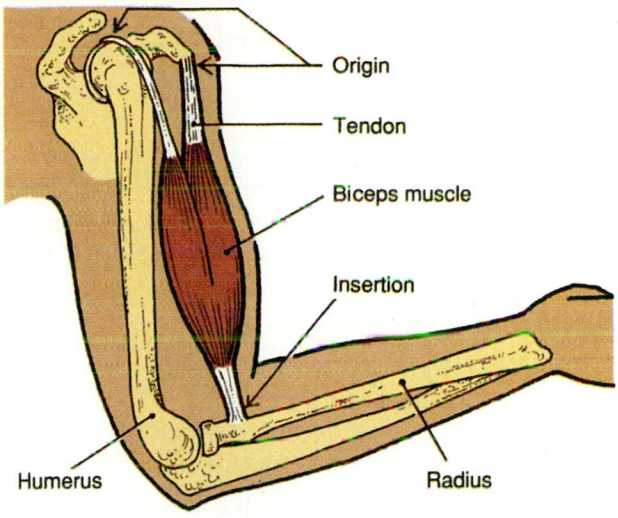

FIGURE 4-28 The biceps muscle causes the elbow to bend when it contracts. Note the points of tendon origin and insertion. As the muscle contracts and shortens, these points are pulled closer together, with motion occurring at the elbow joint.

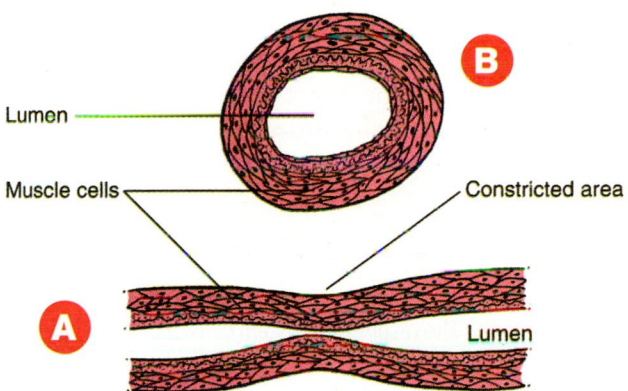

FIGURE 4-29 A: Smooth muscle lines the walls of the tubular structures of the body. **B:** Contraction of the muscles narrows the diameter of the structure, and relaxation allows the diameter to increase in size.

Cardiac Muscle

The heart is a large muscle composed of a pair of pumps of unequal force: one of lower pressure and one of higher pressure. The heart must function continuously from birth to death. It is a specially adapted involuntary muscle with a very rich blood supply and its own electrical system, which makes it different from both skeletal and smooth muscle. Cardiac muscle can tolerate an interruption of its blood supply for only a few seconds. It requires a continuous supply of oxygen and glucose for normal function. Because of its special structure and function, cardiac muscle is placed in a separate category.

The Respiratory System

The **respiratory system** consists of all the structures of the body that contribute to respiration, or the process of breathing (Figure 4-30). It includes the nose, mouth, throat, larynx, trachea, and bronchi, which are all air passages or airways. The system also includes the lungs, where oxygen is passed into the blood and where carbon dioxide is removed from the blood to be exhaled. Finally, the respiratory system includes the diaphragm, the muscles of the chest wall, and the accessory muscles of breathing, which permit normal respiratory movement. In this text, the term "airway" usually refers to the upper airway or the passage above the **larynx** (voice box).

The function of the respiratory system is to provide the body with oxygen and eliminate carbon dioxide. The exchange of oxygen and carbon dioxide takes place in the lungs and in the tissues. It is a complicated process that occurs automatically unless the airways or the lungs become diseased or damaged.

The Upper Airway

The structures of the upper airway are located anteriorly and at the midline. The upper airway includes the nose, mouth, and throat. The nose and mouth lead to the oropharynx (throat). The nostrils lead to the **naso-pharynx** (above the roof of the mouth), and the mouth leads to the oropharynx. The lining of the nasopharynx gives off watery secretions and helps to moisten the air as we breathe. Air enters through the mouth more rapidly and directly. As a result, it is less moist than air that enters through the nose.

Two passageways are located at the bottom of the pharynx: the esophagus behind and the trachea (windpipe) in front. Food and liquids enter the pharynx and pass into the esophagus, which carries them to the stomach. Air and other gases enter the trachea and go to the lungs.

Protecting the opening of the trachea is a thin, leaf-shaped valve called the **epiglottis**. This valve allows air to pass into the trachea but prevents food or liquid from entering the airway under normal circumstances. Air moves past the epiglottis into the larynx and the trachea.

The Lower Airway

The first part of the lower airway is the larynx, a rather complex arrangement of tiny bones, cartilage, muscles, and the two vocal cords. The larynx does not tolerate any foreign solid or liquid material. A violent episode of coughing and spasm of the vocal cords will result from contact with solids or liquids.

FIGURE 4-30 The respiratory system consist of all the structures of the body that contribute to the process of breathing.

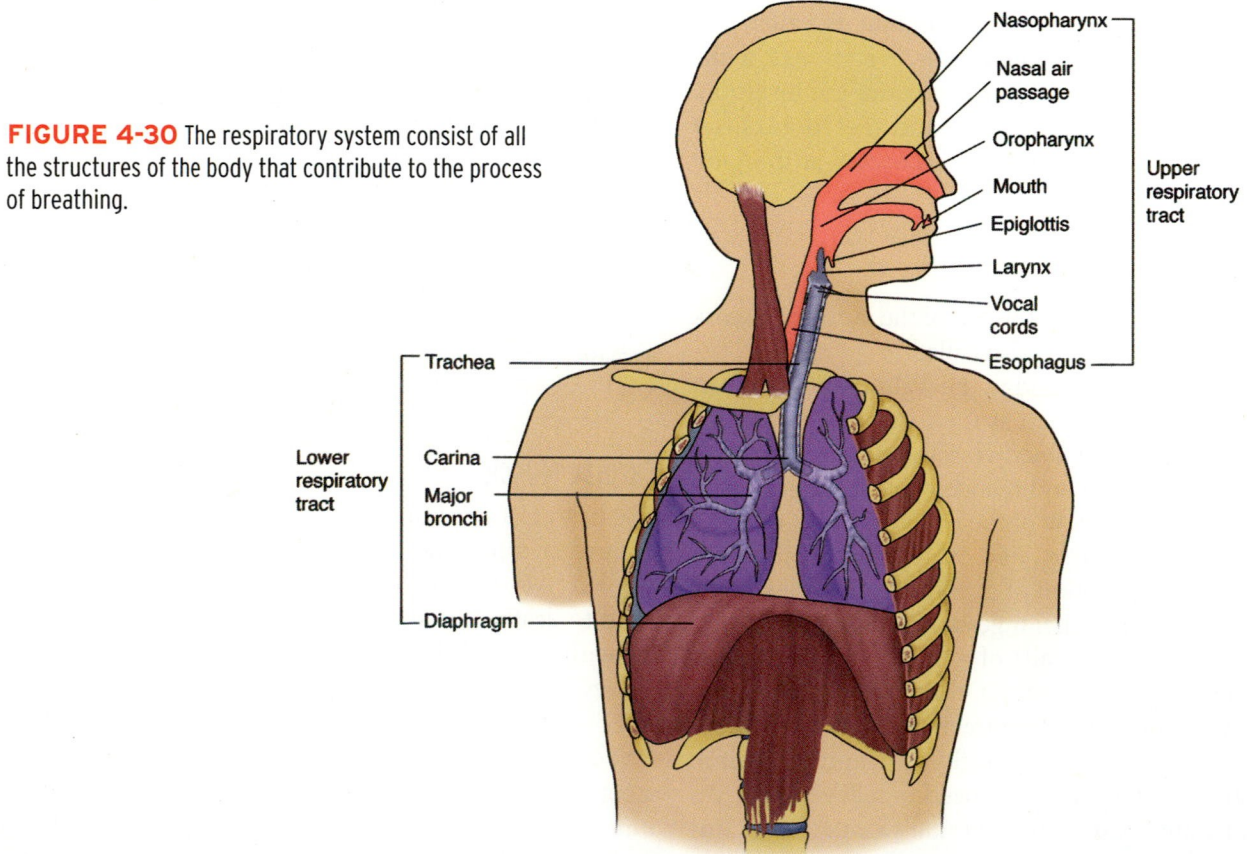

The Adam's apple, or thyroid cartilage, is easily seen in the middle of the front of the neck. The thyroid cartilage is actually the anterior part of the larynx. Tiny muscles open and close the vocal cords and control tension on them. Sounds are created as air is forced past the vocal cords, making them vibrate. These vibrations make the sound. The pitch of the sound changes as the cords open and close. You can feel the vibrations if you place your fingers lightly on the larynx as you speak or sing. The vibrations of air are shaped by the tongue and muscles of the mouth to form understandable sounds. Immediately below the thyroid cartilage is the palpable cricoid cartilage.

Between these two prominences lies the cricothyroid membrane, which can be felt as a depression in the midline of the neck just inferior to the thyroid cartilage. Below the cricoid cartilage is the trachea. The trachea is approximately 5″ long and is a semirigid, enclosed air tube made up of rings of cartilage that are open in the back. This enables food to pass through the esophagus, which lies right behind the trachea. The rings of cartilage keep the trachea from collapsing when air moves into and out of the lungs. The trachea ends at the carina and divides into smaller tubes. These tubes are the right and left main bronchi, which enter the lungs. Each main bronchus immediately branches within the lung into smaller and smaller airways. Within the right lung, three major bronchi are formed. Within the left, there are only two. Each bronchus supplies air to one lobe of the lung.

Lungs

The two lungs are held in place within the chest by the trachea, the arteries and veins that run to and from the heart, and the pulmonary ligaments. Each lung is divided into lobes. The right lung has three lobes: the upper, middle, and lower lobes. The left lung has an upper lobe and a lower lobe. Each lobe is divided further into segments. Also within each lung, the main bronchi divide until they end in very fine airways called bronchioles. The bronchioles end in about 700 million tiny grapelike sacs called **alveoli** (Figure 4-31). The exchange of oxygen and carbon dioxide occurs within these alveoli. The walls of the alveoli contain a network of tiny blood vessels (pulmonary capillaries) that carry the carbon dioxide from the body to the lungs and the oxygen from the lungs to the body.

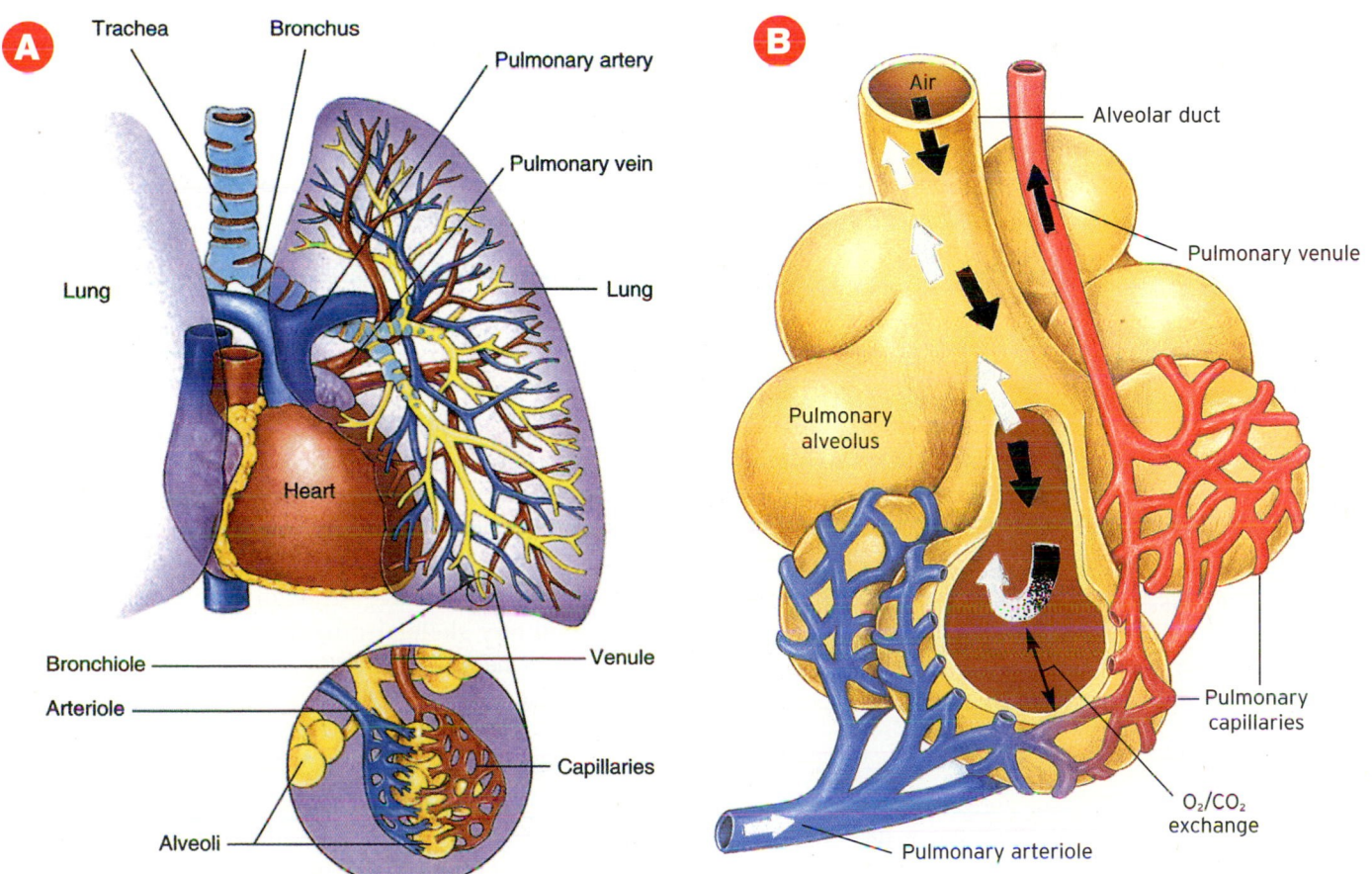

FIGURE 4-31 A: The lungs contain millions of air sacs (alveoli), which lie at the ends of air passages. **B:** The exchange of oxygen and carbon dioxide occurs within the alveoli.

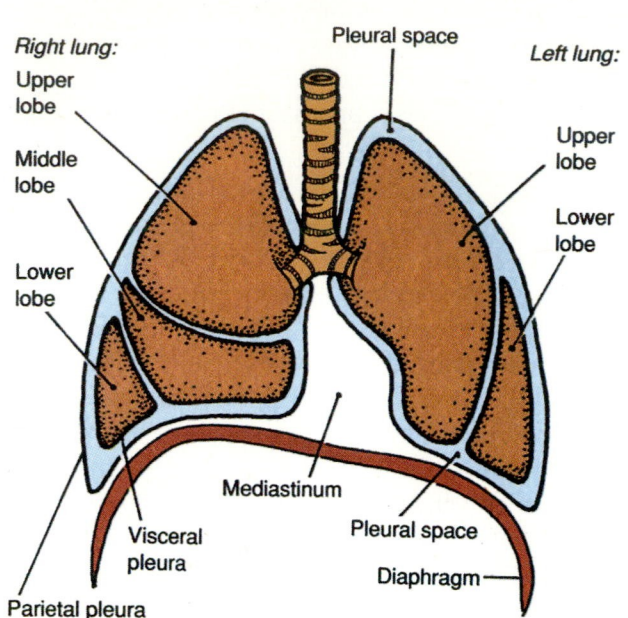

FIGURE 4-32 The pleura lining the chest wall and covering the lungs is an essential part of the breathing mechanism. The pleural space is not an actual space until blood or air leaks into it, causing the pleural surfaces to separate.

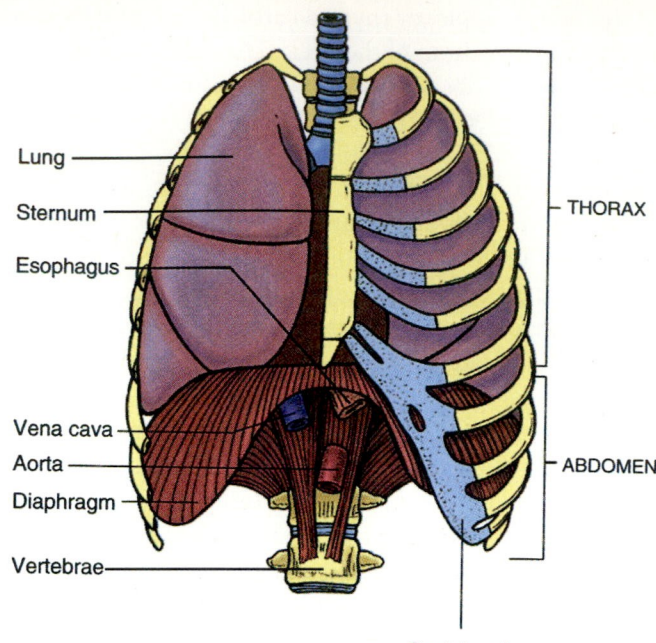

FIGURE 4-33 The dome-shaped diaphragm divides the thorax from the abdomen. It is pierced by the great vessels and the esophagus.

The lungs cannot expand and contract themselves because they have no muscle. There is, however, a very definite mechanism to ensure that they follow the motion of the chest wall and expand or contract with it. Covering each lung is a layer of very smooth, glistening tissue called <u>pleura</u> (Figure 4-32). Another layer of pleura lines the inside of the chest cavity. The two layers are called parietal pleura (lining the chest wall) and visceral pleura (covering the lungs).

Between the parietal pleura and the visceral pleura is the <u>pleural space</u>, which is not a space in the usual sense because normally, these layers are in close contact everywhere. In fact, the layers are sealed tightly against one another by a thin film of fluid. When the chest wall expands, the lung is pulled with it and made to expand by the force exerted through these closely applied pleural surfaces. The pleural space is called a potential space. Normally, the pleural space is quite small and contains only the thin film of plural fluid as each lung entirely fills its chest cavity.

Diaphragm

The diaphragm is unique because it has characteristics of both voluntary (skeletal) and involuntary (smooth) muscle. It is a dome-shaped muscle that divides the thorax from the abdomen and is pierced by the great vessels and the esophagus (Figure 4-33). Under the micro-

scope, it has striations like skeletal muscle. Also, it is attached to the costal arch and the lumbar vertebrae like other skeletal muscles. Thus, in many ways, it looks like a voluntary muscle; however, we do not have complete voluntary control over its function. It acts like a voluntary muscle whenever we take a deep breath, cough, or hold our breath. We control these variations in the way we breathe.

However, unlike other skeletal or voluntary muscles, the diaphragm performs an automatic function. Breathing continues while we sleep and at all other times. Even though we can hold our breath or temporarily breathe faster or slower, we cannot continue these variations in breathing pattern indefinitely. Ultimately, when the concentration of carbon dioxide is close to being disturbed, automatic regulation of breathing resumes. Therefore, although the diaphragm looks like voluntary skeletal muscle and is attached to the skeleton, it behaves, for the most part, like an involuntary muscle.

During inhalation, the diaphragm and intercostal muscles contract. When the diaphragm contracts, it moves down slightly and enlarges the thoracic cage from top to bottom. When the intercostal muscles contract, they raise the ribs up and out. These actions combine to enlarge the chest cavity in all dimensions. Pressure within the cavity falls, and air rushes into the lungs.

The function of the respiratory system is to provide the body with oxygen and eliminate carbon dioxide.

During exhalation, the diaphragm and the intercostal muscles relax. Unlike inhalation, exhalation does not normally require muscular effort. As these muscles relax, all dimensions of the thorax decrease, and the ribs and muscles assume a normal resting position. When the volume of the chest cavity decreases, air in the lungs is compressed into a smaller space. Pressure is increased, and air is pushed out through the trachea.

Respiratory Physiology

Each living cell in the body requires a regular supply of oxygen. Some cells need a constant supply of oxygen to survive. For example, cells in the heart may be damaged if the oxygen supply is interrupted for more than a few seconds. Brain cells and cells in the nervous system may die after as few as 4 to 6 minutes without oxygen. Dead brain and nerve cells can never be replaced. Permanent changes in the body, such as brain damage, result from the damage caused by a lack of oxygen. Other cells in the body are not as vitally dependent on a constant oxygen supply. They can tolerate short periods without oxygen and still survive. Normally, the air that we breathe contains 21% oxygen and 78% nitrogen. Small amounts of other gases make up the remaining 1%.

The exchange of oxygen and carbon dioxide. As blood travels through the body, it gives its oxygen and nutrients to various tissues and cells. Oxygen passes from the blood through the capillaries to tissue cells. In the reverse process, carbon dioxide and cell waste passes from tissue cells through capillaries to the blood (Figure 4-34).

Each time we take a breath, the alveoli receive a supply of oxygen-rich air. The oxygen then passes into a fine network of pulmonary capillaries, which are in close contact with the alveoli. In fact, the capillaries in the lungs are located in the walls of the alveoli. The walls of the capillaries and the alveoli are extremely thin. Thus, the air in the alveoli and the blood in the capillaries are separated by two very thin layers of tissue.

Oxygen and carbon dioxide pass rapidly across these thin tissue layers through diffusion. Diffusion is a passive process in which molecules move from an area with

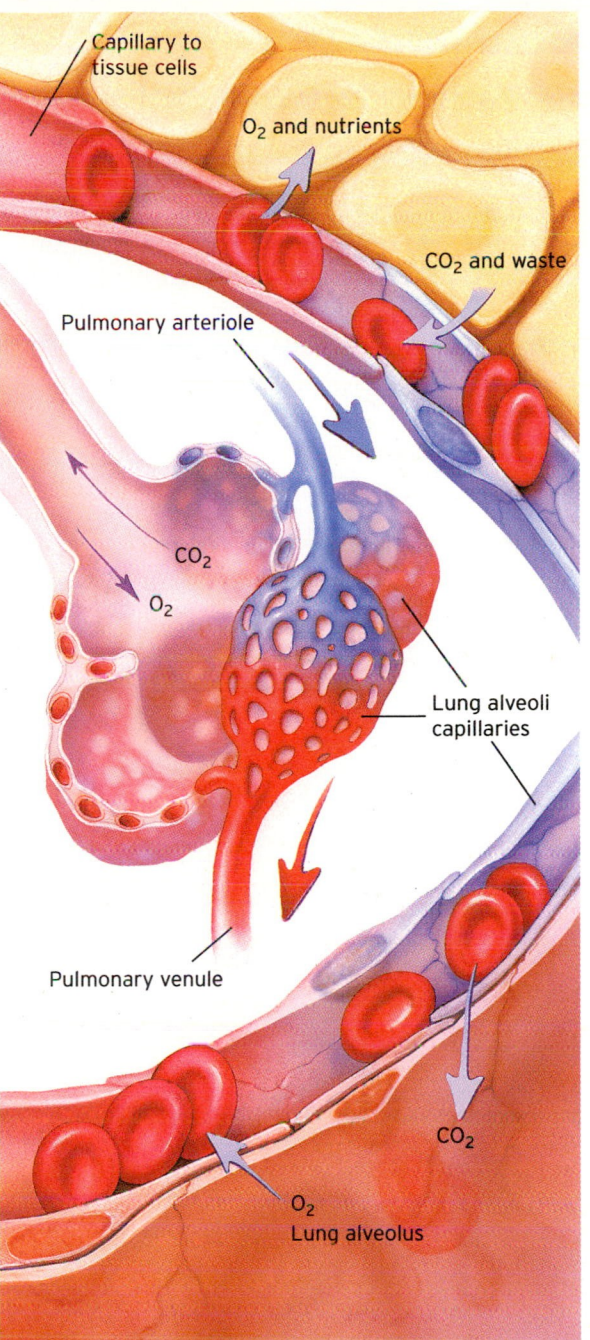

Capillary to tissue cells

O_2 and nutrients

CO_2 and waste

Pulmonary arteriole

CO_2

O_2

Lung alveoli capillaries

Pulmonary venule

CO_2

O_2

Lung alveolus

FIGURE 4-34 In the capillaries of the lungs, oxygen passes from the blood to the tissue cells, and carbon dioxide and waste pass from the tissue cells to the blood.

higher concentration of molecules to an area of lower concentration. For example, a gas such as hydrogen sulfide moves from an area of high concentrations (a rotten egg) by spontaneous movement of the gas molecules until the odor fills the room. There are more oxygen molecules in the alveoli than in the blood. Therefore, the oxygen molecules move from the alveoli into the blood. Because there are more carbon dioxide molecules in the blood than in the inhaled air, carbon dioxide moves from the blood into the alveoli.

caring for kids

The anatomy of the respiratory system in children is proportionally smaller and less rigid than that in an adult (Figure 4-35). A child's nose and mouth are much smaller than those of an adult. The larynx, cricoid cartilage, and trachea are smaller, softer, and more flexible as well. This makes the mechanics of breathing much more delicate. A child's pharynx is also smaller and less deeply curved. The tongue takes up proportionally more space in a child's mouth than in an adult's mouth.

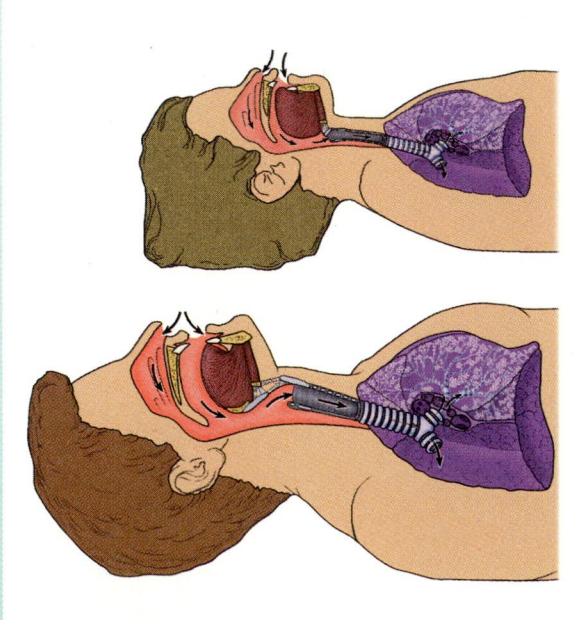

FIGURE 4-35 The respiratory system of a child is proportionally smaller and less rigid than that of an adult.

These anatomic differences are important for your assessment. For example, the smaller larynx of a child becomes obstructed more easily. The chest wall in children is softer. Therefore, children depend more heavily on the diaphragm for breathing. You will notice that the abdomen moves in and out considerably with each breath, especially in an infant. Infants younger than age 1 month do not know how to breathe through the mouth. Therefore, as you assess an infant or a child, you must carefully consider these differences.

The blood does not use all the inhaled oxygen as it passes through the body. Exhaled air contains 16% oxygen and 3% to 5% carbon dioxide; the rest is nitrogen (Figure 4-36). This 16% concentration of oxygen is adequate to support artificial ventilation. So as you provide artificial ventilations to a patient who is not breathing, that patient is receiving 16% concentration of oxygen with each ventilation.

The control of breathing. The brain—or more specifically, an area of the brain stem—controls breathing. This area is in one of the best-protected parts of the nervous system—deep within the skull. The nerves in this area act as sensors of the level of carbon dioxide in the blood. The brain automatically controls breathing if the levels of carbon dioxide or oxygen in the arterial blood are too high or too low. In fact, adjustments can be made in just one breath. For these reasons, you cannot hold your breath indefinitely or breathe rapidly and deeply indefinitely.

When the level of carbon dioxide becomes too high, the brain stem sends nerve impulses down the spinal cord that cause the diaphragm and the intercostal muscles to contract. This increases our breathing, or

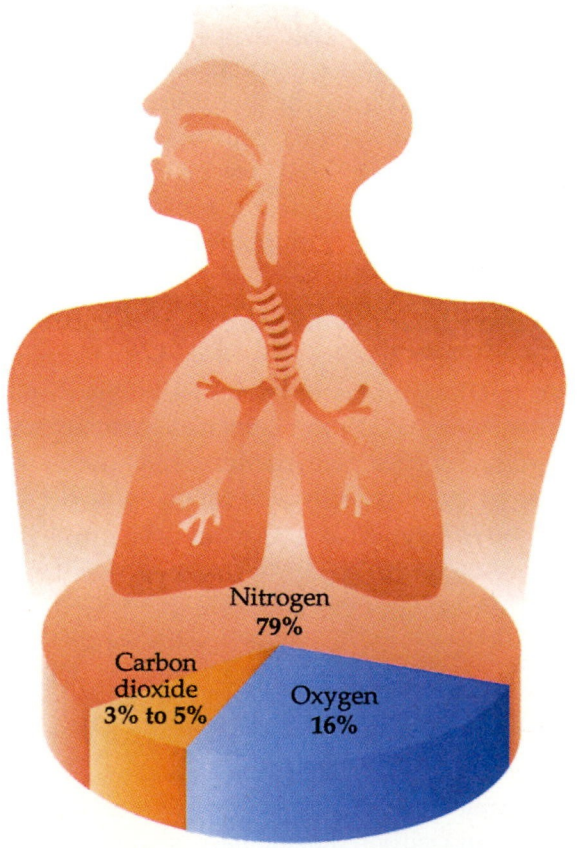

FIGURE 4-36 The components of exhaled air include oxygen, carbon dioxide, and nitrogen.

respirations. The higher the level of carbon dioxide in the blood, the stronger is the impulse to cause breathing. Once the carbon dioxide levels become acceptable, the strength and frequency of respiration decreases.

We also have a "backup system" to control respiration called the hypoxic drive. When oxygen levels fall, this system will also stimulate breathing. There are nerves in the brain, the walls of the aorta, and the carotid arteries that act as oxygen sensors. These sensors are easily satisfied by minimal levels of oxygen in the arterial blood. Therefore, our backup system, the hypoxic drive, is much less sensitive and less powerful than the carbon dioxide sensors in the brain stem.

Characteristics of normal breathing. You can think of a "normal" breathing pattern as a bellows system. Normal breathing should appear easy, not labored. As with a bellows that is used to move air to start a fire, breathing should be a smooth flow of air moving into and out of the lungs. Normal breathing has the following characteristics:

- A normal rate and depth (tidal volume)
- A regular rhythm or pattern of inhalation and exhalation
- Good audible breath sounds on both sides of the chest
- Regular rise and fall movement on both sides of the chest
- Movement of the abdomen

Inadequate breathing patterns in adults. An adult who is awake, alert, and talking to you has no immediate airway or breathing problems. However, you should keep supplemental oxygen on hand to assist with breathing if it should become necessary. An adult who is not breathing well will appear to be working hard to breathe. This type of breathing pattern is called labored breathing. Labored breathing requires effort and may involve the accessory muscles. The person may also be breathing either much slower (fewer than 8 breaths/min) or much faster (more than 24 breaths/min) than normal. An adult who is breathing normally will have respirations of 12 to 20 breaths/min (Table 4-3).

TABLE 4-3	Normal Respiration Rate Ranges
Adults	12 to 20 breaths/min
Children	15 to 30 breaths/min
Infants	25 to 50 breaths/min

With a normal breathing pattern, the accessory muscles are not being used. With inadequate breathing, a person, especially a child, may use the accessory muscles of the chest, neck, and abdomen. Other signs that a person is not breathing normally include the following:

- Muscle retractions above the clavicles, between the ribs, and below the rib cage, especially in children
- Pale or cyanotic (blue) skin
- Cool, damp (clammy) skin
- Tripod position

caring for kids

Normal breathing patterns in infants and children are essentially the same as those in adults. However, infants and children breathe faster than adults. An infant who is breathing normally will have respirations of 25 to 50 breaths/min. A child will have respirations of 15 to 30 breaths/min. Like adults, infants and children who are breathing normally will have smooth, regular inhalation and exhalation, equal breath sounds, and regular rise and fall movement on both sides of the chest.

Breathing problems in infants and children often appear the same as breathing problems in adults. Signs such as faster respirations, an irregular breathing pattern, unequal breath sounds, and unequal chest expansion indicate breathing problems in both adults and children. Other signs that an infant or child is not breathing normally include the following:

- Muscle retractions, in which the muscles of the chest and neck are working extra hard in breathing
- Nasal flaring in children, in which the nostrils flare out as the child breathes
- Seesaw respirations in infants, in which the chest and abdominal muscles alternately contract to look like a seesaw

Exhalation becomes active when infants and children have trouble breathing. Normally, inhalation alone is the active, muscular part of breathing, as described earlier. However, with labored breathing, both inhalation and exhalation are hard work. With labored breathing, exhalation is not passive. Instead, air is forced out of the lungs during exhalation, and the child will often begin to wheeze. This type of labored breathing involves the use of the accessory muscles of breathing.

A patient may also appear to be breathing after the heart has stopped. These occasional, gasping breaths are called <u>agonal respirations</u>. Agonal respirations occur when the respiratory center in the brain continues to send signals to the breathing muscles. These respirations are not adequate, since they are slow and generally shallow. You should assist ventilations of patients with agonal respirations.

The Circulatory System

The <u>circulatory system</u> is a complex arrangement of connected tubes, including the arteries, arterioles, capillaries, venules, and veins (Figure 4-37). The circulatory system is entirely closed, with capillaries connecting arterioles and venules. There are two circuits in the body: the systemic circulation in the body and the pulmonary circulation in the lungs. The systemic circulation, the circuit in the body, carries oxygen-rich

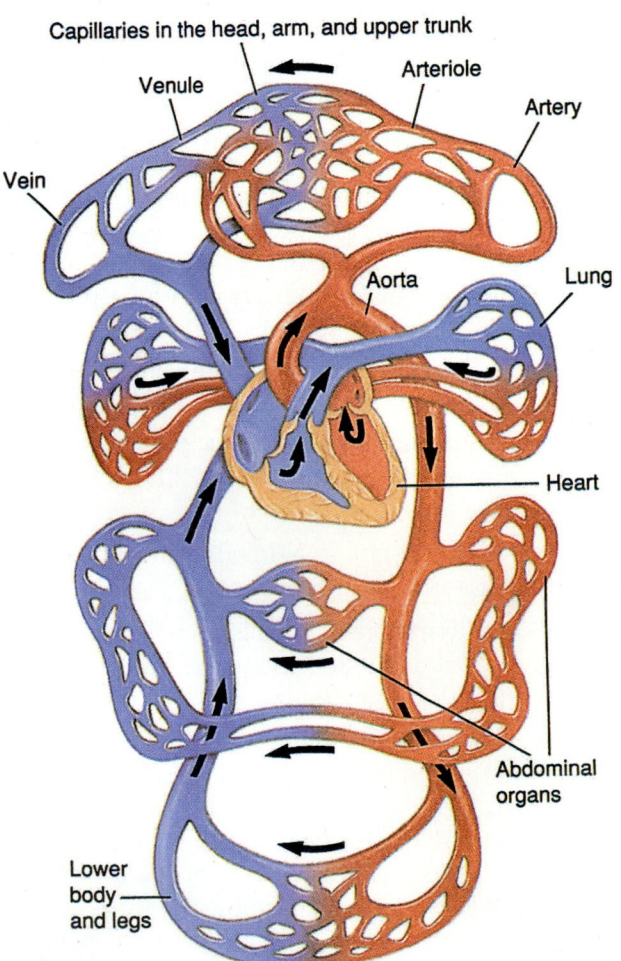

FIGURE 4-37 The circulatory system includes the heart, arteries, veins, and interconnecting capillaries. The capillaries are the smallest vessels and connect with the venules and arterioles.

blood from the left ventricle through the body and back to the right atrium. In the systemic circulation, as blood passes through the tissues and organs, it gives up oxygen and nutrients and absorbs cellular wastes and carbon dioxide. The cellular wastes are eliminated in passages through the liver and the kidneys. The pulmonary circulation, the circuit in the lungs, carries oxygen-poor blood from the right ventricle through the lungs and back to the left atrium. In the pulmonary circulation, as blood passes through the lungs, it is refreshed with oxygen and gives up carbon dioxide.

At the center of the system, and providing its driving force, is the heart. Blood circulates through the body under pressure generated by the two sides of the heart.

Heart

The <u>heart</u> is a hollow muscular organ approximately the size of an adult's clenched fist. It is made of a unique, adapted tissue called cardiac muscle or <u>myocardium</u> and actually works as two paired pumps, the one on the left side being more muscular. A wall called the septum divides the heart down the middle into right and left sides. Each side of the heart is divided again into an upper chamber (<u>atrium</u>) and a lower chamber (<u>ventricle</u>).

The heart is an involuntary muscle. As such, it is under the control of the autonomic nervous system. However, it has its own electrical system and continues to function even without its central nervous system control. It is distinct from skeletal or smooth muscle in its requirement for a continuous supply of oxygen and nutrients.

The heart must function continuously from birth to death and has developed special adaptations to meet the needs of this continuous function. It can tolerate a serious interruption of its own blood supply for only a very few seconds before the signs of a heart attack develop. Thus, its blood supply is as rich and well distributed as possible.

How the heart works. The heart receives the first blood distribution from the aorta. The two main coronary arteries have their openings immediately above the aortic valve at the beginning of the aorta where the pressures are highest (Figure 4-38).

The right side of the heart receives blood from the veins of the body (Figure 4-39). The blood enters from the venae cavae into the right atrium, then fills the right ventricle passing through a valve that closes to prevent backflow after the right atrial muscle contracts. Contraction of the right ventricle causes blood to flow into the pulmonary artery and the pulmonary circulation.

The left side receives oxygenated blood from the lungs through the pulmonary veins into the left atrium where it passes through a valve into the left ventricle. Contraction of this most muscular of the pumping chambers pumps the blood into the aorta and then to the arteries of the body.

The exit of each of the four heart chambers is governed by a one-way valve. The valves prevent the backflow of blood and keep it moving through the circulatory system in the proper direction. When a valve controlling the filling of a heart chamber is open, the other valve allowing it to empty is shut and vice versa. Normally, blood moves in only one direction through the entire system.

When a ventricle contracts, the valve to the artery opens, and the valve between the ventricle and atrium closes. Blood is forced from the ventricle out into the pulmonary artery or aorta. At the end of contraction, the ventricle relaxes. Backpressure causes the valve to the artery to close, and the entry valve to the ventricle opens as the ventricle relaxes. Blood then flows from the atrium into the ventricle. When the ventricle is stimulated to contract, the cycle is repeated.

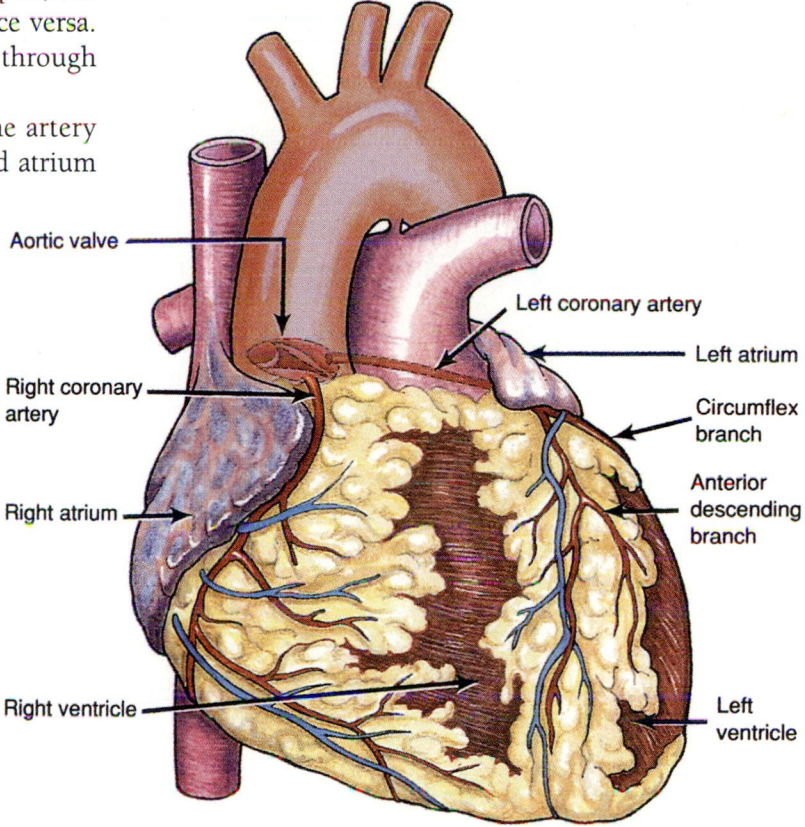

FIGURE 4-38 The two main coronary arteries supply the heart with blood.

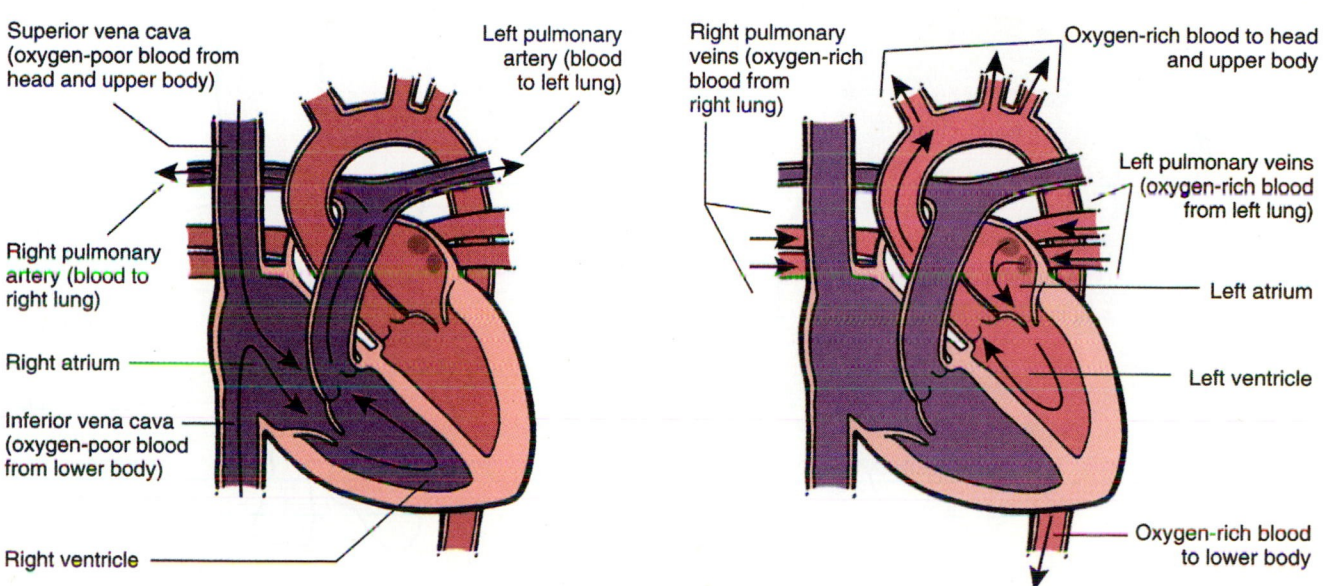

FIGURE 4-39 A: The right side, or lower pressure side, of the heart pumps blood from the body to the lungs.
B: The left side, or higher pressure side, of the heart pumps oxygen-rich blood to all parts of the body.

Normal heartbeat. In the normal adult, the heartbeat may range from 50 to 180 beats/min, depending on the level of activity. A very well-conditioned athlete may have a normal resting <u>heart rate (pulse)</u> of 50 to 60 beats/min. During vigorous physical activity, the heart rate may rise normally to as fast as 180 beats/min. The usual adult resting heart rate is between 60 and 100 beats/min (Table 4-4). At each beat, 70 to 80 mL of blood are ejected from the adult heart. In one minute, the entire blood volume of 5 to 6 L is circulated through all the vessels.

Electrical conduction system. A network of specialized tissue that is capable of conducting electrical current runs throughout the heart (Figure 4-40). The flow of electrical current through this network causes smooth, coordinated contractions of the heart. These contractions produce the pumping action of the heart. Each mechanical contraction of the heart is associated with two electrical processes. The first is depolarization, during which the electrical charges on the surface of the muscle cell change from positive to negative. The second is repolarization, during which the heart returns to its resting state and the positive charge is restored to the surface.

When the heart is working normally, the electrical impulse begins high in the atria at the sinus (SA) node, then travels to the atrioventricular (AV) node, and moves through the Purkinje fibers to the ventricles. This movement produces a smooth flow of electricity through the heart, which depolarizes the muscle and produces a coordinated pumping contraction. The heart's electrical

TABLE 4-4	Normal Heart Rates
Adults	60 to 100 beats/min
Children	80 to 100 beats/min
Toddlers	100 to 120 beats/min

system becomes disturbed if part of the heart is oxygen deficient, is injured, or dies. As a result, the heart may not continue to beat properly. Blood pressure decreases, and a patient may lose consciousness.

Arteries

The arteries carry blood from the heart to all body tissues (Figure 4-41). They branch into smaller arteries and then into arterioles. The arterioles, in turn, branch

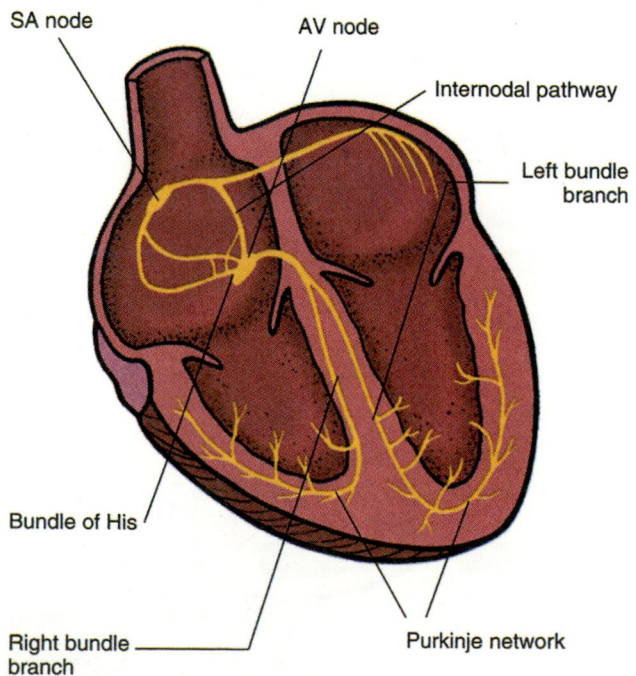

FIGURE 4-40 Electrical current flows through the heart to produce its pumping action.

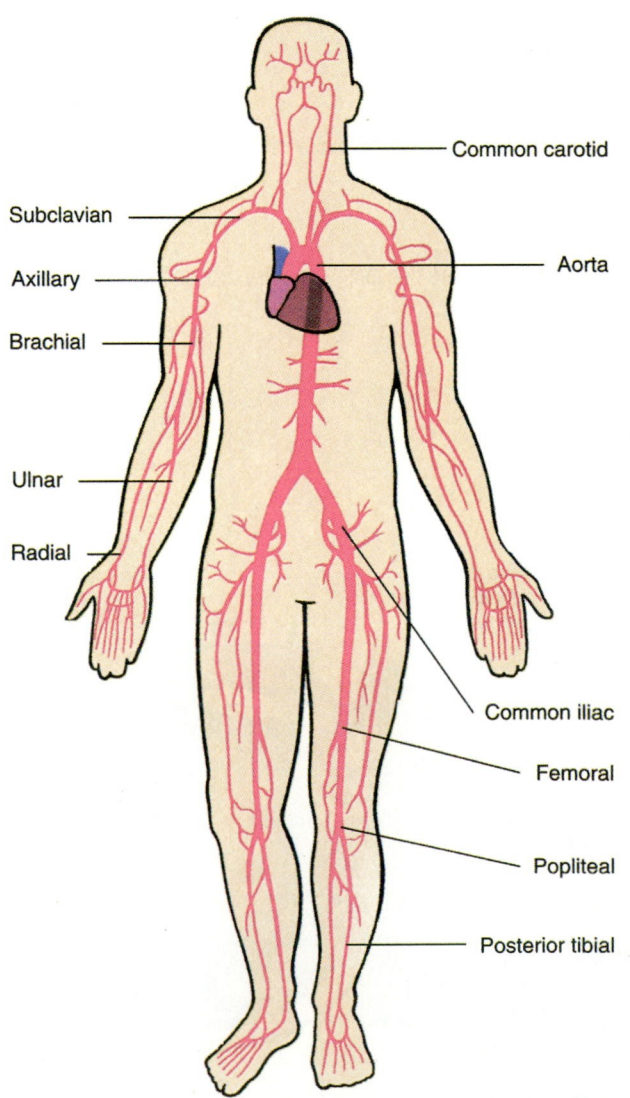

FIGURE 4-41 The principal arteries supply blood to a vast network of smaller arteries and arterioles, which nourish the tissue cells via the capillaries.

into smaller vessels until they connect to the vast network of capillaries. The walls of an artery are made of fine, circular muscle tissue. Some arteries even have elastic tissue.

Arteries contract to accommodate loss of blood volume and also to increase blood pressure. Blood is supplied to tissues as they need it. For example, the digestive system is supplied with more blood after you eat a meal. The leg muscles are supplied as you are jogging. Some tissues need a constant blood supply, especially the heart, the kidneys, and the brain. Other tissues, such as the muscles in the extremities, the skin, and intestines, can function with less blood when at rest.

The **aorta** is the principal artery leaving the left side of the heart; it carries freshly oxygenated blood to the body. This blood vessel is found just in front of the spine in the chest and abdominal cavities. The aorta has many branches that supply the heart, head, neck, arms, and abdominal and thoracic organs before it ends in the lower abdomen. It divides at the level of the umbilicus into the two common iliac arteries that lead to the lower extremities. All of the aorta's branches ultimately become arterioles leading into the body's capillary network.

The **pulmonary artery** begins at the right side of the heart and carries oxygen-poor blood to the lungs. It divides into finer and finer branches until it meets with the pulmonary capillary system located in the thin walls of the alveoli. These arteries are the only ones in the body that carry oxygen-poor blood.

The **carotid artery** is the major artery that supplies blood to the head and brain. The carotid arteries are located on both sides of the neck. You can easily feel the carotid pulse if you place your fingers at the anterior lateral part of the neck. Since the carotid artery is rather close to the heart, you can feel its pulse even after the pulse in the distal extremities is too weak to feel.

The **femoral artery** is the major artery that supplies blood to the lower extremities. It is palpable in the groin. It divides at the level of the knee and supplies blood to the leg. At the ankle, two of these branches are palpable. You can feel a pulse at the **posterior tibial artery**, which is behind the medial prominence of the ankle (medial malleolus). You can also feel a pulse at the **dorsalis pedis artery** on the anterior surface of the foot (dorsum of the foot).

The **brachial artery** is the major vessel in the upper extremity that supplies blood to the arm. It divides into two major branches just below the elbow. This is the artery that is used in assessing blood pressure with a blood pressure cuff and stethoscope.

The **radial artery** is the major artery in the lower arm and is palpable at the wrist on the thumb side (radial side). The **ulnar artery** is also palpable at the wrist on the opposite side (ulnar side), although its pulse is not as strong. Both of these arteries supply blood to the hand.

Arteries branch into smaller arteries and then into arterioles. **Arterioles** are the smallest branches of an artery leading to the vast network of capillaries.

Capillaries

In the body, there are billions of cells and billions of capillaries. **Capillary vessels** are fine end divisions of the arterial system that allow contact between cells of the body tissues and the plasma and the red blood cells. At this level, each individual cell of the body lives. Oxygen and other nutrients pass from blood cells and plasma in the capillaries to the individual tissue cells through the very thin wall of the capillary. Carbon dioxide and other metabolic waste products pass in a reverse direction from the tissue cells to the blood to be carried away. Blood in arteries is characteristically bright red, because its hemoglobin is rich in oxygen. Blood in the veins is dark bluish red, because it has passed through a capillary bed and given up its oxygen to the cells. Capillaries connect directly at one end with the flow regulating arterioles and at the other with the venules.

Veins

Oxygen-poor blood from the capillary system next moves to the venules, which are the smallest branches of the veins. The veins then return blood to the heart.

Once blood passes through the network of capillaries and moves through the venules, it returns to the heart via a network of larger and larger veins (See Figure 4-34). Veins have much thinner walls than arteries and are generally larger in diameter. The veins becomes larger and larger and ultimately form two major vessels. These major vessels, part of the great vessels, are located in the midline, just to the left of the spine and channel blood from the body and collect it just before it enters the heart.

The **superior vena cava** carries blood returning from the head, neck, shoulders, and upper extremities. Blood from the abdomen, pelvis, and lower extremities passes through the **inferior vena cava**. The superior and inferior venae join at the right atrium of the heart. The right ventricle receives blood from the right atrium and pumps it through the pulmonary arteries into the lungs.

The **pulmonary veins** carry oxygen-rich blood from the lungs to the left atrium. The oxygenated blood from the lungs enters the four pulmonary veins that unite at the left atrium. It then passes to the left ventricle and is pumped to the body again.

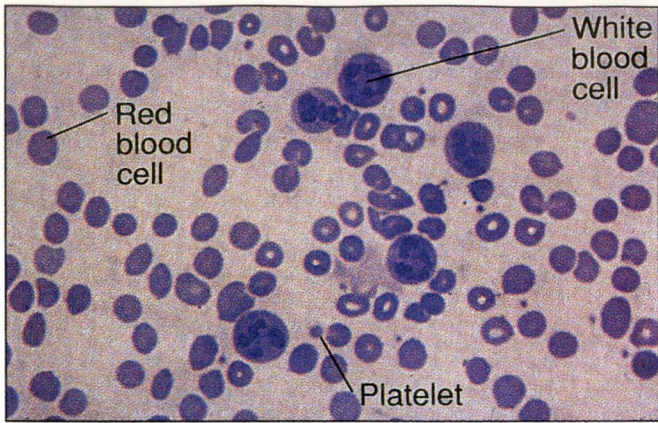

FIGURE 4-42 The components of blood include red blood cells, white blood cells, platelets, and plasma.

Components of Blood

Blood is a complex, thick, red fluid composed of plasma, red blood cells called erythrocytes, white blood cells called leukocytes, and platelets (Figure 4-42).

- <u>Plasma</u> is a sticky, yellow fluid that carries the blood cells and nutrients. It also transports cellular waste material to the organs of excretion. It contains most of the compounds needed to produce a blood clot.

- The iron-containing hemoglobin molecules in <u>red blood cells</u> give color to the blood and carry oxygen.

- <u>White blood cells</u> play a role in the body's immune defense mechanisms against infection.

- <u>Platelets</u> are tiny, disk-shaped elements that are much smaller than the cells. They are essential in the initial formation of a blood clot, the mechanism that stops bleeding.

Blood under pressure will gush or spurt intermittently from an artery and is bright red. From a vein, it will flow in a steady stream and is dark bluish-red. From capillaries, it will ooze at many tiny individual points. Clotting normally takes from 6 to 10 minutes.

Physiology of the Circulatory System

The <u>pulse (heart rate)</u>, which is palpated most easily at the neck, wrist, or groin, is created by the forceful pumping of blood out the left ventricle and into the major arteries. It is present throughout the entire arterial system. It can be felt most easily where the larger arteries are near the skin. The central pulses are the carotid artery pulse, which can be felt at the upper portion of the neck, and the femoral artery pulse, which is felt in the

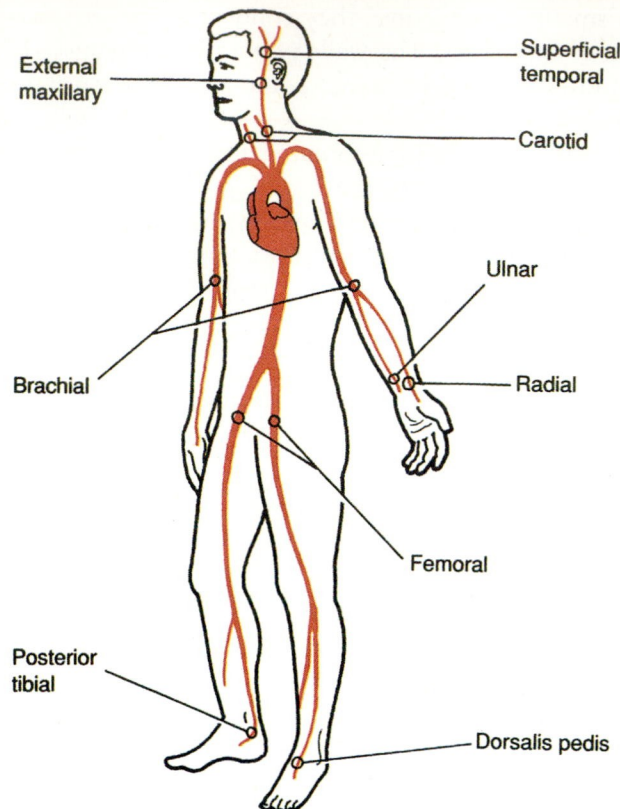

FIGURE 4-43 The central and peripheral pulses can be felt where the large arteries are near the skin.

groin. The peripheral pulses are the radial artery pulse, which is felt at the wrist at the base of the thumb; the brachial artery pulse, which is felt on the medial aspect of the arm, midway between the elbow and shoulder; the posterior artery pulse, which is felt posterior to the medial malleolus; and the dorsalis pedis artery pulse, which is felt on the top of the foot (Figure 4-43).

<u>Blood pressure</u> is the pressure that the blood exerts against the walls of the arteries as it passes through them. When the cardiac muscle of the left ventricle contracts, it pumps blood from the ventricle into the aorta. This muscular contraction phase is called <u>systole</u>. When the muscle of the ventricle relaxes, the ventricle fills with blood. This phase is called <u>diastole</u>. The pulsed forceful ejection of blood from the left ventricle of the heart into the aorta is transmitted through the arteries as a pulsatile pressure wave. This pressure wave keeps the blood moving through the body. The high and low points of the wave can be measured with a sphygmomanometer (blood pressure cuff) and are expressed numerically in millimeters of mercury (mm Hg). The high point is called the systolic blood pressure (measured as the heart muscle is contracting). The low point is called the diastolic blood pressure (measured when the heart muscle is in its relaxation phase).

The average adult has approximately 6 L of blood in the vascular system. Children have less, 2 to 3 L, depending on their age and size. Infants have only about 300 mL. The loss of an amount of blood that may be negligible for an adult could be fatal for an infant.

Normal circulation in adults. In all healthy people, the circulatory system is automatically adjusted and readjusted constantly so that 100% of the capacity of the arteries, veins, and capillaries holds 100% of the blood at that moment. Never are all the vessels fully dilated or constricted. The size of arteries and veins is controlled by the nervous system, according to the amount of blood that is available and many other factors to keep blood pressure normal at all times. Under the condition of normal pressure, with a system that can hold just 100% of the blood available, all parts of the system will have adequate blood supply all of the time.

Perfusion is the circulation of blood within an organ or tissue in adequate amounts to meet the cells' current needs. Blood enters an organ or tissue through the arteries and leaves it through the veins (Figure 4-44). Loss of normal blood pressure is an indication that the blood is no longer circulating efficiently to every organ in the body. There are many reasons for loss of blood pressure. The result in each case is the same: Organs, tissues, and cells are no longer adequately perfused or supplied with oxygen and food, and wastes can accumulate. Under these conditions, cells, tissues, and whole organs may die. The state of inadequate circulation, when it involves the entire body, is called shock.

Inadequate circulation in adults. When a patient loses a small amount of blood, the arteries, veins, and heart automatically adjust to the smaller new volume. The adjustment occurs in an effort to maintain adequate pressure throughout the circulatory system and thereby maintain circulation for every organ. The adjustment occurs very rapidly after the loss, usually within minutes. Specifically, the vessels contract to provide a smaller bed for the reduced volume of blood to fill. And the heart pumps more rapidly to circulate the remaining blood more efficiently. As the blood pressure falls, the pulse increases to attempt to keep the cardiac output constant at 5 to 6 L per minute. If the loss of blood is too great, the adjustment fails, and the patient goes into shock.

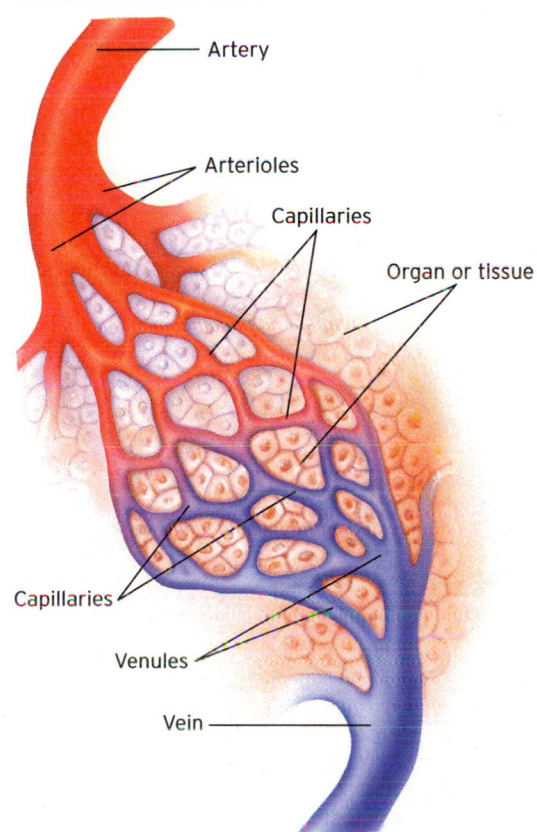

FIGURE 4-44 Blood enters an organ or tissue through the arteries and leaves through the veins. This process, call perfusion, provides adequate blood flow to the tissue to meet the cells' needs.

Artery
Arterioles
Capillaries
Organ or tissue
Capillaries
Venules
Vein

The Nervous System

The nervous system controls virtually all activities of the body, both voluntary and involuntary activities. The somatic nervous system is the part of the nervous system that regulates activities over which there is voluntary control. Such activities include walking, talking, and writing. The autonomic nervous system controls the many body functions that occur without voluntary control. These activities include body functions such as digestion, dilation and constriction of blood vessels, sweating, and all other involuntary actions that are necessary for basic body functions. Anatomically, the nervous system is divided into two parts: the central nervous system and the peripheral nervous system. Thus, the nervous system as a whole can be divided *anatomically* into the central and peripheral nervous systems, and *functionally* into somatic (voluntary) and autonomic (involuntary) components.

The Central Nervous System

The central nervous system (CNS) is made up of the brain and the spinal cord. From a practical point of view, the central nervous system can be considered the

FIGURE 4-45 The brain lies well protected within the skull. Its principal subdivisions are the cerebrum, the cerebellum, and the brain stem.

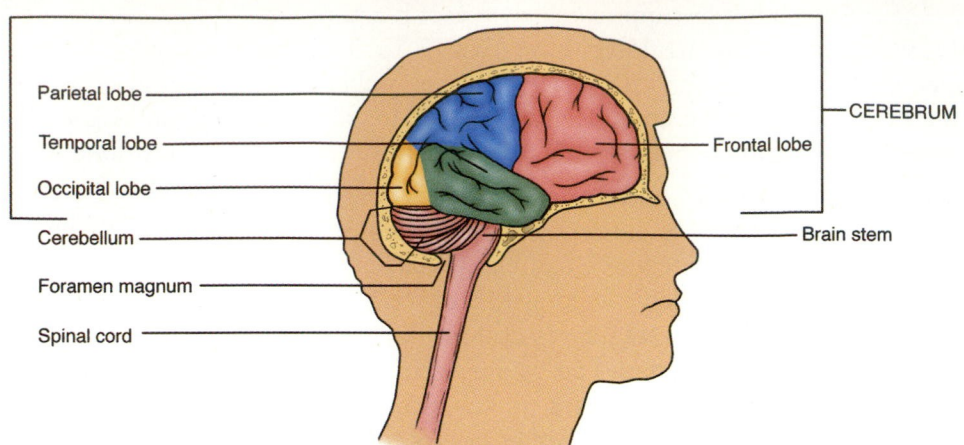

Parietal lobe

Temporal lobe

Occipital lobe

Cerebellum

Foramen magnum

Spinal cord

CEREBRUM

Frontal lobe

Brain stem

part of the nervous system that is covered and protected by bones. The brain is covered by the skull, and the spinal cord is covered by the spinal column. The major parts of most nerve cells (the nucleus and the cell body) lie within the central nervous system.

Brain. The <u>brain</u> is the controlling organ of the body. It is the center of consciousness. It is responsible for all our voluntary body activities, the perception of our surroundings, and the control of our reactions to the environment. In addition, the brain enables us to experience all the fine shadings of thought and feeling that make us individuals. The brain is subdivided into several areas, all of which have specific functions. Three major subdivisions of the brain are the cerebrum, the cerebellum, and the brain stem (Figure 4-45).

The <u>cerebrum</u>, which is the largest part of the brain and is sometimes called the "gray matter," makes up about three fourths of the volume of the brain and is itself composed of four lobes: frontal, parietal, temporal, and occipital. The cerebrum on one side of the brain controls activities on the opposite side of the body. Each lobe of the cerebrum is responsible for a specific function. For example, one group of brain cells in the frontal lobe is responsible for the activity of all the voluntary muscles of the body. Brain cells in this area generate impulses that are sent along nerve fibers that extend from each cell into the spinal cord. Another area in the parietal lobe has cells that receive sensory impulses from the peripheral nerves of the body. Other parts of the cerebrum are responsible for other body functions. For instance, the occipital region, on the back of the cerebrum, receives visual impulses for the eyes; other areas control hearing, balance, and speech. Still other parts of the cerebrum are responsible for emotions preparing other characteristics of an individual's personality.

The <u>cerebellum</u>, which is located underneath the great mass of cerebral tissue, is sometimes called the "little brain." The major function of this area is to coordinate the various activities of the brain, particularly body movements. Without the cerebellum, very specialized muscular activities such as writing or sewing would be impossible.

The <u>brain stem</u> is so called because the brain appears to be sitting on this portion of the central nervous system as a plant sits on its stem. The brain stem is the most primitive part of the central nervous system. It lies deep within the cranium and is the best-protected part of the central nervous system. The brain stem is the controlling center for virtually all body functions that are absolutely necessary for life. Cells in this part of the brain control cardiac, respiratory, and other basic body functions.

The brain has many other anatomic areas, all of which have specific and important functions. The brain receives a vast amount of information from the environment, sorts it all out, and directs the body to respond appropriately. Many of the responses involve voluntary muscle action; others are automatic and involuntary.

The spinal cord. The spinal cord is the other major portion of the central nervous system (Figure 4-46). Like the brain, the spinal cord contains nerve cell bodies, but the major portion of the spinal cord is made up of nerve fibers that extend from the cells of the brain. These nerve fibers transmit information to and from the brain. All the fibers join together just below the brain stem to form the spinal cord. The spinal cord exits through a large opening at the base of the skull called the foramen magnum. It is encased within the spinal canal down to the level of the second lumbar vertebra. The spinal canal is created by the vertebrae, stacked one on another. Each vertebra surrounds the cord, and together the vertebrae form the bony spinal canal.

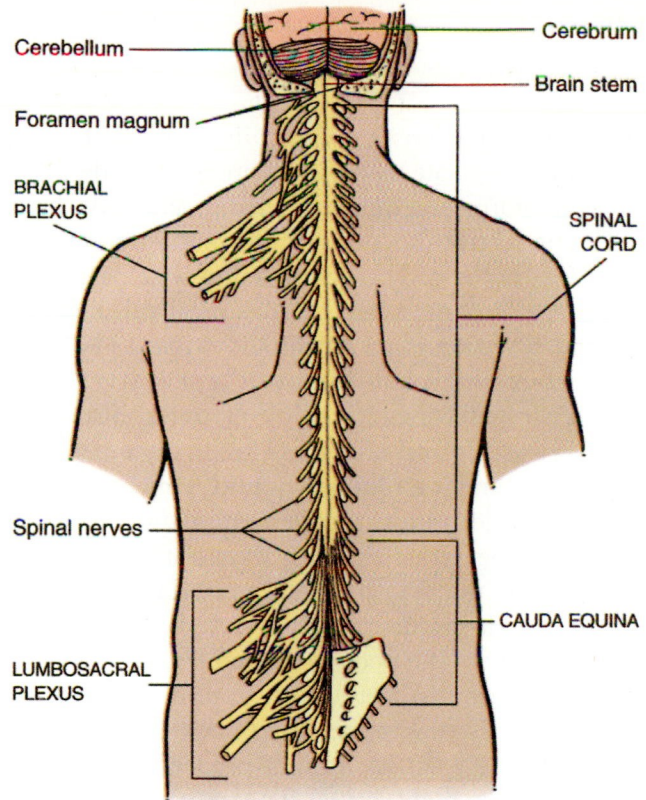

Cerebellum

Cerebrum

Brain stem

Foramen magnum

BRACHIAL PLEXUS

SPINAL CORD

Spinal nerves

CAUDA EQUINA

LUMBOSACRAL PLEXUS

FIGURE 4-46 The spinal cord is a continuation of the brain stem. It exits the skull at the foramen magnum and extends down to the level of the second lumbar vertebra.

The principal function of the spinal cord is to transmit messages between the brain and the body. These messages are passed along the nerve fibers as electrical impulses, just as messages are passed along a telephone cable. The nerve fibers are arranged in specific bundles within the spinal cord to carry the messages from one specific area of the body to the brain and back.

The Peripheral Nervous System

Many of the cells in the central nervous system have long fibers that extend from the cell body out through openings in the bony covering of the spinal canal to form a cable of nerve fibers that link the central nervous system to the various organs of the body. These cables of nerve fibers make up the peripheral nervous system. The three major types of nerves are sensory nerves, motor nerves, and connecting nerves. Sensory nerves carry information from the body to the central nervous system. Motor nerves carry information from the central nervous system to the muscles of the body. Connecting nerves do just what their name implies: They connect the sensory and motor nerves.

The nervous system controls virtually all activities of the body, both voluntary and involuntary activities.

The peripheral nervous system is composed of 31 pairs of peripheral nerves called spinal nerves and 12 pairs called cranial nerves. At each vertebral level from the first cervical to the fifth sacral, on each side of the spinal cord, a spinal nerve exits the spinal cord and passes through an opening in the bony canal. This spinal nerve is composed of nerve fibers from nerve cells that originate within the spinal cord. The nerve fibers conduct sensory impulses from the skin and other organs to the spinal cord. They also conduct motor impulses from the spinal cord to the muscles that are present in that segment of the body. For example, between the seventh and eighth ribs, the spinal nerve carries sensory fibers from the skin between those two ribs and also has motor nerve fibers to innervate the intercostal muscle between the seventh and eighth ribs. This specific arrangement of nerve fibers becomes more complex and confusing in both the cervical and lumbar regions because of the large number of muscles in the arms and legs that must be supplied with nerve fibers. The spinal nerves combine to form a complex nerve network (called a plexus) in these two areas: the brachial plexus for the upper extremity and the lumbosacral plexus for the lower extremity.

The 12 pairs of peripheral nerves that exit the brain through holes in the skull are called the cranial nerves. For the most part, they are very specialized nerves that provide specific functions in the head and face. For example, the facial (seventh cranial) nerves send motor impulses to many of the facial muscles.

Sensory nerves. Sensory nerves of the body are quite complex. There are many different types of sensory cells in the nervous system. One type forms the retina of the eye; others are responsible for the hearing and balancing mechanisms in the ear. Other sensory cells are located within the skin, muscles, joints, lungs, and other organs of the body. When a sensory cell is stimulated, it transmits its own special message to the brain. There are special sensory nerves to detect heat, cold, position, motion, pressure, pain, balance, light, taste, and smell, as well as other sensations. Specialized nerve endings are adapted for each cell so that it perceives only one type of sensation and it transmits only that message.

The sensory impulses constantly provide information to the brain about what the different parts of our body are doing in relation to our surroundings. Thus, the brain is continuously made aware of its surroundings. The cranial nerves supply sensations directly to the brain. Visual sensations (what we see) reach the brain directly by way of the *optic nerve* (the second cranial nerve) in each eye. The nerve endings for the optic nerve lie in the retina of the eye. The nerve endings are stimulated by light, and the impulses are carried along the nerve that passes through a hole in the back of the eye socket and carries impulses to the occipital portion of the brain.

When sensory nerve endings in the extremities are stimulated, the impulses are transmitted along a peripheral nerve to the spinal cord. The cell body of the peripheral nerve lies in the spinal cord. The impulse is then transmitted from that cell body to another nerve ending in the spinal cord. The impulse is then sent up the spinal cord to the sensory area in the parietal lobe of the brain, where the sensory information can be interpreted and acted on by the brain.

Motor nerves. Each muscle in the body has its own motor nerve. The cell body for each motor nerve lies in the spinal cord, and a fiber from the cell body extends as part of the peripheral nerve to its specific muscle. Electrical impulses that are produced by the cell body in the spinal cord are transmitted along the motor nerve to the muscle and cause it to contract. The cell body in the spinal cord is stimulated by an impulse produced in the motor strip of the cerebral cortex. This impulse is transmitted along the spinal cord to the cell body of the motor nerve.

Connecting nerves. Within the brain and the spinal cord are cells with short fibers that connect the sensory nerves with the motor nerves. In the spinal cord, they connect the sensory and motor nerves directly, bypassing the brain. These connecting nerves allow sensory and motor impulses to be transmitted from one nerve to another within the central nervous system.

The connecting nerves in the spinal cord complete a reflex arc between the sensory and motor nerves of the limbs. An irritating stimulus to the sensory nerve, such as heat, will be transmitted from the sensory nerve along the connecting nerve directly to the motor nerve. This will stimulate the sensory nerve. The muscle responds promptly, withdrawing the limb from the irritating stimulus even before this information can be transmitted to the brain. When a physician taps your knee with a rubber hammer, he or she is testing to see whether your reflex arc is intact.

The Skin

The skin, the largest single organ in the body, serves three major functions: to protect the body in the environment, to regulate the temperature of the body, and to transmit information from the environment to the brain.

The protective functions of the skin are numerous. Over 70% of the body is composed of water. The water contains a delicate balance of chemical substances in solution. The skin is watertight and serves to keep this balanced internal solution intact. The skin also protects the body from the invasion of infectious organisms: bacteria, viruses, and fungi. These organisms are everywhere and are routinely found lying on the skin surface and deep in its grooves and glands. However, they never penetrate the skin unless it is broken by injury; thus, the skin provides a constant protection against outside invaders.

The energy of the body is derived from **metabolism** (chemical reactions) that must take place within a very narrow temperature range. If the body temperature is too low, these reactions cannot proceed, metabolism ceases, and the body dies. If the temperature becomes too high, the rate of metabolism increases. Dangerously high temperatures producing too high a metabolic rate can result in permanent tissue damage and death.

Functions of the Skin

The major organ for regulation of body temperature is the skin. Blood vessels in the skin constrict when the body is in a cold environment and dilate when the body is in a warm environment. In a cold environment, constriction of the blood vessels shunts the blood away from the skin to decrease the amount of heat radiated from the body surface. When the outside environment is hot, the vessels in the skin dilate, the skin becomes flushed or red, and heat radiates from the body surface.

Also, in the hot environment, sweat is secreted to the skin surface from the sweat glands. Evaporation of the sweat requires energy. This energy, as body heat, is taken from the body during the evaporation process, which causes the body temperature to fall. Sweating alone will not reduce body temperature; evaporation of the sweat must also occur.

Information from the environment is carried to the brain through a rich supply of sensory nerves that originate in the skin. Nerve endings that lie in the skin are adapted to perceive and transmit information about heat, cold, external pressure, pain, and the position of the body in space. The skin thus recognizes any changes in the environment. The skin also reacts to pressure, pain, and pleasurable stimuli.

Anatomy of the Skin

The skin is divided into two parts: the superficial epidermis, which is composed of several layers of cells, and the deeper dermis, which contains the specialized skin structures (Figure 4-47). Below the skin lies the subcutaneous layer of fat. The cells of the epidermis are sealed to form a watertight protective covering for the body.

The <u>epidermis</u> is actually composed of several layers of cells. At the base of the epidermis is the germinal layer, which continuously produces new cells that gradually rise to the surface. On the way to the surface, these cells die and form the watertight covering. The epidermal cells are held together securely by an oily substance called sebum, which is secreted by the <u>sebaceous glands</u> of the dermis. The outermost cells of the epidermis are constantly rubbed away and then replaced by new cells produced by the germinal layer. The deeper cells in the germinal layer also contain pigment granules that (along with the blood vessels lying in the dermis) produce skin color.

The epidermis varies in thickness in different areas of the body. On the soles of the feet, the back, and the scalp, it is quite thick, but in some areas of the body, the epidermis is only two or three cell layers thick. The watertight seal provided by the epidermis prevents the invasion of bacteria and other organisms.

The deeper part of skin, the <u>dermis</u>, is separated from the epidermis by the layer of germinal cells. Within the dermis lie many of the special structures of the skin: sweat glands, sebaceous (oil) glands, hair follicles, blood vessels, and specialized nerve endings.

<u>Sweat glands</u> produce sweat for cooling the body. The sweat is discharged onto the surface of the skin through small pores, or ducts, that pass through the epidermis onto the skin surface. The sebaceous glands produce sebum, the oily material that seals the surface epidermal cells. The sebaceous glands lie next to hair follicles and secrete sebum along the hair follicle to the skin surface. In addition to providing waterproofing for the skin, sebum keeps the skin supple so that it does not crack.

<u>Hair follicles</u> are the small organs that produce hair. There is one follicle for each hair connected with a sebaceous gland and also with a tiny muscle. The muscle pulls the hair into an erect position when the individual is cold or frightened. All hair grows continuously and is either cut off or worn away by clothing.

Blood vessels provide nutrients and oxygen to the skin. The blood vessels lie in the dermis. Small branches extend up to the germinal layer. There are no blood vessels in the epidermis. A complex array of nerve endings also lie in the dermis. These specialized nerve endings are sensitive to environmental stimuli; they respond to these stimuli and send impulses along the nerves to the brain.

Beneath the skin, immediately under the dermis and attached to it, lies the <u>subcutaneous tissue</u>. The subcutaneous tissue is composed largely of fat. The fat serves as an insulator for the body and as a reservoir to store energy. The amount of subcutaneous tissue varies

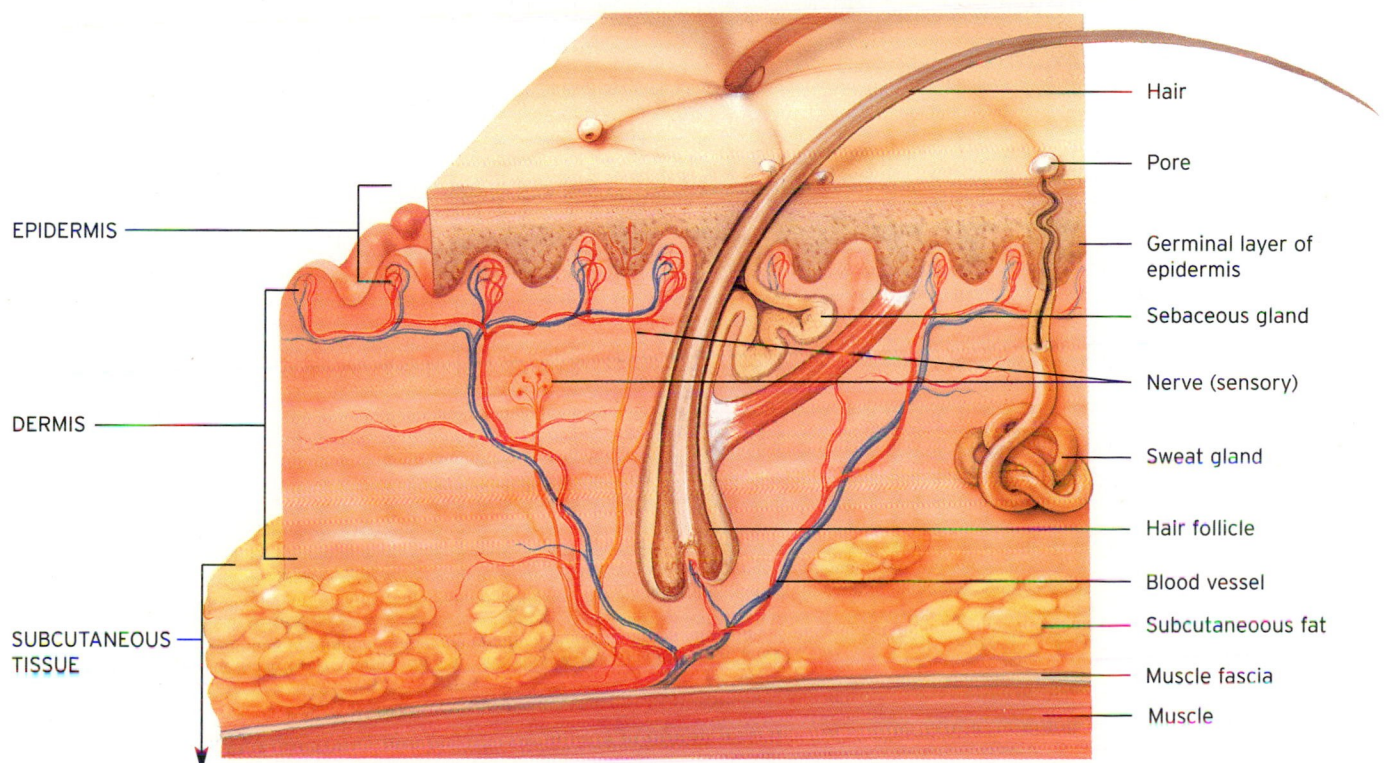

FIGURE 4-47 The skin has two principal layers: the epidermis and the dermis. Below the skin is a layer of subcutaneous fat.

greatly from individual to individual. Beneath the sub-cutaneous tissue lie the muscles and the skeleton.

The skin covers all of the external surface of the body. The various orifices (openings to the body)—including the mouth, nose, anus, and vagina—are not covered by skin. Orifices are lined with mucous membranes. Mucous membranes are quite similar to skin in that they provide a protective barrier against bacterial invasion. Mucous membranes differ from skin in that they secrete mucus, a watery substance that lubricates the openings. Thus, mucous membranes are moist, whereas the skin is dry. A mucous membrane lines the entire gastrointestinal tract from the mouth to the anus.

The Endocrine System

The brain controls the body through both the nervous system and the endocrine system. The endocrine system is a complex message and control system that integrates many body functions. It releases substances called hormones, either by target organs or directly (Figure 4-48). Adrenaline and insulin are examples of hormones. Each endocrine gland produces one or more hormones. Each hormone has a specific effect on some organ, tissue, or process (Table 4-5). The brain controls

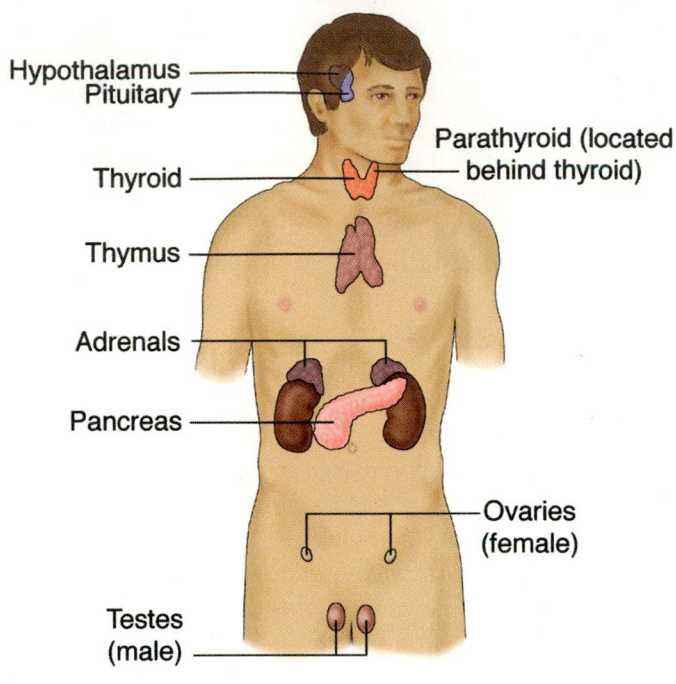

FIGURE 4-48 The endocrine system controls the release of hormones in the body.

TABLE 4-5	Endocrine Glands		
Gland	**Location**	**Function**	**Hormones Produced**
Adrenal	Abdomen	Regulate salt, sugar, and sexual function	Adrenaline (epinephrine) and others
Ovary	Female pelvis (2 glands)	Regulate sexual function, characteristics, and reproduction	Estrogen and others
Pancreas	Abdomen	Regulate glucose metabolism and other functions	Insulin and others
Parathyroid	Neck (behind the thyroid) (3-5 glands)	Regulate serum calcium	Parathormone
Pituitary	Base of skull	Regulate all other endocrine glands	Multiple, very important hormones
Testes	Male scrotum (2 glands)	Regulate sexual function, characteristics, and reproduction	Testosterone and others
Thyroid	Neck (over the larynx)	Regulate metabolism	Thyroxin and others

the release of hormones by the endocrine glands with other (stimulating or inhibiting) hormones. The final effect influences the endocrine glands and the brain. As a result, we have a tightly controlled system with primary and secondary feedback loops to keep body systems in balance (Figure 4-49). For example, when we are frightened, the brain stimulates the adrenal gland through a hormone to release adrenaline (epinephrine). Release of adrenaline increases our blood pressure and heart rate. The resulting increase in blood pressure and heart rate decreases the amount of hormone released by the adrenal gland. The brain then reduces the amount of stimulation to the adrenal gland. Thus, a new steady state is achieved at heightened levels of alertness. Insulin is another hormone that is intimately involved in the control of the blood glucose and metabolism of food.

Excesses or deficiencies in hormones cause various diseases. With endocrine diseases, specific body functions are increased, decreased, or absent. Diabetes mellitus is a common problem. Because production of the hormone insulin is deficient, the body is unable to use glucose normally. This disease also damages the small blood vessels in the body. The tissue damage that results is as much a part of diabetes as is the difficulty in regulating the amount of glucose in the blood.

The Digestive System

The digestive system is composed of the gastrointestinal tract (stomach and intestines), mouth, salivary glands, pharynx, esophagus, liver, gallbladder, pancreas, rectum, and anus. The function of this system is **digestion**: the processing of food that nourishes the individual cells of the body.

How Digestion Works

Digestion of food, from the time it is taken into the mouth until essential compounds are extracted and delivered by the circulatory system to nourish all of the cells in the body, is a complicated chemical process. In succession, different secretions, primarily enzymes, are added to the food by the salivary glands, the stomach, the liver, the pancreas, and the small intestine to convert the food into basic sugars, fatty acids, and amino acids. These basic products of digestion are carried across the wall of the intestine and transported through the portal vein to the liver. In the liver, the products are processed further and then stored or transported to the heart through veins draining that organ. The heart then pumps the blood with these nutrients throughout the

arteries and then to the capillaries, where the nutrients pass through the capillary walls to nourish the body's individual cells.

In normal routine activity, without any food or fluid ingestion at all, between 8 to 10 L of fluid are secreted daily into the gastrointestinal tract. This fluid comes from the salivary glands, stomach, liver, pancreas, and small intestine. In a normal adult, about 7% of the body weight is delivered as fluid daily to the gastrointestinal tract. If significant vomiting or diarrhea occurs for more than 2 or 3 days, the patient will lose a very substantial portion of body composition and become severely ill.

Anatomy of the Digestive System

Mouth. The mouth consists of the lips, cheeks, gums, teeth, and tongue. A mucous membrane lines the mouth. The roof of the mouth is formed by the hard and soft palates. The hard palate is a bony plate lying anteriorly; the soft palate is a fold of mucous membrane and muscle that extends posteriorly from the hard palate into the throat. The soft palate is designed to hold food that is being chewed within the mouth and to help initiate swallowing.

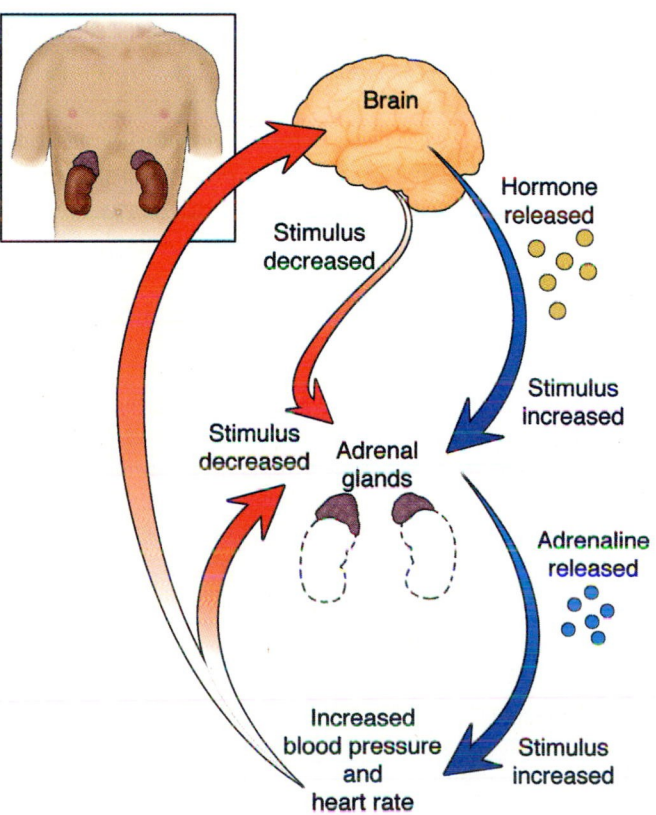

FIGURE 4-49 The endocrine system is tightly controlled with primary and secondary feedback loops to keep body systems in balance.

Salivary glands. There are two salivary glands located under the tongue, one on each side of the lower jaw, and one inside each cheek. They produce nearly 1.5 L of saliva daily. Saliva is approximately 98% water. The remaining 2% is composed of mucus, salts, and organic compounds. Mucus serves as a binder for the chewed food that is being swallowed and as a lubricant within the mouth.

Oropharynx. The oropharynx is a tubular structure about 5″ long that extends vertically from the back of the mouth to the esophagus and trachea. An automatic movement of the pharynx during swallowing lifts the larynx to permit the epiglottis to close over it so that liquids and solids are moved into the esophagus and away from the trachea.

Esophagus. The esophagus is a collapsible tube about 10″ long that extends from the end of the pharynx to the stomach and lies just anterior to the spinal column in the chest. Contractions of the muscle in the wall of the esophagus propel food through it to the stomach. Liquids will pass with very little assistance.

Stomach. The stomach is located in the left upper quadrant of the abdominal cavity, largely protected by the lower left ribs. Muscular contractions in the wall of the stomach and gastric juice, which contains much mucus, convert ingested food to a thoroughly mixed semi-solid mass. The stomach produces approximately 1.5 L of gastric juice daily for this process. The principal function of the stomach is to receive food in large quantities intermittently, store it, and provide for its movement into the small bowel in regular, small amounts. In 1 to 3 hours, the semi-solid food mass derived from one meal is propelled by muscular contraction into the duodenum, the first part of the small intestine.

Pancreas. The pancreas, a flat, solid organ, lies below and behind the liver and stomach and behind the peritoneum on the spine and muscles of the back. It is firmly fixed in position, deep within the abdomen, and is not easily damaged. It contains two kinds of glands. One set of glands secretes nearly 2 L of pancreatic juice daily. This juice contains many enzymes that aid in the digestion of fat, starch, and protein. Pancreatic juice flows directly into the duodenum through the pancreatic ducts. The other kind of gland is the islets of Langerhans, which produces insulin. Insulin regulates the amount of glucose in the blood.

Liver. The liver is a large, solid organ that takes up most of the area immediately beneath the diaphragm in the right upper quadrant. It is the largest solid organ in the abdomen and has several functions. Poisonous substances produced by digestion are brought to the liver and rendered harmless. Factors that are necessary for blood clotting and for the production of normal plasma are formed here. Between 0.5 and 1 L of bile is made by the liver daily to assist in the normal digestion of fat. The liver is the principal organ for the storage of sugar or starch for immediate use by the body for energy. It also produces many of the factors that aid in the proper regulation of immune responses. Anatomically, the liver is a large mass of blood vessels and cells, packed tightly together. It is fragile and, because of its size, relatively easily injured. Blood flow in the liver is high, because all of the blood that is pumped to the gastrointestinal tract passes into the liver, through the portal vein, before it returns to the heart. In addition, the liver has a generous arterial blood supply of its own. Ordinarily, approximately 25% of the cardiac output of blood (1.5 L) passes through the liver each minute.

Bile ducts. The liver is connected to the intestine by the bile ducts. The gallbladder is an outpouching from the bile ducts that serves as a reservoir and concentrating organ for bile produced in the liver. Together, the bile ducts and gallbladder form the biliary system. The gallbladder discharges stored and concentrated bile into the duodenum through the common bile duct. The presence of food in the duodenum triggers a contraction of the gallbladder to empty it. The gallbladder usually contains about 60 to 90 mL of bile.

Small intestine. The small intestine is the major hollow organ of the abdomen. The cells lining the small intestine produce enzymes and mucus to aid in digestion. Enzymes from the pancreas and the small intestine carry out the final processes of digestion. More than 90% of the products of digestion (amino acids, fatty acids, and simple sugars), together with water, ingested vitamins, and minerals are absorbed across the wall of the lower end of the small intestine into veins to be transported to the liver. The small intestine is composed of the duodenum, the jejunum, and the ileum. The duodenum, which is about 12″ long, is the part of the small intestine that receives food from the stomach. Here, food is mixed with secretions from the pancreas and liver for further digestion. Bile, produced by the liver and stored in the gallbladder, is emptied as needed into the duodenum. It is greenish black, but through changes during digestion, it gives feces its typical brown color. Its major function is in the digestion of fat. The jejunum and ileum together measure more than 20′ on average to make up the rest of the small intestine.

Large intestine. The large intestine, another major hollow organ, consists of the cecum, the colon, and the rectum. About 5' long, it encircles the outer border of the abdomen around the small bowel. The major function of the colon, the portion of the large intestine that extends from the cecum to the rectum, is to absorb the final 5% to 10% of digested food and water from the intestine to form solid stool, which is stored in the rectum and passed out of the body through the anus.

Appendix. The appendix is a tube 3" to 4" long that opens into the cecum (the first part of the large intestine) in the right lower quadrant of the abdomen. It may easily become obstructed and, as a result, inflamed and infected. Appendicitis, which is the term for this inflammation, is one of the major causes of severe abdominal distress. The appendix has no known function.

Rectum. The lowermost end of the colon is the rectum. It is a large, hollow organ that is adapted to store quantities of feces until it is expelled. At its terminal end is the anus, a 2" canal lined with skin. The rectum and anus are supplied with a complex series of circular muscles called sphincters that control, both voluntarily and automatically, the escape of liquids, gases, and solids from the digestive tract.

The Urinary System

The urinary system controls the discharge of certain waste materials filtered from the blood by the kidneys. In the urinary system, the kidneys are solid organs; the ureters, bladder, and urethra are hollow organs (Figure 4-50). Ordinarily, we consider the urinary and genital systems together, because they share many organs.

The body has two kidneys that lie on the posterior muscular wall of the abdomen behind the peritoneum in the retroperitoneal space. These organs rid the blood of toxic waste products and control its balance of water and salt. Blood flow in the kidneys is high. Nearly 20% of the output of blood from the heart passes through the kidneys each minute. Large vessels attach the kidneys directly to the aorta and the inferior vena cava. Waste products and water are constantly filtered from the blood to form urine. The kidneys continuously concentrate this filtered urine by reabsorbing the water as it passes through a system of specialized tubes within them. The tubes finally unite to form the renal pelvis, a cone-shaped collecting area that connects the ureter and the kidney. Normally, each kidney drains its urine into one ureter through which the urine passes to the bladder.

A ureter passes from the renal pelvis of each kidney along the surface of the posterior abdominal wall behind the peritoneum to drain into the urinary bladder. The ureters are small (0.2" in diameter), hollow, muscular tubes. Peristalsis, or a muscular contraction, occurs in these tubes to move the urine to the bladder.

The urinary bladder is located immediately behind the pubic symphysis in the pelvic cavity and is composed of smooth muscle with a specialized lining membrane. The two ureters enter posteriorly at its base on either side. The bladder empties to the outside of the body through the urethra. In the male, the urethra passes from the anterior base of the bladder through the penis. In the female, the urethra opens at the front of the vagina. The normal adult forms 1.5 to 2 L of urine every day. This waste is extracted and concentrated from the 1,500 L of blood that circulate through the kidneys daily.

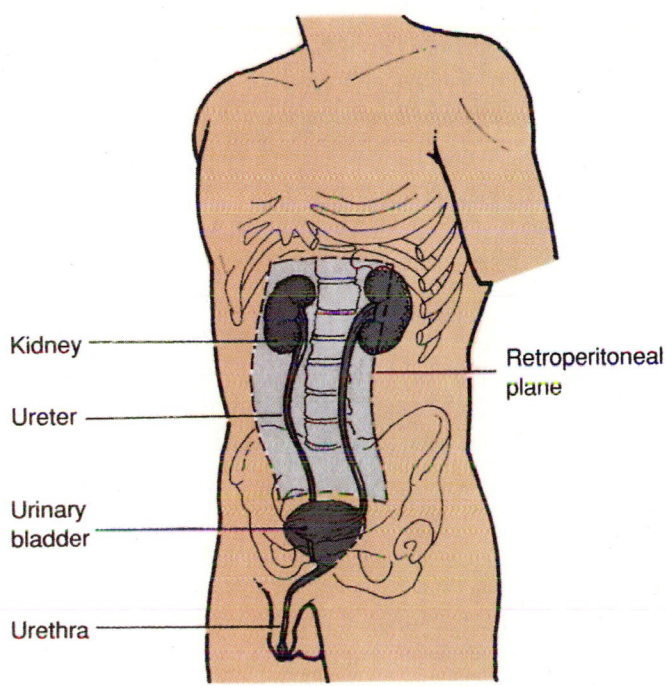

Kidney

Ureter

Urinary bladder

Urethra

Retroperitoneal plane

FIGURE 4-50 The urinary system lies in the retroperitoneal space behind the organs of the digestive system. The kidneys are solid organs; the ureter, bladder, and urethra are hollow organs.

Ordinarily, the urinary and genital systems are considered together because they share many organs.

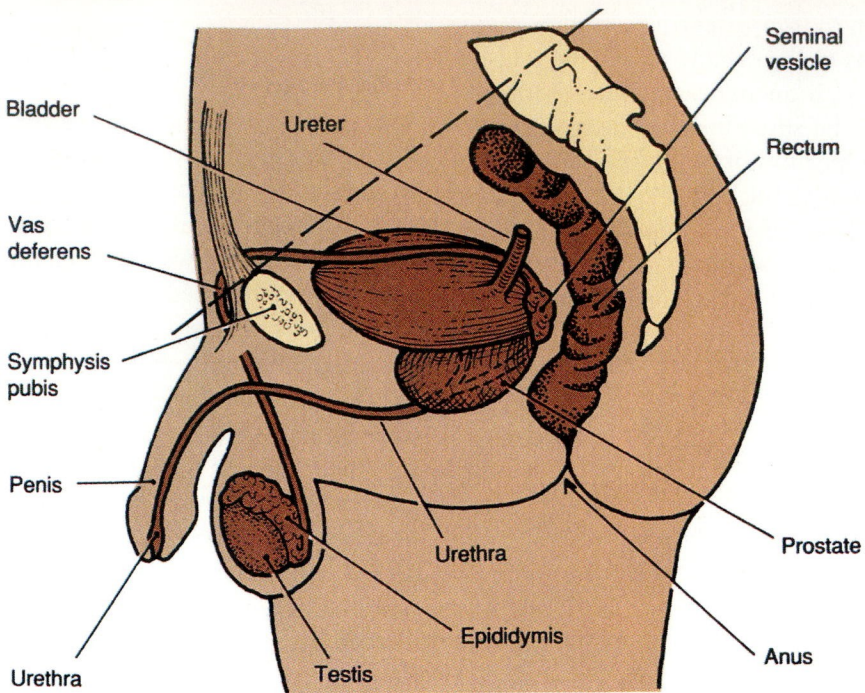

FIGURE 4-51 The male reproductive system consists of the testicles, vasa deferentia, seminal vesicles, prostate gland, urethra, and penis.

The Genital System

The **genital system** controls the reproductive processes by which life is created. The male genitalia, except for the prostate gland and the seminal vesicles, lie outside the pelvic cavity. The female genitalia are contained entirely within the pelvis. The male and female reproductive organs have certain similarities and, of course, basic differences. They allow the production of sperm and egg cells and appropriate hormones and the act of sexual intercourse and reproduction.

The Male Reproductive System and Organs

The male reproductive system consists of the testicles, vasa deferentia, seminal vesicles, prostate gland, urethra, and penis (Figure 4-51). Each **testicle** contains specialized cells and ducts; some of these produce male hormones, and others develop sperm. The hormones are absorbed directly into the bloodstream from the testicles. The **vasa deferentia** travel from the testicles up beneath the skin of the abdominal wall for a short distance. They then pass through an opening into the abdominal cavity and into the prostate gland to connect with the urethra. The vasa deferentia carry the sperm from the testicles to the urethra. The **seminal vesicles** are small storage sacs for sperm and seminal fluid. The vesicles also empty into the urethra.

Semen, also called seminal fluid, contains sperm cells that are carried up each vas from each testicle to be mixed with fluid from the seminal vesicles and prostate gland. The **prostate gland** surrounds the urethra where it emerges from the urinary bladder. Fluids from the prostate gland and from the seminal vesicles mix during sexual intercourse. During intercourse, special mechanisms in the nervous system prevent the passage of urine into the urethra. Only seminal fluid, prostatic fluid, and sperm pass from the penis into the vagina during ejaculation.

The penis contains a special type of tissue called erectile tissue. This specialized tissue is largely vascular and, when filled with blood, causes the penis to distend into a state of erection. As the vessels fill under pressure from the circulatory system, the penis becomes a large, rigid organ that can enter the vagina. Certain spinal injuries and some diseases can cause a painful continuous erection called priapism.

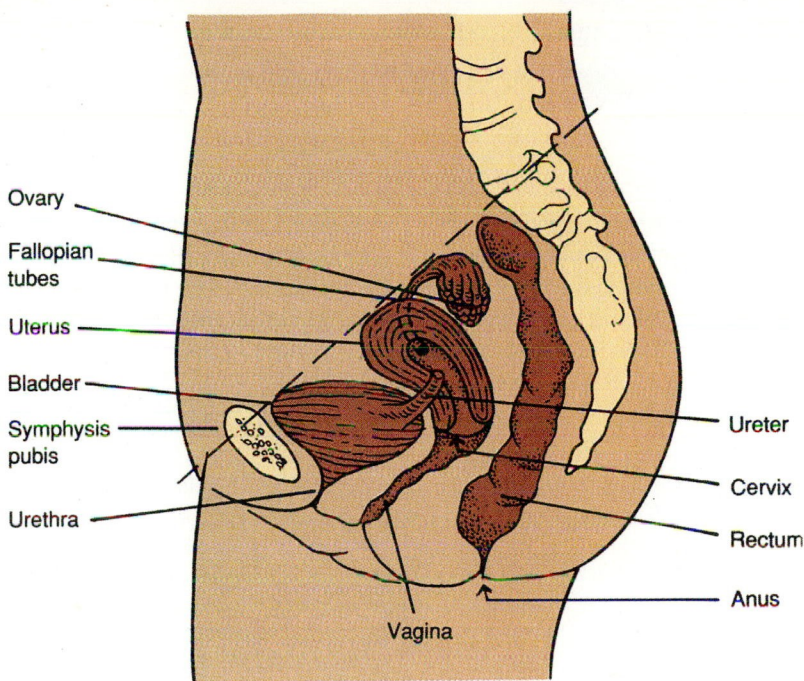

Ovary
Fallopian tubes
Uterus
Bladder
Symphysis pubis
Urethra
Ureter
Cervix
Rectum
Anus
Vagina

FIGURE 4-52 The female reproductive system consists of the ovaries, fallopian tubes, uterus, cervix, and vagina.

The Female Reproductive System and Organs

The female reproductive organs include the ovaries, fallopian tubes, uterus, cervix, and vagina (Figure 4-52). The <u>ovaries</u>, like the testicles, produce sex hormones and specialized cells for reproduction. The female sex hormones are absorbed directly into the bloodstream. A specialized ovum, or egg cell, is produced regularly during the adult female's reproductive years. The ovaries release a mature egg approximately every 28 days. This egg travels through the fallopian tubes to the uterus.

The <u>fallopian tubes</u> connect with the uterus and carry the ovum into the cavity of this organ. The uterus is pear-shaped and hollow, with muscular walls. The narrow opening from the uterus to the vagina is the cervix. The <u>vagina</u> is a muscular distensible tube that connects the uterus with the vulva (the external female genitalia). The vagina receives the penis during sexual intercourse, when semen is deposited in it. The sperm in the semen may pass into the uterus and fertilize an egg, causing pregnancy. Should the pregnancy come to completion at the end of nine months, the baby will pass through the vagina and be born. The vagina also channels the menstrual flow from the uterus out of the body.

prep kit

ready for review

To do your work as an EMT-B, you must have a working knowledge of human anatomy so that you can communicate with hospital personnel and other healthcare providers. You must be able to identify superficial landmarks of the body and know what lies underneath the skin so that you can perform an accurate assessment. Hospital personnel will use these terms to ask you questions about a patient; therefore, it is critical for the well-being of your patient you learn them and can use them correctly.

vital vocabulary

abdomen The second major body cavity that contains the major organs of digestion and excretion.

abduction Motion of a limb away from the midline.

acetabulum The depression in which the femoral head fits snugly.

Adam's apple The firm prominence in the upper part of the larynx formed by the thyroid cartilage. It is more prominent in men than in women.

adduction Motion of a limb toward the midline.

agonal respirations An irregular, gasping respiration, sometimes heard in dying patients.

alveoli The air sacs of the lungs in which the exchange of oxygen and carbon dioxide takes place.

anatomic position The position of reference in which the patient stands facing you, arms at the side, with the palms of the hands forward.

angle of Louis A ridge on the sternum that lies at the level where the second rib is attached to the sternum; provides a constant and reliable bony landmark on the anterior chest wall.

anterior The front surface of the body; the side facing you.

anterior superior iliac spines The hard, bony prominences at the front on each side of the lower abdomen just below the plane of the umbilicus.

aorta The principal artery leaving the left side of the heart and carrying freshly oxygenated blood to the body.

apex (plural: apices) The tip or the topmost portion of a structure.

appendix A small tubular structure that is attached to the lower border of the cecum in the lower right quadrant of the abdomen.

arteriole The smallest branch of an artery leading to the vast network of capillaries.

atrium Upper chamber of the heart.

autonomic nervous system The part of the nervous system that regulates functions, such as digestion and sweating, that are not controlled by a voluntary act of conscious.

ball-and-socket joint A joint that allows internal and external rotation as well as bending.

biceps The large muscle that covers the front of the humerus.

bilateral A body part that appears on either side of the midline.

bile ducts Ducts that convey bile between the liver and the intestine.

blood pressure The pressure that the blood exerts against the walls of the arteries as it passes through them.

brachial artery The major vessel in the upper extremity that supplies blood to the arm.

brain The controlling organ of the body and center of consciousness; functions include perception, control of reactions to the environment, emotional responses, and judgment.

brain stem The area of the brain between the spinal cord and cerebrum, surrounded by the cerebellum; controls functions that are necessary for life, such as respirations.

capillary vessels The fine end divisions of the arterial system that allow contact between cells of the body tissues and the plasma and the red blood cells.

www.emtb.com

carotid artery The major artery that supplies blood to the head and brain.

carpometacarpal joint The joint between the wrist and the metacarpal bones; the thumb joint.

cecum The first part of the large intestine, into which the ileum opens.

central nervous system (CNS) The brain and spinal cord.

cerebellum One of the three major subdivisions of the brain, sometimes called the "little brain"; coordinates the various activities of the brain, particularly body movements.

cerebrum The largest part of the three subdivisions of the brain, sometimes called the "gray matter"; made up of several lobes that control movement, hearing, balance, speech, visual perception, emotions, and personality.

cervical spine The portion of the spinal column consisting of the first seven vertebrae that lie in the neck.

circulatory system The complex arrangement of connected tubes, including the arteries, arterioles, capillaries, venules, and veins, that moves blood, oxygen, nutrients, carbon dioxide, and cellular waste throughout the body.

clavicle The collarbone; it is medial to the sternum and lateral to the scapula.

coccyx The last three or four vertebrae of the spine; the tailbone.

connecting nerves Nerves that connect the sensory and motor nerves.

costal arch A bridge of cartilage that connects the ends of the sixth through tenth ribs with the lower portion of the sternum.

costovertebral angle An angle that is formed by the junction of the spine and the tenth rib.

cranium The area of the head above the ears and eyes; the skull. The cranium contains the brain.

cricoid cartilage A firm ridge of cartilage that forms the lower part of the larynx.

cricothyroid membrane A thin sheet of fascia that connects the thyroid and cricoid cartilages that make up the larynx.

deep Further inside the body and away from the skin.

dermis The inner layer of the skin, containing hair follicles, sweat glands, nerve endings, and blood vessels.

diaphragm A muscular dome that forms the undersurface of the thorax, separating the chest from the abdominal cavity. Contraction of the diaphragm (and the chest wall muscles) brings air into the lungs. Relaxation allows air to be expelled from the lungs.

diastole The dilation, or period of dilatation, of the heart, especially of the ventricles.

digestion The processing of food that nourishes the individual cells of the body.

distal Structures that are nearer to the free end of the extremity.

dorsal The posterior surface of the body, including the back of the hand.

dorsalis pedis artery The artery on the anterior surface of the foot between the first and second metatarsals.

endocrine system The complex message and control system that integrates many body functions, including the release of hormones.

epidermis The outer layer of skin, which is made up of cells that are sealed together to form a watertight protective covering for the body.

prep kit 4

epiglottis A thin, leaf-shaped valve that allows air to pass into the trachea but prevents food or liquid from entering.

esophagus A collapsible tube that extends from the pharynx to the stomach; contractions of the muscle in the wall of the esophagus propel food and liquids through it to the stomach.

extend To straighten.

fallopian tube Long, slender tube that extends from the uterus to the region of the ovary on the same side, and through which the ovum passes from ovary to uterus.

fascia A sheet or band of tough fibrous connective tissue; lies deep under the skin and forms an outer layer for the muscles.

femoral artery The principal artery of the thigh, a continuation of the external iliac artery. It supplies blood to the lower abdominal wall, external genitalia, and legs. It can be palpated in the groin area.

femoral head The proximal end of the femur, articulating with the acetabulum.

femur The thighbone; the longest and one of the strongest bones in the body.

flex To bend.

floating ribs The eleventh and twelfth ribs, which do not attach to the sternum through the costal arch.

foramen magnum A large opening at the base of the skull where the brain connects to the spinal cord.

Fowler's position The position in which the patient is sitting up with the knees bent.

gallbladder A pear-shaped sac on the undersurface of the liver that collects bile from the liver and discharges it into the duodenum through the common bile duct.

genital system The male and female reproductive systems.

greater trochanter A bony prominence on the proximal lateral side of the thigh, just below the hip joint.

hair follicles The small organs that produce hair.

heart A hollow muscular organ that receives blood from the veins and propels it into the arteries.

heart rate (pulse) The wave of pressure that is created by the heart's contracting and forcing blood out the left ventricle and into the major arteries.

hinge joints Joints that can bend and straighten but cannot rotate.

humerus The supporting bone of the arm.

hypoxic drive A "backup system" to control respiration.

iliac crest The rim of the pelvic bone.

ilium One of three bones that fuse to form the pelvic ring.

inferior The part of the body, or any body part, nearer to the feet.

inferior vena cava One of the two largest veins in the body; carries blood from the lower extremities and the pelvic and the abdominal organs into the heart.

inguinal ligament The tough, fibrous ligament that stretches between the lateral edge of the pubic symphysis and the anterior superior iliac spine.

involuntary muscle Muscle that continues to contract, rhythmically, regardless of the conscious will of the individual.

ischium One of three bones that fuse to form the pelvic bones.

joint (articulation) The place where two bones come into contact.

joint capsule The fibrous sac with synovial lining that encloses a joint.

kidneys Two retroperitoneal organs that excrete the end products of metabolism as urine and regulate the body's salt and water content.

large intestine The portion of the digestive tube that encircles the abdomen around the small bowel, consisting of the cecum, the colon, and the rectum.

larynx Voice box: a structure composed of thyroid cartilage on the top and cricoid cartilage on the bottom.

lateral Parts of the body that lie at some distance from the midline. Also called outer structures.

ligaments A band of the fibrous tissue that connect bones to bones. It supports and strengthens a joint.

liver A large solid organ that lies in the right upper quadrant immediately below the diaphragm; it produces bile, stores sugar for immediate use by the body, and produces many substances that help regulate immune responses.

lumbar spine The lower part of the back; formed by the lowest five nonfused vertebrae.

lumbar vertebrae Vertebrae of the lumbar spine.

mandible The bone of the lower jaw.

manubrium The upper quarter of the sternum.

mastoid process A prominent, hard bony mass at the base of the skull behind the ear.

maxillae The upper jawbones that assist in the formation of the orbit, the nasal cavity, and the palate, and lodge the upper teeth.

medial Parts of the body that lie closer to the midline; also called inner structures.

metabolism The sum of all the physical and chemical processes of living organisms; the process by which energy is made available for the uses of the organism.

midaxillary line An imaginary vertical line drawn through the middle of the axilla (armpit), parallel to the midline.

midclavicular line An imaginary vertical line drawn through the middle portion of the clavicle and parallel to the midline.

midline An imaginary vertical line drawn from the middle of the forehead through the nose and the umbilicus (navel) to the floor.

motor nerves Nerves that carry information from the central nervous system to the muscles of the body.

mucous membranes The lining of body cavities and passages that communicate directly or indirectly with the environment outside the body.

mucus The opaque, sticky secretion of the mucous membranes that lubricates the body openings.

musculoskeletal system The bones and voluntary muscles of the body.

myocardium The heart muscle.

nasopharynx The part of the pharynx that lies above the level of the soft palate.

nervous system The system that controls virtually all activities of the body, both voluntary and involuntary activities.

occiput The most posterior portion of the cranium.

orbit The eye socket.

oropharynx A tubular structure that extends vertically from the back of the mouth to the esophagus and trachea.

ovary A female gland that produces sex hormones and ova (eggs).

palmar The front region of the hand.

pancreas A flat, solid organ that lies below the liver and the stomach; it is a major source of digestive enzymes and produces the hormone insulin.

parietal regions The region between the temporal and occiput regions of the cranium.

patella The kneecap; a specialized bone that lies within the tendon of the quadriceps muscle.

perfusion The circulation of blood within an organ or tissue in adequate amounts to meet the cells' current needs.

peripheral nervous system The part of the nervous system that consists of 31 pairs of spinal nerves and 12 pairs of cranial nerves. These peripheral nerves may be sensory nerves, motor nerves, or connecting nerves.

peristalsis The wavelike movement by which the ureters or other tubular organs propel their contents.

pinna The external part of the ear.

plantar The bottom of the foot.

plasma A sticky, yellow fluid that carries the blood cells and nutrients and transports cellular waste material to the organs of excretion.

platelets Tiny, disk-shaped elements that are much smaller than the cells; they are essential in the initial formation of a blood clot, the mechanism that stops bleeding.

pleura The serous membrane covering the lungs and lining the thoracic cavity, completely enclosing a potential space known as the pleural space.

pleural space The potential space between the parietal pleura and the visceral pleura. It is described as "potential" because under normal conditions, the lungs fill this space.

posterior The back surface of the body; the side away from you.

prep kit

4

prep kit

posterior tibial artery The artery just posterior to the medial malleolus; supplies blood to the foot.

prone position The position in which the body is lying face down.

prostate gland A small gland that surrounds the male urethra where it emerges from the urinary bladder; it secretes a fluid that is part of the ejaculatory fluid.

proximal Structures that are closer to the trunk.

pubis One of three bones that fuse to form the pelvic ring.

pulmonary artery The major artery leading from the right ventricle of the heart to the lungs; it carries oxygen-poor blood.

pulmonary veins One of the four veins that return oxygenated blood from the lungs to the left atrium of the heart.

pulse (heart rate) The rate at which the heart is contracting. The normal pulse rate in an adult is 60 to 80 beats/min; for a child, the normal rate is 80 to 100 beats/min.

quadrants The way to describe the sections of the abdominal cavity. Imagine two lines intersecting at the umbilicus dividing the abdomen into four equal areas.

radial artery The major artery in the lower arm; is palpable at the wrist on the thumb side.

radius The bone on the thumb side of the forearm.

rectum The lowermost end of the large intestine.

red blood cells Cells that carry oxygen to the body's tissues; also called erythrocytes.

renal pelvis A cone-shaped collecting area that connects the ureter and the kidney.

respiratory system All the structures of the body that contribute to the process of breathing, consisting of the upper and lower airways.

retroperitoneal Behind the abdominal cavity.

sacrum One of three bones (sacrum and two pelvic bones) that make up the pelvic ring.

salivary glands The glands that produce saliva to keep the mouth and pharynx moist.

scalp The thick skin covering the cranium, which usually bears hair.

scapula The shoulder blade.

sebaceous glands Glands that produce an oily substance called sebum, which discharges along the shafts of the hairs.

semen Seminal fluid ejaculated from the penis and containing sperm.

seminal vesicles Storage sacs for sperm and seminal fluid, which empty into the urethra at the prostate.

sensory nerves The nerves that carry sensations of touch, taste, heat, cold, pain, or other modalities.

shock position The position that has the head and torso (truck) supine and the lower extremities elevated 8" to 12". This helps to increase blood flow to the brain; also referred to as the modified Trendelenburg's position.

shoulder girdle The proximal portion of the upper extremity, made up of the clavicle, the scapula, and the humerus.

skeletal muscle Striated muscle that is attached to bones and usually crosses at least one joint; also called voluntary muscle and striated muscle.

skeleton The framework that gives us our recognizable form; also designed to allow motion of the body and protection of vital organs.

small intestine The portion of the digestive tube between the stomach and the cecum, consisting of the duodenum, jejunum, and ileum.

smooth muscle Nonstriated, involuntary muscle; it constitutes the bulk of the gastrointestinal tract and is present in nearly every organ to regulate automatic activity.

somatic nervous system The part of the nervous system that regulates activities over which there is voluntary control.

spinal cord An extension of the brain, composed of virtually all the nerves carrying messages between the brain and the rest of the body. It lies inside of, and is protected by, the spinal canal.

sternocleidomastoid muscles The muscles on either side of the neck that allow movement of the head.

sternum The breastbone.

striated muscle Muscle that has characteristic stripes, or striations, under the microscope; voluntary, skeletal muscle.

subcutaneous tissue Tissue, largely fat, that lies directly under the dermis and serves as an insulator of the body.

superficial Closer to or on the skin.

superior The part of the body, or any body part, nearer to the head.

superior vena cava One of the two largest veins in the body; carries blood from the upper extremities, head, neck, and chest into the heart.

supine position The position when the body is lying face up.

sweat glands The glands that secrete sweat.

systole The contraction, or period of contraction, of the heart, especially that of the ventricles.

temporal regions The lateral portions on each side of the cranium.

temporomandibular joint The joint that meets with the cranium just in front of each ear.

testicle A male genital gland that contains specialized cells that produce hormones and sperm.

thoracic cage The chest or rib cage.

thoracic spine The 12 vertebrae that lie between the cervical vertebrae and the lumbar vertebrae. One pair of ribs is attached to each of the thoracic vertebrae.

thorax The cavity that contains the heart, lungs, esophagus, and great vessels (the aorta and the two venae cavae).

thyroid cartilage A firm prominence of cartilage that forms the upper part of the larynx; the Adam's apple.

tibia The shinbone, the larger of the two bones of the lower leg.

topographic anatomy The superficial landmarks of the body that serve as guides to the structures that lie beneath them.

torso The trunk without the head and limbs.

trachea The windpipe; the main trunk for air passing to and from the lungs.

Trendelenburg's position The position in which the body is supine with the head lower than the feet.

triceps The muscle in the back of the upper arm.

ulna The inner and larger bone of the forearm, on the side opposite the thumb.

ulnar artery One of the major arteries of the arm; it can be palpated at the medial wrist at the base of the fifth finger.

ureter A small, hollow tube that carries urine from the kidneys to the bladder.

urethra The membranous canal that conveys urine from the bladder to outside the body.

urinary bladder A sac made of smooth muscle that collects and stores urine.

urinary system The organs that control the discharge of certain waste materials filtered from the blood and excreted as urine.

vagina A muscular distensible tube that connect the uterus with the vulva (the external female genitalia); also called the birth canal.

vasa deferentia The spermatic duct of the testicles; also called vas deferens.

ventral The anterior surface of the body.

ventricle The lower chamber of the heart.

voluntary muscle Muscle that is under direct voluntary control of the brain and can be contracted or relaxed at will; skeletal muscle.

white blood cells Blood cells that play a role in the body's immune defense mechanisms against infection.

xiphoid process The narrow, cartilaginous lower tip of the sternum.

zygomas The quadrangular bones of the cheek, articulating with the frontal bone, the maxillae, the zygomatic processes of the temporal bone, and the great wings of the sphenoid bone.

assessment in action

You and your partner are spending a quiet night at the station when you hear gunfire. A neighbor begins banging on the front door to the quarters, yelling, "Come quickly! Someone's been shot!"

Your partner notifies dispatch of the situation and requests law enforcement backup. Once the scene is secured, you and your part-ner move to the front porch and find a 21-year-old man lying on his back. He has one gunshot wound in the right shoulder and one almost directly through the right nipple. He tells you that he "hurts" and is having difficulty breathing.

1. You suspect that the bullet that entered just below the right nipple went straight through the patient before exiting out his back. This path has most likely caused injury to the:
   A. liver.
   B. right lung.
   C. stomach.
   D. spinal cord.

2. On the basis of this injury, you would most likely now suspect that the patient has:
   A. severe internal bleeding.
   B. respiratory compromise.
   C. abdominal pain.
   D. partial paralysis.

3. The patient's pulse rate was very fast on initial assessment. A few minutes later, the pulse is about 70 beats/min. This drop in pulse rate has most likely occurred because the patient has:
   A. some form of CNS depression.
   B. sustained a penetrating injury to the heart.
   C. calmed down after being very frightened.
   D. a history of a major head injury at some time earlier in his life.

4. You look under the pressure dressing over the nipple wound to see whether the bleeding has stopped. Blood squirts out onto your shirt. The bullet has most likely hit:
   A. an artery.
   B. a small vein.
   C. the heart.
   D. a capillary bed.

5. Of the following, which structure is in most need of a steady, uninterrupted supply of oxygen?
   A. Muscles.
   B. Bones.
   C. Brain.
   D. Skin.

points to ponder

Objectives 1–1.8

You respond at 2:00 A.M. to a medical distress call of a 24-year-old woman with acute abdominal pain. The patient describes a burning pain in her lower abdomen. She states that she has had diarrhea for two days now and that her period is due any day. The pain is just superior to her pubic hair. When you palpate the lower quadrants, she complains of pain on both sides.

- Would you expose the area for observation? What organs may be involved? What other questions regarding her body functions would you ask?

online outlook

As an EMT-B, you must have a good understanding of basic human anatomy and physiology. Improve your knowledge by completing Exercise 4 at www.emtb.com.

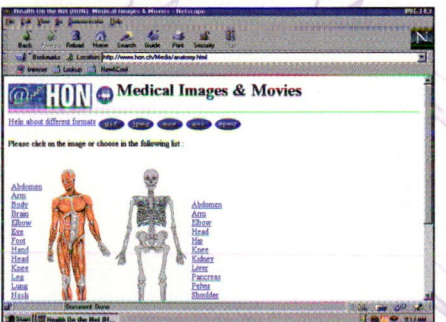

Baseline Vital Signs and SAMPLE History

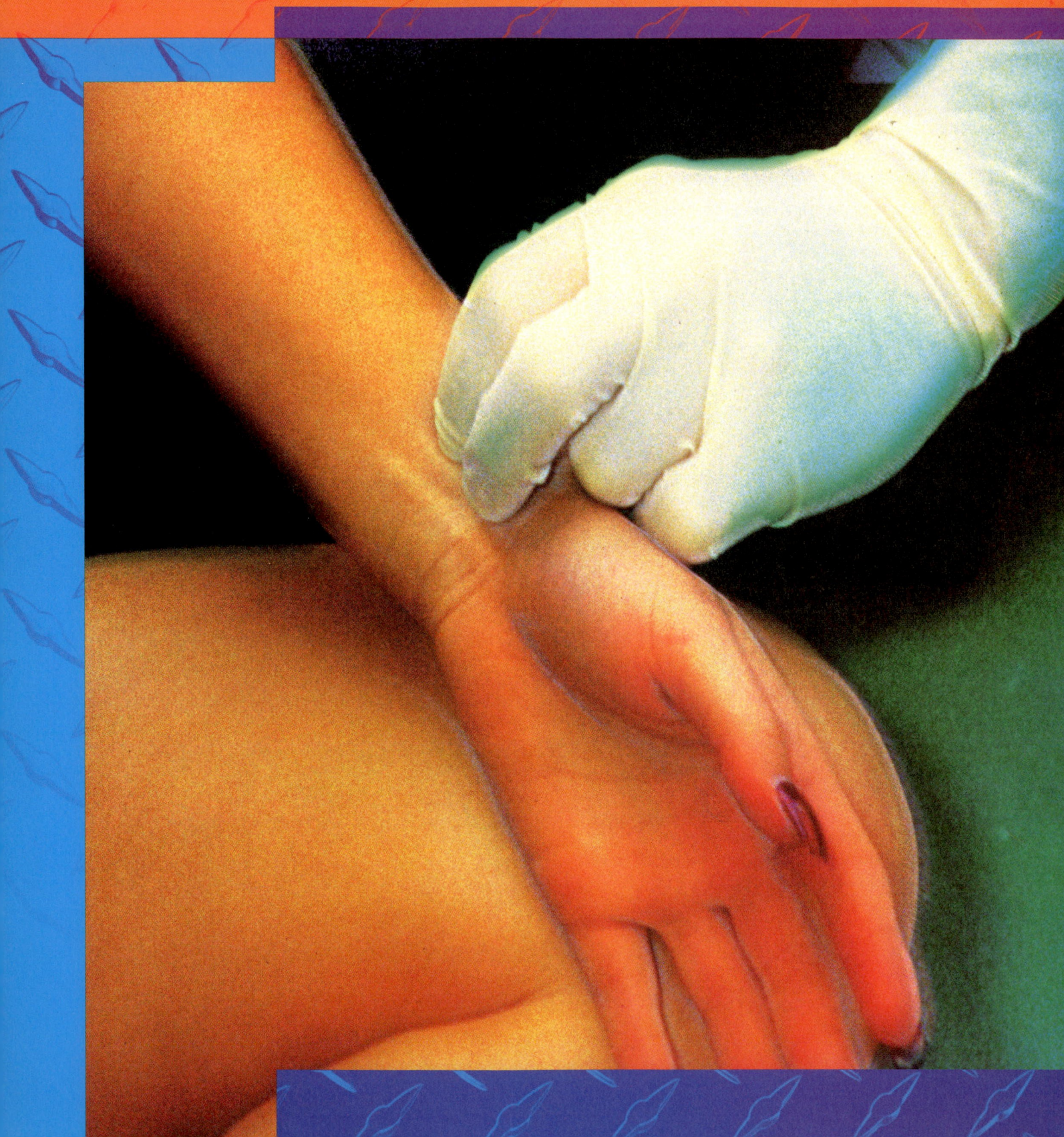

objectives

Cognitive

1. Identify the components of vital signs.

2. Describe the methods to obtain a breathing rate.

3. Identify the attributes that should be obtained when assessing breathing.

4. Differentiate between shallow, labored, and noisy breathing.

5. Describe the methods to obtain a pulse rate.

6. Identify the information obtained when assessing a patient's pulse.

7. Differentiate between a strong, weak, regular, and irregular pulse.

8. Describe the methods to assess the skin color, temperature, condition (capillary refill in infants and children).

9. Identify the normal and abnormal skin colors.

10. Differentiate between pale, blue, red, and yellow skin color.

11. Identify the normal and abnormal skin temperature.

12. Differentiate between hot, cool, and cold skin temperature.

13. Identify normal and abnormal skin conditions.

14. Identify normal and abnormal capillary refill in infants and children.

15. Describe the methods to assess the pupils.

16. Identify normal and abnormal pupil size.

17. Differentiate between dilated (big) and constricted (small) pupil size.

18. Differentiate between reactive and nonreactive pupils and equal and unequal pupils.

19. Describe the methods to assess blood pressure.

20. Define systolic pressure.

21. Define diastolic pressure.

22. Explain the difference between auscultation and palpation for obtaining a blood pressure.

23. Identify the components of the SAMPLE history.

24. Differentiate between a sign and a symptom.

25. State the importance of accurately reporting and recording the baseline vital signs.

26. Discuss the need to search for additional medical identification.

Affective

27. Explain the value of performing the baseline vital signs.

28. Recognize and respond to the feelings patients experience during assessment.

29. Defend the need for obtaining and recording an accurate set of vital signs.

30. Explain the rationale of recording additional sets of vital signs.

31. Explain the importance of obtaining a SAMPLE history.

Psychomotor

32. Demonstrate the skills involved in assessment of breathing.

33. Demonstrate the skills associated with obtaining a pulse.

34. Demonstrate the skills associated with assessing the skin color, temperature, condition, and capillary refill in infants and children.

35. Demonstrate the skills associated with assessing the pupils.

36. Demonstrate the skills associated with obtaining blood pressure.

37. Demonstrate the skills that should be used to obtain information from the patient, family, or bystanders at the scene.

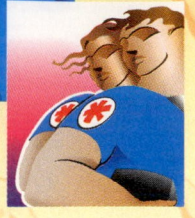

you are the emt

Squad 12, report to Sunnydale Care Facility for a special assignment. You have been assigned to Blood Pressure Day. Your partner groans, "Why are these folks so concerned about their weekly blood pressure check?" "It's good preventive medicine. You have to know the normal pressure to identify the abnormal." Your philosophical answer leaves your partner thinking quietly as you get into your unit to drive to Sunnydale.

This chapter describes the importance of obtaining and evaluating baseline vital signs and the SAMPLE history. It will also help you to answer the following questions:

1. Should vital signs be absolutely accurate, or are approximate readings sufficient?
2. When should you first obtain vital signs? After that, how often should you obtain them?

Baseline Vital Signs and SAMPLE History

As an EMT-B, you must perform a quick but thorough assessment to identify a patient's needs and to provide proper emergency medical care. Patient assessment includes many steps and is the most complex skill that you will learn in the EMT-B course. To make the task easier, it is helpful to identify and discuss the key components and skills of patient assessment before you learn the entire process.

As you begin your assessment, you must gather and record some key information about the patient. You will also need to obtain and evaluate the patient's vital signs. The injuries, illnesses, or symptoms that lead to the call to 9-1-1 and the history of what occurred before and since the call was made are key pieces of information that you will have to obtain by asking a series of questions. You must also learn about the patient's past medical history and overall health.

This chapter begins by defining the chief complaint and signs and symptoms. It then explains what key information about the patient you need to obtain at the start of the assessment and why you need it. It also describes each of the vital signs and provides a step-by-step explanation of how to obtain each. Both normal and abnormal vital signs are discussed. The chapter ends with a description of the SAMPLE history.

Gathering Key Patient Information

During the assessment, you will be using your eyes, ears, nose, hands, and a few basic medical instruments to obtain information about your patient. You will need to know which questions to ask and how to ask them (Figure 5-1). By using your deductive powers, you will be able to interpret the meaning and implications of your findings and the information that you have gathered. When assessing the patient, you will have to look, listen, feel, and think. Your scene size-up or the information that is given to you by a first responder or relative when you arrive at the scene should make it immediately apparent whether you were called to the scene because of an accident with injuries or an acute medical problem.

As you begin the physical examination, you should ask another EMT-B, if available, to obtain the patient's full name, address, age, gender, and race and to record

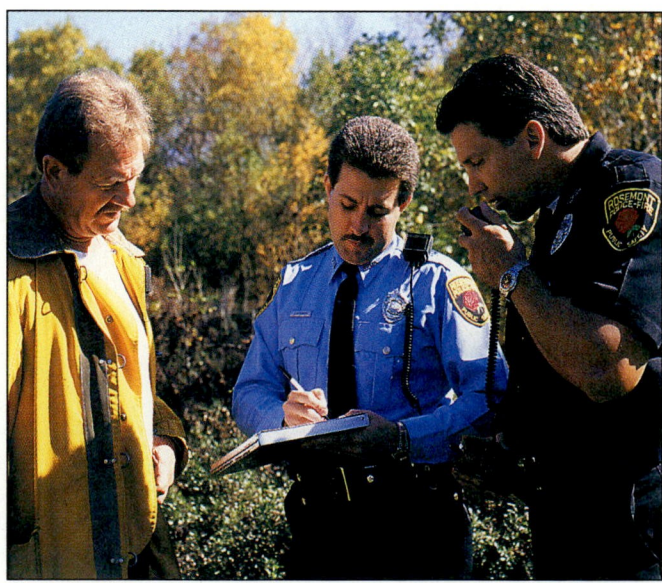

FIGURE 5-1 You must know how to gather information about the scene and the patient by using your senses and by asking relevant questions.

them on the run report. This information may be important if the patient later loses consciousness or becomes disoriented, and it helps the hospital staff to retrieve past medical records. However, *collection of this information is not a priority.* You must not lose sight of the initial assessment and its purpose.

You will also need some of this information in the field. You will need to know the patient's name so that you can properly address the patient. Unless an adult patient is a close friend or relative of yours, you should address him or her as "Mr.," "Ms.," "Miss," or "Mrs.," followed by the patient's last name. You may ask the patient how he or she wishes to be called. Often, relatives or staff members of a nursing home or other extended care facility address elderly patients by their first names. You should not use such a familiar mode of address. If the patient's name is difficult to pronounce, you can simply say "Sir" or "Ma'am" instead, to convey a similar respectful and professional manner.

You should try to address children by their first name, especially the name they are customarily called, such as "Johnny," "Betty," or "Joey." Even infants and toddlers who do not yet respond verbally can recognize their name and may be less anxious when it is used.

If an unaccompanied patient is disoriented or unconscious, you should look in his or her wallet or purse for a driver's license or other piece of identification that will tell you the patient's name. At the same time, you should check for any hospital identification or medical alert card. *Always* look for patient identification in the presence of another EMT or law enforcement officer at the scene.

Age and gender are also important considerations in assessing a patient. Some conditions and illnesses are found predominantly in younger patients; others are commonly found only in older patients. Some conditions are prevalent in a certain age group in adult men but in a different age group in women. Some are more prevalent in one gender, and some are limited exclusively to either male or female patients. In addition, the normal range of some of the vital signs will be different for different age groups of children, adults, and elderly patients.

Chief Complaint/ Mechanism of Injury

The reason that a patient or others call 9-1-1 is vital information. This reason is called the patient's **chief complaint**. In the most literal definition, chief complaints are the major signs and symptoms that the patient reports when asked, "What seems to be the matter?" or "What's wrong?" A patient who responds "My chest hurts" is stating the chief complaint. What you see must also be considered in determining the chief complaint. If the patient's response demonstrates that he or she is having significant difficulty breathing, "difficulty breathing" should be included in the chief complaint as if the patient had reported it verbally. In some protocols, a chief complaint also includes any significant gross, apparent injuries.

The problems or feelings the patients reports to you, such as "I feel dizzy," "My leg hurts," or "Ow, that hurts a lot!" are called **symptoms**. These cannot be felt or observed by others. The severity of a symptom is subjective because it is based on the patient's interpretation and tolerance. **Signs** are conditions that can be seen, heard, felt, smelled, or measured by you or others. Wounds, external bleeding, marked deformities, respirations, and pulse are all signs (Figure 5-2).

Signs and symptoms that occurred before you arrived, such as dizziness that resulted in a loss of consciousness,

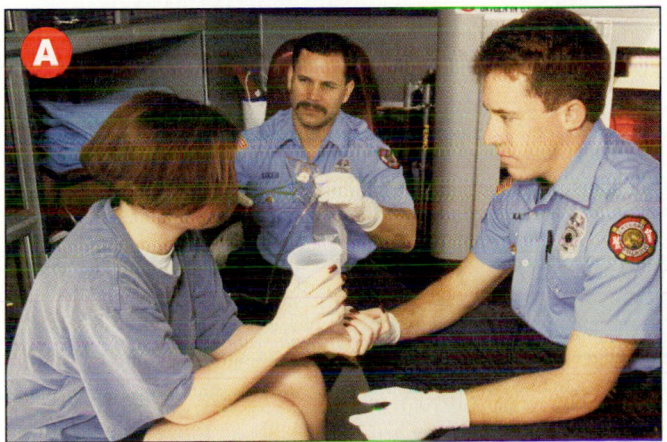
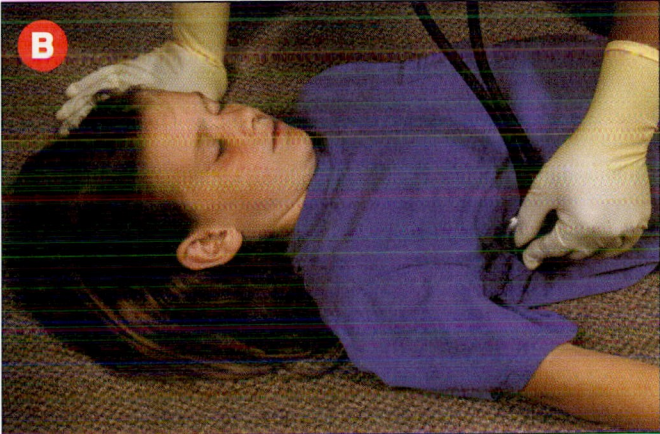

FIGURE 5-2 A: A symptom is a condition that the patient feels and tells you about. **B:** A sign is condition that you can observe about the patient.

may be reported by the patient or others at the scene. Because signs and symptoms are essential to understanding the sequence of events and may include signs that are no longer present, they are important parts of the patient history. You should always report how and/or when the signs and symptoms began. This information is important because the reason that signs and symptoms develop often differs, depending on the situation.

Baseline Vital Signs

The initial assessment is a rapid evaluation of the patient's general condition to identify any potentially life-threatening conditions. The brain and other vital organs require constant oxygen. Significant problems with breathing or circulation must be considered potentially life-threatening conditions. A critical problem or deficit in any of the body's other vital systems or functions will progressively affect and be reflected by changes in the respiratory, circulatory, and central nervous systems. Therefore, the status of these three systems serves as your guideline for evaluating and measuring the patient's general condition.

Vital signs are the key signs that are used to evaluate the patient's initial general condition. The first set of vital signs that you obtain is called the *baseline vital signs*. By periodically reassessing the vital signs and comparing the findings with the baseline set, you will be able to identify any significant trends in the patient's condition, particularly whether the patient's condition is becoming worse (Figure 5-3).

Because key indicators include a quantitative (numeric) objective measurement, you will always include the patient's respirations, pulse, and blood pressure when taking and evaluating the vital signs. Other key indications of the patient's respiratory, cardiovascular, and central nervous system status include evaluation of the following:

- Skin temperature and condition in adults
- Capillary refill in children
- Pupillary reaction
- Level of consciousness

Respirations

A patient who is breathing independently is said to have **spontaneous respirations** or spontaneous ventilations. Each complete breath includes two distinct phases: inspiration and expiration. During inspiration (inhalation), the chest rises up and out, drawing oxygenated air into the alveoli in the lungs. During expiration (exhalation), the chest returns to its original position, releasing air with an increased carbon dioxide level out of the lungs. Inhalation and exhalation times occur in a 1:3 ratio; the active inhalation phase lasts one third the amount of time of the passive exhalation phase.

Breathing is a continuous process in which each breath regularly follows the last with no notable interruption. Breathing is normally a spontaneous automatic process that occurs without conscious thought, visible effort, marked sounds, or pain. You will assess breathing by watching the patient's chest rise and fall, feeling for air through the mouth and nose during exhalation, and listening to breath sounds with a stethoscope over each lung. Chest rise and breath sounds should be equal on both sides of the chest. A conscious patient who is speaking has spontaneous respirations.

When assessing respirations, you must determine the rate, depth, and quality (character) of the patient's breathing.

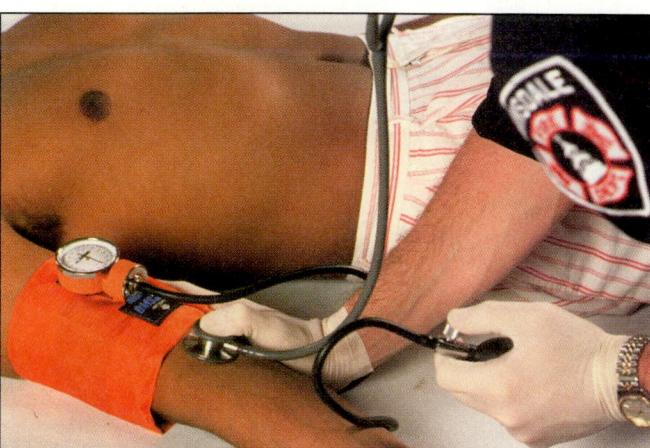

FIGURE 5-3 Baseline vital signs are key signs that are used to evaluate the patient's initial condition.

timing the respirations or pulse rate

When timing a patient's respirations or pulse rate, count the number of breaths or beats in a 30-second period and then multiply by 2. This method produces a significantly more reliable figure than you would get if you counted for only 15 seconds and multiplied by 4. With either method, the result will always be an even number.

You might find it easier to count if you use an analog watch with a sweep second hand or a digital watch with a stopwatch function.

When assessing respirations, you must determine the rate, depth, and quality (character) of the patient's breathing.

Rate. Respirations are determined by counting the number of breaths in a 30-second period and multiplying by 2. The result equals the number of breaths per minute. For accuracy, you should count each breath at the same point in its cycle. This is most easily done by counting each peak chest rise. Although you can see peak chest rise, it is easier to place your hand on the patient's chest and feel it. However, be aware that a conscious patient who knows that you are evaluating his or her breathing will often override the automatic rate and depth by breathing more slowly and deeply. To prevent this from happening, you should check respirations in a conscious, alert patient without making the patient aware of what you are evaluating. This can be easily done by first taking a radial pulse and then, without releasing the wrist or otherwise suggesting a change, counting the chest rise that you see or feel as the patient's forearm rises and falls with the movement of the chest (Figure 5-4). If the patient coughs, yawns, sighs, or talks during the 30-second period, you should wait a few seconds and start again. Table 5-1 shows the normal range of respiratory rates of patients who are at rest.

Normal respirations can vary greatly. In a well-conditioned athlete, normal respirations may be as low as 6 to 8 breaths/min.

Quality. You can determine the quality or character of respirations as you are counting. Table 5-2 shows the four ways in which the quality or character can be described.

Rhythm. While counting the patient's respirations, you should also note the rhythm. If the time from one peak chest rise to the next is fairly consistent, respirations are considered regular. If respirations vary or change frequently, they are considered irregular. When you document the vital signs, be sure to note whether the patient's respirations were regular or irregular.

Depth. The amount of air that the patient is exchanging depends on both the rate and the <u>tidal volume</u>, the amount of air that is exchanged with each breath. The depth of the breath determines whether the tidal volume is normal, less than normal, or more than normal. Respirations are described as shallow when the movement of the chest wall and air that you feel exhaled with each breath is less than normal. Deep respirations occur

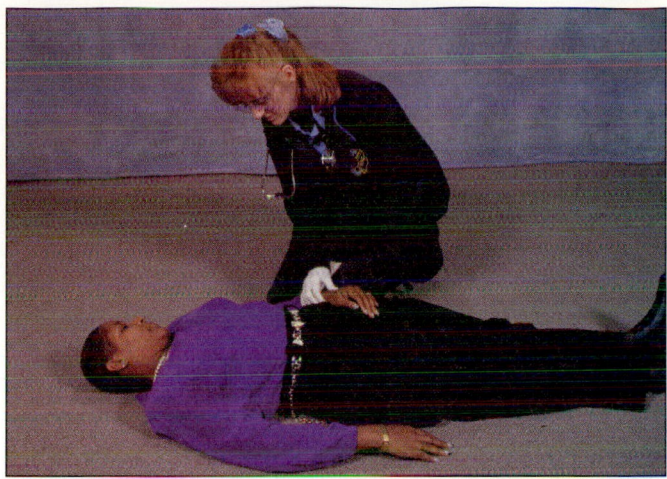

FIGURE 5-4 Assess respirations in a conscious patient by first taking a radial pulse and then, without releasing the patient's wrist, counting the chest rise and fall for 30 seconds.

TABLE 5-1	Normal Ranges for Respirations
Age	**Range**
Adults	12 to 20 breaths/min
Children	15 to 30 breaths/min
Infants	25 to 50 breaths/min

TABLE 5-2	Characteristics of Respirations
Normal	Breathing is neither shallow nor deep
	Average chest wall motion
	No use of accessory muscles
Shallow	Slight chest or abdominal wall motion
Labored	Increased breathing effort
	Grunting, stridor
	Use of accessory muscles
	Possible gasping
	Nasal flaring, supraclavicular and intercostal retractions in infants and children
Noisy	Increase in sound of breathing, including snoring, wheezing, gurgling, and crowing

when chest movement and exhaled air are significantly greater than normal. You should document when the patient's respirations are shallow or deep; however, you do not have to record a normal depth of breathing.

caring for kids

Chest rise in a small child is less marked than that in an adult. However, a small child's abdomen moves more with each breath than an adult's does. Place your hands on the outer margin of the lower anterior chest to feel the chest wall and abdominal movement, and determine whether the depth is normal, shallow, or deep. In a patient of any age, if it is difficult to gauge the depth of breathing from the chest movement, note instead the amount of air that you feel is exhaled with each breath.

Effort. Normally, breathing is an effortless process that does not affect a patient's speech, posture, or positioning. Speech is a good indicator of whether a conscious patient is having difficulty breathing. A patient who can speak smoothly without unusual extra pauses is breathing normally. However, a patient who can speak only one word at a time or must stop every two to three words to catch his or her breath is having significant difficulty breathing. Patients who are having marked difficulty breathing will instinctively assume a posture in which it is easier for them to breathe. This is called the <u>sniffing position</u> or tripod position. In this position, a patient sits unusually upright with the head and chin thrust slightly forward and is having sufficient difficulty breathing that a significant marked conscious effort is required (Figure 5-5) .

Breathing that becomes progressively more difficult requires progressively more effort. When you can see that effort, the patient's breathing is described as <u>labored breathing</u>.

Initially, labored breathing is characterized by the patient's position, concentration on breathing, and the increased effort and depth of each breath. As breathing becomes progressively more labored, accessory muscles in the face and neck are used, and the patient may make some grunting sounds with each breath. In infants and small children, nasal flaring and *supraclavicular* and *intercostal retractions* (indentation above the clavicles and in the spaces between the ribs) are commonly associated with labored breathing. Sometimes, the patient may be gasping.

Infants and small children will continue to have labored breathing for a sustained period, will then often become exhausted, and finally will no longer have the strength to maintain the necessary energy to breathe. These patients will then appear to breathe normally again, even though the amount of ventilation is insufficient; however, their respirations will progressively decline until respiratory arrest develops. In infants and small children, cardiac arrest is generally caused by respiratory arrest.

Noisy breathing. Normal breathing is silent or, in a very quiet environment, accompanied only by the sounds of air movement at the mouth and nose. Through a stethoscope, normal breath sounds include only the sound of air movement through the bronchi accompanied by a soft, low-pitched murmur. Breathing accompanied by other sounds indicates a significant respiratory problem. When the airway is partially obstructed by a foreign body, fluid, or swelling, you may hear <u>stridor</u>, a harsh, high-pitched, crowing sound. If you can hear bubbling or gurgling, the patient probably has fluid in the airway. With a complete airway obstruction, the patient will not be able to pass any air and will no longer be able to cough or talk. You may hear other sounds, including wheezes, snoring, gur-

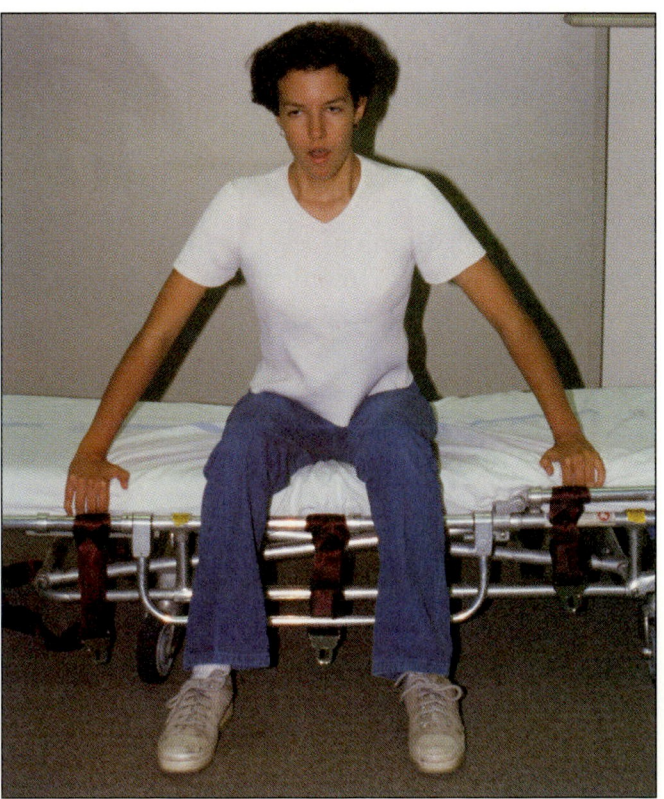

FIGURE 5-5 A patient in a tripod position (also called the sniffing position) will sit unusually upright with the head and chin thrust forward slightly.

gling, or bubbling. The presence of any of these indicates that a serious respiratory problem exists.

A patient who coughs up thick, yellowish or greenish *sputum* (matter from the lungs) most likely has an advanced respiratory infection. A patient with a chest injury may cough up blood or a frothy whitish or pinkish foamlike sputum. A patient with congestive heart failure may also cough up a frothy sputum. The presence of either substance, regardless of its cause, indicates that an urgent, potentially critical cardiovascular and respiratory problem exists. The patient's condition may deteriorate rapidly to a point at which the patient can no longer breathe.

Pulse

With each heartbeat, the ventricles contract, forcefully ejecting blood from the heart and propelling it into the arteries. The **pulse** is the pressure wave that occurs as each heartbeat causes a surge in the blood circulating through the arteries. The pulse is most easily felt at a pulse point where a major artery lies near the surface and can be pressed gently against a bone or solid organ. To *palpate* (feel) the pulse, hold together your index and long fingers and place their tips over a pulse point, pressing gently against the artery until you feel intermittent pulsations. Sometimes, you may have to slide your fingertips a little to each side and press again until you feel a pulse. When palpating a pulse, do not allow your thumb to touch the patient. If you do so, you may mistake the strong pulsing circulation in your thumb for the patient's pulse.

In responsive patients who are older than age 1 year, you should palpate the radial pulse at the wrist (Figure 5-6). In unresponsive patients older than age 1 year, you should palpate the carotid pulse in the neck, which is easier to locate. When palpating the carotid pulse, you should place the fingertips of your index and long fingers along the carotid artery. Use caution when palpating the carotid pulse in a responsive patient, especially an elderly patient. Only gentle pressure on one side of the neck should be used. Never press on the carotid arteries on both sides of the neck at the same time. Doing so can cut off circulation to the brain.

In infants, both the radial and carotid pulses are difficult to locate. Because of the infant's soft, immature trachea, palpating the carotid pulse is not recommended. Palpate the brachial pulse, located at the underside of the upper arm, in children younger than age 1 year (Figure 5-7). With the infant lying supine, you can access the brachial pulse by elevating the arm over the infant's head. Because most infants have

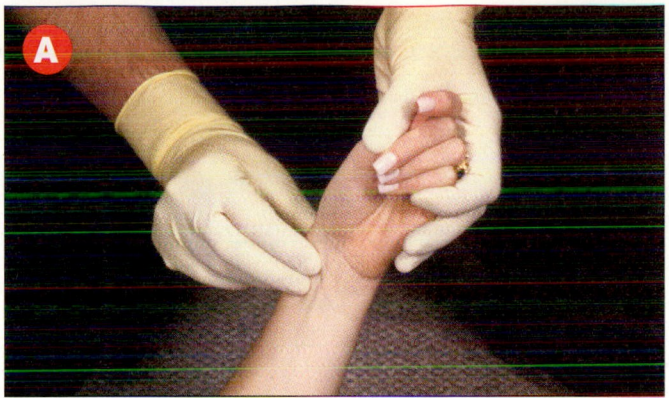
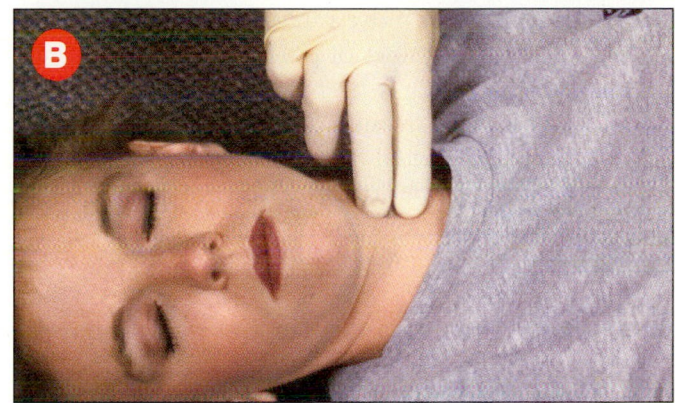

FIGURE 5-6 A: To palpate the radial pulse, place the tips of your first two fingers over the radial artery, pressing gently until you feel intermittent pulsations. **B:** To palpate the carotid pulse, place the tips of your first two fingers over the carotid artery, pressing gently until you feel intermittent pulsations.

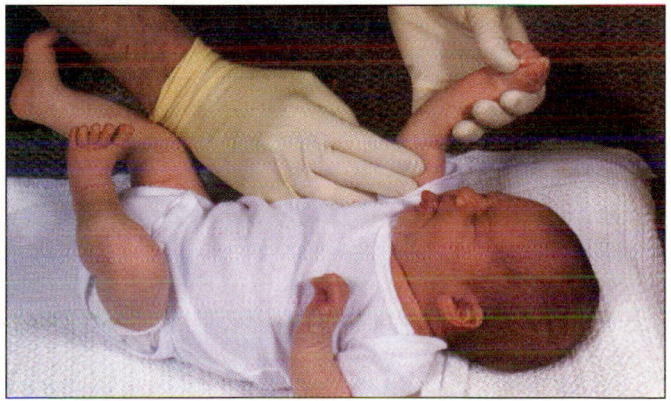

FIGURE 5-7 To palpate the brachial pulse in an infant, press firmly along the brachial artery at the underside of the upper arm.

chubby arms, you need to press your adjacent fingertips firmly along the brachial artery, which lies parallel to the long axis of the upper arm, to be able to palpate the pulse.

Your first consideration when taking a pulse is to determine whether the patient has a palpable pulse or is pulseless. When taking the pulse, you should assess and report its rate, strength, and regularity.

TABLE 5-3	Normal Ranges for Pulse Rate
Age	**Range**
Adults	60 to 100 beats/min
Children	80 to 100 beats/min
Toddlers	100 to 120 beats/min
Newborns	120 to 140 beats/min

Rate. To obtain the pulse rate in most patients, you should count the number of pulses felt in a 30-second period and then multiply by 2. A pulse that is weak and difficult to palpate, irregular, or extremely slow should be palpated and counted for a full minute. A pulse rate is counted as beats per minute; however, in reporting the pulse rate, it is not necessary to state or write "beats per minute" after the number.

The pulse rate in most adults (at rest) averages around 72 beats/min. However, pulse rate can vary significantly from person to person. In the well-conditioned athlete or in individuals taking heart medications such as beta-blockers, the pulse rate may be considerably lower. A pulse rate between 60 and 100 beats/min is considered normal in adults. The average pulse rate in children is generally higher. Table 5-3 shows the normal ranges of pulse rates.

In assessing the pulse rate in an adult patient, a rate that is greater than 100 beats/min is described as **tachycardia**, and a rate of less than 60 beats/min is described as **bradycardia**.

Strength. You should always report the pulse's strength and regularity whenever reporting or recording the pulse. The pulse is generally palpated at the radial or carotid arteries in adults and at the brachial artery in infants, because it is normally strong and easily palpable at these locations. Therefore, if the pulse feels of normal strength, you should describe it as being strong. You should describe a stronger than normal pulse as "bounding" and a pulse that is weak and difficult to feel as "weak" or "thready." With a little experience, you will be able to make the necessary distinctions easily.

Regularity. When assessing the quality of the pulse, you must also determine whether it is regular or irregular. When the interval between each ventricular contraction of the heart is short, the pulse is rapid. When the interval is longer, the pulse is slower. No matter what the rate, the interval between each contraction should be the same, and the pulse that results should occur at a constant, regular rhythm. You should note and document this rhythm as regular.

The rhythm is considered irregular if the heart periodically has a premature or late beat or if a pulse beat is missed. Some individuals have a chronically irregular pulse; however, if an irregular pulse is found in a patient with signs and symptoms that suggest a cardiovascular problem, the patient likely needs advanced cardiac assessment and life support. Therefore, depending on your protocols, you should call for ALS backup, arrange for an intercept, or initiate prompt transport to definitive care.

The Skin

The condition of the patient's skin can tell you a lot about the patient's peripheral circulation and perfusion, blood oxygen levels, and body temperature. When assessing the skin, you should evaluate its color, temperature, and moisture.

Color. Assessing the skin helps you to determine the adequacy of perfusion after trauma. **Perfusion** is the circulation of blood within an organ or tissue. Adequate perfusion meets the cells' current needs; inadequate perfusion will cause cells and tissues to die.

Many blood vessels lie near the surface of the skin. The skin's color is determined by the blood circulating through these vessels and the amount and type of pigment that is present in the skin. Blood is red when it is properly saturated with oxygen. As a result, skin in lightly pigmented individuals is pinkish. The pigmentation in most individuals will not hide changes in the skin's underlying color, regardless of the individual's race. In patients with deeply pigmented skin, changes in color may be apparent only in certain areas, such as the fingernail beds, the mucous membranes in the mouth, the lips, the underside of the arm and palm (which are usually less pigmented), and the conjunctiva of the eyes. In addition, the palms of the hands and soles of the feet should be assessed in infants and children.

Poor peripheral circulation will cause the skin to appear pale, white, ashen or gray, possibly with a waxy translucent appearance like a white candle. Abnormally cold or frozen skin may also appear this way. When the blood is not properly saturated with oxygen, it appears bluish. Therefore, in a patient with insufficient air exchange and low levels of oxygen in the blood, the blood and vessels become bluish, and the lips, mucous membranes, nail beds, and skin over the blood vessels appear blue or gray. This condition is called **cyanosis** (Figure 5-8).

High blood pressure will cause the skin to be abnormally flushed and red. In some patients with extremely high blood pressure, all the visible blood vessels will be so full that the skin will appear to be a dark reddish-

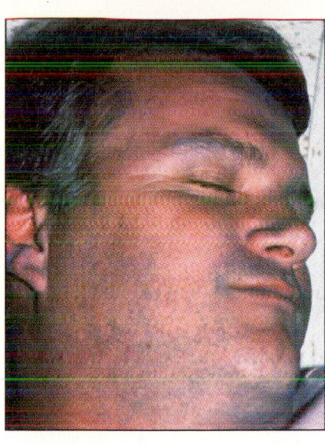

FIGURE 5-8 Cyanosis occurs when the patient has low levels of oxygen in the blood.

purple. A patient with carbon monoxide poisoning or a significant fever, heatstroke, sunburn, mild thermal burns, or other conditions in which the body is unable to properly dissipate heat will also appear to have red skin.

Changes in skin color may also result from chronic illness. Liver disease or dysfunction may cause **jaundice**, resulting in the patient's skin and sclera turning yellow.

Temperature. Normally, the skin is warm to the touch. When the patient has a significant fever, sunburn, or hyperthermia, the skin feels hot to the touch. The skin will feel cool when the patient is in early shock, has exercised and is sweating profusely, or has heat exhaustion. The skin will feel cold when the patient is in profound shock, has hypothermia, or has frostbite.

Body temperature is normally measured with a thermometer in the hospital. However, in the field, feeling the patient's forehead with the back of your hand is usually adequate to determine whether the patient's temperature is elevated or depressed (Figure 5-9).

Moisture. Dry skin is normal. Skin that is wet, moist (often called diaphoretic), or excessively dry and hot suggests a problem. In the early stages of shock, the skin will become slightly moist. Skin that is only slightly moist but not covered excessively with sweat is described as clammy, damp, or moist. When the skin is bathed in sweat, such as after strenuous exercise or when the patient is in the late stages of shock, the skin is described as wet.

Because the skin's color, temperature, and moisture are often related signs, you should consider them together. When recording or reporting your assessment of the skin, you should first describe the color, then the temperature, and last, whether the skin is dry, moist, or wet. For example, you could say or write, "Skin: pale, cool, and clammy."

Capillary Refill

Capillary refill is a test that evaluates the ability of the circulatory system to restore blood to the capillary system. When evaluated in an uninjured limb, capillary refill reflects the patient's perfusion. Capillary refill time is often affected by the patient's body temperature, position, and medications. To test capillary refill, place your thumb on the patient's fingernail with your fingers on the underside of the patient's finger, and gently compress (Figure 5-10). The blood will be forced from the

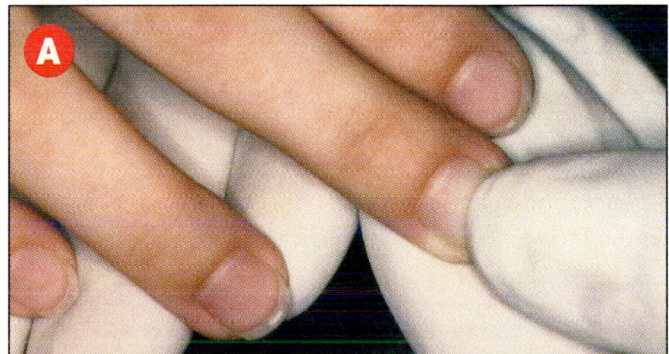

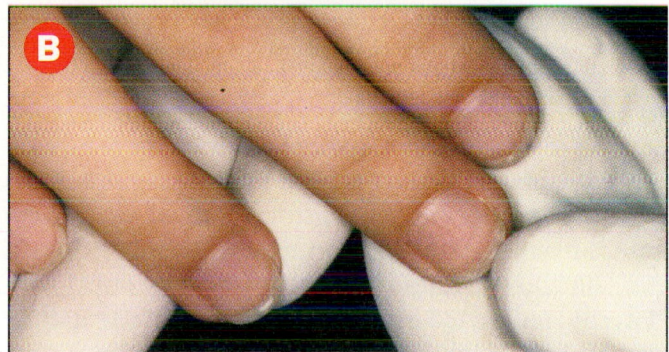

FIGURE 5-10 A: To test capillary refill, gently compress the fingertip until it blanches. **B:** Release the fingertip, and count until it returns to its normal pink color.

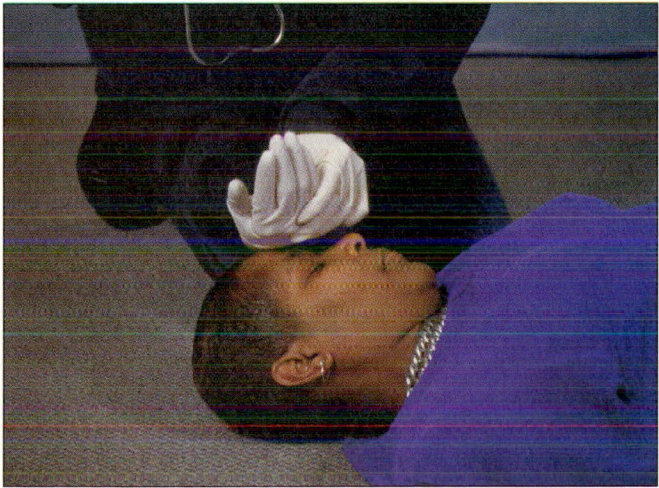

FIGURE 5-9 Assess skin temperature by feeling the patient's forehead with the back of your hand.

capillaries in the nail bed. When you remove the pressure applied against the tip of the patient's finger, the nail bed will remain blanched and white for a brief period. As the underlying capillaries refill with blood, the nail bed will be restored to its normal deep pink color. Capillary refill should be both prompt and pink. With adequate perfusion, the color in the nail bed should be restored to its normal pink within 2 seconds, or about the time it takes to say "capillary refill" at a normal rate of speech. You should report and document the capillary refill as normal. You should suspect poor peripheral circulation when capillary refill takes more than 2 seconds or the nail bed remains blanched. In this instance, you should report and document the capillary refill as delayed.

A bluish color may indicate that the capillaries are refilling with blood drawn from the veins rather than with fresh, oxygenated blood from the arteries, making the test invalid. You should also consider the capillary refill test invalid if the patient is in or has been exposed to a cold environment or if the patient is elderly. In both situations, delayed capillary refill is normal.

To assess capillary refill in infants and children younger than age 6 years, press on the skin or nail bed, and determine how long it takes for the pink color to return. As with adults, normal capillary refill takes less than 2 seconds.

Blood Pressure

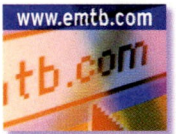

Adequate blood pressure is necessary to maintain proper circulation and perfusion of the vital organ cells. **Blood pressure (BP)** is the pressure of circulating blood against the walls of the arteries. A decrease in the blood pressure may indicate one of the following:

- Loss of blood or its fluid components
- Loss of vascular tone and sufficient arterial constriction to maintain the necessary pressure even without any actual fluid or blood loss
- A cardiac pumping problem

When any of these conditions occurs and results in a small drop in circulation, the body's compensatory mechanisms are activated, the heart and pulse rates increase, and the arteries constrict. Normal blood pressure is maintained, and by decreasing the blood flow to the skin and extremities, available blood volume is temporarily redirected to the vital organs so that they remain adequately perfused. However, as shock progresses, and the body's defense mechanisms can no longer keep up, the blood pressure will fall. *Decreased*

blood pressure is a late sign of shock and indicates that the critical decompensated phase has begun. Any patient with a markedly low blood pressure has inadequate pressure to maintain proper perfusion of all the vital organs and needs to have his or her blood pressure and perfusion restored immediately to a normal level.

When the blood pressure becomes elevated, the body's defenses act to reduce it. Some individuals have chronically high blood pressure from progressive narrowing of the arteries that occurs with age, and during an acute episode, their blood pressure may increase to even higher levels. Head injury or a number of other conditions may also cause blood pressure to rise to very high levels. Abnormally high blood pressure may result in a rupture or other critical damage in the arterial system.

You should measure blood pressure in all patients older than age 3 years. In addition to baseline vital signs, you should note a sick appearance, respiratory distress, or unresponsiveness when evaluating infants and children younger than age 3 years.

Blood pressure contains two key separate components: diastolic pressure and systolic pressure. **Diastolic pressure** is the residual pressure that remains in the arteries during the relaxing phase (diastole) of the heart's cycle, when the left ventricle is at rest. **Systolic pressure** is the increased pressure that is caused along the artery with each contraction (systole) of the ventricle and the pulse wave that it produces. Systolic pressure represents the maximum pressure to which the arteries are subjected, and the diastolic pressure represents the minimum amount of pressure that is always present in the arteries.

Early blood pressure gauges contained a column of mercury and a linear scale that was graduated in millimeters. Even though different gauges are used today, the blood pressure is still measured in millimeters of mercury (mm Hg). Blood pressure is reported as a fraction in the form systolic pressure over diastolic pressure. Therefore, if the patient's systolic pressure is 120 and the diastolic pressure is 78, you would record it as "BP 120/78 mm Hg." You would report the patient's blood pressure verbally as "BP is 120 over 78."

Blood pressure contains two key separate components: diastolic pressure and systolic pressure.

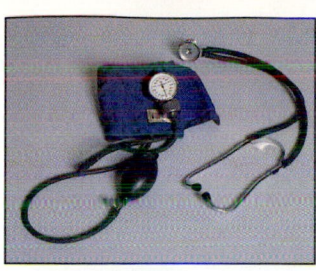

FIGURE 5-11
A blood pressure cuff.

Equipment for measuring blood pressure. You will use a *sphygmomanometer* (blood pressure cuff) to apply pressure against the artery when measuring the blood pressure. The sphygmomanometer contains the following components (Figure 5-11):

- A wide outer cuff designed to be fastened snugly around the entire arm or leg
- An inflatable wide bladder sewn into a portion of the cuff
- A ball-pump with a one-way valve that allows air to enter and a turn-valve that can be closed or, when opened, will allow air to be released at a controlled speed from the cuff
- A pressure gauge calibrated in millimeters of mercury, which indicates the pressure that exists in the cuff that is being applied against the underlying artery

Make sure that you carry at least three sizes of blood pressure cuffs: normal, extra-large, and pediatric (Figure 5-12). The normal size cuff is designed to adjust properly around the upper arm of most adults. Use an extra-large cuff with patients who are obese or have exceptionally well-developed arm muscles or to take the blood pressure of the thigh in patients who have injuries in both arms. Use a narrow, small pediatric cuff with children and exceptionally small adults.

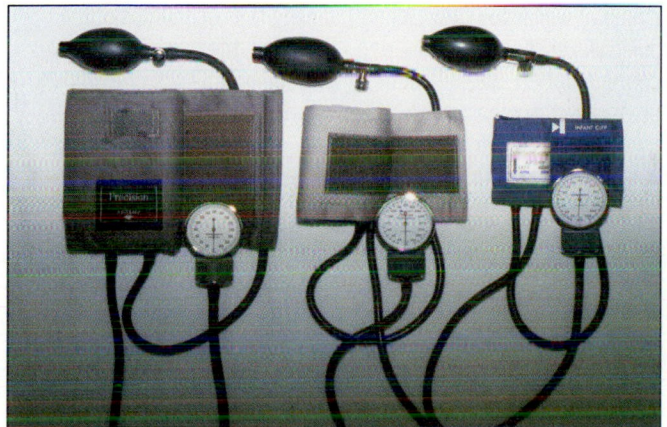

FIGURE 5-12 The three sizes of blood pressure cuffs: extra-large, normal, and pediatric.

You must be sure to select the appropriately sized cuff. A cuff that is too small may result in falsely high readings; a cuff that is too large may result in falsely low readings.

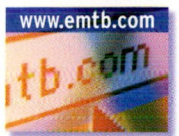

Auscultation. **Auscultation** is the method of listening to sounds within organs with a stethoscope. You will usually measure blood pressure by auscultation (Figure 5-13).

With the patient's arm extended with the palm up, place the cuff so that it lies across the upper arm and is located with its distal edge about 1″ above the crease at the inside of the patient's elbow. Make sure the center of the inflatable bladder, which is usually marked by an arrow on the cuff, lies over the brachial artery. Next, wrap the ends so that the cuff surrounds the upper arm snugly but not tightly. Secure the cuff with the Velcro fastener attached to it, making sure to rub your hand over the entire area where the two sides of the Velcro fastener are in contact. Once the cuff has been properly secured around the upper arm, the arm should be held at about the same level as the heart.

Next, palpate the brachial artery in the antecubital fossa, located at the anterior aspect of the elbow. Place the diaphragm of the stethoscope over the artery, and hold it firmly pressed against the artery with the fingers of your nondominant hand. Hold the rubber ball-pump in the palm of your other hand and the turn-valve between your thumb and first finger. Close the valve tightly, and pump the ball-pump until the gauge indicates that you have reached a pressure of 200 mm Hg. You should hear no pulse sounds. Slowly turn the valve, opening it until air is steadily escaping from the cuff and you see the hand of the gauge slowly drop. Watch the gauge, and listen carefully. Note the patient's systolic pressure as the reading on the gauge at which the "taps" or "thumps" of the pulse waves can first be heard clearly. As the pressure in the cuff is progressively reduced, pulse sounds will continue for a time, then suddenly disappear. Note the patient's diastolic pressure as the reading on the gauge at which the sounds stopped. At the point at which the sound disappears, the pressure that is exerted against the artery is less than the diastolic pressure. When a greater pressure than the patient's systolic pressure is applied against the outside of the arterial wall, blood flow distal to that point will be occluded, and you will not be able to palpate a distal pulse.

As soon as the pulse sounds stop, open the valve, and release the remaining air quickly. Once you have finished measuring the blood pressure, you should document your findings, the time at which the blood pressure was taken, and in which arm it was taken. Blood pressure is most often measured by auscultation with the

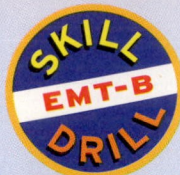

Obtaining a Blood Pressure by Auscultation
Figure 5-13

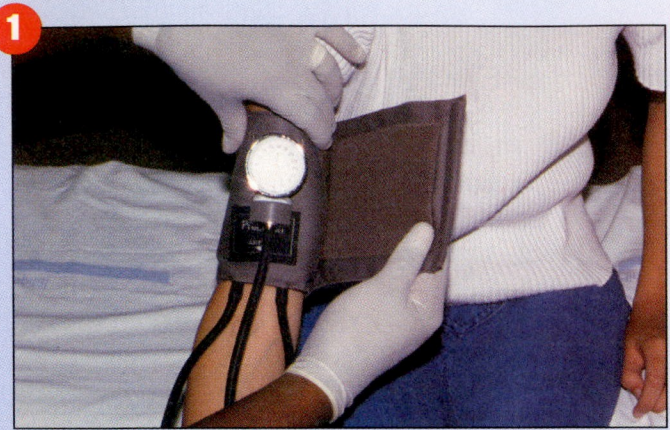

Wrap the cuff snugly around the upper arm, about 1" above the elbow.

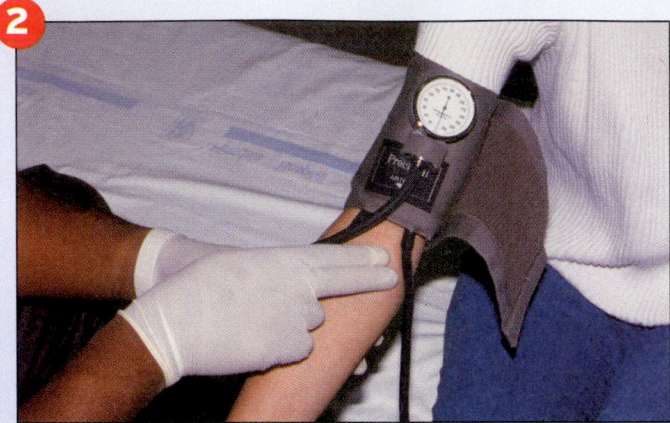

Palpate the brachial pulse to determine where to place the end of the stethoscope.

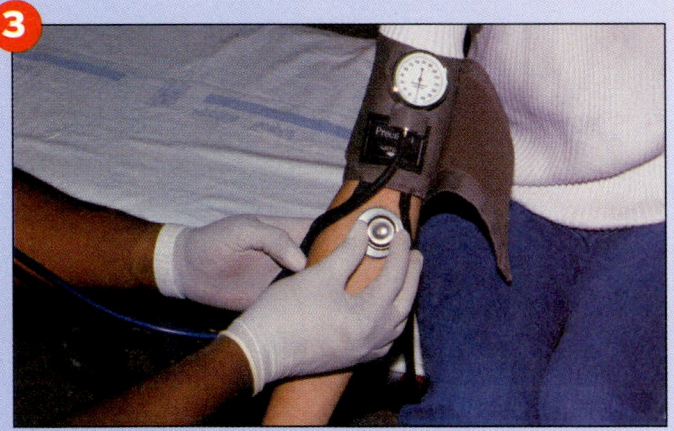

Place the stethoscope over the artery as you hold the ball-pump in your other hand and the turn-valve between your thumb and index finger.

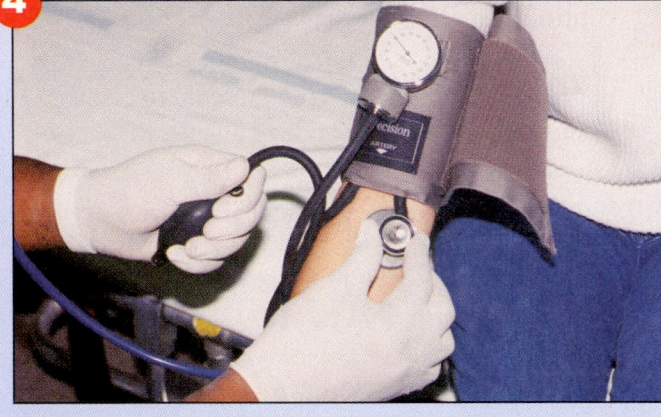

Close the valve, and pump the ball-pump until the gauge reaches 200 mm Hg. At this point, you should hear no sounds. Slowly open the valve until air is steadily escaping from the cuff and you see the pressure dropping. Note the systolic pressure as the reading on the gauge at which you first clearly hear the taps or thumps of the pulse waves. As you continue to release air, the pulse sound will continue for a time and suddenly disappear. Note the diastolic pressure as the reading on the gauge at which the sound stops.

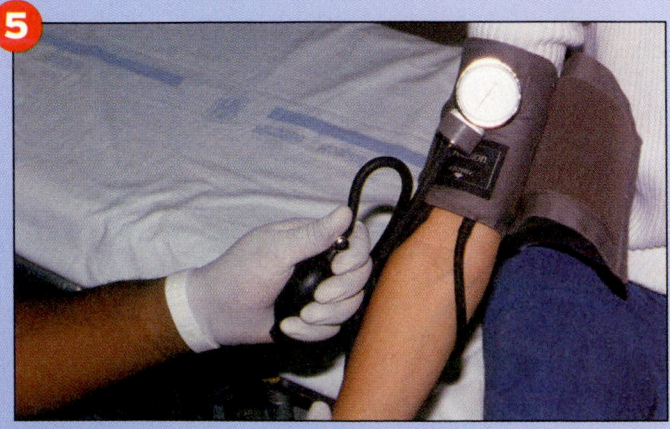

As soon as the sounds stop, open the valve, and release the air quickly.

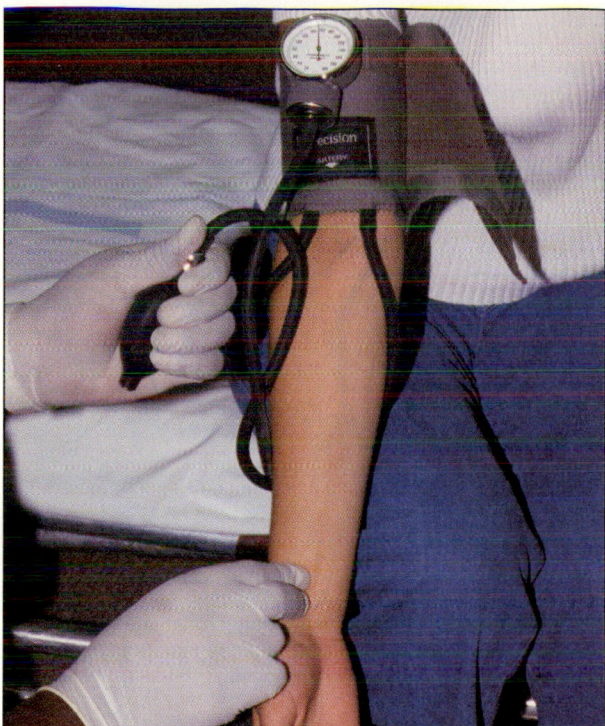

FIGURE 5-14 When obtaining a blood pressure by palpation, you should place your fingertips on the radial artery so that you feel the radial pulse. As you inflate the cuff, you will no longer feel the pulse. Open the turn-valve so that air slowly escapes from the cuff, and watch the gauge. When you can feel the radial pulse again, note the reading on the gauge as the patient's systolic blood pressure.

TABLE 5-4	Normal Ranges for Blood Pressure
Age	**Range**
Adults	90 to 140 mm Hg (systolic) 60 to 90 mm Hg (diastolic)
Children (ages 1 to 8 years)	80 to 110 mm Hg (systolic)
Infants (newborn to age 1 year)	Two times the patient's age, plus 80

TABLE 5-5	Normal Systolic Blood Pressures
Adult Men	Add 100 to the patient's age, up to 150 mm Hg
Adult Women	Add 90 to the patient's age, up to 150 mm Hg
Children	Add 80 to 2 times the patient's age in years

patient in a sitting or semi-sitting position. Be sure to note whether a different method or position was used.

Occasionally, when a patient's blood pressure is very low, you will continue to hear pulse sounds from the reading at which they started all the way until the gauge has reached 0. When this occurs, you should record the diastolic pressure "0" or "all the way down" to indicate that it was not measurable by stethoscope.

Palpation. The auscultation method will be difficult or impossible to use in a very noisy environment and may produce inaccurate findings. The palpation method, which is examination by touch that does not depend on your ability to hear sounds, should be used in these cases.

To measure blood pressure by palpation, secure the appropriately sized cuff around the patient's upper arm in the manner previously described. With your non-dominant hand, palpate the patient's radial pulse on the same arm as the cuff, without moving your fingertips once you have located it, until you have completed taking the blood pressure (Figure 5-14). While holding the ball-pump in your other hand, close the turn-valve and rapidly inflate the cuff to 200 mm Hg. As the cuff inflates, you will no longer feel the pulse under your fin-

gertips. Open the turn-valve so that air slowly escapes from the cuff, and carefully observe the gauge. When you can again feel the radial pulse under your fingertips, you should note the reading on the gauge as the patient's systolic blood pressure. You will not be able to determine the diastolic pressure with this method. Next, open the turn-valve further, and completely deflate the cuff. Document your findings, including the time and in which arm blood pressure was measured, and note that the pressure was taken by palpation. If you are noting the blood pressure in a box on your run form, you can abbreviate it to "120/by palp."

Normal blood pressure. Blood pressure levels vary with age and gender. Table 5-4 serves as a guideline of normal blood pressure ranges.

A patient has **hypotension** when the blood pressure is lower than the normal range and **hypertension** when the blood pressure is higher than the normal range.

Typically, you will see children less frequently than adults; therefore, you might not remember the normal ranges for the various age groups. You might wish to carry a chart in the ambulance and carry-in kit that lists normal blood pressure ranges and other vital sign ranges. Table 5-5 shows rules of thumb that you can also use as a guideline to determine what a patient's systolic pressure should be.

AVPU scale

The **AVPU scale** is a rapid method of assessing the patient's level of consciousness using one of the following four terms:

A   **A**wake and **A**lert
V   Responsive to **V**erbal Stimulus
P   Responsive to **P**ain
U   Unresponsive

You should determine whether a patient who is awake and alert is oriented to person, place, time, and event. A patient who is oriented will know his or her first and last name. A young child will know his or her first name and whom he or she lives with. A patient who is oriented to place will know his or her location. Most patients who are oriented to time will know the year, month, and day. A patient who is oriented to event will know what happened.

In your report, you can note a person who is oriented to person, place, time, and event as "alert and oriented times four" (A & O x 4). If the patient is not oriented to all four conditions, be sure to note which condition(s) the patient is not oriented to.

A patient who is not awake and alert but who is aroused and responds to your voice by opening his or her eyes, moaning, speaking, or moving is responding to verbal stimulus. A patient who does not respond to your normal speaking voice but who responds to your yelled voice is responding to loud verbal stimulus. Be sure to note how the patient responded. Tap a patient who is hearing impaired with your fingers repeatedly. If the patient responds, note that the patient is hearing impaired but responds to being tapped.

To determine whether a patient who does not respond to verbal stimuli will respond to a painful stimulus, you should gently but firmly pinch the patient's skin (Figure 5-15). A patient who moans or withdraws is responding to painful stimulus. Be sure to note the type and location of the stimulus and how the patient responded.

If the patient does not respond to a painful stimulus on one side, try to elicit a response on the other side. Note that a patient who remains flaccid without moving or making a sound is unresponsive.

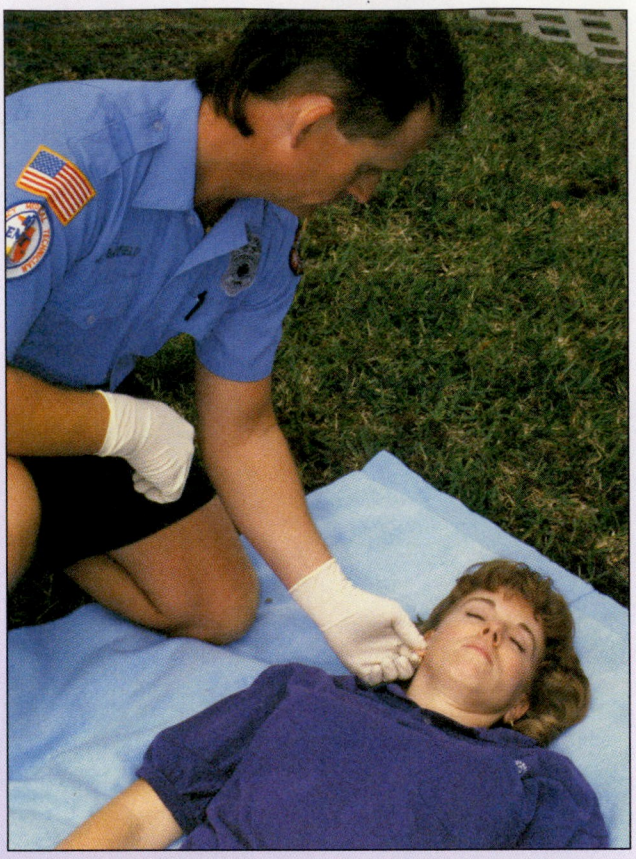

FIGURE 5-15 To assess whether a patient will respond to a painful stimulus, gently, but firmly, pinch the patient's skin. This can be done at the neck or on the earlobe.

TABLE 5-6	Critically Low Systolic Blood Pressures
Male Adults/Adolescents	90 mm Hg or less
Female Adults/Adolescents	80 mm Hg or less
Children	70 mm Hg or less

Critical hypotension. You must assume that a patient who has a critically low blood pressure can no longer compensate sufficiently to maintain adequate perfusion. Table 5-6 shows the point at which blood pressure is considered to be critically low.

In assessing the patient's general circulation, the blood pressure, pulse, skin temperature, and capillary refill should *not* be assessed in an injured limb. However, once you have obtained these vital signs from an uninjured limb, you might wish to compare the distal skin temperature, quality of the distal pulse, and/or capillary refill time in the injured limb with those found on the uninjured side. This information is useful in evaluating whether the injury may have compromised the circulation in the injured limb.

Level of Consciousness

The patient's level of consciousness (LOC) is considered a vital sign because the status of the respiratory, cardiovascular, and central nervous systems are reflected by it. However, in the early assessment, you need to ascertain only the apparent gross level of consciousness by determining whether the patient is awake and alert with an unaltered LOC, conscious but with an altered LOC, or unconscious.

As you assess a patient, you must determine the appropriateness of a response by how well it demonstrates the patient's understanding and mental activity, not how well it reflects your definition of socially acceptable behavior.

When a patient is conscious with a lower level of consciousness, the body's defense mechanisms may no longer be able to compensate adequately, possibly indicating that inadequate perfusion and oxygenation or a chemical or neurologic problem is adversely affecting the brain and its ability to function. A lowered level of consciousness in a conscious patient can also be caused by medications, drugs, alcohol, or poisoning.

Your assessment of a patient who is unconscious when you arrive should be focused initially on ABCD and then on identifying other emergency care that the patient may need. Sustained unconsciousness should warn you that a critical respiratory, circulatory, or central nervous system problem or deficit may exist, and you must assume that the patient has a potentially critical injury or condition. In addition, you must consider the condition of any patient who remains unconscious for a sustained period as grave. Therefore, after rapidly assessing the patient and providing any emergency treatment, you should package the patient and provide prompt transport to the hospital.

The Glasgow Coma Scale is a method of assessing a patient's level of consciousness by scoring the patient's response to eye opening, motor response, and verbal response (Figure 5-16).

GLASGOW COMA SCALE

Eye Opening

Spontaneous	4
To Voice	3
To Pain	2
None	1

Verbal Response

Oriented	5
Confused	4
Inappropriate Words	3
Incomprehensible Words	2
None	1

Motor Response

Obeys Command	6
Localizes Pain	5
Withdraws (pain)	4
Flexion (pain)	3
Extension (pain)	2
None	1

Glasgow Coma Score Total	15

FIGURE 5-16 The Glasgow Coma Scale.

Pupils. The diameter of the patient's pupils reflects the status of the brain's perfusion, oxygenation, and condition (Figure 5-17). The pupil is a circular opening in the center of the pigmented iris of the eye. The pupils are normally round and of approximately equal size and serve as optical diaphragms, adjusting their size depending on the available light. In normal room light, the pupil appears to be midsize. With less light, the pupils dilate, allowing more light to enter the eye, making it possible to see even in dim light. With high light levels or when a bright light is suddenly introduced, the pupils instantly constrict, allowing less light to enter, protecting the sensitive receptors in the inner eye from damage. When a brighter light is introduced into one eye (or higher levels of light enter one eye only), both pupils should constrict equally to the appropriate size for the pupil receiving the most light.

In the absence of any light, the pupils will become fully relaxed and dilated. When light is introduced, each eye sends sensory signals to the brain indicating the level of light it is receiving. Pupil size is regulated by a series of continuous motor commands that the brain automatically sends through the oculomotor nerves to each eye, causing both pupils to constrict to the same appropriate size. Normally, pupil size changes instantly to any change in light level.

You must assume the patient has depressed brain function as a result of either central nervous system depression or injury if the pupils react in any of the following ways:

- Become fixed with no reaction to light
- Dilate with introduction of a bright light and constrict when the light is removed
- React sluggishly instead of briskly
- Become unequal in size
- Become unequal in size when a bright light is introduced into or removed from one eye

Depressed brain function can be produced by the following situations:

- Injury of the brain or brain stem
- Trauma or stroke
- Brain tumor or other growth
- Inadequate oxygenation or perfusion
- Drugs or toxins (central nervous system depressants)

Opiates, which are one category of central nervous system depressants, cause the pupils to constrict so significantly, regardless of light, that they become so small

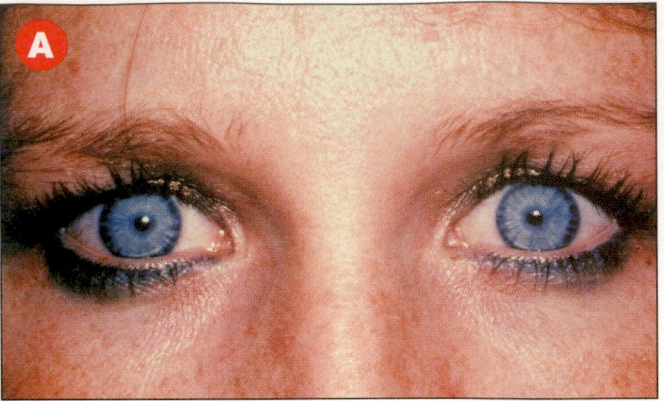
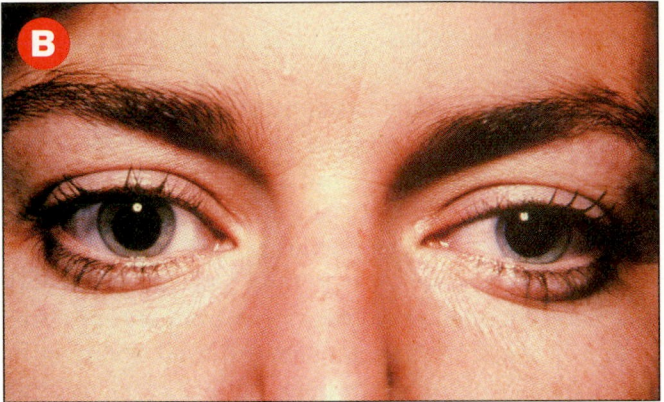
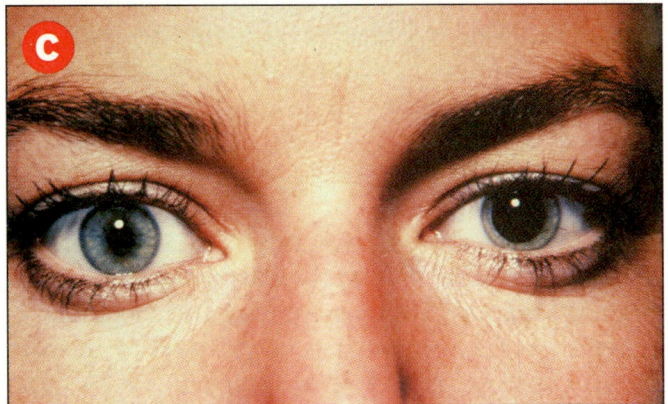

FIGURE 5-17 A: Constricted pupils. **B:** Dilated pupils. **C:** Unequal pupils.

as to be described as pinpoint. Intracranial pressure from intracranial bleeding at the side of the head may cause sufficient pressure against the oculomotor nerve on one side that the motor commands can no longer pass from the brain to that eye. When this occurs, the eye no longer receives commands to constrict, and its pupil becomes fully dilated and fixed. This is described as a blown pupil.

Pupils may be dilated, may be unequal as a result of medication placed into one or both eyes or from an injury or condition of the eye, or may not be reacting appropriately. You cannot determine the cause as you assess the patient. Further examination of the patient in the emergency department will determine the cause.

The letters PEARRL serve as a useful guide in assessing the pupils. They stand for the following:

P = **P**upils

E = **E**qual

A = **A**nd

R = **R**ound

R = **R**egular in size

L = react to **L**ight

You can report patients with normal pupils as "Pupils are equal, round, and regular in size, and react properly to light" or "the patient has PEARRL." Describe any abnormal findings using the longer form, such as "Pupils are equal and round, the left pupil is dilated and fixed, the right pupil is regular in size and reacts to light."

Reassessment of the Vital Signs

The vital signs that you obtain serve two important functions. The first set establishes an important initial measurement of the patient's respiratory and cardiovascular systems and the quality of perfusion and oxygenation of the brain and other vital organs. The initial vital signs also serve as a key baseline.

Throughout your care of the patient, you should monitor the patient's vital signs for any changes from your initial findings. You should reassess and record vital signs at least every 15 minutes in a stable patient and at least every 5 minutes in an unstable patient. You should also reassess and record vital signs following all medical interventions. This ongoing comparative assessment is an important indicator of whether your interventions have restored the patient's vital functions to an acceptable range or are at least preventing further deterioration. Reassessment also indicates whether you should consider more aggressive intervention whenever deterioration continues.

> You should reassess and record vital signs at least every 15 minutes in a stable patient and at least every 5 minutes in an unstable patient.

Obtaining a SAMPLE History

Once you have provided emergency care and are ready to further examine the patient, you should try to obtain a key brief history, or **SAMPLE history**. As part of the assessment of every patient, you should ask the following questions, using the word SAMPLE as a guideline:

- **S**igns and **S**ymptoms of the episode: What signs and symptoms occurred at onset of the incident? Does the patient report pain? If so, where is the pain and how strong is it on a scale of 1 to 10? How often does the pain occur and how long does it last?

- **A**llergies: Is the patient allergic to any medication, food, or other substance? What reactions did the patient have to any of them? If the patient has no known allergies, you should note this on the run report as "no known allergies" or "nka."

- **M**edications: What medications was the patient prescribed? What dosage was prescribed? How often is the patient supposed to take the medication? What prescription and over-the-counter medications has the patient taken in the last 12 hours? How much was taken and when?

- **P**ertinent past history: Does the patient have any history of medical, surgical, or trauma occurrences? Has the patient had a recent accident, fall, blow to the head? Was the patient unconscious at any time before or since the incident occurred?

- **L**ast oral intake: When did the patient last eat or drink? What did the patient eat or drink and how much was consumed? Did the patient take any drugs or drink alcohol? Has there been any other oral intake in the last 4 hours?

- **E**vents leading to the injury or illness: What are the key events that led up to this incident? What occurred between the onset of the incident and your arrival? Has the patient experienced any chest pain? If so, did it occur during exertion or while the patient was at rest?

With practice, you will be able to obtain, document, and report a meaningful brief history. Be sure to ask the patient and bystanders for information. If the patient is unconscious, look for a medical identification tag or for a medical information card in the patient's wallet or purse. *Always* look for patient identification in the presence of another EMT or law enforcement officer at the scene.

prep kit

ready for review

Whenever you are called to the scene of an illness or injury, you should find out the patient's chief complaint. Your assessment of the patient should include rapidly evaluating the patient's general condition and identifying any potentially life-threatening injuries or conditions. Baseline vital signs are the key signs that you will use to evaluate the patient's general condition. You will be assessing the patient's respirations, pulse, skin, capillary refill, blood pressure, level of consciousness, and pupils.

After you have initially assessed the patient and obtained the baseline vital signs, you should reassess the patient for any changes from your initial findings.

In addition to determining the chief complaint and assessing the patient's general condition, you should try to obtain a SAMPLE history from the patient or bystanders. By asking several important questions, you will be able to determine the patient's signs and symptoms, allergies, medications taken, pertinent past history, last oral intake, and the events leading up to the incident.

vital vocabulary

www.emtb.com

auscultation　A method of listening to sounds within an organ with a stethoscope.

AVPU scale　A method of assessing a patient's level of consciousness by determining whether the patient is awake and alert, responsive to verbal stimulus or pain, or unresponsive; used principally in the initial assessment.

blood pressure (BP)　The pressure of circulating blood against the walls of the arteries.

bradycardia　Slow heart rate, less than 60 beats/min.

capillary refill　A test that evaluates the ability of the circulatory system to restore blood to the capillary system.

chief complaint　The reason a patient called for help. Also, the patient's response to questions such as "What's wrong?" or "What happened?"

cyanosis　A bluish, gray skin color that is caused by reduced levels of oxygen in the blood.

diastolic pressure　The component of blood pressure in which pressure remains in the arteries during the relaxing phase of the heart's cycle when the left ventricle is at rest.

Glasgow Coma Scale　A method of assessing a patient's level of consciousness by scoring the patient's response to eye opening, motor response, and verbal response; used primarily in the detailed and ongoing assessment.

hypertension　Blood pressure that is higher than the normal range.

hypotension　Blood pressure that is lower than the normal range.

jaundice　A yellow skin color that is caused by liver disease or dysfunction.

labored breathing　A way in which to describe breathing that requires increased effort; characterized by grunting, stridor, and use of accessory muscles.

perfusion　Circulation of blood within an organ or tissue in adequate amounts to meet the cells' current needs.

pulse　The pressure wave that occurs as each heartbeat causes a surge in the blood circulating through the arteries.

SAMPLE history　A key brief history of a patient's condition to determine signs and symptoms, allergies, medications, pertinent past history, last oral intake, and events leading to the injury or illness.

sign　An objective finding that can be seen, heard, felt, smelled, or measured.

sniffing position　An unusually upright position in which the patient's head and chin are thrust slightly forward; also called a tripod position.

spontaneous respirations　Breathing in a patient that occurs with no assistance.

stridor　A harsh, high-pitched inspiratory sound, such as the sound often heard in acute laryngeal (upper airway) obstruction.

symptom　A subjective finding that the patient feels but that can be identified only by the patient.

systolic pressure　The component of blood pressure in which pressure is increased along an artery with each contraction of the ventricle.

tachycardia　Rapid heart rhythm, more than 100 beats/min.

tidal volume　The amount of air that is exchanged with each breath.

vital signs　The key signs that are used to evaluate the patient's overall condition, including respirations, pulse, blood pressure, level of consciousness, and skin characteristics.

assessment in action

You and your partner are dispatched to a private residence, where you find a 63-year-old woman complaining that she is "dizzy and weak everywhere" and that she has felt this way for almost three weeks. The patient is alert and oriented but looks angry. She demands to know why it took you so long to respond. The patient says that she has no allergies and takes no medications other than an aspirin every day. Your partner obtains baseline vital signs as you interview the patient. She has a blood pressure of 148/82 mm Hg, a regular pulse of 92 beats/min, respirations of 16/min, and warm, dry skin.

1. The "A" in the SAMPLE history refers to:
   A. Age.
   B. Affect.
   C. Attitude.
   D. Allergies.

2. The "M" in the SAMPLE history refers to:
   A. Medications.
   B. Mental status.
   C. Motor response.
   D. Memories of yesterday.

3. The "P" in the SAMPLE history refers to:
   A. Pulse checks.
   B. Pupil status response.
   C. Possible diagnosis.
   D. Past pertinent events.

4. The "L" in the SAMPLE history refers to:
   A. Life history.
   B. Last oral intake.
   C. Length of illness.
   D. Level of consciousness.

5. The "E" in the SAMPLE history refers to:
   A. Ear, nose or throat problems.
   B. Events leading up to the illness or injury.
   C. Exercises that the patient does.
   D. Estimated time since the symptoms started.

points to ponder

Objectives 1-5.28, 1-5.31, 1-1.8, 1-3.9

You have responded to a 34-year-old patient who was in-line skating and fell. The patient has scrapes on both knees and is bleeding from an open fracture of the left ulna. While controlling the bleeding, you begin asking SAMPLE history questions. When you ask about pertinent past history, the patient tells you that he is HIV positive but asks you not to tell anyone. The patient is currently quite healthy and does not want others to know. The patient is also afraid that if you tell the hospital, his insurance carrier will find out.

- Would you record this information and/or pass it on to the hospital? Why or why not?

online outlook

If time permits, you should attempt to learn the patient's SAMPLE history. Improve your ability to identify SAMPLE information by completing Exercise 5 at www.emtb.com.

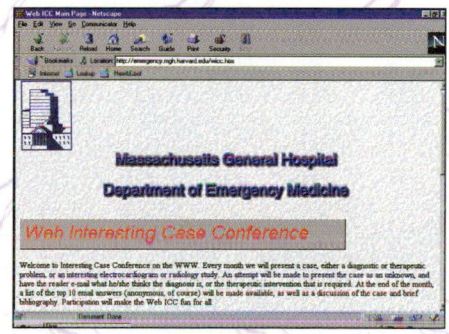

prep kit 5

Lifting and Moving Patients

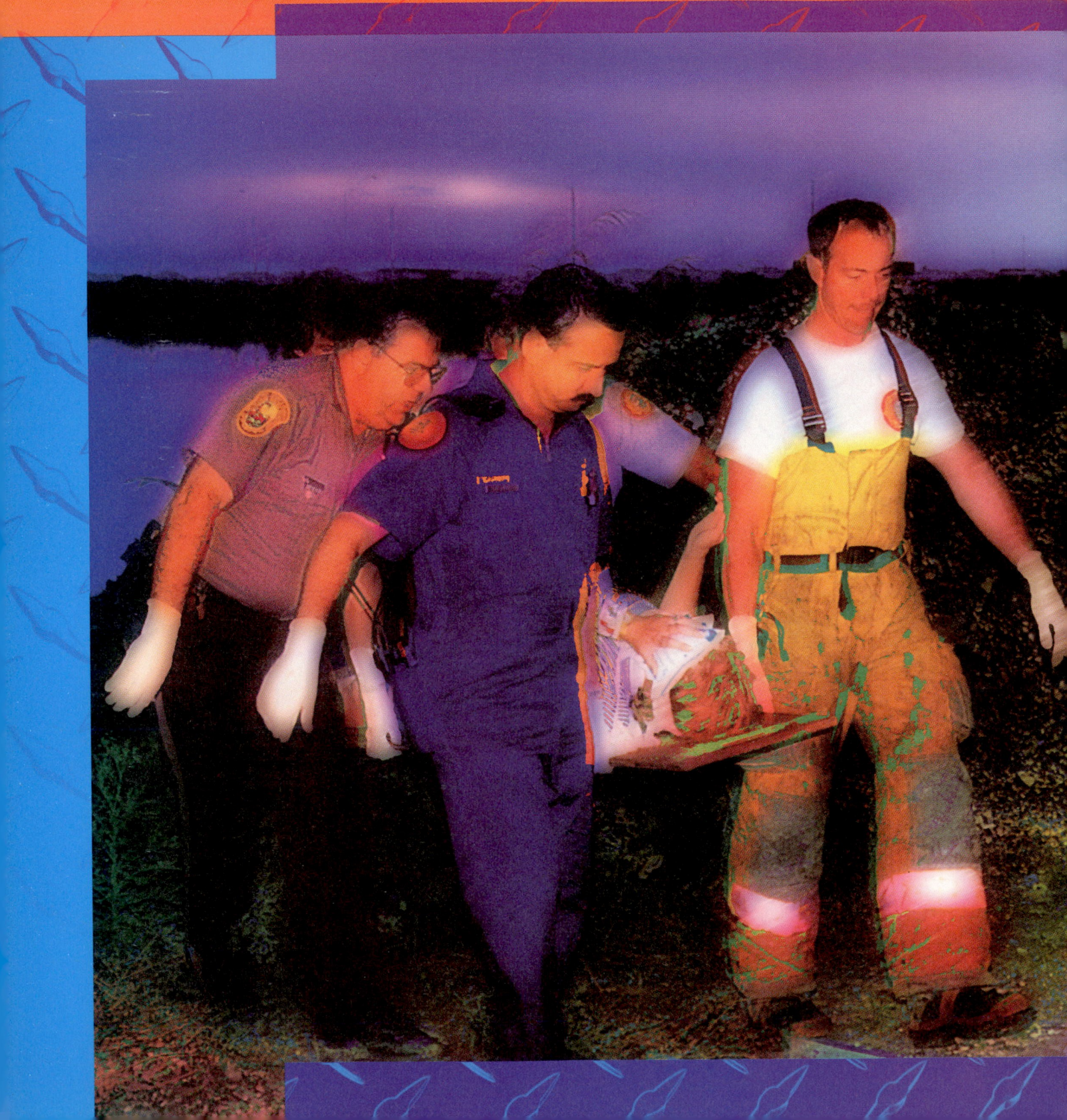

objectives

Cognitive

1. Define body mechanics.

2. Discuss the guidelines and safety precautions that need to be followed when lifting a patient.

3. Describe the safe lifting of cots and stretchers.

4. Discuss the guidelines and safety precautions for carrying patients and/or equipment.

5. Discuss one-handed carrying techniques.

6. Describe correct and safe carrying procedures on stairs.

7. State the guidelines for reaching and their application.

8. Describe correct reaching for log rolls.

9. State the guidelines for pushing and pulling.

10. Discuss the general considerations of moving patients.

11. State three situations that may require the use of an emergency move.

12. Identify the following patient carrying devices:

   • Wheeled ambulance stretcher

   • Portable ambulance stretcher

   • Stair chair

   • Scoop stretcher

   • Long spine board

   • Basket stretcher

   • Flexible stretcher

Affective

13. Explain the rationale for properly lifting and moving patients.

Psychomotor

14. Working with a partner, prepare each of the following devices for use, transfer a patient to the device, properly position the patient on the device, move the device to the ambulance, and load the patient into the ambulance: wheeled ambulance stretcher, portable ambulance stretcher, stair chair, scoop stretcher, long spine board, basket stretcher, and flexible stretcher.

15. Working with a partner, the EMT-B will demonstrate techniques for the transfer of a patient from an ambulance stretcher to a hospital stretcher.

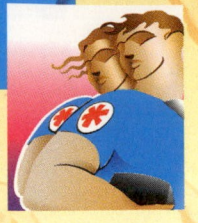

you are the emt

Your ambulance has been out of service for an hour when dispatch finally pages you to report that the emergency repairs to the ambulance cot have been completed and the ambulance is ready to be picked up.

The ambulance cot is one of the most heavily worked pieces of equipment on the ambulance. As such, it needs to be in excellent working condition at all times. This chapter will cover the fundamentals that are involved with the lifting and moving of patients. It will also help you to answer the following questions:

1. Why does every ambulance have such a variety of devices for lifting and moving patients?
2. What is the most common injury incurred by EMS providers?

Lifting and Moving Patients

You will have to move the patient several times to provide emergency medical care in the field and transport the patient to the emergency department. Often, you will have to move the patient into a different position or location. Once you have assessed and provided emergency care, you and your team will have to move the patient onto a long backboard or ambulance cot. Then you must move the patient to the waiting ambulance and load the patient into the patient compartment. After you arrive at the hospital, you must unload the patient, move him or her to the correct examining room, and transfer the patient from the ambulance cot to the emergency department bed. To avoid injury to the patient, yourself, or your partners, you will have to learn how to lift and carry the patient properly, using proper body mechanics and a power grip. To be able to safely and properly move a patient in the various situations that you will encounter in the field, you will have to learn how to perform emergency body drags and lifts, rapidly move a patient from a car onto the ambulance cot, assist a patient from a chair or bed onto the ambulance cot, and lift a patient from the floor onto the ambulance cot. In addition, you will need to move a patient from the bed onto the ambulance cot or carry a patient up or down stairs. You and your team will have to know how to place a patient with a suspected spinal injury onto a long backboard and package patients with and without suspected spinal injury. At times, you and your team will need to move a patient who weighs more than 300 lb or carry a patient on a trail or across rugged terrain. You will need to know the special techniques for loading and unloading the ambulance cot and transferring the patient from the ambulance cot to an examining table or bed in the emergency department.

Lifting and carrying are dynamic processes. To ensure that no individual suddenly bears unexpected, dangerous weight and to reduce the risk of injury to an EMT-B or the patient, you must know where rescuers should be positioned and how to give and receive lifting commands so that all parties act simultaneously. You will also need to know how to prepare patient-moving devices, such as a wheeled ambulance stretcher (also called an ambulance cot or simply "the cot"), stair chair, backboard, scoop stretcher, folding ambulance stretcher, basket stretcher, or flexible stretcher, and when and how to use them. This chapter will cover lifting, carrying, and reaching techniques as well as principles of moving patients, including emergency, urgent, and nonurgent moves. In addition, different types of equipment and patient positioning will be discussed in detail.

Body Mechanics

Anatomy Review

The shoulder girdle rests on the rib cage and is supported by the vertebrae that lie inferior to it. The arms are connected to and hang from the shoulder girdle. When the person is standing upright, the individual weight-bearing vertebrae are stacked on top of each other and aligned over the sacrum. The sacrum is both the mechanical weight-bearing base of the spinal column and the fused central posterior section of the pelvic girdle.

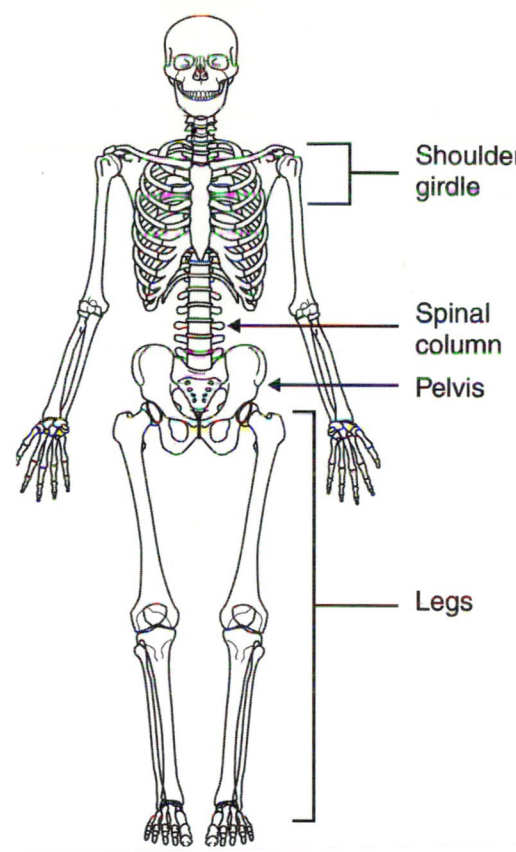

FIGURE 6-1 When you are standing upright, the weight of anything that you lift and carry in your hands is borne by the shoulder girdle, the spinal column, the pelvis, and the legs.

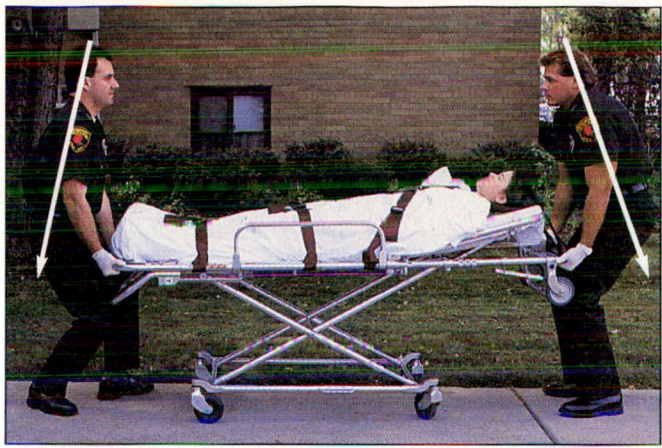

FIGURE 6-2 If your body is properly aligned when you lift, the line of force exerted against the spine occurs in an essentially straight line down the vertebrae. In this way, the strong stacked vertebrae support the lift.

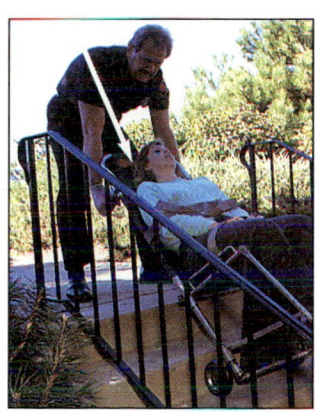

Figure 6-3 You may be injured if you lift with your back curved, as the lifting force is exerted primarily across, rather than down, the spinal column. When this occurs, the muscles of the back, not the vertebrae, are supporting the lift.

When the person is standing upright, the weight of anything being lifted and carried in the hands is reflected onto the shoulder girdle, the spinal column inferior to it, the pelvis, and then the legs (Figure 6-1). In lifting, if the shoulder girdle is aligned over the pelvis and the hands are held close to the legs, the force that is exerted against the spine occurs in an essentially straight line down the strong stacked vertebrae in the spinal column. Therefore, with the back properly maintained in an upright position, very little strain occurs against the muscles and ligaments that keep the spinal column in alignment, and significant weight can be lifted and carried without injury to the back (Figure 6-2). However, you may injure your back if you lift with your back curved or, even if straight, bent significantly forward at the hips. With the back in either of these positions, the shoulder girdle lies significantly anterior to the pelvis, and the force in lifting is exerted primarily across, rather than down, the spinal column. When this occurs, the weight is supported by the muscles of the back and ligaments that run from the base of the skull to the pelvis, keeping the spinal column in alignment, rather than by each vertebral body and disk resting on those

aligned below it (Figure 6-3). In addition, the upper spine and torso serve as a lever so that the force that is exerted against the muscles and ligaments in the lumbar and sacral regions, as a result of the mechanical advantage produced, is many times that of the combined weight of your upper body and the object you are lifting. Therefore, the first key rule of lifting is to always keep the back in a straight, upright (vertical) position and to lift without twisting.

When lifting, you should spread your legs about 15" apart and place your feet so that your center of gravity is properly balanced between them. Then, with the back held upright, bring your upper body down by bending the legs. Once you have properly grasped the patient or litter and made any necessary adjustments in the location of your feet, lift the patient by raising your upper body and arms and by straightening your legs until you are again standing. Because the leg muscles are exercised by walking, climbing stairs, or running, they are well developed and extremely strong. Therefore, as well as being the safest way to lift, lifting by extending the properly placed flexed legs is also the most powerful way to lift. This method is appropriately called a **power lift**.

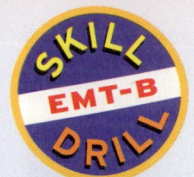

Performing the Power Lift

Figure 6-4

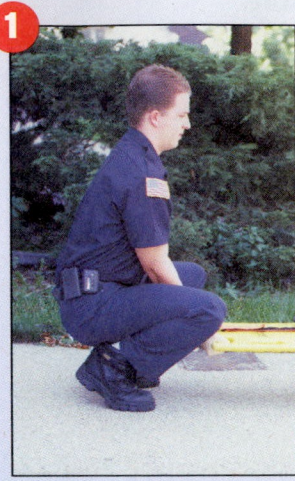

1 Lock your back in its normal upright position. Spread your legs apart about 15", and bend your legs to lower your torso and arms. Grasp the backboard with your hands held palms up and just in front of you. Adjust your orientation and position until the weight is balanced and centered between both arms.

2 Be sure to straddle the object, keep your feet flat, and distribute your weight to the balls of your feet or just behind them.

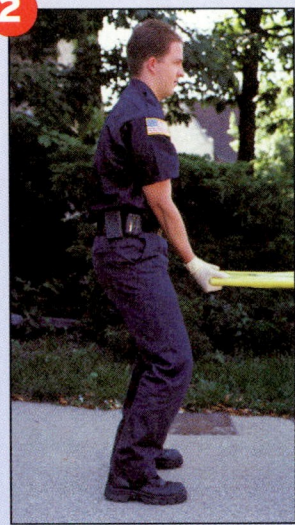

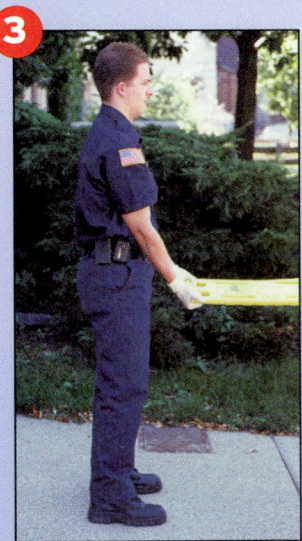

3 With your arms extended down, lift by straightening your legs until you are standing upright. Make sure your back is locked and your upper body comes up before your hips.

The power lift position is also useful for individuals who have weak knees or thighs.

Even if the back is held properly upright, the same adverse force across the spinal column and leverage against the lower back will occur if you lift a heavy object with your arms outstretched so that your hands are significantly anterior to the plane described by the front of the torso. Therefore, you should *never* lift a patient or other heavy object while reaching any significant distance in front of your torso or face. Whenever you are lifting or carrying a patient, be sure to hold your arms so that your hands are almost immediately adjacent to the plane described by your anterior torso (the anterior torso and imaginary lines extended vertically above and below it). Always keep the weight that you are lifting as close to your body as possible.

Lateral force across the spine and sideways leverage against the lower back must also be avoided. If you lift with only one arm or with the arms extended more to one side than the other, more force will be exerted against one side of the shoulder girdle than the other, causing lateral force to be exerted across the spinal column. To prevent this, keep your arms approximately the same distance apart as when hanging at each side of the body, with the weight distributed equally and properly centered between them. If the weight is not balanced between both arms or properly centered between the shoulders when you are preparing to lift, turn your body and/or move to the left or right until the weight is properly balanced and centered. To lift safely and produce the maximal power lift, you should take the following steps (Figure 6-4):

1. **Make sure your back is locked** in its normal curvature and in a slight inward curve.

2. **With your legs apart and your back upright,** bend your legs to lower your torso and arms.

3. **With arms extended down each side of the body,** grasp the litter or backboard with your hands held palm up and just in front of the plane described by the anterior torso and imaginary lines extending vertically from it to the ground.

4. **Adjust your orientation and position** until the weight is balanced and centered between both arms.

5. **Reposition your feet** as necessary so that they are about 15" apart with one slightly farther forward and rotated so that you and your center of

gravity will be properly balanced between them. Be sure to straddle the object, keep your feet flat, and distribute your weight to the balls of the feet or just behind them.

6. **With the arms extended downward,** lift by straightening your legs until you are fully standing. Make sure your back is locked in and that your upper body comes up before your hips.

Reverse these steps whenever you are lowering the stretcher or cot. Always remember to avoid bending at the waist.

Your safety, as well as that of the other EMT-Bs and the patient, depends on the use of proper lifting techniques and having and maintaining a proper hold when lifting or carrying a patient. If you do not have a proper hold of the litter, or of the patient in a body lift, you will not be able to bear a proper share of the weight, and there is an increased chance that you can suddenly lose your grasp with one or both hands. If you temporarily lose your grasp with one or both hands, the position and weight distribution of the litter change suddenly, and the other members of the team must quickly reach beyond a safe distance to avoid dropping the patient. As a result, sudden excessive force may be placed across each one's spine, causing lower back injury.

You should use the **power grip** to get the maximum force from your hands whenever you are lifting a patient (Figure 6-5). The arm and hand have their greatest lifting strength when facing palm up. Whenever you grasp a litter or backboard, your hands should be at least 10" apart. Each hand should be inserted under the handle with the palm facing up and the thumb extended upward. You should then advance the hand until the thumb prevents further insertion and the cylindrical handle lies firmly in the crease of the curved palm. Curl your fingers and thumb tightly over the top of the handle. All your fingers should be at the same angle. To have the proper power grip, make sure that the underside of the handle is fully supported on your curved palm with only the fingers and thumb

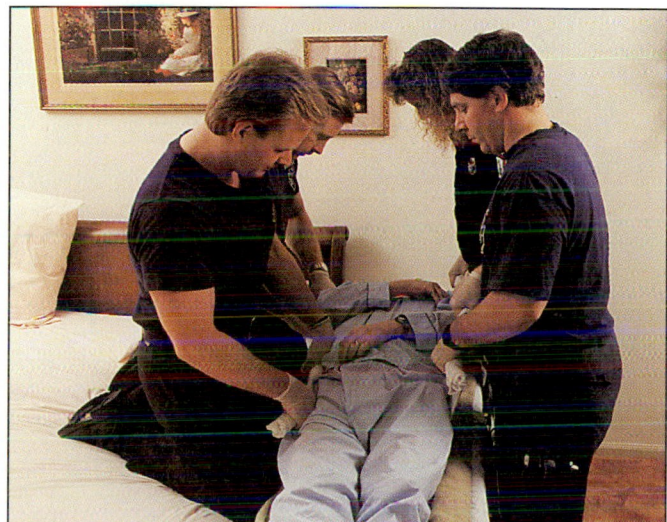

Always keep the weight that you are lifting as close to your body as possible.

preventing it from being pulled sideways or upward out of the palm.

If you must lift the object higher once you have lifted by extending your legs, you will be able to "curl" the object higher by using your biceps to flex the arms while maintaining the power grip and weight supported in the palms.

You should *never* grasp a litter or backboard with the hand placed palm down over the handle. In lifting with the palm down, the weight is supported by the fingers rather than the palm. This hand orientation places the tips of the fingers and thumb under the handle. If the weight forces them apart, your grasp on the handle will be lost.

When lifting a patient by a sheet or blanket, you should center the patient on the sheet and tightly roll up the excess fabric on each side. This produces a cylindrical handle that provides a strong, secure way to grasp the fabric (Figure 6-6).

When directly lifting a patient, you should tightly grip the patient in a place and manner that will ensure that you will not lose your grasp on the patient.

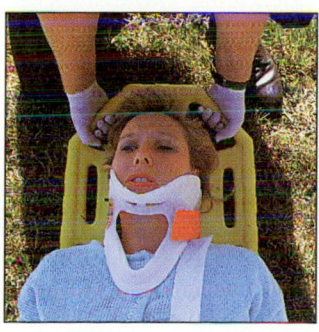

FIGURE 6-5 To perform the power grip, grasp the handle of the backboard with your palms up and your thumb extending up. Make sure your hands are about 10" apart and that your fingers are all at the same angle. The underside of the handle should be fully supported by the palm of your hand.

FIGURE 6-6 When lifting a patient by a bedsheet, you should center the patient on the sheet and tightly roll up the excess fabric on each side. This produces a cylindrical handle that provides a strong way to grasp the fabric.

Weight and Distribution

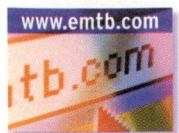

Whenever possible, you should use a device that can be rolled to move a patient. However, in case a wheeled device is not available, you must make sure that you understand and follow certain guidelines for carrying a patient on a stretcher or cot. Table 6-1 shows the guidelines.

If a patient is supine on a backboard or is lying or in a semi-sitting position on the ambulance cot, his or her weight is not equally distributed between the two ends of the device. Between 68% and 78% of the body weight of a patient in a horizontal position is in the torso. Therefore, more of the patient's weight rests on the head half of the device than on the foot half.

A patient on a backboard or stretcher should be lifted and carried by four rescuers in a **diamond carry**, with one EMT-B at the head end of the device, one at the foot end, and one at each side of the patient's torso (Figure 6-7). To best balance the weight, the EMT-Bs at each side should be located so that they are able to grasp the board or stretcher with one hand adjacent to the distal edge of the patient's pelvis and the other midthorax.

The four EMT-Bs should lift the device while facing in toward the patient. Once the patient and device have been lifted, the EMT-B at the foot end should turn around so that he or she is facing forward, and the

TABLE 6-1	Guidelines for Carrying a Patient on a Stretcher

- Be sure that you know or can find out the weight to be lifted and the limitations of the team's abilities.

- Coordinate your movements with those of the other team members while constantly communicating with them.

- Keep the weight that you are carrying as close to your body as possible while keeping your back in a locked-in position.

- Do not twist your body as you are carrying the patient.

- Be sure to flex at the hips, not at the waist, and bend at the knees, while making sure that you do not hyperextend your back by leaning back from your waist.

EMT-B at each side should turn the hand at the torso to palm down and then release the hand holding the board at the patient's pelvis and turn toward the feet. All four should be facing the same direction and will be walking forward when carrying the patient (Figure 6-8). A patient on a backboard or stretcher should be carried feet first to place the lightest load on the EMT-B at the patient's feet, who, to walk forward, must turn and grasp the handles with his or her back to the device. Carrying the patient feet first will also allow a conscious patient to see in the direction of movement.

It is important that you and your team use the correct lifting techniques to lift the stretcher. You must also make sure that your team members are of the same approximate height and strength.

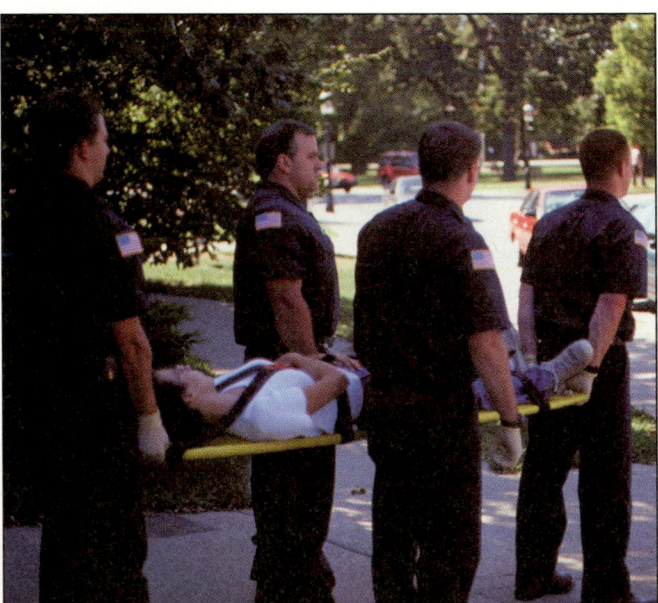

FIGURE 6-7 The diamond carry requires four rescuers, one at the head of the backboard, one at the foot end, and one at each side of the patient's torso.

Between 68% and 78% of the body weight of a patient in a horizontal position is in the torso. Therefore, more of the patient's weight rests on the head half of a carrying device than on the foot half.

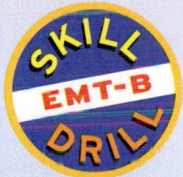

Performing the Diamond Carry
Figure 6-8

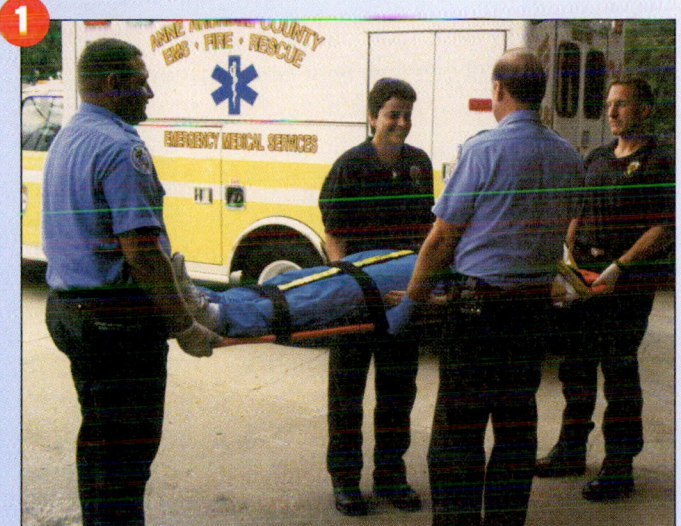

You should lift the backboard while facing in toward the patient.

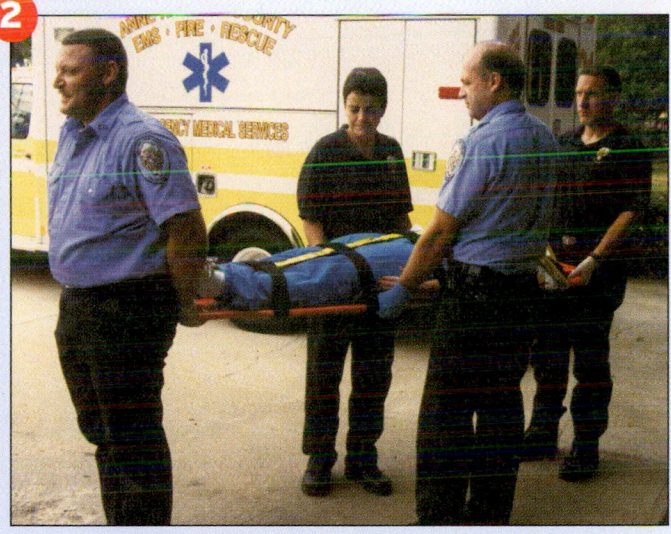

Once the lift is complete, the EMT-B at the foot end should turn around to face forward.

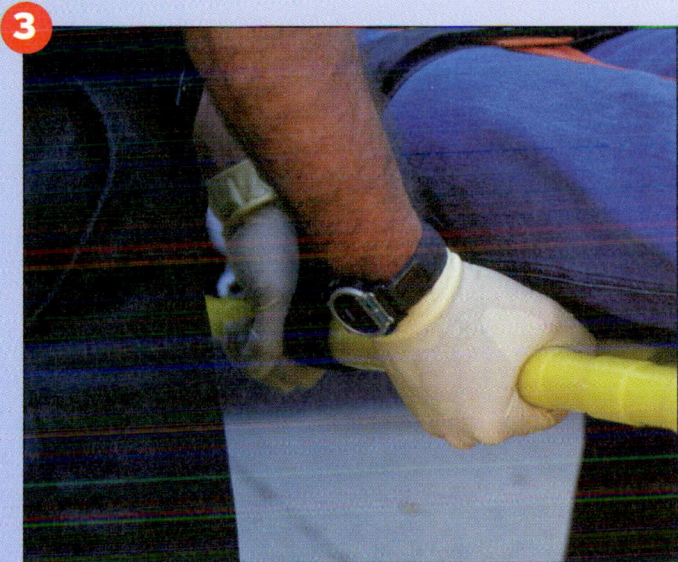

The EMT-Bs at the side should first turn the hand at the patient's head palm down and then release the hand holding the board at the patient's feet.

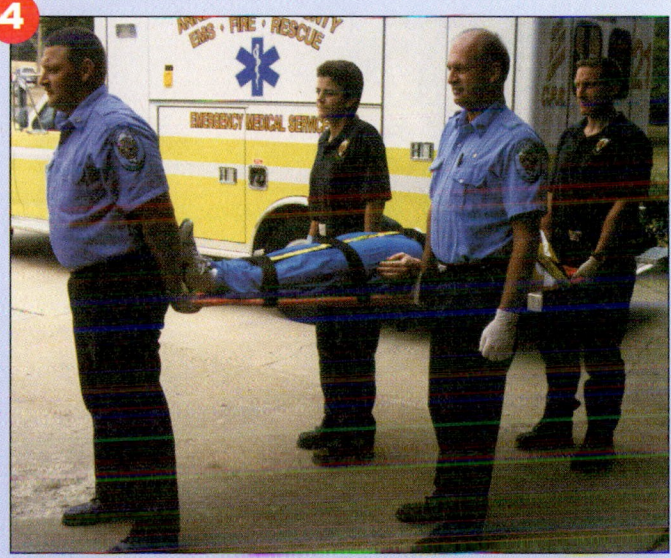

The EMT-Bs at the side should then turn toward the foot end. All four rescuers should be facing in the same direction and will walk forward when carrying the patient.

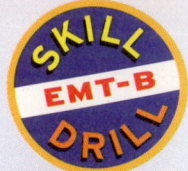

Performing the One-Handed Carrying Technique

Figure 6-9

1

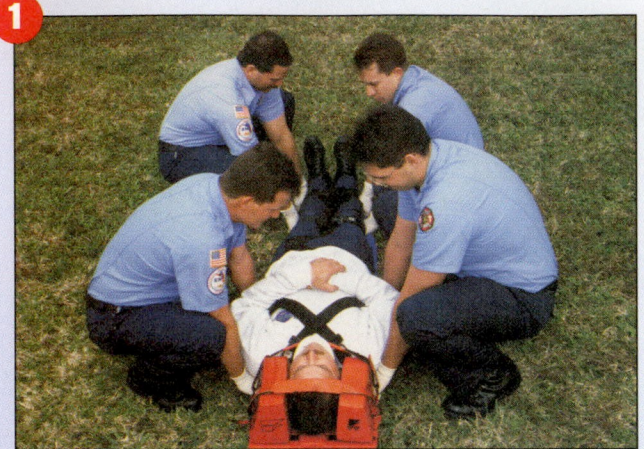

Ensure that two EMT-Bs are on each side of the stretcher facing each other and using both hands.

2

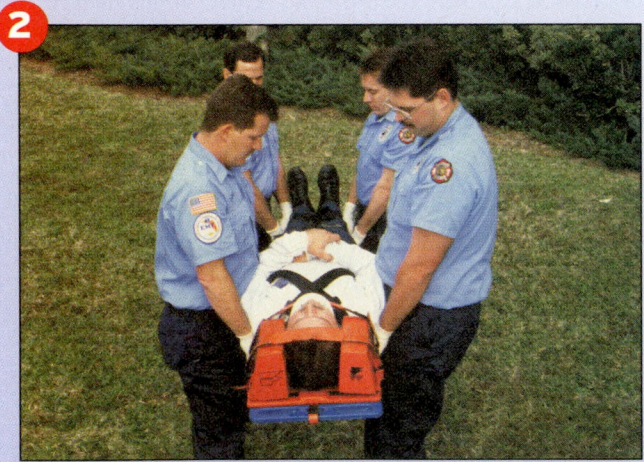

Lift the stretcher to carrying height.

3

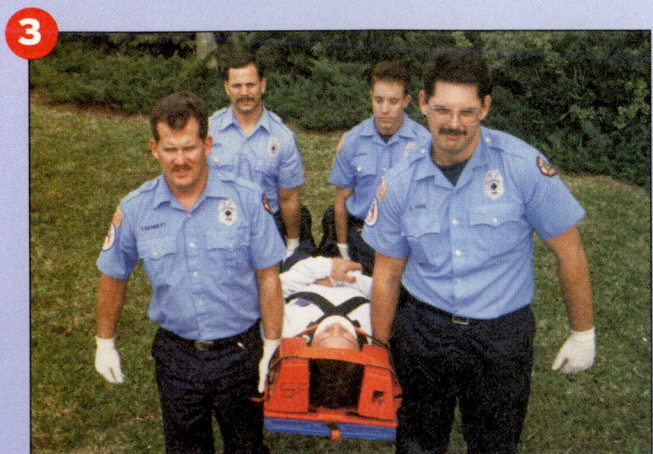

Turn in the direction in which you will be walking, and switch to using one hand.

One method of lifting and carrying a patient on a stretcher is the one-handed carrying technique (Figure 6-9). With this method, four or more EMT-Bs each use one hand to support the stretcher so that they are able to face forward as they are walking. When using this technique to lift the stretcher, be sure that at least two EMT-Bs are on each side of the stretcher facing each other and using both hands. Once you have lifted the stretcher to carrying height, you and your partners can turn in the direction you will be walking and switch to using one hand.

Be sure to pick up and carry the stretcher with your back in the locked-in position. If you need to lean to either side to compensate for a weight imbalance, you have probably exceeded your weight limitation. If this occurs, you may need to add helpers or reevaluate the carry, or you might injure yourselves or drop the patient.

A diamond carry is more stable than a carry in which there are two EMT-Bs at each side of the stretcher with no one at the patient's head or feet. With two EMT-Bs at each side, each EMT-B can only hold the board or stretcher with one hand when turned to face in the same direction. However, both carrying methods are recommended and widely used in the field.

The diamond carry is recommended when a patient must be carried in a building (Figure 6-10). If you must carry a patient through a narrow doorway or hallway, simply stop and have all the EMT-Bs turn until each is again facing in toward the patient. Then, by taking small, slow steps, you can move through the doorway. If the doorway is too narrow for the EMT-Bs at the sides of the stretcher to fit through, have one go through the doorway before the board or stretcher. As the other three EMT-Bs slowly move through the doorway, the EMT-B who walked through before the stretcher should grasp the board from the other side of the doorway before the EMT-B who is still at the side of the board reaches the doorway and must let go.

Sometimes, if a doorway, hallway, or stairwell is very narrow, it will only be possible to carry the backboard or stretcher from the head and foot ends. When this occurs, the EMT-Bs who were lifting and carrying at each side should relocate to help those at each end. One should move next to the EMT-B at the head end and share the load with him or her. The other should move in front of and grasp the belt of the EMT-B carrying the foot end, and steady and guide him or her.

Whenever you must carry a backboard or stretcher up or down a flight of stairs or other significant incline, you must be sure that the patient is so anatomically secured to the device that he or she cannot slide signifi-

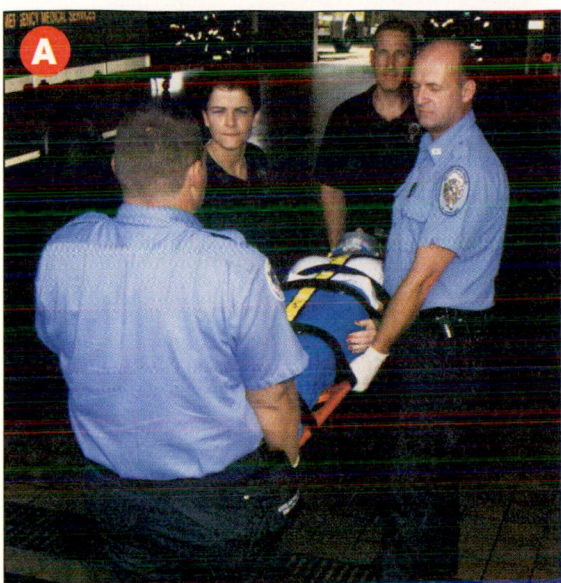

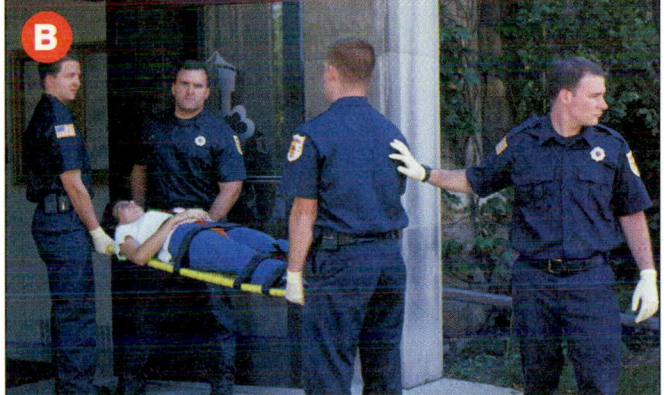

FIGURE 6-10 Carrying a patient through a narrow doorway or hallway. **A:** Stop and turn in to face the patient until you move through the passage. **B:** If the doorway or hallway is very narrow, the EMT-Bs at the side will need to move. One should move next to the EMT-B at the head end and share the load. The other should move in front of and support the back of the EMT-B carrying the foot end to steady and guide him or her through the passage.

cantly when the stretcher is at an angle (Figure 6-11). A strap that passes tightly across the upper torso and through each armpit, but not over the arms, is required to hold the patient in place. The strap is secured to the handles at both sides of the board so that it cannot slide toward the foot end of the board. A pair of groin loops is also recommended. Groin loops are straps that are anchored to each side of the board at the patient's waist and pass under the buttock, through the groin area, and diagonally over the pelvis back to the waist on each side.

When you carry the patient down stairs or an incline, make sure the board or stretcher is carried with the foot end first so that the head end is elevated higher than the foot end. The strap through the armpits and the groin

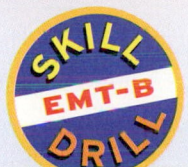

Carrying a Backboard or Stretcher on Stairs
Figure 6-11

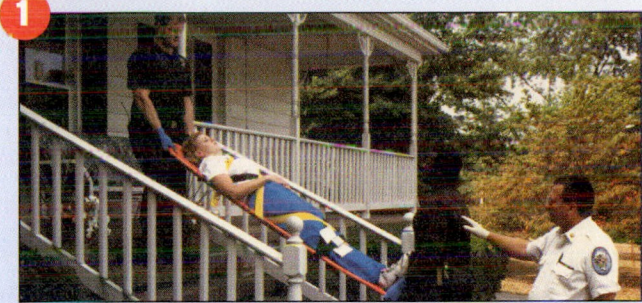

When you carry a backboard or stretcher up or down a flight of stairs, ensure that the patient is properly secured with one strap across the upper torso and through each armpit, leaving the arms free. In addition, groin loops may be used to anchor the patient to the board.

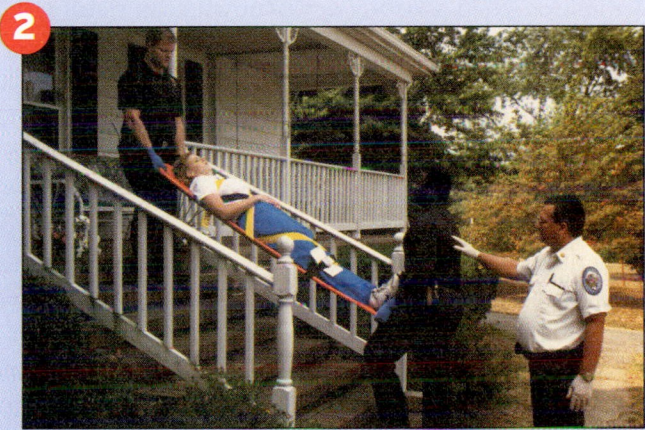

When you carry the patient down the stairs, make sure the board or stretcher is carried with the foot end first so that the head end is elevated higher.

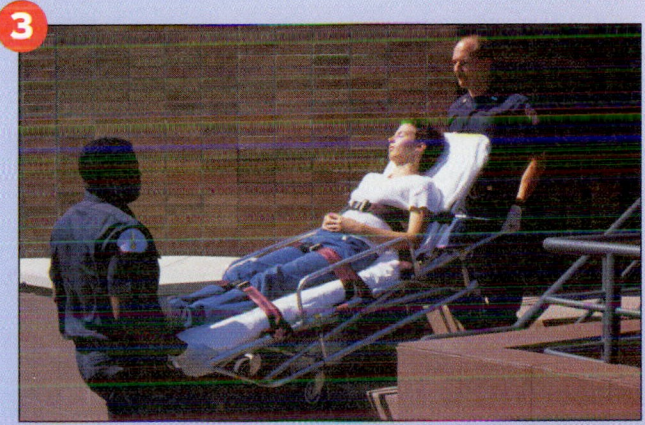

When you carry the patient up a flight of stairs, the elevated head end of the board or stretcher should go first.

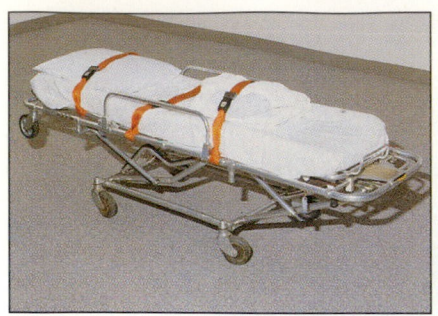

FIGURE 6-12 The wheeled ambulance stretcher is specially designed to roll along the ground.

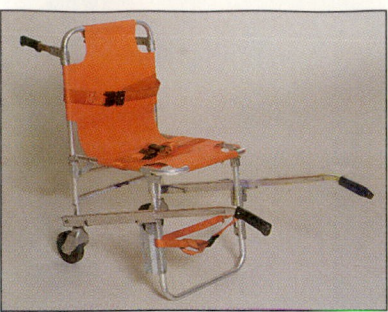

FIGURE 6-13 A wheeled stair chair can be used to transfer a conscious patient up or down a flight of stairs.

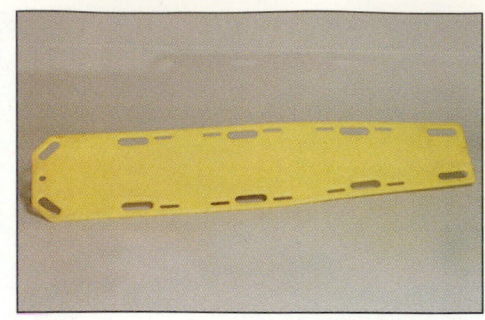

FIGURE 6-14 A backboard is used to transfer patients who must be moved in a supine or immobilized position.

loops (if included) will prevent the patient from sliding down or off the board. Similarly, when you carry a patient up stairs or an incline, the elevated head end of the board or stretcher should go first.

Whenever possible, you should use the patient's armpits as similar anatomic anchors and support points when you use a direct body lift or drag to move the patient or when assisting a patient who can stand.

The **wheeled ambulance stretcher** or cot, which is a specially designed stretcher that can be rolled along the ground, weighs between 40 and 70 lb, depending on its design and features (Figure 6-12). Because its weight must be added to that of the patient, it is generally not taken up or down stairs or to other locations where the patient must be carried rather than rolled for any significant distance. When the patient is upstairs, you should bring the wheeled ambulance stretcher to the ground floor landing and prepare it for the patient. You should then take either a wheeled stair chair or a backboard upstairs. Both of these devices are considerably lighter than a wheeled cot and may be used to carry the patient down to the waiting stretcher. Use a wheeled **stair chair** to bring a conscious patient down to the waiting cot if the patient's condition allows him or her to be placed in a sitting position (Figure 6-13). Once the cot has been reached, transfer the patient from the stair chair onto the cot. When the patient is in cardiac arrest, must be moved in a lying position, or must be immobilized, secure the patient onto a backboard. A **backboard**, which is a device that provides support to patients whom you suspect have hip, pelvic, spinal, or lower extremity injuries, is also called a spine board, trauma board, or longboard (Figure 6-14). You can then carry the patient on the backboard down the stairs to the prepared ambulance cot. Once you reach the ambulance cot, place both the board and patient on the cot and secure them with additional straps.

Directions and Commands

To safely lift and carry a patient, you and your team must anticipate and understand every move, and each move must be executed in a coordinated manner. The team leader should indicate where each team member is to be located and rapidly describe the sequence of steps that will be performed to ensure that the team knows what is expected of it before any lifting is initiated. If you must lift and move the patient through a number of separate stages, the team leader should first give an abbreviated overview of the stages, followed by a more detailed explanation of each stage just before it will occur. Orders that will initiate the actual lifting or moving or any significant changes in movement should be given in two parts: a preparatory command and a command of execution. For example, if the team leader says, "All ready to stop. STOP!," the "All ready to stop" will get your attention, identify who should act, and prepare them to act; the declarative "STOP!" will indicate the exact moment for execution. Commands of execution should be delivered in a louder voice. Often, a countdown is helpful when you need to lift a patient. To avoid confusion in using a countdown, always clarify whether "three" is to be a part of the preparatory command or whether it is to serve as the order to execute. You can say "We're going to lift on three, One-two-THREE!" or "I'm going to count to three and then we're going to lift, One-two-three-LIFT!"

Additional Lifting and Carrying Guidelines

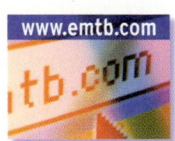

You should find out how much the patient weighs before attempting to lift him or her. Commonly, adult patients weigh between 100 and 210 lb. If you use the correct technique, you and one other EMT-B should be able to safely lift this weight. Depending on your individual strength, you and another EMT-B may be able to safely lift an even heavier patient. However, because it is quite a bit safer to have four rescuers lift, you should try to use four rescuers whenever the available resources allow. *You should know how much you can comfortably and safely lift and should not attempt to lift a proportional weight (the share of the weight that you will bear) that exceeds this amount.* If you find that lifting the patient places strain on you, call for the lifting to be stopped and the patient to be lowered. You should then obtain additional help before again attempting to lift the patient. Be sure to communicate clearly and frequently with your partner and other rescuers whenever you are lifting a patient.

You should *not* attempt to lift a patient who weighs more than 250 lb with fewer than four rescuers, regardless of individual strength. Protocols should include a method to rapidly summon additional help to lift and carry such a patient or, as in the case of a cardiac arrest, provide and maintain the necessary care in the field and when moving and transporting the patient. In addition, you must know, or be able to find out, the weight limitations of the equipment you are using and how to handle patients who exceed the weight limitations. Special techniques, equipment, and resources generally are required to move any patient who weighs more than 300 lb to the ambulance. These resources should be summoned when you arrive.

Because more than half of a patient's weight is distributed to the head end of the backboard or stretcher, the strongest of the available EMT-Bs should be located at the head end of the device. Even with four or more EMT-Bs carrying the patient, the strain on the EMT-B carrying the head end of the device will be increased when you must negotiate a narrow area or flight of stairs. In carrying a patient up or down a flight of stairs, proportionally greater weight will also be distributed to the EMT-B who is carrying the foot end when the backboard or stretcher becomes angled because of the incline. You should anticipate this and, in such cases, make sure the two strongest EMT-Bs are positioned at the head and foot ends of the board. Because of the incline of the stairway, if one of the two EMT-Bs is considerably taller than the other, it will be easier if the shorter of the two is at the head end and the taller is at the foot end.

The dynamics that are involved in carrying a patient down a flight of stairs or for any significant distance will not allow you to carry as much proportional weight as you can to safely lift or support the patient during a move onto a nearby backboard or cot. Therefore, if you feel that you are approaching your maximum lifting capacity as you are moving the patient onto a backboard or cot, you should not attempt to lift and carry the patient for any significant distance or down a flight of stairs. You can again attempt to lift and carry the patient after you have decreased the amount of proportional weight you will be carrying by changing your position on the device or that of the others on the team or have obtained additional help.

You should try to use a stair chair instead of a stretcher, whenever possible, to carry a patient down stairs (Figure 6-15). As with other carries, always remember to keep your back in a locked-in position and to flex at the hips, not the waist. You should also bend at the knees and keep the patient's weight and your arms as close to your body as possible. Try to avoid any unnecessary lifting and carrying of the patient. If an assist, log roll, or body drag will not harm or jeopardize the patient, use one to move the patient onto the backboard, stretcher, or ambulance cot.

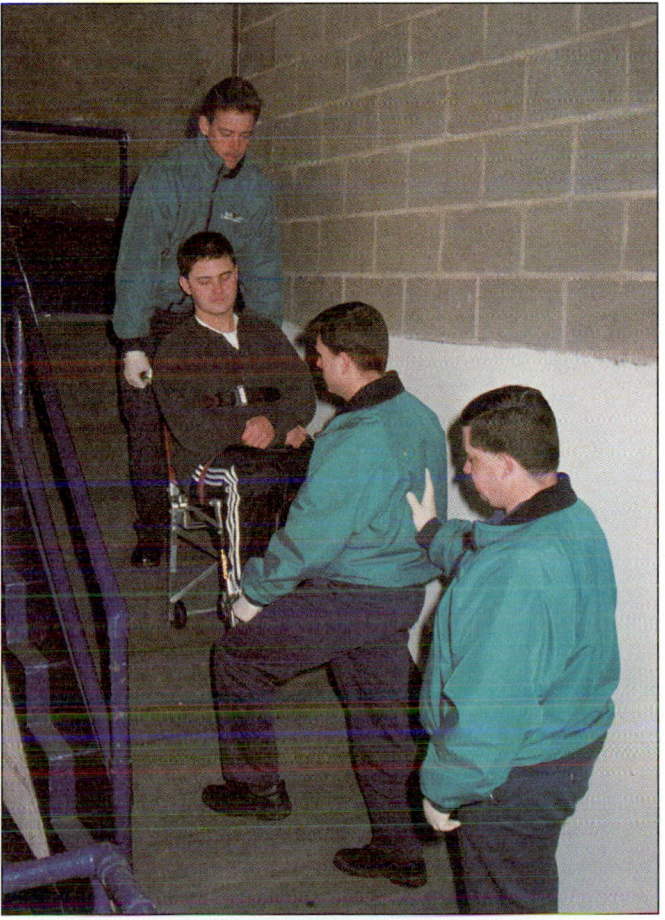

FIGURE 6-15 When using a stair chair instead of a stretcher, remember to keep your back in a locked-in position, and flex at the hips. Bend at the knees, and keep the patient's weight and your arms as close to your body as possible.

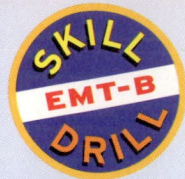

Reaching and Pulling Safely
Figure 6-16

1

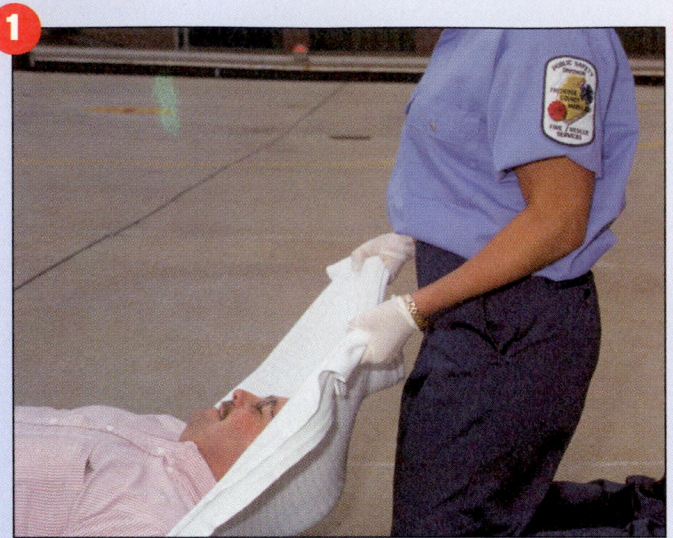

When you are pulling a patient who is on the ground, kneel so that you minimize the distance you will have to lean over.

2

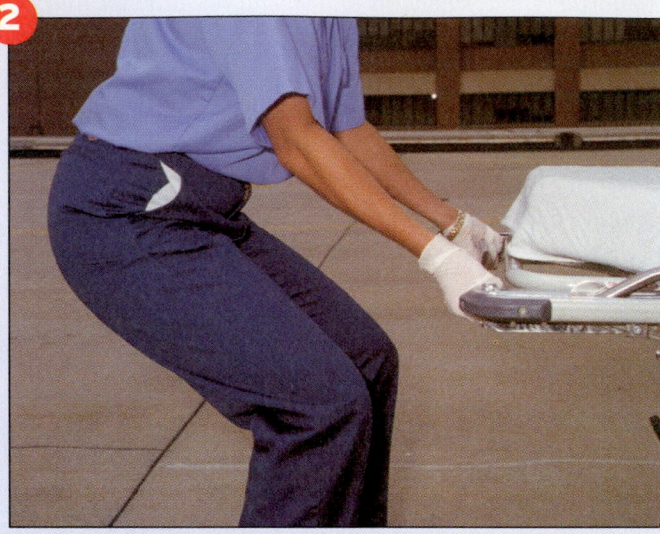

When you are pulling a patient who is at a different height than you, bend your knees until your hips are just below the height of the plane across which you will be pulling the patient.

3

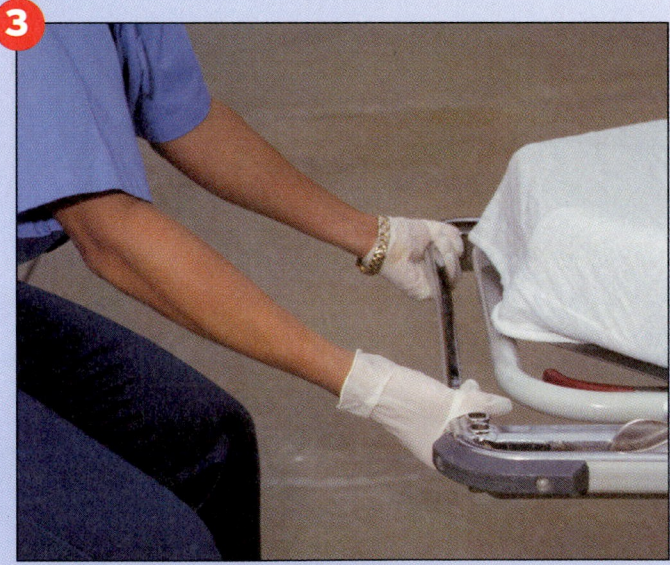

When pulling, extend your arms no more than 15" to 20" in front of your torso. Also make sure that your elbows are just beyond the anterior torso.

4

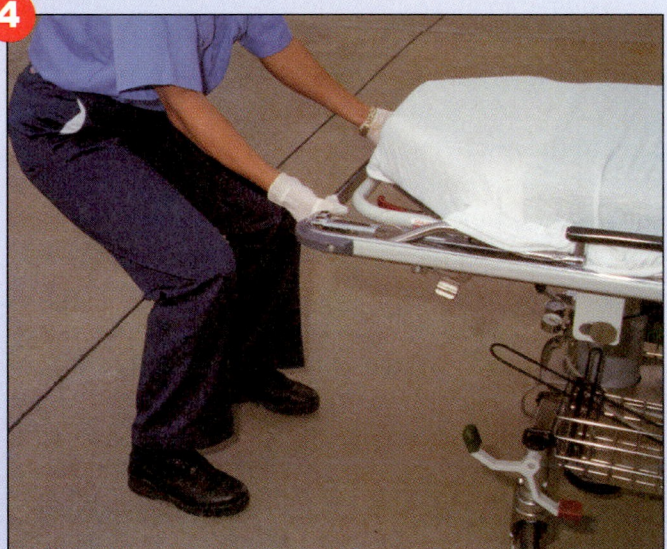

Position your feet (or knees if you are kneeling) so that the force of pull is balanced equally between both arms and the line of pull centered between them.

Principles of Safe Reaching and Pulling

When you use a body drag to move a patient, the same basic body mechanics and principles apply as when lifting and carrying (Figure 6-16). Your back should always be locked and straight, not curved or bent laterally, and you should avoid any twisting so that the vertebrae remain in normal alignment. When reaching overhead, avoid hyperextending your back. When you are pulling a patient who is on the ground, you should always kneel to minimize the distance that you will have to lean over. When pulling a patient who is at a different height from you, bend your knees until your hips are just below the height of the plane across which you will be pulling the patient. When pulling, you should extend your arms no more than about 15" to 20" in front of your torso. To keep your reach within the recommended distance, reach forward and grasp the patient so that your elbows are just beyond the anterior torso. Reposition your feet (or knees, if kneeling) so that the force of pull will be balanced equally between both arms and the line of pull will be centered between them. Pull the patient by slowly flexing your arms. When you can pull no farther because your hands have reached the front of your torso, stop and move back another 15" to 20". Then, when properly positioned, repeat the steps. You should alternate between pulling the patient by flexing your arms and then repositioning yourself so that your arms are again extended with your hands about 15" in front of your torso. By not moving yourself and the patient simultaneously, you will prevent undesirable jostling of the patient and the chance that sudden unscheduled force will occur across your spine. You should also try to prevent injury to yourself by avoiding situations that involve strenuous effort lasting more than 1 minute.

If you must drag a patient for a considerable distance across a bed, you will have to kneel on the bed to avoid reaching beyond the recommended distance. Then follow the steps described above until the patient is within 15" to 20" of the bed's edge. You can then complete the drag while standing at the side of the bed. Rather than dragging the patient by his or her clothing, use the sheet or blanket under the patient for this purpose.

Unless the patient is on a backboard, transfer a patient from the ambulance cot to a bed in the emergency department or the patient's hospital room with a body drag. With the ambulance cot at the same height as the bed and held firmly against its side, you and another EMT-B should kneel on the hospital bed and, in the manner previously described, drag the patient in increments until he or she is properly centered on the bed. When transferring the patient onto a narrow examining table, rather than kneeling on the table, you can usually drag the patient while standing against the opposite side.

Sometimes during a body drag, you and another EMT-B may have to pull the patient with one of you on each side of the patient (Figure 6-17). You will have to alter the usual pulling technique to prevent pulling sideways and producing adverse lateral leverage against your lower back. You should position yourself by kneeling just beyond the patient's shoulder and facing toward his or her groin. By extending one arm across and in front of your chest, you can grasp the armpit and, with the other arm extended in front and to the side of the torso, the patient's belt. Then, by raising your elbows and flexing your arms, you can pull the patient with the line of force at the minimum angle possible.

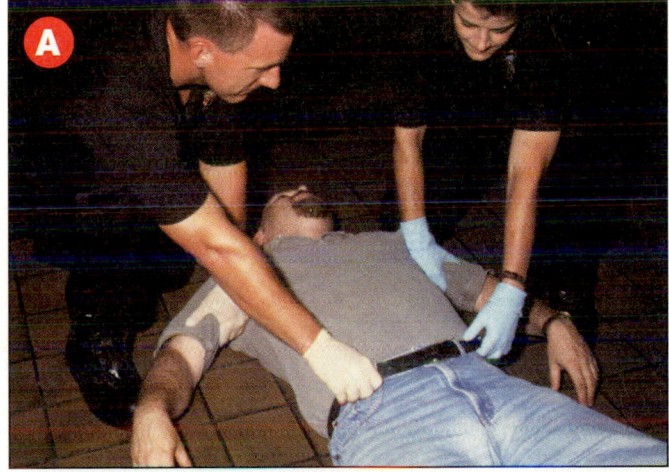

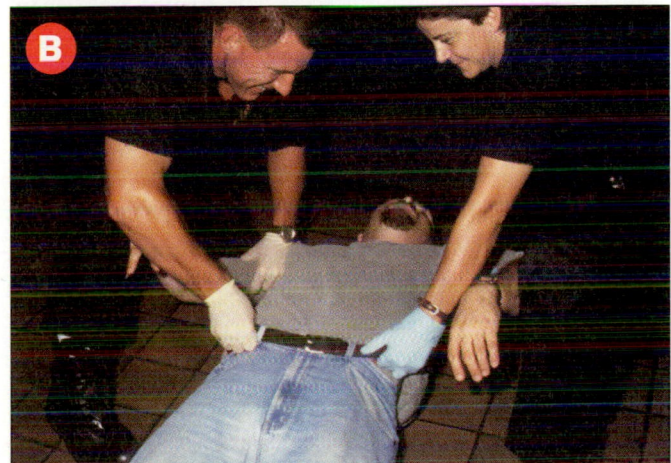

FIGURE 6-17 A body drag with an EMT-B on each side of the patient **A:** Kneel just beyond the patient's shoulder, facing his or her groin. Extend one arm across and in front of your chest, and grasp the armpit. Extend your other arm in front and to the side of the patient's torso, and grasp the patient's belt. **B:** Raise your elbows, and flex your arms to pull the patient.

Generally, when log-rolling a patient onto his or her side, you will initially have to reach farther than 18" (Figure 6-18). To minimize this distance, kneel as close to the patient's side as possible, leaving only enough room so that your knees will not prevent the patient from being rolled. When you lean forward, keep your back straight, and lean solely from the hips. Be sure to use your shoulder muscles to help with the roll. To minimize the amount of time you are extended like this and to support the patient's weight, roll the patient without stopping until the patient is resting on his or her side. Some EMS experts consider that, during a log roll, you should pull rather than push the patient. Local protocols will guide your training in this area.

When rolling the wheeled ambulance stretcher, make sure that it is elevated (Figure 6-19). Pull the stretcher from the foot end. Make sure your arms are held close to your body, and be careful to avoid reaching significantly behind you or hyperextending your back. Your back should be locked, straight, and untwisted. While you are walking and pulling the cot, bend slightly forward at the hips. As you walk, your legs are pulled back with the feet on the ground, your pelvis is moved forward, and the movement of the pelvis is transferred to the cot through your straight torso and firmly held arms. You should try to keep the line of the pull through the center of your body by bending your knees.

A second EMT-B should guide the head end and assist you by pushing with his or her arms held with the elbows bent so that the hands are about 12" to 15" in front of the torso. To protect your elbows from injury, you should never push an object with your arms fully extended in a straight line and the elbows locked. When you push with the elbow bent but firmly held from bending further, the strong muscles of the arm serve as a shock absorber if the wheels or foot end of the cot strikes an obstacle that causes its progress to be suddenly slowed or stopped. You must be sure that you push from the area of your body that is between the waist and shoulder. If the weight you are pushing is lower than your waist, you should push from a kneeling position. Be careful that you do not push or pull from an overhead position.

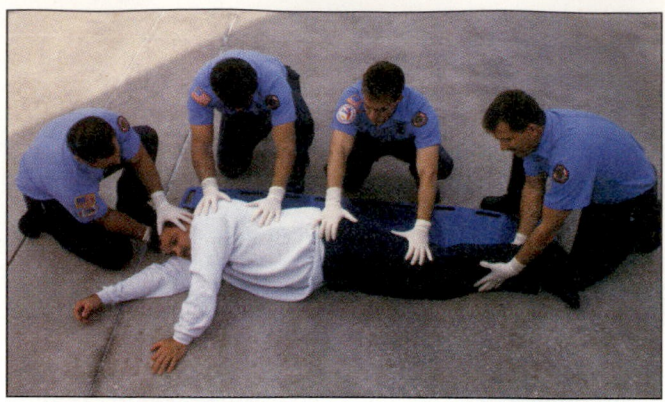

FIGURE 6-18 When placing a patient onto a backboard, roll the patient onto his or her side. Kneel as close to the patient's side as possible leaving only enough room so that your knees will not prevent the patient from being rolled. Lean forward, keeping your back straight and leaning solely from the hips. Use your shoulder muscles to help with the roll.

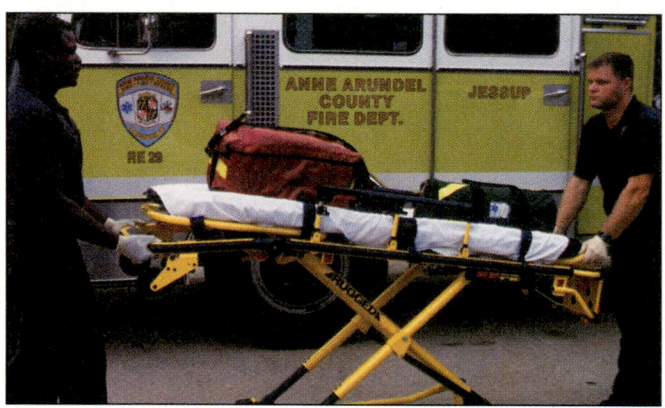

FIGURE 6-19 A wheeled ambulance stretcher should be elevated. You should pull the stretcher from the foot end with your arms held close to your body and without hyperextending your back. A second EMT-B should guide the head, assisting you by pushing with the arms held so that the elbows are bent and the hands 12" to 15" in front of the torso.

General Considerations

Moving a patient should normally be done in an orderly, planned, and unhurried fashion. This approach will protect both you and the patient from further injury and reduce the risk of worsening the patient's condition when he or she is moved. At a minimum, on most calls you will have to lift and carry the patient to the wheeled ambulance stretcher, move the cot and patient to the ambulance, and load the cot into the patient compartment.

You will often have to include several additional steps to place the patient onto a backboard and/or carry him or her down a flight of stairs. You will also have to add a stop at the top of the stairway so that everyone can

> Prevent injury to yourself by avoiding situations that involve strenuous effort lasting more than 1 minute.

reposition for carrying the patient down the stairs. Repositioning usually requires lowering the board to the ground and lifting it again when all EMT-Bs are in their proper places. If you are carrying the patient in a stair chair, the additional step occurs after you have descended the stairs and reached the cot. At that point, you will have to assist or lift the patient from the stair chair onto the ambulance cot.

You should carefully plan ahead and select the methods that will involve the least lifting and carrying. Remember to always consider whether there is an option that will cause less strain to you and the other EMT-Bs.

Emergency Moves

You should use an <u>emergency move</u> to move a patient before initial assessment and care are provided when there is some potential danger, and you and the patient must move to a safe place to avoid possible serious harm or death. The presence of fire, explosives, or hazardous materials and your inability to protect the patient from other hazards or gain access to others in a vehicle who need lifesaving care are all situations in which you should use an emergency move.

The only other time you should use an emergency move is if you cannot properly assess the patient or provide immediate potentially critical emergency care because of the patient's location or position.

If you are alone and danger at the scene makes it necessary for you to use an emergency move, regardless of a patient's injuries, you should use a drag to pull the patient along the long axis of the body. This will help to keep the spinal column in line as much as possible. When performing an emergency move, one of your primary concerns is the danger of aggravating an existing spinal injury. Remember that it is impossible to remove a patient quickly from a vehicle while providing as much protection to the spine as you would give by using an immobilization device. However, if you follow certain guidelines during the move, you can usually move a patient from a life-threatening situation without causing further injury to the patient.

You can move a patient on his or her back along the floor or ground by using one of the following methods (Figure 6-20, see next page):

- Pull on the patient's clothing in the neck and shoulder area.

- Place the patient onto a blanket, coat, or other item that can be pulled.

- Rotate the patient's arms so that they are extended straight on the ground beyond his or her head, grasp the wrists, and, with the arms elevated above the ground, drag the patient.

- Place your arms under the patient's shoulders and through the armpits, and, while grasping the patient's arms, drag the patient backward.

If you are alone and must remove an unconscious patient from a car, you should first move the patient's legs so they are clear of the pedals and are against the seat. Then rotate the patient so that his or her back is positioned facing the open car door. Next, place your arms through the armpits and grasp either the patient's forearms or your own forearms (Figure 6-21). Support the patient's head against your body. While supporting the patient's weight, drag the patient from the seat.

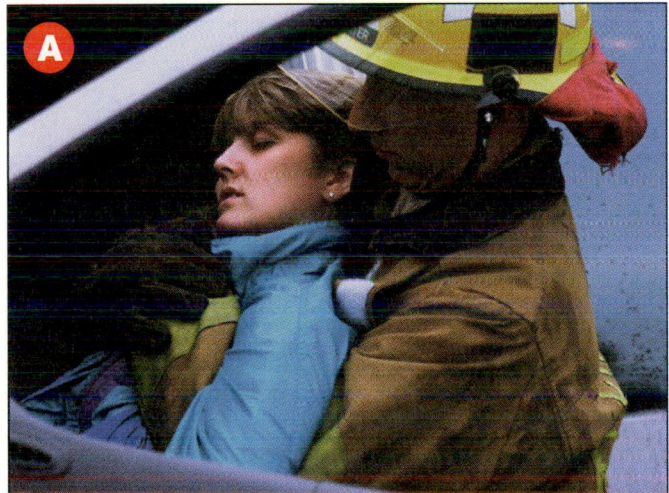

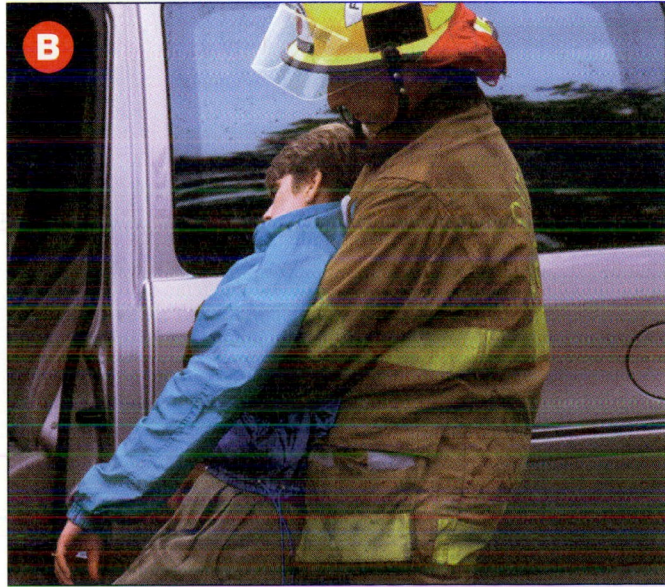

FIGURE 6-21 One-person technique for moving an unconscious patient from a car. **A:** Grasp the patient under the arms. **B:** Pull the patient down into a supine position.

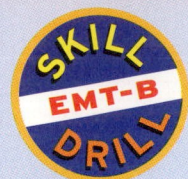

Dragging Methods
Figure 6-20

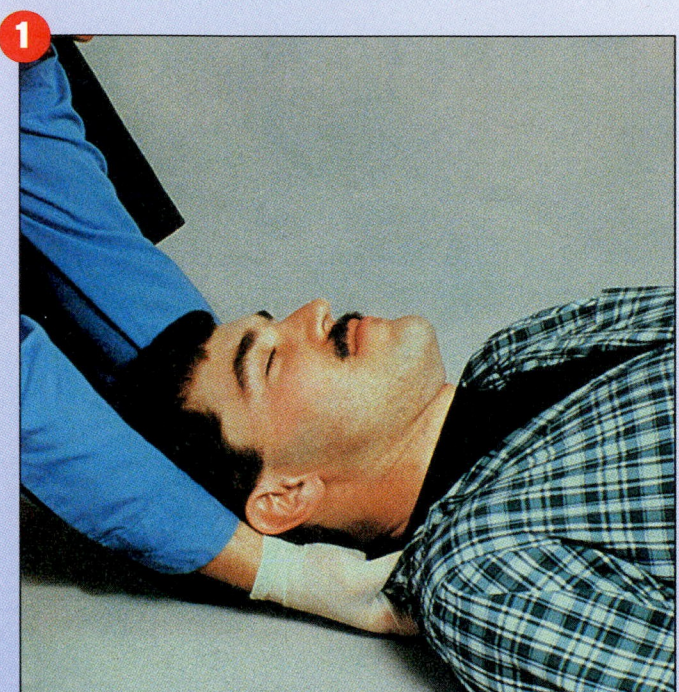

1

Emergency clothes drag.

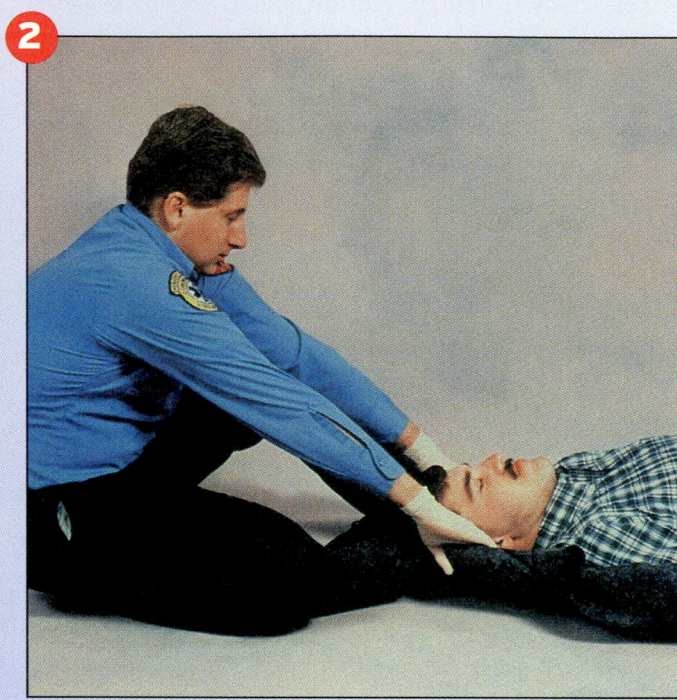

2

Blanket drag.

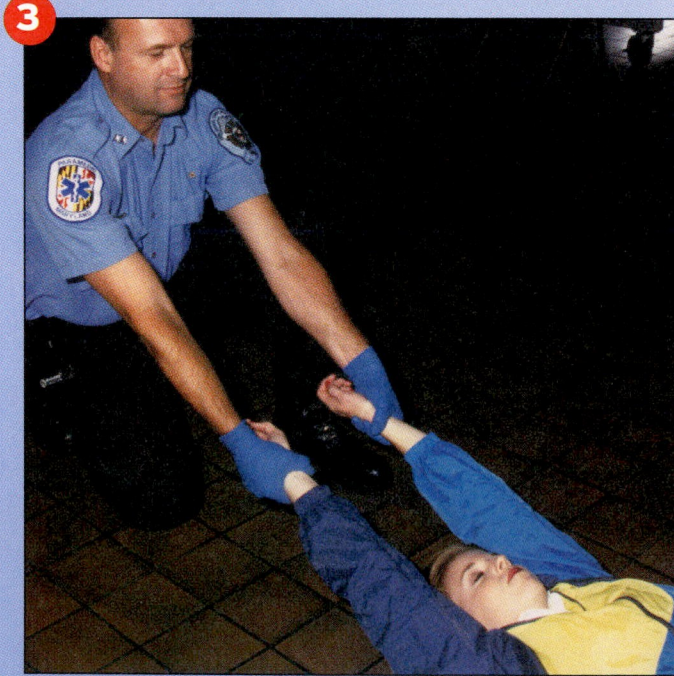

3

Arm drag.

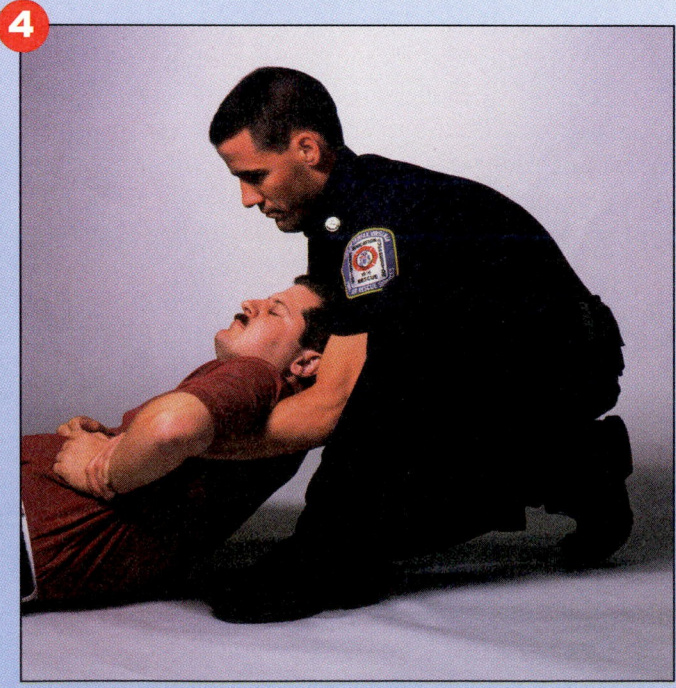

4

Arm-to-arm drag.

If the legs and feet clear the car easily, you can rapidly drag the patient to a safe location by continuing this method. If the legs and feet do not clear the car easily, you can slowly lower the patient until he or she is lying on his or her back next to the car, clear the legs from the vehicle, and, as previously described, use a long-axis body drag to move the patient a safe distance from the vehicle.

You should use one-person techniques to move a patient only if a potentially life-threatening danger exists and you are alone or, because of the pressing nature of the danger, your partner is moving a second patient simultaneously. Additional one-rescuer drags, carries, and lifts are shown in Figure 6-22.

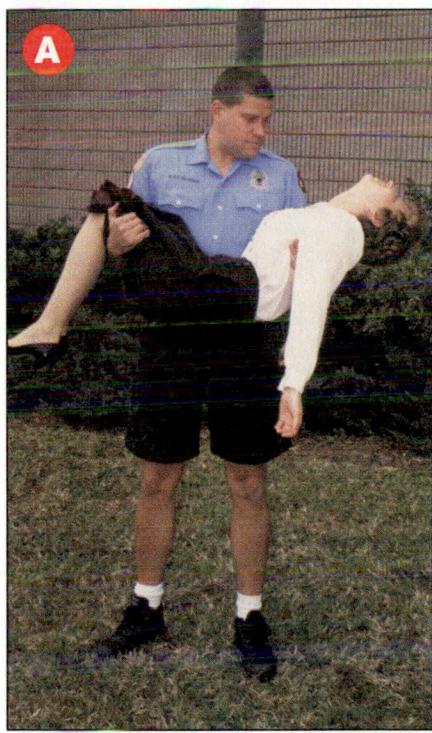

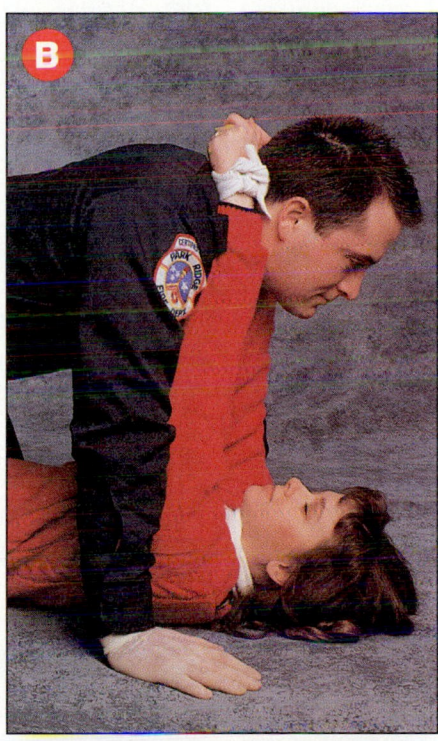

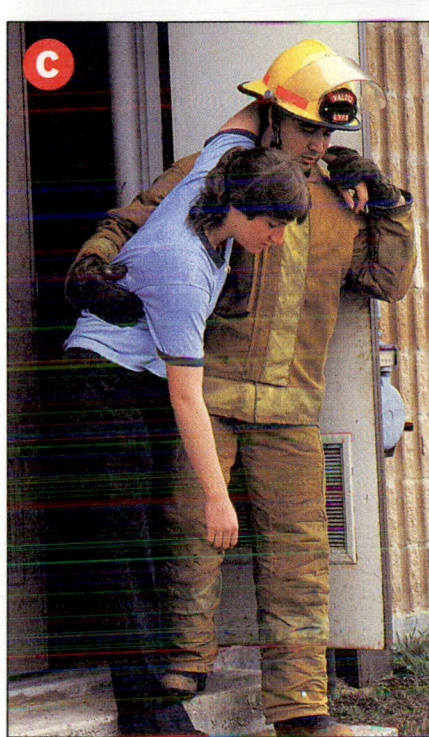

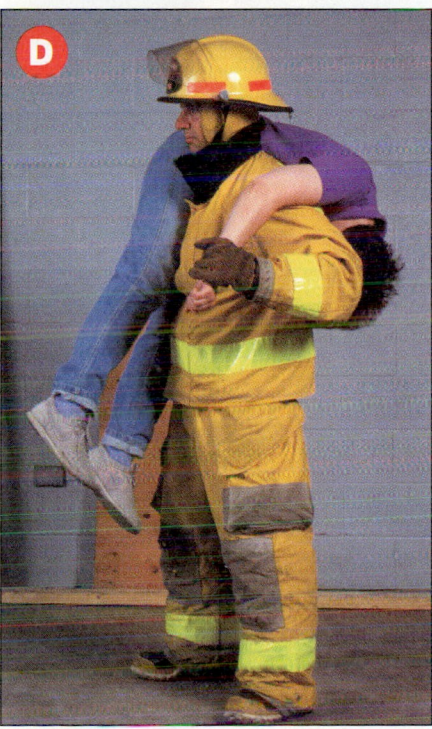

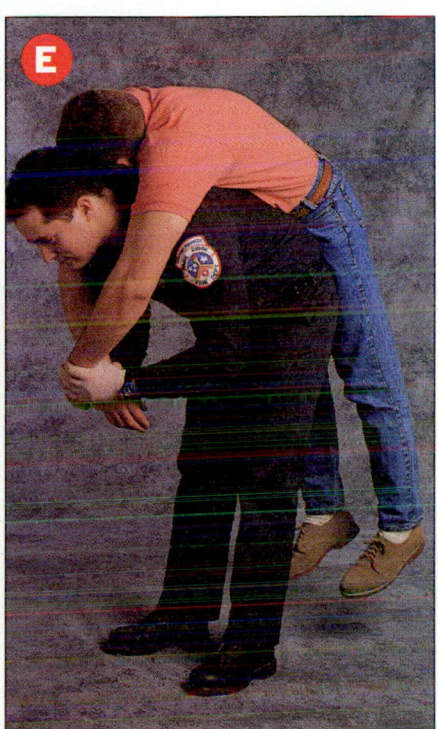

FIGURE 6-22
One-rescuer drags, carries, and lifts.
A: Front cradle.
B: Firefighter's drag.
C: One-person walking assist.
D: Firefighter's carry.
E: Pack strap.

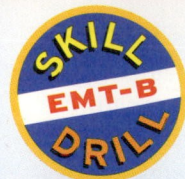

Performing Rapid Extrication Technique
Figure 6-23

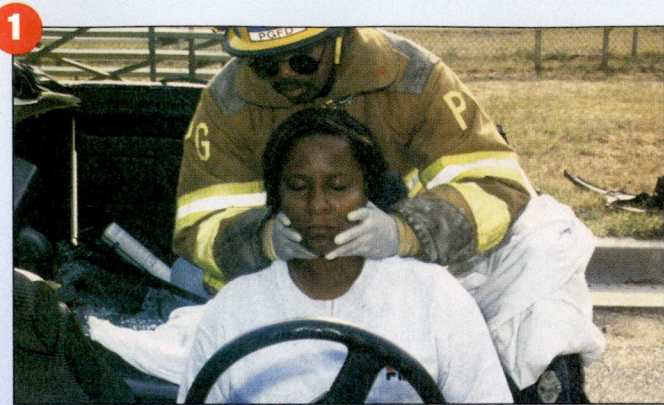

First EMT-B provides in-line manual support of the head and cervical spine from behind.

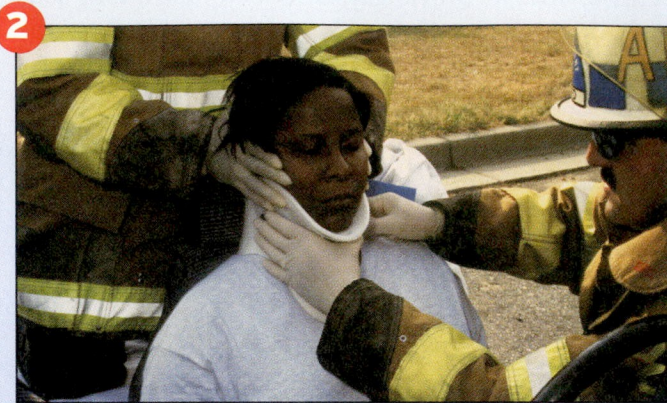

Second EMT-B applies a cervical collar and performs the initial assessment.

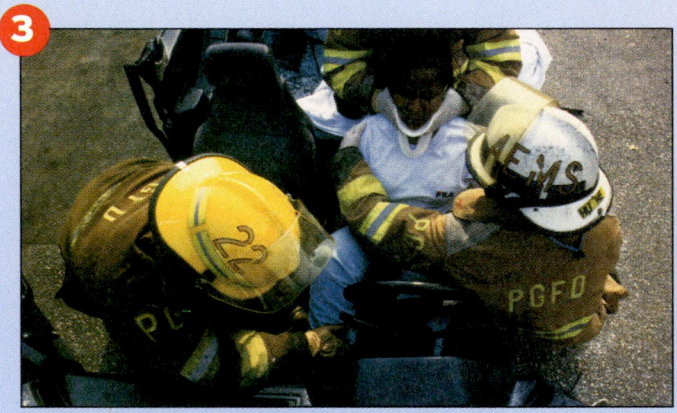

Second EMT-B supports the thorax as Third EMT-B frees the patient's legs from the pedals.

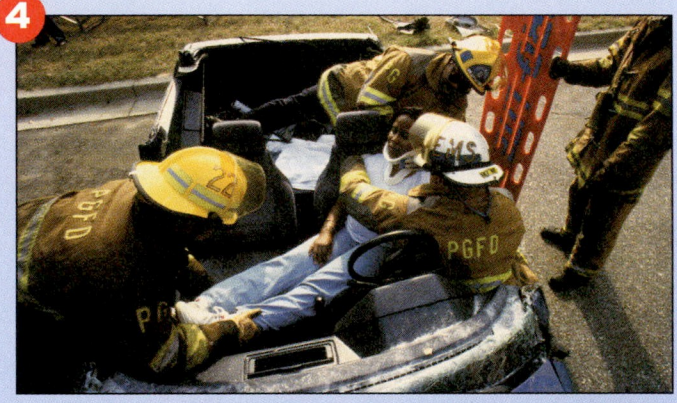

At the direction of the Second EMT-B, he and the Third EMT-B rotate the patient in several short, coordinated moves until the patient's back is in the open doorway and her feet are on the passenger seat.

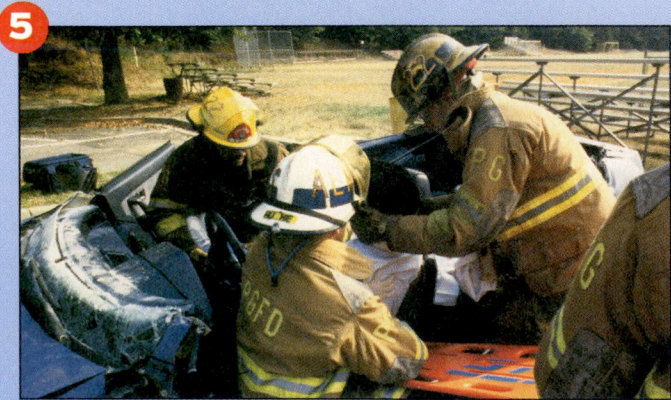

The First EMT-B supports the head and neck while the Second and Third EMT-B's lower the patient onto the long spine board. If the First EMT-B is unable to support the head and neck, another available EMT-B or bystander must take over support.

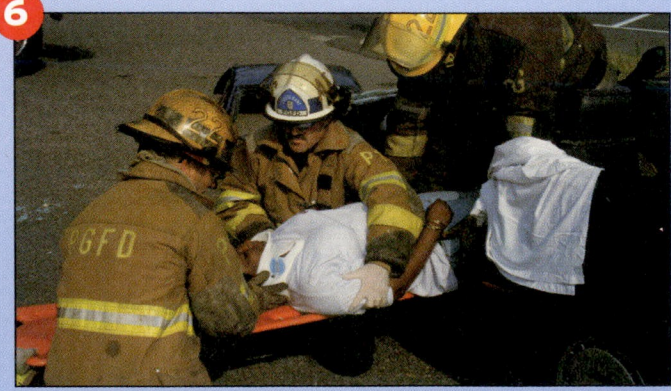

Second EMT-B and Third EMT-B slide the patient along the backboard.

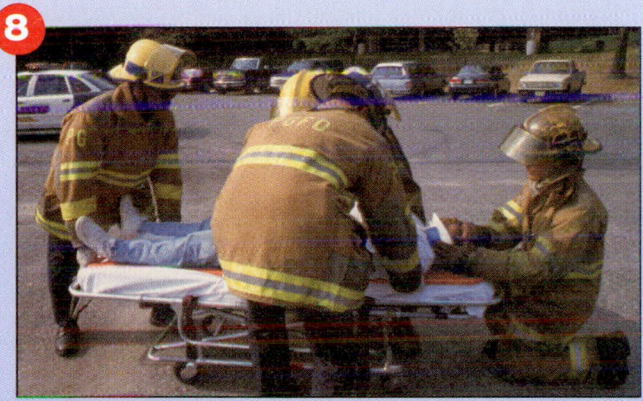

Third EMT-B then gets out of the vehicle and moves to the opposite side of the backboard, across from Second EMT-B. Third EMT-B now controls the shoulders, Second EMT-B moves to the hips, and they continue to slide the patient along until his or her hips rest fully on the backboard.

Fourth EMT-B continues to stabilize the head and neck, while Second EMT-B and Third EMT-B grasp their side of the board and carry the patient away from the vehicle.

TABLE 6-2	Situations in Which to Use the Rapid Extrication Technique

- The vehicle or scene is unsafe.
- The patient cannot be properly assessed before being removed from the car.
- The patient needs immediate intervention that requires a supine position.
- The patient's condition requires immediate transport to the hospital.
- The patient blocks the EMT-B's access to another seriously injured patient.

Urgent Moves

An urgent move may be necessary for moving a patient with an altered level of consciousness, inadequate ventilation, or shock (hypoperfusion). An extreme weather condition may also make an urgent move necessary. In some cases, patients must be urgently moved from the location or position in which they are found. When a patient who is sitting in a car or truck must be urgently moved, you should use the rapid extrication technique.

Rapid Extrication Technique

The long backboard, short backboard, and vest-type devices are known as immobilization devices. Normally, you would use an extrication-type vest or half-backboard device to immobilize a seated patient with a suspected spinal injury before removing the patient from the car. However, using either of these devices usually requires between 6 and 8 minutes, in some cases even longer. By using the **rapid extrication technique** instead, the patient can be moved from sitting in the car to lying supine on a backboard in 1 minute or less. Table 6-2 describes the situations in which you should use the rapid extrication technique.

In such cases, the delay that occurs in applying an extrication-type vest or half-board is contraindicated. However, the manual support and immobilization that you provide when using the rapid extrication technique produce a greater risk of spine movement. You should not use the rapid extrication technique if no urgency exists.

The rapid extrication technique requires a team of three EMT-Bs who are knowledgeable and practiced in the procedure. You should take the following steps when using the rapid extrication technique (Figure 6-23):

1. **First EMT-B applies manual in-line support** of the patient's head and cervical spine from behind. Support may be applied from the side, if necessary, by reaching through the driver's side doorway.

2. **Second EMT-B serves as team leader** and, as such, gives the commands until the patient is supine on the backboard. Because Second EMT lifts and turns the patient's torso, he or she must be physically capable of moving the patient. Second EMT works from the driver's side doorway. If First EMT is also working from that doorway, Second EMT should stand closer to the door hinges toward the front of the vehicle. Second EMT applies a cervical immobilization device.

3. **Second EMT-B provides continuous support** of the patient's torso until the patient is supine on the backboard. Once Second EMT-B takes control of

the torso, usually in the form of a body hug, he or she should not let go of the patient for any reason. Some type of cross-chest shoulder hug usually works well, but you will have to decide what method works best for you on any given patient. You must remember that you cannot simply reach into the car and grab the patient; this will only twist the patient's torso. You must rotate the patient as a unit.

4. **Third EMT-B works from the front passenger's seat** and is responsible for rotating the patient's legs and feet as the torso is turned. If necessary, this position can be filled by an on-scene recruit, such as a firefighter or law enforcement officer. With care, Third EMT-B should first move the patient's nearer leg laterally without rotating the patient's pelvis and lower spine. The pelvis and lower spine rotate only as Third EMT-B moves the second leg during the next step. Moving the nearer leg early makes it much easier to move the second leg in concert with the rest of the body. After Third EMT-B moves the legs together, they should be moved as a unit.

The first four steps of the rapid extrication technique direct the team to their starting positions and responsibilities. First EMT applies in-line support and immobilization of the head and neck. Second EMT gives orders and supports the torso. Third EMT moves and supports the patient's legs. The team is now ready to move the patient.

5. **The patient is rotated 90°** so that his or her back is facing out the driver's door and the feet are on the front passenger's seat. This movement is done in three or four short, quick "eighth turns." Second EMT directs each quick turn by saying, "Ready, turn" or "Ready, move." Hand position changes should be made between moves.

6. **In most cases, First EMT-B will be working from the back seat.** At some point, either because the doorpost is in the way or because he or she cannot reach farther from the back seat, First EMT-B will be unable to follow the torso rotation. At that time, Third EMT should assume temporary in-line support of the head and neck until First EMT can regain control of the head from outside the vehicle. If a fourth EMT-B is present, Fourth EMT-B stands next to Second EMT. Fourth EMT takes control of the head and neck from outside the vehicle without involving Third EMT-B. As soon as the change has been made, the rotation can continue.

7. **Once the patient has been fully rotated,** the backboard should be placed against the patient's buttocks on the seat. Do not try to wedge the backboard under the patient. If only three EMTs are present, be sure to place the backboard within arm's reach of the driver's door before the move so that the board can be pulled into place when needed. In such cases, the far end of the board can be left on the ground. When a fourth EMT-B is available, First EMT-B exits the rear seat of the car, places the backboard against the patient's buttocks, and maintains pressure in toward the vehicle from the far end of the board. (Note: When the door opening allows, some EMT-Bs prefer to insert the backboard onto the car seat before the patient is rotated.)

8. **As soon as the patient has been rotated** and the backboard is in place, Second EMT-B and Fourth EMT-B lower the patient onto the board while supporting the head and torso so that neutral alignment is maintained. First EMT-B holds the backboard until the patient is secured.

9. **Next, Third EMT must move across the front seat** to be in position at the patient's hips. If Third EMT-B stays at the patient's knees or feet, he or she will be ineffective in helping to move the body's weight. The knees and feet follow the hips.

10. **Fourth EMT maintains manual in-line support** of the head and now takes over giving the commands. If a fourth EMT-B is not present, you can direct a volunteer to assist you. Second EMT-B maintains direction of the extrication. Second EMT-B stands with his or her back to the door, facing the rear of the vehicle. The backboard should be immediately in front of Third EMT-B. Second EMT-B grasps the patient's shoulders or armpits. Then, on command, Second EMT-B and Third EMT-B slide the patient 8″ to 12″ along the backboard, repeating this slide until the patient's hips are firmly on the backboard. At that time, Third EMT-B gets out of the vehicle and moves to the opposite side of the backboard, across from Second EMT-B. Third EMT-B now takes control at the shoulders, and Second EMT-B moves back to take control of the hips. On command, these two EMT-Bs move the patient along the board in 8″ to 12″ slides until the patient is placed fully on the board.

11. **Fourth EMT-B continues to maintain manual in-line support** of the head. Second EMT-B and Third EMT-B now grasp their side of the board, and then carry it and the patient away from the vehicle onto the prepared cot nearby.

In some cases, you will be able to rest the head end of the backboard on the ambulance cot while the patient is moved onto the backboard. In others, you will not. Once the backboard and patient have been placed on the ambulance cot, you should begin lifesaving treatment immediately. If you used the rapid extrication technique because the scene was dangerous, you and your team should immediately move the cot a safe distance away from the vehicle before you assess or treat the patient.

The steps of the rapid extrication technique must be considered a general procedure to be adapted as needed. Two-door cars differ from four-door models. Larger cars differ from smaller compact models, pickup trucks, and full-size sedans and four-wheel-drive vehicles. You will handle a large, heavy adult differently from a small adult or child. Every situation will be different—a different car, a different patient, and a different crew. Your resourcefulness and ability to adapt are necessary elements to successfully perform the Rapid Extrication technique.

Nonurgent Moves

When both the scene and the patient are stable, you should carefully plan how to move the patient. If your patient move is rushed or not well planned, it may result in discomfort or injury to the patient, you, and your team. Before you attempt any move, the team leader must be sure that there are enough personnel, any obstacles have been identified or removed, the proper equipment is available, and the procedure and path to be followed have been clearly identified and discussed.

In nonurgent situations, you and your team may choose one of several methods for lifting and carrying a patient. Three general methods are presented here, which may serve as a basis for your plan. You may adapt these procedures to meet your needs on a case-by-case basis.

Direct Ground Lift

The **direct ground lift** is used for patients with no suspected spinal injury who are found lying supine on the ground. You should use this lift when you have to lift and carry the patient some distance to be placed on the stretcher. If you find the patient semi-prone or lying on his or her side, you should first roll the patient onto his or her back. Ideally, the direct ground lift should be performed by three EMT-Bs; however, it can be done with only two. The direct ground lift is performed as follows (Figure 6-24):

1. **Line up on one side of the patient** with First EMT-B at the patient's head, Second EMT-B at the patient's waist, and Third EMT-B at the patient's knees. All EMT-Bs kneel on one knee, preferably the same knee.
2. **The patient's arms should be placed on his or her chest if possible.**
3. **First EMT-B places one arm under the patient's neck and shoulders** and cradles the patient's head. First EMT-B then places the other arm under the patient's lower back.

4. **Second EMT-B places both arms under the waist,** and the other two rescuers slide their arms either up to the midback or down to the buttocks as appropriate.
5. **Third EMT-B places one arm under the patient's knees** and the other above the buttocks.
6. **On command, the team lifts the patient** up to knee level as each EMT-B rests an arm on his or her knee.
7. **As a team and on signal,** each EMT-B rolls the patient in toward his or her chest. Again on signal, the team stands and carries the patient to the ambulance cot.
8. **The steps are reversed** to lower the patient onto the ambulance cot.

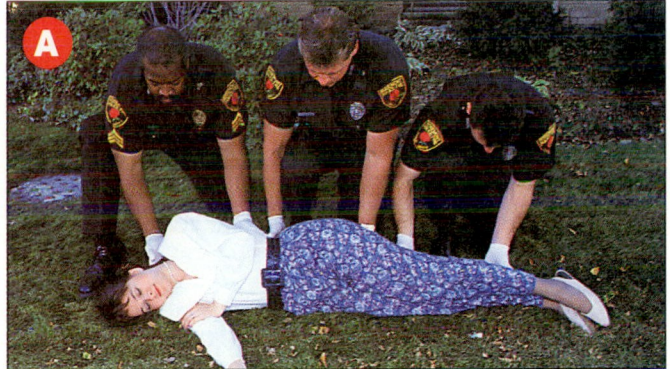

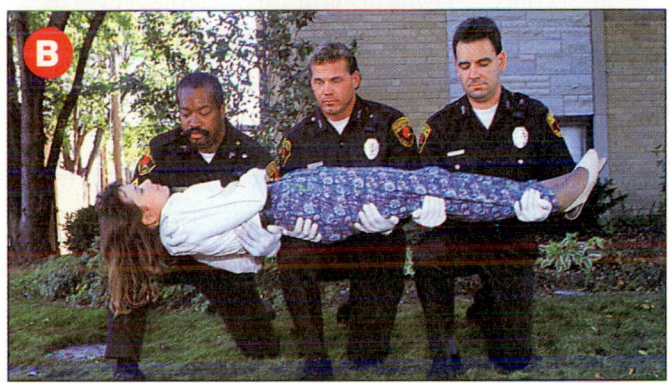

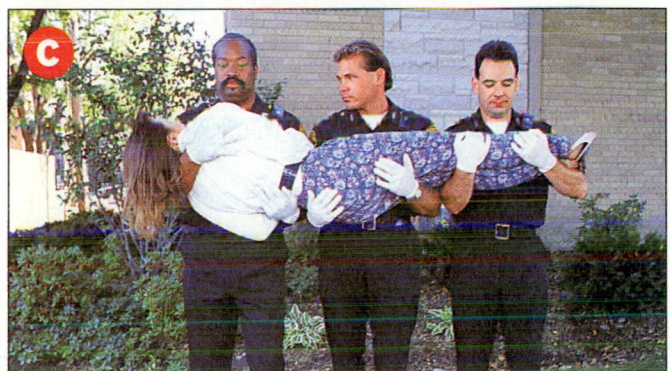

FIGURE 6-24 The direct ground lift. **A:** Line up on one side of the patient, with one EMT-B at the head, one at the waist, and one at the patient's knees. Place the patient's arms on his or her chest. **B:** On command, lift the patient to knee level. **C:** On command, roll the patient toward your chest, then stand and carry the patient to the ambulance cot.

If your patient move is rushed or not well planned, it may result in discomfort or injury to the patient, you, and your team.

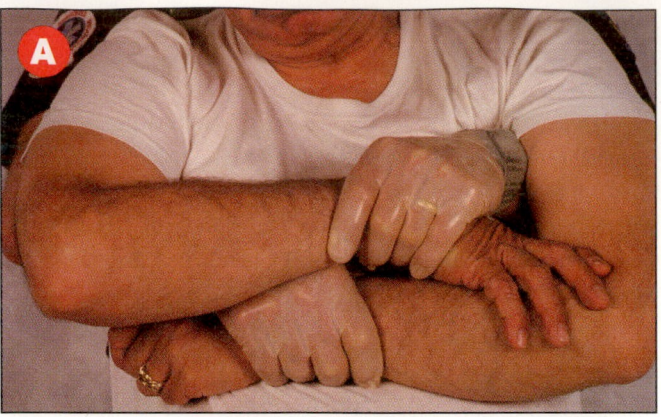

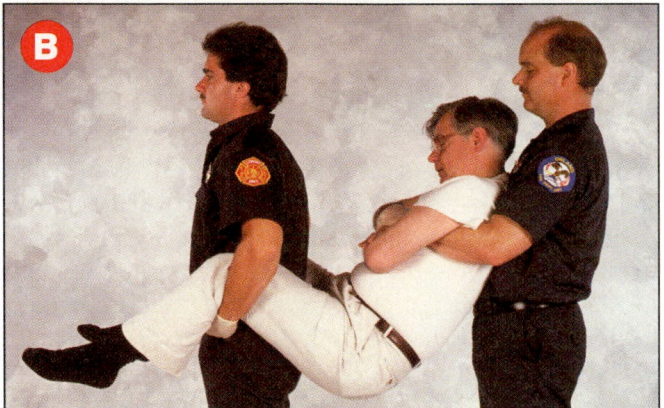

FIGURE 6-25 The extremity lift. **A:** Place your arms through the patient's armpits, and grasp the patient's forearms. **B:** Second EMT-B moves to between the patient's legs, facing in the same direction as the patient, and slips his or her hands under the patient's knees.

Extremity Lift

The extremity lift may also be used for patients with no suspected extremity or spinal injuries who are supine or in a sitting position on the ground. The extremity lift may be especially helpful when the patient is in a very narrow space or there is not enough room for the patient and a team of EMTs to stand side by side.

Communication is the key to success with this lift. You and your partner must coordinate your movements through direct verbal commands. You should perform the extremity lift, as follows:

1. **First EMT-B kneels behind the patient's head** as Second EMT-B kneels at the patient's feet. The two EMTs are facing each other.

2. **The patient's hands should be crossed** over his or her chest.

3. **First EMT-B places one hand** under each of the patient's armpits. Second EMT grasps the patient's wrists. The two EMT-Bs pull and lift the upper torso until the patient is in a sitting position.

4. **First EMT-B reaches his or her arms** through the patient's armpits and grasps the patient's forearms, or his or her own wrists (Figure 6-25).

5. **Second EMT-B moves to a position** between the patient's legs, facing in the same direction as the patient, and slips his or her hands under the patient's knees.

6. **Both EMT-Bs move up to a crouching standing position.**

7. **Both EMT-Bs make sure they are balanced** with a good grip on the patient. On command, both EMT-Bs stand fully upright and move the patient to a stretcher.

You will be less likely to injure yourself if you bend at the hips and knees and use your legs for lifting. However, this lift and carry method increases pressure on the patient's chest, so the patient may be uncomfortable in this position.

Transfer Moves

There are several ways to transfer the patient from a bed onto the ambulance cot.

Direct carry. To transfer a supine patient from a bed to the stretcher using the direct carry method, you should position the stretcher parallel to the bed (Figure 6-26), with the head of the stretcher at the foot of the bed. Be sure that you prepare the stretcher by unbuckling the straps and remove any other items from it. Both you and your partner should face the patient while standing between the bed and the stretcher. You should slide one arm under the patient's neck and cup the patient's shoulder. Your partner should slide his or her hand under the patient's hip and lift slightly. You should then slide your other arm under the patient's back, and your partner should place both arms underneath the patient's hips and calves. Slide the patient to the edge of

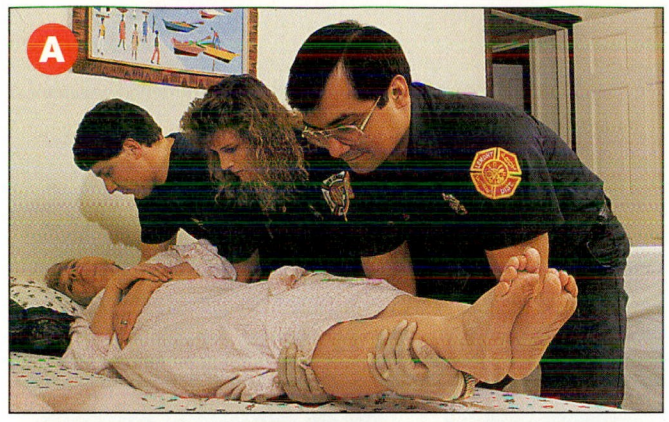

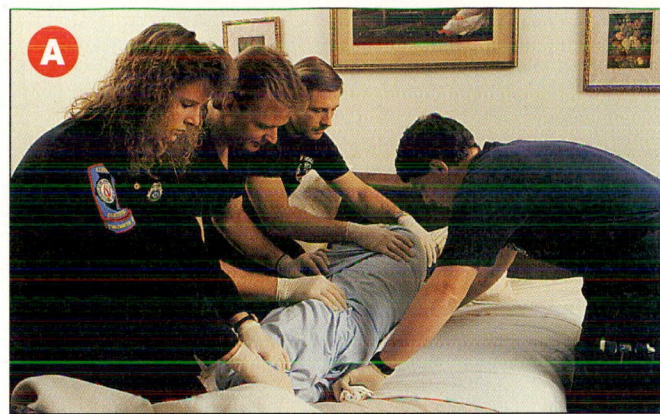

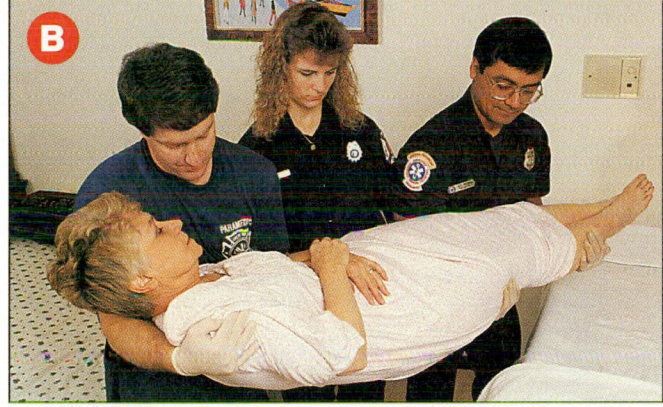

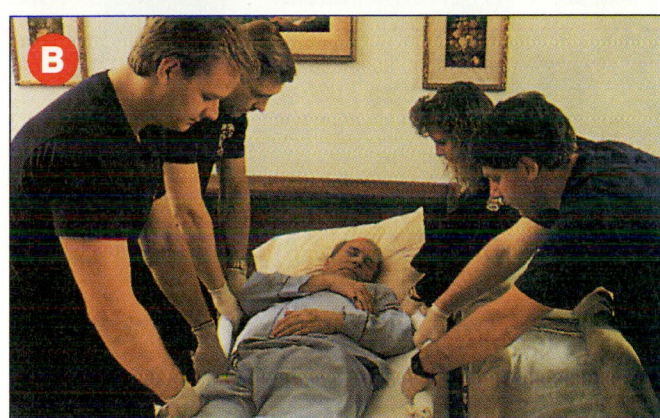

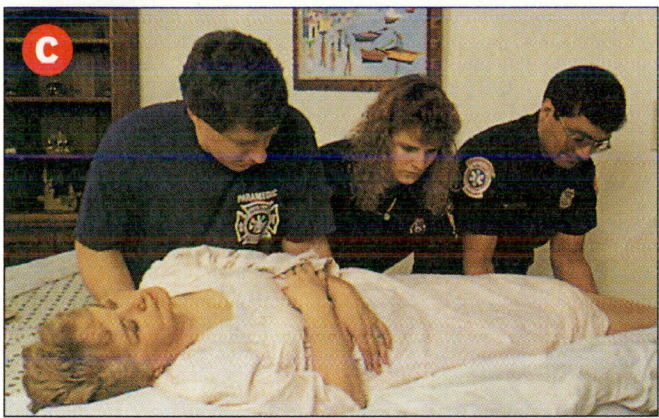

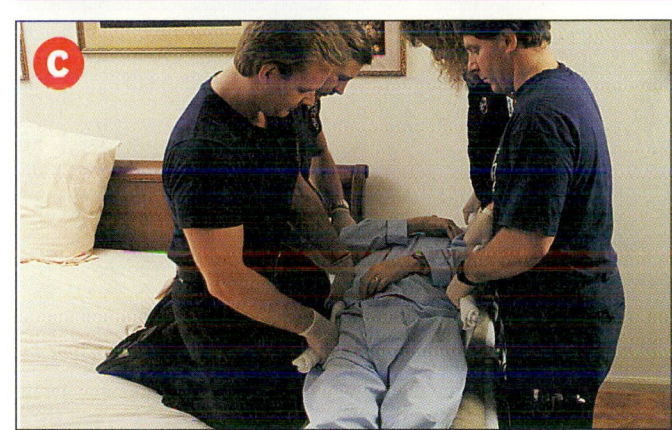

FIGURE 6-26 The direct carry method. **A:** Bring the stretcher in parallel to the bed with the patient's feet facing the head of the stretcher. Secure the stretcher to prevent it from rolling. **B:** Lift the patient in a smooth, coordinated fashion. Slowly walk the patient around, and position him or her over the stretcher. **C:** Slowly and gently lower the patient onto the stretcher.

FIGURE 6-27 The draw sheet method. **A:** Log roll the patient onto a sheet or blanket. **B:** Bring the stretcher in parallel to the bed. Gently pull the patient to the edge of the bed. **C:** Transfer the patient to the stretcher.

the bed, and lift and curl the patient toward your chests. You and your partner should then rotate to the stretcher and gently place the patient onto it.

Draw sheet method. To move the patient onto a stretcher using the draw sheet method, place the ambulance cot next to the bed, making sure it is at the same height as the bed and rails are lowered and straps are unbuckled (Figure 6-27). Be sure to hold the cot to keep it from moving. Loosen the bottom sheet underneath the patient, or log roll the patient onto a blanket. Reach across the cot, and grasp the sheet or blanket firmly at the patient's head, chest, hips, and knees. Gently slide the patient onto the cot.

Other carries. Other carries are performed in the following manner:

- Place a backboard next to the patient and, after using a log roll or slide to move the patient onto the board, secure the patient and lift and carry the backboard to the nearby prepared cot.

- Insert the halves of a scoop stretcher under each side of the patient, and fasten the two sides together. Lift and carry the patient to the nearby prepared cot (Figure 6-28).

- Assist an able patient to the edge of the bed, and, placing the patient's legs over the side, help the

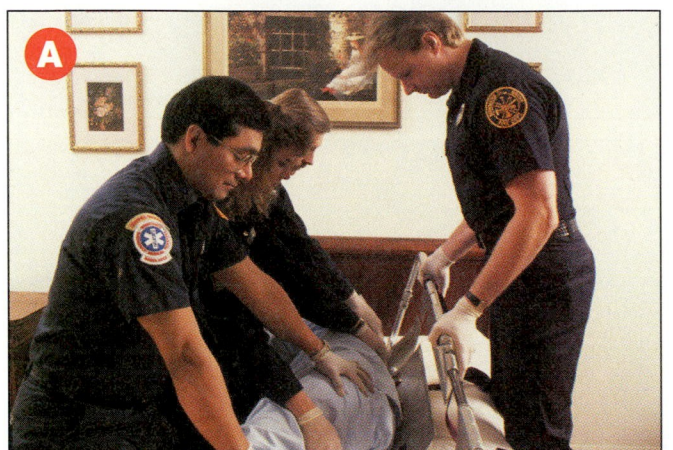

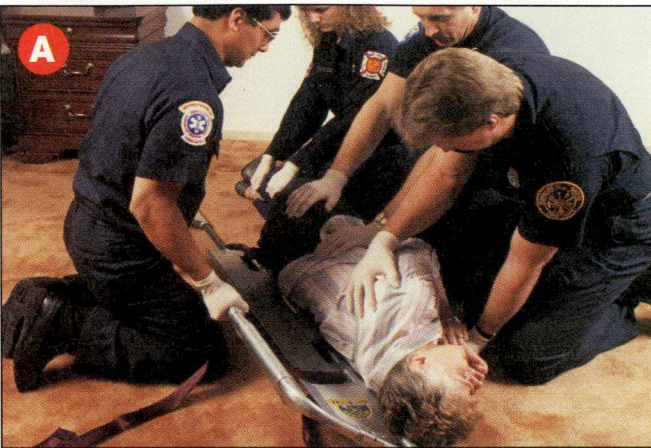

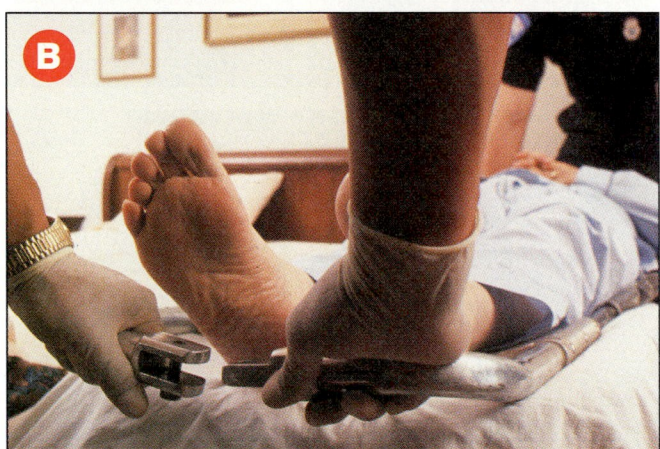

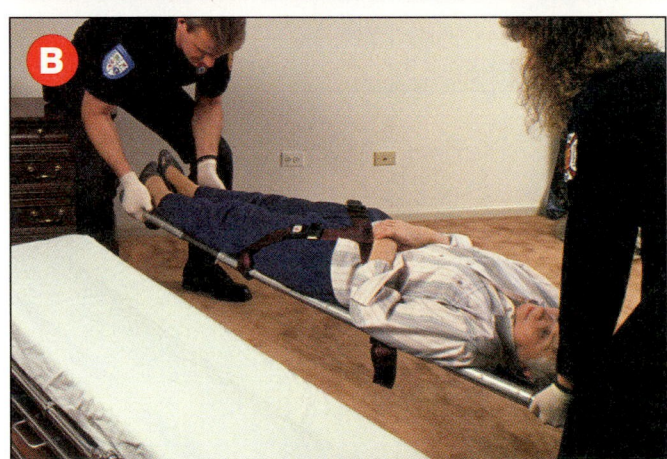

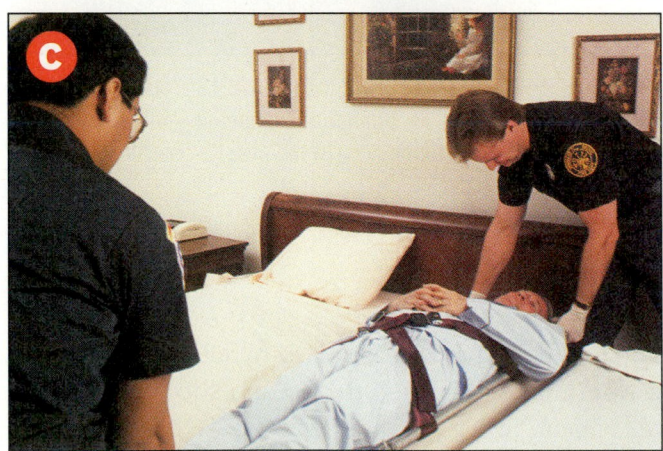

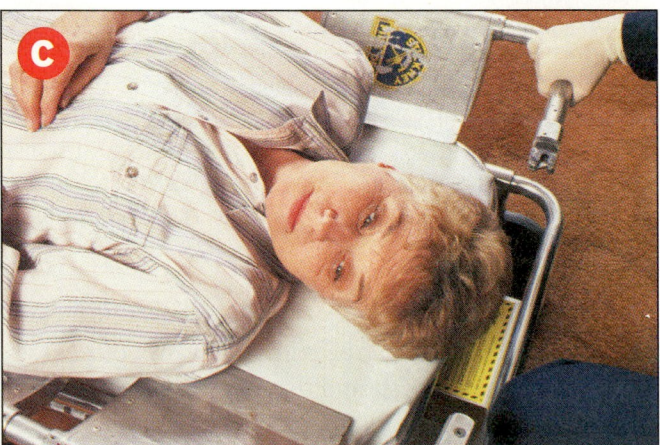

FIGURE 6-28 Using a scoop stretcher for a patient in bed. **A:** Log roll the patient onto the scoop stretcher. **B:** Position the stretcher parallel to the bed, and lock it into position. **C:** Transfer the patient from the bed to the stretcher. Remove the scoop stretcher if desired.

FIGURE 6-29 Using a scoop stretcher for a patient on the ground. **A:** Log roll the patient onto the scoop stretcher. **B:** Lift the scoop stretcher, and transfer the patient to the stretcher. **C:** Remove the scoop stretcher if desired.

patient to sit up. Move the ambulance cot so that its foot end touches the bed near the patient. Help the patient to stand and rotate so that he or she can sit down on the center of the cot. Lift the patient's legs, and rotate them onto the cot while your partner lowers the torso onto the cot.

To avoid the strain of unnecessary lifting and carrying, you should use the draw sheet method or assist an able patient to the cot whenever possible.

To move a patient from the ground or the floor onto the ambulance cot you should use one of the following methods:

- Lift and carry the patient to the nearby prepared cot using a direct body carry.

- Use a log roll or long-axis drag to place the patient onto a backboard, and then lift and carry the backboard to the cot. Place both the backboard and the patient onto the cot.

- Insert the halves of a scoop stretcher under the patient, and, after securing the halves together, lift and carry the stretcher to the prepared cot (Figure 6-29). Separate and remove the scoop stretcher once the patient has been placed on the cot.

- Log roll the patient onto a blanket, centering the patient on the blanket and rolling up the excess material on each side. Lift the patient by the blanket, and carry him or her to the nearby cot (Figure 6-30).

If a patient is sitting in a chair and cannot assist you, transfer the patient from the chair to a wheelchair (Figure 6-31).

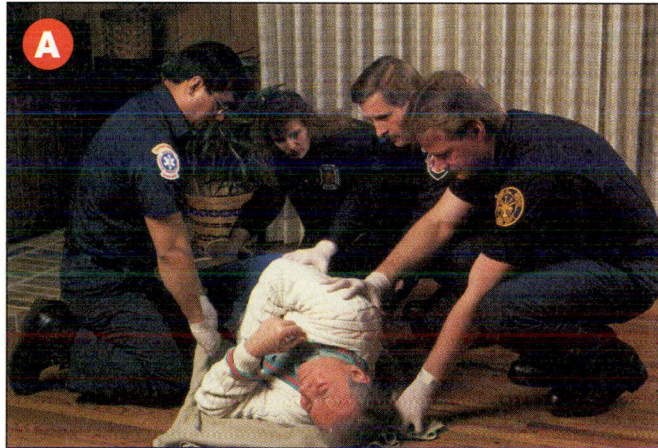

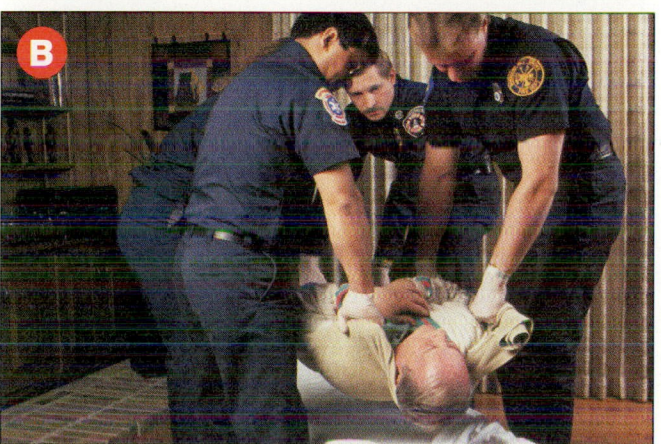

FIGURE 6-30 Log-rolling a patient on the ground. **A:** Log roll the patient onto a blanket. **B:** Lift the blanket and transfer the patient to the stretcher.

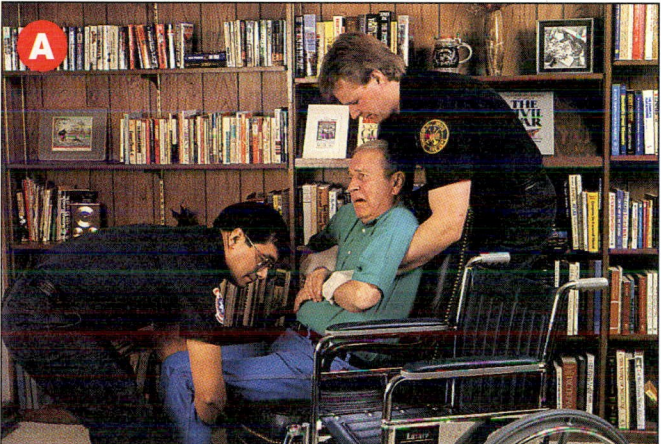

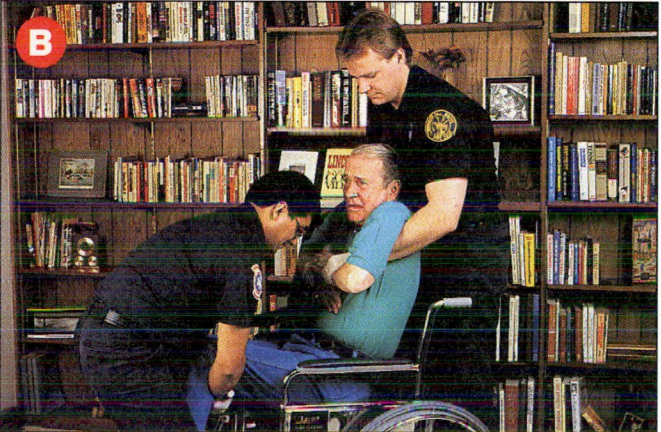

FIGURE 6-31 Moving a patient from a chair to a wheelchair. **A:** Slide your arms through the patient's armpits, and grasp the patient's crossed forearms. Second EMT-B grasps the patient's legs at the knees. **B:** Gently lift the patient into the locked wheelchair.

Patient-Moving Equipment

The Wheeled Ambulance Stretcher

The wheeled ambulance stretcher, or ambulance cot, is the most commonly used device to move and transport patients. Only when you must transport two patients in the same ambulance should it be necessary to transport one patient on a folding stretcher or backboard placed on the long squad bench.

Most patients are placed directly on the ambulance cot. However, you will need to place and secure patients with a possible spinal injury or multiple systems trauma onto a backboard. Patients who may need CPR or must be carried down (or up) a flight of stairs while supine should also be placed on a backboard. The backboard and patient are then secured onto the ambulance cot.

You can use a stair chair to carry a patient who can tolerate being in a sitting position down a flight of stairs to the prepared cot, which is waiting in the lower hallway. You should then transfer the patient from the chair to the cot.

In most instances, it is best if you pull the foot end of the stretcher while your partner guides it from the head end. When the stretcher must be carried, it is best if four rescuers are available to carry it. There is more stability with a four-person carry, and the carry requires less strength. One EMT-B should be positioned at each corner of the stretcher to provide an even lift. A four-person carry is much safer if the stretcher must be moved over rough ground. If only two EMT-Bs are available, or if limited space will allow room for only two EMT-Bs to carry the stretcher, there is risk that the stretcher will become unbalanced. In a two-person carry, the two EMT-Bs should stand facing each other, with one person at the head end of the stretcher and the other at the foot end. With this type of carry, one EMT-B will have to walk backward.

> The wheeled ambulance stretcher, or ambulance cot, is the most commonly used device to move and transport patients.

Features. The modern ambulance cot is available in a number of different models, which may include different features (Figure 6-32). Before going on a call, you should be fully familiar with the specific features of the cot that your ambulance carries. You must know where the controls to adjust and lock each feature are located and how each works.

The ambulance cot has a specific head end and foot end. The cot has a strong horizontal rectangular tubular metal main frame to which all of its other parts are attached. The cot should be pulled, pushed, and lifted only by its main frame or handles, which are attached to the main frame specifically for this purpose.

On most models, a second tubular frame made up of three sections is attached within or above the main frame. A metal plate is fastened to each of the three sections between its sides. This plate serves as the platform on which the cot mattress and patient are supported. The head section runs from the head end of the cot to near the center of the cot, where the patient's hips will be. Hinges at the area where the hips will be allow the head end to be elevated and the patient's back to be positioned at any desired angle from flat to fully upright. The head end of the cot is designed to be elevated or moved down only when a tilt control is purposely released. At all other times, the back will remain locked at the position in which it was placed. The frame and plates that lie from the hips to the foot end of the cot are divided into two hinged sections. These sections may be connected so that the foot end can be drawn in toward the knees, causing the frame and plates to hinge upward under the patient's knees to elevate them as desired. This feature is not found in all models.

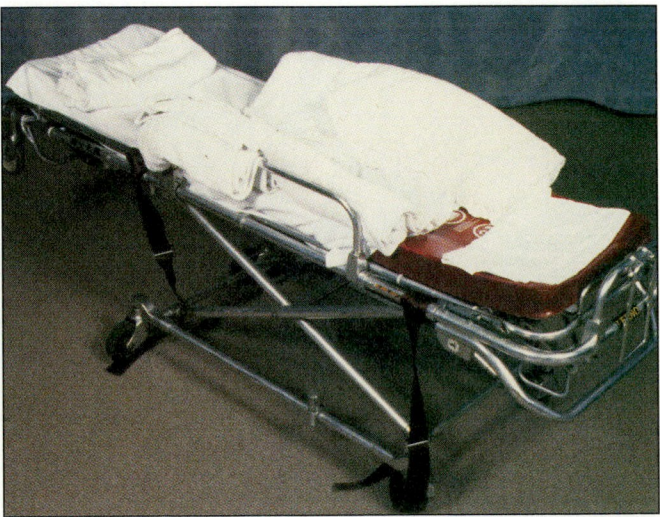

FIGURE 6-32 An ambulance stretcher.

A retractable guardrail is attached along the central portion of the main frame of the cot at each side and is lowered out of the way when a patient is being loaded onto the cot. Once the patient has been properly placed on the cot, the handle is drawn up and locked in an elevated position perpendicular to the surface of the cot. The patient cannot roll off either side of the cot even if a securing strap becomes released. The guardrail at each side can be lowered only if its locking handle is released.

The underside of the main frame of the cot is supported on a folding undercarriage that has a smaller horizontal rectangular frame and four large rubber casters at its bottom end. The folding undercarriage is designed so that the litter can be adjusted to any height from about 12" above the ground, which is the desired height when the stretcher is secured in the ambulance, to 32" to 36" above the ground, which is the desired height when the stretcher is being rolled. Because you are able to lock the cot at any height between its lowest height and its fully extended height, it can be locked at the same height as any bed or examining table to allow the patient to be slid from one to the other. This permits you to transfer the patient without the need for any additional lifting. The controls for folding the undercarriage are designed so that the cot remains locked at its present height when the controls are not being activated. As an additional safety feature on most cots, the main frame must be slightly lifted so that the undercarriage becomes unweighted before it will fold, even if the control is pulled. Therefore, if the handle is accidentally pulled, the elevated cot will not suddenly drop. Controls for elevating and lowering most cots are located at the foot end and at one or both sides. You and your partner must use the proper lifting mechanics to lift the wheeled ambulance stretcher.

The mattress on an ambulance cot must be fluid resistant so that it does not absorb any type of potentially infectious material, including water, blood, or other body fluid.

Moving the stretcher. Whenever a patient has been placed onto the cot, one EMT-B must hold the main frame to make sure that it cannot roll. When the cot is elevated, the main frame and the patient extend considerably beyond the wheels at both the head end and foot end of the cot. Therefore, whenever a patient is on an elevated cot, you must ensure that it is held firmly between two hands at all times so that even if the patient moves, the cot cannot tip (Figure 6-33).

If the loaded cot must be carried down a short flight of steps, be sure to first retract the undercarriage; however, this is not necessary when the cot must be lifted over a curb, single step, or obstacle of a similar height (Figure 6-34). Remember, if the patient must be carried up or down a full flight or several flights of stairs, you should prepare the cot and leave it on the ground floor at the bottom (or top) of the stairs. Use a backboard or stair chair to carry the patient up or down the stairs to the waiting cot.

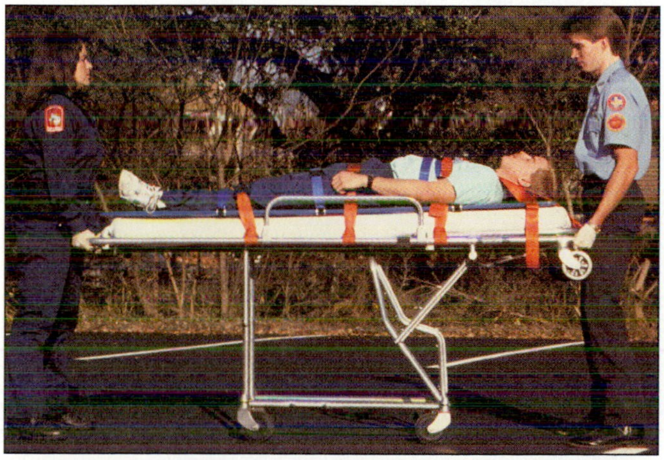

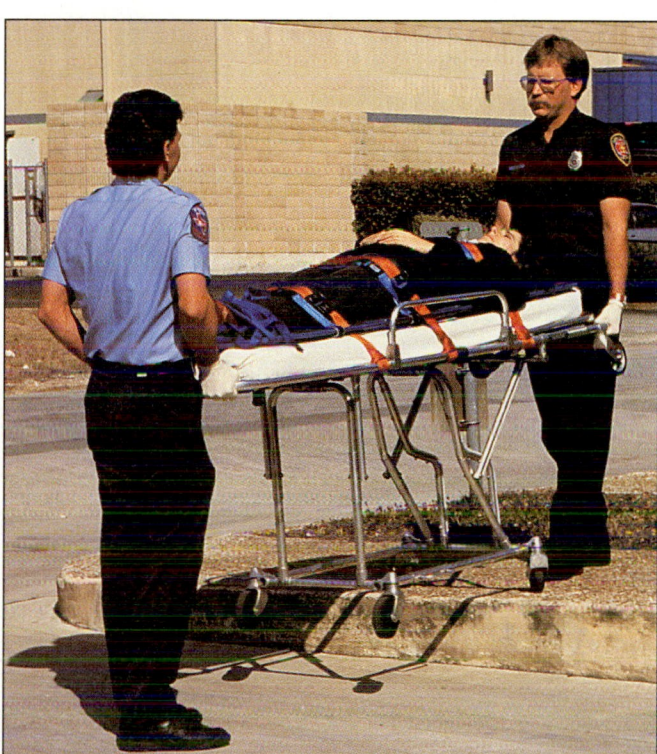

FIGURE 6-33 Make sure that you hold the main frame of the ambulance stretcher when it is elevated so that even when the patient moves, the stretcher does not tip.

FIGURE 6-34 You need not retract the undercarriage of the ambulance stretcher when lifting it over a curb, single step, or obstacle of similar height.

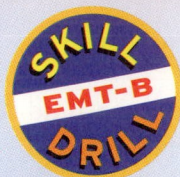

Loading a Stretcher onto an Ambulance
Figure 6-35

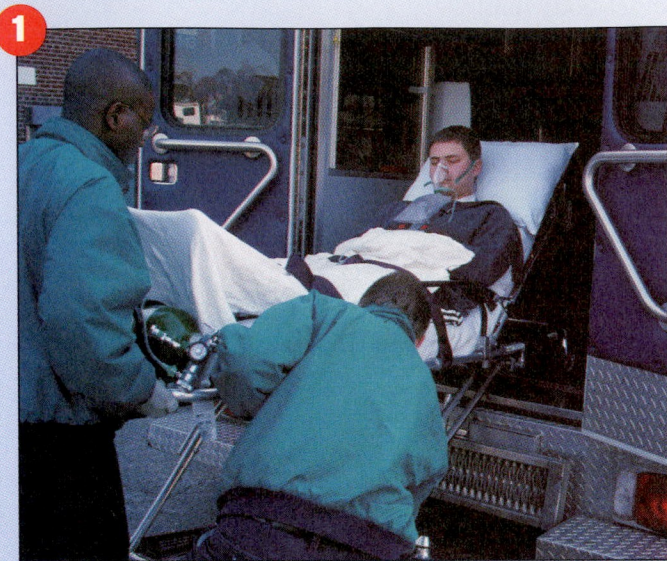

Tilt the head of the stretcher upward, and place it into the patient compartment with the wheels on the floor.

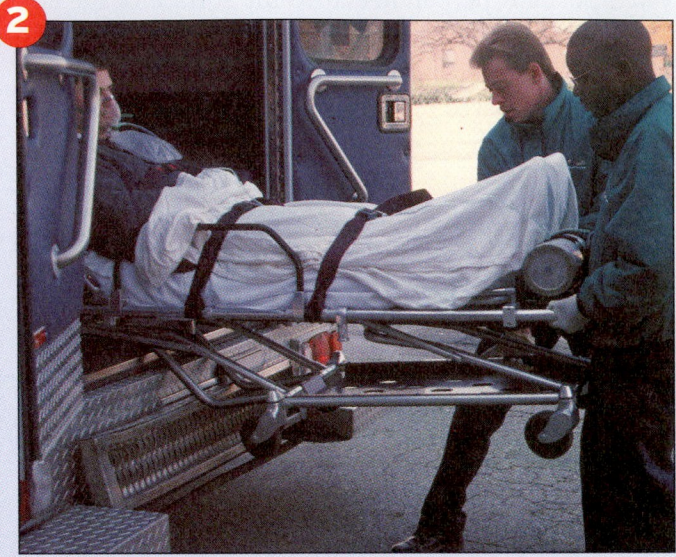

Move to the side of the stretcher, and release the undercarriage lock to lift the undercarriage up to its fully retracted position.

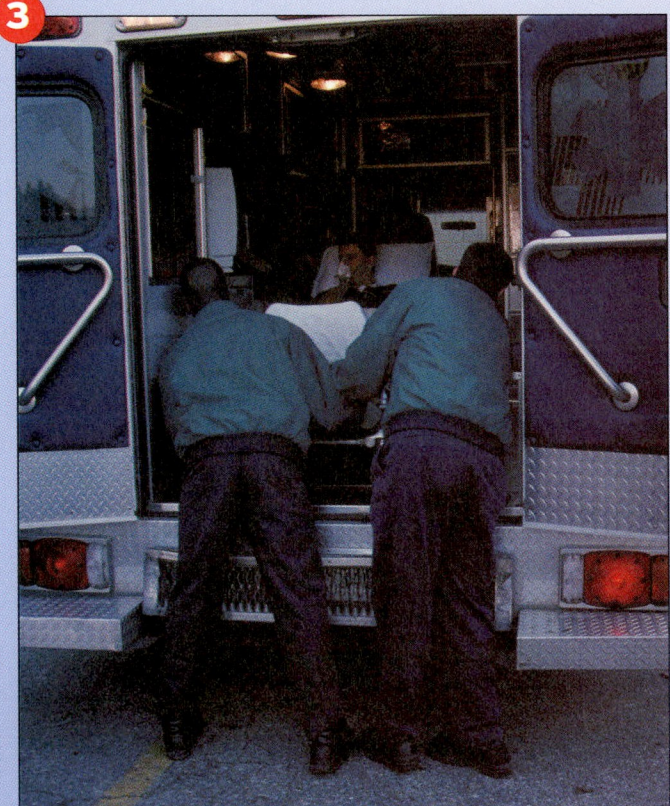

Roll the stretcher into the back of the ambulance.

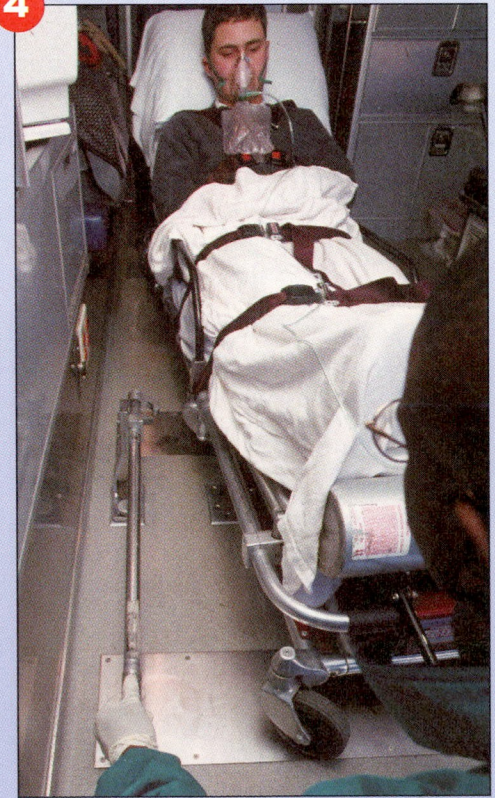

Secure the stretcher by fastening it to the clamps that are located on the floor (or side) of the ambulance.

Two additional wheels that extend just below the head end are attached to the main frame so that when you reach the back of the ambulance, you can tilt the head end of the main frame upward and place it into the patient compartment with the wheels on the floor (Figure 6-35). Then, with the patient's weight supported by these two wheels and the EMT-B at the foot end of the cot, you can move to the side of the main frame and release the undercarriage lock to lift the undercarriage up to its fully retracted position. In this position, the wheels of the undercarriage and the two on the head end of the main frame will be on the same level, so the cot can simply be rolled the rest of the way into the back of the ambulance and rested on all six wheels.

The cot is secured in the ambulance by strong clamps that fasten around the undercarriage when the cot is pushed into them. The clamps are located in a rack on the floor or side of the patient compartment. The clamps will hold the cot in place until they are released at the hospital. You can control and release the clamps with a single handle that is positioned so that you can activate it when standing on the ground at the open back doors of the ambulance when the cot is to be unloaded. The ambulance cot is designed to be rolled on regular flat surfaces. If the patient must be moved over a lawn or other irregular surface, you must lift and carry the cot over the terrain.

An IV pole is attached to many ambulance cots. The IV pole can be unfolded or extended above the main frame to hold an IV bag above the patient while you move the cot to the ambulance. Some wheeled ambulance stretchers even include a carrier to hold an ECG monitor or AED and portable oxygen unit. If the model you use does not include these features, you will have to secure the portable oxygen unit and ECG monitor or AED to the top surface of the cot mattress at the patient's legs.

The extra wheels below the head end of the main frame of the cot are not featured on some older or less expensive wheeled ambulance stretchers. These stretchers are not self-loading. When you reach the back of the ambulance with such a cot, you must lower it until the undercarriage is in its lowest retracted position and

then, with you and your partner at each side of the cot, lift it to the height of the floor of the ambulance and roll it into the track that locks it into place. Table 6-3 shows the guidelines that you must follow to load the stretcher into the ambulance.

Make sure that all stretchers and patients are fully secured before you move the ambulance.

Portable/Folding Stretchers

A portable stretcher is a stretcher with a strong rectangular tubular metal frame and rigid fabric stretched across it (Figure 6-36). Portable stretchers do not have a second multipositioning frame or adjustable undercarriage. Some models have two wheels that fold down about 4″ underneath the foot end of the frame and legs of a similar length that fold down from the head end at each side. The wheels make it easier to move the loaded stretcher. The legs should not be used as handles.

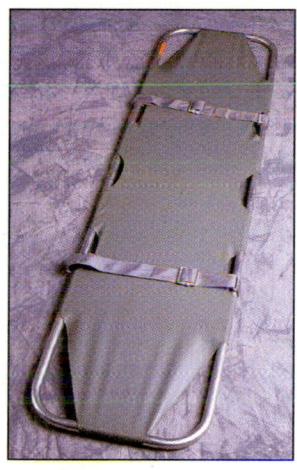
FIGURE 6-36
A portable stretcher.

Some portable stretchers can be folded in half across the center of each side so that the stretcher is only half its usual length during storage. Many ambulances carry a portable stretcher to use if a patient is in an area that is difficult to reach with a wheeled ambulance stretcher or a second patient must be transported on the squad bench of the ambulance.

A portable stretcher weighs much less than a wheeled stretcher and does not have a bulky undercarriage. However, because most models do not have wheels, you and your team must support all of the patient's weight and any equipment along with the weight of the stretcher.

Flexible Stretchers

Several types of flexible stretchers, such as the SKED, Reeves, or Navy stretcher, are available and can be rolled up across either the stretcher's width or, in the case of the SKED, its length so that the stretcher becomes a smaller tubular package for storage and carrying (Figure 6-37). When you must carry the equipment a considerable

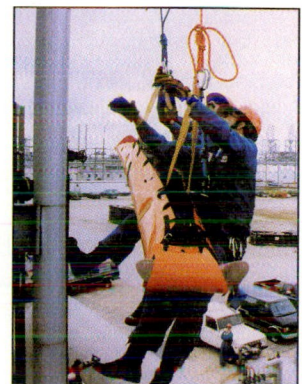
FIGURE 6-37
A flexible stretcher.

TABLE 6-3	Guidelines for Loading the Stretcher into the Ambulance

- Make sure there is sufficient lifting power.
- Follow the manufacturer's directions for safe and proper use of the stretcher.
- Load any hanging stretchers before you load the wheeled stretcher.

distance from the nearest place that the ambulance can be located, this is an important consideration. A flexible stretcher forms a rigid stretcher that conforms around the patient's sides and does not extend beyond them. When these stretchers are extended, they are particularly useful when you must remove a patient from or through a confined space. The SKED stretcher can also be used if the patient must be belayed or rappelled by ropes.

The flexible stretcher is the most uncomfortable of all the various devices; however, it provides excellent support and immobilization. When the stretcher is wrapped around the patient and the straps are secured, the patient is completely immobilized. The stretcher can then be lowered by rope or slid down a flight of stairs by resting it on the front edge of each step.

Backboards

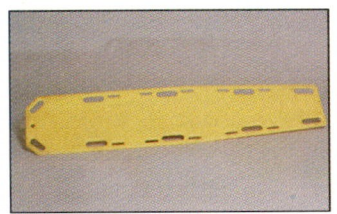

FIGURE 6-38
A long backboard.

Backboards are long, flat boards made of rigid, rectangular material. Backboards were originally made of wood but are now made of other materials as well. They are used to carry patients and to immobilize supine patients with suspected spinal injury or other multiple trauma (Figure 6-38). Backboards can also be used to move patients out of awkward places. They are 6′ to 7′ long and are commonly used for patients who are found lying down. Parallel to the sides and ends of the backboard are a number of long holes that are about ½″ to 1″ from the outer edge. These holes form handles and handholds so that the board can be easily grasped, lifted, and carried. The handles and adjacent holes also allow straps used to secure and immobilize the patient to the board to be secured to each side and end of the board at any needed location.

For many years, backboards were made of thick marine plywood whose surface was sealed with polyurethane or another marine varnish. Wooden backboards are still used in some places. If wooden boards are used, you must follow infectious control procedures before you can reuse the boards. Where wooden boards are no longer used, they have generally been stored so that they will be available in the event of a multiple-casualty situation. Newer backboards are made of plastic materials that will not absorb blood or other infectious substances.

You can use a short backboard, called either a short board or a half-board, to immobilize the torso, head, and neck of a seated patient with a suspected spinal injury

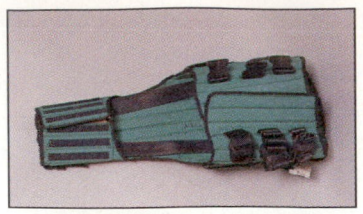

FIGURE 6-39
A vest-type short backboard.

until you can immobilize the patient on a backboard. Short boards are 3′ to 4′ long. The original short wooden backboard has generally been replaced with a vest-type device that is specifically designed to immobilize the patient until he or she is moved from a sitting position to supine on a backboard (Figure 6-39). The vest-type devices are easier to use than the wooden board.

Basket Stretchers

You should use a rigid **basket stretcher**, often called a Stokes litter, to carry a patient across uneven terrain from a remote location that is inaccessible by ambulance or other vehicle (Figure 6-40). If you suspect that the patient has a spinal injury, you should first immobilize him or her on a backboard and then place the backboard into the basket stretcher. Once you have reached the ambulance and wheeled ambulance stretcher, you can remove the patient and backboard from the basket stretcher and place them on the ambulance cot.

Basket stretchers either are made of plastic with an aluminum frame or have a full steel frame that is connected by a woven wire mesh. The wire basket is very uncomfortable for the patient unless the wire is padded. Either type can be used to carry a patient across fields, rough terrain, or trails or on a toboggan, boat, or all-terrain vehicle. Basket stretchers surround and support the patient, yet their design allows water to drain through holes in the bottom. Basket stretchers are also used for technical rope rescues and some water rescues. Not all basket stretchers are rated or appropriate for each of these specialized rescue uses. The types of basket stretchers that are acceptable for specialized rescue must be determined by individuals with additional special training.

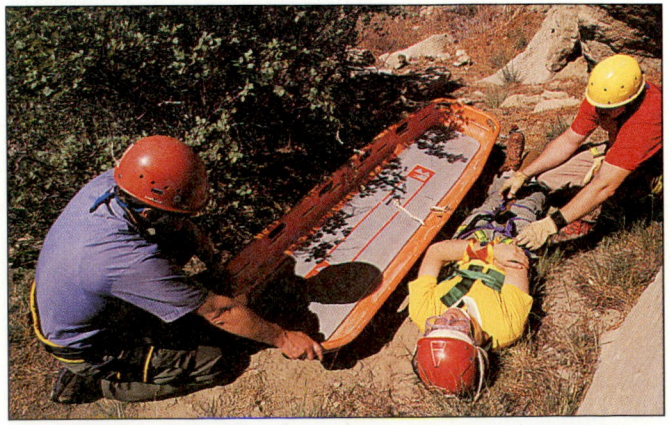

FIGURE 6-40 A basket stretcher.

Scoop Stretcher

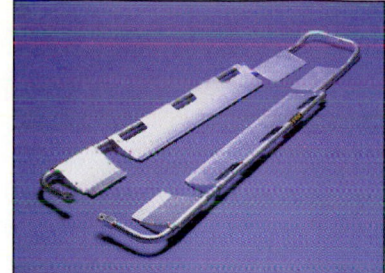

FIGURE 6-41 A scoop stretcher.

The scoop stretcher, or split litter, is designed to be split into two or four pieces (Figure 6-41). These sections are fitted around a patient who is lying on the ground or another relatively flat surface. The parts are reconnected, and the patient is lifted and placed on a long backboard or stretcher. A scoop stretcher may be used for patients who have been struck by a motor vehicle.

A scoop stretcher is efficient; however, both sides of the patient must be accessible. You must also pay special attention to the closure area beneath the patient so that clothing, skin, or other objects are not trapped. As with the long backboard, you must fully stabilize and secure the patient before moving him or her; however, you cannot slip a scoop stretcher under the long axis of the patient's body. Scoop stretchers are narrow, well constructed, and compact and have excellent body support features but are not adequate when used alone for standard immobilization of a spinal injury. You and your team should practice often with a scoop stretcher to be ready for using it with a patient.

Stair Chairs

Stair chairs are folding aluminum frame chairs with fabric stretched across them to form a seat and seat back (Figure 6-42). They have fold-out handles to help you carry their head and foot ends up or down a flight of stairs, and most have rubber wheels at their back with casters in front so that they can be rolled along the floor and make turns. Stair chairs serve as an adjunct for moving a patient up or down stairs to the ground floor, where the prepared wheeled ambulance stretcher is waiting. You can roll the stair chair on the floor until you reach the stairwell, then carry it (rather than roll and bump it) up or down the stairs. Once you reach the ground floor, you can roll it to the waiting cot and assist or lift the patient onto the ambulance cot.

Be sure to follow manufacturer's directions for maintenance, inspection, repair, and upkeep for any device that you use as patient-handling equipment.

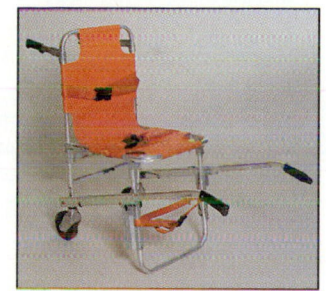

FIGURE 6-42 A stair chair.

Moving and Positioning the Patient

Every time you have to move a patient, you must take special care that neither you, your team, nor the patient is injured. Patient packaging and handling are technical skills that you will learn and perfect through practice and training.

Training and practice are required to use all the equipment that is described in this chapter. You must master the skills necessary for their use and understand the advantages and limitations of each device. Practice each technique with your team often so that when you must move a patient, you can perform the move quickly, safely, and efficiently. After each patient transfer, you and your team should evaluate the appropriateness of the technique that you used, as well as your technical skill in completing the transfer. You must also be sure to maintain your equipment according to the manufacturer's instructions. Using clean, well-maintained equipment is but one part of providing high-quality patient care.

After you deliver the patient to the emergency department, you and your team must begin preparing for your next call. Review the positive points about the transport. Discuss changes that would improve the next run. This process of review and evaluation identifies the following:

- Procedures that need more practice
- Equipment that needs to be cleaned or repaired
- Skills that you need to review or acquire

Most important, a critical review helps you and your team to become more confident and better-skilled EMT-Bs.

Certain patient conditions, such as head injury, shock, spinal injury, and pregnancy, call for special lifting and moving techniques. Patients with chest pain or difficulty breathing should sit in a position of comfort, as long as they are not hypotensive. Patients with suspected spinal injuries must be immobilized on a long backboard. Patients who are in shock should be packaged and moved in a supine position or with their legs elevated 8" to 12". Pregnant patients who are hypotensive should be positioned and transported on their left sides. Move an unresponsive patient with no suspected spinal injury into the recovery position by rolling the patient onto his or her side without twisting the body. Transport a patient who is nauseated or vomiting in a position of comfort, but be sure that you are positioned appropriately to manage the airway.

prep kit

ready for review

The first key rule of lifting is to always keep your back in an upright position and lift without twisting. You can lift and carry significant weight without injury as long as your back is in the proper upright position.

The power lift is the safest and most powerful way to lift. The safety of you, your team, and the patient depends on the use of proper lifting techniques and maintaining a proper hold when lifting or carrying a patient. If you do not have a proper hold, you will not be able to bear your share of the weight, or you may lose your grasp with one or both hands and possibly cause a lower back injury to one or more EMT-Bs.

It is always best to move a patient on a device that can be rolled. However, if a wheeled device is not available, you must understand and follow certain guidelines for carrying a patient on a stretcher or cot. You must constantly coordinate your movements with those of the other team members and make sure that you communicate with them.

When lifting a stretcher, you must make sure that you and your team use correct lifting techniques. You and your team should also be of similar height and strength.

If you must carry a loaded backboard or stretcher up or down stairs or other incline, be sure that the patient is tightly secured to the device to prevent sliding. Be sure to carry the board or stretcher foot end first so that the patient's head is elevated higher than the feet.

Directions and commands are an important part of safe lifting and carrying. You and your team must anticipate and understand every move and execute it in a coordinated manner. The team leader is responsible for coordinating the moves.

You should try to use four rescuers whenever resources allow. You should also know how much you can comfortably and safely lift and not attempt to lift more than this amount. Rapidly summon additional help to lift and carry a weight that is greater than you are able to lift.

The same basic body mechanics apply for safe reaching and pulling as for lifting and carrying. Keep your back locked and straight, and avoid twisting. Do not hyperextend your back when reaching overhead.

You should normally move a patient with nonurgent moves, in an orderly, planned, and unhurried fashion, selecting methods that involve the least amount of lifting and carrying. At times, you may have to use an emergency move to move a patient before providing initial assessment and care. You should perform an urgent move if a patient has an altered level of consciousness, inadequate ventilation, or shock or in extreme weather conditions.

The wheeled ambulance stretcher, or ambulance cot, is the most commonly used device to move and transport patients. Other devices that are used to lift and carry patients include portable stretchers, flexible stretchers, backboards, basket stretchers (Stokes litters), scoop stretchers, and stair chairs.

Whenever you are moving a patient, you must take special care so that neither you, your team, nor the patient is injured. You will learn the technical skills of patient packaging and handling through practice and training. Training and practice are also required to use all the equipment that is available to you. You must practice each technique with your team often so that you are able to perform the move quickly, safely, and efficiently.

vital vocabulary

www.emtb.com

backboard A device that is used to provide support to a patient who is suspected of having a hip, pelvic, spinal, or lower extremity injury. Also called a trauma board or longboard.

basket stretcher A rigid stretcher commonly used in technical and water rescues that surrounds and supports the patient yet allows water to drain through holes in the bottom. Also called a Stokes litter.

diamond carry A carrying technique in which one EMT-B is located at the head end, one at the foot end, and one at each side of the patient; each of the two EMT-Bs at the sides uses one hand to support the stretcher so that all are able to face forward as they walk.

direct ground lift A lifting technique that is used for patients who are found lying supine on the ground with no suspected spinal injury.

emergency move A move in which the patient is dragged or pulled from a dangerous scene before initial assessment and care are provided.

extremity lift A lifting technique that is used for patients who are supine or in a sitting position with no suspected extremity or spinal injuries.

flexible stretcher A stretcher that is a rigid carrying device when secured around a patient but can be folded or rolled when not in use.

portable stretcher A stretcher with a strong rectangular tubular metal frame and rigid fabric stretched across it.

power grip A technique in which the litter or backboard is gripped by inserting each hand under the handle with the palm facing up and the thumb extended, fully supporting the underside of the handle on the curved palm with the fingers and thumb.

power lift A lifting technique in which the EMT-B's back is held upright, with legs bent, and the patient is lifted when the EMT-B raises his or her upper body and arms and straightens his or her legs.

Rapid Extrication Technique A technique that was developed to move a patient from a sitting position inside a vehicle to supine on a backboard in less than 1 minute.

scoop stretcher A stretcher that is designed to be split into two or four sections that can be fitted around a patient who is lying on the ground or other relatively flat surface; also called a split litter.

stair chair A lightweight folding device that is used to carry a conscious, seated patient up or down stairs.

wheeled ambulance stretcher A specially designed stretcher that can be rolled along the ground. A collapsible undercarriage allows it to be loaded into the ambulance. Also called the cot or an ambulance cot.

assessment in action

You have been off work for almost two weeks with a back injury. During a routine carry from an apartment complex, you slipped and fell on a little patch of ice. Fortunately for everyone involved, the patient was not injured during the incident.

The training officer called yesterday to find out how you were doing and to let you know that the continuing education topic this month is on lifting and moving patients. There is little doubt that your fall has prompted this renewed interest in this particular topic.

1. Which of the following is **NOT** considered a guideline for safe lifting and moving?
   A. Accurately estimating or finding out the weight to be lifted
   B. Communicating with your partner throughout the move or lift
   C. Bending at the waist while keeping the legs straight
   D. Keeping the weight to be lifted as close to the body as possible

2. Whenever you have to reach to lift a patient, you should **NOT**:
   A. be in an extended position when you are reaching over your head.
   B. reach more than 15" to 20" in front of your body.
   C. keep your back straight whenever you reach over a patient.
   D. limit lifts involving strenuous effort to less than 1 minute.

3. Which of the following techniques is considered the **LEAST** desirable in lifting and moving a patient?
   A. Pulling the patient whenever possible
   B. Keeping your elbows bent and your arms close to your sides
   C. Lifting with your back straight and your eyes looking forward
   D. Using a squatting position if the patient is below the level of your waist

4. Which of the following statements about making an emergency move is **FALSE**?
   A. The greatest danger to a trauma patient is exacerbating a spinal injury.
   B. The patient should be pulled in the direction of the long axis of the body.
   C. A patient who is found lying on the ground should not be moved unless you can lift the patient over your shoulders and carry him or her.
   D. You cannot manually remove a patient from a vehicle and provide as much stability as when you use a long backboard.

5. Which of the following statements about patient positioning is true?
   A. An unresponsive patient should always be placed in a supine position during transport.
   B. A patient who is having difficulty breathing need not be placed in a position of comfort unless absolutely necessary.
   C. A patient who is showing signs of shock should have his or her head elevated between 8" and 12".
   D. A patient who is believed to have a spinal injury should be immobilized to a long backboard or similar device.

prep **6** kit

points to ponder

You are working transfers and are assigned to transport a 43-year-old man from his home to the hospital for admission. His bedroom is on the second floor, and the stairway has two turns in it that require you to lift the stretcher above the railing to make the turn. When you enter the bedroom, you find that the patient appears to weigh over 400 lb. He has pneumonia and is being hospitalized for treatment. The patient has been able to get up to use the restroom, but only with difficulty. Besides you and your partner, his caretaker, who is of average size, and the patient's 65-year-old mother are present. Protocols are very clear that the patient is to be moved on the stretcher and at no time should walk. It appears to you that the patient is too large to get down the stairs on the stretcher but that, given enough time, he could walk down the stairs. No other units are available at this time.

• How would you deal with this situation? Would you go against protocol? Why or why not? How long would you wait for assistance?

online outlook

Seven patient carrying devices were discussed in this chapter. To improve your knowledge of this equipment, complete Exercise 6 at www.emtb.com.

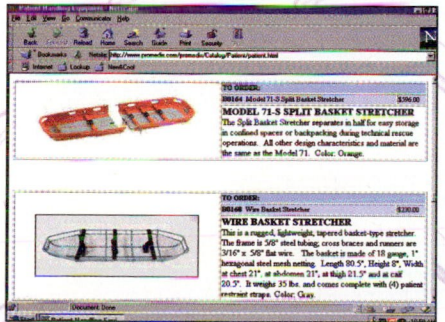

Airway

Alice "Twink" Dalton, RN, MS

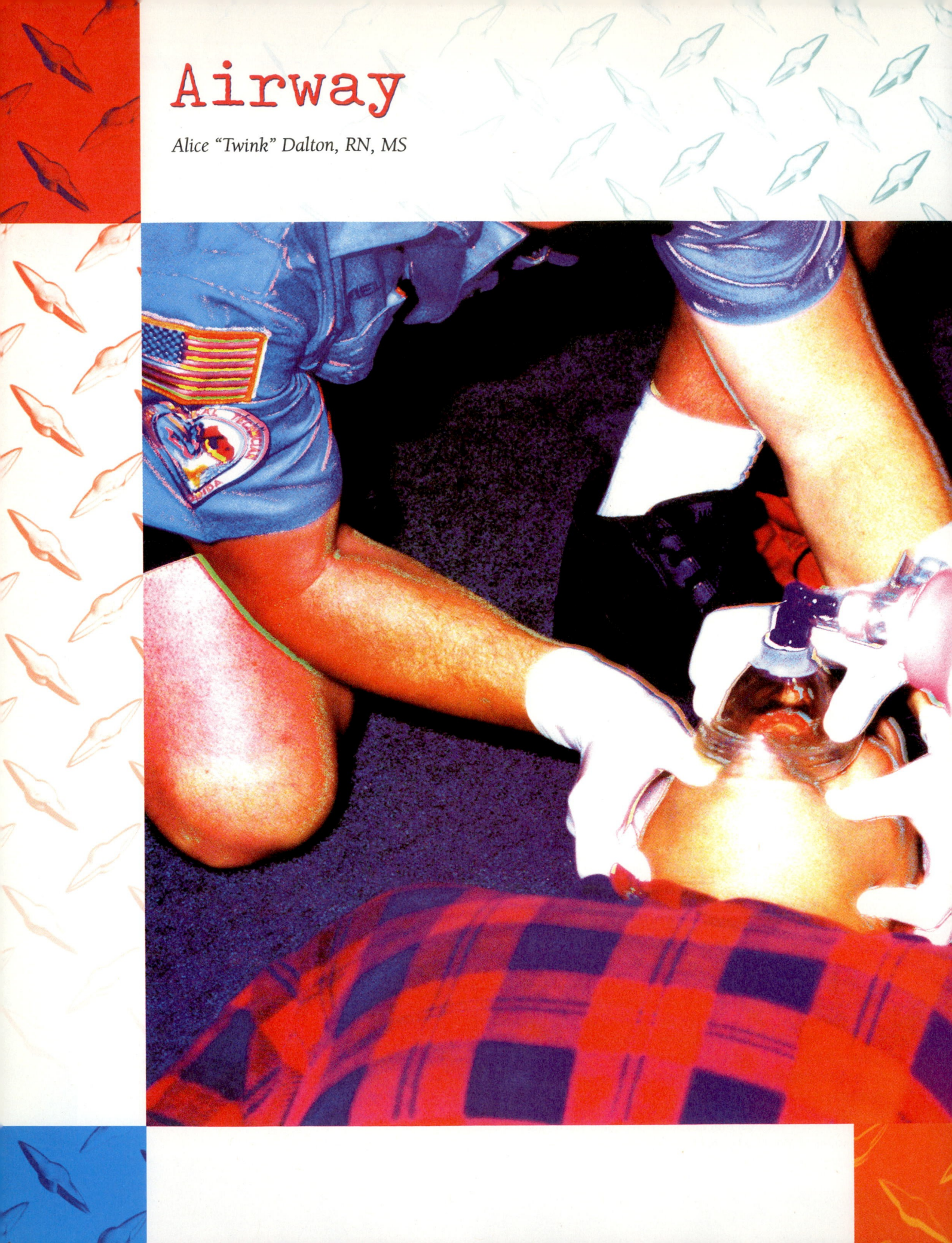

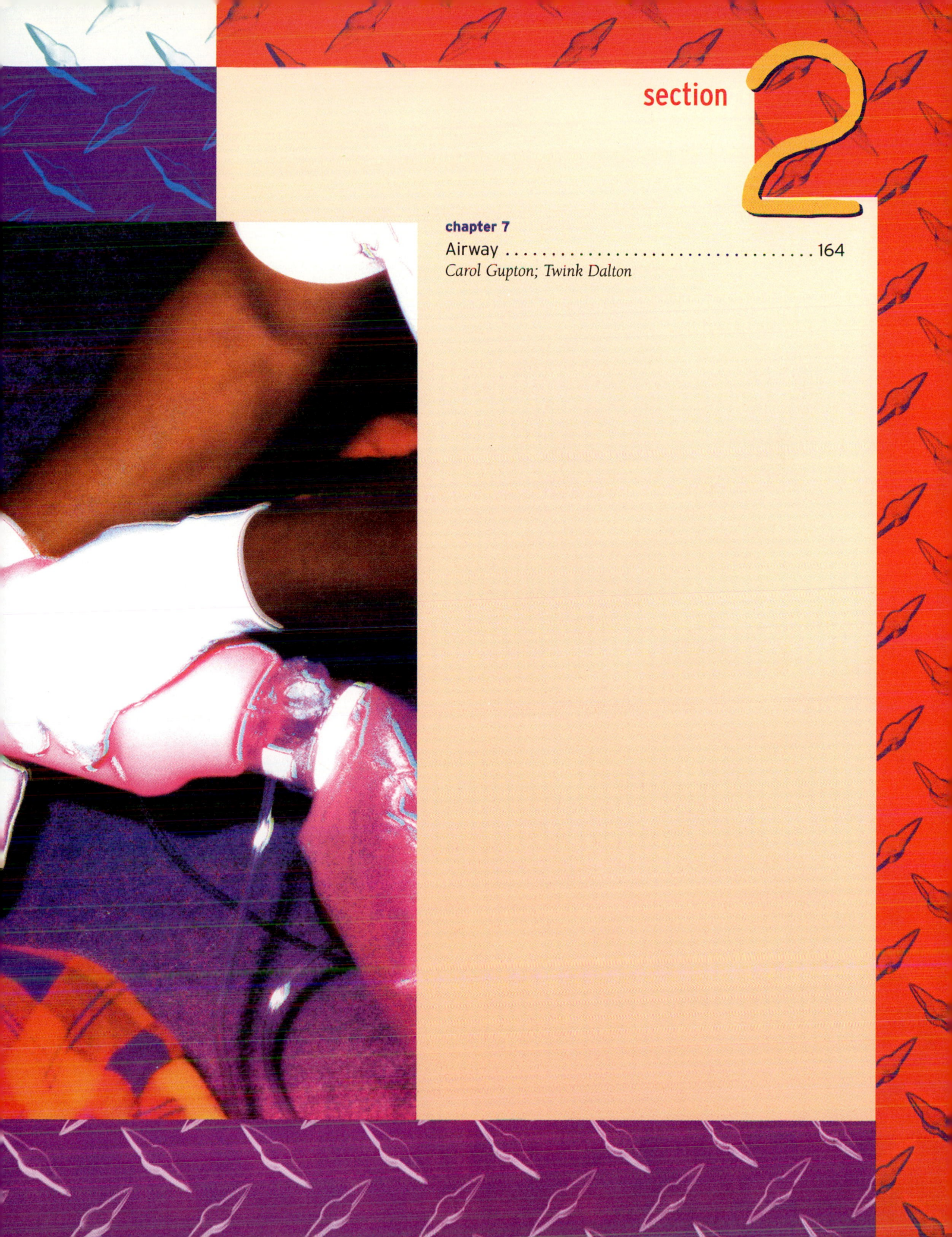

Airway

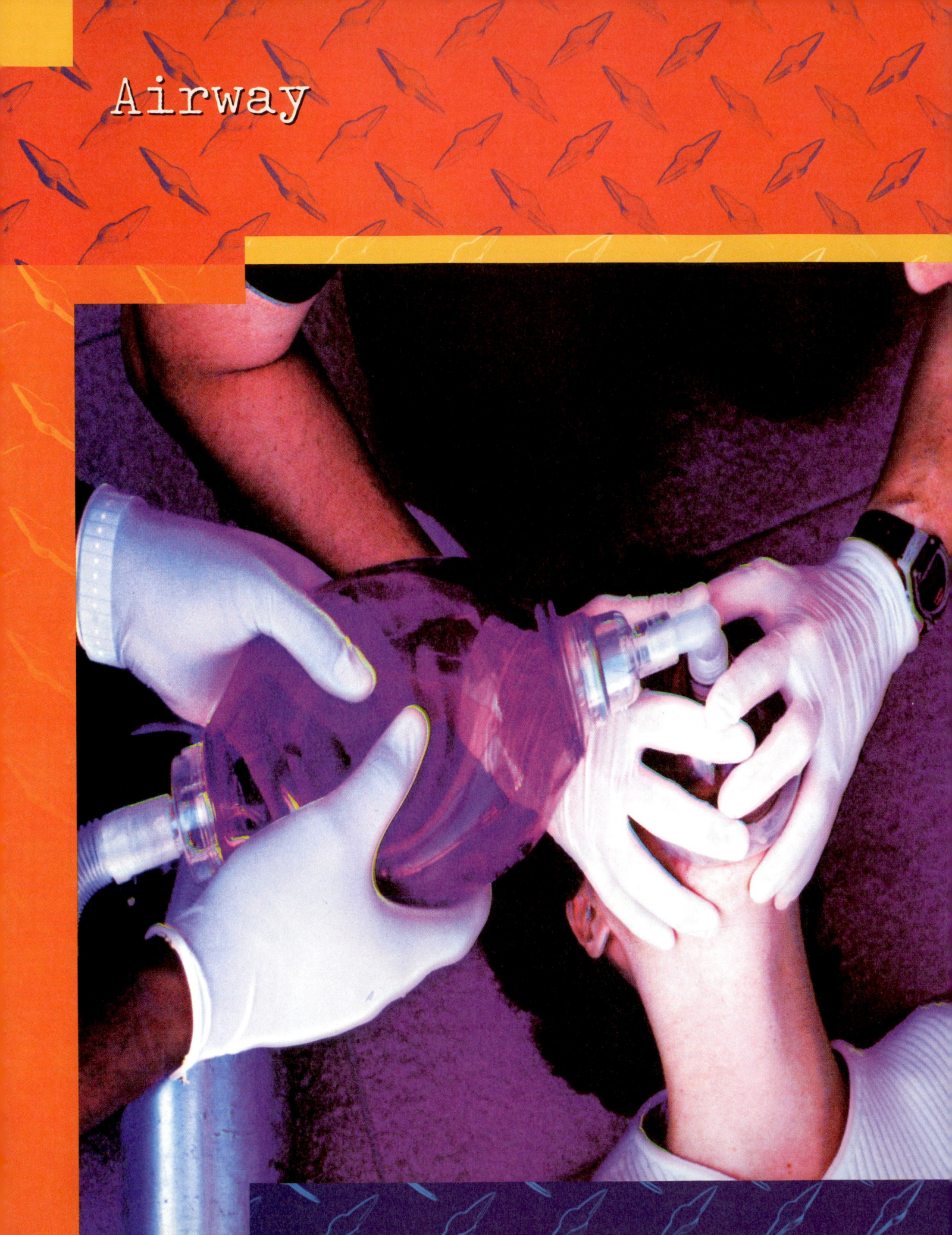

objectives

Cognitive

1. Name and label the major structures of the respiratory system on a diagram.
2. List the signs of adequate breathing.
3. List the signs of inadequate breathing.
4. Describe the steps in performing the head-tilt/chin-lift maneuver.
5. Relate mechanism of injury to opening the airway.
6. Describe the steps in performing the jaw-thrust maneuver.
7. State the importance of having a suction unit ready for immediate use when providing emergency care.
8. Describe the techniques of suctioning.
9. Describe how to artificially ventilate a patient with a pocket mask.
10. Describe the steps in performing the skill of artificially ventilating a patient with a bag-valve-mask while using the jaw-thrust maneuver.
11. List the parts of a bag-valve-mask system.
12. Describe the steps in performing the skill of artificially ventilating a patient with a bag-valve-mask for one and two rescuers.
13. Describe the signs of adequate artificial ventilation using the bag-valve-mask.
14. Describe the signs of inadequate artificial ventilation using the bag-valve-mask.
15. Describe the steps in ventilating a patient with a flow-restricted, oxygen-powered ventilation device.
16. List the steps in performing the actions taken when providing mouth-to-mouth and mouth-to-stoma artificial ventilation.
17. Describe how to measure and insert an oropharyngeal (oral) airway.
18. Describe how to measure and insert a nasopharyngeal (nasal) airway.
19. Define the components of an oxygen delivery system.
20. Identify a nonrebreathing face mask and state the oxygen flow requirements needed for its use.
21. Describe the indications for using a nasal cannula versus a nonrebreathing face mask.
22. Identify a nasal cannula and state the flow requirements needed for its use.

Affective

23. Explain the rationale for basic life support, artificial ventilation, and airway protective skills taking priority over most other basic life support skills.
24. Explain the rationale for providing adequate oxygenation through high inspired oxygen concentrations to patients who, in the past, may have received low concentrations.

Psychomotor

25. Demonstrate the steps in performing the head-tilt/chin-lift maneuver.
26. Demonstrate the steps in performing the jaw-thrust maneuver.
27. Demonstrate the techniques of suctioning.
28. Demonstrate the steps in providing mouth-to-mouth artificial ventilation with body substance isolation (barrier shields).
29. Demonstrate how to use a pocket mask to artificially ventilate a patient.
30. Demonstrate the assembly of a bag-valve-mask unit.
31. Demonstrate the steps in performing the skill of artificially ventilating a patient with a bag-valve-mask for one and two rescuers.
32. Demonstrate the steps in performing the skill of artificially ventilating a patient with a bag-valve-mask while using the jaw-thrust maneuver.
33. Demonstrate artificial ventilation of a patient with a flow-restricted, oxygen-powered ventilation device.
34. Demonstrate how to artificially ventilate a patient with a stoma.
35. Demonstrate how to insert an oropharyngeal (oral) airway.
36. Demonstrate how to insert a nasopharyngeal (nasal) airway.
37. Demonstrate the correct operation of oxygen tanks and regulators.
38. Demonstrate the use of a nonrebreathing face mask and state the oxygen flow requirements needed for its use.
39. Demonstrate the use of a nasal cannula and state the flow requirements needed for its use.
40. Demonstrate how to artificially ventilate the infant and child patient.
41. Demonstrate oxygen administration for the infant and child patient.

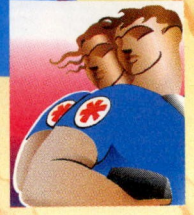

you are the emt

Squad 16 . . . Take a call at the Splash Magic Water Park for "a child not breathing." Gate C-6 is your closest access. Go to the Thunder Tube water slide. Four minutes later, you and your partner are on scene. "I hope whoever dragged the kid out of the water has a clue what they're doing," says your partner.

More than 10% of calls to 9-1-1 are airway-related. You are likely to respond to a call similar to the one described above. This chapter will help to prepare you to care for airway emergencies as well as help you to answer the following questions:

1. Why is it so time consuming to respond to and care for a patient who is experiencing an airway problem?

2. Why are airway calls so common?

Airway

The single most important step in caring for any patient is to make sure that he or she can breathe. The patient who cannot breathe properly is not delivering oxygen to body tissues and cells, which need a constant supply of oxygen to survive. Within seconds of being deprived of oxygen, the heart may not beat normally. After as few as 4 to 6 minutes without oxygen, the brain may be severely or permanently damaged.

Oxygen reaches body tissues and cells through two separate but related processes: breathing and circulation. As we inhale, oxygen moves from the atmosphere into our lungs, then passes from the air sacs in the lungs to the capillaries to oxygenate the blood. The blood, enriched with oxygen, travels through the body by the pumping action of the heart. At the same time, carbon dioxide produced by cells moves from the blood into the air sacs. The carbon dioxide then leaves our bodies as we exhale.

As an EMT-B, you must be able to locate the parts of the respiratory system, understand how the system works, and be able to recognize which patients are breathing adequately and which ones are breathing inadequately.

This chapter will review the anatomy and physiology of the respiratory system, that is, the parts of the system and how they work. It will then describe how to assess patients quickly and carefully to determine their airway and ventilation status. The equipment, procedures, and guidelines that you will need to manage patients' airway and breathing are described in detail. You will learn several ways to open a patient's airway and specific techniques for removing foreign objects or fluids that may be blocking the airway. Because artificial airway equipment can have serious results if used improperly, the chapter will thoroughly discuss airway adjuncts, oxygen therapy devices, and artificial ventilation methods.

Anatomy of the Respiratory System

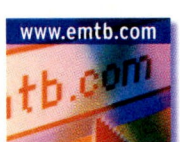

The respiratory system consists of all the structures in the body that help us breathe, or ventilate (Figure 7-1). These include the diaphragm, the muscles of the chest wall, and the accessory muscles of breathing. **Ventilation** is the exchange of air between the lungs and environment. The diaphragm and muscles of the chest wall are responsible for the regular rise and fall of the chest that accompany normal breathing. The term **airway** usually refers to the upper airway or the passage above the larynx (voice box). The upper airway consists of the nose, mouth, and throat (pharynx). The portion of the throat behind the nose is the nasopharynx; the portion behind the mouth is the oropharynx.

The lower airway begins with the larynx (voice box), which is covered by a structure called the epiglottis, a leaf-shaped structure that prevents food and liquid from entering the lower airway during swallowing. Cricoid cartilage is a firm cartilage ring that forms the lower part of the larynx. The trachea is directly connected to the larynx. The main bronchi and other air passages branch off from the trachea, extending into each lung.

The chest (thoracic cage) contains the lungs, one in each half, or hemithorax (Figure 7-2). The lungs hang freely within the chest cavity. Between the lungs, in a space called the mediastinum, lie the heart, the great vessels, the esophagus, the trachea, the major bronchi, and many nerves. The boundaries of the thorax are the rib cage anteriorly, superiorly, and posteriorly and the diaphragm inferiorly.

Because it is attached to the costal arch and the vertebrae, the diaphragm is a skeletal muscle. It is considered a specialized muscle because it functions as both a voluntary and an involuntary muscle. It acts as a voluntary muscle whenever we take a deep breath, cough, or hold

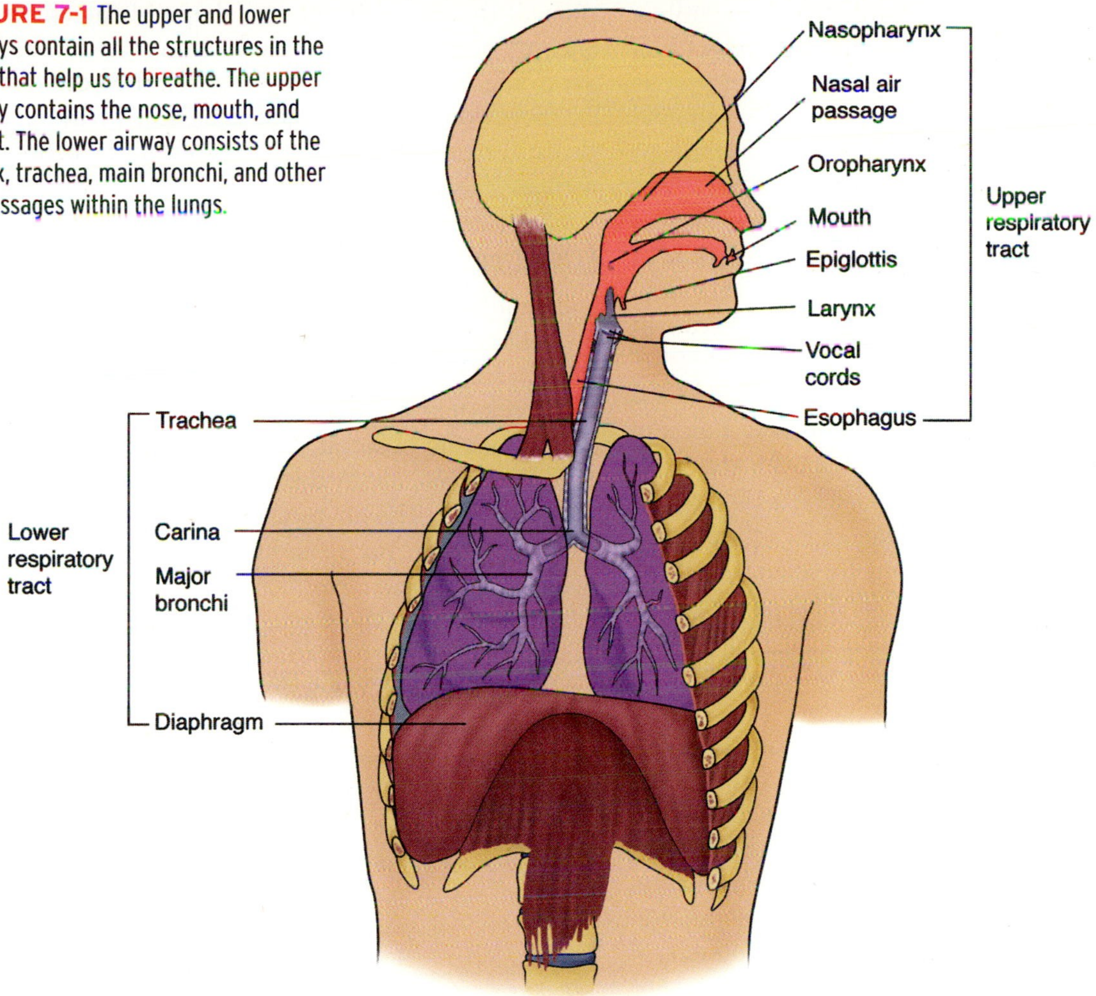

FIGURE 7-1 The upper and lower airways contain all the structures in the body that help us to breathe. The upper airway contains the nose, mouth, and throat. The lower airway consists of the larynx, trachea, main bronchi, and other air passages within the lungs.

Nasopharynx

Nasal air passage

Oropharynx

Mouth

Epiglottis

Larynx

Vocal cords

Esophagus

Upper respiratory tract

Trachea

Carina

Major bronchi

Diaphragm

Lower respiratory tract

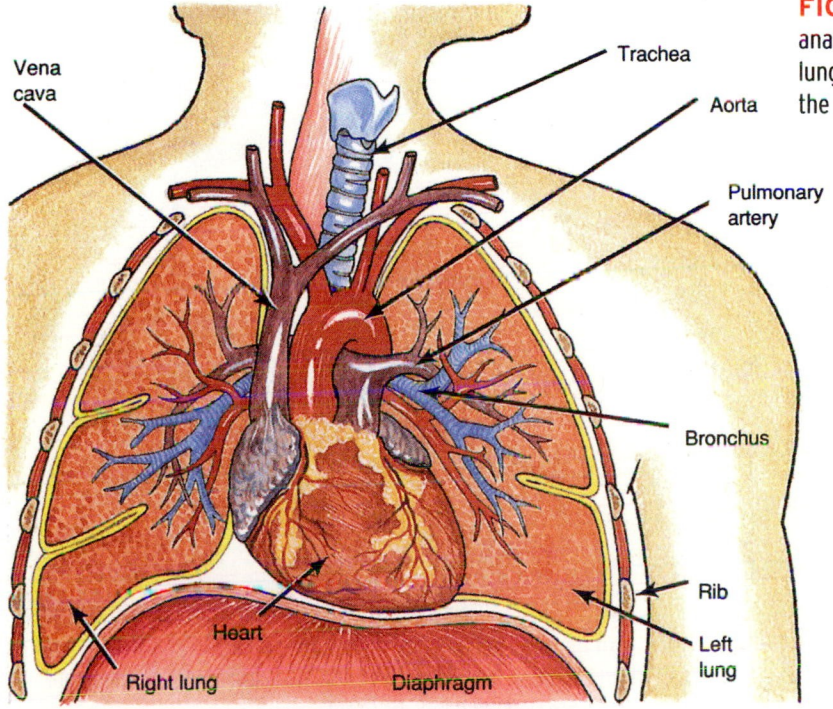

FIGURE 7-2 The thoracic cage contains important anatomic structures for respiration, including the lungs, the heart, the great vessels, the trachea and the major bronchi.

Vena cava

Trachea

Aorta

Pulmonary artery

Bronchus

Rib

Left lung

Heart

Right lung

Diaphragm

our breath, actions that we control. However, unlike other skeletal or voluntary muscles, the diaphragm performs an automatic function. Breathing continues while we sleep and at all other times. Even though we can hold our breath or temporarily breathe more quickly or slowly, we cannot continue these variations in breathing indefinitely. When the concentration of carbon dioxide rises within the blood, the automatic regulation of breathing resumes under the control of the brain stem.

Because they have no muscle tissue, the lungs cannot move on their own. They need the help of other structures to be able to expand and contract as we inhale and exhale. Therefore, the ability of the lungs to function properly is partially dependent on the movement of the chest and supporting structures. These structures include the thorax, the thoracic cage (chest), the diaphragm, the intercostal muscles, the pleura, and the accessory muscles of breathing.

Inhalation

The active muscular part of breathing is called **inhalation**. As we inhale, air enters the body through the trachea. It then travels to and from the lungs, filling and emptying the alveoli. During inhalation, the diaphragm and intercostal muscles contract. When the diaphragm contracts, it moves down slightly and enlarges the thoracic cage from top to bottom. When the intercostal muscles contract, they raise the ribs up and out. As we inhale, the combined actions of these structures enlarge the thorax in all directions. Because the lungs are attached to these structures, the lungs follow the motion of the chest wall exactly. Take a deep breath to see how your chest expands.

The air pressure outside the body, called the atmospheric pressure, is normally higher than the air pressure within the thorax. As we inhale and the thoracic cage expands, the air pressure within the thorax decreases a bit more, creating a slight vacuum. This drives air in through the trachea and fills the lungs. When the air pressure outside equals the air pressure inside, air stops moving. Gases, such as oxygen, will move from an area of high pressure to an area of lower pressure until the pressures are equal. At this point, the air stops moving, and we stop inhaling. **Tidal volume** is the amount of air that is moved during one normal breath. Minute volume is tidal volume times respiratory rate or the amount of air moved through the lungs in 1 minute.

It may help you to understand this if you think of the thoracic cage as a bell jar in which balloons are suspended. In this example, the balloons are the lungs. The base of the jar is the diaphragm, which moves up and down slightly with each breath. The ribs, which are the

sides of the jar, maintain the shape of the chest. The only opening into the jar is a small tube at the top, similar to the trachea. During inhalation, the bottom of the jar moves down slightly and decreases pressure in the jar, creating a slight vacuum. As a result, the balloons fill with air (Figure 7-3).

Exhalation

Unlike inhalation, exhalation does not normally require muscular effort. During **exhalation**, the diaphragm and the intercostal muscles relax. In response, the thorax decreases in size, and the ribs and muscles assume a normal resting position. When the size of the thoracic cage decreases, air in the lungs is compressed into a smaller space. The air pressure within the thorax then becomes higher than the pressure outside, and air is pushed out through the trachea.

Let's return to the example of the bell jar. During exhalation, the bottom of the jar (the diaphragm) moves up, returning to its normal resting position. This movement increases air pressure within the jar. With this increase in pressure, the sides of the jar contract, and the balloons empty.

Remember that air will reach the lungs only if it travels through the trachea. Air may readily pass into

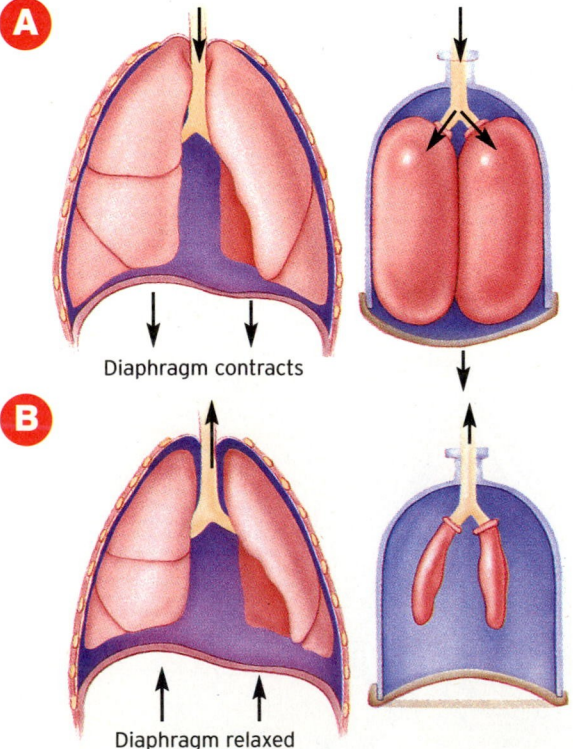

FIGURE 7-3 The mechanisms of respiration can be compared with that of a bell jar. **A:** Inhalation and chest expansion, anatomic (left) and bell jar, (right). **B:** Exhalation and chest contraction, anatomic (left) and bell jar (right).

Diaphragm contracts

Diaphragm relaxed

the chest cavity through another opening in the throat or chest wall as a result of trauma or certain medical conditions, but it will not reach the alveoli. This is why clearing and maintaining an open airway are so important. Clearing the airway means removing obstructing material, tissue, or fluids from the nose, mouth, or throat. Maintaining the airway means keeping the airway open so that air can enter and leave the lungs freely (Figure 7-4).

Physiology of the Respiratory System

All living cells need energy to survive. Cells take energy from nutrients through a series of chemical processes. The name given to these processes as a whole is **metabolism**. During metabolism, each cell combines nutrients and oxygen and produces energy and waste products, primarily water and carbon dioxide.

Each living cell in the body, then, requires a regular supply of oxygen and a means of getting rid of waste (carbon dioxide). The body provides these through respiration. Some cells need a constant supply of oxygen to survive. Other cells in the body can tolerate short periods without oxygen and still survive. For example, cells in the heart may be damaged if their oxygen supply is interrupted for more than a few seconds. After 4 to 6 minutes without oxygen, brain cells and cells in the nervous system may be severely and permanently damaged and may even die (Figure 7-5). Dead brain cells can never be replaced.

Normally, the air that we breathe contains 21% oxygen and 78% nitrogen. Small amounts of other gases make up the remaining 1%.

The Exchange of Oxygen and Carbon Dioxide

As blood travels through the body, it gives oxygen and nutrients to various tissues and cells. Oxygen passes from the blood through the capillaries to tissue cells, while carbon dioxide and cell waste passes in the opposite direction: from tissue cells through capillaries to the blood (Figure 7-6).

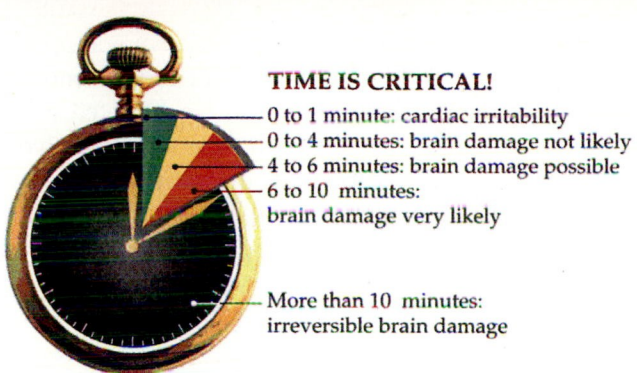

TIME IS CRITICAL!
- 0 to 1 minute: cardiac irritability
- 0 to 4 minutes: brain damage not likely
- 4 to 6 minutes: brain damage possible
- 6 to 10 minutes: brain damage very likely
- More than 10 minutes: irreversible brain damage

FIGURE 7-5 Cells need a constant supply of oxygen to survive. Some cells may be severely and permanently damaged after 4 to 6 minutes without oxygen.

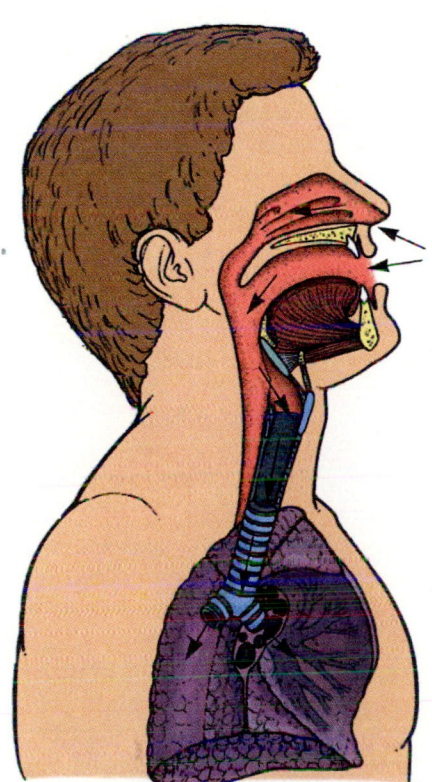

FIGURE 7-4 Air reaches the lungs only if it travels through the trachea. Maintaining the airway means keeping the airway open so that air can enter and leave the lungs freely.

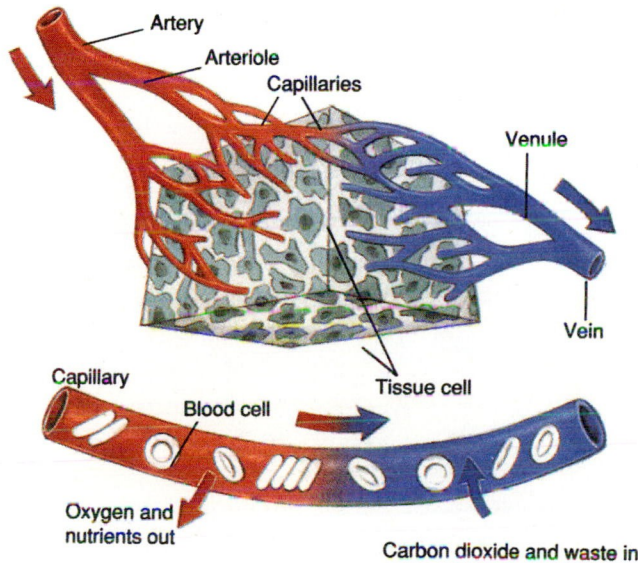

FIGURE 7-6 Oxygen passes from the blood through capillaries to tissue cells. Carbon dioxide passes from tissue cells through capillaries to the blood.

Each time we inhale, the alveoli receive a supply of oxygen-rich air through a network of tiny pulmonary capillaries. These capillaries are, in fact, located in the walls of the alveoli. This means that the air in the alveoli and the blood in the capillaries are separated only by two very thin layers of wall tissue. Each time we exhale, the carbon dioxide from the bloodstream travels across the same two layers of tissue to the alveoli and is expelled into the atmosphere.

Oxygen and carbon dioxide pass rapidly across the walls of the alveoli and the capillaries through diffusion. **Diffusion** is a passive process in which molecules move from an area with higher concentration of molecules to an area of lower concentration. For example, when we walk into a kitchen and it smells like a rotten egg, that is because the molecules of hydrogen sulfide gas have moved spontaneously from an area of high concentration near the egg to fill the whole space. Molecules of oxygen move from the alveoli into the blood because there are fewer oxygen molecules in the blood. In the same way, molecules of carbon dioxide move from the blood into the alveoli because there are fewer carbon dioxide molecules in the alveoli (Figure 7-7).

The blood does not use all the inhaled oxygen as it passes through the body. So the air that we exhale contains 16% oxygen and 3% to 5% carbon dioxide; the rest is nitrogen (Figure 7-8). Therefore, when you provide artificial ventilations to a patient who is not breathing, that patient is receiving a 16% concentration of oxygen with each of your exhaled breaths.

The Control of Breathing

The area of the brain stem that controls breathing is deep within the skull, in one of the best-protected parts

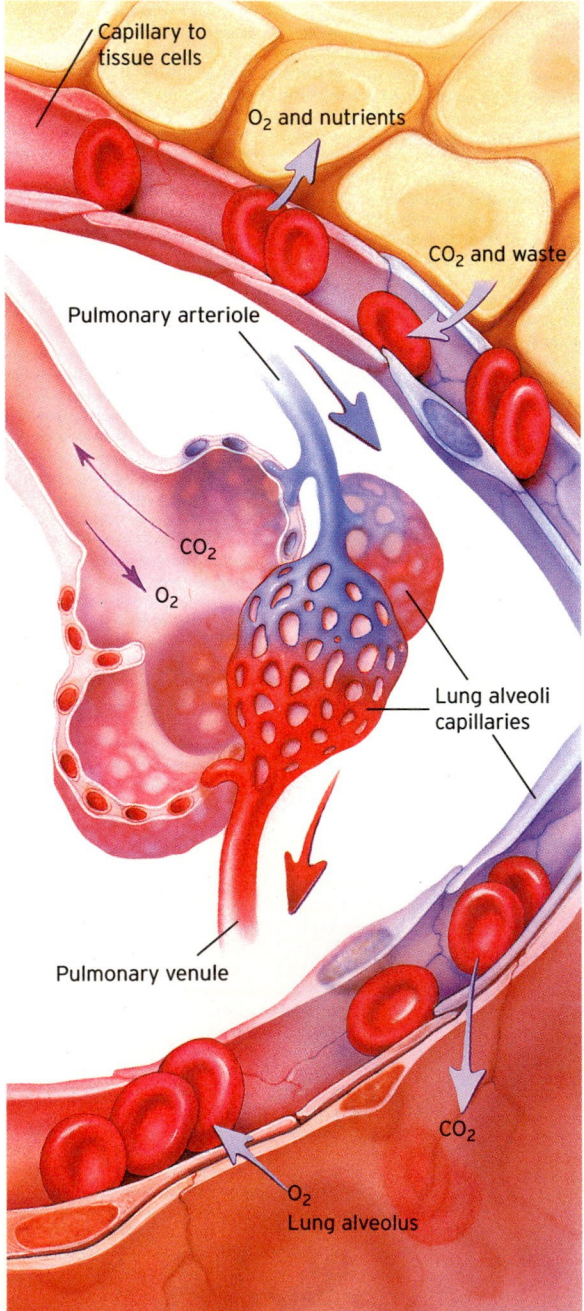

FIGURE 7-7 With diffusion, molecules of oxygen move from the alveoli into the blood, because there are fewer oxygen molecules in the blood. Similarly, molecules of carbon dioxide move from the blood into the alveoli, because there are fewer carbon dioxide molecules in the alveoli.

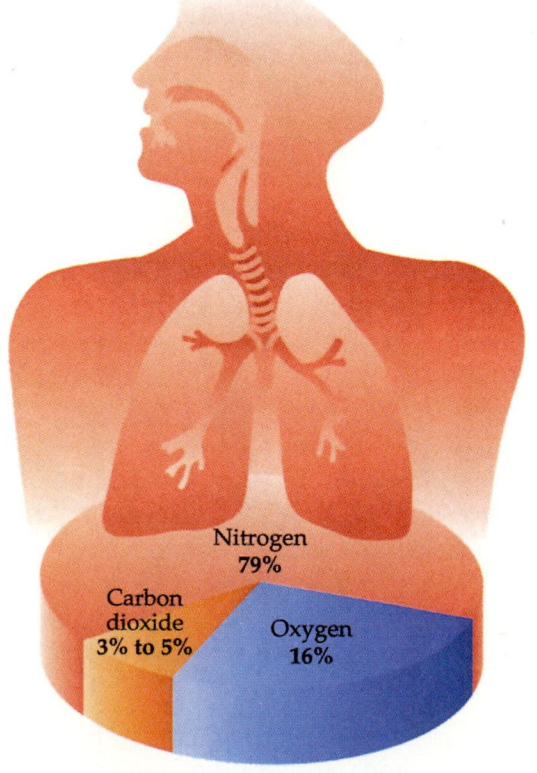

Components of Exhaled Air

FIGURE 7-8 Exhaled air contains 16% oxygen, and 3% to 5% carbon dioxide; the rest is nitrogen.

of the nervous system. The nerves in this area act as sensors, reacting primarily to the level of carbon dioxide in the arterial blood. If the levels of carbon dioxide are too high or too low, the brain automatically adjusts breathing. This happens very quickly, in just one breath. Again, this is why you cannot hold your breath indefinitely or breathe rapidly and deeply for very long. In a healthy person, the stimulus to breathe is referred to as the normal respiratory drive.

When the level of carbon dioxide becomes too high, the brain stem sends nerve impulses down the spinal cord that cause the diaphragm and the intercostal muscles to contract. This increases our breathing, or respirations. The higher the level of carbon dioxide in the blood, the stronger the impulses to cause breathing. Once the carbon dioxide returns to an acceptable level, the strength and frequency of respiration decrease.

We also have a "backup system" to control respiration, called the hypoxic drive. This system stimulates breathing when oxygen levels fall. However, the nerves in the brain, the walls of the aorta, and the carotid arteries that act as oxygen sensors are easily satisfied with minimal levels of oxygen. Therefore, the hypoxic drive is much less sensitive and less powerful than the carbon dioxide sensors in the brain stem.

Hypoxia. Hypoxia is an extremely dangerous condition in which the body's tissues and cells do not have enough oxygen; unless it is reversed, patients may die in a matter of moments. Hypoxia develops quickly in the vital organs of patients who are not breathing adequately, as well as those who are not breathing at all. Inadequate breathing means that the person cannot move enough air into the lungs with each breath to meet the body's needs.

Patients who are breathing inadequately will show varying signs of hypoxia. The onset and the degree of tissue damage will depend on the quality of ventilations. The signs of hypoxia may include mental status changes, the use of accessory muscles for breathing, difficulty breathing, possibly chest pain, and, late in the process, cyanosis. Early signs include nervousness, irritability, apprehension, tachycardia (fast heart rate), and fear. Conscious patients will complain of shortness of breath and may not be able to talk in complete sentences. The best time to give a patient oxygen is before any symptoms appear.

The following conditions are commonly associated with hypoxia:

- **Myocardial infarction (heart attack).** Ischemia within the heart muscle from myocardial infarction occurs when there is inadequate circulation of oxygen-carrying blood to the tissues of the heart.

- **Pulmonary edema.** Fluid accumulates in the lungs, making the transfer of oxygen to the blood from the alveoli less efficient.

- **Acute narcotic overdose.** Respirations may become infrequent and shallow.

- **Inhalation of smoke and/or toxic fumes.** These substances cause pulmonary edema and destroy lung tissue, causing problems with gas exchange.

- **Stroke (cerebrovascular accident).** The cause of hypoxia in a stroke patient may be due to facial paralysis and poor control of respirations and heart rhythms by the brain.

- **Chest injury.** Pain interferes with full chest wall expansion, thus limiting the amount of gases that are exchanged. Lung damage can also prevent efficient gas exchange.

- **Shock (hypoperfusion).** Shock often occurs as a result of injuries involving substantial blood loss. With the loss of the red blood cells' hemoglobin, not enough oxygen is available to the tissues. Certain other types of shock will lead to inefficient gas exchange from the slowing of respiratory system function.

- **Chronic obstructive pulmonary disease (COPD and emphysema).** Chronic irritation of the lungs and air passages produces alveolar damage and poor gas exchange.

All hypoxic patients, whatever the cause of their condition, should be treated with high-flow supplemental oxygen. The method of oxygen delivery will vary, depending on the cause and the severity of the hypoxia.

Patient Assessment

Recognizing Adequate Breathing

Earlier, we compared breathing to an expandable bell jar with a movable bottom. You can also think of a normal breathing pattern as a bellows system. Breathing should appear easy, not labored. As with a bellows used to move air to start a fire, breathing should be a smooth flow of air moving into and out of the lungs. Normal, or adequate, breathing has the following characteristics:

- A normal rate and depth (between 12 and 20 breaths/min) for adults

- A regular pattern of inhalation and exhalation

- Clear and equal lung sounds on both sides of the chest (bilateral)

- Regular and equal chest rise and fall (chest expansion)

- Adequate depth (tidal volume)

Recognizing Inadequate Breathing

An adult who is awake, alert, and talking to you has no immediate airway or breathing problems. However, you should always have supplemental oxygen close at hand to assist with breathing if this becomes necessary. An adult who is breathing normally will have respirations of 12 to 20 breaths/min (Table 7-1). The adult patient who is breathing either much slower (fewer than 8 breaths/min) or much faster (more than 24 breaths/min) should be evaluated for inadequate breathing.

A patient with inadequate breathing may appear to be working hard to breathe. This type of breathing pattern is called <u>labored breathing</u>. It requires effort and, especially among children, may involve the accessory muscles. Accessory muscles are secondary muscles of respiration. They include the sternocleidomastoid (neck) muscles, the pectoralis major (chest) muscles, and the abdominal muscles (Figure 7-9). These muscles are not used in normal breathing.

Other signs that a person is not breathing normally include the following:

- Accessory muscles being used in the neck (muscle retractions above the clavicle), intercostal retractions (muscle retractions between the ribs), or abdominal breathing (muscle retractions of the diaphragm)
- Cyanotic (blue) skin, usually seen first around the lips and mouth; remember, this is a late sign of hypoxia
- Cool, damp (clammy) skin
- Irregular (uneven) pattern of inhalation and exhalation
- Lung sounds that are decreased, unequal, or "wet"
- Shallow and/or uneven chest rise and fall

You should also be aware that a patient may appear to be breathing after the heart has stopped. These occa-

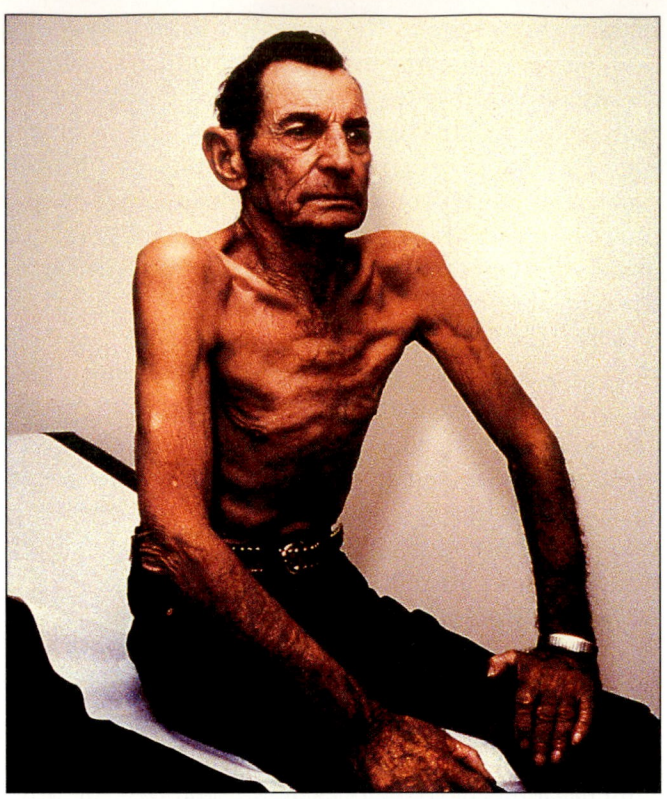

FIGURE 7-9 The accessory muscles of breathing are used when a patient is having difficulty breathing, not for normal breathing. These include the sternocleidomastoid, pectoralis major, and abdominal muscles.

sional, gasping breaths are called <u>agonal respirations</u>. They occur when the respiratory center in the brain continues to send signals to the breathing muscles. These respirations are not adequate, since they are slow and generally shallow. You should always assist ventilations of patients with agonal respirations.

Some patients may have irregular respiratory breathing patterns that are related to a specific patient condition. Examples include Cheyne-Stokes respirations, often seen in patients with stroke, and central neurogenic hyperventilation, often associated with patients with head injuries. Cheyne-Stokes respirations are an irregular respiratory pattern in which the patient breathes with an increasing rate and depth of respiration that is followed by a period of apnea, or lack of spontaneous breathing, followed again by the pattern of increasing rate and depth. Central neurogenic hyperventilation is an abnormal respiratory pattern in which the patient's respirations are rapid and deep.

Patients with inadequate breathing have inadequate minute volume and need to be treated immediately. This is most easily recognized in patients who are unable to speak in complete sentences when at rest. Emergency medical care includes airway management, supplemental oxygen, and ventilatory support.

TABLE 7-1	Normal Respiration Rate Ranges
Adults	12 to 20 breaths/min
Children	15 to 30 breaths/min
Infants	25 to 50 breaths/min

To obtain the breathing rate in a patient, count the number of breaths in a 30-second period and multiply by 2. To prevent influencing the rate, avoid letting the patient know that you are counting.

Positioning Patients for BLS and CPR

Your initial assessment of a patient should identify whether breathing problems are present. If breathing is absent, you should begin treatment with BLS measures immediately. The outstanding advantage of BLS is that it permits the earliest possible treatment of airway obstruction, respiratory arrest, or cardiac arrest without initially needing specialized equipment or material. It may be that once you open or clear the airway, the patient will be able to breathe. If not, you may have to begin artificial ventilation. If a patient stops breathing before his or her heart stops, there may be enough oxygen in the lungs to maintain life for several minutes. You will know that your efforts are successful when you see the following:

- The regular rise and fall of the chest with each ventilation

- A regular rate of ventilations, appropriate for the age of the patient

- A resumption of the regular heart rate

If the patient's heart does not resume a regular, coordinated pumping action, you may have to begin CPR. For an unconscious patient who needs CPR, try to find out what happened. Was the patient hit in the head? Does he or she have a spinal injury? Neither a head injury nor a spinal injury should keep you from starting BLS. It simply means that you must perform BLS within certain specific physical limits and with extra care, taking care during CPR to protect the spinal cord from injury.

Use the following steps to reposition an unconscious adult patient who needs airway management and has a suspected cervical spine injury (Figure 7-10).

1. **Kneel beside the patient.** Have your partner kneel far enough away that the patient, when rolled toward you, does not come to rest in your lap.

2. **Rapidly straighten the patient's legs,** and move the nearer arm across the patient's chest to minimize movement.

3. **Place your hands behind the back of the patient's head and neck** to maintain the cervical spine. Have your partner place his or her hands on the distant shoulder and hip.

4. **Turn the patient toward you** by pulling on the distant shoulder and hip. Control the head and neck so that they move as a unit with the rest of the torso. In this way, the head and neck stay in

the same vertical plane as the back. This single motion will minimize aggravation of any spinal injury. At this point, you should apply a cervical collar.

5. **Replace the patient's farther arm back** at his or her side.

If possible, log roll the patient onto a long spine board. This device will provide support during transport and emergency department care.

Now you can easily assess the patient's airway, breathing, and circulation and start BLS, if necessary. The few seconds it takes to position the patient properly will greatly improve the delivery of CPR.

Opening the Airway

Emergency medical care for patients begins with ensuring an open airway. The patient's airway and breathing status are the first steps in your initial assessment for a very good reason: Unless you can immediately open a compromised airway, you cannot give appropriate patient care.

In an unconscious patient, the most common airway obstruction is the patient's own tongue, which falls back into the throat when the muscles of the throat and tongue relax (Figure 7-11). Dentures (false teeth), blood, vomitus, mucus, food, or other foreign objects may also create a blockage. Therefore, you should always have a suction device available to help open and maintain the airway.

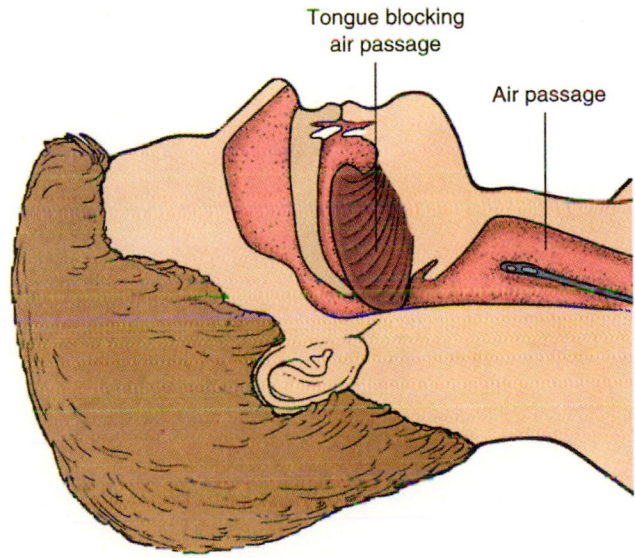

FIGURE 7-11 The most common airway obstruction is the patient's tongue, which can fall back into the throat when the muscles of the throat and tongue relax.

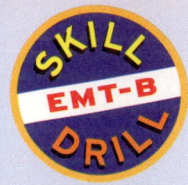

Repositioning an Unconscious Adult
Figure 7-10

Steps for repositioning an unconscious adult who needs airway management and has a suspected spinal injury.

1

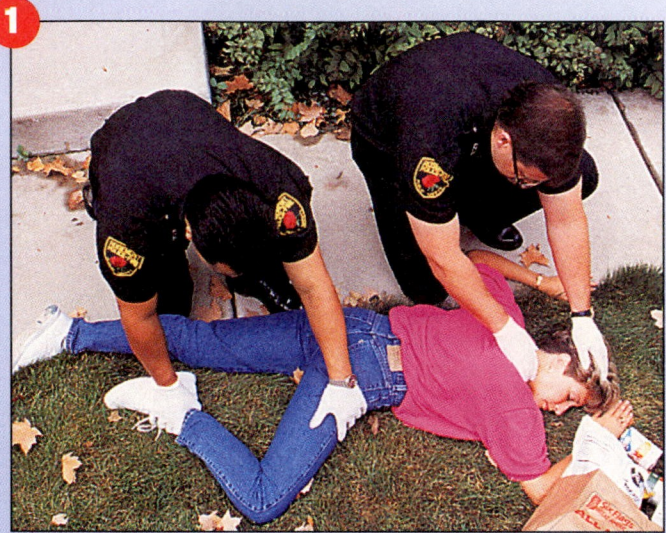

Maintain in-line stabilization of the head while your partner straightens the patient's legs. Ask a third person to move the backboard in position.

2

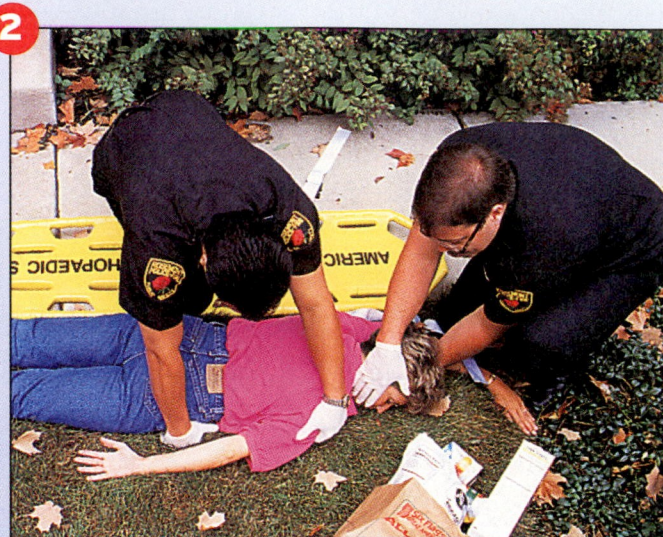

Have your partner grab the patient's far shoulder and hips.

3

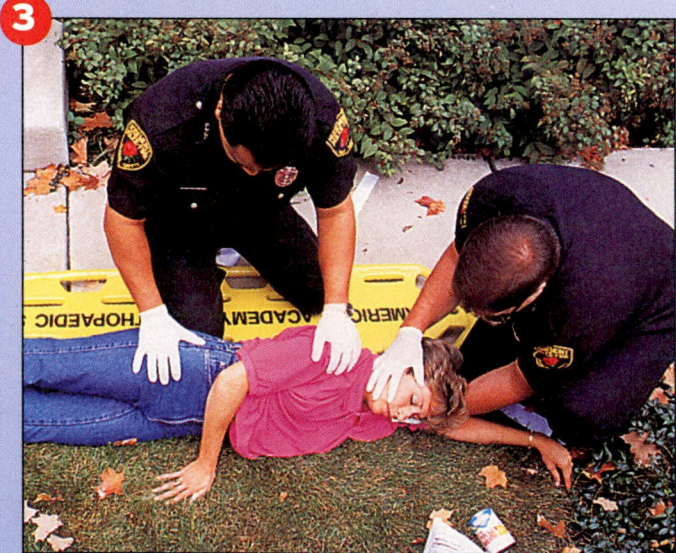

Roll the patient as a unit, with the person at the head calling the count to control moving the patient.

4

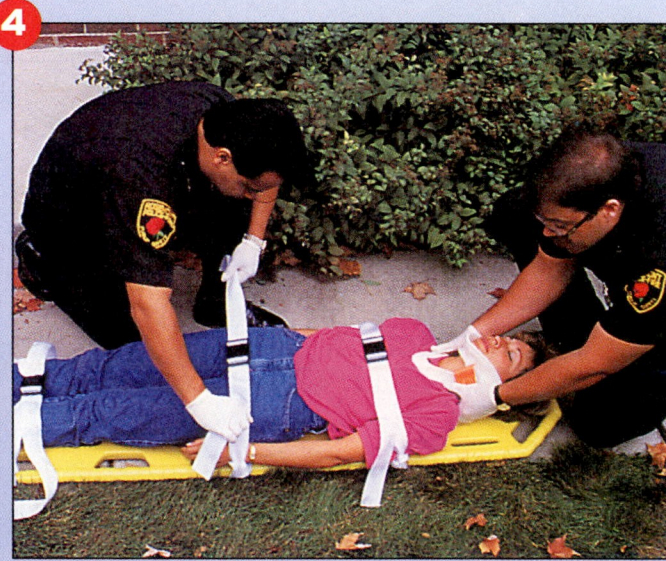

Secure the body first and then secure the head.

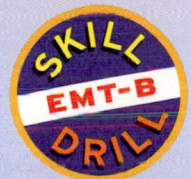

Performing Head-Tilt/Chin-Lift Maneuver

SKILL DRILL EMT-B

Figure 7-12

The head-tilt/chin-lift maneuver is a simple technique for opening the airway in a patient who does not have a cervical spine injury.

2

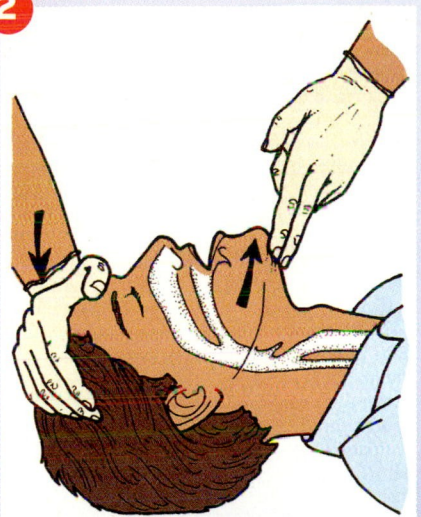

Place the tips of your fingers of your other hand under the bony part of the chin, although you may find it takes more than two fingers to accomplish this task. Lift the chin upward, bringing the entire lower jaw with it, helping to tilt the head back.

1

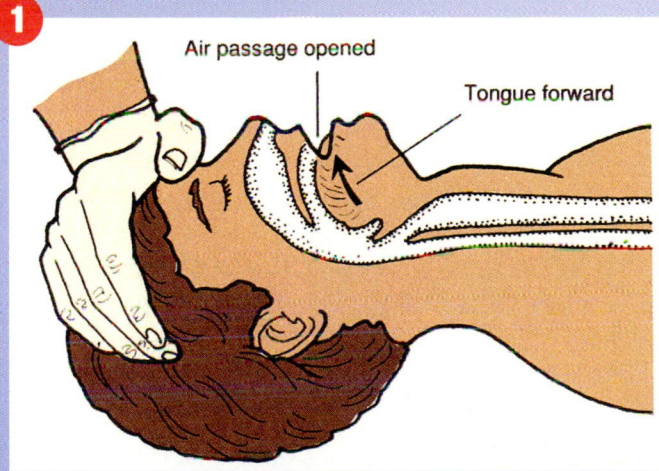

Air passage opened

Tongue forward

Place one hand on the patient's forehead, and apply firm backward pressure with your palm. Move the patient's head back as far as possible.

3

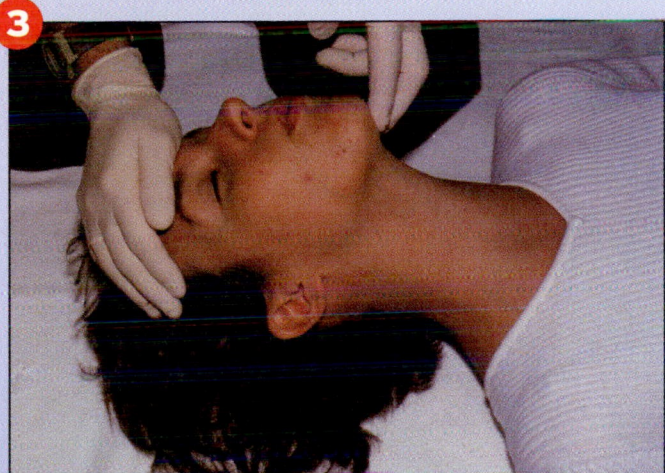

The completed maneuver.

Airway problems can be especially challenging in patients with serious facial injuries. Because the blood supply in the face is so rich, blunt injuries to the face can result in severe tissue swelling and bleeding into the airway.

Head-Tilt/Chin-Lift Maneuver

Opening the airway to relieve an obstruction can often be done quickly and easily by simply tilting the patient's head back and lifting the chin in what is known as the head-tilt/chin-lift maneuver. For patients who have not sustained trauma, this simple maneuver is sometimes all that is needed for the patient to resume breathing. If the patient has any foreign material or vomitus in the mouth, you should quickly remove it. Wipe out any liquid materials from the mouth with a piece of cloth held by your index and middle fingers; use your hooked index finger to remove any solid material.

You should perform the head-tilt/chin-lift maneuver in the following way (Figure 7-12).

1. **Make sure the patient is supine.** Kneel close beside the patient.
2. **Place one hand on the patient's forehead,** and apply firm backward pressure with your palm to tilt the patient's head back. This extension of the neck will move the tongue forward, away from the back of the throat, and clear the airway if the tongue is blocking it.
3. **Place the tips of the fingers of your other hand under the lower jaw** near the bony part of the chin. Do not compress the soft tissue under the chin, as this would block the airway.

Performing Jaw-Thrust Maneuver
Figure 7-13

1

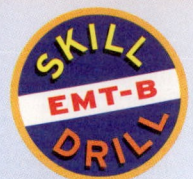

Use your thumbs to pull the patient's lower jaw down, to allow breathing through the mouth as well as the nose.

2

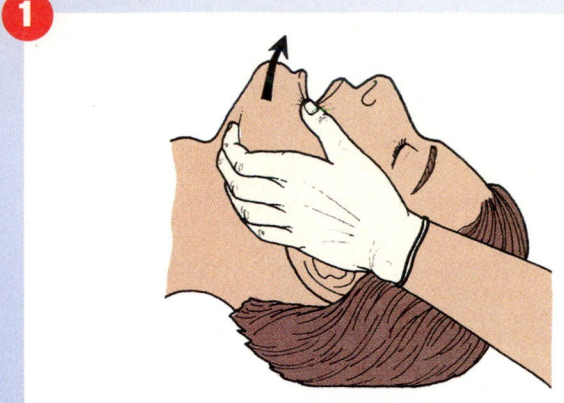

The completed maneuver should look like this.

3

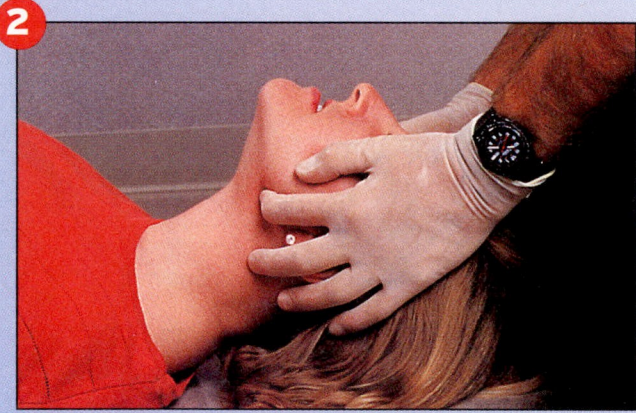

With the modified jaw-thrust maneuver, use your thumbs to seal the nose while your index and long fingers thrust the jaw anteriorly.

4. **Lift the chin upward,** bringing the entire lower jaw with it, helping to tilt the head back. Do not use your thumb to lift the chin. Lift so that the teeth are nearly brought together, but avoid closing the mouth completely. Continue to hold the forehead to maintain the backward tilt of the head.

Loose dentures can be held in place with the chin lift, making obstruction by the lips less likely. Performing mouth-to-mask ventilation is much easier when dentures are in place. However, loose dentures make it much harder to perform mouth-to-mask ventilation. Therefore, dentures that do not stay in place should be removed. The same is true of any dental appliances, including crowns, bridges, or even braces. Partial dentures (plates) may come loose following an accident or as you are providing care. Check patients with partial dentures periodically to make sure their plates are firmly in place.

Jaw-Thrust Maneuver

The head-tilt/chin-lift will open the airway in most patients. In some cases, however, forward movement of the lower jaw may be needed. The <u>jaw-thrust maneuver</u> is a technique to open the airway by placing the fingers behind the angle of the jaw and lifting the jaw upward.

Perform the jaw-thrust maneuver in an adult in the following way (Figure 7-13):

1. **Kneel above the patient's head.** Place your fingers behind the angles of the patient's lower jaw, and forcefully move the jaw upward.

2. **Use your thumbs to open the patient's mouth** to allow breathing through the mouth as well as the nose.

If you suspect a cervical spine injury, you can modify this maneuver to keep the head in a neutral position as you move the jaw forward and open the mouth. However, only an unconscious patient will tolerate this form of the maneuver. You can easily seal a mask around the mouth while doing the jaw-thrust maneuver. With the modified jaw-thrust maneuver, you can use your thumbs to seal the nose closed while your index and long fingers thrust the jaw anteriorly.

Once the airway has been opened by one of these techniques, the patient may start to breathe on his or her own. Assess whether breathing has returned by bending over and placing your ear about 1" above the patient's nose and mouth. Listen carefully for sounds of breathing (Figure 7-14). Can you feel and hear movement of air? Turn your head to watch the patient's chest and abdomen. If you can see the patient's chest and abdomen

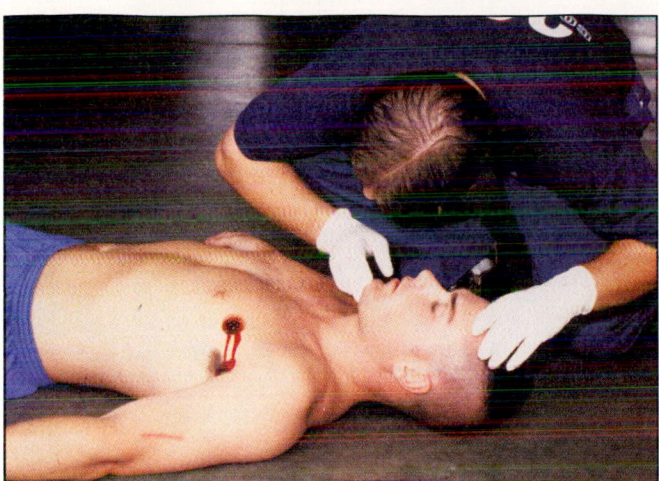

FIGURE 7-14 The Look, Listen, and Feel technique is used to assess whether breathing has returned spontaneously. When supporting the lower jaw, you should use care to avoid exerting pressure on the soft tissue.

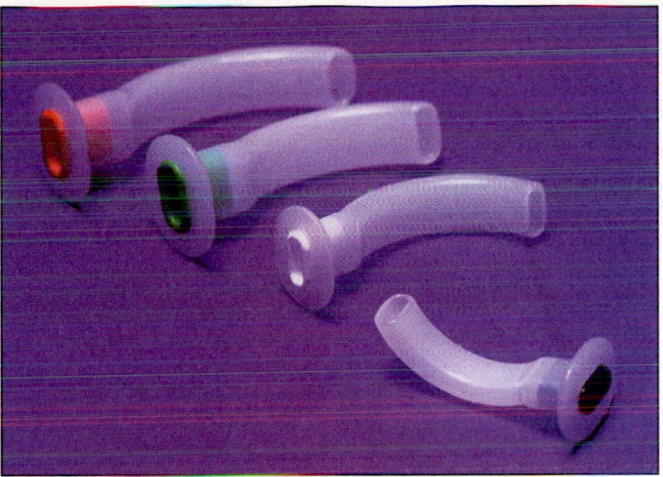

FIGURE 7-15 An oral airway is used for unconscious patients who have no gag reflex. It works to keep the tongue from blocking the airway and to make suctioning the airway easier. Note that the opening in the middle and along the side of the airway allows for both functions.

move with each breath, breathing has returned. However, feeling and hearing the actual movement of air are more important than seeing the chest and abdomen move. You may also place your hand on the patient's chest to feel for movement.

With complete airway obstruction, there will be no movement of air. However, you may see the chest and abdomen rise and fall considerably with the patient's frantic attempts to breathe. Observing chest and abdominal movement is often difficult with a fully clothed patient. You may see little, if any, chest movement, even with normal breathing. This is particularly true in some patients with chronic lung disease. You must begin artificial ventilation immediately if you use the three-part approach—look, listen, and feel—and discover that there is no movement of air.

Basic Airway Adjuncts

The primary function of an artificial airway is to prevent obstruction of the upper airway by the tongue and allow the passage of air and oxygen to the lungs.

Oropharyngeal Airways

An oropharyngeal (oral) airway has two principal purposes. The first is to keep the tongue from blocking the upper airway. The second is to make it easier to suction the airway if necessary. Both functions are made possible by an opening down the center or along either side of the oropharyngeal airway (Figure 7-15). This type of airway is often used in conjunction with bag-valve-mask (BVM) ventilation.

An oropharyngeal airway should be inserted promptly in unconscious patients who have no gag reflex. These patients may or may not be breathing on their own. The gag reflex is a normal reflex mechanism that causes retching when the soft palate or the back of the throat is touched. If you try to insert an oropharyngeal airway in a patient with a gag reflex, the result may be vomiting or a spasm of the vocal cords. An oropharyngeal airway is also a safe, effective way to maintain the airway of the patient with a possible spinal injury. Constant use of the head-tilt/chin-lift or other maneuvers for patients may not be necessary.

You must be very clear on when and how this device is used. If the oropharyngeal airway is not the proper size or is inserted incorrectly, it could actually push the tongue back into the pharynx, blocking the airway. To select the proper size, measure from the patient's earlobe to the corner of the mouth on the side of the face. When inserted properly, the airway will rest in the mouth with the curvature of the airway following the contour of the tongue. The flange should rest against the lips or teeth, the other end opening into the pharynx.

The primary function of an artificial airway is to prevent obstruction of the upper airway by the tongue and allow the passage of air and oxygen to the lungs.

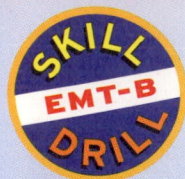

Inserting an Oral Airway
Figure 7-16

1

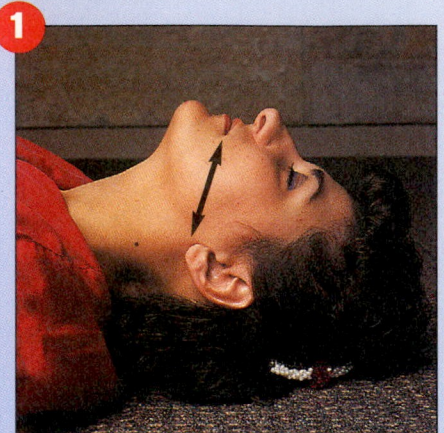

Size the airway by measuring from the patient's earlobe to the corner of the mouth.

2

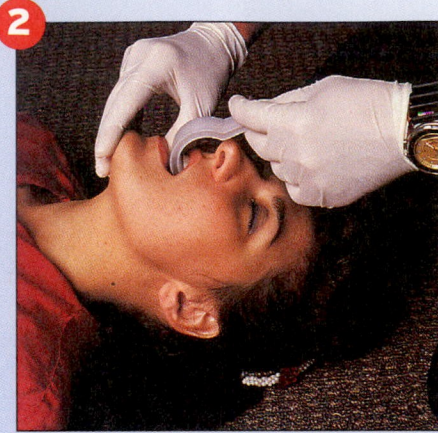

Insert the airway with the tip facing the roof of the patient's mouth.

3

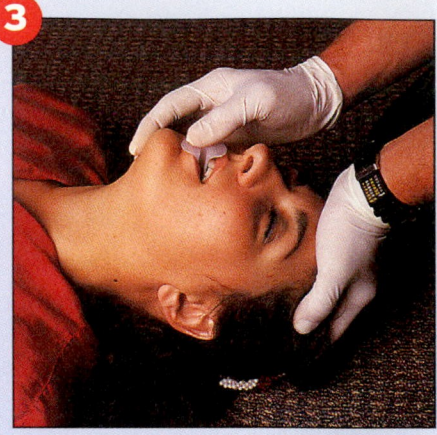

Rotate the airway 180° until the flange rests on the patient's lips and teeth. In this position, the airway will hold the tongue forward.

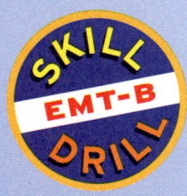

Inserting a Nasal Airway
Figure 7-18

1

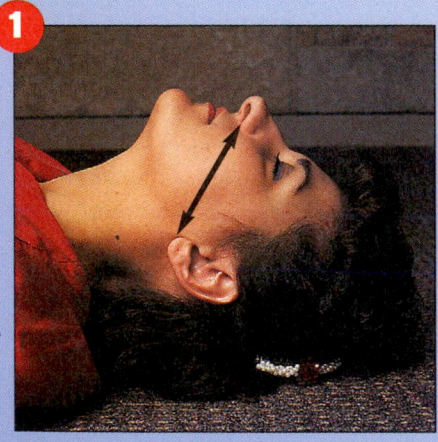

Size the airway by measuring from the tip of the nose to the patient's earlobe.

2

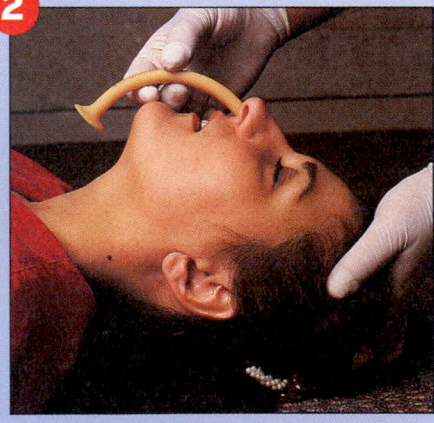

Insert the nasal airway with the bevel facing the septum and curvature following the floor of the nose.

3

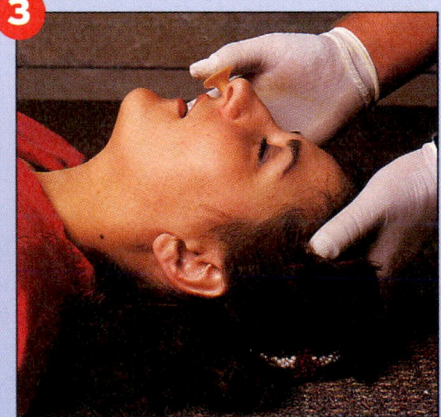

Gently insert the airway until the flange rests against the patient's nose.

Follow these steps to insert an oropharyngeal airway (Figure 7-16):

1. **Select the proper sized airway,** as described above.

2. **Open the patient's mouth** with one hand.

3. **Hold the airway upside down** with your other hand. Insert it into the patient's mouth with the tip facing the roof of the patient's mouth.

4. **Rotate the airway 180°** until the flange (the trumpet-shaped flare) comes to rest on the patient's lips and/or teeth. In this position, the airway will hold the tongue forward.

If you are having trouble inserting the airway, you may use a tongue blade to hold the tongue out of the way while you insert the airway.

Take care to avoid injuring the hard palate as you insert the airway. Roughness can cause bleeding, which may aggravate airway problems or even cause vomiting.

In some instances, a patient may become responsive and regain the gag reflex after you have inserted the oropharyngeal airway. If this occurs, you should gently remove the airway by pulling it out, following the normal curvature of the mouth and throat. Be prepared for the patient to vomit. Have suction available, and log roll the patient onto his or her side to allow any fluids to drain out.

Nasopharyngeal Airways

A **nasopharyngeal (nasal or trumpet) airway** is usually used with a conscious patient who is not able to maintain an airway (Figure 7-17). Patients with an altered mental status or those experiencing a seizure may also benefit from this type of airway. If a patient has had severe trauma to the head or face, you should consult medical control before inserting a nasopharyngeal airway. Extreme care must be used with such trauma patients. If the airway is accidentally pushed through the hole caused by a fracture of the base of the skull, it may penetrate through the cranium and into the brain.

This type of airway is usually well tolerated by patients who have an intact gag reflex. It is not as likely as the oropharyngeal airway to cause vomiting. You should coat the airway well with a water-soluble lubricant, such Lubafax or KY gel, before inserting it. Be aware that slight bleeding may occur even when the airway is inserted properly. However, you should never force the airway into place.

One disadvantage to the nasopharyngeal airway is that it usually does not allow for adequate suctioning. The diameter of the airway is not large enough for a standard suction tip or large suction catheter. You may also need to perform a head-tilt/chin-lift or some other maneuver when using this airway.

Before inserting the airway, be sure you have selected the proper size. Measure from the tip of the nose to the earlobe. In almost all individuals, one nostril is larger than the other. The airway should be placed in the larger nostril, with the curvature of the device following the curve of the floor of the nose. The flange rests against the nostril. The other end of the airway opens into the posterior pharynx.

Follow these steps to insert an nasopharyngeal airway (Figure 7-18):

1. **Select the proper sized airway,** as described above. Make sure you coat the tip with a water-soluble lubricant, such as Lubafax or KY gel.

2. **Gently stretch the nostrils open** with your thumb.

3. **With the bevel toward the septum, gently insert the airway** through the larger nostril until the flange rests against the skin. If you feel any resistance or obstruction, remove the airway and insert it into the other nostril.

If the patient becomes intolerant of the nasal airway, you may have to remove it. Gently withdraw the airway from the nasal passage.

Suctioning

You must keep the airway clear so that you can ventilate the patient properly. If a patient has a mouth full of foreign material, whether broken teeth, food, or vomitus, it must be removed before ventilation. Otherwise, you will force the material into the lungs and possibly cause a complete airway obstruction. Therefore, suctioning is your next priority. If you have any doubt about the situation, remember this rule: *If you hear gurgling, the patient needs suctioning!*

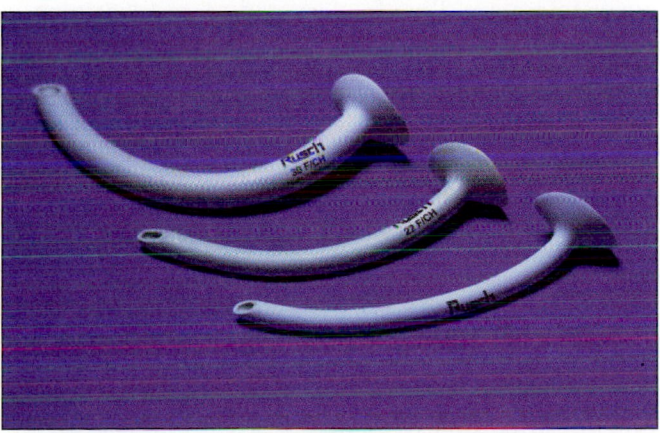

FIGURE 7-17 A nasal airway is typically used for conscious patients who have an intact gag reflex.

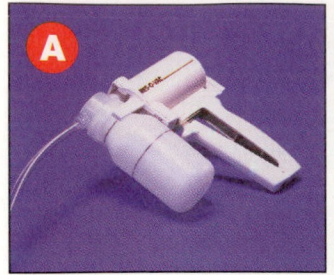
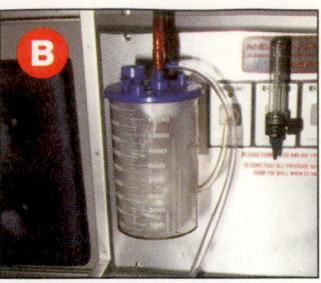
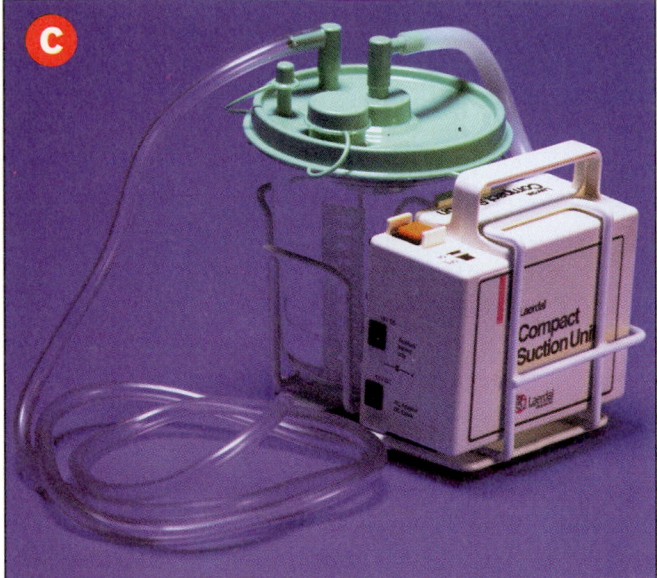

FIGURE 7-19 Suctioning equipment is essential for resuscitation. **A:** Hand operated. **B:** Fixed unit. **C:** Portable unit.

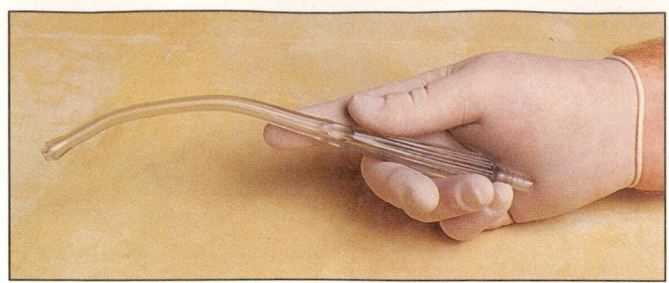

FIGURE 7-20 Tonsil-tip catheters are the best for suctioning, as they have wide diameter tips and are somewhat rigid.

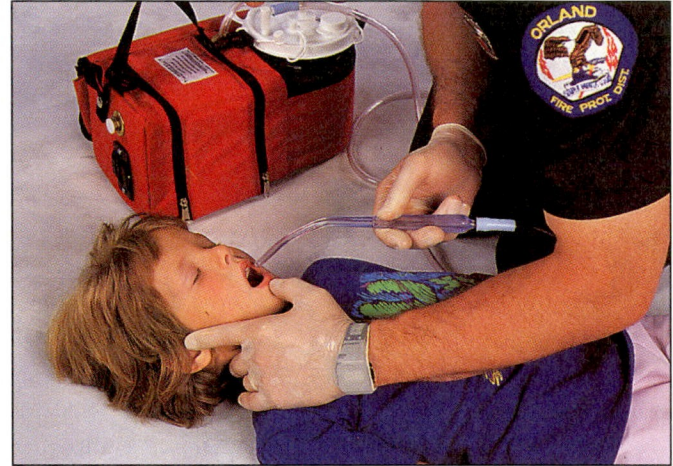

FIGURE 7-21 Use extreme caution when suctioning; ensure that you insert the tip only as far as you can visualize.

Make sure that you keep the airway clear so that you can ventilate the patient properly. Always follow BSI techniques when suctioning.

Suctioning Equipment

Portable and fixed (mounted) suctioning equipment is essential for resuscitation (Figure 7-19). A portable suctioning unit must provide enough vacuum pressure and flow to allow you to effectively suction the mouth and oropharynx. Hand-operated suctioning units with disposable chambers are reliable, effective, and relatively inexpensive. A fixed suctioning unit should generate air flow of more than 30 L/min and a vacuum of more than 300 mm Hg when the tubing is clamped.

A suctioning unit should be fitted with the following:

- Wide-bore, thick-walled, nonkinking tubing
- Plastic, semi-rigid pharyngeal suction tips, called **tonsil tips** or Yankauer tips
- Nonrigid plastic catheters, called French or whistle-tip catheters
- A nonbreakable, disposable collection bottle
- A supply of water for rinsing the tips

You should make sure that the suction yoke, the collection bottle, water for rinsing, and the suction tube are easily accessible at the patient's head.

A **catheter** is a hollow, cylindrical structure that drains or delivers fluids. Tonsil tips are the best kind of catheter for suctioning the pharynx in adults, children, and infants. These plastic tips have a large diameter and are somewhat rigid, so they do not collapse. Tips with a curved contour allow for easy and rapid placement in the pharynx (Figure 7-20). Be careful not to touch the back of the airway. This can activate the gag reflex, cause vomiting, and increase the possibility that contents from the stomach will get into the lungs.

You should use extreme caution when suctioning a conscious or semi-conscious patient. Put the tip in only as far as you can visualize (Figure 7-21). Be aware that suctioning may induce vomiting in these patients.

Soft plastic, nonrigid catheters, sometimes called French or whistle-tip catheters, are used to suction the nose and liquid secretions in the back of the mouth and in situations in which you cannot use a rigid catheter, such as for a patient with a stoma (Figure 7-22). For example, a patient who has clenched teeth

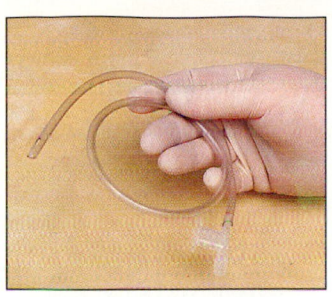

FIGURE 7-22 French, or whistle-tip, catheters are used in situations in which rigid catheters cannot be used, such as with a patient who has a stoma or if the patient's teeth are clenched.

could break off a tooth trying to bite a rigid catheter, whereas a flexible catheter may be worked in without injury. Before you insert any catheter, make sure to measure for the proper size. Use the same technique as you would use when measuring for an oropharyngeal or nasopharyngeal airway. Never insert a catheter past the base of the tongue, as this may result in gagging and vomiting.

You should clean and decontaminate your suctioning equipment according to the manufacturer's guidelines after each use. You should also inspect this equipment regularly to make sure it is in proper working condition. Switch on the suction, clamp the tubing, and make sure that the unit generates a vacuum of more than 300 mm Hg. Check that a battery-charged unit has charged batteries.

Techniques of Suctioning

Follow these steps to operate the suction unit:

1. **Check** the unit for proper assembly of all its parts.

2. **Turn on** the suctioning unit.

3. **Select and attach** the appropriate catheter to the tubing. Use a bulb suction or soft catheter set at the low to medium setting when suctioning the nose.

4. **Remember to measure** the catheter as you would an oropharyngeal or nasopharyngeal airway to ensure that you do not allow it to be inserted too deeply.

5. **Open the patient's mouth** using the jaw-thrust maneuver.

6. **Insert the suction tip,** with its convex side along the roof of the mouth, until you reach the pharynx. Do not use suction unless it is absolutely necessary. Insert the tip only to the base of the tongue.

7. **After the tip is in place, release** the clamp on the tube, and suction as you withdraw the suction tip from the pharynx and mouth. Move the suction tip from side to side.

8. **Never suction for more than 15 seconds** at one time. Suctioning removes oxygen from the airway along with obstructive material.

9. **Rinse the catheter** and tubing with water to prevent clogging of the tube with dried vomitus or other secretions.

10. **Repeat suctioning** only after the patient has been ventilated and re-oxygenated.

At times, a patient may have secretions or vomitus that cannot be suctioned quickly and easily. There are also some suction units that are unable to effectively remove solid objects such as teeth, foreign bodies, and food. In these instances, you should remove the catheter from the patient's mouth, log roll the patient to the side, and then clear the mouth carefully with your gloved finger. A patient may also produce frothy secretions as quickly as you can suction them from the airway. In this situation, you might need to alternate hyperventilation with suctioning. However, note that hyperventilation is not appropriate if vomitus or other particles are present.

Maintaining the Airway

The **recovery position** is used to help maintain a clear airway in a patient who has not had traumatic injuries and is breathing on his or her own with a normal rate and adequate tidal volume (depth of breathing). Take the following steps to put the patient in the recovery position:

1. **Roll the patient onto the left or right side** so that head, shoulders, and torso move at the same time without twisting.

2. **Place the patient's hands under his or her cheek** (Figure 7-23).

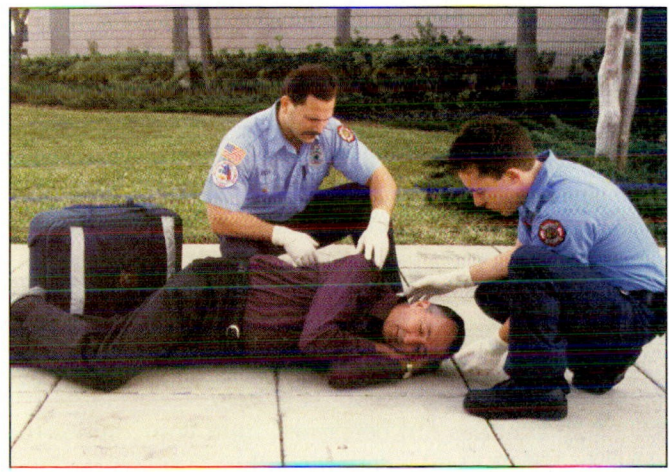

FIGURE 7-23 In the recovery position, the patient is rolled onto the side, and the hands are placed under the cheek.

Once patients have resumed spontaneous breathing after being resuscitated, the recovery position will prevent the aspiration of vomitus. However, this position is not adequate for adult patients who are unconscious and require airway management. You must reposition such patients to provide access to the airway.

Supplemental Oxygen

You should always give supplemental oxygen to patients who are not breathing on their own and to those who are not breathing well enough to supply adequate oxygen to the lungs.

Some tissues and organs, such as the heart, the central nervous system, lungs, kidneys, and liver, need a constant supply of oxygen to function normally. Never withhold oxygen from any patient who may benefit from it, even if you must assist ventilations.

All patients in cardiac arrest should be given oxygen. This may speed recovery from hypoxia. Use high-concentration oxygen in any arrest situation, whether the patient is an infant or an adult. These patients are dying and need as much oxygen as possible. Do not worry about problems resulting from an excess of oxygen; these develop only after several days of more than 50% inspired oxygen delivered at higher than normal pressures.

Supplemental Oxygen Equipment

In addition to knowing when and how to give supplemental oxygen, you must understand how oxygen is stored and the various hazards associated with its use.

Oxygen cylinders. The oxygen that you will give to patients is usually supplied as a compressed gas in green, seamless steel or aluminum cylinders. Some bottles may be silver or chrome with a green area around the valve stem on top. Newer bottles are often made of lightweight aluminum or spun steel; older bottles are much heavier.

Check to make sure that the cylinder is labeled for medical oxygen. You should look for letters and numbers stamped into the metal on the collar of the cylinder (Figure 7-24). Of particular importance are the month and year stamps, which indicate when the bottle was last tested.

Oxygen cylinders are available in several sizes. The two sizes that you will most often use are the D (or super D) and M cylinders (Figure 7-25). The D (or super D) cylinder can be carried from your unit to the patient. The M tank remains on board your unit as a main supply tank. Other sizes that you will see are A, E, G, H, and K (Table 7-2).

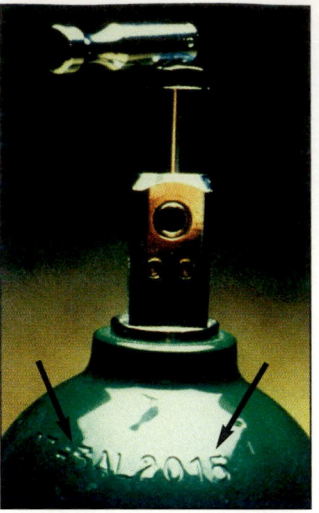

FIGURE 7-24 Oxygen tanks for medical use will have a series of letters and numbers stamped into the metal on the collar of the cylinder.

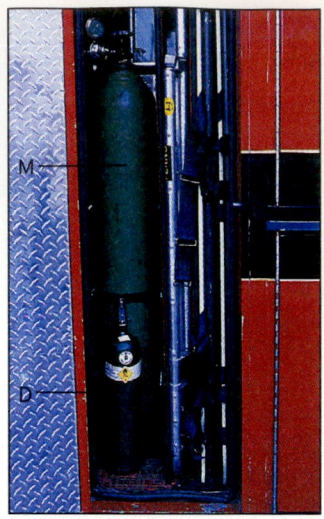

FIGURE 7-25 The cylinders that are most commonly found on an ambulance are the D (or super D) and M size cylinders.

TABLE 7-2	Oxygen Cylinder Sizes Carried on the Ambulance
Size	**Volume**
D	350 L
Super D	500 L
E	625 L
M	3,000 L
G	5,300 L
H, A, K	6,900 L

Safety considerations. Compressed gas cylinders must be handled very carefully because their contents are under pressure. Cylinders are fitted with pressure regulators to make sure that patients receive the right amount and type of gas. Make sure that the correct pressure regulator is firmly attached before you transport the cylinders. A puncture or hole in the tank can cause the cylinder to become a deadly missile. Do not handle a cylinder by the neck assembly alone. Cylinders should be secured with mounting brackets when they are stored on the ambulance. Oxygen cylinders that are in use during transport should be positioned and secured to prevent the tank from falling or from damage occurring to the valve-gauge assembly.

Pin-indexing system. The compressed gas industry has established a <u>pin-indexing system</u> for portable cylinders to prevent an oxygen regulator from being

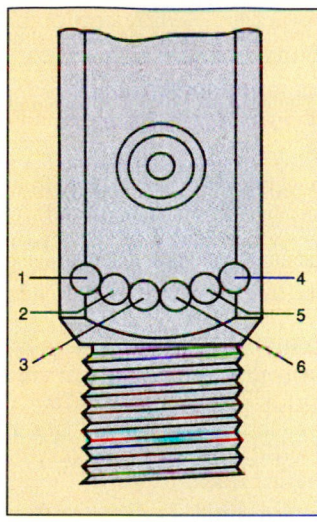

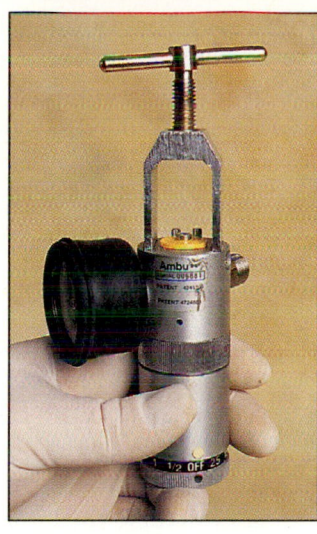

FIGURE 7-26 The locations of the pin-indexing safety system holes in a cylinder valve face. Each cylinder of a specific gas has a given pattern and a given number of pins.

FIGURE 7-27 A yoke-type pressure-reducing gauge is used with a small oxygen cylinder.

Pressure regulators. The pressure of gas in a full oxygen cylinder is 2,100 psi. This is far too much pressure to be safe or useful for your purposes. Pressure regulators reduce the pressure to a more useful range, usually 40 to 70 psi. Most pressure regulators that are in use today reduce the pressure in a single stage, although multi-stage regulators do exist. A two-stage regulator will reduce the pressure first to 700 psi and then to 40 to 70 psi.

After the pressure is reduced to a workable level, the final attachment for delivering the gas to the patient is usually through one of the following ways:

- A quick-connect female fitting that will accept a quick-connect male plug from a pressure hose or ventilator or resuscitator
- A flowmeter that will permit the regulated release of gas measured in liters per minute

Humidification. Some EMS systems provide humidified oxygen to patients during transport (Figure 7-28). However, humidified oxygen is usually indicated only for long-term oxygen therapies. Dry oxygen is not considered harmful for short-term use. Therefore, many EMS systems do not use humidified oxygen in the prehospital setting. Always refer to medical control or local protocols for guidance involving patient treatment issues.

Flowmeters. Flowmeters are usually permanently attached to pressure regulators on emergency medical equipment. The two types of flowmeters that are commonly used are pressure-compensated flowmeters and Bourdon-gauge flowmeters.

A pressure-compensated flowmeter incorporates a float ball within a tapered calibrated tube. The float rises or falls according to the gas flow within the tube. The flow of gas is controlled by a needle valve located

connected to a carbon dioxide cylinder, a carbon dioxide regulator from being connected to an oxygen cylinder, and so on. In preparing to administer oxygen, always check to be sure that the pinholes on the cylinder exactly match the corresponding pins on the regulator.

The pin-indexing system features a series of pins on a yoke that must be matched with the holes on the valve stem of the gas cylinder. The arrangement of the pins and holes varies for different gases according to accepted national standards (Figure 7-26). Other gases that are supplied in portable cylinders, such as acetylene, carbon dioxide, and nitrogen, use regulators and flowmeters that are very similar to those used with oxygen. Each cylinder of a specific gas has a given pattern and a given number of pins. These safety measures make it impossible for you to attach a cylinder of nitrous oxide to an oxygen regulator. The oxygen regulator will not fit.

The outlet valves on D size or smaller cylinders are designed to accept yoke-type pressure-reducing gauges, which conform to the pin-indexing system (Figure 7-27). The safety system for large cylinders is known as the <u>American Standard System</u>. In this system, cylinders larger than D sizes are equipped with threaded gas outlet valves. The inside and outside thread sizes of these outlets vary depending on the gas in the cylinder. The cylinder will not accept a regulator valve unless it is properly threaded to fit that regulator. The purpose of these safety devices is the same as in the pin-indexing system: to prevent the accidental attachment of a regulator to a wrong cylinder.

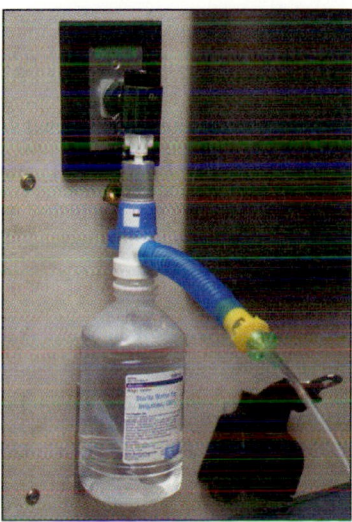

FIGURE 7-28 Giving humidified oxygen may be preferred with long transport times. However, the use of this type of oxygen delivery system is not universal for all EMT-Bs.

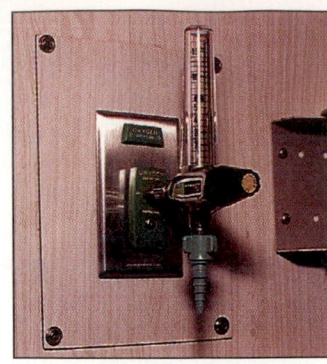

FIGURE 7-29 Pressure-compensated flowmeters contain a float ball that rises or falls according to the gas flow within the tube. It must be maintained in an upright position for an accurate reading.

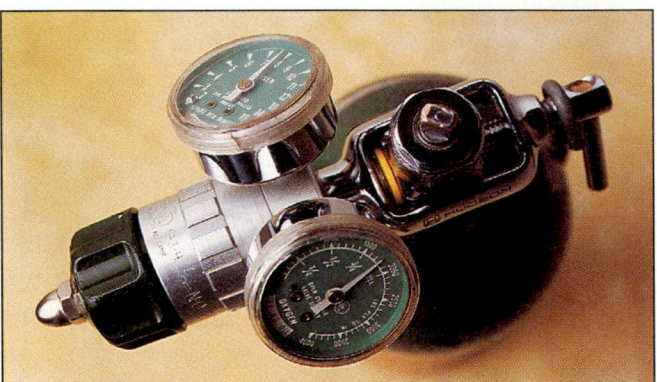

FIGURE 7-30 The Bourdon-gauge flowmeter is not affected by gravity and can be used in any position.

downstream from the float ball. This type of flowmeter is affected by gravity and must always be maintained in an upright position for an accurate flow reading (Figure 7-29).

The Bourdon-gauge flowmeter is commonly used because it is not affected by gravity and can be used in any position. It is actually a pressure gauge that is calibrated to record flow rate (Figure 7-30). The major disadvantage of this flowmeter is that it does not compensate for backpressure. Therefore, it will usually record a higher flow rate when there is any obstruction to gas flow downstream.

Operating Procedures

Take the following steps when placing an oxygen cylinder into service (Figure 7-31):

1. **Inspect the cylinder and its markings.** If the cylinder was commercially filled, it will have a plastic seal around the valve stem covering the opening in the stem. Remove the seal, and inspect the opening to make sure that it is free of dirt and other debris. The valve stem should not be sealed or covered with adhesive tape or any petroleum-based substances. These can contaminate the oxygen and can contribute to spontaneous combustion when mixed with the pressurized oxygen.

2. **"Crack" the cylinder,** by quickly opening and then reclosing the valve, to help make sure that dirt particles and other possible contaminants do not enter the oxygen flow. *Never face the tank toward you or others when cracking the cylinder.* Open the tank by attaching a tank key to the valve and rotating the valve counterclockwise. You should be able to clearly hear the rush of oxygen coming from the tank. Close the tank by rotating the valve clockwise.

3. **Attach the regulator/flowmeter to the valve stem** after clearing the opening. On one side of the valve stem, you will find three holes. The larger one, on top, is a true opening through which the oxygen flows. The two smaller holes below it do not extend to the inside of the tank. They provide stability to the regulator. Following the design of a pin-indexing system, these two holes are very precisely located in positions that are unique to oxygen cylinders.

   Above the pins on the inside of the collar is the actual port through which oxygen flows from the cylinder to the regulator. A metal or plastic O-ring is placed around the oxygen port to maximize the airtight seal between the collar of the regulator and the valve stem.

   Place the regulator collar over the cylinder valve, with the oxygen port and pin-indexing pins on the side of the valve stem that has the three holes. Open the screw bolt just enough to allow the collar to fit freely over the valve stem. Move the regulator so that the oxygen port and the pins fit into the correct holes on the valve stem. The screw bolt on the opposite side should be aligned with the dimpled depression. As you hold the regulator securely against the valve stem, tighten the screw bolt until the regulator is firmly attached to the cylinder. At this point, you should not see any open spaces between the sides of the valve stem and the interior walls of the collar.

4. **With the regulator firmly attached, open the cylinder** and read the pressure level on the regulator gauge. Most portable cylinders have a maximum pressure of 2,100 psi. Most EMS services consider a cylinder with less than 500 psi to be too low to keep in service. Learn your department's policies in this regard.

5. The flowmeter will have either a second gauge or a selector dial that indicates the oxygen flow rate. Several popular types of devices are widely used. **Attach the selected oxygen device to the flowmeter** by connecting the universal oxygen connective tubing to the "Christmas tree" nipple

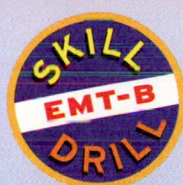

Placing an Oxygen Cylinder Into Service
Figure 7-31

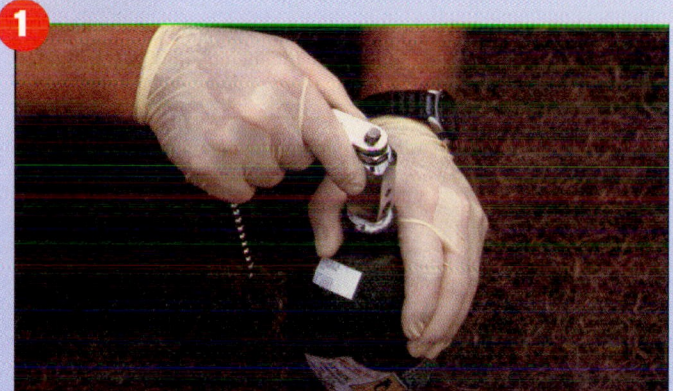

1 Using an oxygen wrench, turn the valve counterclockwise to "crack" the cylinder.

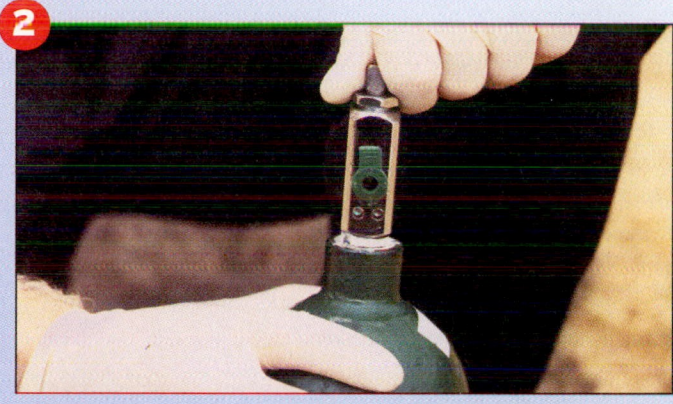

2 Check for the two pin-indexing holes and make sure that the washer is in place over the large hole.

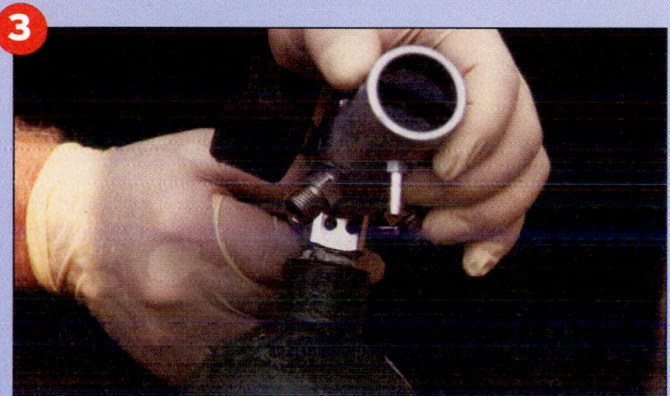

3 Align the regulator so that the pins fit snugly into the correct holes on the valve stem and hand tighten the regulator.

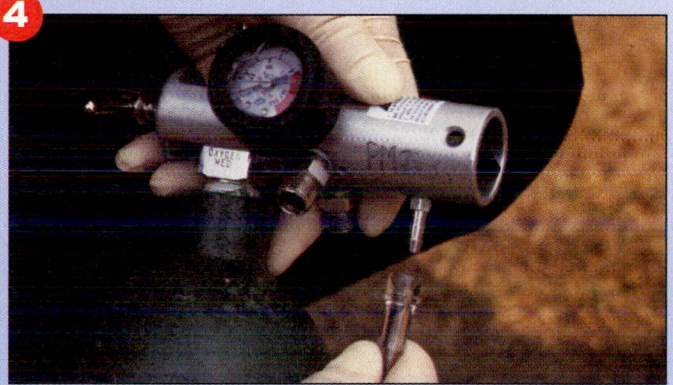

4 Attach the oxygen connective tubing to the flowmeter.

on the flowmeter. Most oxygen delivery devices come with this tubing permanently attached. Some oxygen masks do not. You must add this tubing to the oxygen delivery device if it is not attached.

6. **Open the flowmeter to the desired flow rate.** This is done differently on different devices. *Remember that you must be completely familiar with the equipment before attempting to use it on a patient.*

7. **Once the oxygen is flowing at the desired rate, apply the oxygen device** to the patient and make any necessary adjustments. Monitor the patient's reaction to the oxygen and to the oxygen device, and periodically recheck the regulator gauge to make sure there is sufficient oxygen in the cylinder.

8. **Disconnect the tubing from the flowmeter nipple and turn off the cylinder valve** when oxygen therapy is complete, or when the patient has been transferred to the hospital and has been switched to the hospital's oxygen system. In a few seconds, the sound of oxygen flowing from the nipple will cease. This indicates that all the pressurized oxygen has been removed from the flowmeter.

9. **Turn off the flowmeter.** The gauge on the regulator should read zero with the tank valve closed. This confirms that there is no pressure left above the valve stem. *As long as there is a pressure reading on the regulator gauge, it is not safe to remove the regulator from the valve stem.*

Hazards of Supplemental Oxygen

Oxygen does not burn or explode. However, it does support combustion. The more oxygen is around, the faster the combustion process. A small spark, even a glowing cigarette, can become a flame in an oxygen-rich atmosphere. Therefore, you must keep any possible source of fire away from the area while oxygen is in use. Make sure the area is adequately ventilated, especially in industrial settings where hazardous materials may be present and where sparks are easily generated. Be extremely cautious in any enclosed environment in which oxygen is being administered, as an oxygen-rich environment increases the chance of fire if a spark or flame is introduced. A bystander who is smoking or sparks from a vehicle extrication are possible ignition sources.

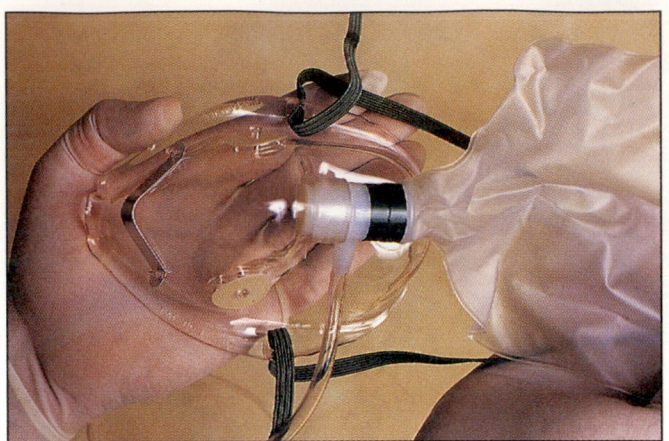

FIGURE 7-32 The nonrebreathing mask is similar to a face mask but contains flapper valve ports at the cheek areas of the mask to prevent the patient from rebreathing exhaled air.

Oxygen Delivery Equipment

In general, the oxygen delivery equipment that is used in the field should be limited to nonrebreathing masks and nasal cannulas, depending on local protocol. However, you may encounter other devices during transports between medical facilities.

Nonrebreathing Mask

The **nonrebreathing mask** is the preferred way of giving oxygen in the prehospital setting. With a good mask-to-face seal, it is capable of providing up to 90% inspired oxygen.

The nonrebreathing mask is a combination mask and reservoir bag system. The mask is similar to a simple face mask. Oxygen fills a reservoir bag that is attached to the mask by a one-way valve. The system is called a nonrebreathing mask because the exhaled gas escapes through flapper valve ports at the cheek areas of the mask (Figure 7-32). The valve also prevents the patient from rebreathing exhaled gases as the gas in the reservoir bag flows into the mask during inhalation.

Oxygen concentrations of more than 60% inspired air can be delivered with a partial rebreathing mask. In this system, you must be sure that the reservoir bag is full before the mask is placed on the patient. Adjust the flow rate so that the bag does not fully collapse when the patient inhales. This is about two thirds of the bag volume or 15 L/min. Use a smaller reservoir bag with infants and children, as they will inhale a smaller volume.

Nasal Cannula

A **nasal cannula** delivers oxygen through two small, tubelike prongs that fit into the patient's nostrils (Figure

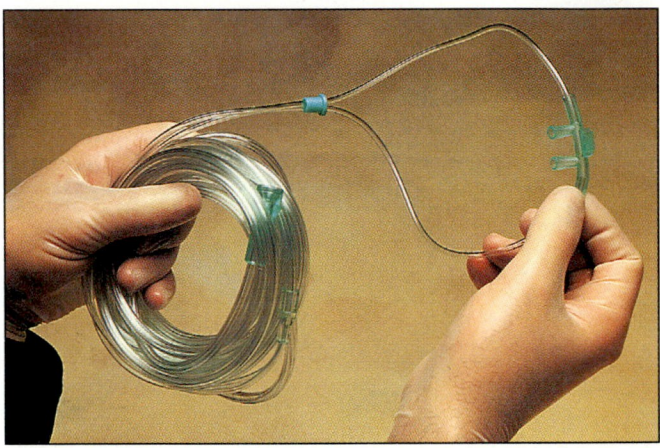

FIGURE 7-33 The nasal cannula delivers oxygen directly through the nostrils.

7-33). This device can provide 35% to 50% inspired oxygen if the flowmeter is set at 6 L/min. The nasal cannula delivers dry oxygen directly into the nostrils. Therefore, when you anticipate a long transport time, you should consult medical control about humidification.

A nasal cannula has limited use in the prehospital care setting. For example, a patient who breathes through the mouth or who has a nasal obstruction will get little or no benefit from a nasal cannula. You may consider using this device with patients who you believe to be stable and not hypoxic, but use a nonrebreathing mask instead with patients in unstable condition who are breathing on their own. *Always try to give high-flow oxygen through a nonrebreathing mask if you suspect that a patient may have hypoxia, coaching him or her as necessary.* However, if the patient will not tolerate this device, you will have to use a nasal cannula, which some patients find more comfortable. As always, a good assessment of your patient will guide your decision.

Artificial Ventilation

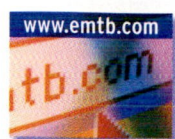

Obviously, a patient who is not breathing needs artificial ventilation and supplemental oxygen. But the same is true of patients who are breathing inadequately, that is, fewer than 8 breaths/min or more than 24 breaths/min. The literature varies regarding the number of breaths/min that is considered inadequate; however, most sources state that fewer than 8 breaths/min or more than 24 to 30 breaths/min are considered inadequate. Keep in mind that fast, shallow breathing can be as dangerous as very slow breathing. Fast, shallow breathing moves air primarily in the larger airway passages (dead space air) and does not allow for adequate exchange of air and carbon dioxide in the alveoli. Although you do not need any special equipment to provide simple artificial ventilation, remember to follow BSI techniques as needed.

You should note that patients who are short of breath or cyanotic with cool, clammy skin need oxygen. Although you must be careful when administering oxygen to patients with COPD or newborns, be sure that patients who present with cyanosis and cool, clammy skin are given high-concentration oxygen.

Once you determine that a patient is not breathing or needs assisted ventilations, you should begin artificial ventilation immediately. With a patient who is not breathing, there are several ways to do this, some of which do require equipment. The methods that an EMT-B may use to provide artificial ventilation include the two-person bag-valve-mask (BVM), mouth-to-mask ventilation, an oxygen-powered manually triggered breathing device, or a one-person BVM. Note, however, that mouth-to-mask ventilation is now being used less often than it was in the past.

Mouth-to-Mouth and Mouth-to-Mask Ventilation

As you learned in your CPR course, mouth-to-mouth ventilations are now routinely done with a barrier device, such as a mask. A **barrier device** is a protective item that features a plastic barrier placed on a patient's face with a one-way valve to prevent the back flow of secretions, vomitus, and gases. Barrier devices provide adequate BSI. Mouth-to-mouth ventilations without a barrier device should be provided only in extreme conditions. Performing mouth-to-mask ventilations with a pocket mask with a one-way valve is a better way to prevent possible disease transmission (Figure 7-34).

A mask with an oxygen inlet provides oxygen during mouth-to-mask ventilation to supplement the air from

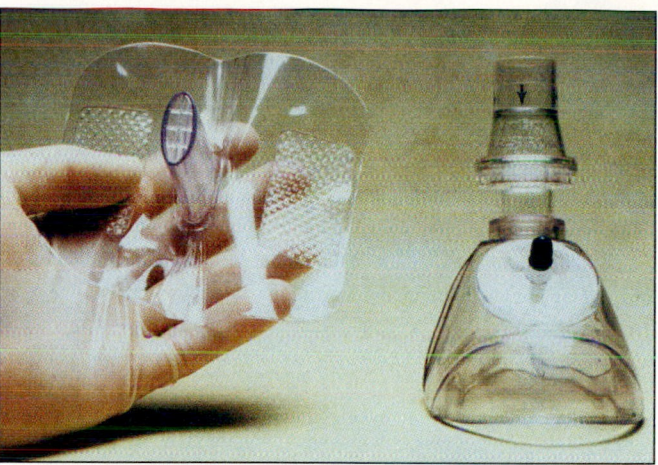

FIGURE 7-34 Barrier devices such as a plastic shield or a pocket mask with a one-way valve provide adequate BSI.

your own lungs. Remember that the gas you exhale contains 16% oxygen, more than enough to maintain the patient's life. With the mouth-to-mask system, however, the patient gets the additional benefit of significant oxygen enrichment with inspired air. This system also frees both your hands to help keep the airway open and helps you to provide a better seal between the mask and the face.

The mask may be shaped like a triangle or a doughnut, with the apex (top) placed across the bridge of the nose. The base (bottom) of the mask is placed in the groove between the lower lip and the chin. In the center of the mask is a chimney with a 15-mL connector.

Follow these steps to use mouth-to-mask ventilation (Figure 7-35):

1. **Kneel at the patient's head.** Open the airway using the head-tilt/chin-lift maneuver or the jaw-thrust maneuver if indicated.

2. **Connect the one-way valve** to the face mask.

3. **Place the mask on the patient's face.** Make sure the top is over the bridge of the nose and the bottom is in the groove between the lower lip and the chin.

4. **Grasp the patient's lower jaw** with your first three fingers on each hand. Place your thumbs on the dome of the mask. Make an airtight seal by applying firm pressure between the thumbs and the fingers.

5. **Maintain an upward and forward pull** on the lower jaw with your fingers to keep the airway open.

6. **Take a deep breath** and exhale through the open port of the one-way valve. Breathe slowly into the patient's mask for $1\frac{1}{2}$ to 2 seconds.

7. **Remove your mouth,** and watch the patient's chest fall during passive exhalation.

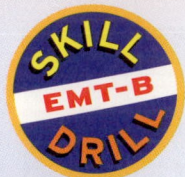

Performing Mouth-to-Mask Ventilation

Figure 7-35

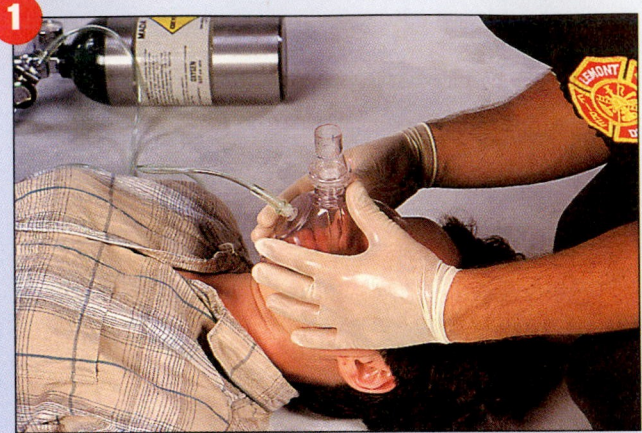

Once the patient's head is properly positioned, place the mask on the patient's face. Seal the mask to the face using both hands.

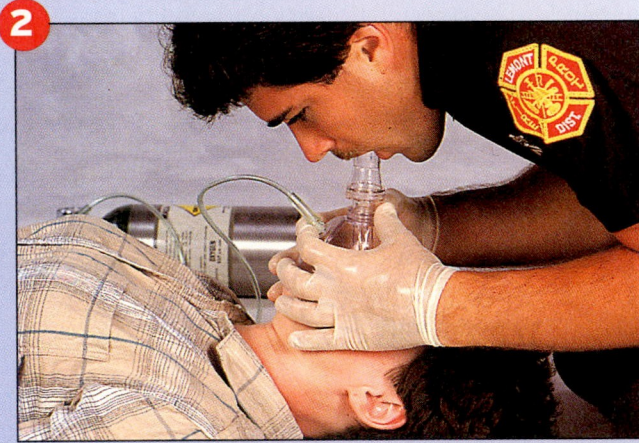

Exhale slowly into the open port of the one-way valve for 1½ to 2 seconds.

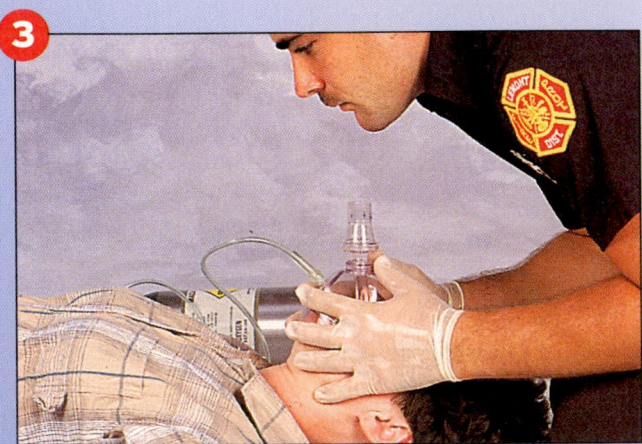

Remove your mouth, and watch for the patient's chest to fall during passive exhalation.

You know that you are providing adequate ventilations if you see the patient's chest rise and fall. Feel for resistance of the patient's lungs as they expand. You should also hear and feel air escape as the patient exhales. Make sure that you are providing the correct number of breaths/min. for the patient's age.

To increase the oxygen concentration, give high-flow oxygen at 15 L/min through the oxygen inlet valve. This, when combined with your exhaled breath, will give the patient 55% oxygen.

The mask also works well for patients breathing on their own who need supplemental oxygen but not full ventilatory assistance. The mask may have an elastic strap for use with these patients.

The Bag-Valve-Mask Device

Both mouth-to-mouth and mouth-to-mask ventilations can provide large volumes of inspired air-up to 4 L per breath. But with mouth-to-mouth ventilation, the concentration of oxygen delivered to the patient is only 16%. With mouth-to-mask ventilation connected to high-flow oxygen, the concentration of oxygen, at best, is only 55%.

At the same oxygen flow rate (10 to 15 L/min) as the mask alone, a **bag-valve-mask (BVM) device** with an oxygen reservoir can deliver more than 90% oxygen (Figure 7-36). Most BVM devices on the market today include modifications or accessories (reservoirs) that permit the delivery of oxygen concentrations approaching 100%. However, the device can deliver only as much gas as you can squeeze out of the bag by hand. The BVM device provides less tidal volume than mouth-to-mask ventilation; however, use of the BVM device is more widespread than use of mouth-to-mask ventilation. An experienced EMT-B will be able to supply adequate tidal volumes with a BVM device. Be sure to practice on ventilation manikins several times before using a BVM device on a real patient.

A BVM device should be used when you need to deliver high oxygen concentrations to patients who are not ventilating adequately. The device is also used for patients with respiratory arrest or severe respiratory failure. You will typically use an oropharyngeal or nasopharyngeal airway with the BVM device.

Components. All BVM devices should have the following components:

- A self-refilling bag that is either disposable or easily cleaned and sterilized

- No pop-off valve

- A true valve for nonrebreathing

- A transparent self-inflating, deflatable reservoir bag or tube to allow for high concentrations of oxygen

- A one-way, no-jam valve that incorporates the following: the exhalation port oxygen inflow at a maximum of 15 L/min a standard 15/22 mm connection between the face mask and the bag and an attachment for the transparent reservoir bag or tube

- A transparent face mask (available in five sizes: adult, child, and three infant sizes, including a "preemie" size)

- Ability to perform under extreme heat or cold

The total amount of gas in the reservoir bag of an adult BVM device is usually 1,200 to 1,600 mL. The pediatric bag contains 500 to 700 mL, and the infant bag holds 150 to 240 mL. A volume of 10 to 15 mL/kg should be delivered over 2 seconds.

Technique. Whenever possible, you and your partner should work together to provide BVM ventilation. One person secures the mask to the face with two hands while the other squeezes the bag. It may be very difficult for one EMT-B to maintain a proper seal between the mask and face with one hand and get adequate air into the patient with the other, although you can do so effectively with enough practice.

Follow these steps to use the BVM technique:

1. **Kneel above the patient's head.** If possible, your partner should be at the side of the head to bag the patient while you hold a seal between the mask and the patient's face with two hands. (This assumes that you have enough personnel to do everything else that needs to be done at the same time, such as chest compressions, putting the stretcher in place, or helping to lift the patient onto the stretcher.)

2. **Maintain the patient's neck in an extended position** unless you suspect a cervical spine injury. In that case, you should immobilize the patient's head and neck. Have your partner hold the head, or, if you are alone, use your knees to immobilize the head.

3. **Open the patient's mouth,** and suction as needed. Insert an oropharyngeal or nasopharyngeal airway to maintain an open airway.

4. **Select the proper mask size.**

5. **Place the mask on the patient's face.** Make sure the top is over the bridge of the nose and the bottom is in the groove between the lower lip and the chin. If the mask has a large, round cuff around the ventilation port, center the port over the patient's mouth. Inflate the collar to obtain a better fit and seal to the face.

6. **Bring the lower jaw up to the mask** with your ring finger and little finger. This will help to maintain an open airway. If you think the patient may have a spinal injury, make sure your partner immobilizes the cervical spine as you move the lower jaw.

7. **Hold the mask in position** by placing the thumbs over the top part of the mask and the index and middle fingers over the bottom half. Make sure you do not grab the fleshy part of the neck, as you may compress structures and create an airway obstruction.

8. **Connect the bag to the mask** if you have not already done so.

9. **Hold the mask in place** while your partner squeezes the bag with two hands until the patient's chest rises. Continue squeezing the bag once every 5 seconds for adults and once every 3 seconds for infants and children (Figure 7-37).

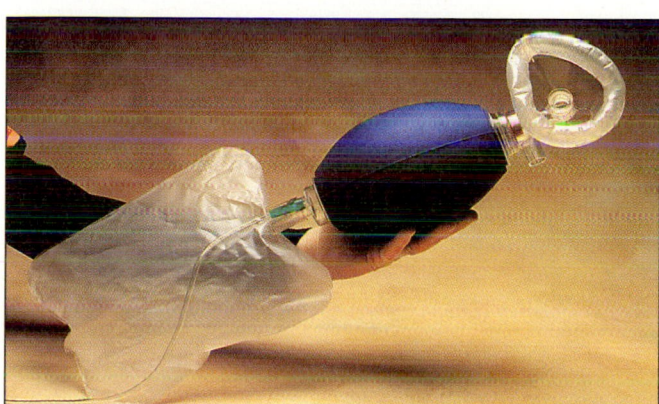

FIGURE 7-36 A bag-valve-mask (BVM) device with an oxygen reservoir can deliver more than 90% oxygen.

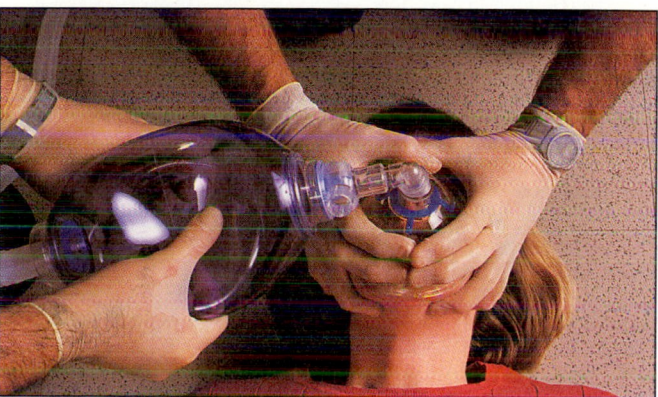

FIGURE 7-37 With two-person BVM ventilation, you should hold the mask in place while your partner squeezes the bag with two hands until the patient's chest rises.

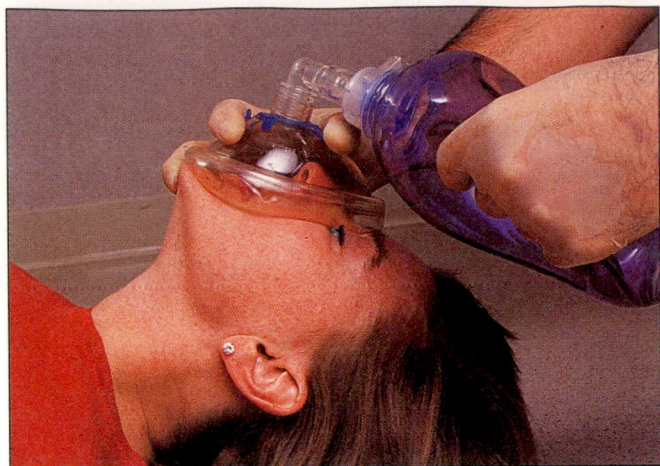

FIGURE 7-38 Maintain the seal of the mask to the face using the C-clamp if you must do BVM ventilations alone.

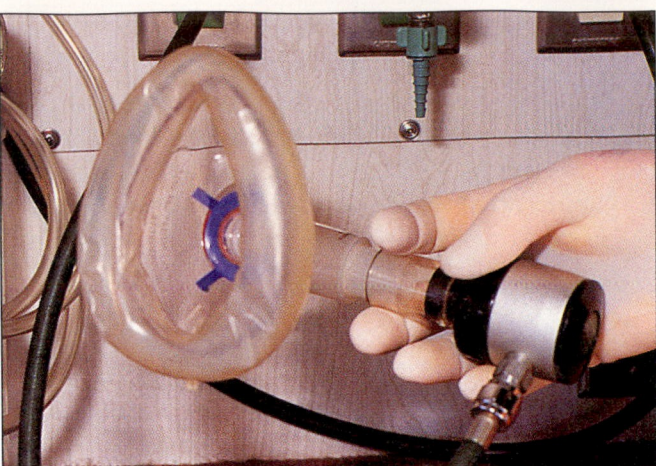

FIGURE 7-39 A flow-restricted oxygen-powered ventilation device can provide up to 100% oxygen.

10. **If you are alone, hold your index finger** over the lower part of the mask, and secure the upper part of the mask with your thumb. This is known as the C-clamp and will maintain the seal. Use the head-tilt/chin-lift maneuver to make sure the neck is extended. Make sure the fourth and fifth fingers do not exert pressure on the neck, to avoid stimulating the vagus nerve, which could cause the heart rate to drop. Squeeze the bag in a rhythmic manner once every 5 seconds with your other hand. Continue squeezing the bag once every 5 seconds for adults and once every 3 seconds for infants and children (Figure 7-38).

When using the device to assist respirations, you should deflate the bag as the patient tries to breathe in, ideally achieving a more normal rate and depth of respiration.

As you are assisting ventilations with a BVM device, you should evaluate how well the patient is breathing. You will know that artificial ventilation is not adequate if the patient's chest does not rise and fall with each ventilation, the breathing rate is too slow or too fast, or the heart rate does not produce a palpable pulse. If the patient's chest does not rise and fall, you may need to reposition the head or use an airway adjunct. If the patient's stomach seems to be rising and falling, you should reposition the head. In a patient with possible spinal injury, you should reposition the jaw rather than the head. If too much air is escaping from under the mask, reposition the mask for a better mask seal. If after these corrections, the patient's chest still does not rise and fall, you should try another airway device, such as mouth-to-mask ventilation or an oxygen-powered manually triggered breathing device. Make sure you recheck the airway for any obstruction.

The BVM device may also be used in conjunction with an endotracheal tube or with other airway adjunct devices such as the Esophageal Tracheal Combitube, the Pharyngeotracheal Lumen Airway, and the Trachlight.

Flow-Restricted, Oxygen-Powered Ventilation Devices

A third method of providing artificial ventilation is with flow-restricted, oxygen-powered ventilation devices. These devices are widely available but should not be used on infants and children or on patients with suspected cervical spine or chest injury.

Components. Flow-restricted, oxygen-powered ventilation devices should have the following components (Figure 7-39):

- A peak flow rate of 100% oxygen at up to 40 L/min
- An inspiratory pressure safety release valve that opens at approximately 60 cm of water and vents any remaining volume to the atmosphere or stops the flow of oxygen

A BVM device should be used when you need to deliver high oxygen concentrations to patients who are not ventilating adequately.

- An audible alarm that sounds whenever you exceed the relief valve pressure

- The ability to operate satisfactorily under normal and varying environmental conditions

- A trigger (or lever) positioned so that both your hands can remain on the mask to provide an airtight seal while supporting and tilting the patient's head and keeping the jaw elevated

Learning how to use these devices correctly requires proper training and considerable practice. As with BVM devices, you must make sure there is an airtight fit between the patient's face and mask. You must also be alert for **gastric distention**, a condition in which air fills the stomach, as a result of such a high flow rate. The amount of pressure that is necessary to ventilate a patient adequately will vary according to the size of the patient, the patient's lung volume, and the condition of the lungs. A patient with COPD will need greater pressure to receive a given volume than would be necessary for a patient with normal lungs. Pressures that are too great can blow out a lung. Flow-restricted, oxygen-powered ventilation devices are not recommended for use on patients with COPD, chest injury, or on infants and children. Always follow local medical protocols carefully when you use these devices.

Technique. Perform ventilations with a flow-restricted, oxygen-powered ventilation device as follows:

1. **Open the patient's airway,** and suction as needed. Insert an oropharyngeal or nasopharyngeal airway.

2. **Place your thumbs over the top half of the mask** and your index and middle fingers over the bottom half.

3. **Place the top of the mask over the bridge of the nose,** and then lower the mask over the mouth and upper chin.

4. **Bring the lower jaw up to the mask** with your ring finger and little finger. This will help to maintain an open airway.

5. **Trigger the device's demand valve** until the patient's chest rises (Figure 7-40).

6. **Ventilate at the appropriate rate** for the patient situation. In most cases, this will be once every 3 to 5 seconds.

7. **If the chest does not rise,** the patient is not being ventilated effectively. At this point, you need to consider the following possible problems:

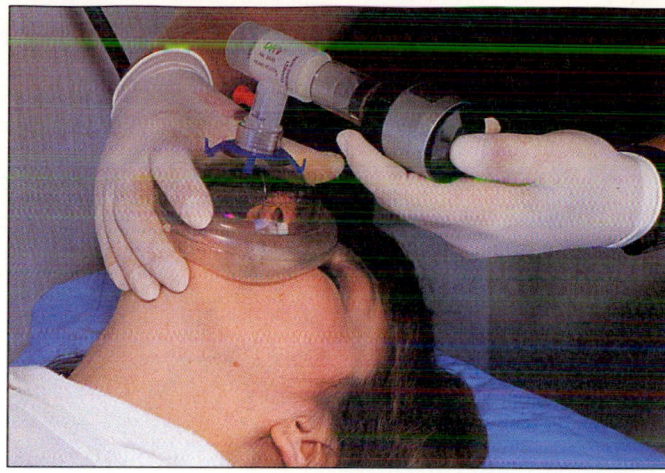

FIGURE 7-40 With a flow-restricted oxygen-powered ventilation device, you should ensure that there is a good seal between the mask and the patient, allowing you to trigger the device's demand valve until the patient's chest rises.

   a. If the abdomen rises, reposition the patient's head.

   b. If air is leaking from under the mask, reposition your fingers to create a better mask-to-face seal.

   c. If the above two methods fail to fix the problem, consider using techniques for complete airway obstruction. You may also consider alternative methods of providing artificial ventilations.

8. **If necessary, use the flow-restricted,** oxygen-powered ventilation device with an endotracheal tube or with other airway adjuncts such as the Esophageal Tracheal Combitube, the Pharyngeotracheal Lumen Airway, and the Trach-light.

Special Considerations

Gastric Distention

Gastric distention occurs when artificial ventilation fills the stomach with air. Although it most commonly affects children, it also affects adults. Gastric distention is most likely to occur when you blow too forcefully or too often in artificial ventilation or when the airway is obstructed as a result of a foreign body or improper head position. For this reason, you are instructed to give slow, gentle breaths during artificial ventilation. Slight gastric distention is not of concern; however, severe inflation of the stomach is dangerous because it causes vomiting during CPR. Gastric distention can also reduce the lung volume by elevating the diaphragm.

If the patient's stomach becomes distended as a result of rescue breathing, you should recheck and reposition the airway and then watch for rise and fall of the chest wall as you perform rescue breathing. Continue slow rescue breathing without attempting to expel the stomach contents. Applying manual pressure over the patient's upper abdomen will likely result in vomiting. If vomiting does occur, turn the patient's entire body to the side, suction and/or wipe out the mouth with your gloved hand, and return the body back to a supine position so that you can continue CPR.

If gastric distention makes ventilation impossible, despite the above precautions, consider applying manual pressure, but remember that the patient is likely to vomit. Be ready to turn the patient and suction or wipe the mouth before you resume CPR.

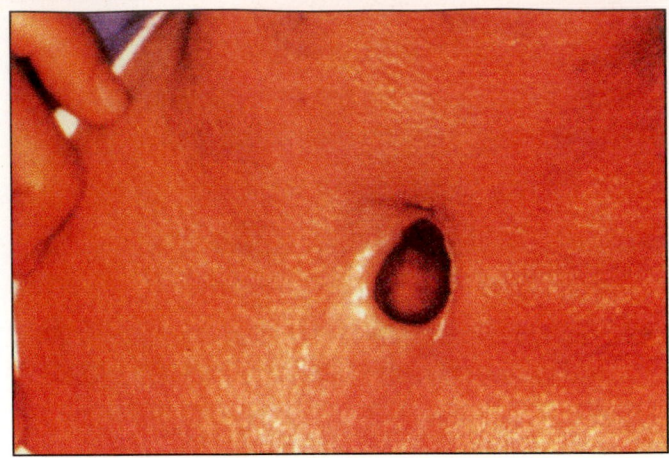

FIGURE 7-41 A tracheal stoma typically lies in the midline of the neck. The midline opening is the only one that can be used to deliver oxygen to the patient's lungs.

Stomas

BVM ventilation must also be used for patients who have had a laryngectomy (surgical removal of the larynx). These patients have a permanent tracheal **stoma** (an opening in the neck that connects the trachea directly to the skin) (Figure 7-41). It may be seen as an opening at the center, at the front and base of the neck. Many of these patients will have other openings in the neck, according to the type of operation done. You should ignore any opening other than the midline tracheal stoma. The midline opening is the only one that can be used to put air into the patient's lungs. In general, other neck openings will lie to one side or the other but not in the midline.

Neither the head-tilt/chin-lift nor the jaw-thrust maneuver is required for ventilating a patient with a stoma. If the patient has a tube in the stoma, you should ventilate through the tube (Figure 7-42). Use an infant or child mask to make a seal. Seal the patient's mouth and nose with one hand to prevent a leak of air up the trachea when you ventilate through a tracheal tube or stoma. Release the seal of the patient's mouth and nose for exhalation. This allows the air to exhale through the upper airway.

If you are unable to ventilate a patient who has a stoma, try suctioning the stoma and the mouth with a soft or satin tip catheter before giving the patient artificial ventilation through the mouth and nose. If you seal the stoma during ventilations, the ability to artificially ventilate the patient in this way may be improved, or it may help to clear any obstructions.

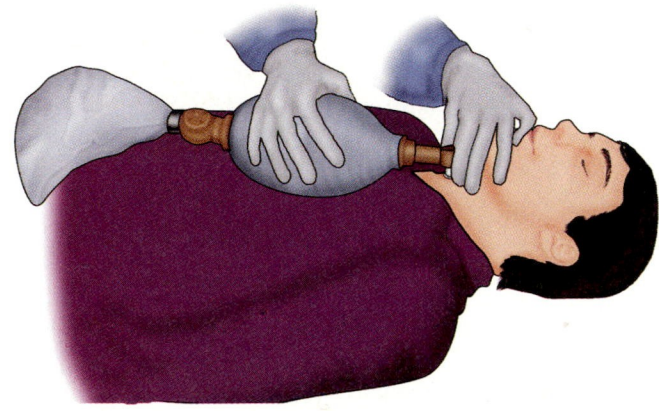

FIGURE 7-42 Use a BVM device to ventilate a patient with a stoma.

Foreign Body Obstruction

Causes

The presence of one or more of the following conditions can cause foreign body airway obstruction to occur (Figure 7-43):

- Relaxation of the tongue and throat tissues in an unconscious patient
- Vomited stomach contents
- Blood clots, bone fragments, or damaged tissue after an injury
- Foreign objects, such as dentures, food, and small toys

Tongue Blocking Airway

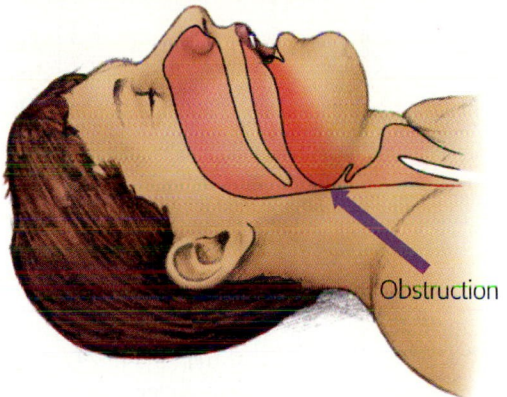

Obstruction

Injury

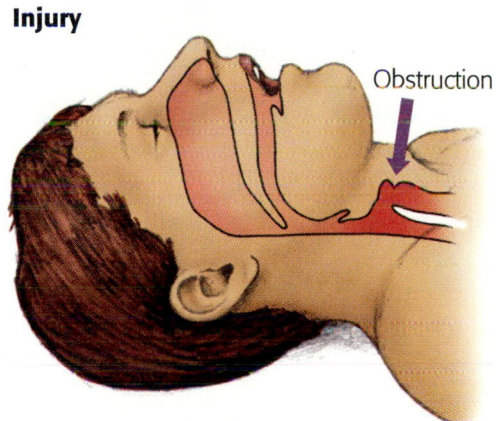

Obstruction

Swelling

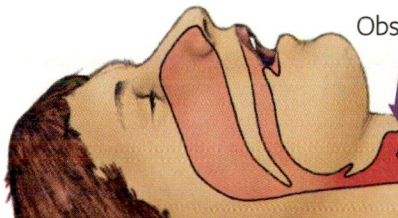
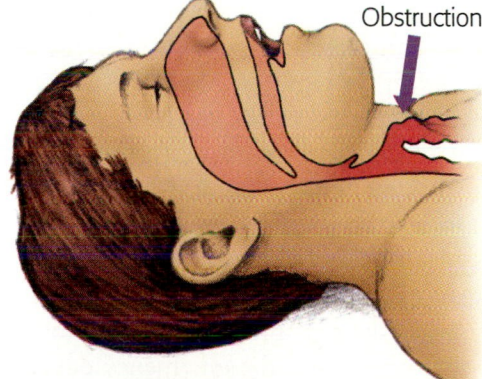

Obstruction

Foreign Object

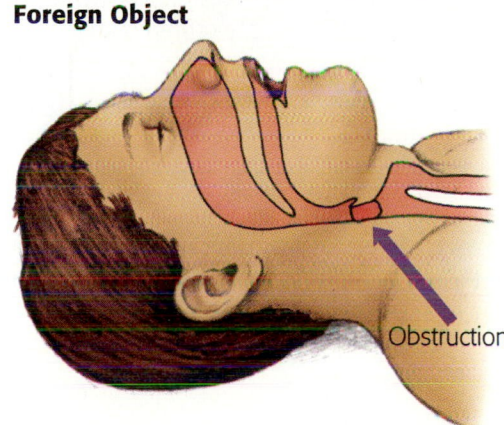

Obstruction

FIGURE 7-43 Airway obstruction is commonly caused by relaxation of the tongue into the throat, tissue damage and swelling following an injury or due to a medical condition, or the presence of a foreign body lodged in the throat.

In an adult, sudden airway obstruction by a foreign object usually occurs during a meal. In a child, it occurs while eating, playing with small toys, or crawling about the house. An otherwise healthy child who has sudden difficulty breathing has probably aspirated a foreign object. *The earlier you recognize airway obstruction, the better.* You must learn to recognize the difference between airway obstruction caused by a foreign object and that resulting from a medical condition. Airway obstruction in a child is usually caused by a foreign object or an infection, resulting in swelling and narrowing of the airway. With infection, attempts at clearing the airway will not be helpful and can be dangerous. These attempts will result in delaying transport.

One sure sign of an obstruction is a sudden inability to speak or cough during or immediately after eating. The person may grasp his or her throat, begin to turn blue, and have extreme difficulty breathing (Figure 7-44). There is little or no air movement. At first, the person will remain conscious and be able to signal to you what is wrong. Make sure you ask, "Are you choking?" If the patient nods "yes," then you know to act. If you do not clear the airway quickly, the oxygen in the lungs will be used up. Unconsciousness and death will follow.

When you find a patient unconscious, you will not know the cause of the unconsciousness at first. The unconsciousness may have been caused by an airway obstruction, a heart problem, or any number of other problems. Any patient you find unconscious must be managed as if he or she is in cardiac arrest. You must

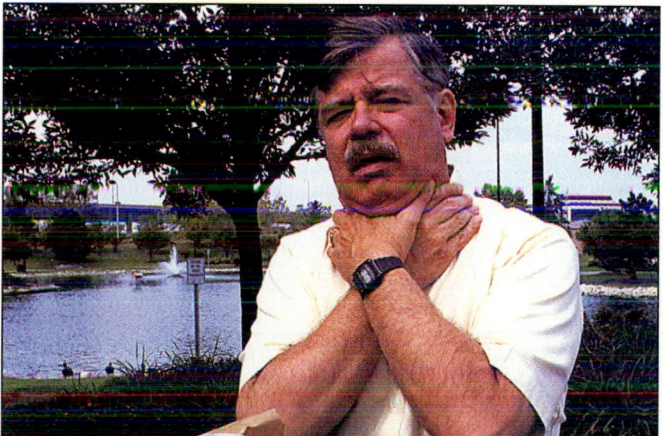

FIGURE 7-44 The universal sign of choking is a person who grasps his or her throat, begins to turn cyanotic, and has difficulty breathing.

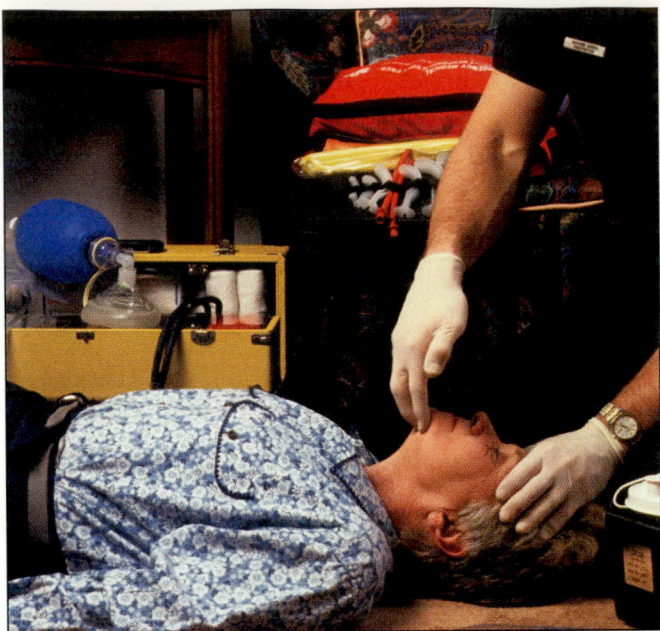

FIGURE 7-45 Securing and maintaining the airway and assuring adequate breathing are the first, most important steps in caring for an unconscious patient.

first open the airway and then provide artificial ventilation as you would for CPR (Figure 7-45). If, after opening the airway, you feel resistance after ventilating the patient's lungs, or pressure is felt (poor lung compliance), you should consider the possibility of airway obstruction. Lung compliance is defined as the ability of the alveoli to expand when air is drawn in on inhalation; poor lung compliance is the inability of the alveoli to fully expand on inhalation.

Removal Techniques

You should use the Heimlich maneuver (abdominal thrusts) followed by finger sweeps and manual removal of the object to relieve complete airway obstruction.

The Heimlich maneuver is the most effective method of dislodging and forcing an object out of the airway.

> In an adult, sudden airway obstruction by a foreign object usually occurs during a meal. In a child, it occurs while eating, playing with small toys, or crawling about the house.

Residual air, which is always present in the lungs, is compressed upward and used to expel the object. BLS techniques are reviewed in detail in Chapter 39.

You should perform the head-tilt/chin-lift maneuver to clear an obstruction that is caused by the tongue and throat muscles relaxing back into the airway. Loose dentures and large pieces of vomited food, mucus, or blood clots in the mouth should be swept forward and out of the mouth with your gloved index finger. Once it becomes available, suctioning should be used to maintain a clear airway. On occasion, a large foreign object will be aspirated and block the upper airway. In these instances, you should perform three cycles of the Heimlich maneuver. If you are not successful in dislodging the object, transport the patient and continue your efforts to clear the airway en route.

Occasionally, a patient will be able to exchange air in the lungs but will still have some degree of respiratory distress. This condition is called a **partial airway obstruction**. The patient will be breathing noisily and may be coughing. With good air exchange, the patient can cough forcefully, although there may be wheezing between coughs. As long as the patient can breathe, cough, or talk, you should not interfere with the patient's attempts to expel the foreign object. Abdominal thrusts are not usually effective for dislodging a partial obstruction. Manual removal is dangerous because the object could be forced farther down the airway, causing a complete obstruction. You must take great care to prevent a partial airway obstruction from becoming a complete airway obstruction.

With a partial airway obstruction, the head-tilt/chin-lift or jaw-thrust maneuvers should be performed to support the airway in its most efficient position. You should also give 100% supplemental oxygen and then provide transport. Of course, if air movement stops completely, you should immediately perform the Heimlich maneuver. Notify the emergency department personnel of the problem and the expected time of arrival.

Dental Appliances

Many dental appliances can cause airway obstruction. Always check the airway for any foreign object or substance. If a dental appliance, such as a crown or bridge or even a piece or section of braces, has become loose, you should remove it before assisting ventilations to avoid an obstruction.

prep kit

ready for review

The respiratory system includes the diaphragm, the muscles of the chest wall, and the accessory muscles of breathing. The term "airway" usually means the upper airway, including the nose, mouth, and throat. Clearing the airway means removing obstructing material; maintaining the airway means keeping it open. Patients who are breathing inadequately show signs of hypoxia, a dangerous condition in which the body's tissues and cells do not have enough oxygen. Adequate breathing features a normal rate of 12 to 20 breaths/min., a regular pattern of inhalation and exhalation, bilateral lung sounds, and regular and equal chest rise and fall. Patients with inadequate breathing need to be treated immediately. Emergency medical care includes airway management, supplemental oxygen, and ventilatory support.

Basic techniques for opening the airway include the head-tilt/chin-left maneuver and the jaw-thrust maneuver. One basic airway adjunct is the oropharyngeal airway, which keeps the tongue from blocking the airway in unconscious patients with no gag reflex. If the oropharyngeal airway is not the proper size or is inserted incorrectly, it can actually push the tongue back into the pharynx. Another basic airway adjunct is the nasopharyngeal airway, which is usually used with a conscious patient. Unlike the oropharyngeal airway, the nasopharyngeal airway does not allow for adequate suctioning.

Suctioning is the next priority after opening the airway. Semi-rigid tonsil tips are the best catheters to use when suctioning the pharynx; soft plastic catheters are used to suction the nose and liquid secretions in the back of the mouth. The recovery position is used to help maintain the airway in patients without traumatic injuries who are breathing on their own.

You should always give supplemental oxygen to patients who are not breathing on their own or not breathing adequately, including patients in cardiac arrest. Handle compressed gas cylinders very carefully; their contents are under pressure. Always make sure the correct pressure regulator is firmly attached before transporting a cylinder. The pin-indexing safety system features a series of pins on a yoke that must be matched with the holes on the valve stem of the gas cylinder. Pressure regulators reduce the pressure of gas in an oxygen cylinder to between 40 and 70 psi. Pressure- compensated flowmeters and Bourdon-gauge flowmeters permit the regulated release of gas measured in liters per minute. When oxygen therapy is complete, disconnect the tubing from the flowmeter nipple and turn off the cylinder valve, then turn off the flowmeter; as long as there is a pressure reading on the regulator gauge, it is not safe to remove the regulator from the valve stem. Keep any possible source of fire away from the area while oxygen is in use.

Nasal cannulas and the far more effective nonrebreathing masks are used most often to deliver oxygen in the field; always try to use the latter with patients who you suspect may have hypoxia. Nonrebreathing masks can provide up to 95% inspired oxygen, compared with 60% with a partial rebreathing mask.

The methods of providing artificial ventilation include two-person bag-valve-mask, mouth-to-mask ventilation, oxygen-powered manually triggered breathing device, and one-person bag-valve-mask. Combined with your own exhaled breath, mouth-to-mask ventilation will give up to 55% oxygen; a BVM device with an oxygen reservoir can deliver more than 90% oxygen.

When providing artificial ventilations, remember that blowing too forcefully can cause gastric distention. Slow, gentle breaths during artificial ventilation can help to prevent gastric distention. Also consider patients who have a tracheal stoma. You will need to ventilate such a patient through the stoma.

Foreign body airway obstruction usually occurs during a meal in an adult, or while a child is eating, playing with small objects, or crawling about the house. The earlier you recognize any airway obstruction, the better. You must learn to recognize the difference between airway obstruction caused by a foreign object and that caused by a medical condition.

A complete airway obstruction can be removed by the Heimlich maneuver or by finger sweeps and manual removal of the object. Perform the head-tilt/chin-lift or jaw-thrust maneuver in a patient with a partial airway obstruction, provide 100% supplemental oxygen, and transport.

Check for loose dental appliances in a patient before assisting ventilations. Loose appliances should be removed to prevent them from obstructing the airway.

prep kit 7

prep kit

vital vocabulary

www.emtb.com

agonal respirations Occasional, gasping breaths that occur after the heart has stopped.

airway The upper airway tract or the passage above the larynx, which includes the nose, mouth, and throat.

American Standard System A safety system for size D or larger oxygen cylinders, designed to prevent the accidental attachment of a regulator to a wrong cylinder.

bag-valve-mask (BVM) device A device with face mask attached to a bag containing a reservoir and connected to oxygen; delivers more than 90% supplemental oxygen.

barrier device A protective item, such as a pocket mask with a valve, that limits exposure to a patient's body fluids.

catheter A hollow, cylindrical structure that drains or delivers fluids.

diffusion A process in which molecules move from an area of higher concentration of molecules to an area of lower concentration.

exhalation Part of the breathing process in which the diaphragm and the intercostal muscles relax.

gag reflex A normal reflex mechanism that causes retching and is activated by touching the soft palate or the back of the throat.

gastric distention A condition in which air fills the stomach as a result of high volume and pressure during artificial ventilation.

head-tilt/chin-lift maneuver A combination of two movements to open the airway by tilting the forehead back and lifting the chin.

hypoxia A dangerous condition in which the body tissues and cells do not have enough oxygen.

inhalation The active muscular part of breathing that occurs as we inhale.

jaw-thrust maneuver Technique to open the airway by placing the fingers behind the angle of the jaw and bringing the jaw forward.

labored breathing Breathing that requires more than normal effort; may be slower or much faster than normal.

metabolism The chemical processes that provide the cells with energy from nutrients.

nasal cannula An oxygen delivery device in which oxygen flows through two small, tubelike prongs that fit into the patient's nostrils.

nasopharyngeal (nasal or trumpet) airway Airway adjunct inserted into the nostril of a conscious patient who is not able to maintain a natural airway.

nonrebreathing mask A mask and reservoir bag system that is the preferred way to give oxygen in the prehospital setting; delivers up to 90% inspired oxygen.

oropharyngeal (oral) airway Airway adjunct inserted into the mouth to keep the tongue from blocking the upper airway and to make suctioning the airway easier.

partial airway obstruction Condition in which the patient is able to exchange air in the lungs but has some degree of respiratory distress.

pin-indexing system A system established for portable cylinders to ensure that a regulator is not connected to the wrong cylinder.

recovery position A position in which the patient lies on the right or left side, with hands under the lower cheek; used to maintain a clear airway following resuscitation in patients without traumatic injuries.

stoma Opening in the neck that connects the trachea directly to the skin.

tidal volume Depth of breathing.

tonsil tip A large, somewhat rigid suction tip recommended for suctioning the pharynx.

ventilation Exchange of air between the lungs and the air of the environment, either spontaneously by the patient or with assistance from an EMT-B.

prep kit 7

assessment in action

Dispatch receives a call from a frantic caller who screams, "It's an emergency! Please hurry!" Seconds later, your and your partner are dispatched to a grocery store, where you find an 80-year-old woman who has collapsed in the vegetable section. She is lying supine on the floor and is unresponsive to any stimuli. A store employee is attempting to provide ventilations with a pocket mask. You note that the patient's skin is cool, moist, and still cyanotic. You ask the employee to stop the rescue breathing so that you can assess the patient. The patient is still not breathing but has a radial pulse of 68 beats/min.

1. Of the following interventions, which would be is the **LEAST** appropriate at this time?
   A. Initiate CPR immediately.
   B. Open and assess the patient's airway.
   C. Insert a properly sized oropharyngeal airway.
   D. Begin assisting ventilations with a BVM device.

2. Which of the following statements about mouth-to-mouth ventilations is true?
   A. ALS providers are the only rescuers who are qualified to perform this technique.
   B. Creating an airtight seal is not possible with this technique.
   C. You cannot provide adequate tidal volume in adult patients.
   D. The risk of infection is increased in using this technique.

3. You attempt to deliver a rescue breath but notice that the patient's cheeks flutter, air leaks out around her lips, and her chest does not rise. You reposition the airway, but you still cannot ventilate the patient. The next step would be to:
   A. move the patient outside into the fresh air.
   B. provide high-flow oxygen via nonrebreathing mask.
   C. deliver chest compressions and try ventilations again later.
   D. perform five abdominal thrusts.

4. The patient gasps, and you now see what appear to be chunks of chocolate in her mouth that need to be removed. As you prepare to suction the patient, you know that you should insert the catheter:
   A. inside the nose.
   B. as far into the throat as possible.
   C. only to the base of the tongue.
   D. only after you have turned on the suctioning unit.

5. One sign that your attempts to provide respiratory support have **NOT** been effective is that you:
   A. feel air escaping after each rescue breath.
   B. see that the patient's skin appears to be pink.
   C. see that the patient's pupils are fixed and dilated.
   D. see that the patient's chest rises and falls with each breath.

points to ponder

You are working a motor vehicle crash, and your patient is unresponsive but breathing and has a pulse. You have her head stabilized and are controlling bleeding on an open fracture of her clavicle. A paramedic comes to assist you and decides to intubate the patient. The paramedic's technique appears somewhat clumsy, but being a rookie, you just do what you are told. Your partner needs some help with extrication of other patients, and the paramedic tells you to go. At the hospital, you find out that your original patient died and that the endotracheal tube had been removed before she got to the hospital. You suspect that the patient was improperly intubated.

• Who would you tell about this problem and your suspicions? Why?

online outlook

The respiratory system is a very important part of the body. It delivers oxygen to the lungs and allows carbon dioxide to be removed. To learn more about the anatomy and physiology of the respiratory system, complete Exercise 7 at www.emtb.com.

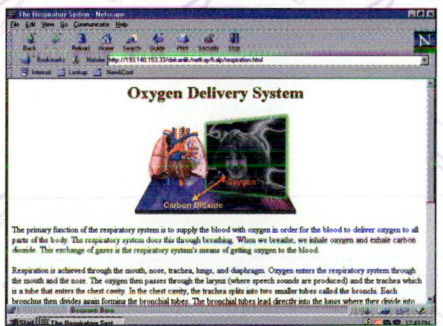

Patient Assessment

Mike Smith, MICP

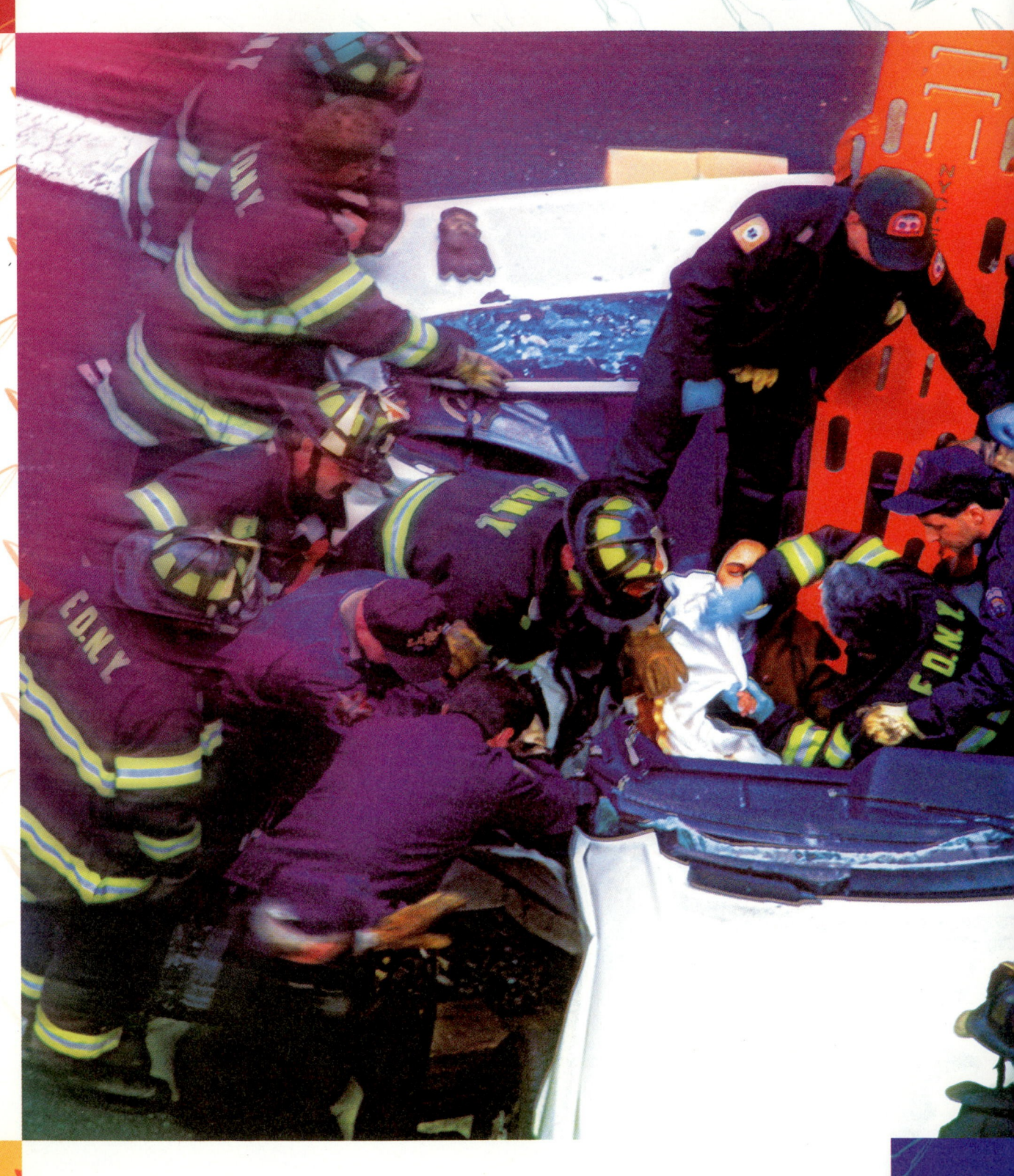

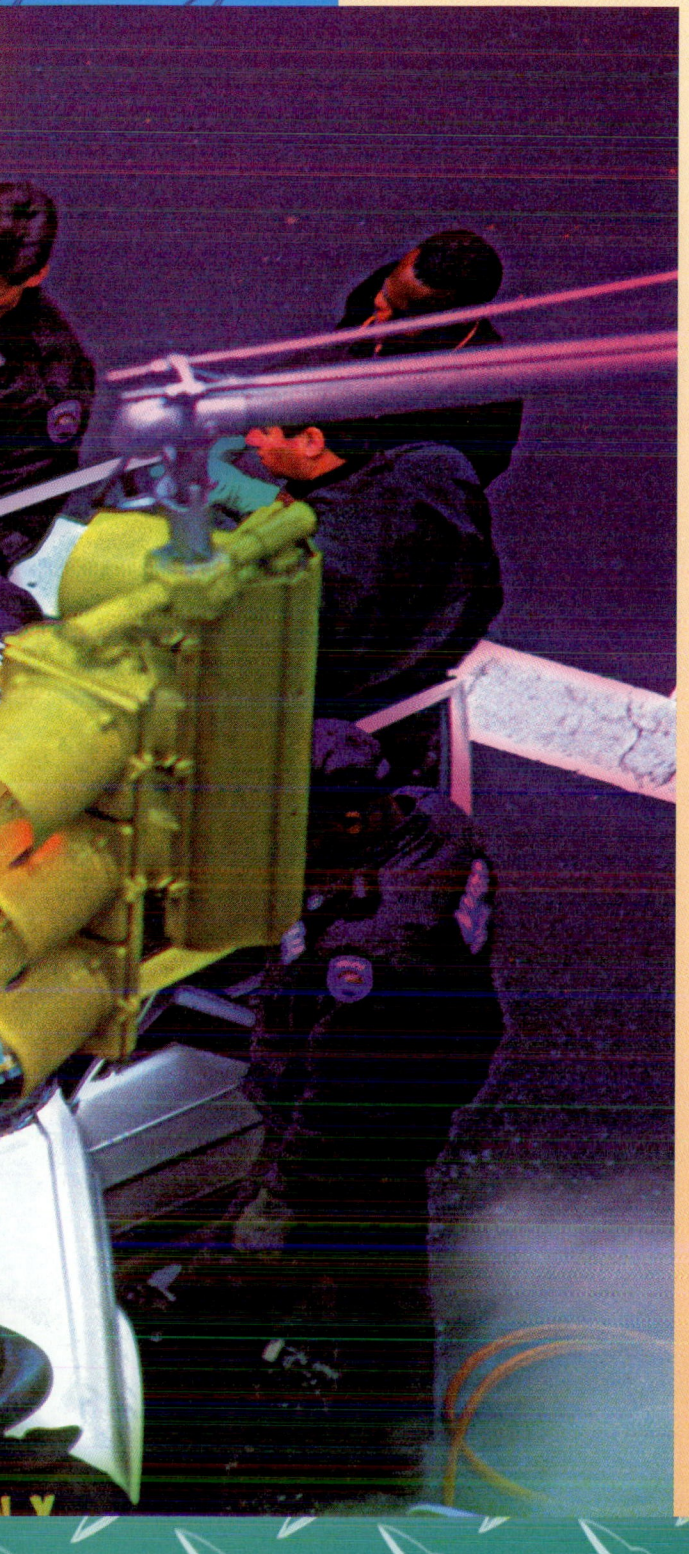

Patient Assessment

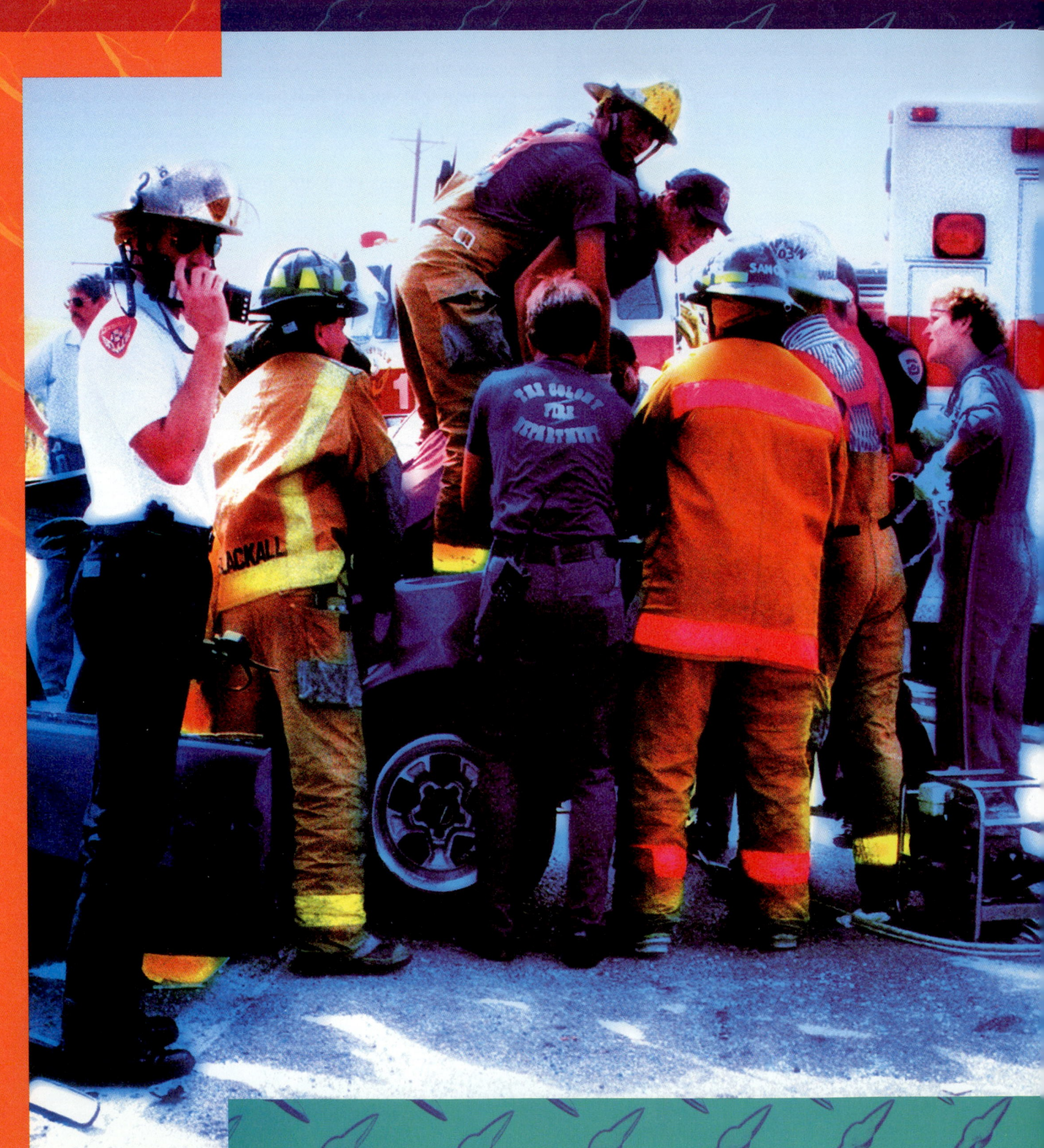

objectives

| Scene Size-Up | Initial Assessment |

Cognitive

1. Recognize hazards/potential hazards.

2. Describe common hazards found at the scene of a trauma and a medical patient.

3. Determine if the scene is safe to enter.

4. Discuss common mechanisms of injury/nature of illness.

5. Discuss the reason for identifying the total number of patients at the scene.

6. Explain the reason for identifying the need for additional help or assistance.

Affective

7. Explain the rationale for crew members to evaluate scene safety prior to entering.

8. Serve as a model for others explaining how patient situations affect your evaluation of mechanism of injury or illness.

Psychomotor

9. Observe various scenarios and identify potential hazards.

Cognitive

1. Summarize the reasons for forming a general impression of the patient.

2. Discuss methods of assessing altered mental status.

3. Differentiate between assessing the altered mental status in the adult, child, and infant patient.

4. Discuss methods of assessing the airway in the adult, child, and infant patient.

5. State reasons for management of the cervical spine once the patient has been determined to be a trauma patient.

6. Describe methods used for assessing if a patient is breathing.

7. State what care should be provided to the adult, child, and infant patient with adequate breathing.

8. State what care should be provided to the adult, child, and infant patient without adequate breathing.

9. Differentiate between a patient with adequate and inadequate breathing.

10. Distinguish between methods of assessing breathing in the adult, child, and infant patient.

11. Compare the methods of providing airway care to the adult, child, and infant patient.

12. Describe the methods used to obtain a pulse.

13. Differentiate between obtaining a pulse in an adult, child, and infant patient.

14. Discuss the need for assessing the patient for external bleeding.

15. Describe normal and abnormal findings when assessing skin color.

16. Describe normal and abnormal findings when assessing skin temperature.

17. Describe normal and abnormal findings when assessing skin condition.

(Continued)

objectives—cont'd.

18. Describe normal and abnormal findings when assessing skin capillary refill in the infant and child patient.

19. Explain the reason for prioritizing a patient for care and transport.

Affective

20. Explain the importance of forming a general impression of the patient.

21. Explain the value of performing an initial assessment.

Psychomotor

22. Demonstrate the techniques for assessing mental status.

23. Demonstrate the techniques for assessing the airway.

24. Demonstrate the techniques for assessing if the patient is breathing.

25. Demonstrate the techniques for assessing if the patient has a pulse.

26. Demonstrate the techniques for assessing the patient for external bleeding.

27. Demonstrate the techniques for assessing the patient's skin color, temperature, condition, and capillary refill (infants and children only).

28. Demonstrate the ability to prioritize patients.

Focused History and Physical Exam: Trauma Patients

Cognitive

1. Discuss the reasons for reconsideration concerning the mechanism of injury.

2. State the reasons for performing a rapid trauma assessment.

3. Recite examples and explain why patients should receive a rapid trauma assessment.

4. Describe the areas included in the rapid trauma assessment and discuss what should be evaluated.

5. Differentiate when the rapid assessment may be altered in order to provide patient care.

6. Discuss the reason for performing a focused history and physical exam.

Affective

7. Recognize and respect the feelings that patients might experience during assessment.

Psychomotor

8. Demonstrate the rapid trauma assessment that should be used to assess a patient based on mechanism of injury.

Focused History and Physical Exam: Medical Patients

Cognitive

1. Describe the unique needs for assessing an individual with a specific chief complaint with no known prior history.

2. Differentiate between the history and physical exam that are performed for responsive patients with no known prior history and responsive patients with a known prior history.

3. Describe the unique needs for assessing an individual who is unresponsive.

4. Differentiate between the assessment that is performed for a patient who is unresponsive or has an altered mental status and other medical patients requiring assessment.

Affective

5. Attend to the feelings that these patients might be experiencing.

Psychomotor

6. Demonstrate the patient care skills that should be used to assist a patient who is responsive with no known history.

7. Demonstrate the patient care skills that should be used to assist a patient who is unresponsive or has an altered mental status.

Detailed Physical Exam

Cognitive

1. Discuss the components of the detailed physical exam.

2. State the areas of the body that are evaluated during the detailed physical exam.

3. Explain what additional care should be provided while performing the detailed physical exam.

4. Distinguish between the detailed physical exam that is performed on a trauma patient and that of the medical patient.

Affective

5. Explain the rationale for the feelings that these patients might be experiencing.

Psychomotor

6. Demonstrate the skills involved in performing the detailed physical exam.

Ongoing Assessment

Cognitive

1. Discuss the reason for repeating the initial assessment as part of the ongoing assessment.

2. Describe the components of the ongoing assessment.

3. Describe trending of assessment components.

Affective

4. Explain the value of performing an ongoing assessment.

5. Recognize and respect the feelings that patients might experience during assessment.

6. Explain the value of trending assessment components to other health professionals who assume care of the patient.

Psychomotor

7. Demonstrate the skills involved in performing the ongoing assessment.

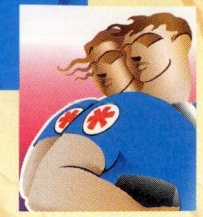

you are the emt

Squad 7 . . . Stop at the county jail lockup for "an unresponsive man." Upon arrival, you find a 24-year-old man who was thrown in the "drunk tank" last night. It's 8:00 A.M., and the patient cannot be aroused. Another man in the cell with him states that his friend had two beers and cannot be drunk. You assess the patient and find a Medic-Alert bracelet that indicates he has insulin-dependent diabetes mellitus. He most likely would have died had you not performed a thorough assessment.

Patient assessment is a skill that you will continue to refine and improve upon throughout your EMS career. This chapter will present information that you will need to build this foundation for your practice as well as help you to answer the following questions:

1. What are the goals of the initial assessment, of the focused history and physical examination, and of the ongoing examination?

2. Is an assessment really needed for all patients or only for those who appear to be really sick or badly hurt?

About This Chapter

This chapter will provide a clear and comprehensive approach to Patient Assessment. A flowchart has been developed to provide a quick, visual reference to guide you through the patient assessment process. The chapter has been divided into 6 sections. Every section is color coded and numbered for easy reference. The Patient Assessment Flowchart is repeated at every section to show you "at a glance" where you are in the patient assessment process.

Special care has been taken to reflect the EMT-Basic National Standard Curriculum, but enhancement information will prepare you for your work in the field.

| Scene Size-Up |
| Initial Assessment |
| Focused History and Physical Exam: Trauma Patients |
| Focused History and Physical Exam: Medical Patients |
| Detailed Physical Exam |
| Ongoing Assessment |

Patient Assessment

From a practical point of view, prehospital emergency care is simply a series of decisions about treatment and transport. The process that guides decision making in EMS is based on your patient assessment findings. For you to make good decisions about how to best care for your patient, you must start by gathering information as you progress through the Patient Assessment process, as listed below:

- Perform the scene size-up.
- Perform an initial assessment.
- Provide spinal immobilization if necessary.
- Identify and treat life-threatening conditions.
- Perform a focused history and physical exam.
- Provide transport for a patient with an obvious life-threatening condition.
- Perform a detailed physical exam on the scene on a patient with no life-threatening conditions.
- Reassess vital signs.
- Perform ongoing assessments.

Scene Size-Up

1

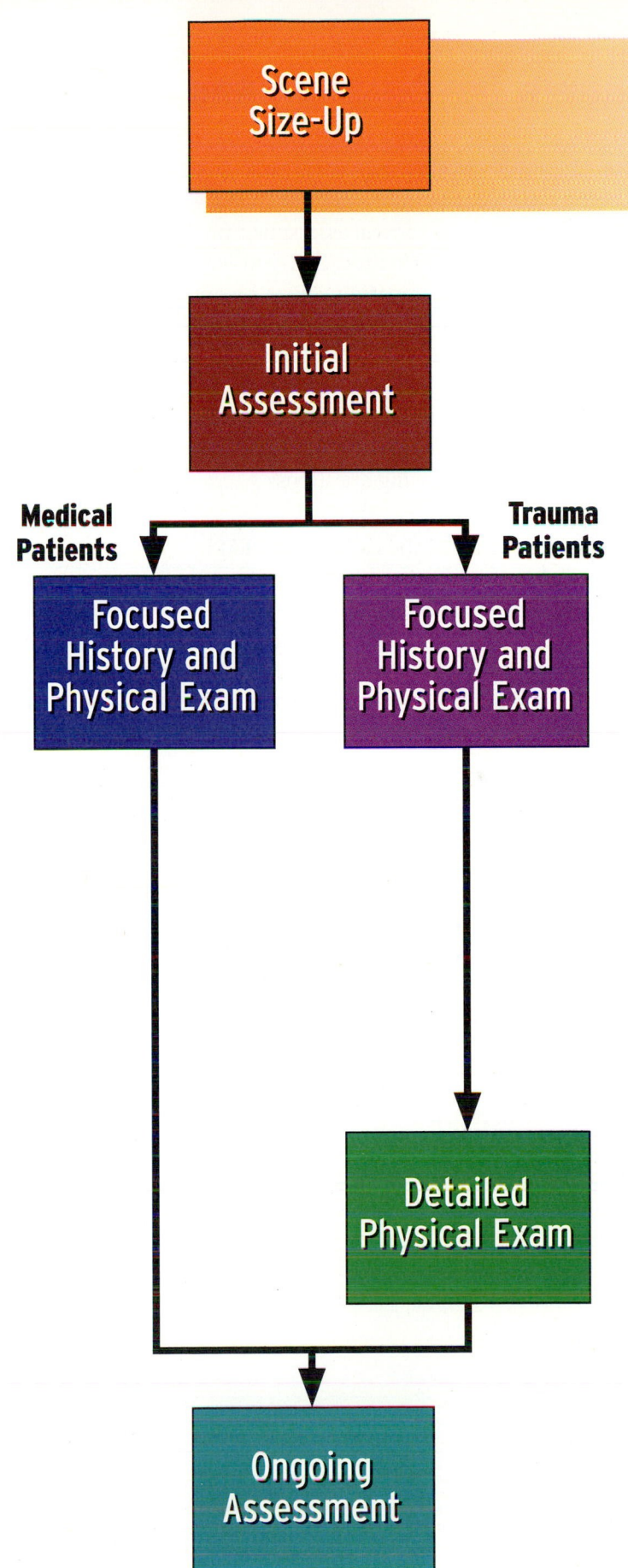

Dispatch Information and Mental Preparation

You should begin the assessment process long before you ever actually make contact with the patient. This *prearrival* assessment process includes using information that you learned from dispatch, as well as preparing yourself mentally to handle the call. Therefore, your first step on any call is to evaluate whatever dispatch information is available, including the location, the nature of the call, and the age and gender of the patient. While not always accurate, dispatch information may provide some insight into the following questions:

1. **What is the nature of the call and has EMS responded to the location before?** For instance, the call may be to a blind curve where head-on collisions are common. Or it may be to a long-term care facility, leading you to expect medical or traumatic problems that are common to geriatric patients.

2. **What are the likely problems based on the patient's age or gender?** These factors may help you to mentally plan ahead. For example, if you are responding to a child with chest pain, you might anticipate a traumatic injury, since this is a likely cause of chest pain in children; the same chest pain call in a 60-year-old man will likely be related to cardiac problems.

3. **What equipment or additional personnel are needed?** Often, dispatch information will help you to select the type of equipment to take to the scene. For instance, taking a backboard would be a good choice for a fall, whereas a suctioning unit may be useful for a patient with nausea and vomiting. Dispatch to a three-car motor vehicle accident could prompt a call for additional EMS or rescue resources.

4. **What are the potential hazards?** Dispatch information can provide valuable information regarding potential hazards that you may encounter on the scene. For instance, calls related to traffic collisions may present a risk because of heavy traffic on a busy highway. Calls involving fires or toxic spills can present a very real danger to rescuers through exposure to smoke or toxic chemicals. Consider these risks as you travel to the scene, and prepare accordingly. When appropriate, consider calling for additional resources to stabilize the scene.

What Is the Nature of the Call?

Suppose you are called to a long-term care facility for a woman who has fallen. On arrival, you and your partner find a 93-year-old woman sitting in her bed. The long-term care facility staff report that the woman fell against a door handle in the hall on her way back from lunch. A large laceration is obvious on the back of the woman's head. Given this dispatch information, you should ask yourself the following questions:

- What questions would you ask the patient first?

- What assessment should be performed at this time?

- What decisions need to be made in this situation?

What should you do in this situation? What should you expect? You will be confronted with the simple question of "what to do" on every call, every day.

What Are the Likely Problems?

Although it is impossible to predict what you will find with any certainty, several factors should be considered. As you learn more about different medical and trauma conditions, you will be better able to anticipate potential problems. In the above case, the patient is elderly. With that in mind, how should you prepare mentally? Next, consider possible events that might cause an elderly woman to fall, including a simple slip and fall, fainting (syncope), a cerebrovascular accident (CVA), a cardiac event, or inadequate oxygen to the brain caused by a respiratory problem.

Once you have considered the causes, think about the consequences of a fall. The patient could have fractured her leg, hip, pelvis, or even spine. She could have also hit her head and/or sustained a closed head injury or a soft-tissue injury such as a laceration. Given this information, you might mentally review the signs, symptoms, and treatment of CVA, cardiac event, or shortness of breath, as well as fractures and soft-tissue injury.

What Equipment Is Needed?

Given the information supplied by dispatch, you might take the following equipment into the long-term care facility with you:

- A blood pressure cuff and stethoscope to obtain vital signs and evaluate respirations

- A backboard in case CPR or spinal immobilization is required

- Oxygen and a BVM device in case oxygen is necessary or the patient is in cardiac arrest

- Bandaging supplies, gloves, and masks in case the patient has open wounds

What Are the Hazards?

Finally, consider potential hazards. For the most part, long-term care facilities are usually fairly safe locations to work. Traffic should not be a problem, and—unless it is part of the nature of the call—hazardous materials should not be a problem. However, the potential for exposure to blood may present a hazard, as could angry, uncooperative family members. In all situations, you should wear gloves, gowns, or masks as necessary and dictated by protocol to protect yourself against exposure to blood or other body substances.

Mental preparation is an essential part of the patient assessment process because it helps you to focus so that you are ready for any situation or circumstances at the scene. In many cases, chaos and inappropriate equipment on a scene can be traced to poor mental preparation. So use the time traveling to the scene to consider and prepare for what you are likely to find when you arrive.

Scene Size-Up

1

Upon arriving at the scene, it is essential to perform a scene size-up. The <u>scene size-up</u> is a quick assessment of the scene and the surroundings that will provide you and your partner with as much information as possible about the safety of the scene, any mechanism of injury, and the nature of the illness before you enter and begin patient care. Table 8-1 lists the components of the scene size-up. Your first step at any scene is to make sure that you and your partner are safe. Never become a victim yourself.

TABLE 8-1 Components of the Scene Size-Up

Safety of the Scene

- Make sure you and your partner are safe:
  Reduce your risk of exposure to communicable disease by following BSI techniques.
  Watch for possible dangers outside the ambulance, such as traffic, leaking fuel, downed electrical lines, fire, hazardous materials.
  Consider your ambulance to be a relatively safe haven if you are responding to a crime scene.

- Make sure the patient and bystanders are safe:
  Move bystanders to a safe area.
  Ask bystanders to help with or perform a specific task.
  Ask for more help if you need it.

Nature of the Illness/Chief Complaint

- Ask the patient, family members, or law enforcement why EMS was called.

Mechanism of Injury

- Use the mechanism of injury as a guide to predict the potential for serious injury:
  How much force was applied to the body?
  How long was the force applied?
  What area of the body was involved?

Multiple Patients

- Call for additional EMS units.

- Begin triage.

  Call for additional resources such as law enforcement, the fire department, rescue units, HazMat teams, and utility companies.

Body Substance Isolation

On every emergency call, you need to be sure to wear the proper protective equipment since this equipment will reduce your risk of exposure to communicable disease. The best way to reduce your risk of exposure is to follow <u>body substance isolation (BSI)</u> techniques. The concept of BSI assumes that all body fluids present a possible risk for infection.

Before you step out of the unit, you and your partner must be wearing the proper protective equipment. Vinyl or latex gloves are always indicated. Eye protection, masks, and gowns may also be indicated if there is a lot of blood or other body fluids in the patient area (Figure 8-1). Eye protection is needed when there may be a risk that blood or other body fluids will splatter or become airborne. You should put on a mask and gown, if needed and dictated by your protocol, before you enter the area immediately around the patient. If the scene involves hazardous materials or fire, wear the appropriate gear for the situation or do not enter the scene.

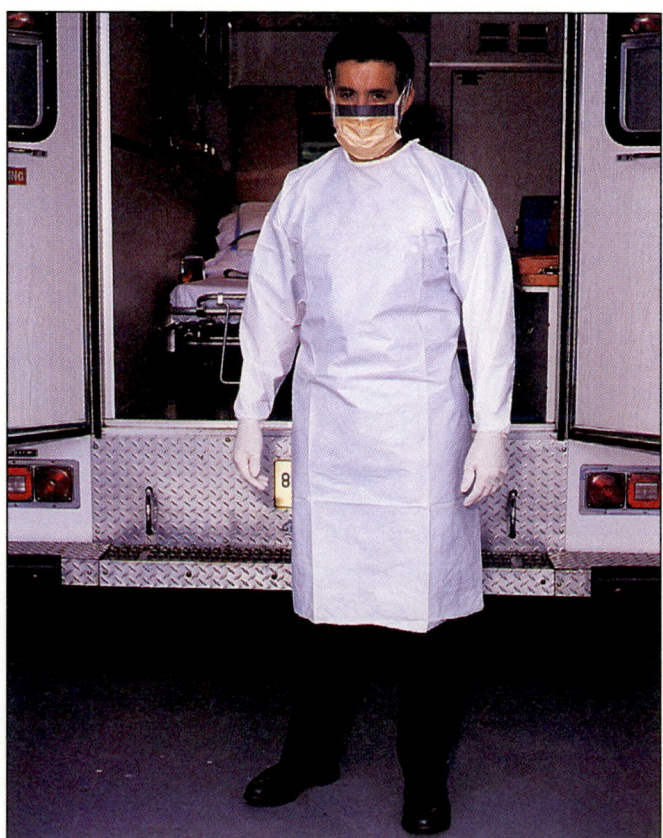

FIGURE 8-1 Proper protective equipment is vital when you are called to a scene in which there is a lot of blood or other body fluids.

Scene Safety

Scene safety is an assessment focused on ensuring the well-being of the EMT-B. You cannot help your patient if you become a victim yourself.

Personal Protection

Look for the following possible dangers before you step out of the unit (Figure 8-2):

- Oncoming traffic
- Unstable surfaces (e.g., wet or icy patches, loose gravel, slopes)
- Leaking gasoline or diesel fuel
- Downed electrical lines
- Hostile bystanders/potential for violence
- Fire or smoke
- Possible hazardous or toxic materials
- Other dangers at crash or rescue scenes
- Crime scenes

You should park your unit in a place that will offer you and your partner the greatest safety but also rapid access to the patient and your equipment (Figure 8-3). In many instances, law enforcement will be at the scene before you arrive. If that is the case, you should talk with them before entering the scene. Make sure to follow local protocol if the scene is a crime scene. Also be sure to have law enforcement accompany you if the patient is a suspect in the crime. Consider your unit a safe haven. You are no help to the patient if you enter the scene without first protecting yourself and your partner.

Your next concern is the safety of the patient(s) and bystanders. This is not an easy task. Bystanders can become a problem when they try to help or direct your care. Protect yourself and bystanders alike by moving them to a safe area or assigning them a specific task.

Making an Unsafe Scene Safe

Occasionally, you and your partner will not be able to safely enter a scene. This may be due to the need for extrication, possible hazardous conditions, or the presence of more patients than you can handle alone. These situations seem very difficult when you want to provide medical care to sick or injured patients. However, your safety and that of your partner are more important. If you need more help, do not hesitate to ask for it. Be as specific as possible about the type of help

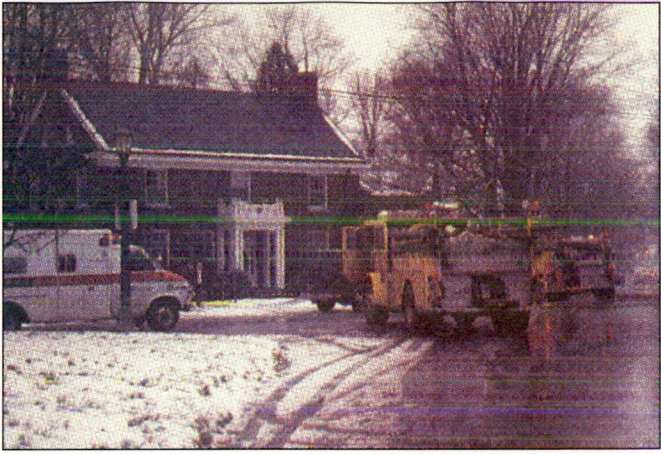

FIGURE 8-2 Before you step out of your unit, be sure to evaluate the scene for any hazards.

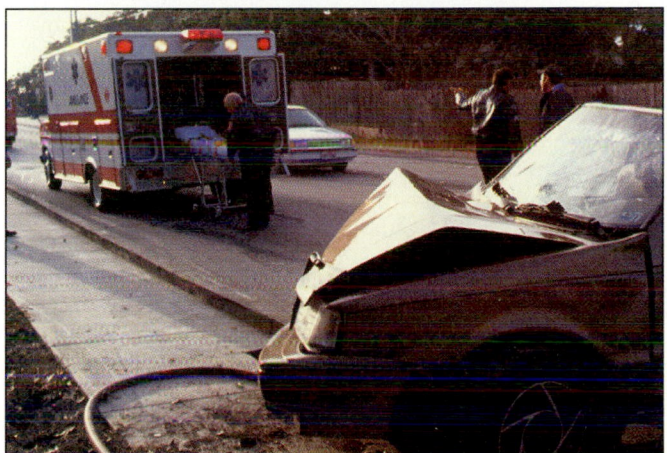

FIGURE 8-3 Park your unit in a place that is safe, yet allows for rapid access to the patient and your equipment. If law enforcement is already on the scene, make sure to check in with them first.

you need. Remember, though, it takes time for additional resources, such as an extrication team, law enforcement, or another EMS unit, to arrive at the scene.

Goals of Scene Size-Up

As an EMT-B, you must ask some standard questions in all cases, whether the problem appears to be traumatic or medical in origin. Then, depending on the answers to these questions, you will ask other questions and follow other leads. But how do you begin? Prehospital assessment has four primary goals. You achieve these four goals by asking questions, obtaining answers, and responding to the information obtained. Table 8-2 lists the four goals, and the standard questions that will help you to achieve them, in order of importance and urgency.

1

TABLE 8-2	The Four Goals of Prehospital Assessment

The Four Goals	How to Achieve Them
1. **To identify immediately life-threatening conditions.** These conditions, such as airway obstruction, inadequate breathing, poor circulation, or grossly abnormal brain function, may kill your patient quickly. Once you identify any of these problems, you must correct them immediately before you perform any additional assessments.	1. **Does the patient have an immediately or potentially life-threatening condition?** If the answer is "yes," you need to start treatment by addressing the life-threatening condition and then provide immediate transport. The goal for any patient with an immediately or potentially life-threatening condition is a time-on-scene of less than 10 minutes.
2. **To identify potentially life-threatening conditions.** Potentially life-threatening conditions may seriously impair or kill a patient, although they have not become serious yet. Examples include swelling in the neck that may cause airway obstruction, a respiratory condition that may worsen, or significant bleeding that—if left uncontrolled—may result in inadequate circulation. Any potentially life-threatening conditions should be closely monitored throughout the call.	2. **Is this patient sick or injured enough to require treatment?** In most cases, the answer is yes—that is why you were called. Your next step is to perform further assessment to determine what type of treatment is necessary. However, in some cases, you are called to situations that do not require emergency care. When this happens, you may simply need to provide transport. In other cases, depending upon your local protocols, you may actually leave the patient at the scene.
3. **To identify and monitor abnormalities in the patient's current condition.** Abnormalities are deviations from normal that do not present any immediately or potentially life-threatening condition—for example, a fast pulse but a very low blood pressure. You might not identify these abnormalities initially, since your focus is on the life-threatening conditions.	3. **Does the patient require transport?** If the answer is yes, you will need to ask and answer additional questions to determine the most appropriate destination for the patient. You will also need to decide how urgently you should initiate transport.
4. **To provide information from the prehospital assessment to compare with later results.** This information is the first that you gather about the patient's condition. Your initial assessment of the patient is important because, in most cases, you are the first to evaluate a patient. All other assessments of the patient, whether they are done in the field, the emergency department, or the hospital, will be compared with this initial assessment. Changes or trends in the patient's condition may be significant in identifying developing problems. As a result, the information from the prehospital assessment often serves as a basis for making changes in treatment throughout the patient's hospital stay.	4. **How did the patient respond to treatment?** To answer this question, you must continue with your ongoing assessments. Once some form of care has been initiated, it is essential for you to reassess the patient. If the patient improves with treatment, you might wish to continue treatment as started. However, if the patient's condition becomes worse, you need to determine, through additional assessment, whether you need to change your approach to treatment.

Mechanism of Injury/
Nature of Illness

One of the great dangers in performing the prehospital assessment is giving in to the temptation to categorize your patient immediately *as either a trauma patient or a medical patient*. Remember, the fundamentals of good patient assessment do not change, despite the unique aspects of trauma and medical care. Careful evaluation of the scene, including the possible mechanism of injury and/or the nature of illness, along with the other information that you gather will help you to lean in one direction or the other. Family members, bystanders, and law enforcement can often tell you what prompted the call to 9-1-1. After you have completed your assessment, you will come to a conclusion as to whether your patient's main problem is medical or traumatic.

Determine from the patient why EMS was activated. You might also rely on information provided by family or bystanders.

Determine how many patients are involved. If there are more patients than your unit can effectively handle, initiate a mass-casualty plan. Call for additional help before making contact with patients or beginning triage. You are less likely to call for help once you are involved in patient care.

Mechanism of Injury

As an EMT-B, you will be called to motor vehicle crashes or other situations in which patients may have sustained life-threatening traumatic injuries. To care for these patients properly, you must understand how traumatic injuries occur, or the **mechanism of injury**. With a traumatic injury, the body has been exposed to some

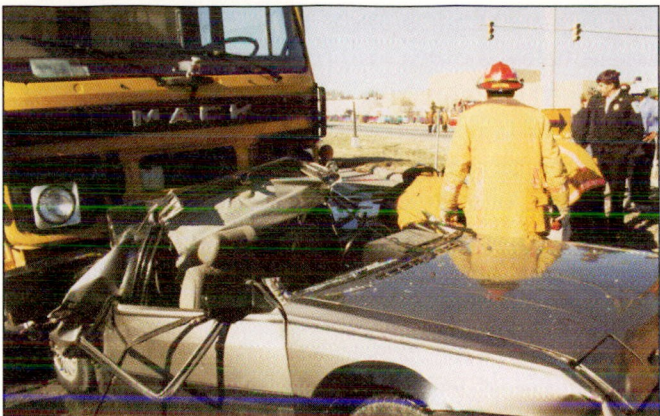

FIGURE 8-4 With traumatic injuries, the patient has been exposed to some force or energy that results in injury or even possibly death. You can learn a great deal about that force by simply looking at the mechanism of injury.

force or energy that has resulted in a temporary injury, permanent damage, or even death (Figure 8-4).

As you might expect, some parts of the body are more easily injured than others. The brain and the spinal cord are very fragile and easy to injure. Fortunately, they are protected anatomically by the skull, the vertebrae, and several layers of soft tissues. The eyes are also easily injured. Even small forces on the eye may result in serious injury. The bones and certain organs are hardier and can absorb small forces without resulting injury. The net result of this information is that you can use the mechanism of injury as a kind of guide to predict the potential for a serious injury by evaluating three factors: the amount of force applied to the body, the length of time the force was applied, and the areas of the body that is involved.

You will commonly hear the terms "blunt trauma" and "penetrating trauma" (Figure 8-5). With **blunt trauma**, the force of the injury occurs over a broad area, and the

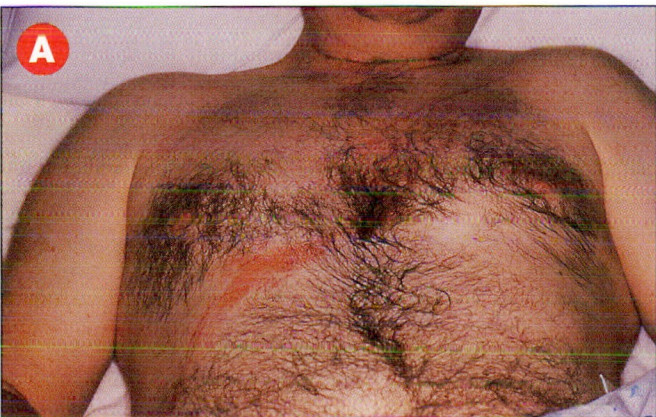

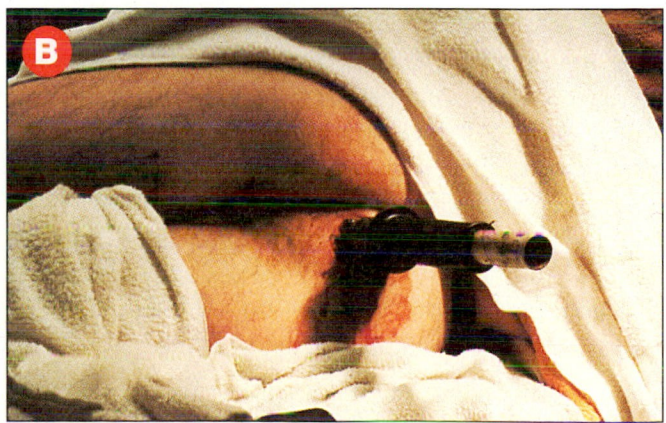

FIGURE 8-5 A: With blunt trauma, the force of injury occurs over a broad area, and the skin is not broken.
B: With penetrating trauma, an object pierces the skin and creates an open wound.

skin is usually not broken. However, the tissues and organs below the area of impact may be damaged. With **penetrating trauma**, the force of the injury occurs at a small point of contact between the skin and the object. The object pierces the skin and creates an open wound. The degree of injury depends on the characteristics of the penetrating object, the amount of force or energy, the part of the body affected, and the likelihood of infection.

Motor vehicle crashes. In motor vehicle crashes, the amount of force that is applied to the body is directly related to the speed of the crash. As the speed of a crash increases, the forces that are exerted on the patients increase as well. Therefore, patients should be evaluated according to the area of the body that was most likely injured. Your evaluation should also be based, to some extent, on the patient's position in the car, the use of seat belts, and how the patient's body shifts during the crash (Figure 8-6). Drivers are typically at higher risk for serious injury than passengers because of the potential for striking the steering wheel with the chest, abdomen, or head. Front seat passengers may also be injured by striking the dashboard.

Risk for serious injury also varies depending on whether seat belts are used and whether they are worn properly. Unbelted victims are at much higher risk for a number of other injuries because they may be catapulted throughout the car. As they go "up and over" or "down and under," they may strike the sides, ceiling, floor, dashboard, steering wheel, or windshield. Even worse, the unrestrained victim may be ejected from the vehicle, dramatically increasing the risk of head injury, spinal cord injury, and possibly death.

Falls. In falls, the amount of force that is applied to the body is directly related to the distance fallen. However, the area of the body injured is very hard to predict. Long falls are high-force falls, and patients should be evaluated accordingly. Any patient who has fallen more than three times his or her own height, or greater than 20′, should be considered at risk for serious injury. With children, a fall of 10′ or more is potentially lethal.

If the patient's condition is stable, you should attempt to determine exactly what happened during the fall. When possible, you should also identify what the patient landed on and how he or she landed. This information, which may be gleaned from the patient and/or bystanders, will help you to predict what areas of the body might be involved.

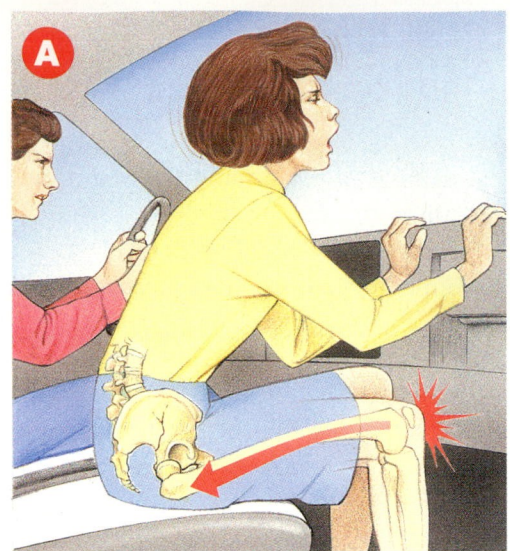

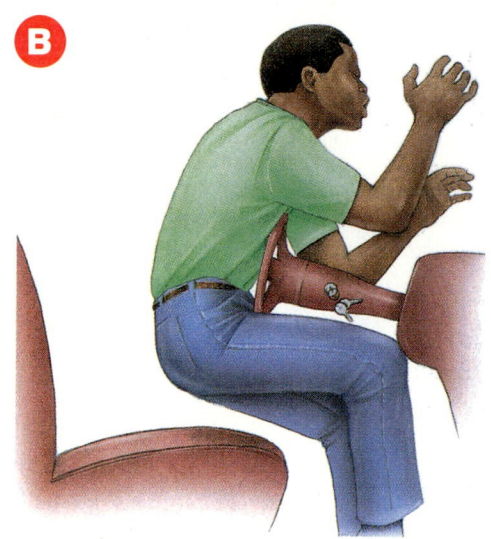

FIGURE 8-6 A: Injury to the lower extremities and pelvis can occur when the knee strikes the dashboard. **B:** Injury to the chest and abdomen occurs when the patient's chest and/or abdomen strikes the steering wheel.

Gunshot and stab wounds. Penetrating trauma, often the result of a gunshot or stab injury, is also very difficult to evaluate because there is little external evidence of the actual damage. The amount of force that is applied to the body in a gunshot wound is most directly related to the caliber of the weapon and the distance the weapon was from the patient when it was fired. Point-blank or high-caliber gunshot wounds are high-force injuries. By comparison, the force that is exerted on the patient in stab injuries is minimal, even though these injuries can still be lethal.

The area of the body that is involved in penetrating trauma may be very difficult to predict. In gunshot wounds, the area that is involved may be predicted by

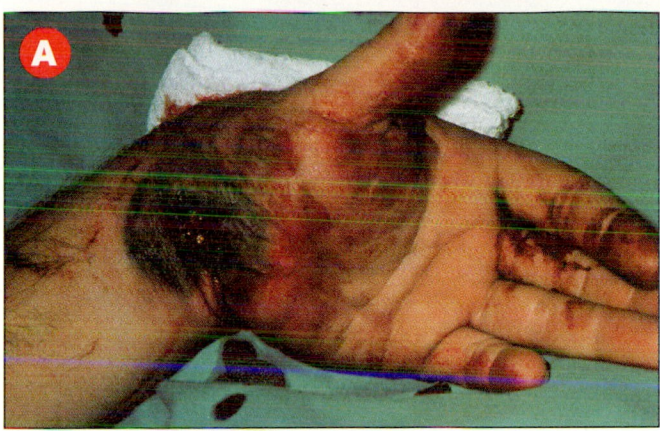

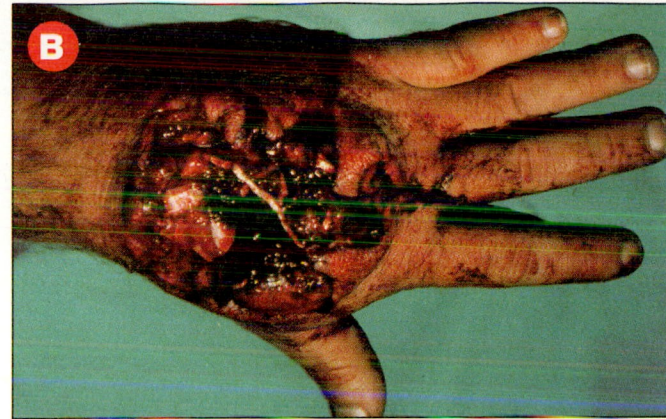

FIGURE 8-7 **A:** Entrance wound from a gunshot. **B:** Exit wound from a gunshot.

creating an imaginary line between the **entrance wound** and the **exit wound**, if one exists, although this is only an approximation at best (Figure 8-7). However, it is important to remember that bullets may bounce off dense bones or organs in the body, making the exact path almost impossible to determine. Some bullets are even designed to tumble or break apart after they enter the body.

In stab wounds, the body area that is involved can be estimated by looking at the location of entrance and the length of the instrument that was used in the stabbing, if known. Remember that you can only estimate the extent of the injury. An assailant may have moved the weapon in a back-and-forth motion after it entered the patient.

Number of patients. As part of your scene size-up, it is essential that you accurately determine the total number of patients. This determination is critical for your estimate of the need for additional resources, such as the HazMat team or a specialized rescue group. You should ask yourself the following questions when considering the need for additional resources:

- How many patients are there?
- What is the nature of their condition?
- Who contacted EMS?
- Is this a possible crime scene in which evidence may need to be preserved?
- Are hazardous materials, such as chemicals or leaking fuel, involved?
- Does the scene pose a threat to your or your patient's safety?

When there are multiple patients, you should call for additional units immediately and then begin triage

(Figure 8-8). **Triage** is a process of identifying the severity of each patient's condition. Once that is accomplished, you can begin to establish treatment and transport priorities. One EMT-B, usually the most experienced, should be assigned to perform triage. This process will help you to provide care and allocate your personnel and equipment resources most effectively and efficiently in a multiple-patient situation. If there is a large number of patients or if patient needs are greater than the available resources, put your local mass-casualty plan into action.

In these situations, you should always call for additional resources, such as law enforcement, the fire department, rescue units, ALS, and even utilities as soon as possible. It is never wrong to call for backup, even if the extra units are sent back. Remember, you are less likely to ask for help after you begin patient care because at that point, you are part of the scene, particularly at a motor vehicle crash in which patients require spinal immobilization.

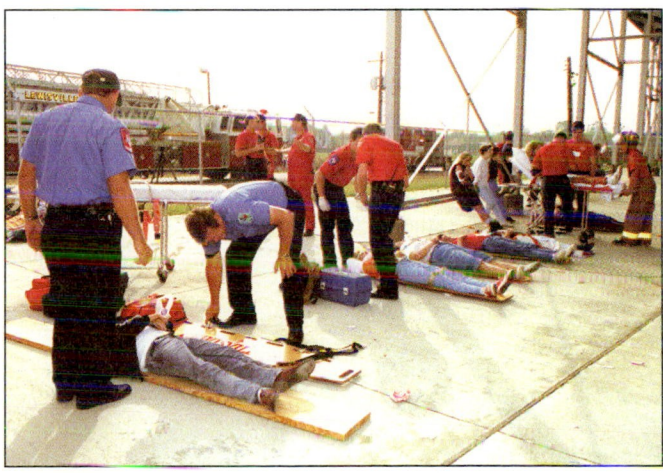

FIGURE 8-8 With multiple patients, you should call for additional resources and then begin triage.

Initial Assessment

During the prearrival and scene size-up phases, you speculated about the patient's condition, based on dispatch information, and asked and answered questions about scene safety. These steps are critically important, particularly in light of their role in ensuring your safety. However, patient assessment actually begins when you come into contact with the patient.

The patient assessment process consists of four steps:

1. The **initial assessment** helps you to identify any immediately or potentially life-threatening conditions and then begin appropriate treatment.

2. The **focused history and physical exam** help you to further evaluate the patient's major complaints or any problems that are immediately evident.

3. During the **detailed physical exam**, you gather information in situations in which the problem cannot be readily identified or you need more specific information about problems that were identified in the focused history and physical exam.

4. The **ongoing assessment** helps you to monitor problems that have already been identified and to assess the patient's response to treatment.

The <u>initial assessment</u> has a single, critical, all-important goal: to identify and initiate treatment of immediately or potentially life-threatening conditions. Information concerning life-threatening conditions comes from a variety of places, such as the visual appearance of the patient, the patient's chief complaint, or the nature of the patient's accident when trauma is involved. Remember that you should have mastered the components of basic life support before this so that you can draw on that knowledge as you provide life-saving care to treat immediately and potentially life-threatening conditions.

Table 8-3 (on page 216) lists the components of the initial assessment.

General Impression of the Patient

As you approach the scene and, ultimately, the patient, you will form a general impression of the patient. The <u>general impression</u> is based on your immediate assessment of the environment, the patient presenting signs and symptoms, and the patient's chief complaint.

Priorities of Care

This impression is important, because it helps you to determine the priorities of care, the mechanism of injury (if trauma was involved), the potential for life-threatening conditions, and the reliability of the information the patient is providing (Figure 8-9).

As you approach the scene, check to see whether the patient is moving or still, awake or unconscious, bleeding or not. Look for the mechanism of injury or the nature of the illness. Listen to what the patient and bystanders have to say. Make note of odors that suggest chemical hazards, smoke, or alcohol on the patient's breath. You can feel for pulses, pain, and deformities when you reach the patient. If the patient is responsive, try to learn as much as possible about what is wrong before you begin your examination. At this time, you should tell the patient your name, identify yourself as an EMT, and explain that you are there to help. You should learn the patient's age, race, gender, and chief complaint and continue to ask questions and talk to a responsive patient throughout the entire assessment.

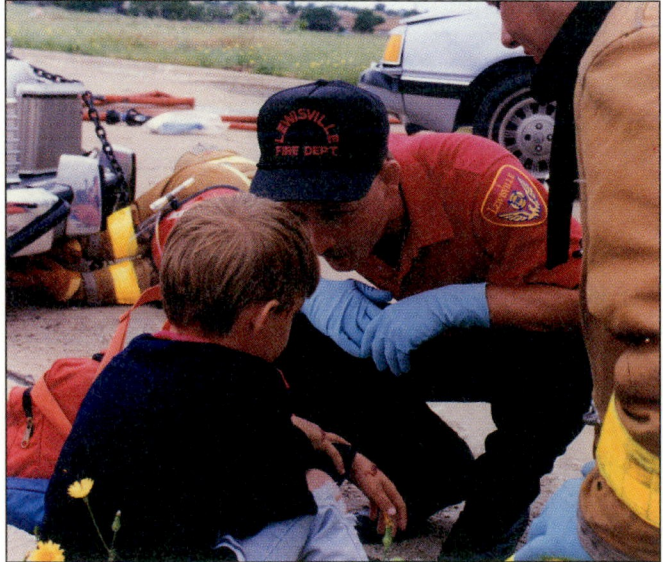

FIGURE 8-9 As you approach the patient, form a general impression of his or her overall condition.

PATIENT ASSESSMENT FLOWCHART

Initial Assessment

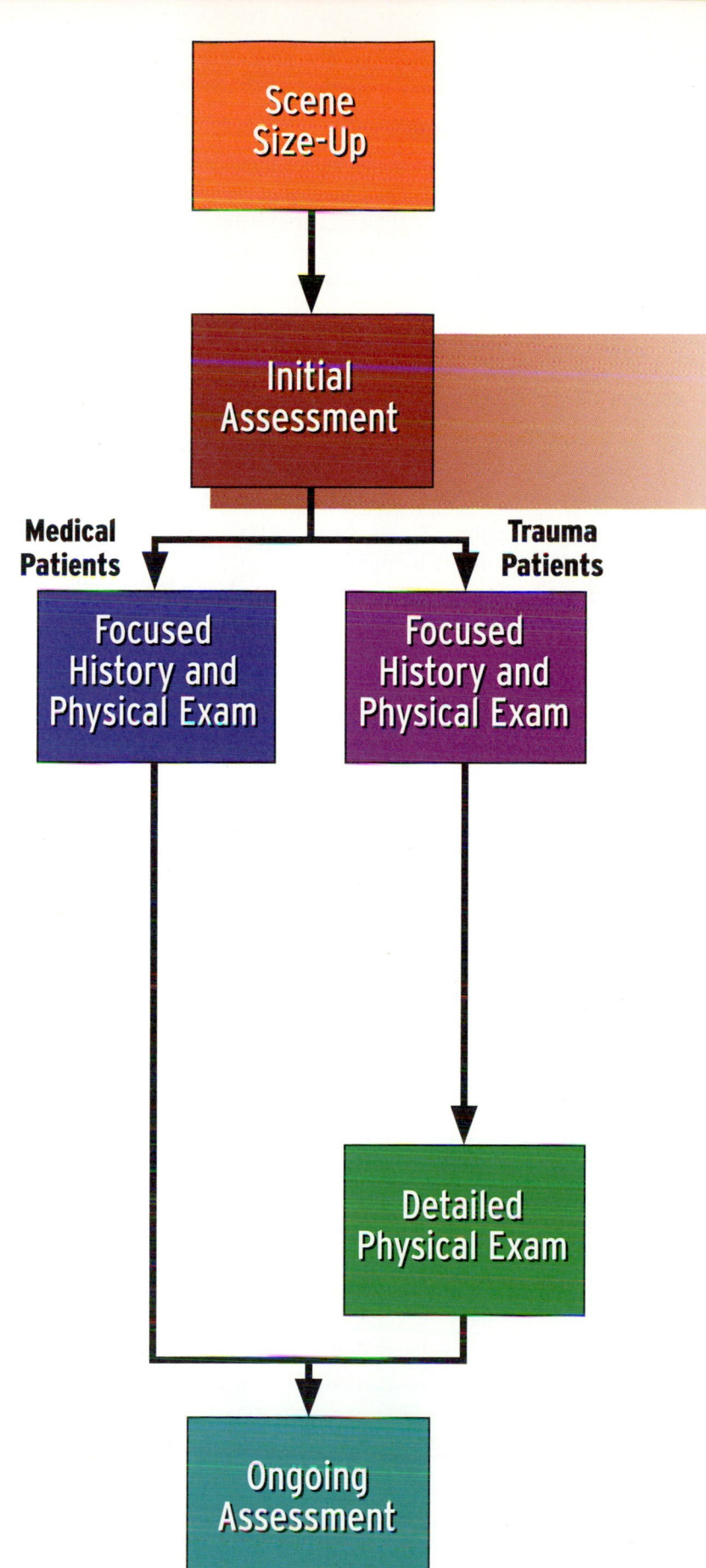

2

2

TABLE 8-3   Components of the Initial Assessment

Develop a General Impression

- Use the general impression as an overview of the relationship between the mechanism of injury or the nature of the illness, the chief complaint, how the patient presents, and the reliability of the information the patient has given you.
- Assess the patient for a life-threatening condition.

Assess Mental Status (in adults)

- Test for responsiveness:
  Check the patient's response to verbal, tactile, and painful stimuli.
- Test for orientation:
  Check the patient's memory of person, place, time, and event (referred to as alert and oriented times 4).
- Use the AVPU scale to describe patient responsiveness.

Assess Mental Status (in children)

- Determine whether the child is alert:
  Alert infants should track you with their eyes.
  Alert children older than age 2 years should know their own name and that of their parents.
  Alert school-age children should be able to tell you about holidays, school activities, and teachers' names.

Assess Airway

- Responsive patients—Clear airway:
  Talking or crying
- Responsive patients—Partially obstructed airway:
  Speaking only two to three words before each breath
  Retractions or use of accessory muscles
  Nasal flaring (in children)
  Labored breathing

Be prepared to open the airway, administer supplemental oxygen, assist ventilations, and initiate transport.

- Unresponsive patients—Partially obstructed airway:
  Any obvious trauma
  Noisy breathing
  Shallow or absent breathing

Open the airway using the head-tilt/chin-lift or jaw-thrust maneuver.

Assess the Adequacy of Breathing

- Shallow or deep respirations?
- Is the patient choking?
- Is the patient cyanotic?
- Is air moving into and out of the lungs?

If the patient has trouble breathing, make sure the airway is open, and give supplemental oxygen via nonrebreathing mask at 15 L/min. For patients who are breathing at less than 8 breaths/min or more than 24 breaths/min, administer a high concentration of oxygen and consider assisting ventilations. Consider a spinal injury in an unresponsive patient who has sustained a traumatic injury, and assist breathing with the proper airway adjunct if the patient is breathing at less than 8 breaths/min or more than 24 breaths/min.

Assess Circulation

- Assess the pulse.
- Identify any external bleeding.
- Evaluate the skin temperature, color, moisture.
- Check capillary refill.

Control external bleeding, assist ventilations, and perform CPR (in an unresponsive patient with no pulse). Consider an AED in an unresponsive patient with no obvious traumatic cause of cardiac arrest.

Identify Priority Patients for Immediate Care and Transport

- Consider:
  Poor general impression
  Unresponsive, with no gag or cough reflexes
  Responsive but unable to follow commands
  Difficulty breathing
  Pale skin/poor perfusion
  Complicated childbirth
  Uncontrolled bleeding
  Severe pain in any area of the body
  Steadily decreasing levels of consciousness
  Severe chest pain, with systolic blood pressure less than 100 mm Hg

Initiate transport as soon as is practical. Consider ALS backup.

You must answer the following questions to begin to form your general impression:

- Does the patient appear to have a life-threatening emergency? Clues could include unconsciousness, obvious difficulty breathing, and either cyanotic (blue) or very pale skin color. If you suspect a life-threatening condition, provide immediate care and transport.

- Was the patient in an accident? If so, what was the mechanism of injury? On the basis of the mechanism of injury, would you expect the patient to be severely injured? If so, assume the worst and begin treatment, including spinal immobilization.

- Does the patient appear coherent and able to answer questions? If not, you need to rely more heavily on your own assessment skills and/or the information that you can learn from others.

Distinguishing Medical and Trauma Patients

Remember that as an EMT-B, you will be called to treat an almost infinite number of different patient problems. Some patients will have a problem that is not related to an accident or trauma; these patients are typically referred to as medical patients. Others will have been injured in an incident such as a fall, a motor vehicle crash, or a shooting. These patients are usually considered trauma patients. In some situations, this distinction will be obvious. If the primary problem appears to be traumatic in origin, you will want to assume the worst and begin treatment, including spinal immobilization. However, quite frequently, it will not. For instance, a patient who falls at a long-term care facility could simply be treated as a trauma patient; however, it is also possible that the fall was caused by a medical condition such as an episode of fainting, a stroke, or even a heart attack. You will learn that it is not usually easy or prudent to label patients as medical or trauma until you have finished your assessment. *In many cases, medicine and trauma go hand in hand.*

For this reason, the assessment process does not encourage you to immediately differentiate between medical and trauma patients. Rather, the assessment process begins by assuming that all patients may have both medical and trauma aspects to their condition. Through the assessment process, you will develop an understanding of the patient's problems, both medical and traumatic, and will begin treatment on the basis of that understanding. This approach is both simpler and safer than an approach that starts with an unsupported assumption that the patient is either medical or trauma. As each call unfolds, your patient's primary problem will become apparent.

This rather general assessment is your opportunity to evaluate "the big picture" before you focus on the patient's specific needs, so use all of your senses in observing the scene and patient.

The first steps in caring for any patient focus on finding and treating the most life-threatening illnesses and injuries (Figure 8-10). Through all of these avenues, you need to ask and get answers to the following questions:

- Does the patient have an altered level of consciousness?

- Does the patient have an obstructed airway?

- Does the patient have inadequate breathing?

- Does the patient have inadequate circulation?

- Does the patient have the potential to develop any of these problems?

- Does the patient have the potential for a spinal cord injury?

If the answer to any of these questions is "yes," you need to take immediate action to resolve or prevent the life-threatening condition by doing one of the following: opening the airway, assisting ventilation, giving supplemental oxygen, stopping severe bleeding, performing spinal immobilization, providing transport, or calling for an ALS unit to assist or assume responsibility for patient care.

Approach to the Assessment Process

Remember, after developing a general impression of the patient, you should begin your assessment and care in this order of importance:

A = Airway

B = Breathing

C = Circulation

D = Disability (includes mental status)

E = Expose

In all cases, your assessment of the patient's airway, breathing, circulation, and disability (ABCD) will govern the extent of your treatment at the scene. In addition, particularly in the trauma patient, it is important to expose (E) the patient's body completely as soon as possible to facilitate a complete exam. Always give priority to emergency care of the ABCD to ensure life- and limb-saving treatment. Remember to assess the nature of the illness or the mechanism of injury as part of the assessment process.

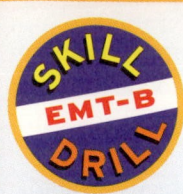

Performing the Initial Assessment
Figure 8-10

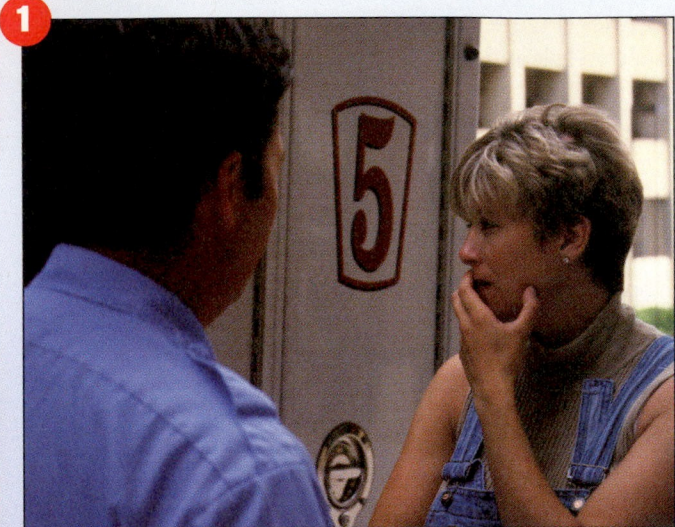

Observe the patient to form a general impression.

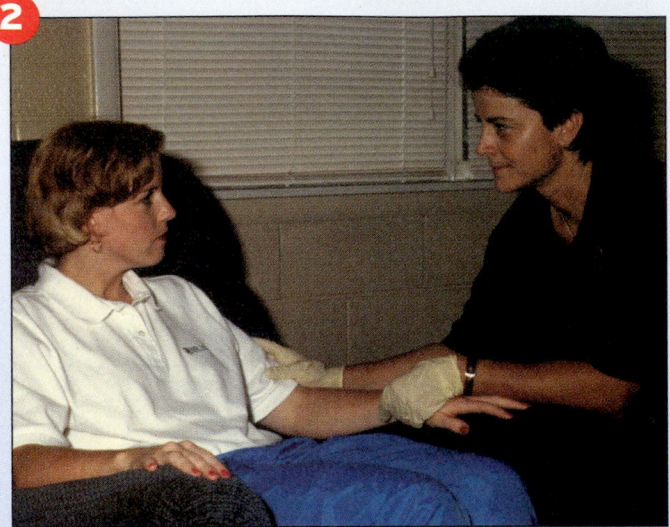

Assess the patient's mental status.

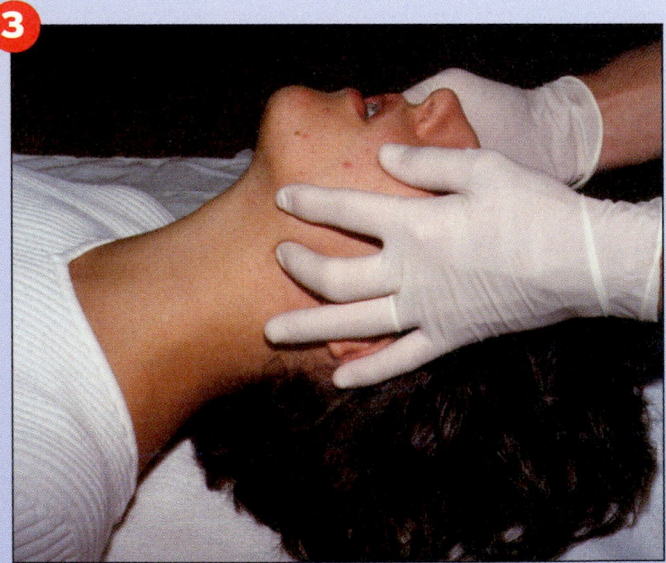

To open the airway of a trauma patient use a jaw-thrust or modified jaw-thrust maneuver, both of which are spine-sparing techniques. Manual immobilization may also be indicated.

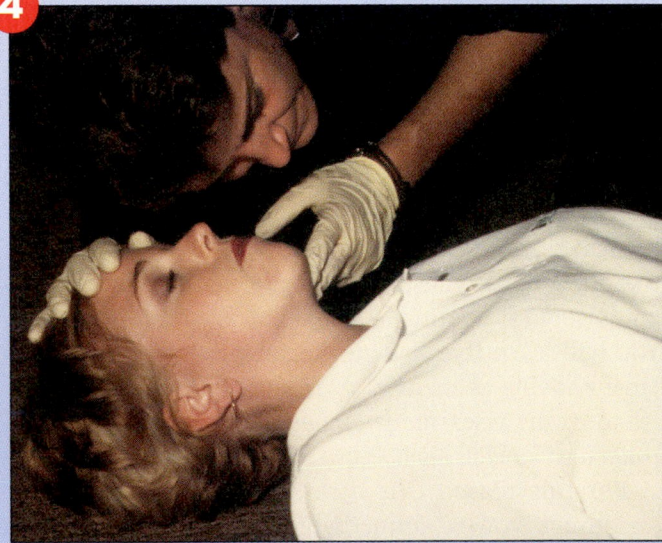

Assess breathing using the Look, Listen, and Feel technique. Give supplemental oxygen if necessary.

2

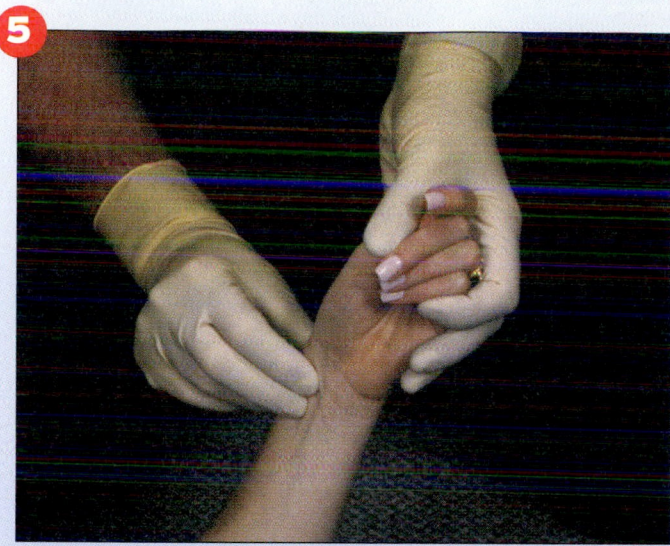

Assess the circulation by taking the pulse, and evaluating skin temperature and condition:

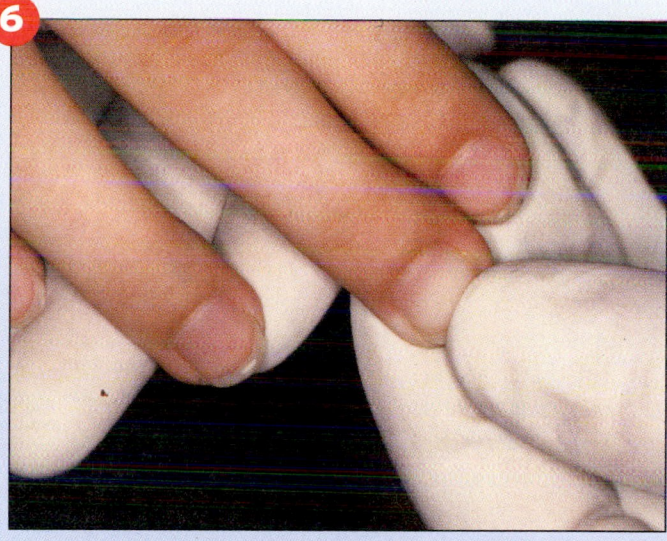

In children, test capillary refill to evaluate circulation.

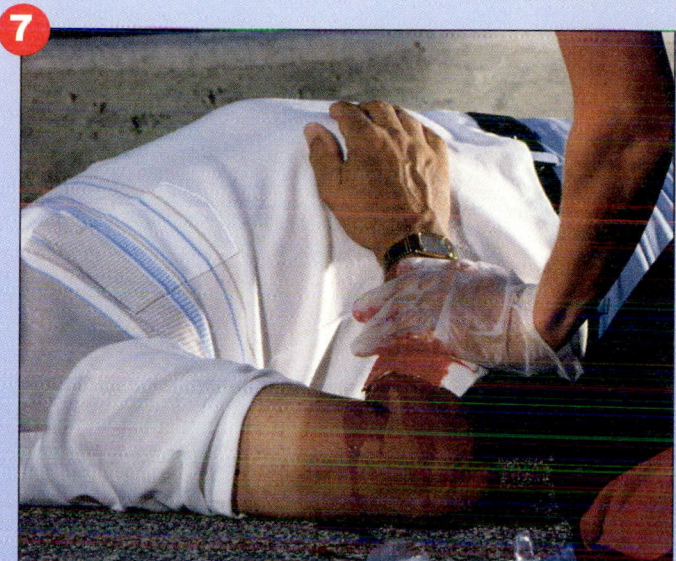

Assess for and control major bleeding.

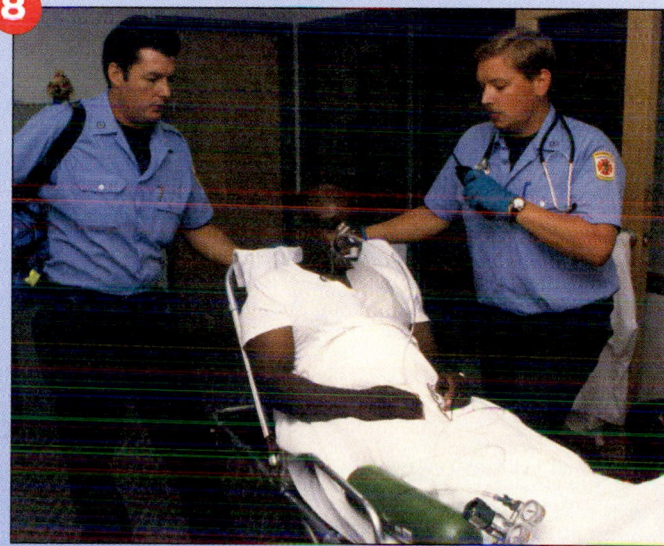

Prepare to treat or immediately transport the patient.

communication tip

People call 9-1-1 during some of the most difficult times of their lives. In some cases, they call because of a serious illness or injury. In others, they call because the patient or family is frightened, overwhelmed, or unable to cope with a more minor problem any longer. The patient is often fatigued, sick, frightened, angry, or sad, and the family often shares some or all of these feelings. Regardless of the exact nature of the call, the patient, family, and bystanders expect you to bring comfort, control, and resolution of these problems—emotional and physical.

In many ways, good communication skills are as important as technical proficiency, if not more so. Each step in the assessment process can be impeded by poor communication, and each can be immeasurably benefited by a good connection between you and the patient and family. Here are five tips that can vastly improve your communication skills during the assessment process:

1. **Do whatever you can, quickly, to make yourself and the patient comfortable.** Patients are uncomfortable communicating with someone who is standing over them, pacing, or looking away. When time permits, sit down and/or position yourself near the patient, introduce yourself, and ask the patient's name (Figure 8-11). This simple action signals the patient that you have time to talk; it opens the channels

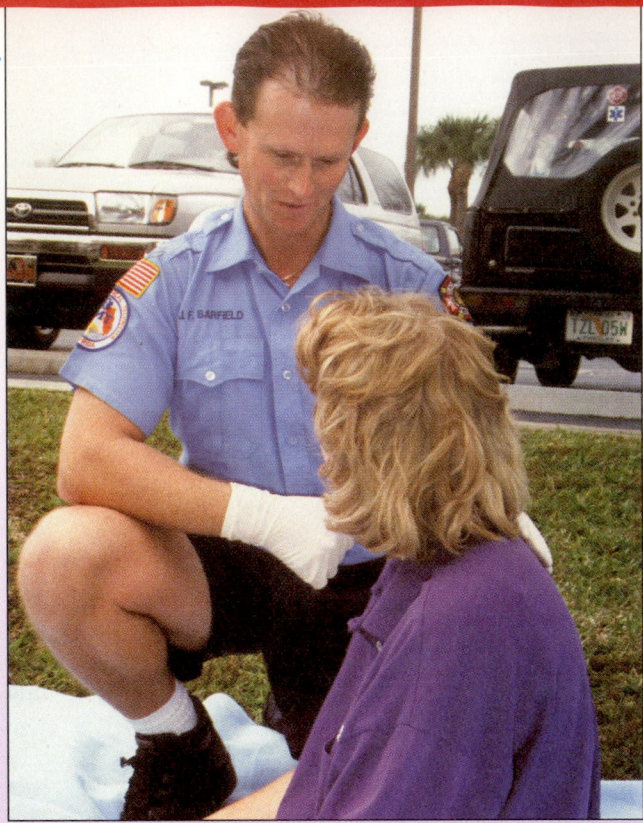

FIGURE 8-11 Position yourself near the patient, at eye level when possible, to begin to establish a relationship with the patient.

of communication as nothing else will. At the same time, be conscious of the patient's personal space. Do not move in too quickly. Ask the patient whether there is something you can do to make him or her more comfortable. Caring gestures and good body language are a visible demonstration of your care and concern.

Assessing Mental Status

Evaluating a patient's mental status and level of consciousness is an important part of the initial assessment because the mental status reflects the functioning of the brain. Remember to maintain spinal immobilization if needed. Many conditions may alter brain function and hence the level of consciousness. You will learn about many of these conditions as you progress through the EMT-B course.

Mental status and level of consciousness can be evaluated in just a few seconds by using two separate tests: responsiveness and orientation. The test for <u>responsiveness</u> assesses how well a patient responds to external stimuli, including verbal stimuli (sound), and tactile stimuli (touch). For a patient who is alert and responding to verbal stimuli, you should next evaluate orientation. <u>Orientation</u> tests assess mental status by checking the patient's memory of person (his or her name), place (the current location), time (the current year, month, and approximate date), and event (what happened). These four questions were not selected at random. They evaluate long-term memory (name and place if the patient is at home), intermediate-term memory (place and time), and short-term memory (event). If the patient knows these facts, the patient is said to be "alert and oriented times four" ("times four" refers to person, place, time, and event). An example of a patient who is not fully oriented would be one who is "alert and oriented times two, disoriented to time and event." Loss of intermediate- and long-term memory (person and place) is thought to be

2. **Actively listen to the patient.** In many cases, patients will be able to tell you what is wrong with them if you are paying attention and are truly listening. You can use several skills to actively listen, including leaning in toward the patient, taking selective notes, and periodically repeating back important points to the patient to ensure that you understood correctly. Active listening is often more difficult than it might seem, because scenes are often noisy and chaotic, and you will be receiving information from the patient, the family, your partner, and other EMS, fire, or law enforcement individuals on the scene. Try to screen them out for a few minutes so that you can truly listen to the patient; it will pay big dividends.

3. **Make eye contact with the person with whom you are speaking.** Eye contact signals that you are listening, so the patient is more likely to open up. An added benefit is that you will see facial expressions that, in some cases, communicate more clearly than the patient's words. For instance, you might see a facial grimace of pain or the averted eyes indicating embarrassment. Note that some cultures are uncomfortable with or offended by direct eye contact. Be sure to be familiar with the customs of people in your area.

4. **Base your initial questions on the patient's complaints.** No one likes to think that he or she is "just another patient." But that is what you communicate if you always ask the same questions of every patient, regardless of their complaints. If you ask questions about their Medicare number while they are trying to tell you about their pain, you are communicating that you are not really interested in their problem. Talk about their problem first, then ask paperwork questions.

5. **Before you start treatment, stop for a moment and mentally summarize what you have learned and what you are going to do, then tell the patient.** By providing necessary information to the patient and family, you help to relieve their anxiety and fear. This will also give them an opportunity to give you additional information if you have missed something.

You should spend your entire EMS career fine-tuning your patient assessment skills, as they are the cornerstone of high-quality prehospital care. A poor assessment almost always results in substandard patient care. Be sure to focus some of your energy on improving the communication process. You will make it easier for patients to feel comfortable around you, which will help them to give honest, direct answers to your questions. As a result, you will get better assessment information in less time.

related to more severe problems than loss of short-term memory. Collectively, your evaluation of the patient's responsiveness and orientation will paint a picture of the overall mental status.

Responsiveness can be evaluated by using the **AVPU** scale:

- **Alert.** The patient's eyes open spontaneously as you approach, and the patient appears aware of and responsive to the environment. The patient appears to follow commands, and the eyes visually track people and objects.

- **Responsive to Verbal Stimulus.** The patient's eyes do not open spontaneously. However, the patient's eyes do open to verbal stimuli, and the patient is able to respond in some meaningful way when spoken to.

caring for kids

Mental status may be difficult to evaluate in children. First, determine whether the child is alert. Even infants should be alert to your presence and should follow you with their eyes (a process called "tracking"). Ask the parent whether the child is behaving normally, particularly as regards alertness. All children older than age 2 years should know their own name and the names of their parents and siblings. Evaluate mental status in school-age children by asking about holidays, recent school activities, or teacher's names.

2

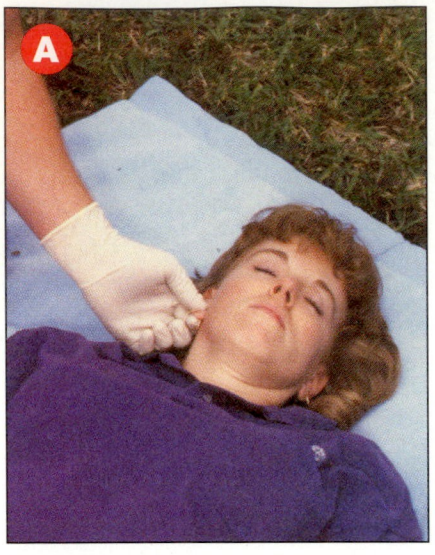
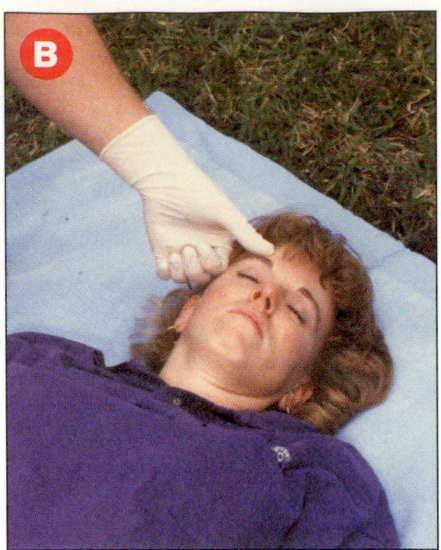
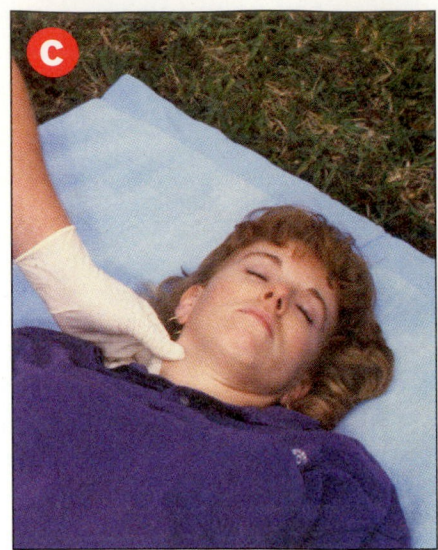

FIGURE 8-12 A: Gently but firmly pinch the patient's earlobe. **B:** Press down on the bone above the eye. **C:** Pinch the muscles of the neck.

- **Responsive to <u>P</u>ain.** The patient does not respond to your questions but moves or cries out in response to a painful stimulus. This response is tested by gently but firmly pinching the patient's earlobe, by pressing down on the bone above the eye, or by pinching the muscles of the neck (Figure 8-12). The sternal rub, although advocated in CPR training, is not recommended because it may be inaccurate in patients with cervical spine injuries. The use of ammonia "smelling salts" is also not recommended. An appropriate response is moaning or pushing away or withdrawing from the pinch. Use of extremely painful stimuli is never appropriate.

- **<u>Unresponsive.</u>** The patient does not respond to any stimuli.

If you are in doubt about whether a patient is truly unconscious, assume the worst and treat appropriately.

An abnormal mental status may be caused by a wide variety of conditions, including head trauma, hypoxemia, hypoglycemia, stroke, cardiac problems, or drug use. If the patient has an abnormal mental status, you should rapidly complete the initial assessment and be prepared to give high-flow supplemental oxygen, consider spinal immobilization if trauma is suspected, and initiate transport. Support the ABCD as required, and continually reassess for changes in the patient's condition.

> Airway obstruction in an unconscious patient is most commonly due to relaxation of the tongue muscles back into throat.

Assessing the Airway

As you move through the steps of assessment, you must always be alert for signs of respiratory compromise or airway obstruction. Regardless of the cause, airway obstruction may result in inadequate or absent air flow into and out of the lungs, which may cause permanent damage to the brain, heart, and lungs or may even result in death.

Responsive Patients

Patients of any age who are responsive and are talking or crying have an open airway. However, watching and listening to how patients speak, particularly those with respiratory problems, may provide important clues about the adequacy of their airway and breathing status.

If you identify an airway problem, stop the assessment process, and open the airway using the head-tilt/chin-lift or jaw-thrust maneuver. Although airway and breathing problems are not the same, their signs and symptoms often overlap. A patient who can speak only two to three words without pausing to take a breath, a condition known as <u>two- to three-word dyspnea</u>, has a severe airway obstruction (a narrowing of the airways caused by trauma or disease) or other breathing problem. The presence of retractions or the use of the <u>accessory muscles</u> of respiration is also a sign of airway obstruction. <u>Nasal flaring</u> and use of the accessory muscles indicate that a child has an airway obstruction. Finally, obviously labored breathing is also a sign of airway or breathing difficulties.

Any of these signs may signal an immediate or pending airway and/or breathing problem. You should be prepared to open the airway, administer supplemental oxygen, assist ventilation, and initiate transport.

Unresponsive Patients

With an unresponsive patient or one with diminished responsiveness, you should immediately assess the patency of the airway. If it is clear, you can continue your assessment. If the airway is not clear, your next priority is to open it using the head-tilt/chin-lift or jaw-thrust maneuver. Airway obstruction in an unconscious patient is most commonly due to relaxation of the tongue muscles back into throat. Dentures, blood clots, vomitus, mucus, food, or other foreign objects may also create a blockage. Signs of airway obstruction in an unconscious patient include the following:

- Obvious trauma, blood, or other obstruction
- Noisy breathing, such as bubbling, gurgling, crowing, or other abnormal sounds (Normal breathing is quiet.)
- Extremely shallow or absent breathing (Airway obstruction may cause impaired breathing.)

To open the airway, positioning depends on the patient's age and size. For medical patients, perform the head-tilt/chin-lift maneuver. For trauma patients or those with illness of an unknown nature, the cervical spine should be stabilized and immobilized, and, if necessary, the jaw-thrust maneuver should be performed.

Assessing Breathing

As you assess the patient's breathing, look at how much work it takes for the patient to breathe. Normal respirations are not unusually shallow or excessively deep, and their rate varies widely in adults, anywhere from 12 to 20 breaths/min. Shallow respirations can be identified by movement of the chest wall. Conversely, deep respirations cause a great deal of chest wall rise and fall and often can be heard as large volumes of air moving into and out of the patient's lungs. As you assess the patient, ask yourself the following questions:

- Are the patient's respirations shallow or deep?
- Does the patient appear to be choking?
- Is the patient cyanotic (blue)?
- Is the patient moving air into and out of the lungs as the chest rises and falls?

If a patient seems to have difficulty breathing, you should immediately reevaluate the airway. Once the airway is open, you should consider assisting ventilation with a BVM device for all patients with respirations greater than 24/min or less than 8/min.

Any patient with a decreased level of consciousness, respiratory distress, or poor skin color should also receive high-flow oxygen. If there is no risk of spinal cord injury, the patient should remain in a comfortable position that supports breathing; this is typically sitting up with the legs dangling. In any patient who has a possible risk for spinal injury, you should immobilize the spine, ensuring that respirations are not compromised while you restrict spinal motion.

You should give supplemental oxygen via a nonrebreathing mask at 15 L/min. Any patient whom you identify as having immediate or potential airway or breathing problems should be given supplemental oxygen. Never withhold oxygen from any patient at the scene!

Use the Look, Listen, and Feel technique to evaluate how well an unconscious patient is breathing. If the patient does not appear to be breathing or has an inadequate airway, start airway management immediately, and assist ventilation. This technique is equally effective in most patients, although it may be more difficult in infants and small children because they have so little chest wall movement during respirations.

In most cases, a spinal injury should be considered a possibility for any unresponsive trauma patient. These patients must be rolled or moved as a single unit onto a flat surface or backboard. The timing for this maneuver depends on the patient's position when you find him or her. If the patient must be moved to access the face or manage the airway, it should be done immediately. Otherwise, you should log roll the patient after you attend to ABCD. Remember, you must move the head, neck, torso, and legs as a unit without any unnecessary bending or twisting.

Once the patient is properly positioned and the airway is opened, you may begin to support the patient's breathing. For patients with respirations of 24/min or more, or 8/min or less (i.e., inadequate breathing), you should assist breathing with the proper airway adjunct.

If the patient is not breathing, open and maintain the airway and provide rescue breathing using the appropriate airway adjunct. In all cases, supplemental oxygen should be given.

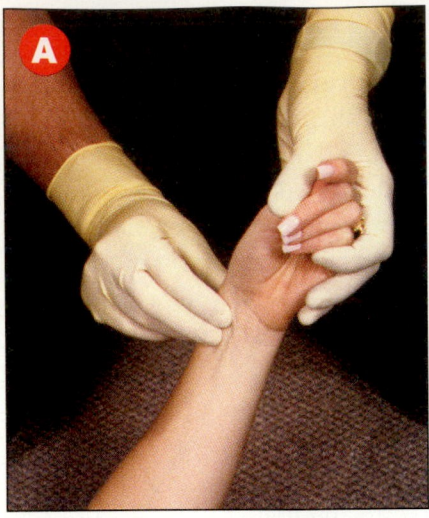
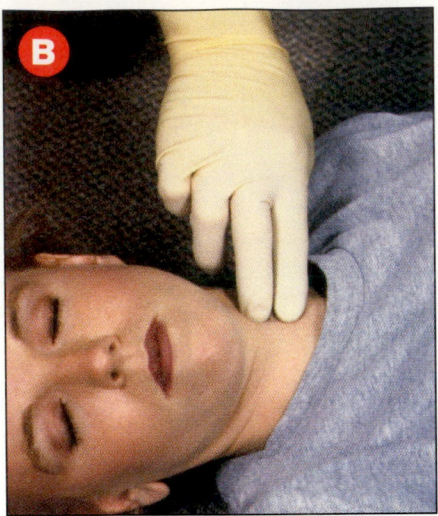
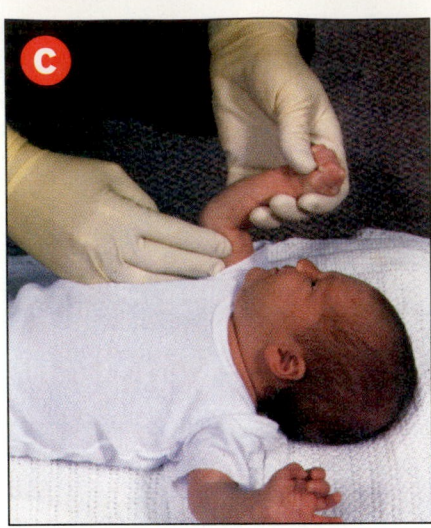

FIGURE 8-13 A: Palpate the radial artery to initially evaluate the pulse. **B:** Palpate the carotid artery if you cannot feel a pulse at the radial artery. **C:** In infants palpate the brachial artery to evaluate the pulse.

Assessing Circulation

Assessing circulation helps you to evaluate how well blood is circulating to the major organs, including the brain, lungs, heart, kidneys, and rest of the body. A variety of problems can impair circulation, including blood loss, shock, conditions that affect the heart, and conditions that affect the major blood vessels. Circulation is evaluated by assessing the presence and qualities of the pulse, identifying external bleeding, and evaluating skin condition.

If the patient has a pulse but is still not breathing, continue rescue breathing at a rate of 12 to 20 breaths/min for an adult, or 20 to 25 breaths/min for a child, until the patient begins breathing adequately again. You should assess the pulse to determine whether rescue breathing has been effective in an unresponsive patient. When rescue breathing is not done properly, the pulse will stop, and the patient will soon go into cardiac arrest. If this occurs, you should begin CPR immediately.

Assessing the Pulse

The rate, rhythm, and strength of the patient's pulse will give you a rough idea of the overall status of the patient's cardiac function. The pulse is one of the vital signs that you should monitor continuously in most patients, even en route to the hospital. Pulse rate is measured by palpating (feeling) an artery at a pulse point, which is an area where an artery lies close to the surface of the skin (Figure 8-13) and is expressed in terms of beats per minute. As you evaluate the pulse, note whether it is strong or weak and whether it is regular or irregular. For an alert, responsive patient, the

contact from your hands taking the pulse can be a very reassuring gesture.

The most common place to **palpate** (examine by touch) for the pulse in an adult patient is at the wrist, along the radial artery. If you cannot feel a pulse at either wrist, you should try to find it in the neck at the carotid artery. The carotid pulse is easier to locate than the radial pulse, especially if the patient has low blood pressure. The carotid pulse is most easily located by first finding the patient's Adam's apple at the front of the neck. You should then slide your index and middle fingers along one side of the neck until you feel the pulse. The carotid pulse can be felt along a groove between the larynx (voice box) and one of the neck muscles. In an unresponsive patient, you should always palpate the carotid pulse. Although the normal pulse rate varies depending upon the patient's underlying physical conditions, most sources suggest that a pulse rate of 60 to 100 beats/min is normal in adults.

If you do not find a pulse, even at the carotid artery, you must take immediate action. For a medical patient over 8 years old or greater than 55 lb, start CPR and apply an AED. For a medical patient under 8 or who weighs less than 55 lb, start CPR. For a trauma patient of any age in cardiac arrest, start CPR.

Assessing and Controlling External Bleeding

The next step is to identify any major external bleeding. In some instances, blood loss can be very rapid and can quickly result in shock and even death. Therefore, this step demands your immediate attention as soon as the patient's airway is secured and breathing is stabilized. Signs of blood loss include active bleeding from wounds

caring for kids

You can feel the pulse of a child at the carotid artery, as in an adult. However, palpating this pulse in an infant may present a problem. Because an infant's neck is often very short and fat, and its pulse is often quite fast, you may have a hard time finding the carotid pulse. Therefore, in infants younger than one year of age, you should palpate the brachial artery to assess the pulse. Normal pulse rates for children are shown in Table 8-4.

TABLE 8-4	Normal Pulse Rates in Infants and Children
Age	**Range**
Newborn	120 to 160
Infant	120 to 140
1 to 3 years	100 to 110
3 to 5 years	90 to 100
5 to 10 years	80 to 100
10 to 15 years	60 to 90
Over 15 years	Adult normal ranges

and/or evidence of bleeding such as blood on the clothes or near the patient. Serious bleeding from a large vein may be characterized by steady blood flow. Bleeding from an artery is characterized by a spurting flow of blood. When you evaluate an unconscious patient, do a sweep for blood by quickly and lightly running your gloved hands from head to toe, pausing periodically to see whether your gloves are bloody.

Controlling external bleeding is often very simple. In almost all instances, direct pressure with your gloved hand and a sterile bandage over the bleeding site will control bleeding. This pressure stops the flow of blood and helps the blood to **coagulate**, or clot naturally. Remember that you must follow BSI techniques whenever you may be exposed to blood or other body fluids.

Most often, bleeding can be adequately controlled by using direct pressure over the bleeding site, along with elevating the extremity if bleeding is on the arms or legs. When direct pressure and elevation are not successful, you may apply pressure directly over arterial pressure points. Another option to control bleeding is use of the pneumatic antishock garment (PASG) for widespread bleeding over the legs and/or pelvic region. However, there are a number of precautions regarding the PASG; these, along with specific information on bleeding control, are described in Chapters 24 and 25 on bleeding and shock.

Evaluating Skin Color, Temperature, and Condition

Assessing the skin is one of the most important and most readily accessible ways of evaluating circulation. You should assess the patient's skin color, temperature, and moisture, as well as look for bleeding.

Color. Skin color depends on pigmentation and blood oxygen levels, as well as the amount of blood circulating through the vessels of the skin. For this reason, skin color is a valuable assessment tool. The normal skin color of lightly pigmented people is pinkish. Deeply pigmented skin may hide color changes that result from illness or injury. Therefore, you should look for changes in color in areas of the skin that have less pigment: the fingernail beds, the sclera (white of the eyes), the conjunctiva (lining of the eyelid), and the mucous membranes of the mouth. Normal skin color, particularly of the conjunctivae and mucous membranes, is pinkish. Skin colors that should alert you to possible medical problems include cyanosis (blue), flushed (red), pale (white), and jaundice (yellow).

Temperature. The skin is actually an organ, and like all other organs, it has many functions. It helps maintain the water content of the body, acts as insulation and protection from infection, and also plays a role in regulation of body temperature. Normal body temperature is 98.6°F (37°C), but it can change as a result of illness or injury. Assess the skin temperature by touching the patient's skin with your wrist or the back of your hand (Figure 8-14).

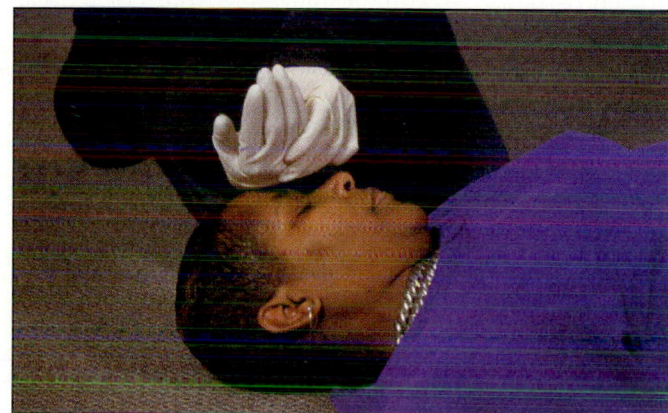

FIGURE 8-14 Assess skin temperature by touching the patient's skin with the back of hand.

2

When rescue breathing
is not done properly, the pulse will stop,
and the patient will soon
go into cardiac arrest.

Condition. Finally, determine whether the patient's skin is dry or moist. The skin is normally warm and dry. Cool or cold, moist, clammy skin suggests shock. Hot skin may indicate an abnormally elevated body temperature.

Evaluating capillary refill. Another way to assess circulation is to check capillary refill, especially in infants and children. <u>Capillary refill</u> is the ability of the circulatory system to restore blood to the capillaries after circulation has been interrupted. You test capillary refill by squeezing the patient's fingernail bed until the area blanches (turns white) (Figure 8-15). Next release the fingernail bed, and watch for it to return to a normal color. The area should return to its normal color within two seconds. If the area remains white or becomes blue, you know that circulation is inadequate, at least in the area being tested.

Capillary refill can be checked in children by squeezing the entire arm or leg at a distal point and observing the return to normal color. Although capillary refill is a quick and very general way to evaluate circulation, it is important to remember that other conditions, not related to the body's circulation, may also slow capillary refill. These conditions include the patient's age and gender, as well as exposure to a cold environment (<u>hypothermia</u>), frozen tissue (<u>frostbite</u>), or injuries to bones or muscles that cause local circulatory compromise.

Restoring circulation. If a patient has inadequate circulation, you must take immediate action to restore or improve circulation, stop severe bleeding, and improve oxygen delivery to the tissues. The apparent *absence* of a palpable pulse in a *responsive* patient is not caused by cardiac arrest. Therefore, do not begin CPR in a responsive patient. However, if you cannot feel a pulse in an unresponsive adult patient, you should immediately begin CPR and, whenever possible and indicated, prepare to defibrillate. Remember to follow BSI techniques, which may include use of a barrier device for ventilation, gloves, and perhaps goggles. Follow these

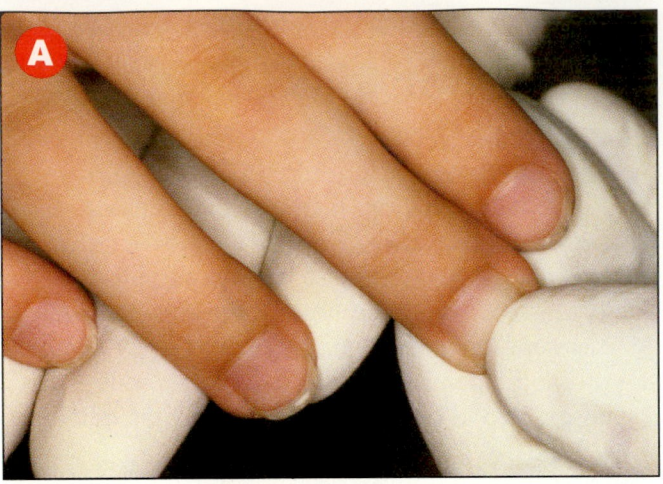

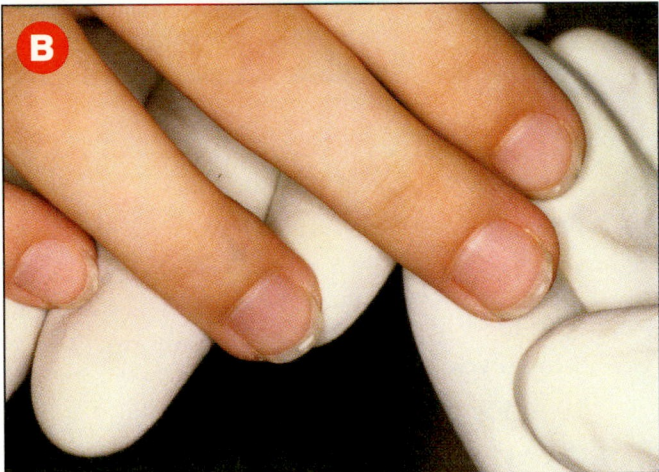

FIGURE 8-15 A: Test capillary refill by squeezing the patient's fingernail bed until the area blanches. **B:** Release the fingernail and watch for it to return to its normal color.

five steps in a patient who has no pulse and is unresponsive:

1. **Immediately begin CPR** if no automated external defibrillator (AED) is available. If an AED is readily available, apply it first.

2. **Prepare to deliver AED** if the patient is older than 8 years of age or weighs more than 55 lb and has no obvious traumatic cause of cardiac arrest. Local protocols may vary on the age and weight requirements for AED use.

3. **If the cardiac arrest is associated** with an obvious, apparently catastrophic traumatic event, perform CPR without preparing for use of the AED. Traumatic arrests do not typically respond to defibrillation. Treatment should include initiation of airway control, ventilation, and chest compressions, followed by transport to the

hospital. If time allows application of the AED, it should be done by briefly stopping the ambulance. Immediate transport to the hospital, preferably a trauma center, is the most valuable therapy for the patient in traumatic cardiac arrest.

4. **Initiate use of the AED** in association with CPR, if in doubt about a traumatic origin of the arrest.

5. **Prepare for immediate transport** to an appropriate facility.

Continued impaired circulation is devastating to the body's cells because it denies them vital oxygen, which is necessary for cell function. CPR and bleeding control are intended to maintain or improve circulation. Oxygen delivery is improved through the administration of supplemental oxygen. Any patient with impaired circulation should receive high-flow oxygen via a non-rebreathing mask or assisted ventilations to improve oxygen delivery at the cellular level.

Identifying Priority Patients

Once you have completed the initial assessment, you have to make some decisions about patient care. You should have already addressed life-threatening injuries and/or illnesses as they are found. Next, you must identify priority patients, or those who need other interventions and/or immediate transport.

Patients with one of the following conditions should be given priority care and/or immediate transport or be considered for ALS backup:

- Poor general impression
- Unresponsive with no gag or cough reflexes
- Responsive but unable to follow commands
- Difficulty breathing
- Pale skin or other signs of poor perfusion
- Complicated childbirth
- Uncontrolled bleeding
- Severe pain in any area of the body
- Severe chest pain, especially when the systolic blood pressure is less than 100 mm Hg
- Inability to move any part of the body

Correct identification of high-priority patients is an essential aspect of the initial assessment and helps to improve patient outcome.

While initial treatment is important, it is essential to remember that immediate transport is one of the keys to the survival of any high priority patient. Transport should be initiated as soon as is practical and possible. Once you have completed the initial assessment, you can turn to the focused history and physical exam.

From here you proceed to the appropriate focused history and physical exam based on your current assessment of whether the patient you are treating has problems of traumatic origin, medical origin, or both.

Focused History and Physical Exam: Trauma Patients

You now have dispatch information and information from both the scene size-up and initial assessment. These have provided you with valuable information about the scene, allowing you to anticipate what you will find and prepare for hazards. If your patient had problems with ABCD, you have stabilized any life-threatening conditions, perhaps provided spinal immobilization, and initiated transport.

How do you proceed now? Your patient may have, almost literally, one or more of a million different problems. How do you identify, prioritize, and treat this variety of potential problems?

Goals of the Focused History and Physical Exam

The <u>focused history and physical exam</u> help you to focus on specific problems. They have three goals:

1. Identify the patient's chief complaint.
   - What happened to this patient?
2. Understand the specific circumstances surrounding the chief complaint.
   - What circumstances were associated with the event?
   - Is the mechanism of injury a high risk for serious injuries?
   - Has this happened before? What were the cause and treatment then?
3. Direct further physical examination.
   - What problems can be identified through the physical exam?

The focused history and physical exam, like the entire assessment process, guide you to take actions that will stabilize or relieve the patient's problems. Depending on the answers to these questions, you should be prepared to return to the initial assessment if potentially life-threatening conditions are identified, perform spinal immobilization, provide transport or coordinate transfer of the patient to an ALS unit, and/or treat problems that you identify during the exam.

Patients who call 9-1-1 following an acute event may have any number of problems-medical, traumatic, or a combination of both. Unfortunately, patients do not wear signs identifying them as "medical" or "trauma." Furthermore, the circumstances surrounding the event may ultimately identify medical causes of trauma or traumatic problems that worsened a medical condition. For this reason, to consider any patient strictly as "medical" or "trauma" is difficult and often inaccurate. Rather, you should assess and manage all patients in the same systematic fashion. However, as each case unfolds, it will often become apparent that the call is predominantly traumatic or medical in nature. When this occurs, you should focus your assessment on the medical or traumatic aspects of the case.

Once you have identified that a patient has sustained a traumatic injury, you need to rapidly make some important treatment and transport decisions. This is because some traumatic injuries are life-threatening and cannot be treated in the field. These patients have the best chance for survival if they arrive at an appropriate hospital, usually a trauma center if available, for definitive care within 60 minutes of the time of injury. You will often hear this period of time called the Golden Hour. The <u>Golden Hour</u> is the time during which treatment of shock or traumatic injuries is most critical and survival potential is the best (Figure 8-16). After the first 60 minutes, the body has increasing difficulty in compensating for traumatic injuries.

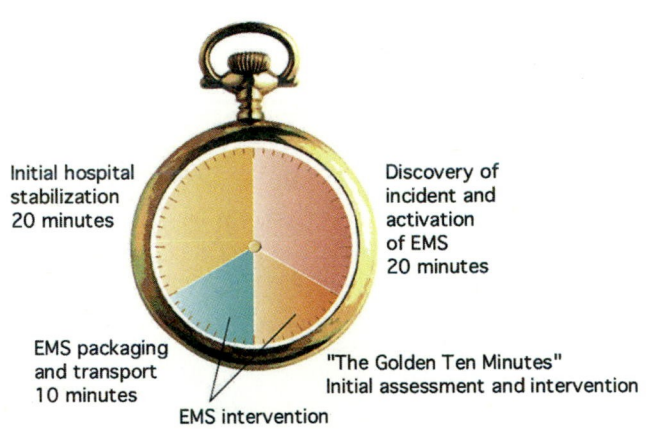

FIGURE 8-16 The Golden Hour is the time during which treatment of shock or traumatic injuries is most critical and the potential for survival is best.

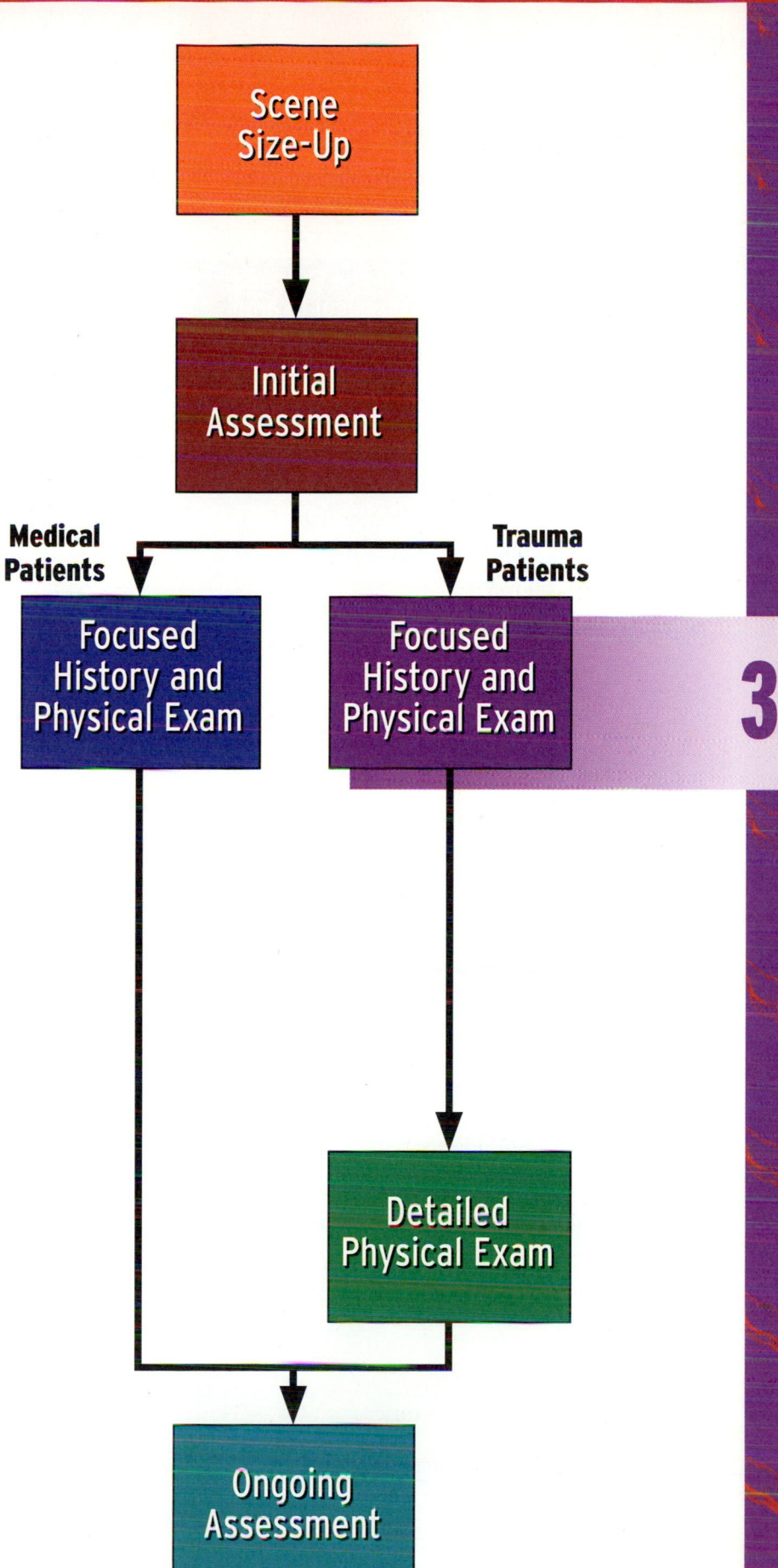

3

For this reason, you should spend as little of the Golden Hour as possible on the scene with patients who have sustained significant or severe trauma. Table 8-5 lists the components of the focused history and physical exam for the trauma patient.

TABLE 8-5	**Components of the Focused History and Physical Exam: Trauma Patient**

Significant Mechanism of Injury

- Ejection from a vehicle
- A death in the passenger compartment
- A fall greater than 20′ (greater than 10′ for children)
- Vehicle rollover
- High-speed vehicle collision
- Medium-speed vehicle collision (for children)
- Vehicle-pedestrian collision
- Motorcycle accident
- Bicycle collision (for children)
- Unresponsiveness or altered mental status
- Hidden injuries from seat belts, airbags, etc.

Reconsider the Mechanism of Injury

- Perform a rapid trauma assessment (on either a responsive or unresponsive patient).
- Take a set of baseline vital signs.
- Obtain a SAMPLE history.

No Significant Mechanism of Injury

- Assess the chief complaint.
- Perform a focused assessment.
- Take a set of baseline vital signs.
- Obtain a SAMPLE history.

Reconsider the Mechanism of Injury

As part of the scene size-up, you evaluated the mechanism of injury before you began treatment. At this point in the assessment process, you should look at the mechanism again to ensure that you have not missed important information. Understanding the mechanism of injury helps you to understand the severity of the patient's problem and provide invaluable information to hospital staff as well. Some patients have experienced a significant mechanism of injury; others clearly have not.

Significant Mechanisms of Injury

Significant mechanisms of injury include the following:

- Ejection from a vehicle
- A death in the passenger compartment
- Fall greater than 20′
- Vehicle rollover
- High-speed vehicle collision
- Vehicle-pedestrian collision
- Motorcycle crash
- Unresponsiveness or altered mental status
- Penetrating head, chest, or abdominal trauma
- Hidden injuries from seat belts, airbags, etc.

Infant and Child Considerations

Significant mechanisms of injury for children include the above with the following additions or modifications:

- Fall greater than 10′
- Bicycle crash
- Medium-speed vehicle collision

Hidden Injuries

Seat belts and airbags have significantly reduced the death and disability that are associated with motor vehicle accidents. However, you should be aware that seat belts and airbags can also cause injuries. When evaluating a patient who was involved in a motor vehicle crash, you should ask questions to determine whether seat belts and/or an airbag was involved.

Seat belts. Seat belts have prevented many thousands of injuries and have saved countless thousands of lives. Patients who otherwise would have been thrown out of a smashed car owe their lives to seat belts. However, if the force of a crash is great enough, patients can have bruises

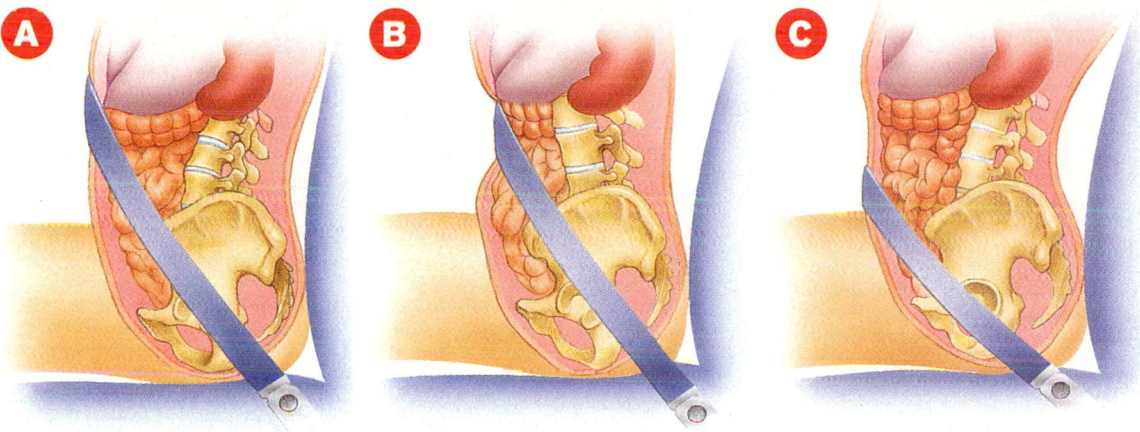

FIGURE 8-17 A: Injury may occur if the seat belt is placed too far above the iliac crest. **B:** A sudden stop could cause compression of the organs between the belt and the spine. **C:** The proper location of the seat belt is at the hip joints.

under the seat belts and possible internal injuries, although these injuries are less severe than the injuries the patients would have if they had not been wearing seat belts. Seat belts that are worn improperly across the abdomen rather than across the pelvic bones increase the potential for internal injuries (Figure 8-17). Lap seat belts must be worn so that they lie below the iliac crests, snugly up against the hip joints. If the seat belt is worn too high, sudden slowing or an abrupt stop might result in abdominal injuries. Occasionally, injuries of the lumbar spine can occur, even if the patient is wearing the seat belt properly.

Lap belts and shoulder belts are now commonly combined into a single unit. Some cars still have separate lap and shoulder belts. Used alone, shoulder belts can cause injuries of the chest, ribs, and liver.

Airbags. Airbags represent a great advance in automotive safety. Before airbags were common, individuals in head-on crashes would have significant facial injuries and bleeding—clear, visible signs that they had been injured. With airbags, patients occasionally have facial burns or respiratory problems from the chemical process that causes the airbag to expand, or they may have abrasions from the airbag itself. However, with airbags and seat belts, patients may or may not have visible injuries. Remember, while patients who have been involved in serious accidents may look fine, they may have internal injuries.

When an airbag deploys, a patient who is not wearing a seat belt can still go up and over, or down and under, the steering column. You should always look under a deployed air bag to see whether the steering wheel is bent or deformed in any way (Figure 8-18). Remove the patient from the car, using spinal precautions if indicated by patient complaint or mechanism of injury. If the wheel is bent or deformed in any way, you should

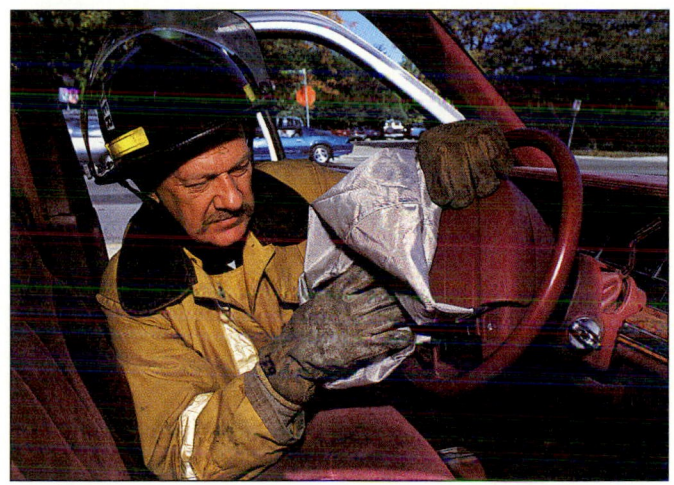

FIGURE 8-18 If an airbag has deployed, you should lift the airbag and check the steering wheel to see whether it is bent.

suspect possible internal injuries. Internal injuries may also be possible if the steering wheel is not bent or deformed. The general health of the patient, the patient's age, and other factors can also impact the likelihood for internal injuries.

During your hand-off report at the hospital, make sure that you tell hospital personnel whether seat belts were worn—and if so, whether they were worn correctly (if you can tell)—and whether the airbag deployed.

> Understanding the mechanism of injury helps you to estimate the severity of the patient's problem.

Trauma Patients With Significant Mechanism of Injury

The rapid trauma assessment should be performed on any patient with significant mechanism of injury, to identify life-threatening injuries. The purpose of this assessment is to zero in on the patient's problems, and identify potentially life-threatening conditions, which will direct your physical exam. The rapid trauma assessment should be performed on responsive and unresponsive patients alike. Remember, you can use a responsive patient as a resource; you should ask him or her about symptoms throughout your assessment.

An integral part of this assessment is evaluation using the simple mnemonic "DCAP-BTLS." For each area of the body, you should quickly look for Deformities, Contusions, Abrasions, Punctures/Penetrations, Burns, Tenderness, Lacerations, and Swelling (DCAP-BTLS). Remember, you should interrupt your assessment to stabilize any immediately or potentially life-threatening conditions. Once these conditions have been stabilized, you may continue with your assessment.

Patient Assessment Process

Trauma Patient with a Significant Mechanism of Injury	Trauma Patient with No Significant Mechanism of Injury

Scene Size-Up

Initial Assessment

Focused History/Physical Exam*

• Reconsider mechanism of injury	• Assess chief complaint
• Rapid trauma assessment	• Focused assessment of area of complaint
• Baseline vital signs	• Baseline vital signs
• SAMPLE history	• SAMPLE history

Detailed Physical Exam

• Area by area exam*	• Area by area exam*

On-Going Assessment*

* If appropriate

Rapid Trauma Assessment

The steps of the rapid assessment for the trauma patient with a significant mechanism of injury are as follows (Figure 8-19, page 234):

1. **Check the patient's ABCD** for any changes in status since the initial assessment.
2. **Continue spinal stabilization.**
3. **Assess mental status.**
4. **Reconsider your transport decision.**
5. **Consider a request for ALS backup.**
6. **Assess the head,** looking for DCAP-BTLS and crepitus.
7. **Assess the neck,** looking for DCAP-BTLS, jugular vein distention, and crepitus.
8. **Apply a cervical spinal immobilization collar.**
9. **Assess the chest,** looking for DCAP-BTLS, paradoxical motion, and crepitus. You should also assess for breath sounds in the apices, at the midclavicular line bilaterally, at the bases, and at the midaxillary line bilaterally.
10. **Assess the abdomen,** looking for DCAP-BTLS, rigidity (firm or soft), and distention.
11. **Assess the pelvis,** looking for DCAP-BTLS. If there is no pain, gently compress the pelvis downward or inward to determine tenderness or instability.
12. **Assess all four extremities,** looking for DCAP-BTLS. Also assess and compare bilaterally for distal pulses, sensation, and motor function.
13. **Roll the patient with spinal precautions,** and assess the posterior aspect of the body, looking for DCAP-BTLS.
14. **Assess baseline vital signs.**
15. **Assess the SAMPLE history.**

Recognizing a possible spinal injury is one of your principal responsibilities as an EMT-B. You should assume a spinal injury in any patient who has a mechanism that reflects or suggests a significant history of trauma, is intoxicated and may have been traumatized, is unconscious, complains of neck/spine pain following a traumatic event, or cannot move or feel in any or all four extremities following a traumatic event. Immediately begin manual immobilization of the spine. Consider requesting ALS backup or transporting the patient with priority status. Also reevaluate the patient's mental status. Table 8-6 lists the conditions for which you should assess in addition to DCAP-BTLS during the rapid trauma assessment.

Head, Neck, and Cervical Spine

Look for abnormalities of the head, neck, and cervical spine. Gently feel the head and the back of the neck for deformity, tenderness, or crepitus, also checking as you feel for any bleeding. <u>Crepitus</u> is the crackling sound that is often heard when two ends of a broken bone rub together or when there are air bubbles under the skin. Ask a responsive patient if he or she feels any pain or tenderness. Next, check the neck for signs of trauma, swelling, or bleeding. Feel the skin of the neck for air under the skin, known as <u>subcutaneous emphysema</u>, as well as any abnormal lumps or masses. It is particularly important to evaluate the neck before covering it with a cervical collar. Also look for pronounced or distended jugular veins. This is normal in a patient who is lying down; however, their presence in the patient who is sitting up suggests some problem with blood returning to the heart. Report and record your findings carefully. Do not move on to the next step until you are sure that the airway is secure and you have initiated or continued spinal immobilization.

Chest

Next, look at and feel over the chest area for injury or signs of trauma, including bruising, tenderness, or swelling. Watch the chest rise and fall with breathing.

Normal breathing causes both sides of the chest to rise and fall together. Look for abnormal breathing signs, including <u>retractions</u> (when the skin pulls in around the ribs during inspiration) or <u>paradoxical motion</u> (when only one side rises on inspiration while another area of the chest falls).

Retractions indicate that the patient has some condition, usually medical, that is impairing the flow of air into and out of the lungs. Paradoxical motion is associated with a fracture of several ribs, causing a section of chest to move independently from the rest of the chest. Feel for grating of bones as the patient breathes. Crepitus is associated with rib fractures. Feel over the chest for subcutaneous emphysema, especially in cases of severe blunt chest trauma.

If the patient reports difficulty breathing or has evidence of trauma to the chest, listen to <u>breath sounds</u>. This helps you to evaluate air movement in and out of the lungs. To listen, you need a stethoscope. Make sure that you place the earpieces facing forward in your ears. The position of the patient will determine the way you proceed to check for breathing (Figure 8-20).

TABLE 8-6	Using DCAP-BTLS in the Rapid Trauma Assessment
Part of the Body	**Look for DCAP-BTLS and the Following:**
Head	• Crepitus
Neck	• Jugular vein distention • Crepitus
Chest	• Paradoxical motion • Crepitus • Quality of breath sounds
Abdomen	• Rigidity • Distention
Pelvis	• Tenderness • Instability
Extremities	• Distal pulses • Sensation • Motor function
Back	

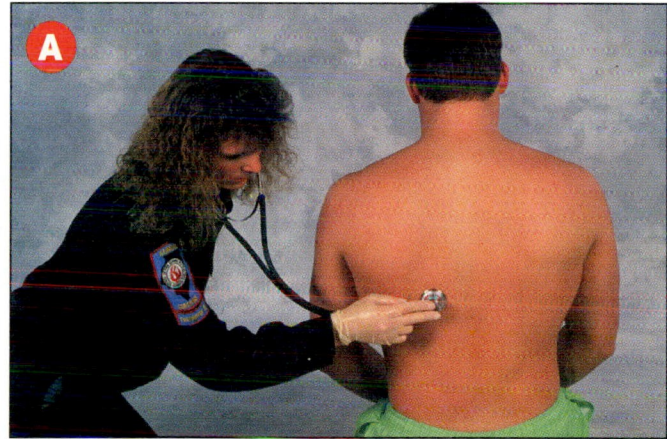

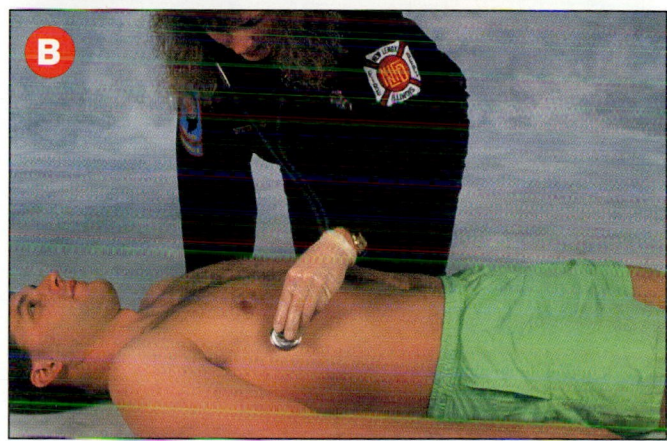

FIGURE 8-20 A: Listen to breath sound from the patient's back if possible, over the apices, the bases, and the major airways. **B:** If the patient is immobilized or in a supine position, listen from the front.

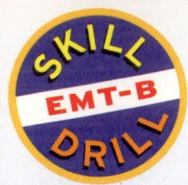

Performing a Rapid Trauma Assessment
Figure 8-19

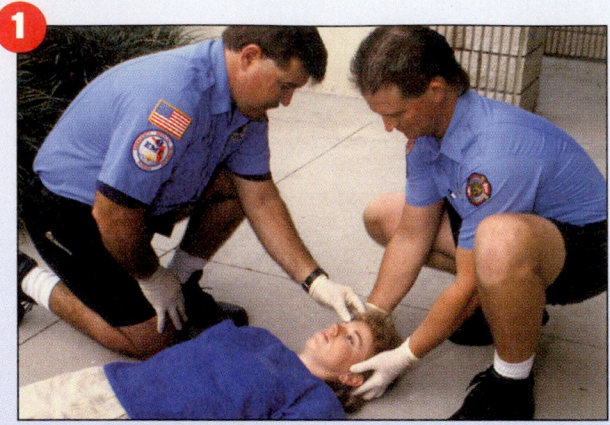

1 Assess the head for DCAP-BTLS and crepitation. Continue spinal stabilization

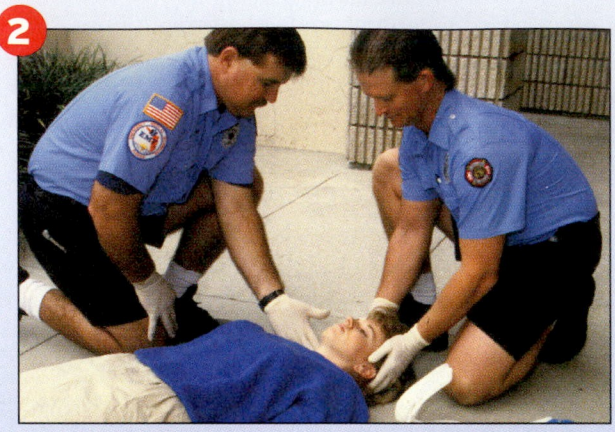

2 Assess the neck for DCAP-BTLS, jugular vein distention, and crepitation.

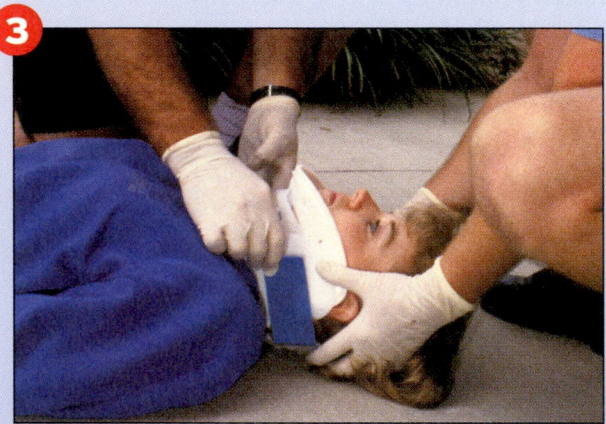

3 Place a cervical collar on the patient.

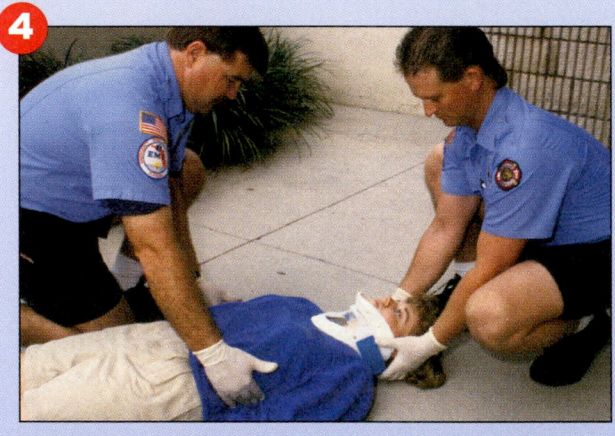

4 Assess the chest for DCAP-BTLS, paradoxical motion, and crepitus. Also assess for breath sounds.

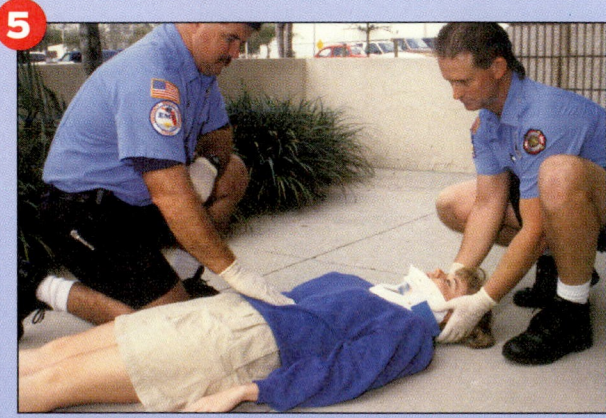

5 Assess the abdomen for DCAP-BTLS, rigidity, and distention.

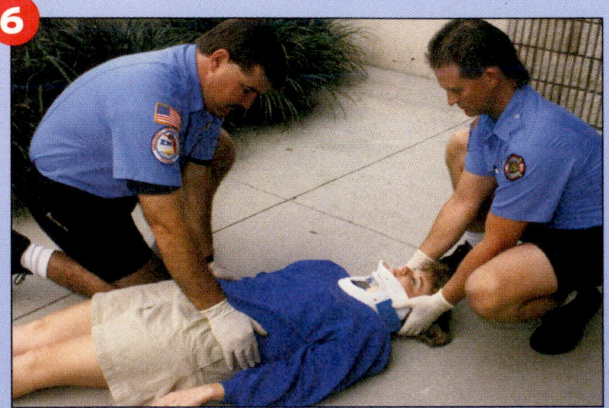

6 Assess the pelvis for DCAP-BTLS.

3

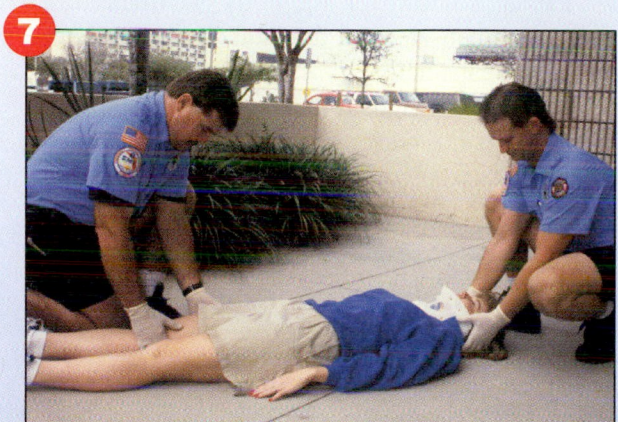

Assess all four extremities for DCAP-BTLS.

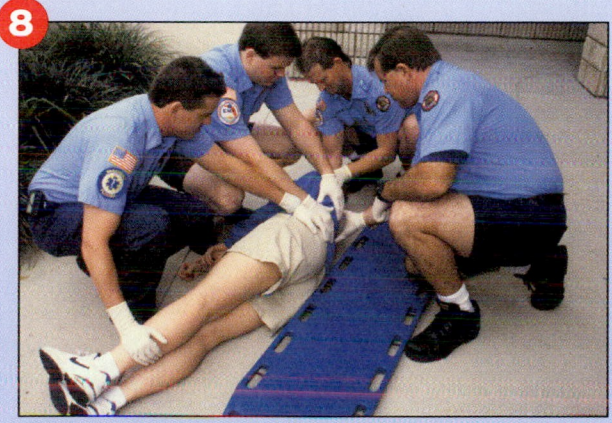

Roll the patient with spinal precautions, and assess the back for DCAP-BTLS.

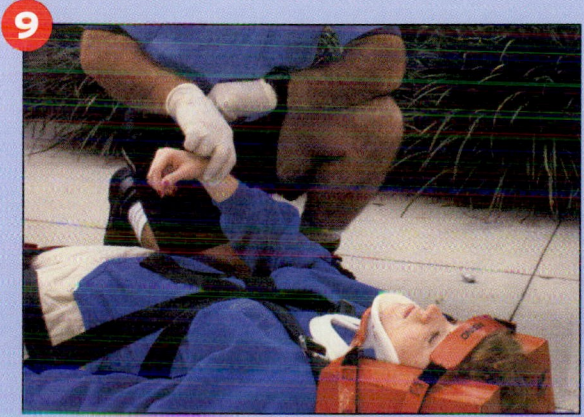

Assess baseline vitals and SAMPLE history.

Here's how and where to listen:

- First, remember that you can almost always hear breath sounds better from the patient's back. So if the patient's back is accessible, listen there. If you have immobilized the patient or if the patient is in a supine position, listen from the front.

- Listen over the upper lungs (apices), the lower lungs (bases), and over the major airways (midclavicular and midaxillary lines).

- Lift the clothing, or slide the stethoscope under the clothing. When you listen over clothing, you are hearing primarily the sound of the stethoscope sliding over the fabric, because the breath sounds are muted by the clothing.

- Place the diaphragm of the stethoscope firmly to best hear the breath sounds.

What are you listening for? Your goal is to hear and document the presence or absence of breath sounds in the three regions described. If you believe that the breathing is abnormal, recheck the initial assessment for breathing, and ensure that the patient is receiving oxygen and, if appropriate, assisted ventilation.

Abdomen

Look at the abdomen for any obvious injuries, bruising, and bleeding. Be sure to feel over both the front and the back of the abdomen, evaluating for tenderness and any bleeding. As you feel all around the abdomen, use the terms "firm," "soft," "tender," or "distended" (swollen) to report your findings. If the patient is awake and alert, ask about pain as you perform the exam. Do not palpate obvious soft-tissue injuries, and be careful not to palpate too hard.

Pelvis

Look for any signs of obvious injury, bleeding, or deformity. If the patient reports no pain, gently press inward and downward on the pelvic bones. Do not rock the pelvis, since this motion may move an unstable spine. If you feel any movement or crepitus, or the patient reports pain or tenderness, it may indicate severe injury. Injuries to the pelvis and surrounding abdomen may bleed profusely, so continue to monitor the patient's skin color, and be sure that you are giving supplemental oxygen.

Extremities

Look for cuts, bruises, swelling, obvious injuries, and bleeding. Next, feel along each extremity for deformities. Ask the patient about any tenderness or pain.

3

As you evaluate the extremities, check for circulation, sensation, and movement:

- **Circulation:** Evaluate the skin color in the hands or feet. Is it normal? How does it compare with the skin color of the other extremities? Pale or cyanotic skin may indicate poor circulation in the extremity. Check the distal pulses on the foot (dorsalis pedis or posterior tibial) and wrist (radial).

- **Sensation:** Evaluate normal feeling in the extremity by asking the patient to close his or her eyes. Gently squeeze or pinch a finger or toe, and ask the patient to identify what you are doing. The inability to feel sensation in the extremity may indicate a local nerve injury. Inability to feel in several extremities may be a sign of spinal cord injury. Recheck to be sure that you have begun and/or are maintaining spinal immobilization.

- **Movement:** Ask the patient to wiggle his or her fingers or toes. An inability to move a single extremity can be the result of a bone, muscle, or nerve injury. Inability to move several extremities may be a sign of a brain abnormality or spinal cord injury. Recheck to be sure that you have initiated spinal immobilization.

Back

Feel the back for tenderness, deformity, and open wounds. If you are placing the patient on a backboard, it is particularly important that you check the back as you log roll the patient onto the backboard. Ensure that you keep the spine in line at all times as you log roll the patient onto his or her side. Carefully palpate the spine from the neck to the pelvis for tenderness or deformity, and visualize for obvious injuries, including bruising.

Baseline Vital Signs and SAMPLE History

After you have completed the rapid assessment, it is time to obtain baseline vital signs and a <u>SAMPLE history</u>.

The baseline vital signs provide useful information about the overall functions of the patient's heart and lungs. They may be an important part of the focused examination if your patient appears to have problems related to blood loss, circulation, or breathing. In other cases, you may simply document the vital signs as baseline information. If the patient's condition is stable, you should reassess the vital signs every 15 minutes until you reach the emergency department. If the patient is unstable, you should reassess at a minimum of every 5 minutes, or as often as the situation permits, looking for trends in the patient's condition. Tables 8-7 through 8-12 provide more information on baseline vital signs.

Do not be falsely reassured by apparently normal vital signs. The body has amazing abilities to compensate for severe injury or illness, especially in children and young adults. Even patients with severe medical or traumatic conditions may initially present with fairly normal vital signs. However, the body eventually loses its ability to compensate, and the vital signs may deteriorate rapidly, especially in children. In fact, this tendency for the vital signs to fall rapidly as the patient decompensates is the reason that it is important to frequently recheck and record the vital signs.

TABLE 8-7	Determining the Quality of Breathing
Normal	• Breathing is neither shallow nor deep. • Average chest wall motion • No use of accessory muscles
Shallow	• Slight chest or abdominal wall motion
Labored	• Increased breathing effort • Grunting, stridor • Use of accessory muscles • Gasping for air • Nasal flaring, supraclavicular and intercostal retractions (in infants and children)
Noisy	• Increase in sound of breathing, including snoring, wheezing, gurgling, and crowing

TABLE 8-8	Normal Respiration Rates
Adults	12 to 20 breaths/min
Children	15 to 30 breaths/min
Infants	25 to 50 breaths/min

TABLE 8-9	Average Pulse Rates
Adults	60 to 100 beats/min
Children	80 to 100 beats/min
Toddlers	100 to 120 beats/min

TABLE 8-10   Assessing the Skin

Color	Possible Cause
Pink	• Normal color
Ashen/White Face and/or Skin on Extremities	• Hypovolemia
Gray-Blue (cyanotic)	• Insufficient air exchange • Low blood oxygen levels
Flushed	• High blood pressure • Carbon monoxide poisoning • Significant fever • Heatstroke • Sunburn • Mild thermal burns
Jaundice	• Liver disease or dysfunction

Temperature/Moisture	Possible Cause
Warm	• Normal condition
Hot	• Significant fever • Sunburn • Hyperthermia
Cool	• Early shock • Heavy exercise/sweating • Heat exhaustion
Cold	• Profound shock • Hypothermia • Frostbite
Dry	• Normal condition
Clammy, Damp, or Moist	• Early shock
Wet	• Profound shock

TABLE 8-11   Systolic Blood Pressure Readings

Expected Readings		Critically Low Readings	
Adult Men	Add 100 to the patient's age, up to 150 mm Hg	Male Adults/Adolescents	90 mm Hg or less
Adult Women	Add 90 to the patient's age, up to 150 mm Hg	Female Adults/Adolescents	80 mm Hg or less
Children	Add 80 to 2 times the patient's age in years	Children	70 mm Hg or less

TABLE 8-12   Pupillary Reactions

Appearance	Possible Cause
Round/equal size	Normal condition
Fixed with no reaction to light	Depressed brain function
Fully dilated and fixed (blown pupil)	Intracranial bleeding
Dilate with bright light, constricted with low light	Depressed brain function
Constricted	Opiates in system
Sluggish reaction	Depressed brain function
Unequal in size	Depressed brain function Medication placed in eye Injury or condition of the eye
Unequal in size when bright light is introduced	Depressed brain function or removed from one eye

For many EMT-Bs, taking the patient history seems to be a bewildering series of questions that seem to bear little or no relationship to the patient's need for help. This becomes worse with patients who have had many medical problems; taking their history is time consuming and often yields little or no information that is useful to you. However, this does not need to be the case. Remember that the mnemonic SAMPLE includes the following elements:

Signs and **S**ymptoms of the episode

Allergies, particularly to medications

Medications, including prescription, over-the-counter, and recreational (illicit) drugs

Past history, particularly involving similar episodes in the past

Last oral intake, including food and/or drinks. This is particularly important if the patient may need surgery

Events leading up to the episode, which may include precipitating factors

Trauma Patients With No Significant Mechanism of Injury

You will not need to perform such a complete exam on most of your patients. After you have completed the initial assessment and care for any actual or potentially life-threatening conditions, you should focus on anything associated with the patient's chief complaint.

Assess the Chief Complaint

Once you are sure that the ABCD is stable, move to the patient's specific injury site or **chief complaint**: the patient's description of "what is wrong." In many cases, especially with trauma, this is logical. For example, if the patient reports ankle pain, you should check the ankle. Note, though, that nontraumatic complaints may be a little less obvious. Here are some things to assess with some common chief complaints:

- **Chest pain:** Evaluate the skin color, pulse, and blood pressure. Look for injuries to the chest and listen to the breath sounds.

- **Shortness of breath:** Evaluate the skin color, pulse, blood pressure, and rate and depth of respirations. Look for signs of airway obstruction, as well as trauma to the neck and chest. Listen carefully to the breath sounds.

- **Abdominal pain:** Evaluate the skin color, pulse, and blood pressure. Look for trauma to the abdomen, and palpate the abdomen to identify any particularly tender spots.

- **Any pain associated with bones or joints:** Evaluate the skin color, movement, and sensation adjacent to and below the affected area.

- **Dizziness:** Evaluate the skin color, pulse, blood pressure, and rate and quality of respirations. Monitor the level of consciousness and orientation carefully. Check the head for signs of trauma.

Next, examine anything that has a noticeable abnormality. Sometimes, during the initial assessment and focused history, you will see something that is obviously abnormal. It may be a cut, a deformed bone, a weakness on one side, abnormal eyes, or some other large abnormality. Avoid being distracted by these conditions; it is easy to let a big cut or deformity draw your attention away from more important, potentially life-threatening problems.

However, once you have evaluated and treated life-threatening conditions and have examined chief complaints, you can come back to any minor problems you found previously. Be sure to ask the patient questions about the abnormality while you are evaluating it. In some cases, deformities or abnormalities may be long-term and unrelated to the patient's present condition. For example, a patient who has had a stroke may have a weakness on one side for months following the stroke; it is not a new problem, and it is not likely to be related to the patient's current call for EMS.

Perform a Focused Assessment

Once you have assessed for problems that are potentially life-threatening, related to the chief complaint or specific injury site, and obviously abnormal, you may begin to perform the focused assessment. As we have noted before, plan ahead for BSI; if bleeding is possible (and it is for most patients), be sure your gloves are on before you begin the focused examination. Next, follow the order and components of the rapid trauma assessment, focusing on the specific area of injury or complaint.

Obtain Baseline Vital Signs and SAMPLE History

As you know, baseline vital signs provide useful information about the overall functions of the patient's heart and lungs. Remember, if the patient's condition is stable, you should reassess the vital signs every 15 minutes until you reach the emergency department. If the patient is unstable, you should reassess at a minimum of every 5 minutes, or as often as the situation permits. Also obtain a SAMPLE history if possible.

Documentation

Baseline findings during this examination document how the patient looked during your assessment. Your written report should include documentation of the following:

- The skin color, temperature, and moisture

- Findings from the initial assessment

- Baseline vital signs (pulse, blood pressure, respirations, temperature) and SAMPLE history

- The circulation sensation and movement in all extremities

- Breath sounds

Other Considerations

Remember, for many patients, you will need to assess the entire body because of the potential severity of their condition. The following patients require a complete rapid trauma assessment, coupled with short scene time and immediate transport to the hospital:

- Any patients who experienced a significant mechanism of injury

- Any patients who are unresponsive or disoriented, since they cannot contribute to the focused history or exam

- Any patients who are extremely intoxicated from drugs or alcohol and cannot reliably contribute to the focused history or exam

Any patients with a complaint that cannot be identified or clearly understood by using a focused exam should receive a more complete exam.

Focused History and Physical Exam: Medical Patients

Early in the assessment process, you need to begin evaluating the patient's problem. In most cases, the patient is alert and able to discuss the problem with you. However, in some cases, the patient may be confused, intoxicated, unable to speak your language, or unconscious. In such a situation, you should immediately proceed to the rapid medical assessment.

When the patient can tell you about his or her problem, the response to general questions such as "What's wrong?" or "What happened?" is called the chief complaint. This is what drives your assessment of the history of the present illness. The chief complaint is typically the problem that is bothering the patient the most, and the question "What's wrong?" or "What happened?" is one of the most critical questions you can ask.

Be careful not to jump to conclusions regarding the chief complaint because of what you have seen or heard about the patient. In many cases, the chief complaint will not be obvious; it may even be different from what the dispatcher reported. When this occurs, stay flexible.

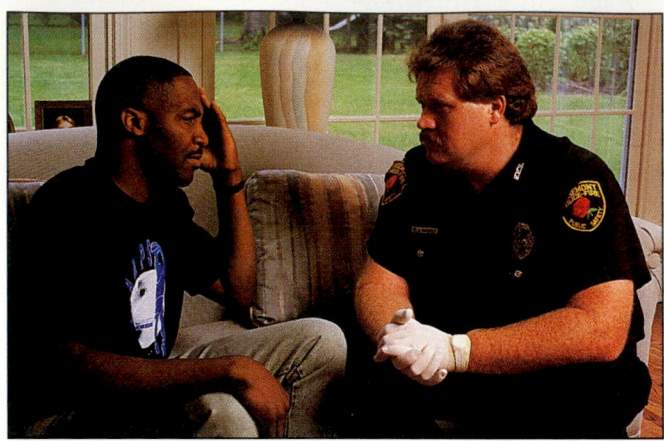

FIGURE 8-21 The patient's initial response to the question "What's wrong?" is the chief complaint.

Treat the patient's problem rather than simply reacting to the dispatch report. Nevertheless, the chief complaint represents what is bothering the patient and will help you to focus your history and physical exam.

Assessing the Responsive Patient

The key to truly understanding a patient's chief complaint is to ask open-ended questions such as "What seems to be the problem?" or "What's wrong?" and then listening (Figure 8-21). This is where good communication skills really pay off. If possible, take the time to sit down and help the patient to get comfortable. Now is the time to listen, as you develop an increased understanding of the patient's real problems. If the patient cannot tell you what is wrong, perhaps because of a language barrier, altered mental status, or severe respiratory difficulty, you may learn the chief complaint from a family member or bystander or from your observations of the scene and patient actions. However, remember that information directly from the patient is far more valuable. You should try, whenever possible, to speak directly to the patient.

As you listen to the patient, you might want to make some brief notes to aid your memory and assist with documentation after the call. You should attempt to record the chief complaint in a few of the patient's own words. Be sure to note if your information comes from someone other than the patient.

4

Patient Assessment Process

Medical Patient Who Is Responsive	Medical Patient Who Is Not Responsive

Scene Size-Up

Initial Assessment

Focused History/Physical Exam*

• Assess chief complaint	• Rapid medical assessment
• O-P-Q-R-S-T	• Baseline vital signs
• Focused physical exam	• SAMPLE history (from family or bystanders)
• Baseline vital signs	

Detailed Physical Exam

• Area by area exam*	• Area by area exam*

On-Going Assessment*

* If appropriate

Focused History and Physical Exam: Medical Patients

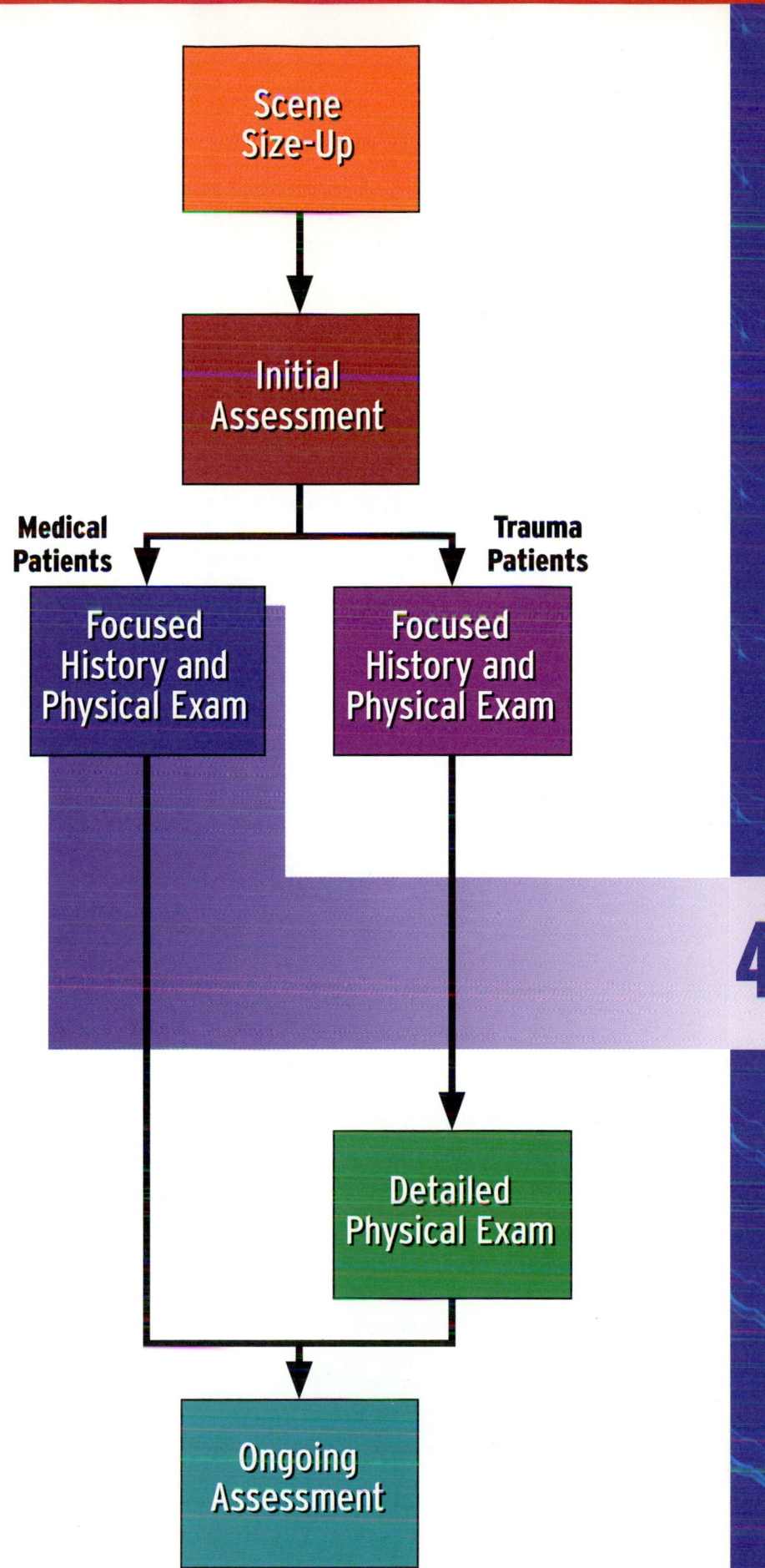

4

OPQRST

As you learn about the chief complaint, you should broaden your knowledge to include the circumstances surrounding the complaint. You can remember the six most important circumstances by using the letters OPQRST, which stand for **O**nset, **P**rovoke, **Q**uality, **R**adiation, **S**everity, **T**ime and **T**reatment. Table 8-13 lists the components of the focused history and physical exam for the medical patient.

Onset. The onset refers to when the patient's problem first began. You should ask the patient when the problem first started or when the accident occurred and how long ago the patient first noticed the problem. If the patient reports that the problem started a long time ago (days or weeks), you should also ask, "What made you finally call now?" In most cases, the patient will note a sudden worsening of the problem or an additional problem that compounded the first one. For example, a patient who has experienced shortness of breath for the past 3 days may have called because of an onset of chest pain an hour ago. You often will not learn about this second problem unless you ask.

For patients with traumatic problems, there may be a delay between when they were hurt and when they called. Again, ask them why they delayed, and what finally caused them to call. The information that they give you may be valuable to you or the hospital staff.

Provoking factors. Learning about provoking factors can be extremely helpful in determining the cause and severity of problems. Provoking factors include anything that seems to bring on the problem or that seems to makes the problem worse. Find out what the patient was doing when the problem started, what he or she thinks caused the problem, and why he or she thinks the accident occurred if trauma is involved. You should also ask the patient what makes the problem better or worse.

The answer to these questions often helps you to appreciate the potential cause. For instance, shortness of breath that started when the patient climbed a set of stairs may be respiratory or cardiac in origin. However, shortness of breath that started after the patient was struck in the chest by a baseball might be the result of fractured ribs or internal injury. These questions are

---

TABLE 8-13   Components of the Focused History and Physical Exam: Medical Patient

Responsive Patient	**Unresponsive Patient**

• Use OPQRST to gather a history of the patient's problem:
  Onset
  Provoking factors
  Quality of pain
  Region and radiation of pain
  Severity
  Time and treatment
	• Perform a rapid medical assessment:
	  Head
	  Neck
	  Chest
	  Abdomen
	  Pelvis
	  Extremities
	  Back

• Obtain a SAMPLE history:
  Signs and symptoms
  Allergies
  Medications
  Past history
  Last oral intake
  Events leading up to the episode
	• Obtain baseline vital signs.
	
	• Provide emergency medical care and transport:
	  Ask the family about the chief complaint, and take a SAMPLE history from the family while en route.

• Perform a focused history:
  Potentially life-threatening conditions
  Chief complaint
  Noticeable abnormalities
	• Document your findings:
	  Skin
	  Initial assessment
	  Baseline vital signs
	  Breath sounds

• Obtain baseline vital signs:
  Reassess every 15 minutes in a stable patient
  Reassess every 5 minutes in an unstable patient	

4

often the clues to hidden medical problems in traumatic incidents, such as the patient who reports that she fell down the stairs because she felt "real dizzy."

Quality of pain. The patient's description of pain may be very useful to hospital staff who are trying to determine the cause. For instance, patients who are having a heart attack classically describe their chest pain as "squeezing" or "pressure," although they may also say things like, "I feel funny," for lack of having a better description. To learn about the quality of pain, ask the patient to describe the pain or explain what the pain feels like to them.

Patients will often initially say, "I don't know," or "It's hard to describe." Once again, the key is for you to be patient. If you wait, most patients will ultimately describe the quality of their pain. Carefully document the patient's own words; these may be very significant to other providers who become involved in the patient's care. If the patient still cannot describe the pain, or if the patient cannot speak, you might consider offering several descriptions of pain and letting the patient choose. For instance, you might ask, "Which of these words best describes your pain: Sharp or dull? Burning, stabbing, crushing, or throbbing?"

Region and radiation of pain or discomfort. Patients can often provide clues about the cause of their problems by describing the region or location of any pain or discomfort (Figure 8-22). <u>Radiation</u> refers to any additional area where the pain or discomfort may also be present. The presence of radiating pain will not alter your treatment very much; however, physicians and nurses caring for the patient in the hospital may be very interested in hearing about areas of radiation. For example, a patient who is having a heart attack may report chest pain that radiates to the left arm and jaw. Document carefully what you learn.

Some patients have limited vocabulary when it comes to their bodies; it may be best to let them simply point to their pain, rather than describe it. Ask patients to point to the area of pain, describe the area of pain, or describe pain anywhere else associated with the problem.

You can learn a great deal about the patient's problem through these questions. For instance, a patient who points to a single place for his or her pain has what is known as <u>focal pain</u>. Many problems, such as fractures or inflammations, are classically focal. However, some patients cannot point to a single location. Instead, they often move their finger around in a circle as they are asked to point to their pain. These patients are experiencing <u>diffuse pain</u>. A number of conditions, including heart attack and internal bleeding, are typically diffuse.

Be careful how you ask about radiation of pain. Most patients will not understand if you ask, "Does your pain radiate anywhere else?" And asking, "Does your pain go (or travel) anywhere else?" might confuse the patient. After all, who ever heard of pain "traveling"? The best way to ask patients about radiation is to ask, "Do you have pain or discomfort anywhere else?"

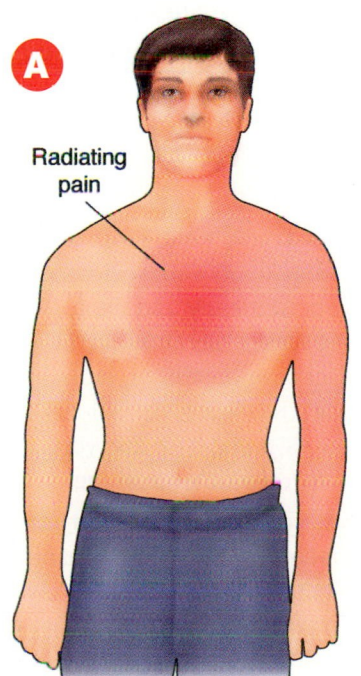
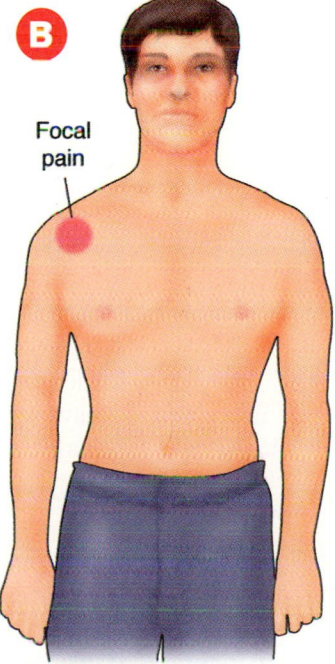
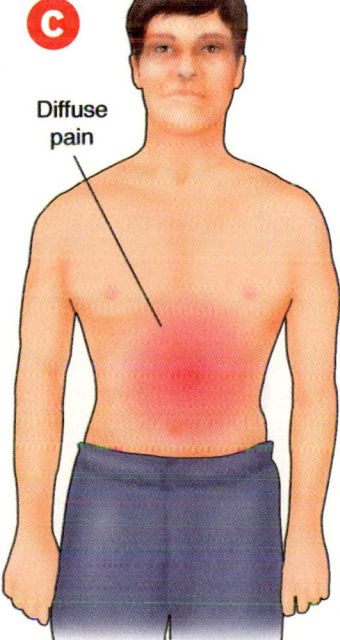

FIGURE 8-22 A: Radiating pain. **B:** Focal pain. **C:** Diffuse pain.

Severity. Severity refers to the patient's perception of "how bad" the current incident is in comparison to others. In some cases, particularly when the patient has experienced the problem before, his or her perception provides extremely useful information. For example, a patient with asthma may be very helpful by comparing this episode with other previous asthma attacks. However, if the problem has never occurred, the patient's perception may not be very useful except as a guide to whether it is getting worse or better during transport. To assess severity, you may ask the following questions:

- "How bad is this episode in comparison to previous ones?" (if the problem is chronic or recurring).

- "What happened the last time you had an episode this bad?" (if the problem is chronic or recurring).

- "How would you rate this problem in numbers, if 1 is normal and 10 is the worst pain or discomfort you can imagine?"

For patients with chronic problems, obtaining the answer to the question "What happened the last time you had an episode this bad?" is invaluable. In most cases, patients have been found to be very accurate in their self-assessments of severity. For instance, a patient with asthma might tell you that the last time he had an attack this bad, he was in the hospital for two weeks, with one week in the intensive care unit. The patient's comments tell you that this episode is extremely serious and that you should complete your assessment and provide immediate transport. At the other extreme, the patient might tell you that he was kept in the emergency department for about an hour and then discharged. Obviously, these two episodes are very different in urgency, and you can adjust your plans for treatment and transport accordingly.

Another way to evaluate changes in the patient's condition during your treatment and transport is to use a numerical score system. For example, a patient with an apparent broken leg might initially tell you that the pain is an 8 on a scale of 1 to 10. After you splint the leg and begin transport, you should recheck the patient's perception. If the pain is now a 9, you might consider changing the position of the leg or using an ice pack. However, if the pain level is now reportedly a 5, you know that the treatment is effective, at least for now. Remember, patients perceive pain in different ways, so it is inappropriate to compare one patient's numerical score with another patient's score.

Time and treatment. The final set of questions provides information about the previous time the patient has experienced the problem and what treatment he or she has tried. You might want to find out whether the problem has been constant or intermittent. If the patient states that the problem is intermittent, ask about what seemed to make it better or worse. You might also ask what the patient has done independently to make it feel better. Did the patient's interventions help?

The answers to these questions will further help you and other health professionals involved with the patient's care to understand the nature of the problem. Some conditions, such as those involving abdominal organs, have classically intermittent pain. Other problems, such as fractures, typically have constant pain. Learning what the patient tried doing to make the problem better might also be very insightful. For instance, some patients smear butter on burns. The greasy wetness of the butter may make the burn look worse than it really is, and the salt in the butter usually intensifies the pain. Also, some patients may take too much medication to try to relieve pain. This may signal another problem: a potential overdose.

Other Questions to Consider

After you have evaluated the chief complaint using OPQRST, you need to ask three more questions pertaining to the chief complaint. Often, because of the intensity of a particular complaint, patients may be unaware or fail to mention other problems. These omissions are usually not serious. However, if the patient fails to mention a potentially life-threatening problem, you could miss an important symptom. For this reason, you should conclude your evaluation of the chief complaint by asking the following three questions:

1. **"Are you sure that you never passed out or were knocked out?"** Changes in mental status are serious signs associated with brain injury or trauma. Try to make sure the patient never lost consciousness before, during, or after the injury or illness.

2. **"Are you sure that you aren't having any difficulty breathing?"** Most patients with shortness of breath will complain about it early and often. However, patients are occasionally unaware of, or fail to mention, their difficulty in breathing, especially if they are in extreme pain. Respiratory problems may have severe consequences, so be sure that your patient is not having any difficulty breathing.

3. **"Are you certain that you have not experienced any chest pain or discomfort?"** As with respiratory problems, most patients with chest pain will report it to you. However, some patients either do not complain about pain or are not aware of their chest discomfort. Yet chest pain may be a symptom of a serious cardiac problem, so it is essential that you do not miss it.

additional follow-up questions

If you have time, you might find it helpful to ask this series of additional questions.

- **"Has this ever happened before?"** This question is very useful in that many patient will be experiencing flare-ups of previously existing problems. If the answer to this question is "yes," you should follow up with additional questions to understand the nature of this episode.

- **"Did you see the doctor or go to the hospital when it happened before?** If so, did the doctor tell you the name of what was wrong? What was it?" The goal here is to learn the patient's diagnosis.

- **"Do you take any medications for this problem?"** If the answer is "yes," then you might want to ask additional questions to determine what prescription and/or over-the-counter medications the patient is taking for the condition. Also ask to see the bottles or containers so that you can take them with you to the emergency department.

You need to ask questions about alcohol and illicit drug use, no matter where you work in EMS. Alcoholism and drug addiction affect all populations, from the wealthiest executive to the poorest of the poor. All races and ethnic groups are affected, too. How you ask these questions will vary from place to place, depending on the patient population that you serve. It is essential that you know the local culture and the terms that are used for alcohol and drug use. Learn how to ask these questions by watching and learning the approach that is used by other EMTs, paramedics, nurses, and doctors in your community. You are trying to obtain important information by asking the following questions:

- **"Are you a heavy alcohol user?** If so, when was your last drink?" Intoxication affects all other aspects of the history and physical exam. The symptoms of alcohol withdrawal are also important to note in conjunction with the patient's presentation.

- **"Do you use illicit drugs?** Which ones?" If the answer is yes, when was the patient's last "high"? Is he or she high now? These findings affect the remainder of the exam. Symptoms of drug withdrawal may complicate the patient's clinical picture by presenting different symptoms. Remember, your role is not law enforcement. You must gain the patient's trust so that you can provide the necessary emergency medical care. Assure the patient that your communication is confidential but that you need this information so that you can fully understanding his or her medical problem.

- **"Do you have any other problems I should know about?"** This question is handy to ask whether the patient has ever had this problem or not. It gives the patient an opportunity to tell you something about apparently unrelated previous medical problems. In most cases, the answer will serve as useful background information. Occasionally, it will provide you and the hospital with essential information.

The SAMPLE History

Once you have obtained a clearer picture of the patient's chief complaint and have explored it using the OPQRST questions, you should obtain a SAMPLE history. Recall that the purpose of this history is to gather information about the patient's past medical experiences. The elements of the SAMPLE history are repeated below for your review.

- **S**igns and **S**ymptoms of the episode
- **A**llergies, particularly to medications
- **M**edications, including prescription, over-the-counter, and recreational (illicit) drugs

- **P**ast history, particularly involving similar episodes in the past
- **L**ast oral intake, including food and/or drinks. This is particularly important if the patient may need surgery.
- **E**vents leading up to the episode, which may include precipitating factors

You should also ask whether the patient has any other problems that you should know about. This question is useful in that it provides the patient with an opportunity to tell you something about apparently unrelated previous medical problems. In most cases, this will serve as

4

SKILL DRILL EMT-B

Performing a Focused Exam: Medical Patient
Figure 8-23

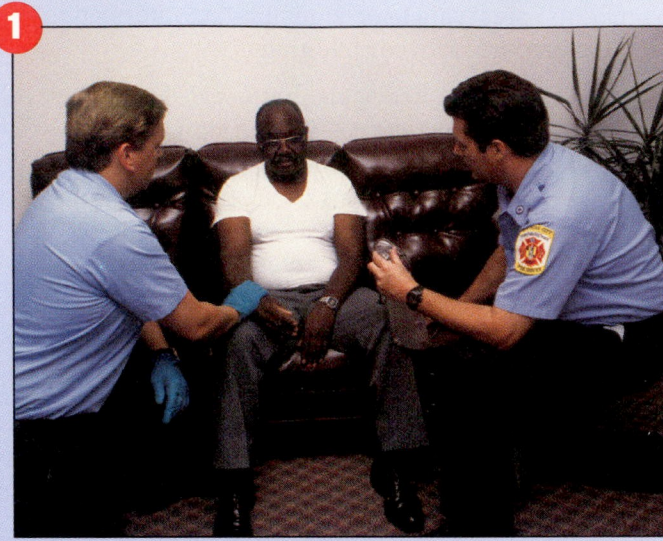

Assess for any immediately or potentially life-threatening conditions, followed by problems associated with the chief complaint.

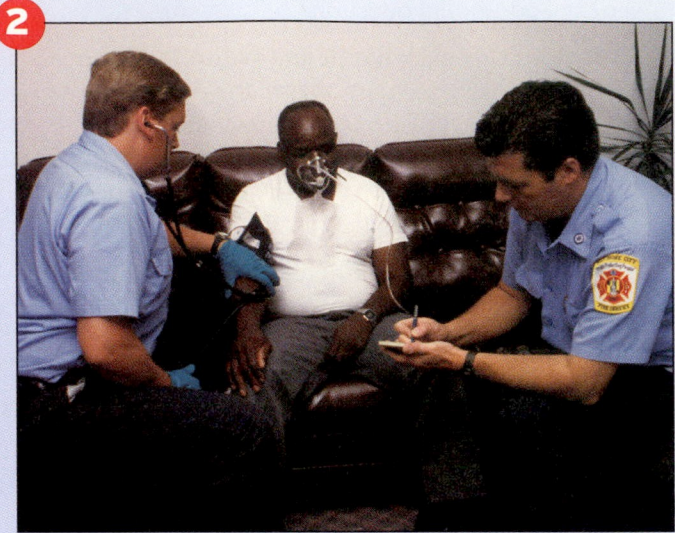

Obtain baseline vital signs, and document your findings.

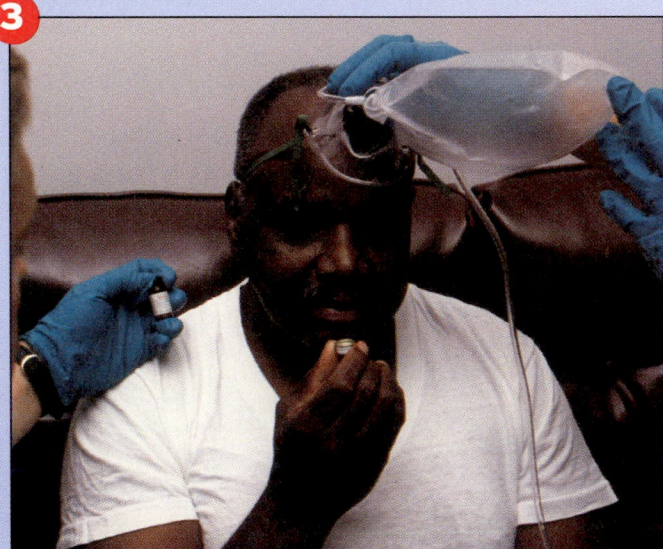

Provide emergency care for life-threatening conditions and then for the chief complaint.

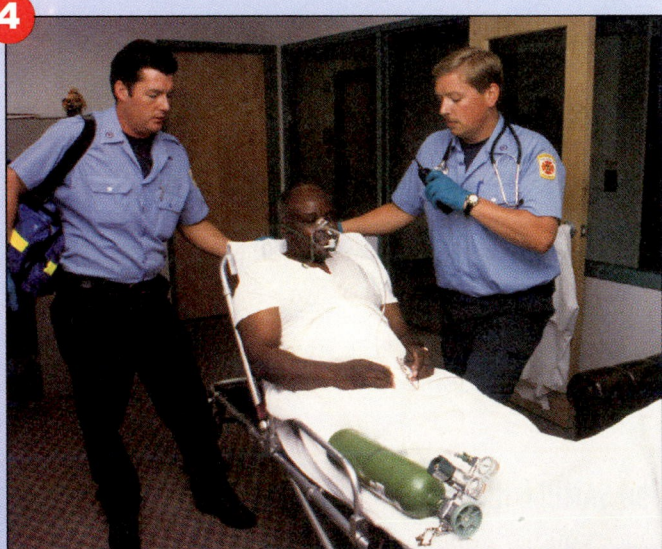

Transport the patient.

useful background information. Occasionally, it will provide you and hospital staff with essential information, such as when you discovered that the patient who fell for no apparent reason has a history of diabetes. This information suggests the possibility that the fall was caused by a complication of the diabetes.

No matter what you have learned about the patient's past history, you need to be aware of certain medical problems that the patient may have forgotten to mention. These conditions might help to explain the current episode or could affect your treatment decisions or those made by ALS or at the hospital. As you conclude the SAMPLE history, ask the patient the following questions:

1. "Have you ever been told that you have a heart condition?"

2. "Have you ever been told that you have asthma, emphysema, or any other problems with your lungs?"

3. "Have you ever been told that you have seizures?"

These three questions will prevent you from missing important, potentially life-threatening cardiac, respiratory, or neurologic conditions. If the patient answers "yes" to any of these three questions, reevaluate the chief complaint in light of this new information. If you have time, return to the history questions to learn more about the nature of the problem.

The Focused Physical Exam

Now that you have learned about the chief complaint, using OPQRST, and have obtained a thorough history, you should perform a focused exam (Figure 8-23).

The key to this examination is to emphasize the priorities that you learned during the history. Be logical, and investigate problems that you identified during the initial assessment and focused history.

This exam has four priorities:

1. Examine anything associated with an actual or potentially life-threatening condition.

2. Examine anything associated with the patient's chief complaint.

3. Examine anything that has a noticeable abnormality.

4. Evaluate the patient as necessary to provide baseline information.

Potential or immediate life threats. You should think back to the initial assessment. Did you find any immediately or potentially life-threatening conditions? If so, now is the time to follow up with an exam. Here are some areas to recheck:

- **Abnormal level of consciousness.** Check the head for trauma, and evaluate the breathing and circulation for adequacy.

- **Obstructed airway.** Look inside the mouth and at the back of the throat for foreign bodies, blood, vomitus, or any other substance that might obstruct the airway. Check the neck for signs of trauma.

- **Inadequate or labored breathing.** Check the airway for obstruction, and evaluate the neck for signs of trauma. Check the chest for trauma, and consider listening to the breath sounds. Evaluate the skin color for signs of pallor.

- **Inadequate circulation.** Look for blood loss, and evaluate the pulse and blood pressure. Check the neck, chest, and abdomen for signs of trauma.

- **Pale skin.** Look for blood loss, and evaluate the pulse and blood pressure to identify signs of shock.

Chief complaint. Once you know that the ABCD is stable, move to the patient's chief complaint. Remember to carefully assess the following chief complaints, as described previously:

- **Chest pain.** Evaluate the skin color, pulse, and blood pressure. Look for trauma to the chest, and consider listening to the breath sounds.

- **Shortness of breath.** Evaluate the skin color, pulse, blood pressure, and rate and depth of respirations. Look for airway obstruction, as well as trauma to the neck and chest. Listen carefully to the breath sounds.

- **Abdominal pain.** Evaluate the skin color, pulse, and blood pressure. Look for trauma to the abdomen, and palpate the abdomen to identify any particularly tender spots.

- **Any pain associated with bones or joints.** Evaluate the skin color, movement, and sensation adjacent to and below the affected area.

- **Dizziness.** Evaluate the skin color, pulse, blood pressure, and adequacy of respirations. Monitor the level of consciousness and orientation carefully. Check the head for signs of trauma.

Abnormalities. Next, examine anything that has a noticeable abnormality. Sometimes, during the initial assessment and focused history, you will see something that is obviously abnormal. It may be a cut, a deformed bone, a weakness on one side, abnormal eyes, or some other abnormality. Avoid being distracted by these conditions; it is easy to let a big cut or deformity draw your attention away from more important, potentially life-threatening problems.

However, once you have evaluated and treated life-threatening conditions and have examined chief complaints, you can come back to these. Be sure to ask the patient questions about the abnormality while you are evaluating it. Remember that deformities or abnormalities may be long-term and unrelated to the patient's present condition. For example, a patient who has had a stroke may have a weakness on one side for months after the stroke; it is not a new problem, and it is not likely to be related to the patient's current call for EMS.

Baseline Vital Signs

As you know, baseline vital signs provide useful information about the overall functions of the patient's heart and lungs. Remember that if the patient's condition is stable, you should reassess the vital signs every 15 minutes until you reach the emergency department. If the patient is unstable, you should reassess at a minimum of every 5 minutes, or as often as the situation permits.

Emergency Medical Care and Transport

Your next steps are to provide the necessary emergency medical care addressing the chief complaint and then to provide transport to the emergency department.

Documentation

Documenting your assessment findings helps identify and track trends in the patient's condition and to help hospital staff provide definitive treatment. Your report should include documentation of the following:

- The skin color, temperature, and moisture
- Findings from the initial assessment
- Baseline vital signs (pulse, blood pressure, respirations, temperature) and SAMPLE history
- The sensation and movement in all extremities
- Breath sounds

Assessing the Unresponsive Patient

Sometimes, new EMT-Bs ask how to assess the chief complaint and history in an unresponsive patient (Figure 8-24). The answer is simple: You cannot.

With unresponsive patients, you never get to that part of the focused history and physical exam. Instead, you should focus your attention on opening and maintaining the airway, immobilizing the spine, assisting with ventilations, administering supplemental oxygen,

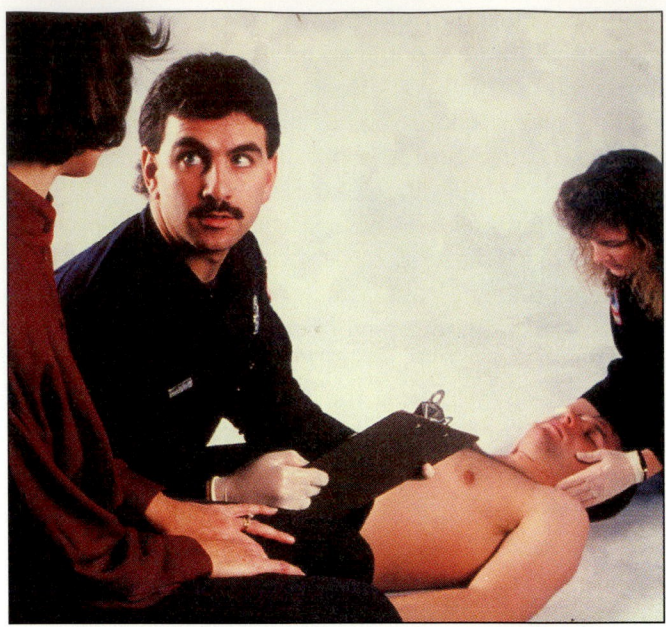

FIGURE 8-24 If the patient is unresponsive, obtain the chief complaint and any other pertinent history from family or bystanders.

controlling bleeding, providing CPR if necessary, and providing immediate transport to an appropriate facility. These priorities reflect the importance of the ABCD approach to the initial assessment.

If you have successfully stabilized the ABCD, you ask chief complaint and SAMPLE history questions of a family member or bystander while en route to the hospital. Never delay transport of a critical patient to take a history from family members (or from the patient, for that matter) at the scene.

The Rapid Medical Assessment

If you have successfully stabilized ABCD on any patient who is unconscious, confused, or unable to adequately relate the chief complaint, you should perform a rapid assessment, using the mnemonic "DCAP-BTLS" and following the order of the rapid trauma assessment. The purpose of the rapid medical assessment is to quickly identify existing or potentially life-threatening conditions. Briefly, the sequence of the assessment is as follows (Figure 8-25):

1. Head
2. Neck
3. Chest
4. Abdomen
5. Pelvis
6. Extremities
7. Back

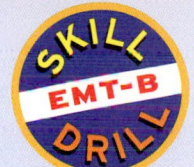

Performing a Rapid Medical Assessment: Unresponsive Patient

Figure 8-25

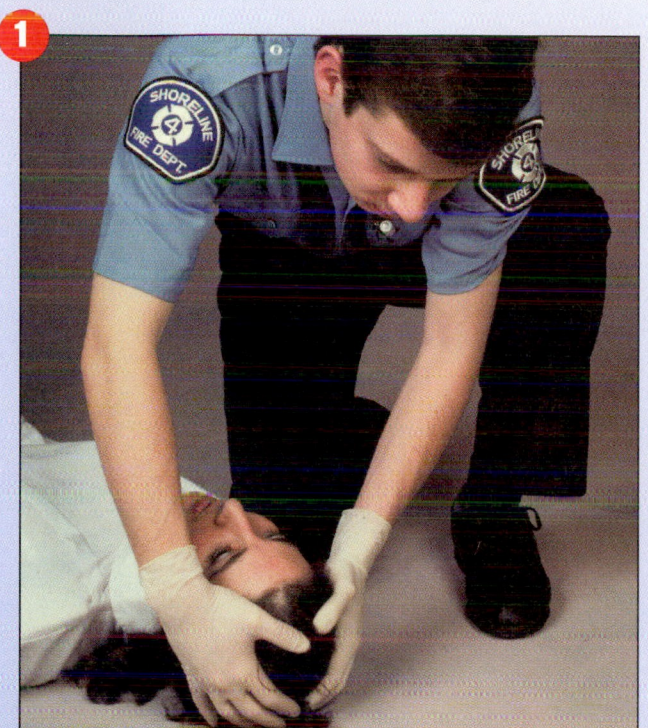

1. Assess the head for DCAP-BTLS and crepitation.

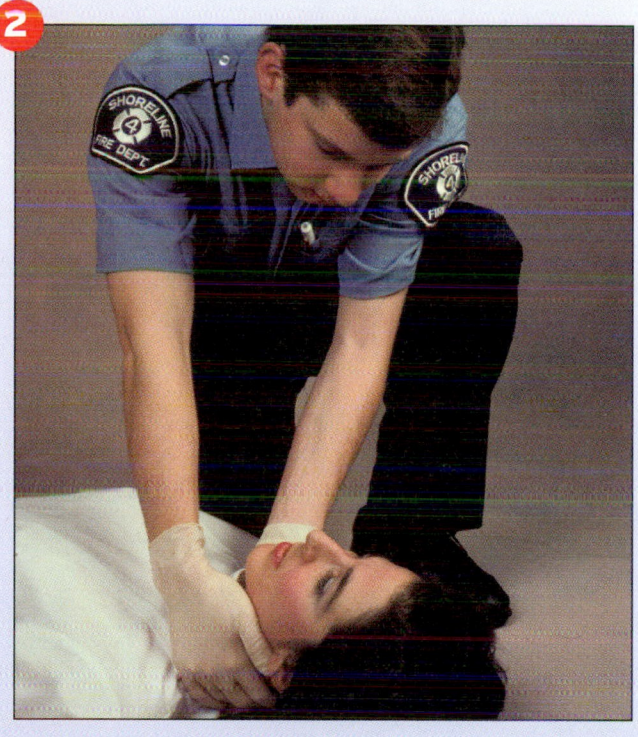

2. Assess the neck for DCAP-BTLS, jugular vein distention, and crepitus.

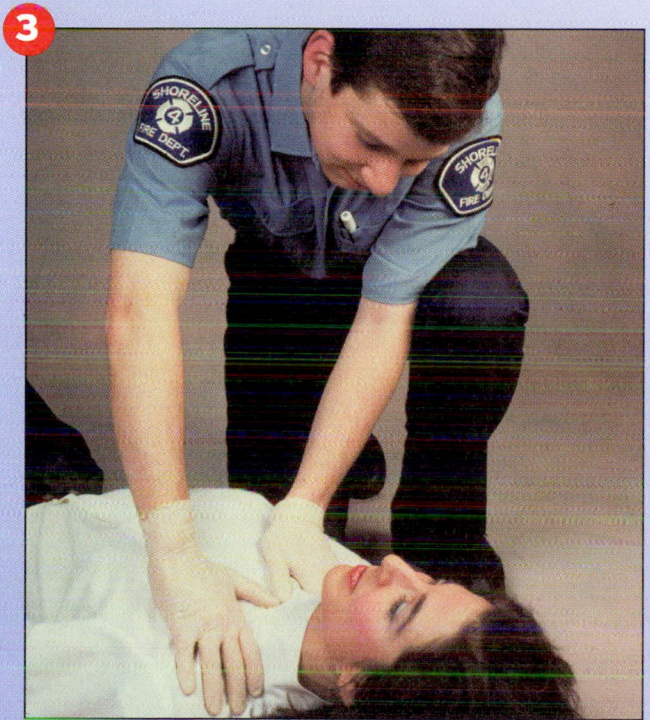

3. Assess the chest for DCAP-BTLS, paradoxical motion, and crepitation.

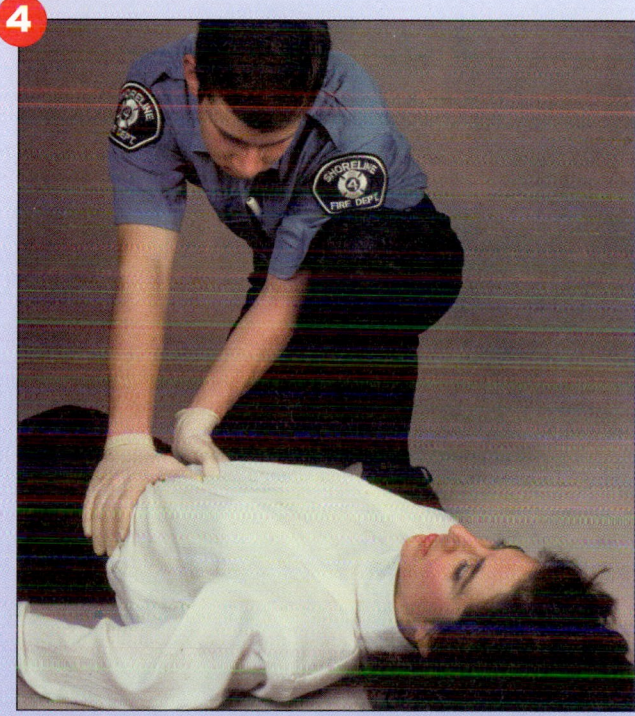

4. Assess the abdomen for DCAP-BTLS, rigidity, and distention.

(Continued)

SKILL DRILL EMT-B

Performing a Rapid Medical Assessment: Unresponsive Patient—cont'd.
Figure 8-25

5

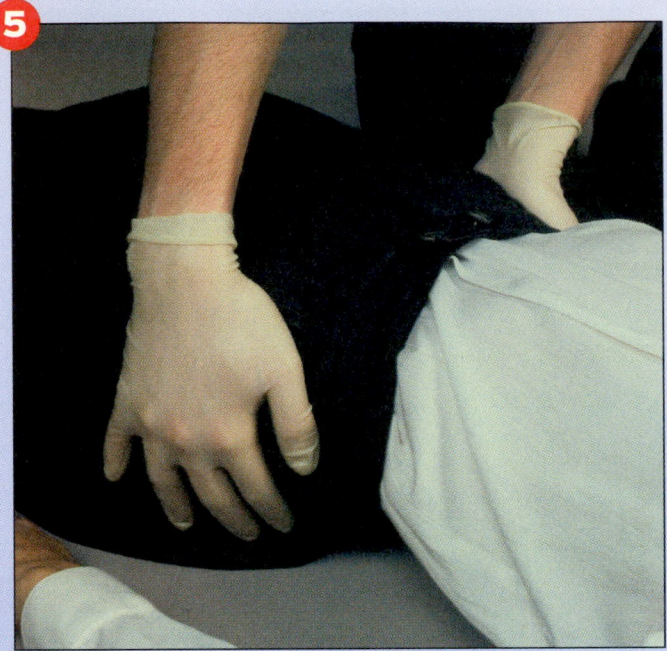

Assess the pelvis for DCAP-BTLS.

6

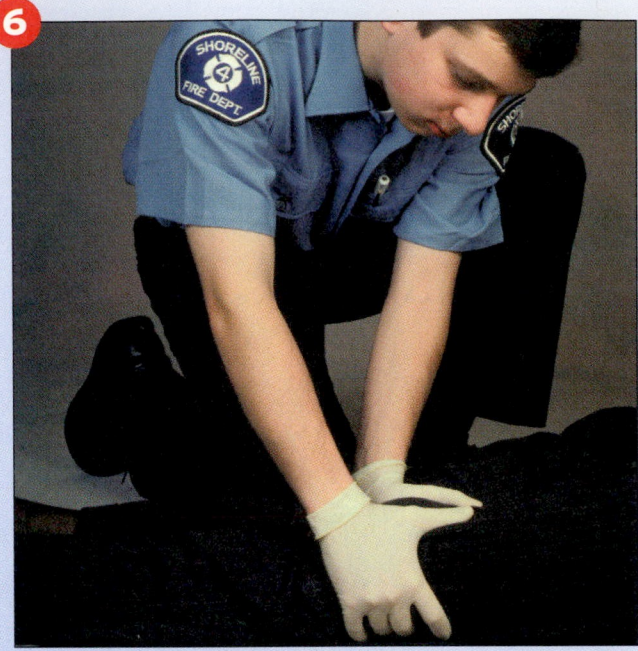

Assess all four extremities for DCAP-BTLS.

7

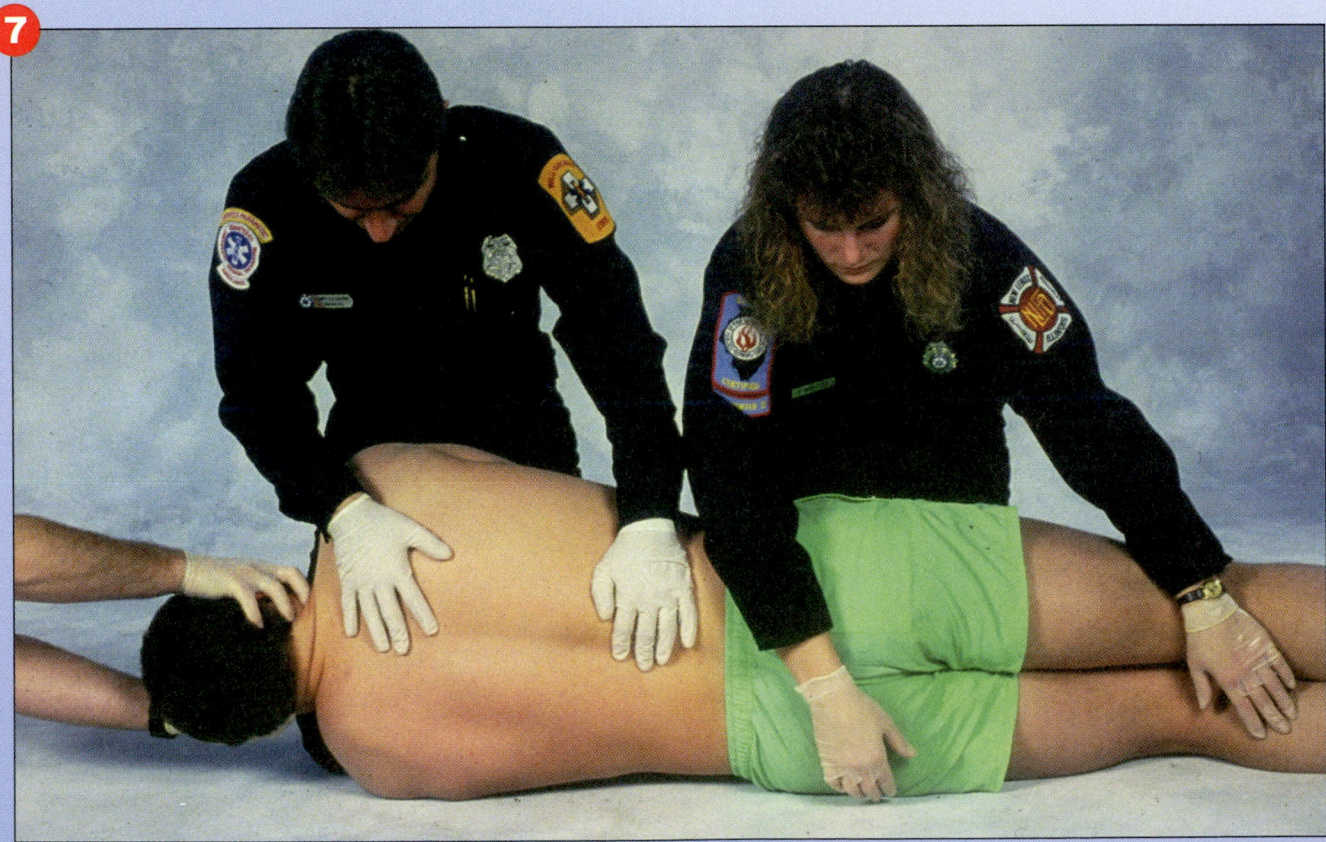

Assess the back for DCAP-BTLS.

Baseline Vital Signs

Baseline vital signs should be obtained after this exam to provide information for trending. Remember, if the patient's condition is stable, you should reassess the vital signs every 15 minutes until you reach the emergency department. If the patient is unstable, you should reassess at a minimum of every 5 minutes, or as often as the situation permits, looking for trends in the patient's condition.

Emergency Medical Care and Transport

Your next steps are to provide the necessary emergency medical care addressing the chief complaint and then to provide transport to the emergency department. Remember, the patient's spine should be immobilized if you suspect significant trauma or if there is a mechanism of injury that would make you suspect a spinal injury.

Documentation

Documenting your baseline findings during this examination is important to track trends in the patient's condition and to help hospital staff provide definitive treatment. Your report should include documentation of the following:

- The skin color, temperature, and moisture
- Findings from the initial assessment
- Baseline vital signs (pulse, blood pressure, respirations, temperature) and SAMPLE history (from bystanders)
- Breath sounds

4

Detailed Physical Exam

Recall that the assessment process began with anticipation and hazard preparation when you received the dispatch information and performed the scene size-up. Then you performed the initial assessment, in which you identified and treated life-threatening conditions. If trauma was a factor in your patient's situation, you also initiated spinal immobilization. When indicated, you followed up on the initial assessment by performing a focused history and a rapid assessment. You also provided transport if your patient had an obvious life-threatening condition. On the basis of what you learned from the history, you assessed selected areas of the patient's body. You have also taken at least one set of vital signs.

In many, if not most, cases, you are already en route to the hospital. If you are still on the scene, it is because the patient does not have any life-threatening conditions and you have not found the cause for the patient's complaints. The patient is in stable condition, and you still have unanswered questions, or you are en route with a long transport time. This is the time to perform the detailed physical exam. The goals of this exam are to further explore problems that were identified during the focused history and physical exam and to possibly identify the cause of complaints that were not identified during the focused history and physical exam.

To achieve these goals, you must simply ask and answer one question: "What additional problems can be identified through a detailed physical exam?" The detailed physical exam will provide you with more information about the nature of the patient's problem. Depending on what is learned, you should be prepared to do the following:

- Return to the initial assessment if a potentially life-threatening condition is identified. (This is unlikely this late in the exam, but it is always possible. Remember, stay focused on the ABCD.)

- Perform spinal immobilization if neck or back pain or abnormality in sensation or movement is identified. (Again, this is unlikely this late in the exam.)

- Modify any treatment that is underway on the basis of any new information.

- Provide treatment for problems that were identified during the exam.

- Provide transport to an appropriate facility, or call for ALS backup.

Goals of the Detailed Physical Exam

The <u>detailed physical exam</u> is a more in-depth examination that builds on the focused physical exam. The patient and the particular injury will determine the need for this exam. Many of your patients will not receive a detailed physical exam, either because it will be irrelevant or unnecessary or because it is not possible given the time constraints.

Most patients have isolated problems that can be adequately evaluated earlier in the assessment process. You will identify the problem and treat it, making a more detailed physical exam of the entire body unnecessary. If you do perform a detailed physical exam in these patients, it will be to further explore what you learned during the rapid assessment.

A few patients will have life-threatening conditions that were identified during the initial assessment. You may spend all of your time with these patients, stabilizing ABCD, which means you will never have a chance to perform a detailed assessment.

You will perform a detailed exam only on stable patients with problems that cannot be identified earlier in the patient assessment process. In most cases, these patients have extremely minor, obscure, or isolated problems, which is why you did not identify them earlier. Regardless of the exact situation, the detailed physical exam is usually performed en route to the hospital, since you could literally spend hours on the scene trying to identify these problems.

Sequence of the Detailed Physical Exam

Here, organized by body region, are some additional assessments that you might want to perform during the detailed exam. As you evaluate each region, visualize and palpate to find evidence of signs of injury, again using the mnemonic "DCAP-BTLS" (Figure 8-26). Table 8-14 lists the components of the detailed physical exam.

Head, Neck, and Cervical Spine

A more detailed exam of these areas could include a careful check of the head, face, scalp, ears, eyes, nose, and mouth for abrasions, lacerations, and contusions.

5

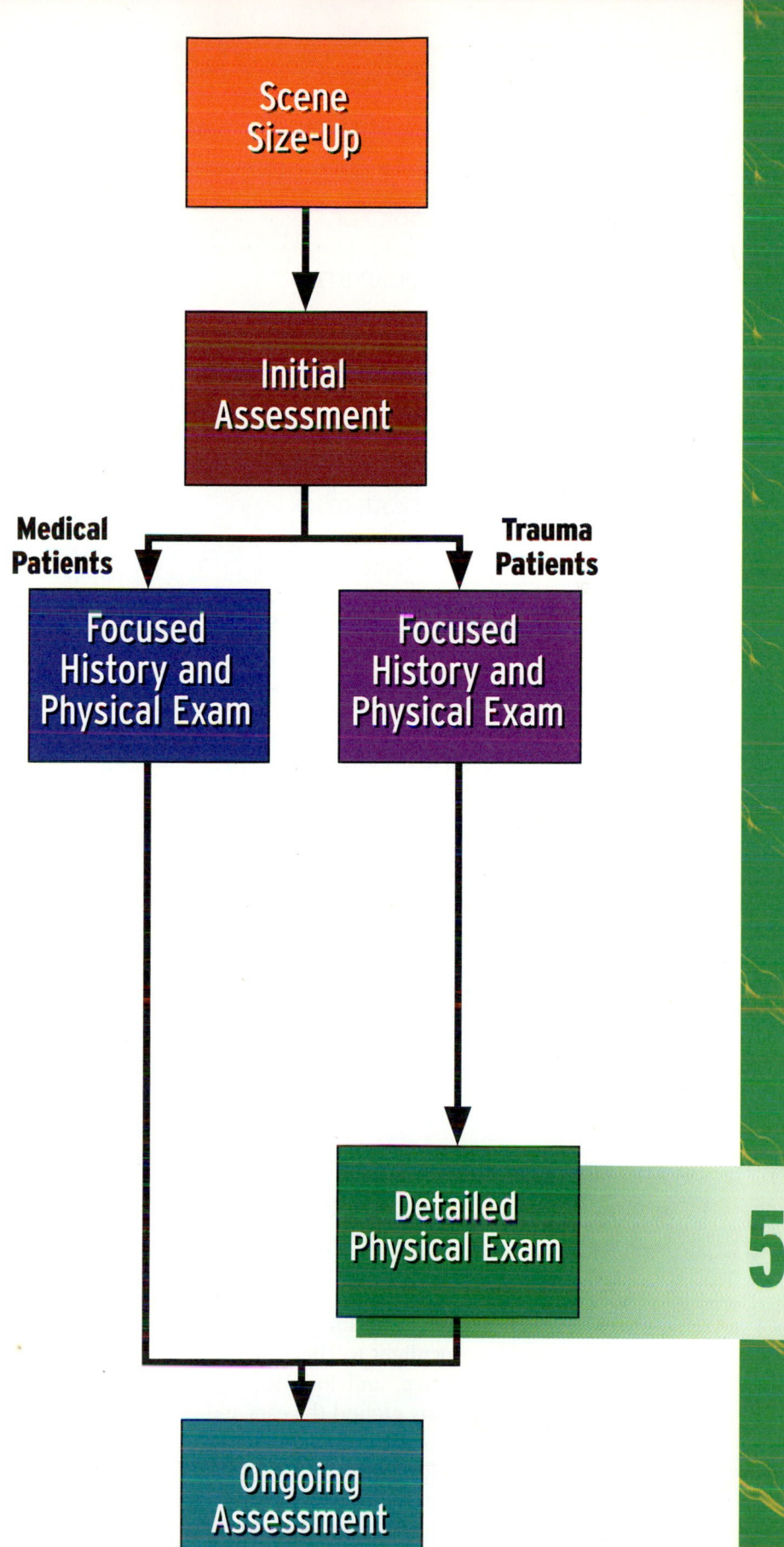

TABLE 8-14 Components of the Detailed Physical Exam

As you inspect and palpate, look and/or feel for the following examples of injuries or signs of injuries: DCAP-BTLS

Assess	Look For	Assess	Look For
Head	• DCAP-BTLS	Chest	• DCAP-BTLS • Crepitus • Paradoxical motion • Breath sounds
Face	• DCAP-BTLS		
Ears	• DCAP-BTLS • Drainage • Bruising or discoloration (Battle's sign)	Abdomen	• DCAP-BTLS • Firmness • Softness • Tenderness • Distention
Eyes	• DCAP-BTLS • Redness • Contact lenses • Equal and reactive pupils • Fluid and drainage • Foreign objects • Bruising or discoloration (raccoon eyes)	Pelvis	• DCAP-BTLS • Pain • Tenderness • Instability • Crepitus
Nose	• DCAP-BTLS • Drainage • Bleeding	Extremities	• DCAP-BTLS • Distal circulation • Sensation • Movement
Mouth	• DCAP-BTLS • Broken or missing teeth or a foreign object • Obstructions • Swollen or lacerated tongue • Unusual breath odors • Discoloration	Back	• DCAP-BTLS (roll with spinal precautions)
Neck	• DCAP-BTLS • Subcutaneous emphysema • Jugular vein distention • Crepitus		

5

Examine the eyes and eyelids, checking for redness and for contact lenses. Use a penlight to check whether the pupils are equal and reactive, and look for any fluid drainage or blood, particularly around the ears and nose. Also check for foreign objects and/or blood in the anterior chamber of the eye. Look for bruising or discoloration around the eyes (raccoon eyes) or behind the ears (Battle's sign); these signs may be associated with head trauma.

Next, palpate gently but firmly around the face, scalp, eyes, ears, and nose for tenderness, deformity, or insta-

bility. Tenderness or abnormal movement of bones often signals a serious injury and may cause upper airway obstruction. Monitor the airway carefully in these patients. Look and feel inside the mouth next. Loose or broken teeth or a foreign object may block the airway. Remember, be cautious when inserting your fingers into a patient's mouth. It's much safer if a bite block is used. You should also look for lacerations, swelling, bleeding, and any discoloration in the mouth and the tongue. Smell the patient's breath. Any unusual odors, such as

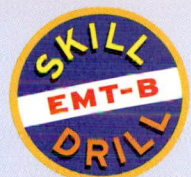

Performing the Detailed Physical Exam
Figure 8-26

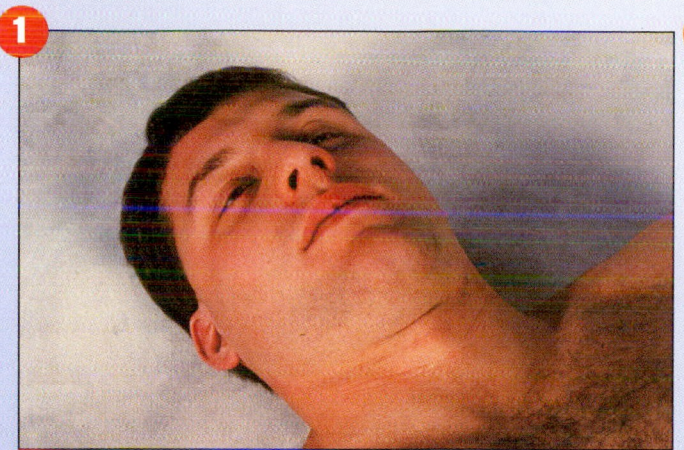

1 Look at the face for obvious lacerations, bruises, or deformities.

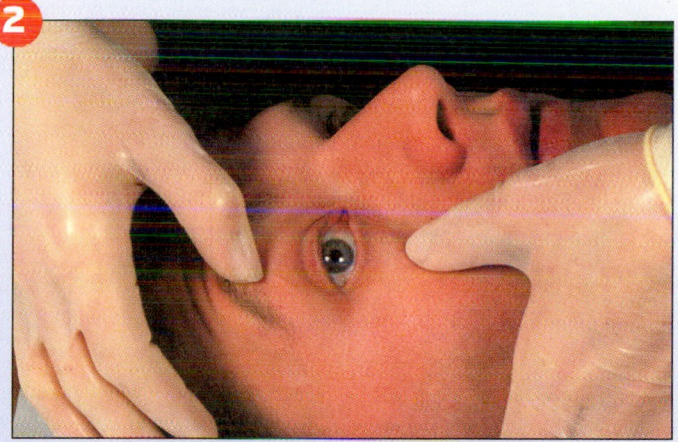

2 Inspect the area around the eyes and eyelids.

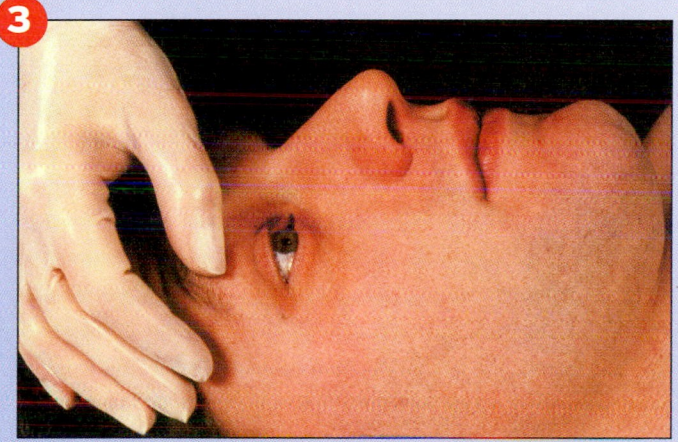

3 Examine the eyes for redness and for contact lenses. Assess the pupils using a penlight.

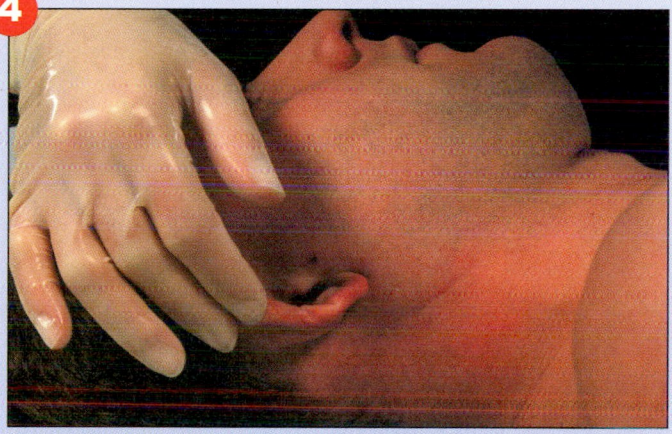

4 Pull the patient's ear forward to assess for bruising (Battle's sign).

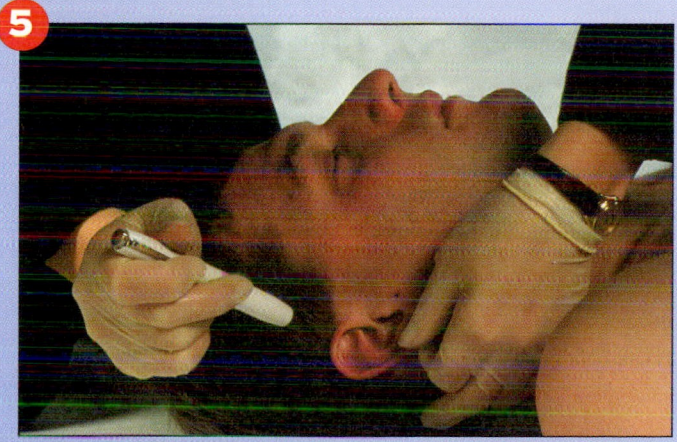

5 Use the penlight to look for drainage or blood in the ears.

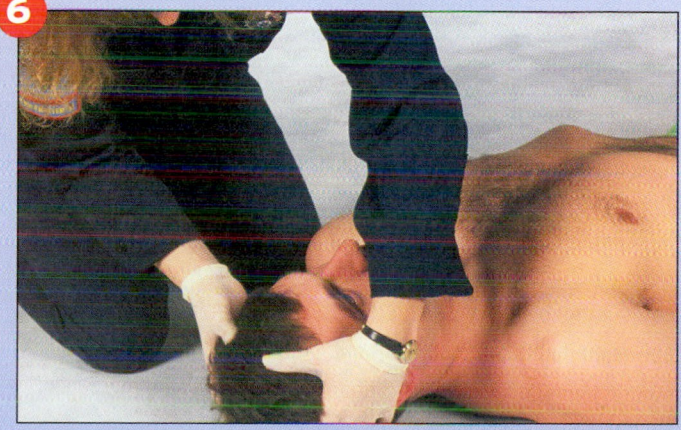

6 Look for bruising and lacerations about the head. Palpate for tenderness, depressions of the skull, and deformities.

(Continued)

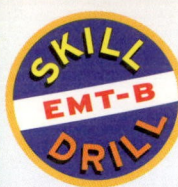

Performing the Detailed Physical Exam—cont'd.
Figure 8-26

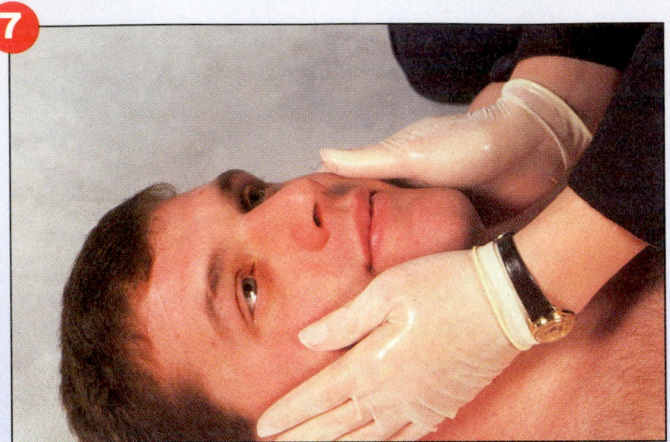

Palpate the zygomas for tenderness or instability.

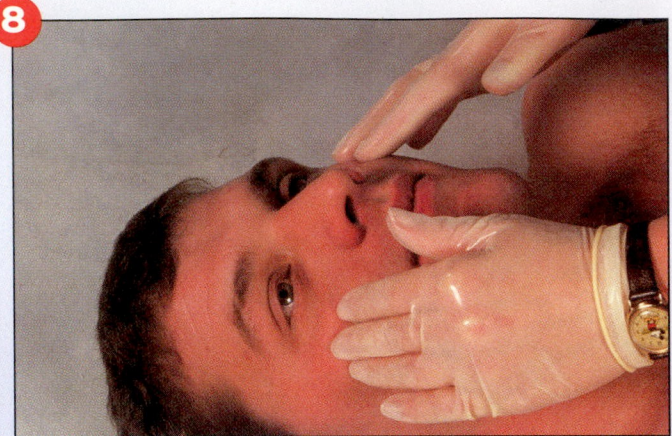

Palpate the maxillae.

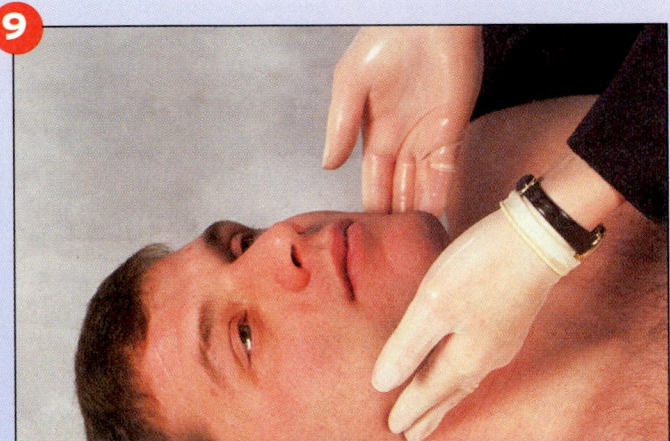

Palpate the mandible.

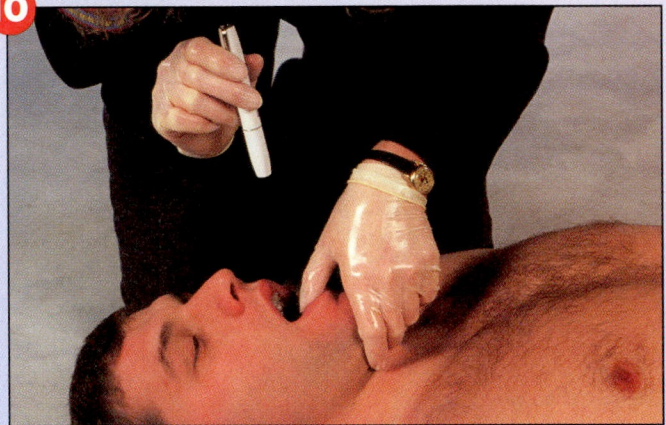

Assess the mouth for cyanosis, foreign bodies (including loose teeth or dentures), bleeding, lacerations, or deformities.

5

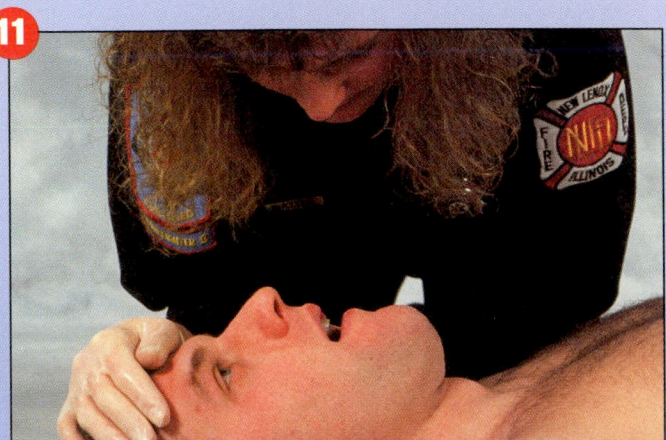

Check for unusual odors on the patient's breath.

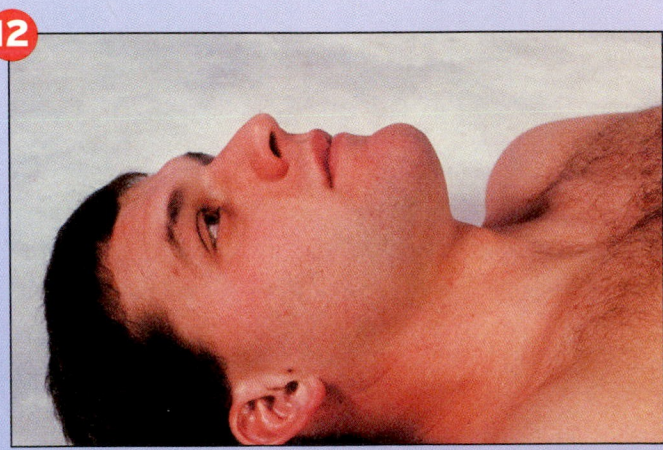

Look at the neck for obvious lacerations, bruises, and deformities.

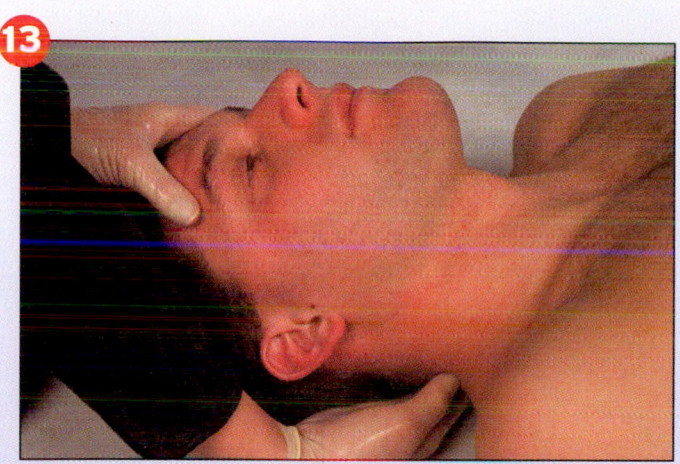

Palpate the front and the back of the neck for tenderness and deformity.

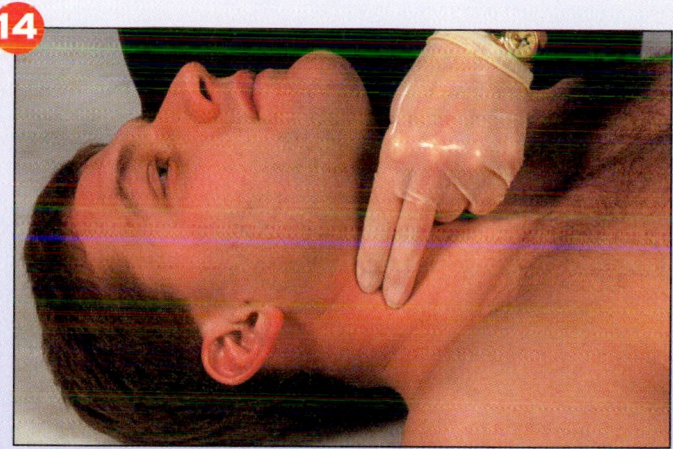

Look for distended jugular veins. Note that distended neck veins are not necessarily significant in a patient who is lying down.

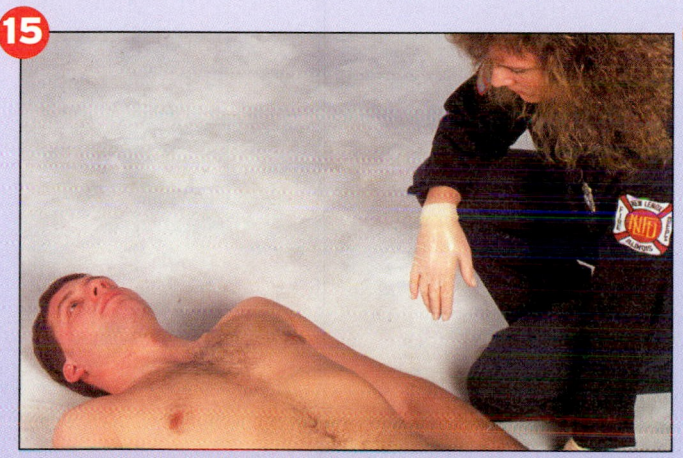

Look at the chest for obvious signs of injury before you begin palpation. Be sure to watch for movement of the chest with respirations.

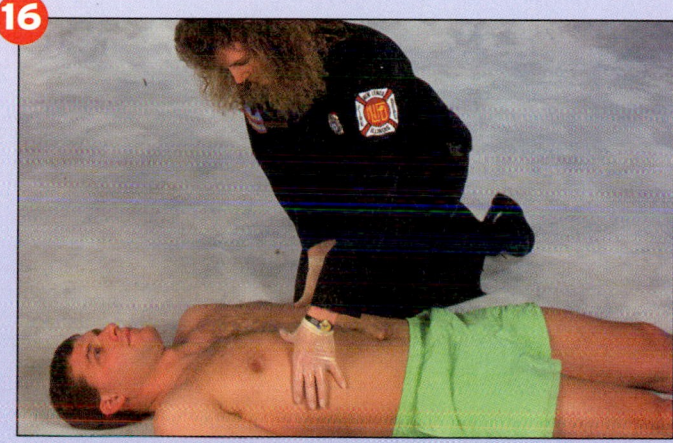

Gently palpate over the ribs to elicit tenderness. Avoid pressing over obvious bruises or fractures.

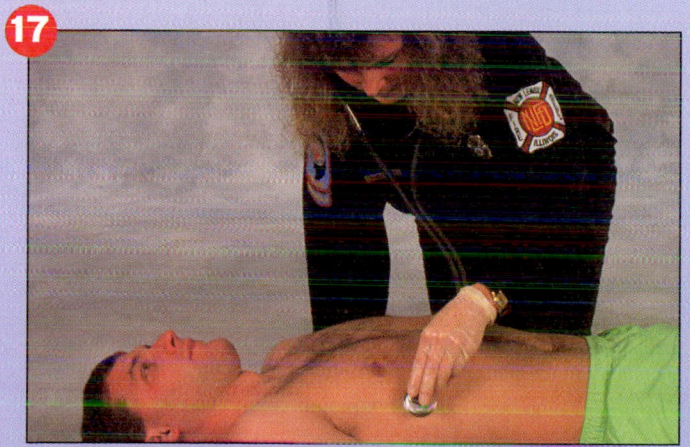

Listen for breath sounds over the midaxillary and midclavicular lines.

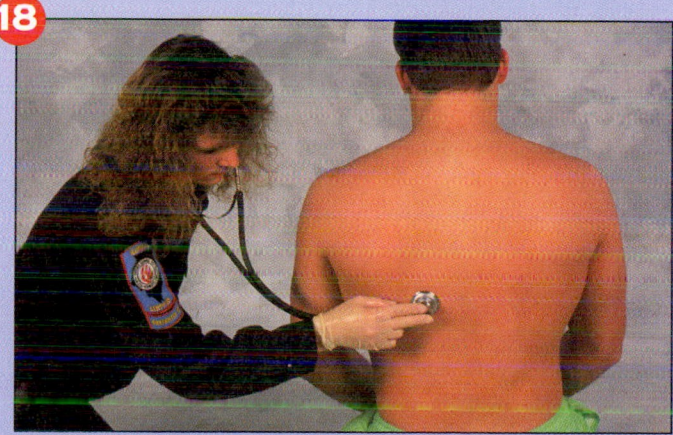

Listen also at the bases and apices of the lungs.

(Continued)

5

Performing the Detailed Physical Exam—cont'd.
Figure 8-26

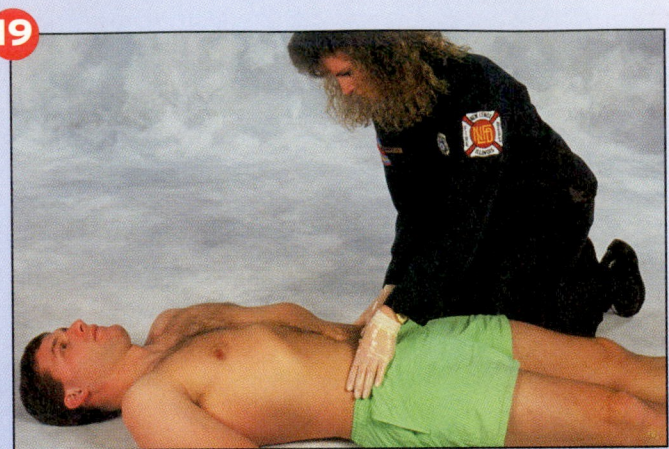

Look at the abdomen and pelvis for obvious lacerations, bruises, and deformities.

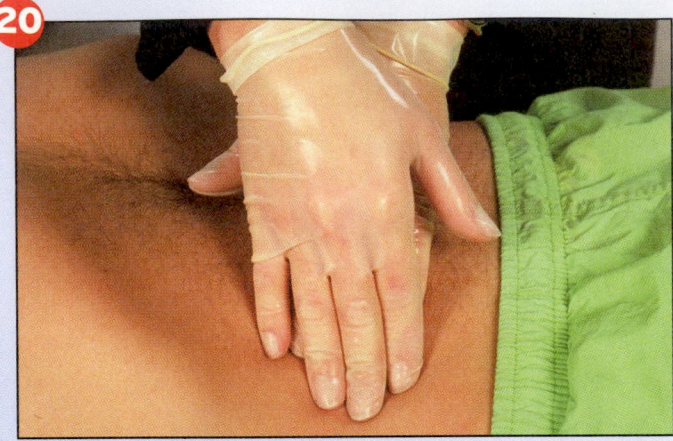

Gently palpate the abdomen for tenderness. If the abdomen is unusually tense, you should describe the abdomen as rigid.

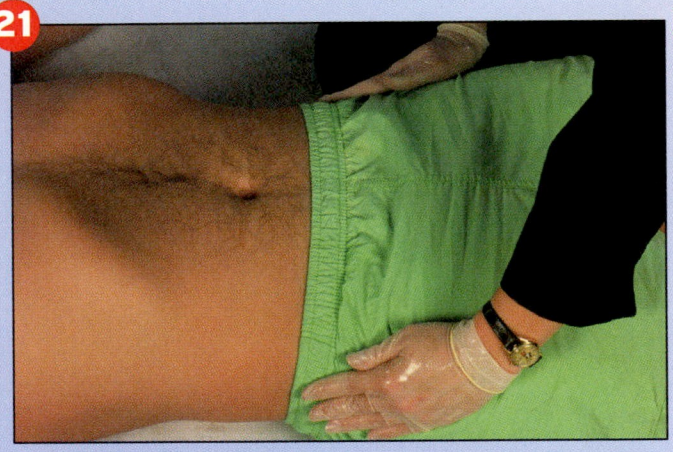

Gently compress the pelvis from the sides to assess for tenderness.

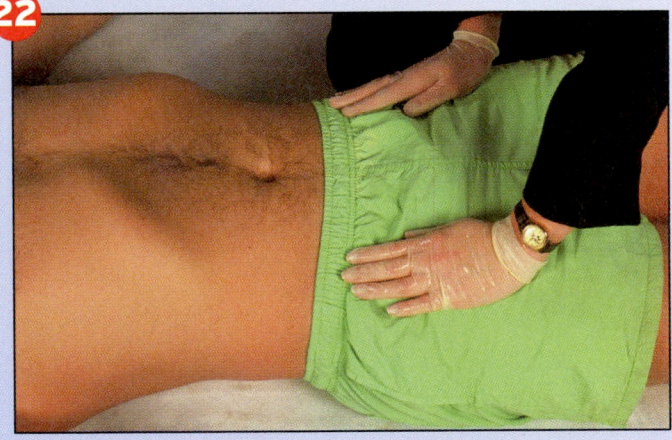

Gently press the iliac crests to elicit instability, tenderness, or crepitus.

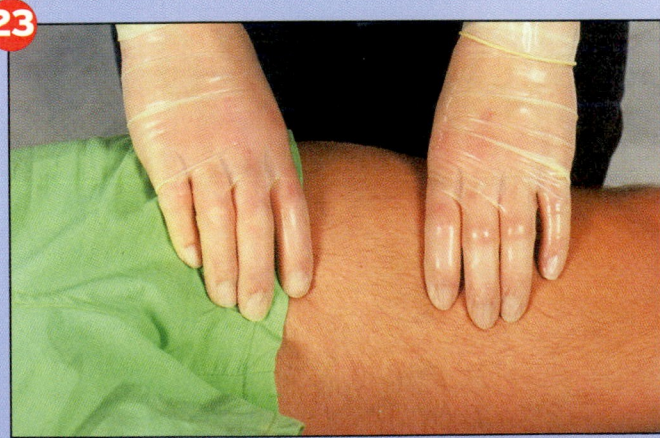

Inspect all four extremities for lacerations, bruises, swelling, and deformities. Also assess distal circulation, sensation, and movement in all extremities.

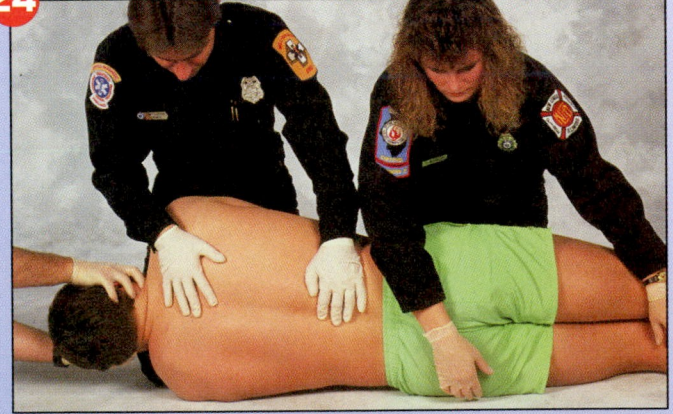

Assess the back for tenderness or deformities. Remember, if you suspect a spinal cord injury, use spinal precautions as you log roll the patient.

a strong alcohol odor or fruity breath odor, should be reported and recorded.

Palpate the front and back of the neck for tenderness and deformity. The sensation of crackling or popping, not unlike palpating the bubbles in bubble-pack packing material, is called subcutaneous emphysema; it indicates that air is leaking into the space under the skin. Usually, this means that the patient has a pneumothorax or has damaged the larynx. Also look for pronounced or distended jugular veins. This is normal in a patient who is lying down; however, their presence in the patient who is sitting up may suggest some type of damage to the heart.

Chest

Throughout the patient assessment process, you should monitor the patient's breathing. If you have not already done so, you should carefully palpate the patient's chest. Feel for crepitus, as this occurs with a ruptured airway or pneumothorax. Also evaluate the movement of the chest wall during breathing. Paradoxical motion of the chest wall means that your patient has a flail chest and might need supplemental oxygen and/or assisted ventilation. You might also wish to perform a more detailed evaluation of the patient's breath sounds. Listening at the apices, at the midclavicular lines bilaterally, at the bases, and at the midaxillary lines bilaterally, check for the specific sounds of breathing. You may be able to identify one of the following:

- Normal breath sounds. These are clear and quiet on both inspiration and expiration.

- Wheezing breath sounds. These suggest an obstruction of the lower airways. Wheezing is a high-pitched squeal that is most prominent on expiration.

- Wet breath sounds. These may indicate cardiac failure. A moist crackling, usually on both inspiration and expiration is called **rales**, or crackles.

- Congested breath sounds. These may suggest the presence of mucus in the lungs. Expect to hear a low-pitched, noisy sound that is most prominent on expiration. This sound may be referred to as **rhonchi**, or "low wheezing." The patient often reports a productive cough associated with this sound.

- A crowing sound. This is often heard without a stethoscope and may indicate that the patient has an airway obstruction in the neck or upper part of the chest. Expect to hear a brassy, crowing sound that is most prominent on expiration. This sound may be referred to as **stridor**.

Abdomen

During the detailed physical exam, you may perform a more complete examination of the abdomen. As you feel all around the abdomen, use the terms firm, soft, tender, or distended (swollen) to report your findings. Some patients may tense the abdomen as you feel it. This reaction may be caused by a ticklish or overly sensitive patient or may be a condition known as **guarding**, which is often associated with damage to organs within the abdomen.

Pelvis

If you have not previously identified any abnormality, recheck the pelvis to identify pain, tenderness, instability, and crepitus; all may indicate a fractured pelvis and the potential for shock.

Extremities

If you have not already done so, you should carefully evaluate the extremities for any signs of trauma, again using the DCAP-BTLS method. You should also evaluate the distal circulation, sensation, and movement. If you have already identified an injury, regular evaluation of the circulation, sensation, and movement below the injury will allow you to be sure that the injury has not compromised circulation.

Back

During the rapid assessment, you should have visualized and palpated the patient's back for signs of trauma, especially near the spine. You must use spinal precautions when rolling the patient for assessment of back injuries. The presence of spinal deformity or pain suggests that—if you have not already done so-the patient requires spinal immobilization. Look for and document any other abnormalities that you find on the back.

Assess Baseline Vital Signs

Sometimes, you will be so busy establishing and maintaining the ABCD that you will not have a chance to get the patient's vital signs. That is as it should be. Nothing should take priority over the airway, breathing, and circulation. However, whenever possible, it is important to get a set of baseline vitals at some time during your patient encounter. If you have not assessed the vital signs, now is the time.

5

Ongoing Assessment

Unlike the detailed physical exam, <u>**ongoing assessment**</u> is performed on all patients during transport. Its purpose is to ask and answer the following questions:

- Is treatment improving the patient's condition?
- Has an already identified problem gotten better? Worse?
- What is the nature of any newly identified problems?

The ongoing assessment helps you to monitor changes in the patient's condition. If the changes are improvements, simply continue whatever treatment you are providing. However, in some instances, the patient's condition will become worse. When this happens, you should be prepared to modify treatment as appropriate and then begin new treatment on the basis of the problem identified.

Steps of the Ongoing Assessment

The procedure for the ongoing assessment is simply to repeat the initial assessment and the focused assessment and to check the intervention steps that pertain to the problems you are treating. These steps should be repeated and recorded every 15 minutes for a stable patient and every 5 minutes for an unstable patient (Figure 8-27). Remember to use your judgment when timing the ongoing assessments. Some patients may require more frequent assessments.

The steps of the ongoing assessment are as follows:

1. Repeat the initial assessment.
   - Reassess mental status.
   - Maintain an open airway.
   - Monitor the patient's breathing.
   - Reassess pulse rate and quality.
   - Monitor skin color and temperature.
   - Reestablish patient priorities.
2. Reassess and record vital signs.
3. Repeat your focused assessment regarding patient complaint or injuries, including questions about the patient's history.
4. Check interventions.
   - Ensure adequacy of oxygen delivery/artificial ventilation.
   - Ensure management of bleeding.
   - Ensure adequacy of other interventions.

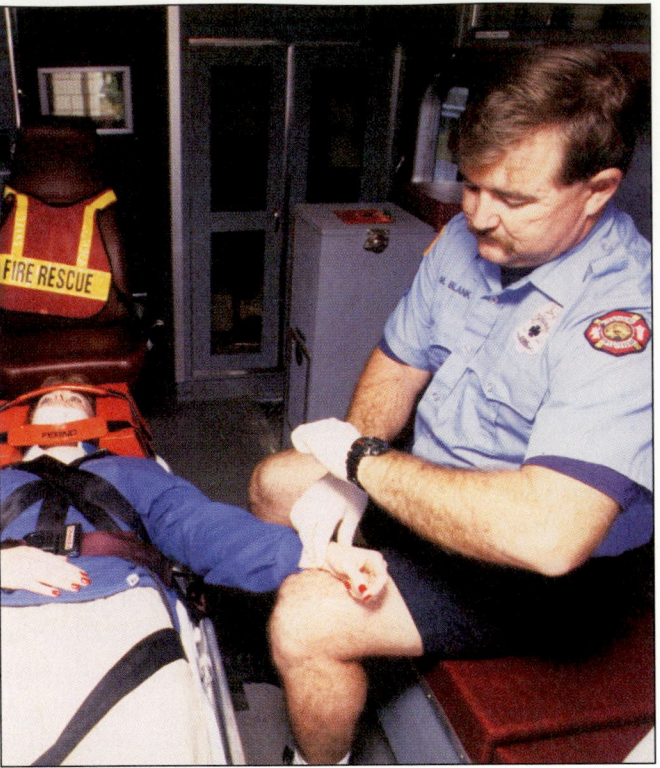

FIGURE 8-27 During the ongoing assessment, repeat your initial assessment, recheck vital signs, and recheck interventions every 5 minutes if the patient is unstable and every 15 minutes if the patient is stable.

Repeat the Initial Assessment

The first step is to repeat the initial assessment. If you have been treating the ABCD, you need to continue monitoring these essential functions. It is particularly important to reassess mental status; changes can be initially subtle and then rapid.

Reevaluate any problems that you have been treating. Reassess the patient's skin color, wound, or anything for which you have begun treatment. If the patient's condition remains stable, great. But, you may discover a need to change a dressing, tighten a strap, or turn up the oxygen. Do it now.

Reassess and Record Vital Signs

Be sure that the patent's vital signs have not changed. Record these so that your documentation is accurate and complete. If the vital signs have changed, evaluate what may have happened and what you should do about it.

PATIENT ASSESSMENT FLOWCHART

Ongoing Assessment

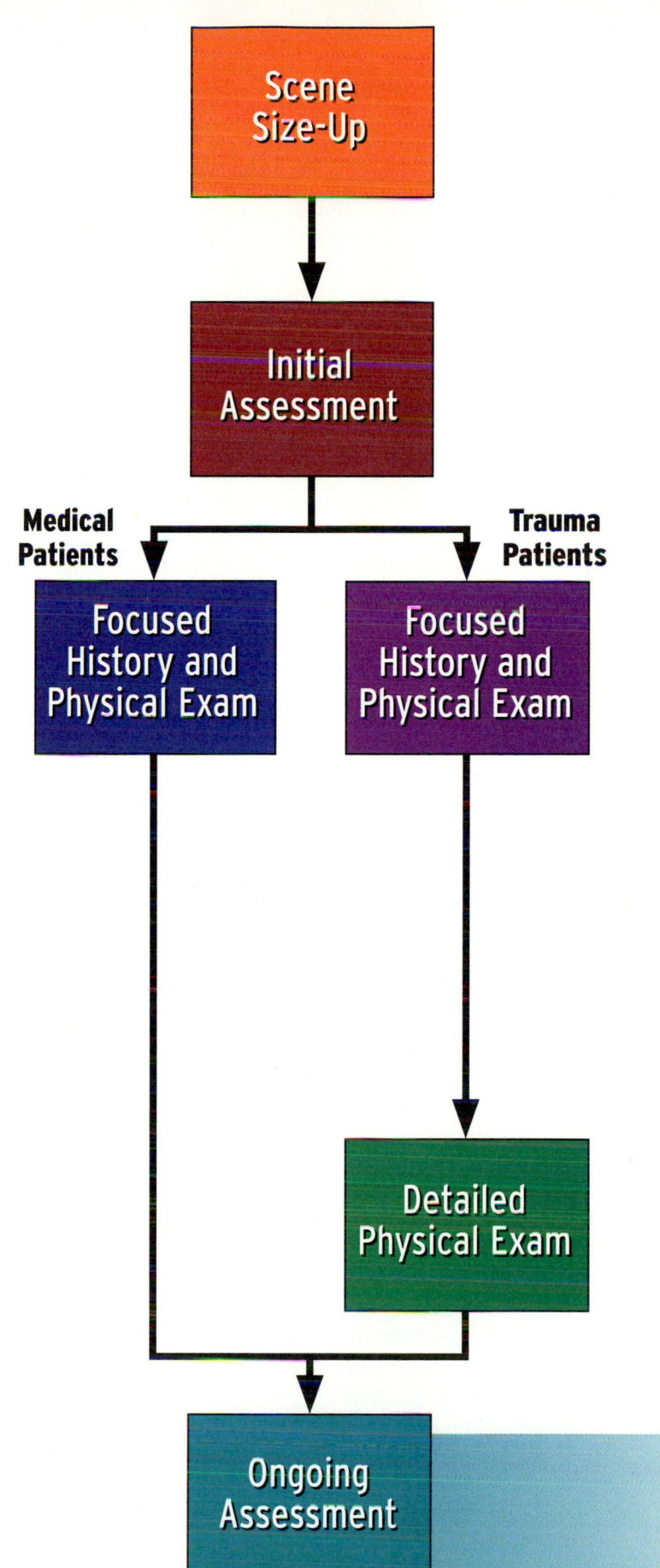

Scene Size-Up

Initial Assessment

Medical Patients

Trauma Patients

Focused History and Physical Exam

Focused History and Physical Exam

Detailed Physical Exam

Ongoing Assessment

6

becoming an expert

You may notice at times that experienced EMT-Bs and paramedics seem to have a "sixth sense" when it comes to some patients. They seem to be able to recognize severe problems even before they have completed their initial assessment. This clinical intuition is one of the hallmarks of the expert EMT that you can develop as you progress through your career—if you pay attention and work at it.

The aspects of clinical intuition include the following:

- **The ability to recognize patterns.** Intuitive EMTs immediately recognize clinical patterns that they have seen before. For example, you may immediately recognize that a pale, diaphoretic patient looks like another patient you have seen in severe shock.

- **Common sense understanding.** Experienced, intuitive EMTs who use their knowledge and experience also use common sense in their assessment and treatment. For instance, they refrain from starting CPR on a responsive patient even though they cannot feel a pulse.

- **The ability to sense what is important.** Good EMTs know how to track problems that are truly important. They avoid the tendency to get lost in unimportant problems and stay focused on the ones that truly matter. For instance, a forehead laceration will not distract them from the serious cardiac problem that caused a fall.

- Deliberate rationally. Good EMTs use their intuition to help them make decisions, but they always temper it by asking, "What if I'm wrong?" For example, a patient who was in a serious motor vehicle accident but has no complaints and appears normal is probably fine. An experienced EMT-B might believe that the patient has no serious injuries and probably does not require spinal immobilization. However, the answer to the question "What if I'm wrong?" could be "Disastrous: permanent spinal cord injury and paralysis." The experienced EMT-B decides to immobilize.

How can you improve your own intuitive powers? First, you need some experience. The truth is that you will not become intuitive until you have been involved in patient care for some time and have evaluated and treated a number of patients.

By following a systematic approach to patient assessment, using your intuition and common sense, and really listening to the patient, you will learn to make good decisions about the treatment and transport of the many patients you will care for in your career.

Repeat Focused Assessment

As you transport your patient, remember to ask the patient about the chief complaint. Is the chest pain getting better or worse? Is leg pain improving with treatment or staying about the same? If you asked the patient to rate symptoms on a 1 to 10 scale, ask for another rating. Remember that this is the reason the patient called 9-1-1.

Check Interventions

Reevaluate any interventions you started. Take a moment to make certain that the oxygen is still flowing, that the backboard straps are still tight, that the bleeding has been controlled, and that the airway is still open. Things often change in the uncontrolled prehospital environment, so this is a good time to be sure that your treatments are still "working" the way you expect.

prep kit

ready for review

The assessment process begins with evaluation of the dispatch information, which often includes the nature of the call and an early report on the chief complaint. The dispatch information may also provide clues to potential hazards to be found on the scene.

The scene size-up identifies real or potential hazards. The patient should not be approached until these hazards have been dealt with in a way that eliminates or minimizes risk to both the EMTs and the patient(s).

The initial assessment is performed on all patients. It identifies any life-threatening conditions to the airway, breathing, circulation, and disability. Any abnormalities that are found must be treated before moving to the next step of the assessment.

The rapid assessment is performed quickly on any patient who is unconscious or unable to articulate the nature of the problem to identify injuries or illnesses. When abnormalities are found, they should be prioritized and treated as appropriate.

The focused history and physical exam are performed on all patients once their ABCD is stabilized. The focused history and physical exam identify potentially life-threatening conditions and help you to identify and explore the patient's chief complaint. In most cases, the focused history and physical exam will provide adequate information to enable you to initiate treatment.

The detailed physical exam is performed on a select group of patients. It helps you to further understand problems that were identified during the focused exam and may also be used to evaluate problems that cannot be identified using the focused exam. The detailed physical exam should be performed en route to the hospital.

The ongoing assessment is also performed on all patients. It gives you an opportunity to reevaluate problems that are being treated and to recheck treatments to be sure that they are still being delivered correctly. Information from the ongoing assessment may be used to change treatment plans.

As you can see, the assessment process is both systematic and dynamic. All patients will be evaluated by using these same steps. However, because of the ability of the focused history and physical exam to center your actions on the major problems, each of your assessments will be slightly different, depending on the needs of the patient. The result will be a process that will enable you to quickly identify and treat the needs of all patients, both medical and traumatic, in a way that meets their unique needs.

Patient Assessment Process

Trauma Patient with a Significant Mechanism of Injury	Trauma Patient with No Significant Mechanism of Injury	Medical Patient Who Is Responsive	Medical Patient Who Is Not Responsive
Scene Size-Up			
Initial Assessment			
Focused History/Physical Exam*			
• Reconsider mechanism of injury	• Assess chief complaint	• Assess chief complaint	• Rapid medical assessment
• Rapid trauma assessment	• Focused assessment of area of complaint	• O-P-Q-R-S-T	• Baseline vital signs
• Baseline vital signs	• Baseline vital signs	• Focused physical exam	• SAMPLE history (from family or bystanders)
• SAMPLE history	• SAMPLE history	• Baseline vital signs	
Detailed Physical Exam			
• Area by area exam*	• Area by area exam*	• Area by area exam*	• Area by area exam*
On-Going Assessment*			

* If appropriate

prep kit

vital vocabulary

accessory muscles The secondary muscles of respiration.

AVPU A method of assessing a patient's level of consciousness by determining whether a patient is awake and alert, responsive to verbal stimulus or pain, or unresponsive; used principally in the initial assessment.

blunt trauma A mechanism of injury in which force occurs over a broad area and the skin is not usually broken.

body substance isolation (BSI) An infection control concept and practice that assumes that all body fluids are potentially infectious.

breath sounds An indication of air movement in the lungs.

capillary refill A test that evaluates the function of the circulatory system at the distal points in the body.

chief complaint The reason a patient called for help. Also, the patient's response to general questions such as "What's wrong?" or "What happened?"

coagulate Formation of clots to plug openings in injured blood vessels and stop blood flow.

conjunctiva The delicate membrane that lines the eyelids and covers the exposed surface of the eye.

crepitus A grating or grinding sensation caused by fractured bone ends or joints rubbing together. Also air bubbles under the skin, giving the skin a crinkly feeling.

cyanosis Blueish-gray skin color that is caused by reduced oxygen levels in the blood.

DCAP-BTLS A mnemonic for assessment in which each area of the body is evaluated for Deformities, Contusions, Abrasions, Punctures/Penetrations, Burns, Tenderness, Lacerations, and Swelling.

detailed physical exam The part of the assessment process in which a detailed area-by-area exam is performed on patients whose problems cannot be readily identified or when more specific information about problems identified in the focused history and physical exam is necessary.

diffuse pain Pain that is not identified as being specific to a single location.

entrance wound The area of the body where a penetrating trauma occurs. In knife or gunshot wounds, this would be the area where the bullet or blade entered. Also seen in serious electrical injuries.

exit wound The area of the body where a penetrating trauma exited. In gunshot wounds, this would be the area where the bullet exited.

focal pain Pain that is easily identified as being specific to a single location.

focused history and physical exam The part of the assessment process in which the patient's major complaints or any problems that are immediately evident are further and more specifically evaluated.

frostbite Damage to tissues as the result of exposure to cold; frozen or partially frozen body parts.

general impression The overall initial impression that determines the priority for patient care. It is based on the patient's surroundings, the mechanism of injury, or the patient's chief complaint.

Golden hour The period of time during which treatment of a patient in shock or with traumatic injuries is most critical. This period of time is generally thought to be the first 60 minutes after injury.

guarding Involuntary muscle contraction of the abdominal wall in an effort to protect the inflamed abdomen.

hypothermia A condition in which the internal body temperature falls below 95°F (35°C) after exposure to a cold environment.

initial assessment The part of the assessment process that helps you to identify any immediately or potentially life-threatening conditions so that you can initiate lifesaving care.

jaundice A yellow skin color that is seen in patients with liver disease or dysfunction.

mechanism of injury The way in which traumatic injuries occur; the forces that act on the body to cause damage.

nasal flaring Flaring out of the nostrils, indicating that there is an airway obstruction.

ongoing assessment The part of the assessment process in which problems are reevaluated and responses to treatment are assessed.

orientation The mental status of a patient; the patient's memory of person (his or her name), place (the current location), time (the current year, month, and approximate date), and event (what happened).

OPQRST The six pain questions: Onset, Provoke, Quality, Radiation, Severity, Time and Treatment.

palpate Examine by touch.

paradoxical motion The motion of the chest wall that is detached in a flail chest; the motion is exactly the opposite of normal motion during breathing; that is, it is in during inhalation, out during exhalation.

penetrating trauma A mechanism of injury in which force occurs in a small point of contact between the skin and the object. The skin is broken and the potential for infection is high.

radiation A continuation of an area of pain or discomfort distal to the site of the origin of the pain.

rales Cracking, rattling breath sound that signals fluid in the air spaces of the lungs. Also called *crackles*.

responsiveness The way in which a patient responds to external stimuli, including verbal stimuli (sound), tactile stimuli (touch), and painful stimuli.

retractions Movements in which the skin pulls in around the ribs during inspiration.

rhonchi Coarse breath sounds heard in patients with chronic mucus in the airways.

SAMPLE history A key brief history of a patient's condition to determine Signs/Symptoms, Allergies, Medications, Pertinent past history, Last oral intake, and Events leading to the illness/injury.

scene size-up The part of the assessment process in which a quick assessment of the scene and the surroundings is made to provide as much information as possible about the safety of the scene.

sclera The white portion of the eye; the tough outer coat of the eye that gives protection to the delicate, light-sensitive inner layer.

stridor A harsh, high-pitched inspiratory sound, such as the sound that is often heard in acute laryngeal (upper airway) obstruction.

subcutaneous emphysema The presence of air in soft tissues, causing a characteristic crackling sensation on palpation.

triage The process of establishing treatment and transportation priorities according to severity of injury and medical need.

two- to three-word dyspnea A condition in which a patient can speak only two to three words at a time without pausing to take a breath.

assessment in action

Moments after the fire department is called about a water flow alarm at the local high school, you and your partner are dispatched to the same address. Firefighters take only a few minutes to isolate the bathroom with the flaming wastebasket and put out the fire. They also find an 18-year-old man in one of the stalls, where he apparently sought refuge from the smoke and flames.

1. Which of the following terms would best describe the patient's current level of consciousness?
   A. Alert and oriented
   B. Responsive to pain
   C. Semi-conscious
   D. Unresponsive

2. Which of the following characteristics of the patient's skin would suggest that the patient is not getting adequate oxygen?
   A. Pale
   B. Cyanotic
   C. Warm
   D. Moist

3. High-concentration supplemental oxygen would be best delivered to the patient by a:
   A. BVM device at 2 L/min.
   B. nasal cannula at 24 L/min.
   C. nonrebreathing mask at 15 L/min.
   D. pocket mask with connector tubing at 4 L/min.

The firefighter who found him said that the patient was initially unresponsive and even now responds only by moaning when you pinch his arm. His pupils are dilated and barely reactive. His skin is warm, moist, and light gray-blue. He has a blood pressure of 104/66 mm Hg, a regular pulse of 130 beats/min, and respirations of 26/min.

4. Which of the following statements about assisted ventilations is true?
   A. An unresponsive patient who has adequate respirations must receive assisted ventilations with a BVM device.
   B. An unresponsive patient with respirations of 4/min should receive high-flow oxygen via nasal cannula.
   C. A patient who has inadequate respirations should receive highflow oxygen and receive assisted ventilations.
   D. A patient who is not breathing should receive 12 to 15 L of oxygen via a nonrebreathing mask.

5. Which of the following conditions is **NOT** considered to be a treatment priority in an adult patient?
   A. Unconscious and unresponsive to any form of stimuli
   B. Difficulty breathing and an altered level of consciousness
   C. Responsive only to pain and does not follow commands
   D. A systolic blood pressure of more than 120 mm Hg and leg pain

points to ponder

Objectives 3-2.5, 3-2.14, 3-2.19, 3-2.21

You and your partner arrive at the scene of a single-car rollover accident. You are first on the scene and find five victims. As you approach the vehicle, you stop at a patient who was thrown from the vehicle. This patient (patient A) has a weak pulse and irregular breathing and is missing about a third of her skull, with obvious brain damage. You continue to the car and find the driver (patient B) holding his arm, which is obviously fractured at midshaft humerus and is very painful. The next two patients are in the back seat. An approximately 10-year-old boy (passenger C) is unresponsive, and you can hear gurgling sounds when he breathes in. The other passenger in the back seat (passenger D) is an elderly woman with an open fracture of her femur, which is bleeding profusely. The last patient is an infant (passenger E), who has somehow become trapped under the front seat of the car. The infant is not making any noise and is not moving, but you are unable to access it quickly to check pulse or breathing. You complete your initial patient assessment and find no significant problems other than the ones listed above. Just you and your partner are present.

- In what order would you treat these patients, and why? Justify the order for each patient.

online outlook

During the initial assessment (ABCD), life-threatening conditions are identified and their management is begun. You can learn more about the initial assessment by following the Trauma Assessment link at www.emtb.com.

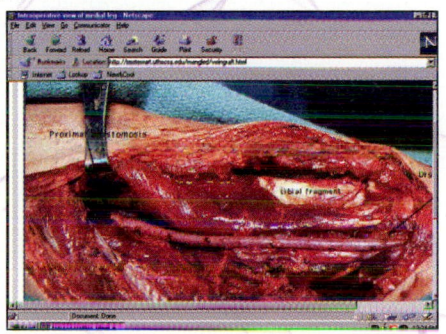

Communications and Documentation

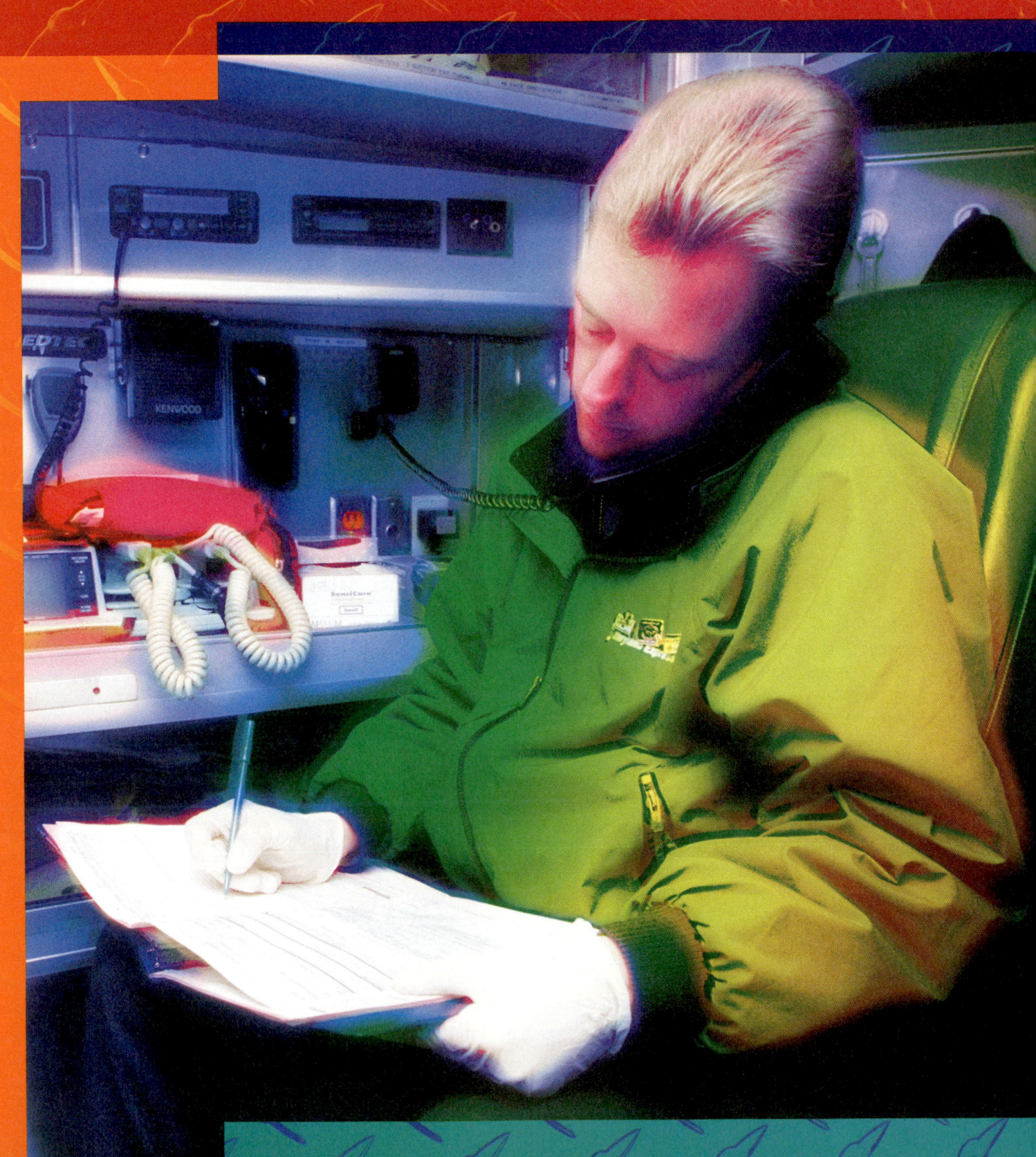

objectives

Cognitive

1. List the proper methods of initiating and terminating a radio call.

2. State the proper sequence for delivery of patient information.

3. Explain the importance of effective communication of patient information in the verbal report.

4. Identify the essential components of the verbal report.

5. Describe the attributes for increasing effectiveness and efficiency of verbal communications.

6. State legal aspects to consider in verbal communication.

7. Discuss the communication skills that should be used to interact with the patient.

8. Discuss the communication skills that should be used to interact with the family, bystanders, individuals from other agencies while providing patient care and hospital personnel, and the difference between skills used to interact with the patient and those used to interact with others.

9. List the correct radio procedures in the following phases of a typical call:
   - To the scene
   - At the scene
   - To the facility
   - At the facility
   - To the station
   - At the station

10. Explain the components of the written report and list the information that should be included on the written report.

11. Identify the various sections of the written report.

12. Describe what information is required in each section of the prehospital care report and how it should be entered.

13. Define the special considerations concerning patient refusal.

14. Describe the legal implications associated with the written report.

15. Discuss all state and/or local record and reporting requirements.

Affective

16. Explain the rationale for providing efficient and effective radio communications and patient reports.

17. Explain the rationale for patient care documentation.

18. Explain the rationale for the EMS system gathering data.

19. Explain the rationale for using medical terminology correctly.

20. Explain the rationale for using an accurate and synchronous clock so that information can be used in trending.

Psychomotor

21. Perform a simulated, organized, concise radio transmission.

22. Perform an organized, concise patient report that would be given to the staff at a receiving facility.

23. Perform a brief, organized report that would be given to an ALS provider arriving at an incident scene at which the EMT-B was already providing care.

24. Practice completing a prehospital care report.

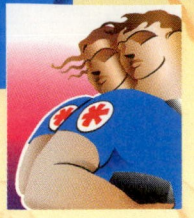
Communications and Documentation

Effective communication is an essential component of prehospital care. Radio and telephone communications link you and your team with other members of the EMS, fire, and law enforcement communities. This link helps the entire team to work together more effectively and provides an important layer of safety and protection for each member of the team. You must know what your system can and cannot do, and you must be able to use your system efficiently and effectively. You must be able to send precise, accurate reports about the scene, the patient's condition, and the treatment that you provide.

Verbal communications are also a vital skill for EMT-Bs. Your verbal skills will enable you to gather information from the patient and bystanders. They will also make it possible for you to effectively coordinate the variety of responders who are often present at the scene. Excellent verbal communications are also an integral part of transferring the patient's care to the nurses and physicians at the hospital. You must possess good listening skills to fully understand the nature of the scene and the patient's problem. You must also be able to organize your thoughts to quickly and accurately verbalize instructions to the patient, bystanders, and other responders. Finally, you must be able to organize and summarize the important aspects of the patient's presentation and treatment when reporting to the hospital staff.

Written communications complete the process. Written communications, in the form of a written patient care report, provide you with an opportunity to communicate the patient's story to others who may participate in the patient's care in the future. Adequate reporting and accurate records ensure the continuity of patient care. Complete patient records also guarantee proper transfer of responsibility, comply with the requirements of health departments and law enforcement agencies, and fulfill your organization's administrative needs. Reporting and record-keeping duties are an essential aspect of patient care, although they must be performed only after the patient's condition has been stabilized.

This chapter describes the skills that you need to be an effective communicator. It begins by identifying the kinds of equipment that are used, along with standard radio operating procedures and protocols. Next, the roles of the Federal Communications Commission (FCC) in EMS are described. The chapter concludes with a discussion of a variety of effective methods of verbal communications and guidelines for appropriate written documentation of patient care.

Communications Systems and Equipment

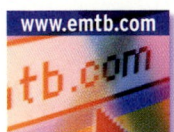
As an EMT-B, you must be familiar with two-way radio communications and have working knowledge of the mobile and hand-held portable radios that are used in your unit. You must also know when to use them and what to say when you are transmitting.

Base Station Radios

The dispatcher usually communicates with field units by transmitting through a fixed radio base station that is controlled from the dispatch center. A **base station** is any radio hardware containing a transmitter and receiver that is located in a fixed place (Figure 9-1). The base station may be used in a single place by an operator speaking into a microphone that is connected directly to the equipment. It also works remotely through telephone lines or by radio from a communications center. Base stations may include dispatch centers, fire stations, ambulance bases, or hospitals.

A two-way radio consists of two units: a transmitter and a receiver. Some base stations may have more than one transmitter and/or more than one receiver. They may also be equipped with one multi-channel transmitter and several single channel receivers. A **channel** is an assigned frequency or frequencies that are used to carry voice and/or data communications. Regardless of the number of transmitters and receivers, they are commonly called base radios or stations. Base stations usually have more power (often 100 watts or more) and higher, more efficient antenna systems than mobile or portable radios. This increased broadcasting range allows the base station operator to communicate with field units and other stations at much greater distances.

The base radio must be physically close to its antenna. Therefore, the actual base station cabinet and hardware are commonly found on the roof of a tall building or at the bottom of an antenna tower. The base station operator may be miles away in a dispatch center or hospital, communicating with the base station radio by dedicated lines or special radio links.

> A two-way radio consists of two units: a transmitter and a receiver.

A **dedicated line**, also known as a hot line, is always open or under the control of the individuals at each end. This type of line is immediately "on" as soon as you lift the receiver and cannot be accessed by outside users.

Mobile and Portable Radios

In the ambulance, you will use both mobile and portable radios to communicate with the dispatcher and/or medical control. An ambulance will often have more than one mobile radio, each on a different frequency (Figure 9-2). One radio may be used to communicate with the dispatcher or other public safety agencies. A second radio is often used for communicating patient information to medical control.

A mobile radio is installed in a vehicle and usually operates at lower power than a base station. Most **VHF (very high frequency)** mobile radios operate at 100 watts of power. Radios that operate at 800 MHz of power are very common in EMS systems. **UHF (ultra-high frequency)** mobile radios usually have only 40 watts of power. Cellular telephones operate on 3 watts of power or less. Mobile antennas are much closer to the ground than base station antennas, so communications from the unit are typically limited to 10 to 15 miles over average terrain.

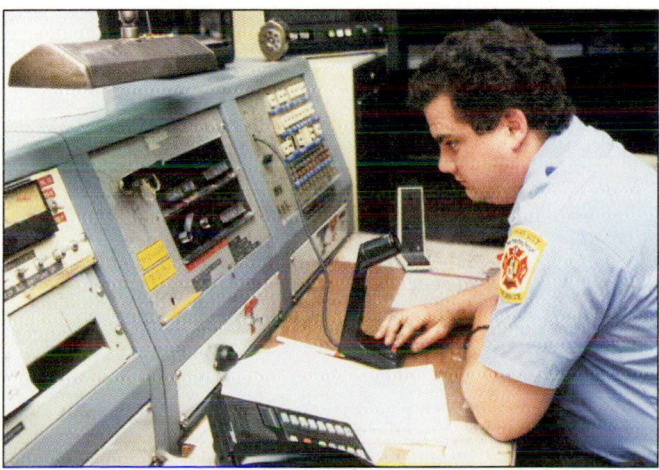

FIGURE 9-1 A base station consists of radio hardware containing a transmitter and a receiver that is located in a fixed place. Some have more than one transmitter and/or more than one receiver.

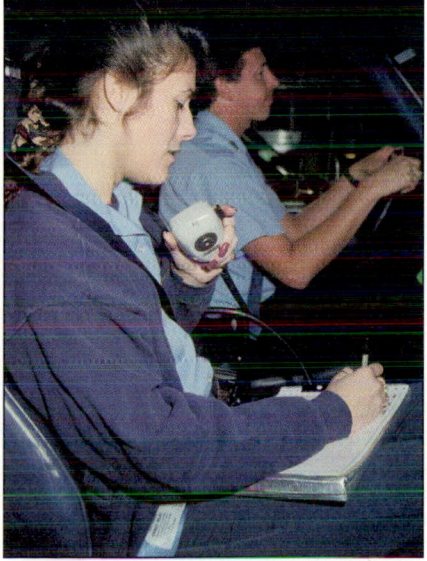

FIGURE 9-2 Some ambulances have more than one mobile radio, each on a different frequency.

Portable radios are hand-carried or hand-held devices that operate at 1 to 5 watts of power (Figure 9-3). Since the entire radio can be held in your hand, when in use the antenna is often no higher than the EMT who is using the radio. The transmission range of a portable radio is more limited than that of mobile or base station radios. Portable radios are essential in helping to coordinate EMS activities at the scene of a multiple-casualty incident. They are also helpful when you are away from the ambulance and need to communicate with dispatch, another unit, or medical control.

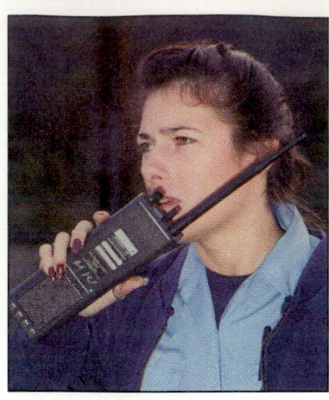

FIGURE 9-3 A portable radio is essential if you need to communicate with the dispatcher or medical control when you are away from the ambulance.

Repeater-Based Systems

A **repeater** is a special base station radio that receives messages and signals on one frequency and then automatically retransmits them on a second frequency. Because a repeater is a base station (with a large antenna), it is able to receive lower-power signals, such as those from a portable radio, from a long distance away. The signal is then rebroadcast with all the power of the base station (Figure 9-4). EMS systems that use repeaters usually have outstanding system-wide communications and are able to get the best signal from portable radios.

Digital Equipment

Although most people think of voice communications when they think of two-way radios, digital signals are also a part of EMS communications. Some EMS systems use telemetry to send an ECG from the unit to the hospital. With **telemetry**, electronic signals are converted into coded, audible signals. These signals can then be transmitted by radio or telephone to a receiver at the hospital with a decoder. The decoder converts the signals back into electronic impulses that can be displayed on a screen or printed. Another example of telemetry is a fax message.

Digital signals are also used in some kinds of paging and tone alerting systems because they transmit faster than spoken words and allow more choices and flexibility.

Cellular Telephones

Cellular telephones are becoming more common in EMS communications systems (Figure 9-5). These telephones are simply low-power portable radios that communicate through a series of interconnected repeater stations called "cells" (hence the name "cellular"). Cells are linked by a sophisticated computer system and connected to the telephone network. Cellular telephones are also popular with other public safety agencies, particularly as more cell sites are constructed in rural areas.

Unlike typical two-way mobile communications, which have free access, a cellular system charges fees for its use. Your system can buy portable or mobile radios on the local EMS frequency and use them at no cost. However, buying a cellular telephone is only half of the process of being able to use it. A cellular telephone cannot simply access the telephone network. The user must be assigned a specially coded number that the cellular system's computers will recognize. It is that access and the amount of time a user spends on the telephone for

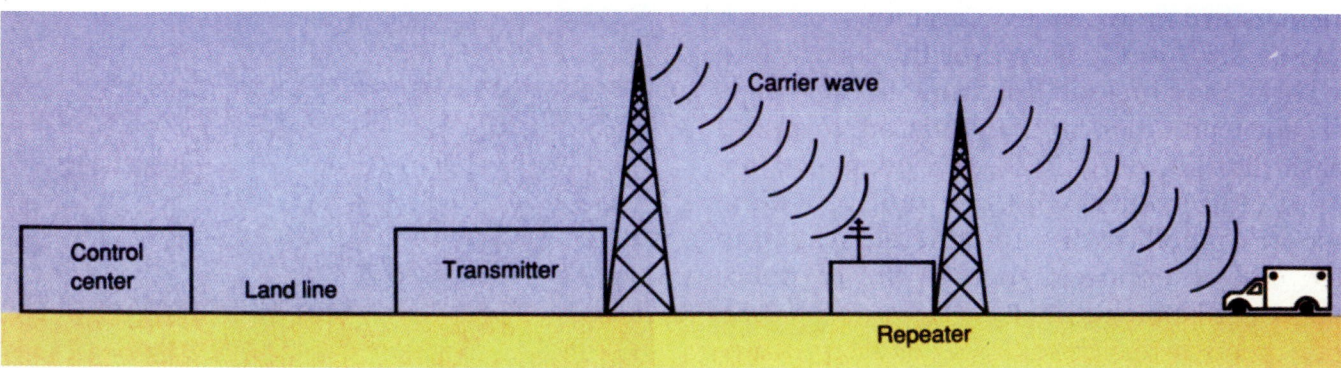

FIGURE 9-4 A message is sent from the control center by a land line to the transmitter. The radio carrier wave is picked up by the repeater for rebroadcast to outlying units. Return radio traffic is picked up by the repeater and rebroadcast to the control center.

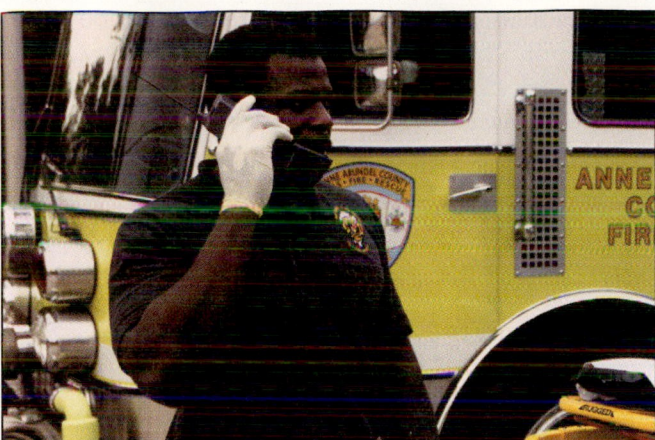

FIGURE 9-5 Use of cellular phones is becoming more common in EMS communications systems.

which the cellular system charges. However, once you are connected to the network, you can call any other telephone in the world and can send voice, data, and telemetry signals.

Many cellular systems make equipment and air time available to EMS services at little or no cost as a public service. The public is often able to call 9-1-1 or other emergency numbers on a cellular telephone free of charge. However, this easy access may result in overloading and jamming of cellular systems in mass-casualty and disaster situations.

As with all repeater-based systems, a cellular telephone is useless if the equipment fails, loses power, or is damaged by severe weather or other circumstances. Like all voice radio communications systems, cellular telephones can be easily overheard on scanners. A scanner is a radio receiver that searches or "scans" across several frequencies until the message is completed. Although cellular telephones are more private than most other forms of radio communications, they can still be overheard. Therefore, you must always speak in a professional manner every time you use the EMS communications system.

Other Communications Equipment

Ambulances and other field units are usually equipped with an external public address system. This system may be a part of the siren or the mobile radio. The intercom between the cab and the patient compartment may also be a part of the mobile radio. These components do not involve radio wave transmission, but you must understand how they work and practice using them *before* you really need them.

EMS systems may use a variety of two-way radio hardware. Some systems operate VHF equipment in the

simplex (push to talk, release to listen) mode. In this mode, radio transmissions can occur in either direction but not simultaneously in both. When one party transmits, the other can only receive and then wait for the other party to finish before he or she can reply. Other systems conduct duplex (simultaneous talk-listen) communications on UHF frequencies and also use cellular telephones. In the full duplex mode, radios can transmit and receive communications simultaneously on one channel. This is sometimes called "a pair of frequencies." A number of VHF and UHF channels, commonly called MED channels, are reserved exclusively for EMS use. However, hundreds of other commercial, local government, and fire services frequencies are also used for EMS communications.

Some EMS systems rely on dedicated lines (hot lines) as control links for their remotely located base stations and antennas. Other systems are more simply configured and require no off-site control links. No matter what type of equipment is used, all EMS communications systems have some basic limitations. Therefore, you must know what your equipment can and cannot do.

The ability for you to communicate effectively with other units or medical control depends on how well the weaker radio can "talk back." Base and repeater station radios often have much greater power and higher antennas than mobile or portable units do. This increased power affects your communications in two ways. First, their signals are generally heard and understood from a much greater distance than the signal produced from a mobile unit. Second, their signals are received clearly from a much greater distance than is possible with a mobile or portable unit. *Remember, when you are at the scene, you may be able to clearly hear the dispatcher or hospital on your radio, but you may not be heard or understood when you transmit.*

Even small changes in your location can significantly affect the quality of your transmission. Also remember that the location of the antenna is critically important for clear transmission. Commercial aircraft flying at 37,000' can transmit and receive signals over hundreds of miles, yet their radios have only a few watts of power. The "power" comes from their 37,000-foot-high antenna!

> You must always speak in a professional manner every time you use the EMS communications system.

At times, you may be able to communicate with a base station radio but you will not be able to hear or transmit to another mobile unit that is also communicating with that base. Repeater base stations eliminate such problems. They allow two mobile or portable units that cannot reach each other directly to communicate through the repeater, using its greater power and antenna.

The success of communications depends on the efficiency of your equipment. A damaged antenna or microphone often prevents high-quality communications. Check the condition and status of your equipment at the start of each shift, and then correct or report any problems.

Radio Communications

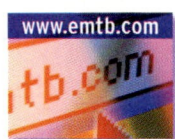 All radio operations in the United States, including those used in EMS systems, are regulated by the <u>Federal Communications Commission (FCC)</u>. The FCC has jurisdiction over interstate and international telephone and telegraph services and satellite communications—all of which may involve EMS activity.

The FCC has five principal EMS-related responsibilities:

1. **Allocating specific radio frequencies for use by EMS providers.** Modern EMS communications began in 1974. At that time, the FCC assigned 10 MED channels in the 460- to 470-MHz (UHF) band to be used by EMS providers. These UHF channels were added to the several VHF frequencies that were already available for EMS systems. However, these VHF frequencies had to be shared with other "special emergencies" uses, including school buses and veterinarians. In 1993, the FCC created an EMS-only block of frequencies in the 220-MHz portion of the radio spectrum.

2. **Licensing base stations and assigning appropriate radio call signs for those stations.** An FCC license is usually issued for 5 years, after which time it must be renewed. Each FCC license is granted only for a specific operating group. Often, the longitude and latitude (locations) of the antenna and the address of the base station determine the call signs.

3. **Establishing licensing standards and operating specifications for radio equipment used by EMS providers.** Before it can be licensed, each piece of radio equipment must be submitted by its manufacturer to the FCC for type acceptance, based on established operating specification and regulations.

4. **Establishing limitations for transmitter power output.** The FCC regulates broadcasting power to reduce radio interference between neighboring communications systems.

5. **Monitoring radio operations.** This includes making spot field checks to help ensure compliance with FCC rules and regulations.

The FCC's rules and regulations fill many volumes and are written in technical and legal language. Only a very small section (part 90, subpart C) deals with EMS communication issues. You are not responsible for reading these detailed and often confusing documents. For appropriate guidance on technical issues, contact your EMS system supervisor. In fact, many EMS systems look to radio and telephone communications experts for advice on technical issues.

Responding to the Scene

EMS communication systems may operate on several different frequencies and may use different frequency bands. Some EMS systems may even use different radios for different purposes. However, all EMS systems depend on the skill of the dispatcher. The dispatcher, who is usually not an EMT-B, receives the first call to 9-1-1 (Figure 9-6). You are part of the team that responds to calls once the dispatcher notifies your unit of an emergency.

The dispatcher has several important responsibilities during the alert and dispatch phase of EMS communications. The dispatcher must do all of the following:

- Properly screen and assign priority to each call (according to predetermined protocols)

- Select and alert the appropriate EMS response unit(s)

- Dispatch and direct EMS response unit(s) to the correct location

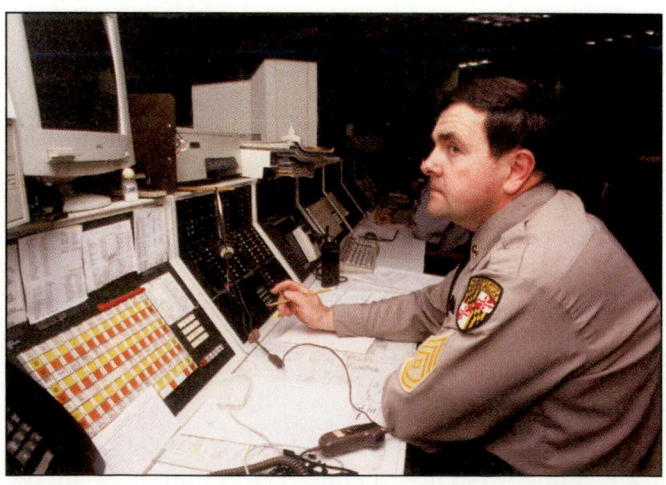

FIGURE 9-6 The dispatcher receives the first call to 9-1-1.

- Coordinate EMS response unit(s) with other public safety services until the incident is over

- Provide emergency medical instructions to the telephone caller so that essential care (e.g., CPR) may begin before the EMTs arrive (according to predetermined protocols).

When the first call to 9-1-1 comes in, the dispatcher must try to judge its relative importance to begin the appropriate EMS response using emergency medical dispatch protocols. First, the dispatcher must find out the exact location of the patient and the nature and severity of the problem. Next, some description of the scene, such as the number of patients or special environmental hazards, is needed. Then, if possible, the dispatcher should ask for the caller's telephone number, the patient's age and name, and other information, as directed by local protocol.

From this information, the dispatcher will assign the appropriate EMS response unit(s) on the basis of the following:

- The dispatcher's perception of the nature and severity of the problem

- The anticipated response time to the scene

- The level of training (first responder, BLS, ALS) of available EMS response unit(s)

- The need for additional EMS units, fire suppression, rescue, a HazMat team, air medical support, or law enforcement

The dispatcher's next step is to alert the appropriate EMS response unit(s) (Figure 9-7). Alerting these units may be done in a variety of ways. The dispatch radio system may be used to contact units that are already in service and monitoring the channel. Dedicated lines (hot lines) between the control center and the EMS station may also be used.

The dispatcher may also page EMS personnel. Pagers are commonly used by both volunteer and full-time EMS personnel. **Paging** involves the use of a coded tone or digital radio signal and a voice or display message that is transmitted to pagers (beepers) or desktop monitor radios. Paging signals may be sent to alert only certain personnel or may be blanket signals that will activate all the pagers in the EMS service. Pagers and monitor radios are convenient because they are usually silent until their specific paging code is received. Alerted personnel contact the dispatcher to confirm the message and receive details of their assignments.

Once EMS personnel have been alerted, they must be properly dispatched and sent to the incident. Every EMS system should use a standard dispatching procedure.

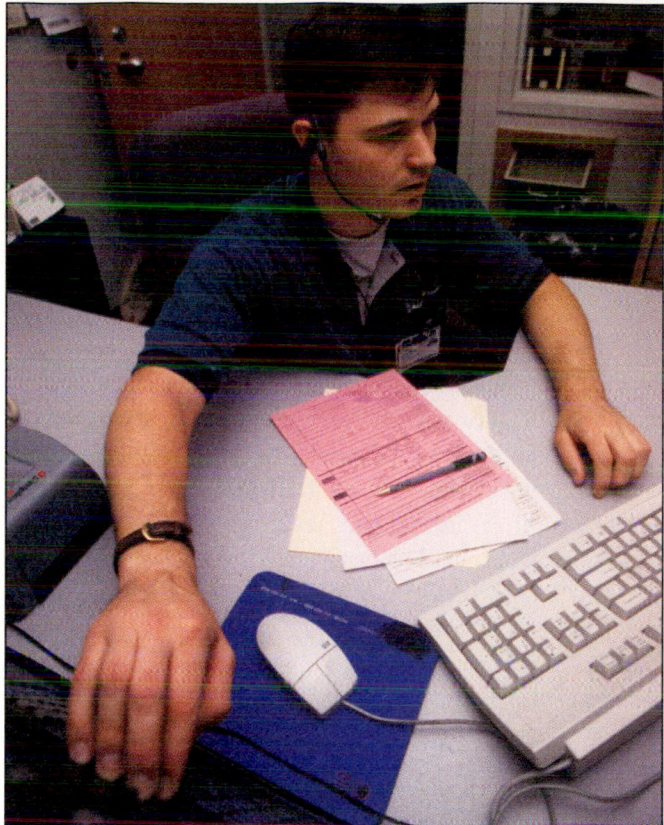

FIGURE 9-7 You will be assigned to a scene by the dispatcher.

The dispatcher should give the responding unit(s) the following information:

- The nature and severity of the injury, illness, or incident

- The exact location of the incident

- The number of patients

- Responses by other public safety agencies

- Special directions or advisories, such as adverse road or traffic conditions or severe weather reports

- The time at which the unit or units are dispatched

Your unit must confirm to the dispatcher that you have received the information and that you are en route to the scene. Local protocol will dictate whether it is the job of the dispatcher or your unit to notify other public safety agencies that you are responding to an emergency. In some areas, the emergency department is also notified whenever an ambulance responds to an emergency.

You should report any problems during your run to the dispatcher. You should also inform the dispatcher that you have arrived at the scene. The arrival report to the dispatcher should include any obvious details that you see during scene size up. For example, you might say, "Dispatcher, Medic One is on scene at Main Street with a two-vehicle collision."

All radio communications during dispatch, as well as other phases of operations, must be brief and easily understood. Although speaking in plain English is best, many areas find that 10 codes are shorter and simpler for routine communications. The development and use of such codes require strict discipline. When used improperly or not understood, codes create rather than clear up confusion.

Communicating with Medical Direction and Hospitals

The principal reason for radio communication is to facilitate communication between you and medical control (and the hospital). Medical control may be located at the receiving hospital, another facility, or sometimes even in another city or state. You must, however, consult with medical control to notify the hospital of an incoming patient, to request advice or orders from medical control, or to advise the hospital of special situations.

It is important to plan and organize your radio communication before you push the transmit button. *Remember, a concise, well-organized report demonstrates your competence and professionalism in the eyes of all who hear your report.* Well-organized radio communications with the hospital will engender confidence in the receiving facility's physicians and nurses, as well as others who are listening. In addition, the patient and family will be comforted by your organization and ability to communicate clearly. A well-delivered radio report puts you in control of the information—which is where you want to be.

Hospital notification is the most common type of communication between you and the hospital. The purpose of these calls is to notify the receiving facility of the patient's complaint and condition (Figure 9-8). On the basis of this information, the hospital is able to appropriately prepare staff and equipment to receive the patient.

Giving the patient report. The patient report should follow a standard format established by your EMS system. The patient report commonly includes the following seven elements:

1. **Your unit identification and level of services.** Example: "Brimfield Medical 71-BLS."

2. **The receiving hospital and your estimated time of arrival.** Example: "Robinson Memorial Hospital, ETA 10 minutes."

3. **The patient's age and gender.** Example: "A 33-year-old woman." The patient's name should not be given over the radio because it may be overheard. This is an invasion of the patient's privacy.

4. **The patient's chief complaint or your perception of the problem and its severity.** Example: "The patient complains of pain in the right lower leg."

5. **A brief history of the patient's current problem.** Example: "The patient fell down the steps." Other important history information that may pertain to the current problem should also be included, such as "The patient has diabetes and takes insulin."

6. **A brief report of physical findings.** This report should include level of consciousness, the patient's general appearance, pertinent abnormalities noted, and vital signs. Example: "The patient is alert and oriented and has normal color and warm skin. Her right lower leg is swollen and tender. Her blood pressure is 132 over 84, pulse is 72, and ventilations 14."

7. **A brief summary of the care given and any patient response.** Example: "We have immobilized the injured leg in a padded cardboard splint. The patient is now on a backboard. She still has motor, sensory, and circulatory function distal to the injured area. She also reports a decrease in pain since the splint was applied."

Be sure that you report all patient information in an objective, accurate, and professional manner. People with scanners are listening. You could be successfully sued for slander if you describe a patient in a way that injures his or her reputation.

The role of medical control. The delivery of EMS involves an impressive array of assessments, stabilization, and treatments. In some cases, you may assist patients in taking medications. Intermediate and advanced EMTs go beyond this level by initiating medication therapy based on the patient's presenting signs. For logical, ethical, and legal reasons, the delivery of such sophisticated care must be done in association with physicians. For this reason, every EMS system needs input and involvement from physicians. One or

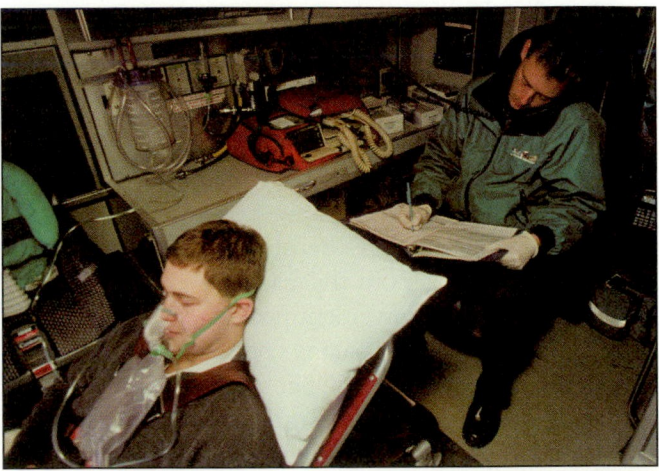

FIGURE 9-8 Giving the patient report should be done in an objective, accurate, professional manner.

more physicians, including your system or department medical director, will provide medical direction (medical control) for your EMS system. Medical control guides the treatment of patients in the system through protocols, direct orders and advice, and post-call review.

Depending upon how the protocols are written, you may need to call medical control for direct orders (permission) to administer certain treatments, to determine the transport destination of patients, or to be allowed to stop treatment and/or not transport a patient. In these cases, the radio or cellular phone provides a vital link between you and the expertise available through the base physician.

To maintain this link 24 hours a day, 7 days a week, medical control must be readily available on the radio at the hospital or on a mobile or portable unit when you call (Figure 9-9). In most areas, medical control is provided by the physicians who work at the receiving hospital. However, many variations have developed across the country. For example, some EMS units receive medical direction from one hospital even though they are taking the patient to another hospital. In other areas, medical direction may come from a free-standing center or even from an individual physician. Regardless of your system's design, your link to medical control is vital to maintain the high quality of care that your patient requires and deserves.

Calling medical control. You can use the radio in your unit or a portable radio to call medical control. A cellular telephone can also be used. Regardless of the type of radio, you should use a channel that is relatively free of other radio traffic and interference. There are a number of ways to control access on ambulance-to-hospital channels. In some EMS systems, the dispatcher monitors and assigns appropriate, clear medical control channels. Other EMS systems rely on

special communications operations, such as CMEDs (Centralized Medical Emergency Dispatch) or resource coordination centers, to monitor and allocate the medical control channels.

Because of the large number of EMS calls to medical control, your radio report must be well organized and precise and must contain only important information. In addition, because you need specific directions on patient care, the information that you provide to medical control must be accurate. *Remember, the physician on the other end bases his or her instructions on the information that you provide.*

You should never use codes when communicating with medical control unless you are directed by local protocol to do so. You should use proper medical terminology when giving your report. Never assume that medical control will know what a "10-50" or "Signal 70" means. Medical control handles many different EMS systems and will most likely not know your unit's special codes or signals.

To ensure complete understanding, once you receive an order from medical control, you must repeat the order back, word for word, and then receive confirmation. Whether the physician gives an order for medication or a specific treatment or denies a request for a particular treatment, you must repeat the order back word for word. This "echo" exchange helps to eliminate confusion and the possibility of poor patient care. *Orders that are unclear or seem inappropriate or incorrect should be questioned.* Do not blindly follow an order that does not make sense to you. The physician may have misunderstood or may have missed part of your report. In that case, he or she may not be able to respond appropriately to the patient's needs.

Information about special situations. Depending on your system's procedures, you may initiate communication with one or more hospitals to advise them of an extraordinary call or situation. For instance, a small rural hospital may be better able to respond to multiple victims of a highway crash if it is notified when the ambulance is first responding. At the other extreme, an entire hospital system must be notified of any disaster, such as a plane or train crash, as early as possible to enable activation of its staff call-in system. These special situations might also include HazMat situations, rescues in progress, multiple-casualty incidents, or any other situation that might require special preparation on the part of the hospital. In some areas, mutual aid frequencies may be designated in multiple-casualty incidents so that responding agencies can communicate with one another on a common frequency.

When notifying the hospital(s) of any special situations, keep the following in mind: The earlier the

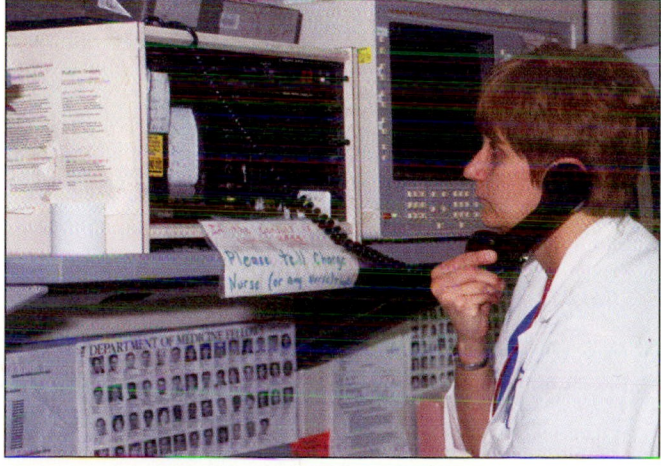

FIGURE 9-9 Medical control must be readily available on the radio at the hospital.

notification, the better. You should ask to speak to the charge nurse or physician in charge, as he or she is best able to mobilize the resources necessary to respond. Also, whenever possible, provide an estimate of the number of individuals who may be transported to the facility. Be sure to identify any special needs the patient(s) might have, such as burns or hazardous materials exposure, to assist the hospital in preparation. In many cases, hospital notification is part of a larger disaster or HazMat plan. Follow the plan for your system.

Standard Procedures and Protocols

You must use your radio communications system effectively from the time you acknowledge a call until you complete your run. Standard radio operating procedures are designed to reduce the number of misunderstood messages, to keep transmissions brief, and to develop effective radio discipline. Standard radio communications protocols help both you and the dispatcher to communicate properly (Table 9-1). Protocols should

TABLE 9-1	Guidelines for Effective Radio Communication

1. **Monitor the channel before transmitting** to avoid interfering with other radio traffic.

2. **Plan your message** before pushing the transmit switch. This will keep your transmissions brief and precise. You should use a standard format for your transmissions.

3. **Press the push-to-talk (PTT) button** on the radio, then wait for 1 second before starting your message. Otherwise, you might cut off the first part of your message before the transmitter is working at full power.

4. **Hold the microphone 2″ to 3″** from your mouth. Speak clearly, but never shout into the microphone. Speak at a moderate, understandable rate, preferably in a clear, even voice.

5. **Identify the person or unit you are calling** first, then identify your unit as the sender. You will rarely work alone, so say "we" instead of "I" when describing yourself.

6. **Acknowledge a transmission** as soon as you can by saying, "Go ahead" or whatever is commonly used in your area. You should say, "Over and out," or whatever is commonly used in your area when you are finished. If you cannot take a long message, simply say, "Stand by" until you are ready.

7. **Use plain English.** Avoid meaningless phrases ("Be advised"), slang, or complex codes. Avoid words that are difficult to hear, such as "yes" and "no." Use "affirmative" and "negative."

8. **Keep your message brief.** If your message takes more than 30 seconds to send, pause after 30 seconds and say, "Do you copy?" The other party can then ask for clarification if needed. Also, someone else with emergency traffic can break through if necessary.

9. **Avoid voicing negative emotions,** such as anger or irritation, when transmitting. Courtesy is assumed, making it unnecessary to say "please" or "thank you," which wastes air time. Listen to other communications in your system to get a good idea of the common phrases and their uses.

10. **When transmitting a number** with two or more digits, say the entire number first and then each digit separately. For example, say, "sixty-seven," followed by "six-seven."

11. **Do not use profanity on the radio.** It is a violation of FCC rules and can result in substantial fines and even loss of your organization's radio license.

12. **Use EMS frequencies** for EMS communications. Do not use these frequencies for any other type of communications.

13. **Reduce background noise** as much as possible. Move away from wind, noisy motors, or tools. Close the window if you are in a moving ambulance. When possible, shut off the siren during radio transmissions.

include guidelines specifying a preferred format for transmitting messages, definitions of key words and phrases, and procedures for troubleshooting common radio communications problems.

The "call up" from one unit to another begins by identifying the called unit first, followed by the unit calling, such as "Dispatch, this is Medic One." This exchange alerts the dispatcher to listen for both the identity of the unit calling and the message.

Reporting Requirements

Proper use of the EMS communications system will help you to do your job more effectively. From acknowledgment of the call until you are cleared from the medical emergency, you will use radio communications. You must report in to dispatch at least six times during your run:

1. **To acknowledge the dispatch** information and to confirm that you are responding to the scene

2. **To announce your arrival** at the scene

3. **To announce that you are leaving** the scene and are en route to the receiving hospital. (At this point, you typically should also state the number of patients being transported, your estimated arrival time at the hospital, and the run status.)

4. **To announce your arrival** at the hospital or facility

5. **To announce that you are clear** of the incident or hospital and available for another assignment

6. **To announce your arrival** back at quarters or other off-the-air location

While en route to and from the scene, you should report to the dispatcher any special hazards or road conditions that might affect other responding units. Report any unusual delay, such as road blocks or elevated bridges. Once you are at the scene, you may request additional EMS or other public safety assistance and then help to coordinate their response.

During transport, you must periodically reassess the patient's overall condition, vital signs, and response to care provided. You should immediately report any significant changes in the patient's condition, especially if the patient seems worse. Medical control can then give new orders and prepare to receive the patient.

Maintenance of Radio Equipment

Like all other EMS equipment, radio equipment must be serviced by properly trained and equipped personnel. Remember that the radio is your lifeline to other public safety agencies (who function to protect you), as well as

medical control, and it must perform under emergency conditions. Radio equipment that is operating properly should be serviced at least once a year. Any equipment that is not working properly should be immediately removed from service and sent for repair.

Sometimes, radio equipment will stop working during a run. In the worst-case scenario, it will stop just as you are trying to consult with medical control about treatment orders. Your EMS system must have several backup plans and options. The goal of a backup plan is to make sure that you can maintain contact with medical control when the usual procedures do not work. There are quite a few options.

The simplest backup plan relies on written standing orders. **Standing orders** are written documents that have been signed by the EMS system's medical director (Figure 9-10). These orders outline specific directions, permissions, and sometimes prohibitions regarding patient care. By their very nature, standing orders do not require direct communication with medical control. When properly followed, standing orders or formal protocols have the same authority and legal status as orders given over the radio. They exist to one extent or another in every EMS system and can be applied to all levels of EMS providers.

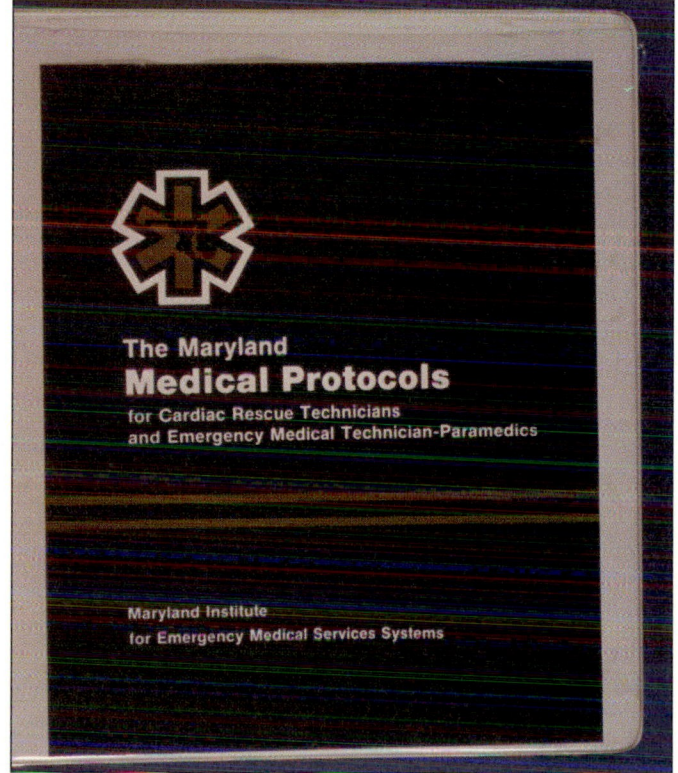

FIGURE 9-10 Standing orders are developed by the medical director and outline specific directions, permissions, and prohibitions regarding patient care.

Verbal Communications

As an EMT-B, you must master many communication skills, including radio operations and written communications. Verbal communications with the patient, the family, and the rest of the health care team are an essential part of high-quality patient care. And as an EMT-B, you must be able to find out what the patient needs and then tell others. *Never forget that you are the vital link between the patient and the remainder of the health care team.*

Communicating with Other Health Care Professionals

EMS is the first step in what is often a long and involved series of treatment phases. Effective communication between the EMT-B and health care professionals in the receiving facility is an essential cornerstone of efficient, effective, and appropriate patient care.

Your reporting responsibilities do not end when you arrive at the hospital. In fact, they have just begun. The transfer of care officially occurs during your oral report at the hospital, not as a result of your radio report en route. Once you arrive at the hospital, a hospital staff member will take responsibility of the patient from you (Figure 9-11). Depending on the hospital and the condition of the patient, the training of the person who takes over the care of the patient varies. However, you may transfer the care of your patient only to someone with at least your level of training. Once a hospital staff member is ready to take responsibility for the patient, you must provide that person with a formal oral report of the patient's condition.

Giving a report is a longstanding and well-documented part of transferring the patient's care from one provider to another. Your oral report is usually given at the same time that the staff member is doing something for the patient. For example, a nurse or physician may be

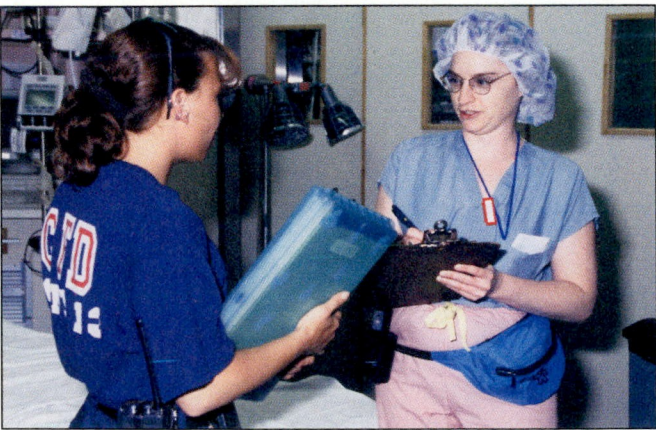

FIGURE 9-11 Once you arrive at the hospital, a staff member will take responsibility for the patient from you.

looking at the patient, beginning assessment, or helping you to move the patient from the stretcher to an examination table. Therefore, you must report important information in a complete, precise way. The following six components must be included in the oral report:

1. **The patient's name** (if you know it) and the chief complaint, nature of illness, or mechanism of injury. Example: "This is Mr. Campbell. His wife told us that he has been acting confused all day."

2. **A summary of the information** that you gave in your radio report. Example: "He has a history of high blood pressure and had a stroke 4 years ago. He has little permanent damage from the stroke. His wife states that he is usually alert and oriented."

3. **Any important history** that was not given already. Example: "His wife told us that he takes his medicine regularly. On the way in, she told us that Mr. Campbell's medicine was just changed 2 days ago."

4. **The patient's response to treatment** given en route. It is especially important to report any changes in the patient or the treatment provided since your radio report. Example: "We started oxygen by face mask at 10 L/min. His LOC improved, and he started to fight the mask. We were able to get him to hold the mask next to his mouth and nose for the rest of the trip."

5. **The vital signs assessed** during transport and after the radio report. Example: "His vitals during transport were blood pressure 184 over 110, pulse 96, ventilations 22. They are generally unchanged since we reported earlier."

6. **Any other information** that you may have gathered that was not important enough to report sooner. Information that was gathered during transport, any patient medications you have brought with you, and any other details about the patient that was provided by family members or friends may be included. Example: "Mrs. Jones's husband rode in with us. Her daughter is coming from home and should be here soon."

Communicating with Patients

Your communication skills will be tested when you communicate with patients and/or families. Remember that someone who is sick or injured is scared and might not understand what you are doing and saying. Therefore, your gestures, body movements, and attitude toward the patient are critically important in gaining the trust of both patient and family. These *Ten Golden Rules* will help you to calm and reassure your patients:

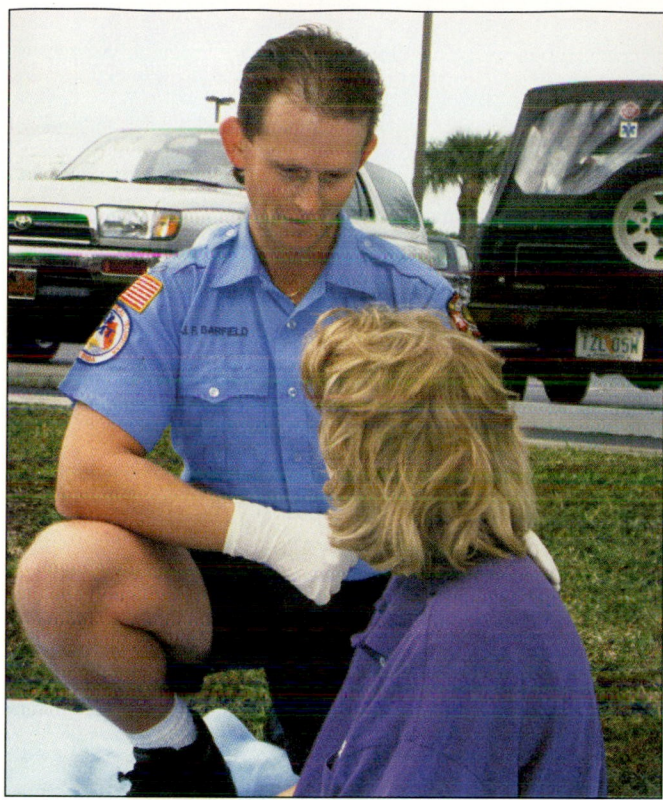

FIGURE 9-12 Maintaining eye contact with your patient builds trust and lets patient know that he or she is your first priority.

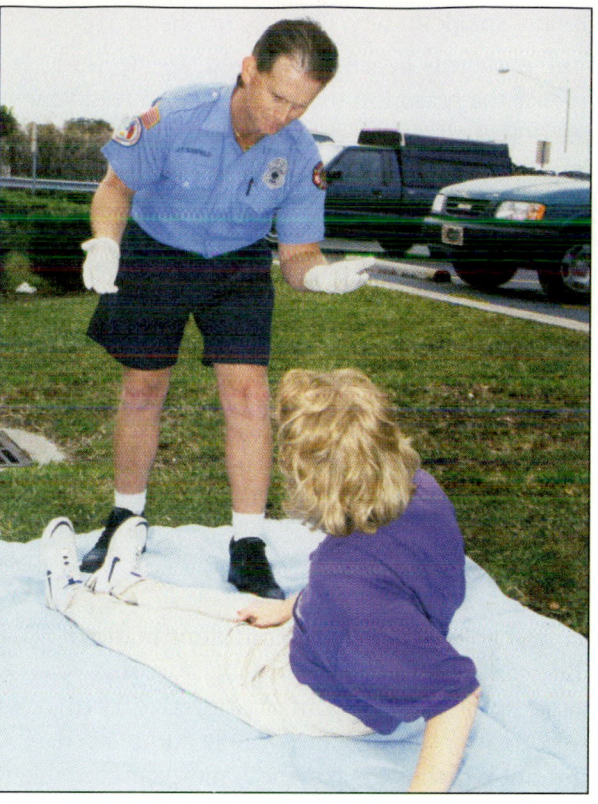

FIGURE 9-13 Watch your body language, as patients may misinterpret your gestures, movements, and stance.

1. **Make and keep eye contact** with your patient at all times (Figure 9-12). Give the patient your undivided attention. This will let the patient know that he or she is your top priority. Look the patient straight in the eye to establish **rapport**. Establishing rapport is building a trusting relationship with your patient. This will make the job of caring for the patient much easier for both you and the patient.

2. **Use the patient's proper name** when you know it. Ask the patient what he or she wishes to be called. Do not use terms such as "Pops," "Lady," "Kid," or "Dear." Avoid using a patient's first name unless the patient is a child or the patient asks you to use his or her first name. Rather, use a courtesy title, such as "Mr. Peters," "Mrs. Smith," or "Ms. Butler."

3. **Tell the patient the truth.** Even if you have to say something very unpleasant, telling the truth is better than lying. Lying will destroy the patient's trust in you and decrease your own confidence. You might not always tell the patient everything, but if the patient or a family member asks a specific question, you should answer truthfully. A direct question deserves a direct answer. If you do not know the answer to the patient's question, say so. For example, a patient may ask, "Am I having a heart attack?" "I don't know" is an adequate answer.

4. **Use language that the patient can understand.** Do not talk up or down to the patient in any way. Avoid technical medical terms that the patient might not understand. For example, ask the patient whether he or she has a history of "heart problems." This will usually result in more accurate information than if you ask about "previous episodes of myocardial infarction" or a "history of cardiomyopathy."

5. **Be careful of what you say** about the patient to others. A patient might hear only part of what is said. As a result, the patient might seriously misinterpret (and remember for a long time) what was said. Therefore, assume that the patient can hear every word you say, even if you are speaking to others and even if the patient appears to be unconscious or unresponsive.

6. **Be aware of your body language** (Figure 9-13). Nonverbal communication is extremely important in dealing with patients. In stressful situations, patients may misinterpret your gestures and movements. Be particularly careful not to appear threatening. Instead, position yourself at a lower level than the patient when practical. Remember that you should always, always conduct yourself in a calm, professional manner.

7. **Always speak slowly,** clearly, and distinctly.

8. **If the patient is hearing impaired,** speak clearly, and face the person so that he or she can read your lips. Do not shout at a person who is hearing impaired. Shouting will not make it any easier for the patient to understand you. Instead, it may frighten the patient and make it even more difficult for the patient to understand you. Never assume that an elderly patient is hearing impaired or otherwise unable to understand you. Also, never use baby talk with elderly patients or with anyone but babies.

9. **Allow time for the patient to answer** or respond to your questions. Do not rush a patient unless there is immediate danger. Sick and injured people may not be thinking clearly and may need time to answer even simple questions. This is especially true in treating elderly patients.

10. **Act and speak in a calm, confident manner** while caring for the patient. Make sure that you attend to the patient's pains and needs. Try to make the patient physically comfortable and relaxed. Find out whether the patient is more comfortable sitting or lying down. Is the patient cold or hot? Does the patient want a friend or relative nearby?

Patients literally place their lives in your hands. They deserve to know that you can provide medical care and that you are concerned about their well-being.

Communicating with Elderly Patients

By the year 2000, about 13% of the U.S. population will be considered geriatric, or over age 65 years. A person's actual age might not be the most important factor in making him or her "elderly." It is more important to determine a person's functional age. The functional age relates to the person's ability to function in daily activities, the person's mental state, and activity pattern.

Most elderly people think clearly, can give you a clear medical history, and can answer your questions (Figure 9-14). *Do not assume that an elderly patient is senile or confused.* Remember, though, that communicating with some elderly patients is extremely difficult. Some may be hostile, irritable, and/or confused. Others may have difficulty hearing or seeing you. You need great patience and compassion when you are called upon to care for such a patient. Think of the patient as someone's grandmother or grandfather—or even as yourself when you reach that age.

Approach an elderly patient slowly and calmly. Allow plenty of time for the patient to respond to your questions. Watch for signs of confusion, anxiety, or impaired

> **Patients deserve to know that you can provide medical care and that you are concerned about their well-being.**

hearing or vision. The patient should feel confident that you are in charge and that everything possible is being done for him or her.

Elderly patients often do not feel much pain. An elderly person who has fallen or been injured may report no pain. In addition, elderly patients might not be fully aware of important changes in other body systems. As a result, be especially vigilant for objective changes—no matter how subtle-in their condition. Even minor changes in breathing or mental state may signal major problems.

Remember to attend to an elderly patient's family members and friends. Seeing a loved one taken away in an ambulance can be a particularly frightening experience. Take a few minutes to explain to an elderly patient's spouse or family what is being done and why such action is being taken. When possible (which is more often than you'd think), give the patient some time to pack a few personal items before leaving for the hospital. Be sure to get any hearing aids, glasses, or dentures packed before departure; it will make the patient's hospital stay much more pleasant. You might want to document on the prehospital care report that these items accompanied the patient to the hospital and were given to a specific staff person in the emergency department.

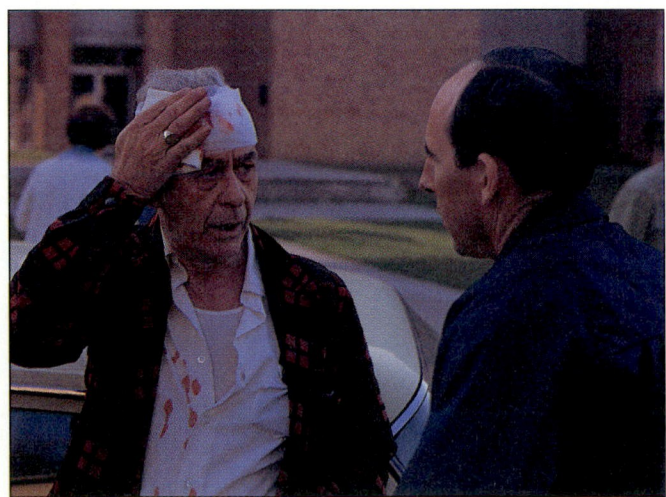

FIGURE 9-14 You need a great deal of compassion and patience when caring for the elderly, but do not assume that the patient is senile or confused.

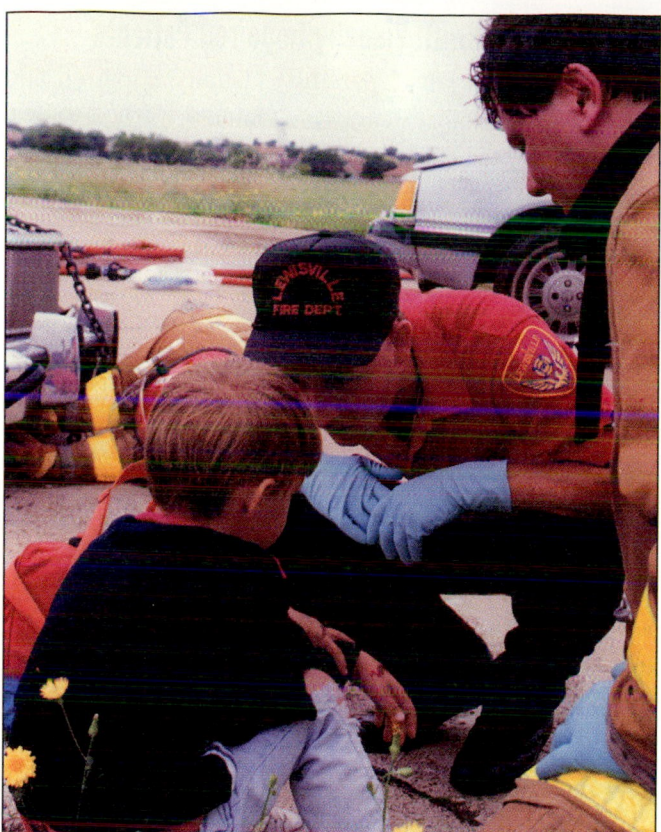

FIGURE 9-15 Maintain eye contact with a child to let the child know that you are there to help and that you can be trusted.

Communicating with Children

Everyone who is thrust into an emergency situation becomes frightened to some degree. However, fear is probably most severe and most obvious in children. Children may be frightened by your uniform, the ambulance, and the number of people who have suddenly gathered around. Even a child who says little may be very much aware of all that is going on.

Familiar objects and faces will help to reduce this fright. Let a child keep a favorite toy, doll, or security blanket to give the child some sense of control and comfort. Having a family member or friend nearby is also helpful. When not contraindicated by the child's condition, it is often helpful to let the parent or an adult friend hold the child during your evaluation and treatment. However, you will have to make sure that this person will not upset the child. Sometimes, adult family members are not helpful because they become too upset by what has happened. An overly anxious parent or relative can make things worse. Be careful about selecting the proper adult for this role.

Children can easily see through lies or deceptions, so you must always be honest with them. Make sure that you explain to the child over and over again what and why certain things are happening. If treatment is going to hurt, such as applying a splint, tell the child ahead of time. Also tell the child that it will not hurt for long and that it will help "make it better."

Respect a child's modesty. Both little girls and little boys are often embarrassed if they have to undress or be undressed in front of strangers. This phobia further intensifies during adolescence. When a wound or site of injury has to be exposed, try to do so out of sight of strangers. Again, it is extremely important to tell the child what you are doing and why you are doing it.

You should speak to a child in a professional yet friendly way. A child should feel reassured that you are there to help in every way possible. Maintain eye contact with a child, as you would with an adult, to let the child know that you are helping and that you can be trusted (Figure 9-15). It is helpful to position yourself at their level so that you do not appear to tower above them.

Communicating with Hearing-Impaired Patients

Patients who are hearing impaired or deaf are usually not ashamed or embarrassed by their disability. Often, it is the people around a deaf or hearing-impaired person who have the problem coping. Remember that you must be able to communicate with hearing-impaired patients so that you can provide necessary or even lifesaving care.

First, you should always assume that hearing-impaired patients have normal intelligence. These patients can usually understand what is going on around them, provided that you can successfully communicate with them. Second, most patients who are hearing impaired can read lips to some extent. Therefore, you should place yourself in a position so that the patient can see your lips. Third, many hearing-impaired patients have hearing aids that may have been lost in an accident or fall. Hearing aids may also be forgotten if the patient is confused or ill. Look around, or ask the patient or the family about a hearing aid.

Remember the following five steps to help you efficiently communicate with patients who are hearing impaired:

1. **Have paper and a pen available.** This way, you can write down questions and the patient can write down answers if necessary. Be sure to print so that your handwriting is not a communications barrier.

2. **If the patient can read lips,** you should face the patient and speak slowly and distinctly. Do not cover your mouth or mumble. If it is night or dark, consider shining a light on your face.

3. **Never shout!**

4. **Be sure to listen carefully,** ask short questions, and give short answers. Remember that although many hearing-impaired patients can speak distinctly, some cannot.

5. **Learn some simple phrases** in sign language. For example, knowing the signs for "sick," "hurt," and "help" may be useful if you cannot communicate in any other way (Figure 9-16).

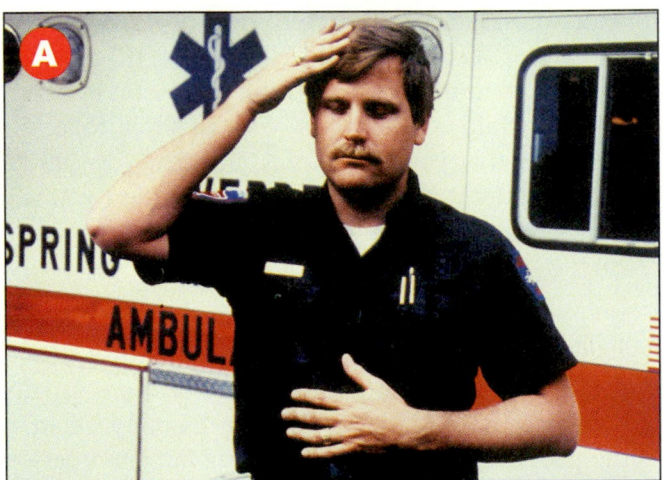

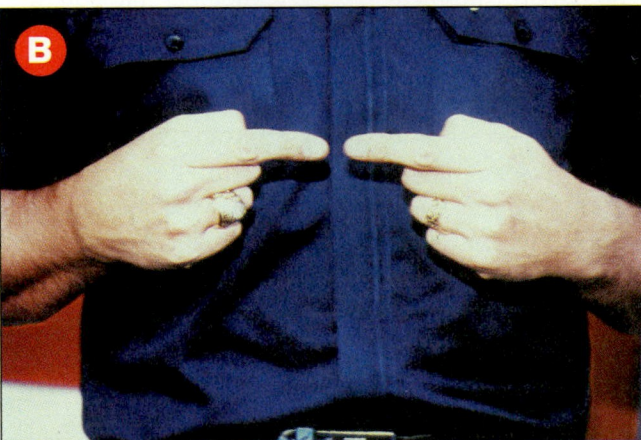

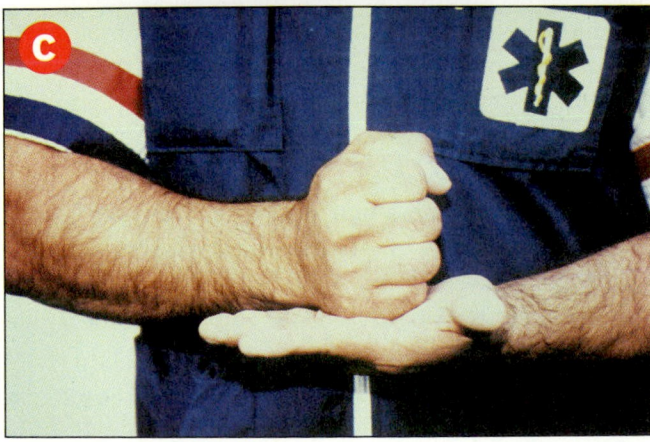

FIGURE 9-16 Learn simple phrases in sign language. **A:** Sick. **B:** Hurt. **C:** Help.

Communicating with Visually Impaired Patients

Like hearing-impaired patients, visually impaired and blind patients have usually accepted and learned to deal with their disability. Of course, not all visually impaired patients are completely blind. Many can perceive light and dark or can see shadows or movement. Ask the patient whether he or she can see at all. Also remember that, as with other patients who have disabilities, you should expect that visually impaired patients have normal intelligence.

As you begin caring for a visually impaired patient, explain everything that you are doing in detail as you are doing it. Be sure to stay in physical contact with the patient as you begin your care. Hold your hand lightly on the patient's shoulder or arm. Try to avoid sudden movements. If the patient can walk to the ambulance, place his or her hand on your arm, taking care not to rush. Transport any mobility aids, such as a cane, with the patient to the hospital. A visually impaired person may have a guide dog. Guide dogs are easily identified by their special harnesses. They are trained not to leave their masters and not to respond to strangers (Figure 9-17). A visually impaired patient who is conscious can tell you

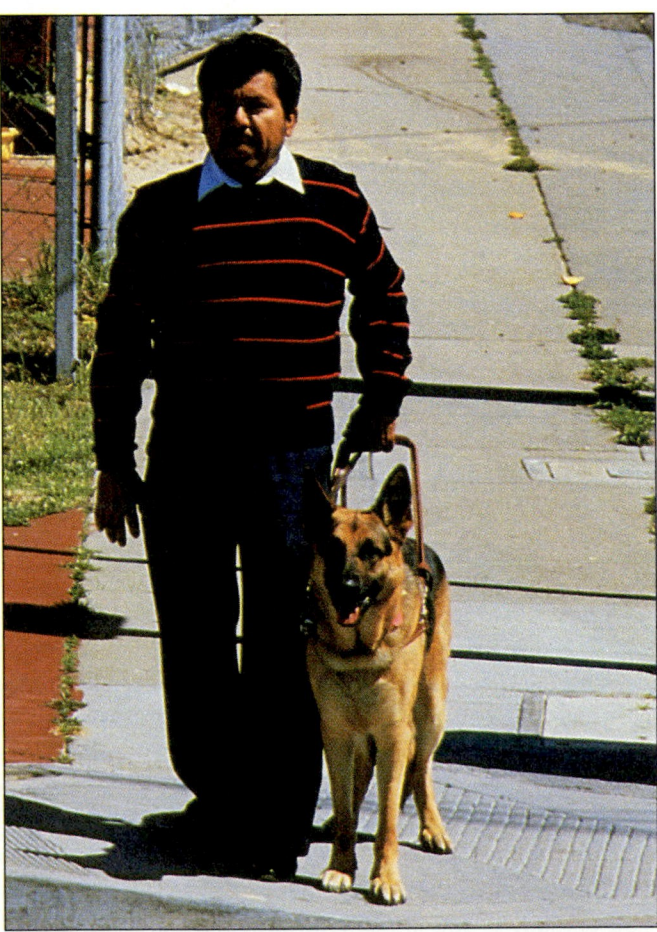

FIGURE 9-17 A guide dog is easily identified by its special harness.

about the dog and give instructions for its care. If circumstances permit, bring the guide dog to the hospital with the patient. If the dog has to be left behind, you should arrange for its care.

Communicating with Non-English-Speaking Patients

As part of the focused physical exam, you must obtain a medical history from the patient. You cannot skip this step simply because the patient does not speak English. Most patients who do not speak English fluently will still know certain important words or phrases.

Your first step is to find out how much English the patient can speak. Use short, simple questions and simple words whenever possible. Avoid difficult medical terms. You can help patients to better understand if you point to specific parts of the body as you ask questions.

In many areas, particularly large urban centers, major segments of the population do not speak English. Your job will be much easier if you learn some common words and phrases in their language, especially common medical terms. Pocket cards are available that show the pronunciation of these terms. If the patient does not speak any English, find a family member or friend to act as an interpreter.

Written Communications and Documentation

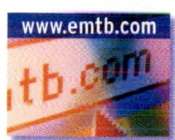

Along with your radio report and oral report, you must also complete a formal written report about the patient before you leave the hospital. You might be able to do the written report en route, if the trip is long enough and the patient needs minimal care. Usually, you will finish the

written report after you have transferred the care of the patient to a hospital staff member. Be sure to leave the report at the hospital before you leave.

Minimum Data Set

The information that you collect during a call becomes part of the data set. The minimum data set includes both patient information and administrative information (Figure 9-18). The patient information that is included in the minimum data set should be as follows:

- Chief complaint
- Level of consciousness (AVPU) or mental status

FIGURE 9-18 The minimum data set includes both patient information and administrative information.

- Systolic blood pressure for patients older than age 3 years
- Capillary refill for patients younger than age 6 years
- Skin color and temperature
- Pulse
- Respirations and effort

The administrative information that is included in the minimum data set should be as follows:

- The time that the incident was reported
- The time that the EMS unit was notified
- The time that the EMS unit arrived at the scene
- The time that the EMS unit left the scene
- The time that the EMS unit arrived at the receiving facility
- The time that patient care was transferred

You will begin gathering the patient information as soon as you reach the patient. Continue collecting information as you provide care until you arrive at the hospital.

Prehospital Care Report

Prehospital care reports help to ensure efficient continuity of patient care. This report describes the nature of the patient's injuries or illness at the scene and the initial treatment you provide. Although this report might not be read immediately at the hospital, it may very well be referred to later for important information. The prehospital care report serves the following six functions:

1. Continuity of care
2. Legal documentation
3. Education
4. Administrative
5. Research
6. Evaluation and continuous quality improvement

A good prehospital care report documents the care that was provided and the patient's condition on arrival at the scene. It also documents any changes in the patient's condition upon arrival at the hospital. The information in the report also proves that you have provided proper documentation. In some instances, it also shows that you have properly handled unusual or uncommon situations. Both objective and subjective information is included in this report. *It is critical that you document everything in the clearest manner possible.* If a patient brings legal action against you, you and your prehospital care report will have to go to court.

These reports also provide valuable administrative information. For example, the report provides information for patient billing. It can also be used to evaluate response times, equipment usage, and other areas of administrative responsibility.

Data may be obtained from the prehospital care forms to analyze causes, severity, and types of illness or injury requiring emergency medical care. These reports may also be used in an ongoing program for evaluation of the quality of patient care. All records are reviewed periodically by your system. The purpose of this review is to make sure that trauma triage and/or other prehospital care criteria have been met.

There are many requirements on a prehospital care report (Table 9-2). Often, these requirements vary from jurisdiction to jurisdiction, mainly because so many agencies obtain information from them. There is no universally accepted form.

Types of Forms

You will most likely use one of two types of forms. The first type is the traditional written form with check boxes and a narrative section. The second type is a computerized version in which you fill in information using an electronic clipboard or similar device (Figure 9-19). If your service uses written forms, be sure to fill in the boxes completely, and avoid making stray marks on the sheet. Make sure that you are familiar with the specific procedures for collecting, recording, and reporting the information in your area.

If you must complete a narrative section, be sure to describe what you see and what you do. Be sure to include significant negative findings and important observations about the scene. Do not record your conclusions about the incident. For example, you may write, "The patient's breath smelled of alcohol." This is a clear description that does not make any judgments about the patient's condition. However, a report that says, "The patient was drunk," makes a conclusion about the patient's condition. Also avoid radio codes, and use only standard abbreviations. When information is of a sensitive nature, note the source of the information. Be sure to spell words correctly, especially medical terms. If you do not know how to spell a particular word, find out how to spell it, or use another word. Also be sure to record the time with all assessment findings.

TABLE 9-2	Components of Prehospital Care Report

- Patient's name, gender, date of birth, and address

- Nature of the call

- Mechanism of injury

- Location of the patient when first seen (including specific details, especially if the incident is a car accident or criminal activity is suspected)

- Rescue and treatment given before your arrival

- Signs and symptoms found during your patient assessment

- Care and treatment given at the site and during transport

- Baseline vital signs

- SAMPLE history changes in vital signs and condition

- Date of the call

- Time of the call

- Location of the call

- Time of dispatch

- Time of arrival at the scene

- Time of leaving the scene

- Time of arrival at the hospital

- Patient's insurance information

- Names and/or certification numbers of the EMT-Bs who responded to the call

- Name of the base hospital involved in the run

- Type of run to the scene: emergency or routine

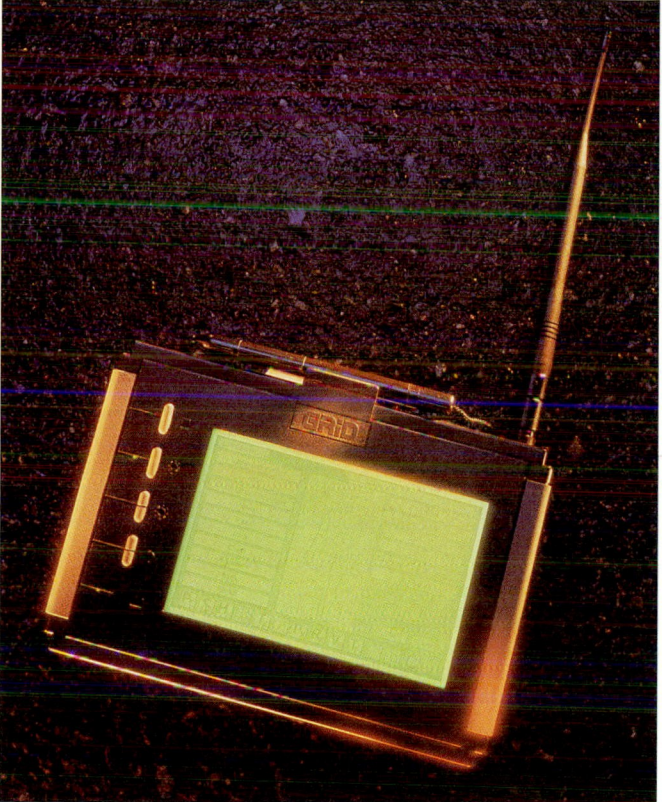

FIGURE 9-19 Your service may use an electronic clipboard, which is a computerized version of the traditional written form.

Remember that the report form itself and all the information on it are considered confidential documents. Be sure that you are familiar with state and local laws concerning confidentiality. All prehospital forms must be handled with care and stored in an appropriate manner once you have completed them. After you have completed a report, distribute the copies to the appropriate locations, according to state and local protocol. In most instances, a copy of the report will remain at the hospital and will become a part of the patient's record.

Reporting Errors

Everyone makes mistakes. If you leave something out of a report or record information incorrectly, do not try to cover it up. Rather, write down what did or did not happen and the steps that were taken to correct the situation. Falsifying information on the prehospital report may result in suspension and/or revocation of your certification/license. More important, falsifying information results in poor patient care, because other health care providers have a false impression of assessment findings or the treatment given. Document only

Falsifying information on the prehospital report may result in suspension and/or revocation of your certification/license.

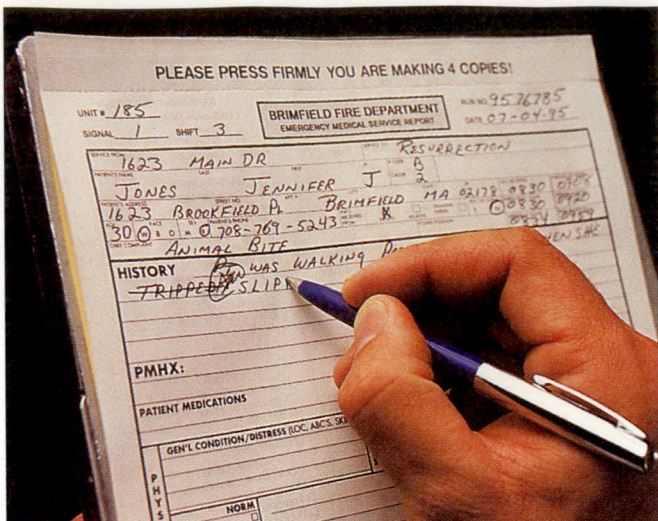

FIGURE 9-20 If you make a mistake in writing your report, the proper way to correct it is to draw a single horizontal line through the error, initial it, and write the correct information next to it.

the vital signs that were actually taken. If you did not give the patient oxygen, do not chart that the patient was given oxygen.

If you discover an error as you are writing your report, draw a single horizontal line through the error, initial it, and write the correct information next to it (Figure 9-20). Do not try to erase or cover the error with correction fluid. This may be interpreted as an attempt to cover up a mistake.

If an error is discovered after you submit your report, draw a single line through the error, preferably in a different color ink, initial it, and date it. Make sure to add a note with the correct information. If you left out information accidentally, add a note with the correct information, the date, and your initials.

When you do not have enough time to complete your report before the next call, you will need to fill it out later.

Usually, you will finish the written report after you have transferred the care of the patient to a hospital staff member. Be sure to leave the report at the hospital before you leave.

Documenting Right of Refusal

Competent adult patients have the right to refuse treatment (Figure 9-21). If you are faced with this situation, you must inform medical control immediately. Before you leave the scene, try to persuade the patient to go to the hospital, and consult medical direction as directed by local protocol. Also make sure that the patient is able to make a rational, informed decision and is not under the influence of alcohol or other drugs or the effects of an illness or injury. Explain to the patient why it is important to be examined by a physician at the hospital. Also explain what may happen if the patient is not examined by a physician. If the patient still refuses, suggest other means for the patient to obtain proper care. Explain that you are willing to return. If the patient still refuses, document any assessment findings and emergency medical care given, then have the patient sign a refusal form. You must also have a family member, police officer, or bystander sign the form as a witness. If the patient refuses to sign the refusal form, have a family member, police officer, or bystander sign the form verifying that the patient refused to sign.

Be sure to complete the prehospital report, including the patient assessment findings. Also include a description of the care that you wished to provide for the patient. You must also include a statement explaining that you informed the patient of the possible consequences of failure to accept care, including potential death, and alternative methods of obtaining the care that you suggested.

Special Reporting Situations

In some instances, you may be required to file special reports with appropriate authorities. These may include incidents involving gunshot wounds, dog bites, certain infectious diseases, or suspected physical, sexual, or substance abuse. Learn your local requirements for reporting these incidents. Failure to report them may have legal consequences. It is important that the report be accurate, objective, and submitted in a timely manner. Also remember to keep a copy for your own records.

Another special reporting situation is a multiple-casualty incident (MCI). The local MCI plan should have some means of recording important medical information temporarily (such as a triage tag that can be used later to complete the form). The standard for completing the form in an MCI is not the same as for a typical call. Your local plan should have specific guidelines.

RELEASE FROM RESPONSIBILITY WHEN PATIENT REFUSES IV THERAPY

This is to certify that I, _____ , am refusing IV treatment. I acknowledge
patient's name

that I have been informed of the risk involved and hereby release the emergency medical services

provider(s), the physician consultant, and the consulting hospital from all responsibility for any ill

effects which may result from this action.

Witness _____   Signed _____
patient name or nearest relative

Witness _____   _____
relationship

RELEASE FROM RESPONSIBILITY WHEN PATIENT REFUSES SERVICE

This is to certify that I, _____ , am refusing the services offered by the
patient's name

emergency medical services provider(s). I acknowledge that I have been informed of the risk

involved and hereby release the emergency medical services provider(s), the physician consultant,

and the consulting hospital from all responsibility for any ill effects which may result from this action.

Witness _____   Signed _____
patient name or nearest relative

Witness _____   _____
relationship

RELEASE FROM RESPONSIBILITY WHEN PATIENT REFUSES SERVICES
BUT ACCEPTS TRANSPORT

This is to certify that I, _____ , am refusing _____
patient's name

_____ . I acknowledge that I have been informed of the risk involved

and hereby release the emergency medical services provider(s), the physician consultant, and the

consulting hospital from all responsibility for any ill effects which may result from this action.

However, I do accept transportation to a medical facility.

Witness _____   Signed _____
patient name or nearest relative

Witness _____   _____
relationship

FIGURE 9-21 A competent adult patient has the right to refuse medical treatment and must sign a refusal form.

prep kit

ready for review

Excellent communication skills are crucial in relaying pertinent information to the hospital before arrival. Radio and telephone communication links you and your team to other members of the EMS, fire, and law enforcement communities. This enables your entire team to work together more effectively. It is your job to know what your communication system can and cannot handle. You must be able to communicate effectively by sending precise, accurate reports about the scene, the patient's condition, and the treatment that you provide.

There are many different forms of communication that an EMT-B must understand and be able to use. First, you must be familiar with two-way radio communications and have a working knowledge of mobile and hand-held portable radios. You must know when to use them and what type of information you can transmit. Remember, the lines of communication are not always exclusive; therefore, you should speak in a professional manner at all times.

In addition to radio and oral communications with hospital personnel, EMT-B's must have excellent person-to-person communication skills. You should be able to interact with the patient and any family members, friends, or bystanders. It is important for you to remember that people who are sick or injured may not understand what you are doing or saying. Therefore, your body language and attitude are very important in gaining the trust of both the patient and family. You must also take special care of individuals such as children, the elderly, and hearing-impaired, visually impaired, and non-English-speaking patients.

Along with your radio report and oral report, you must also complete a formal written report about the patient before you leave the hospital. This is a vital part of providing emergency medical care and ensuring the continuity of patient care. This information guarantees the proper transfer of responsibility, complies with the requirements of health departments and law enforcement agencies, and fulfills your administrative needs. Reporting and record-keeping duties are essential, but they should never come before the care of a patient.

vital vocabulary

www.emtb.com

base station Any radio hardware containing a transmitter and receiver that is located in a fixed place.

cellular telephone A low-power portable radio that communicates through an interconnected series of repeater stations called "cells."

channel An assigned frequency or frequencies that are used to carry voice and/or data communications.

dedicated line A special telephone line that is used for specific point-to-point communications; also known as a "hot line."

duplex The ability to transmit and receive simultaneously.

Federal Communications Commission (FCC) The federal agency that has jurisdiction over interstate and international telephone and telegraph services and satellite communications, all of which may involve EMS activity.

MED channels VHF and UHF channels that the FCC has designated exclusively for EMS use.

paging The use of a radio signal and a voice or digital message that is transmitted to pagers ("beepers") or desktop monitor radios.

rapport A trusting relationship that you build with your patient.

repeater A special base station radio that receives messages and signals on one frequency and then automatically retransmits them on a second frequency.

scanner A radio receiver that searches or "scans" across several frequencies until the message is completed; the process is then repeated.

simplex Single-frequency radio; transmissions can occur in either direction but not simultaneously in both; when one party transmits, the other can only receive, and the party that is transmitting is unable to receive.

standing orders Written documents, signed by the EMS system's medical director, that outline specific directions, permissions, and sometimes prohibitions regarding patient care; also called protocols.

telemetry A process in which electronic signals are converted into coded, audible signals; these signals can then be transmitted by radio or telephone to a receiver at the hospital with a decoder.

UHF (ultra-high frequency) Radio frequencies between 300 and 3,000 MHz.

VHF (very high frequency) Radio frequencies between 30 and 300 MHz; the VHF spectrum is further divided into "high" and "low" bands.

prep kit

9

assessment in action

You are transporting a patient from an extended care facility to the hospital. You obtain baseline vital signs and then contact medical control at the receiving facility to give your radio report. Once you have completed the report, you check to make certain that the patient is still resting comfortably. You then begin to write up the run report. The remainder of the call is uneventful.

1. How close should you hold the microphone to your lips for your voice to be picked up clearly and with minimal interference?

   A. Pressed right against the microphone
   B. 2" to 3"
   C. 10" to 12"
   D. At arm's length

2. Which of the following findings would **NOT** be considered an essential component of your radio report?

   A. A complete family history of illnesses and injuries
   B. The patient's chief complaint and response to treatment
   C. The patient's level of responsiveness and vital signs
   D. The treatment that has been provided for the patient

3. All of the following would be considered a part of the prehospital care communications system **EXCEPT**:

   A. a portable radio.
   B. a cellular telephone.
   C. a repeater/base station.
   D. a patient billing form.

4. You must ensure that your run report is written in:

   A. black ink.
   B. 15 minutes or less.
   C. precise, organized fashion, according to local protocols.
   D. complete detail, including everything that happened on the call.

5. A run report is **NOT** considered:

   A. part of the patient's medical record.
   B. a legal document.
   C. a document that needs a signature.
   D. necessary for nonemergency runs.

prep kit 9

points to ponder

A lawsuit has been filed against you, your partner, and the ambulance service that you work for. It alleges negligence for your treatment of a 15-year-old patient. When your run report is pulled, it is incomplete, and your notes are very sketchy. You were providing patient care, and your partner filled out the report, but both of you signed it, as is normal protocol. In reviewing the case, you and your partner remember many of the issues differently from one another.

- How would you come to agreement on what was done? Would you complete the report now? What other records may be available to help clear up your differences? How could this have been prevented?

online outlook

The Federal Communications Commission (FCC) has five main EMS-related responsibilities. To learn more about the FCC's role in EMS, complete Exercise 9 at www.emtb.com.

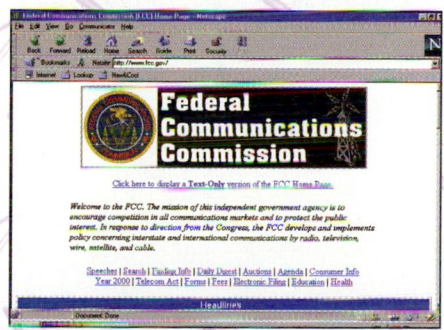

Geriatric Assessment and Transfer

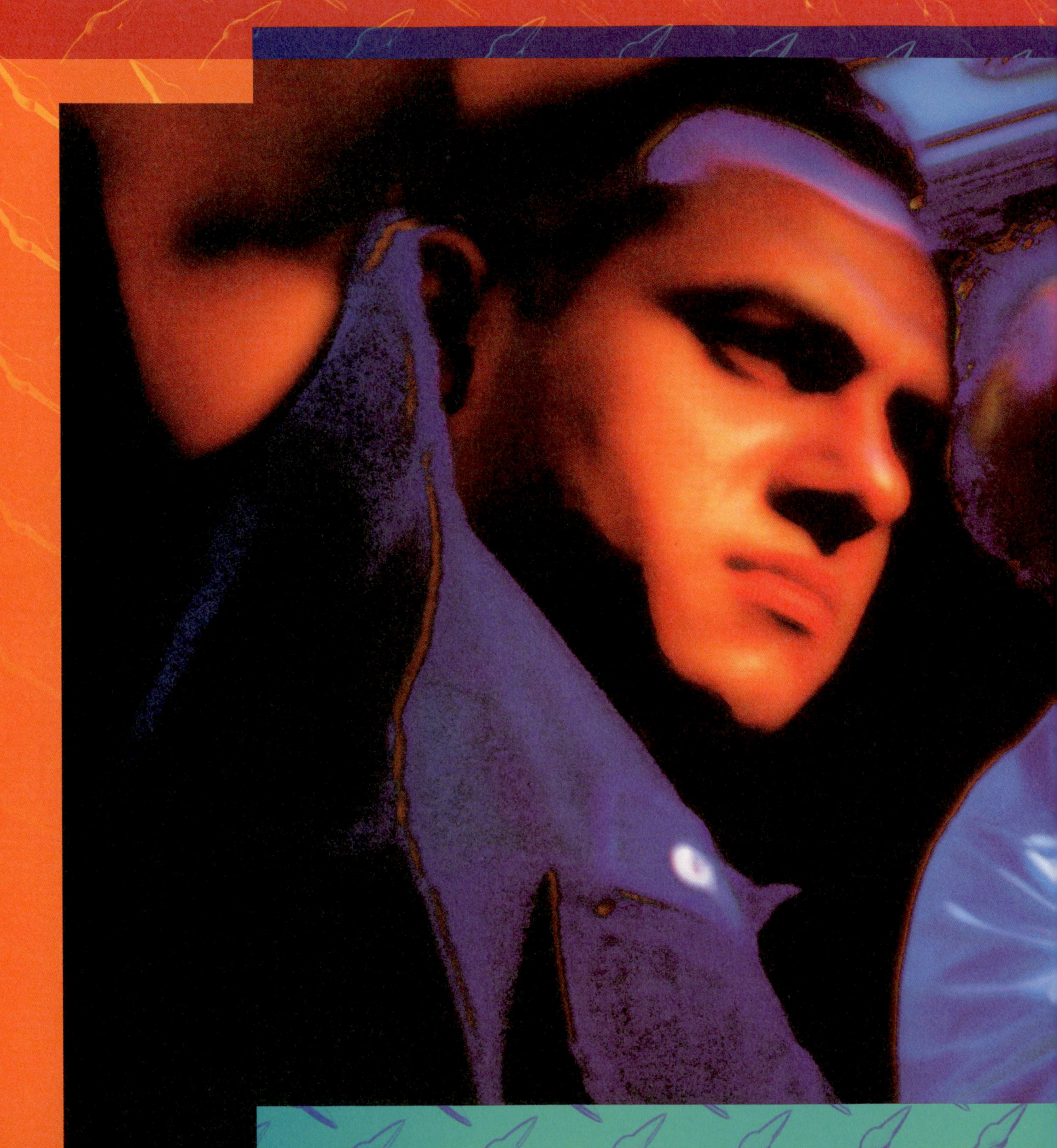

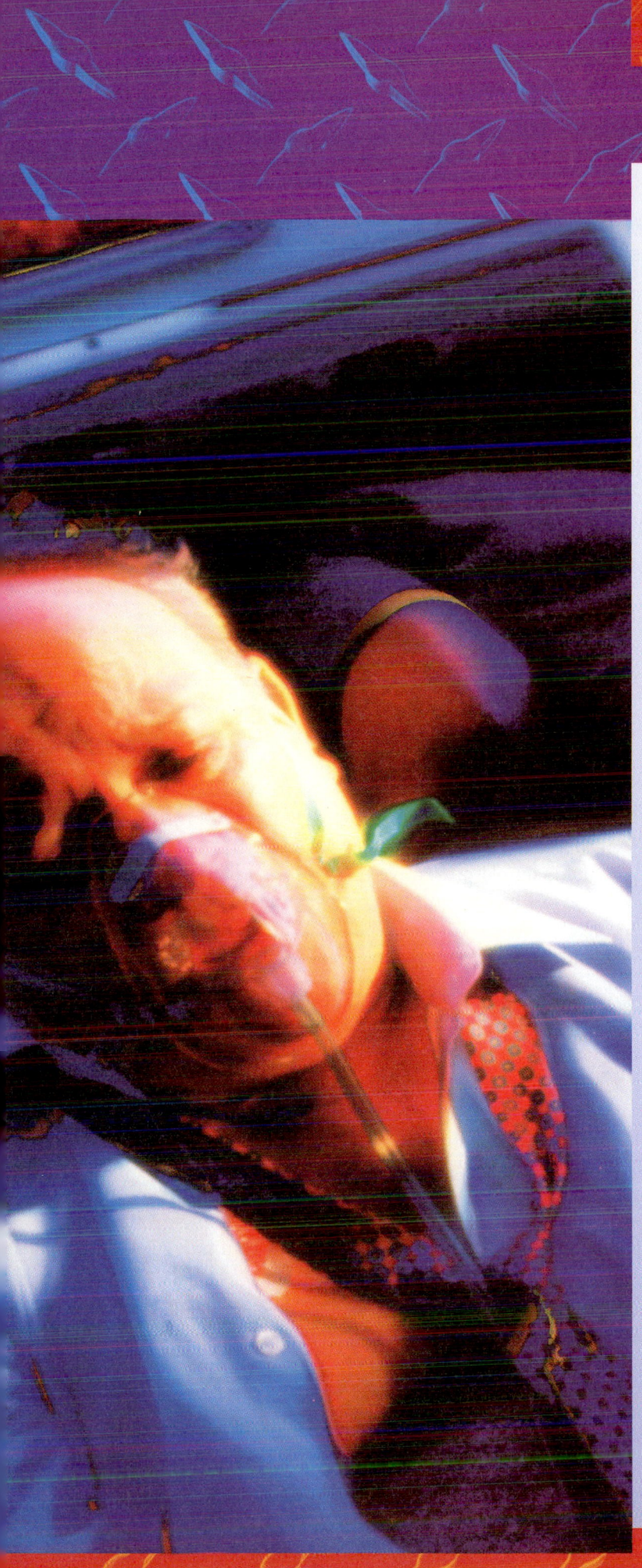

objectives*

Cognitive

1. Define the term "elderly."

2. State the leading causes of death of the elderly.

3. Describe the physiologic changes of aging.

4. Describe the following basics of patient assessment for the elderly:
   • Scene size-up
   • Initial assessment
   • Focused history and physical exam

5. Discuss response to elderly patients in nursing and skilled care facilities.

6. Describe trauma assessment in the elderly.

7. Describe acute illness assessment in the elderly for the following conditions:
   • Cardiovascular emergencies
   • Dyspnea
   • Syncope and altered mental status
   • Acute abdomen

8. State the principles and use of advance directives involving elderly patients.

9. Define elder abuse.

10. Discuss the causes of elder abuse.

11. Discuss why the extent of elder abuse is not well known.

Affective

12. Explain why the special needs of the elderly and the changes that the aging process brings about in physical structure, body composition, and organ function provide a fundamental knowledge base for maintenance of life support functions.

Psychomotor

13. Demonstrate the patient assessment skills that should be used to care for an elderly patient.

* These are non-curriculum objectives.

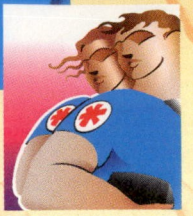

you are the emt

Rescue 6 please respond to Larson General Hospital to transfer a patient to Prairie View Nursing Home at 3200 Potter Road.

Although you may have taken the EMT course expecting to spend your days saving lives, many EMT-Bs who are new to the job will realize quickly that most EMS calls are for non-life-threatening emergencies or situations. Geriatric-related calls constitute a large portion of these calls, and the frequency of this type of call continues to increase. This chapter will prepare you to provide care for this challenging segment of society. It will also help you to answer the following questions:

1. Why do the signs, symptoms, and presentations of the ill or injured geriatric patient differ from those of other adults with similar problems?

2. What are some special transport considerations that might help to make the transfer of a geriatric patient an easier and less stressful experience?

Geriatric Assessment and Transfer

Geriatric or elderly patients are individuals who are older than age 65 years. No one relishes the thought of growing old, but the reality is that we all will, and the elderly will continue to make up a larger percentage of the population beyond the year 2000. According to the *1990 U.S. Census Data*, slightly more than 32 million individuals were older than age 65 years. By the year 2000, the elderly population will be roughly 35 million, and it is projected that by the year 2030, the elderly population will be greater than 70 million. This is a very significant evolutionary trend for the EMT-B because the elderly are major users of EMS and the health care system in general. The elderly use a disproportionate percentage of health care services and are more likely to call EMS. When they do call, their condition is likely to be serious, and they may not have the same type of "classic" presentation as younger patients. Their altered physiology may mask serious conditions. Elderly patients may also have a number of chronic medical problems and be taking numerous medications for their illnesses. Providing effective treatment for this growing number of patients will require that all EMT-Bs have an increased understanding of geriatric care issues and that they modify some of their assessment and treatment approaches.

While many EMT-Bs may relish the action of high-profile "knife-and-gun-club" calls, the reality is that the majority of your patient contacts will involve the elderly.

Lifesaving interventions for geriatric patients may be as simple as noting the home environment, preventing falls, and making referrals to appropriate social services agencies. EMT-Bs who respond to the homes of elderly patients are in an ideal position not only to provide immediate help, but also to provide key information to others in the health care and social services systems. Often, simple preventive measures can help the elderly to avoid further injury, costly medical treatment, and death. The EMT-B is on the front line of helping to prevent and treat geriatric emergencies.

Leading Causes of Death

The leading cause of death in the elderly involves disease associated with the cardiovascular system, including heart disease and strokes. Trauma deaths among the elderly are usually associated with blunt trauma (motor vehicle crashes, motor vehicle versus pedestrians, falls) and penetrating trauma (gunshot wounds, knife wounds).

Table 10-1 shows the risk factors that affect mortality in elderly patients.

The elderly are more susceptible to disease and injury than are younger individuals. Acute illness or trauma is more likely to be accompanied by a chronic disease. In addition, acute illness and trauma are more likely to alter organ systems beyond those initially involved. For example, an elderly patient who has fallen and fractured a hip may also have a lung disorder.

TABLE 10-1	Risk Factors Affecting Mortality in Elderly Patients

- Age greater than 75 years
- Living alone
- Recent death of a significant other
- Recent hospitalization
- Incontinence (inability to hold urine or feces)
- Immobility
- Unsound mind

Physiologic Changes That Accompany Age

As we get older, our physiology changes. In general, a 65-year-old person cannot expect to have the same degree of physical performance as when he or she was 30 years old. By the time a person reaches age 65 years, the amount of total body water and the number of total body cells have decreased by as much as 30%. Generally, after age 30 years, organ systems begin to deteriorate at roughly 1% per year. However, the aging process does not necessarily mean disease.

As we age, even the very fit will experience the loss of ability to perform as well as they did when they were younger. The elderly can continue to stay fit and active even though they will not be able to perform at the same level as they did in their youth (Figure 10-1). Common stereotypes about the elderly include the presence of mental confusion, illness, a sedentary lifestyle, and immobility. Although these perceptions are common, they are usually very far from the norm. Most elderly individuals lead very active lives, participating in sports and in the community, and they are generally healthy in spite of the aging process. What happens when we age?

Skin

Collagen, which is the chief component of connective tissue and bones, is lost as we age, making the skin wrinkled, thinner, and more susceptible to injury. There are also fewer sweat glands, and the skin feels dry. Because it is less elastic, skin is more prone to laceration and bruising and generally takes longer to heal.

Senses

The pupils of the eyes begin to lose the ability to handle changes in light and require more time to adjust, which

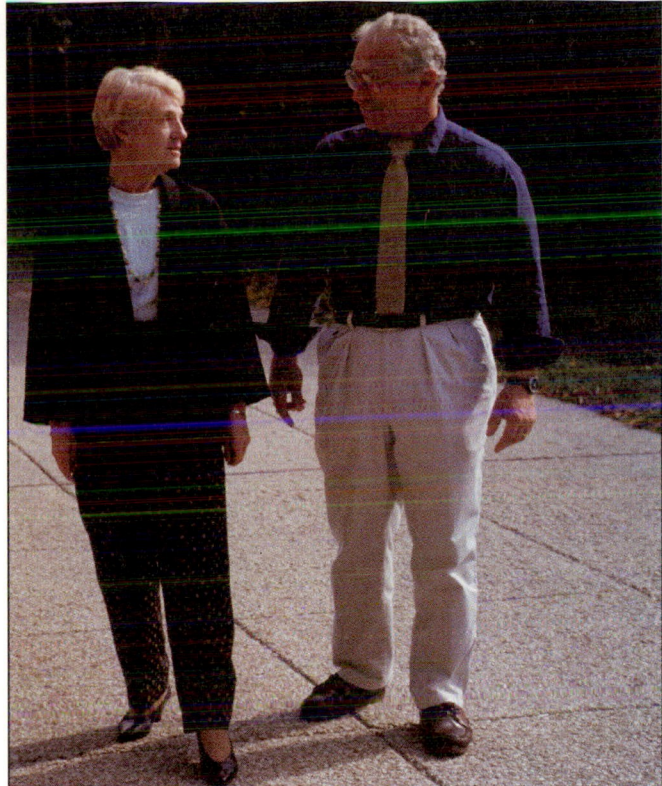

FIGURE 10-1 The elderly can continue to stay fit and active.

can make driving and walking more hazardous. Light changes can cause problems of visual acuity and depth perception. Cataracts, or clouding of the lenses, interfere with vision and make it difficult to distinguish colors and see clearly, increasing the likelihood of falls and accidents, as well as mistakes in taking various medications. Changes in the inner ear make hearing high-frequency sounds difficult; these changes can also cause problems with balance and make falls more likely. Changes in appetite may occur because of a decrease in the number of taste buds.

Respiratory System

Decreased elasticity in the lung tissue and a decreased lung surface area result in a decreased ability to exchange oxygen and carbon dioxide. In addition, the bronchial tree does not move mucous as well, increasing the chances of infection.

Cardiovascular System

Decreased cardiac output, an increased workload on the heart, and an accompanying decrease in the tolerance for exercise generally occur in the elderly. Many elderly patients are at risk for atherosclerosis, which is a disease of large- and medium-sized arteries in which fatty material is deposited and accumulates in the innermost

Generally, after age 30 years, organ systems begin to deteriorate at roughly 1% per year.

layer of the arteries. Major complications of atherosclerosis include myocardial infarction and stroke. The presence of **arteriosclerosis**, which is a disease that causes the arteries to thicken and harden, and calcification make stroke, heart disease, hypertension, and bowel infarction more likely. The elderly are also at an increased risk for **aneurysm**, an abnormal blood-filled dilation of the wall of a blood vessel, and catastrophic blood loss.

Renal System

Kidney function begins to decline because of a 30% to 40% decrease in functioning nephrons. With a decrease in renal function, electrolyte disturbances are more likely to occur. There is also a decrease in the amount of total body water.

Nervous System

The number of brain cells in some areas may decrease by as much as 45%. A 6% to 7% reduction in brain weight can result in memory impairment, a decrease in the ability to perform psychomotor skills, or slower reflex time. Brain shrinkage also makes the elderly individual more prone to head injury when a fall occurs.

Musculoskeletal System

The disks between the vertebrae begin to narrow, and a decrease in height of between 2″ and 3″ may occur. A decrease in the amount of muscle mass often results in less strength, and fractures are more likely to occur because of a decrease in bone density. Posture also changes as flexion at the knees, hips, and spine is more pronounced, making immobilization of the elderly more challenging.

Gastrointestinal System

A decrease in the volume of saliva and gastric juices causes a dry mouth, making it harder to chew and digest foods. Decreased liver function makes it harder to detoxify and eliminate substances such as drugs and alcohol.

Patient Assessment

Any time you assess a patient, you use the same basic approach: scene size-up, initial assessment, and a focused history and physical exam. Assessing an elderly patient is really no different. However, there are some issues that may indicate that you should modify your approach to the initial assessment or become more aware of some conditions that may affect the elderly patient.

The Basics

Your assessment of an elderly patient should include interviews with family members, friends, caretakers, senior citizen center workers, or significant others (Figure 10-2). You should remember that assessment of an elderly patient often takes longer and may be more difficult than that of a younger patient because of communication problems such as visual impairment, hearing loss, fatigue, and distractions in the immediate environment.

During assessment of an elderly patient, remember that the patient may have impaired hearing, sight, comprehension, and mobility. Try always to make eye contact, and grasp the patient's hand to feel for temperature, grip, and skin condition (Figure 10-3). Address the patient by his or her last name, using courtesy titles such as "Mr.," "Mrs.," or "Ms." Minimize noise, distractions, and interruptions.

During the assessment, you should observe the patient's behavior, dress and grooming, ease of rising and sitting, and fluency of speech. Watch for involuntary movement, cranial nerve dysfunction, and difficult respiration. Note whether the patient's movement is easy, unsteady, or unbalanced and whether the patient looks well nourished, thin, or emaciated.

Assessment of the elderly requires using different assessment skills than you would use for younger patients. Ask for specific rather than general information; the elderly tend to respond "yes" to all questions during the assessment process. Although asking open-ended questions is a useful tool when you are evaluating most patients, you may have to help an elderly patient by providing specific details to choose from. For example, "Describe the pain in your hip" and "Describe your chest pain " are open-ended and may lead to imprecise responses from the patient.

The following questions are more specific and may help the patient to give you better information:

- Is the pain in your hip sharp, stabbing, or dull?
- On a scale of 1 to 5, with 5 being the most intense pain, what number describes your pain?

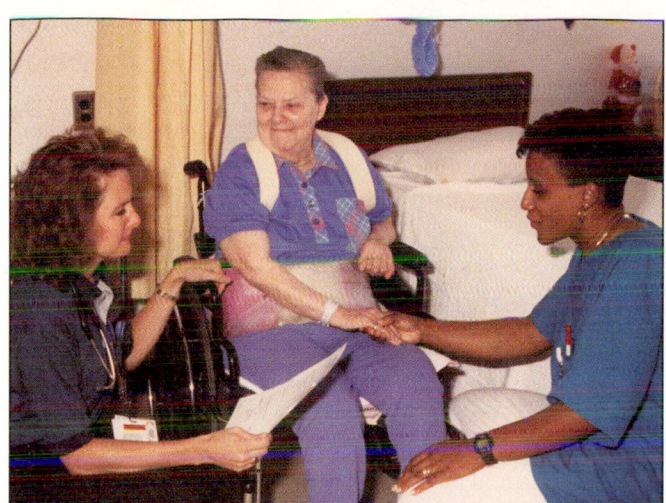

FIGURE 10-2 Interview family members, friends, and caretakers as part of your assessment of an elderly patient.

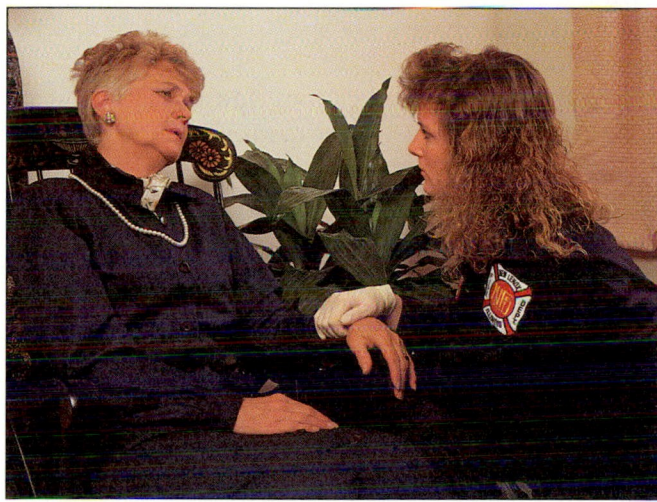

FIGURE 10-3 As you assess an elderly patient, make eye contact, and grasp the patient's hand to feel for temperature, grip, and skin condition.

Scene Size-Up

As you approach any scene, you must be keenly aware of the environment and the reason you were called. Activities of daily living such as the ability to move around, talk on the phone, prepare meals and eat, perform basic cleaning skills, and attend to personal hygiene are essential for continued health in all individuals. For the elderly, the aging or a disease process may make activities of daily living difficult and cause a spiral of problems. For example, suppose that a 70-year-old woman who trips on a loose floorboard is unable to regain her balance, falls, and dislocates her shoulder. She lives alone and has no one to help her with cooking and other daily activities. Her arm is treated, but in the following months of therapy, she becomes weaker and begins to have some difficulty walking, lifting even small

objects, shopping, and making meals. She loses some weight and becomes weaker and is eventually forced to move to an adult care facility because of her need for constant help. All this was the result of a simple fall.

When you first arrive at a patient's residence, you should look for important clues to determine not only your safety, but also that of the occupant. The environment will provide a great deal of important information if you know what to look for.

The general condition of the home will give you some important clues. Is it being kept up, or are some serious repairs needed? Are there hazards, such as steep stairs, missing handrails, or other things that could cause a fall? Is it evident that the person may be having difficulty keeping the house clean? Is there some evidence of adequate food, water, heat, lights, and ventilation? Are there many pill bottles around, indicating treatment for some type of disease process? Does someone else live there who can help to answer questions? These are very important scene clues that can provide much information before you even contact the patient.

Initial Assessment

The sequence of the initial assessment is the same for pediatric, adult, and geriatric patients. However, you should not make any assumptions about an elderly patient's level of consciousness. Never assume that an altered mental status is normal. Altered mental status indicates some level of brain dysfunction and is a serious problem. The best rule of thumb is to always compare the patient's current level of consciousness or ability to function with the level or ability before the problem began. Do not assume that confusion or unresponsiveness is normal behavior for anyone. In many cases, you will have to rely on a family member or caretaker to help establish what the patient's baseline level of consciousness was before the complaint began.

During the initial assessment, you will assess the patient's complaint and ABCD. If a life-threatening condition exists, you will have to perform emergency treatment before continuing your assessment. The initial assessment sets the tone and helps you to decide whether the patient requires a rapid resuscitative approach or a slower, contemplative one. In most cases, the slower, contemplative approach is all that is needed.

Focused History and Physical Exam

It is often said that 80% of a medical diagnosis is based on the patient's history. The history is usually the key in helping to assess a patient's problem. In addition to clearing the airway and managing the ABCD, obtaining a coherent history is one of the most important things you can do. An inaccurate or inadequate history can cause you to make incorrect presumptions and pursue a flawed treatment plan.

To obtain an accurate history, patience and good communication skills are essential. An elderly patient's diminished sight, hearing, and speaking ability may hamper communications. If possible, take a few moments to get the patient's dentures, glasses, or hearing aid. All of these items can help the patient to communicate with you more effectively.

A poor history-gathering technique can hamper communications. You must be able to gain a patient's confidence, which is best accomplished by treating the patient with respect, taking a slow deliberate approach, and explaining what you are doing. First, ask the patient what his or her name is, and then use the patient's name. Avoid being overly familiar with the patient, and do not use any nicknames. Address the patient using courtesy titles, such as "Mr.," "Mrs.," or "Ms.," and his or her last name.

When there are multiple responders, there is a natural tendency to obtain a history "by committee." Everyone asks questions, sometimes several at a time. This is a poor technique that results in a haphazard history regardless of the patient's age. For elderly patients who may have communication or perceptual problems, it makes obtaining a coherent history almost impossible. In addition, many individuals are reluctant to discuss their problems in front of a crowd. Be sure to have one EMT-B obtain the patient's history, one question at a time, providing as much privacy as possible (Figure 10-4).

Reassure the patient, and use your best professional demeanor. Look at the patient when you are speaking, and be sure that the patient can see your lips. Use a normal tone of voice, especially if the patient is wearing a hearing aid. A loud tone may actually cause sound distortion in the hearing aid and make communication worse. Ask as many open-ended questions as possible, and use closed-ended questions to clarify points. While taking the history, write down any key points on a notepad so that you do not ask the same question repeatedly because you forgot the answer. Ask family members or caretakers to clarify what you just learned from the patient. Taking a few minutes to obtain an accurate history saves time in the long run by providing information on which accurate decisions can be based.

Past medical conditions can provide information about the patient's current problem. If possible, enlist a family member or caretaker to write down the patient's past history. Elderly patients often suffer from more than one disease process at a time, and the symptoms of one disease may make the assessment of another more difficult.

Obtain a list of medications and dosages. Elderly patients are often prescribed multiple medications. Information about which medications are currently being taken is vital. In addition, find out whether the patient has recently started or stopped taking any of the medications. Medication interactions and noncompliance with instructions for taking prescribed drugs are common and may contribute to the patient's symptoms or problem.

Be aware that the sensation of pain may be diminished in an elderly patient, leading you to underestimate the severity of a condition. For example, 20% to 30% of elderly patients have "silent" heart attacks, without the typical symptom of chest pain. In addition, fear of hospitalization often causes the patient to either understate or minimize symptoms.

During the focused physical examination, be aware that elderly people are more prone to hypothermia than younger people are. Be sure to keep the patient warm and maintain the body temperature. Inspection and palpation can be hampered by multiple layers of clothing. Remove only the clothing that is necessary for examining the patient, and cover the patient back up when you are finished.

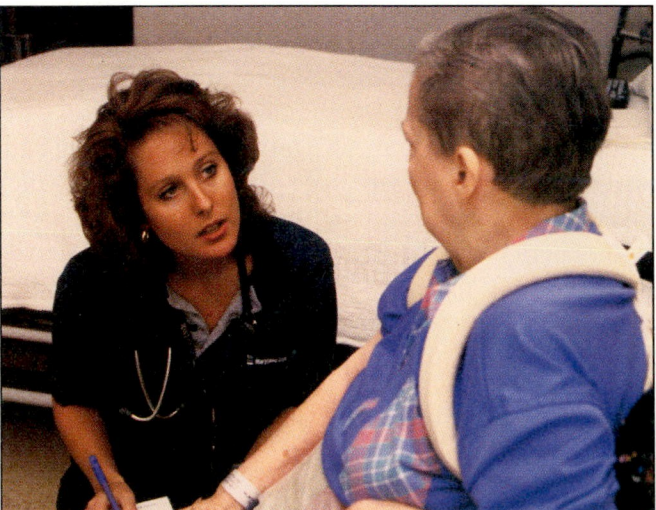

FIGURE 10-4 A slow, deliberate approach to the patient history, with one EMT-B asking the questions, is generally the best strategy in assessing an elderly patient.

To obtain an accurate history, patience and good communication skills are essential.

Response to Nursing and Skilled Care Facilities

Responding to a nursing home or skilled care facility is a common patient contact for EMT-Bs. Before you provide transport for the patient, you should find out the following critical information from the nursing staff:

- What is the patient's chief complaint today?
- What initial problem caused the patient to be admitted to the facility?

To determine the nature of the problem, you will usually have to compare the patient's present condition with his or her condition before onset of the symptoms. Ask the staff about the patient's mobility, activities of daily living, and ability to speak. This will help to paint a picture of the patient's baseline condition and indicate whether today's behavior differs from it.

Many facilities that are transferring patients will include a transfer record that contains the patient's history, medication lists and dosages, previous diagnosis, vital signs, allergies, and so on (Figure 10-5). These records provide members of the medical team with essential information and save time, especially when the patient cannot speak for himself or herself. Be sure to obtain this essential record before leaving for the hospital, and relay it to the hospital staff when giving your verbal report.

Trauma

Mechanism of Injury

Falls are the leading cause of trauma death and disability in the elderly. Most patients survive; however, a significant number require hospitalization. Motor vehicle trauma is the second leading cause of trauma death in the geriatric population. An elderly patient is five times more likely than a younger patient to be fatally injured in a car crash, even though excessive speed is rarely a causative factor in the older age group. Pedestrian accidents and burns are also common mechanisms of injury in elderly patients, resulting in death, serious injury, or disability.

Systemic Impact of Isolated Simple Trauma

You must also consider the body's decreasing ability to isolate simple trauma when you are assessing and caring for an elderly patient. An isolated hip fracture in a healthy 25-year-old adult is rarely associated with systemic decline. However, the same injury in an 85-year-old patient can produce a systemic impact that results in deterioration, shock, and life-threatening **hypoxia**, a dangerous condition in which the body tissues and cells do not have enough oxygen. Although an injury may be considered isolated and not alarming in most adults, an elderly patient's overall physical condition may have lowered the body's normal defenses

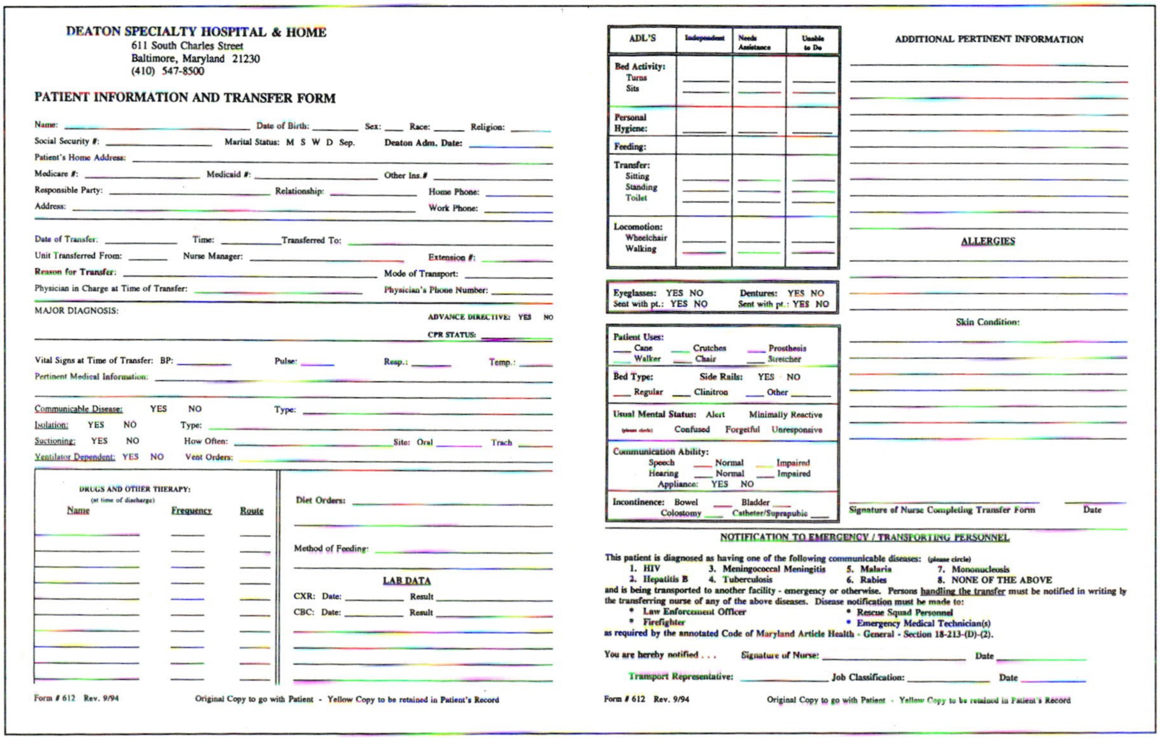

DEATON SPECIALTY HOSPITAL & HOME
611 South Charles Street
Baltimore, Maryland 21230
(410) 547-8500

PATIENT INFORMATION AND TRANSFER FORM

Name: ______ Date of Birth: ______ Sex: ___ Race: ___ Religion: ______
Social Security #: ______ Marital Status: M S W D Sep. Deaton Adm. Date: ______
Patient's Home Address: ______
Medicare #: ______ Medicaid #: ______ Other Ins.# ______
Responsible Party: ______ Relationship: ______ Home Phone: ______
Address: ______ Work Phone: ______

Date of Transfer: ______ Time: ______ Transferred To: ______
Unit Transferred From: ______ Nurse Manager: ______ Extension #: ______
Reason for Transfer: ______ Mode of Transport: ______
Physician in Charge at Time of Transfer: ______ Physician's Phone Number: ______

MAJOR DIAGNOSIS:
ADVANCE DIRECTIVE: YES NO
CPR STATUS: ______

Vital Signs at Time of Transfer: BP: ______ Pulse: ______ Resp.: ______ Temp.: ______
Pertinent Medical Information: ______

Communicable Disease: YES NO Type: ______
Isolation: YES NO Type: ______
Suctioning: YES NO How Often: ______ Site: Oral ______ Trach ______
Ventilator Dependent: YES NO Vent Orders: ______

DRUGS AND OTHER THERAPY:
(at time of discharge)

Name	Frequency	Route

Diet Orders: ______
Method of Feeding: ______

LAB DATA
CXR: Date: ______ Result ______
CBC: Date: ______ Result ______

Form # 612 Rev. 9/94 Original Copy to go with Patient - Yellow Copy to be retained in Patient's Record

ADL'S	Independent	Needs Assistance	Unable to Do
Bed Activity: Turns, Sits			
Personal Hygiene:			
Feeding:			
Transfer: Sitting, Standing, Toilet			
Locomotion: Wheelchair, Walking			

Eyeglasses: YES NO Dentures: YES NO
Sent with pt.: YES NO Sent with pt.: YES NO

Patient Uses:
___ Cane ___ Crutches ___ Prosthesis
___ Walker ___ Chair ___ Stretcher

Bed Type: Side Rails: YES NO
___ Regular ___ Clinitron ___ Other ______

Usual Mental Status: Alert Minimally Reactive
(please circle) Confused Forgetful Unresponsive

Communication Ability:
Speech ___ Normal ___ Impaired
Hearing ___ Normal ___ Impaired
Appliance: YES NO

Incontinence: Bowel ___ Bladder ___
Colostomy ___ Catheter/Suprapubic ___

ADDITIONAL PERTINENT INFORMATION

ALLERGIES

Skin Condition:

Signature of Nurse Completing Transfer Form ______ Date ______

NOTIFICATION TO EMERGENCY / TRANSPORTING PERSONNEL

This patient is diagnosed as having one of the following communicable diseases: (please circle)
1. HIV 3. Meningococcal Meningitis 5. Malaria 7. Mononucleosis
2. Hepatitis B 4. Tuberculosis 6. Rabies 8. NONE OF THE ABOVE
and is being transported to another facility - emergency or otherwise. Persons handling the transfer must be notified in writing by the transferring nurse of any of the above diseases. Disease notification must be made to:
- Law Enforcement Officer
- Rescue Squad Personnel
- Firefighter
- Emergency Medical Technician(s)

as required by the annotated Code of Maryland Article Health - General - Section 18-213-(D)-(2).

You are hereby notified . . . Signature of Nurse: ______ Date ______
Transport Representative: ______ Job Classification: ______ Date ______

Form # 612 Rev. 9/94 Original Copy to go with Patient - Yellow Copy to be retained in Patient's Record

FIGURE 10-5 A transfer record from a long-term care facility contains vital information for members of the medical team.

what do you think?

A cleaning service and a social worker sent by the city find an 80-year-old man, John, frozen to death in his second-floor apartment. For months, John's neighbors tried to help him because he did not seem to be able to care for himself. Neighbors gave him money for food and ran an extension cord to his apartment when his electricity was turned off. When John was found dead, the radiator in his apartment was working, but most of the heat was being lost through a broken window. The apartment was so cold that a half-empty can of beer near the window was frozen. Filthy clothing and sheets, soiled mattresses, and paint chips littered the apartment.

Jane is a 75-year-old woman with Alzheimer's disease who is confined to her apartment, where she lives with her husband, son, and daughter-in-law, Gail. Gail works full time as a waitress and provides most of Jane's support. Jane's 77-year-old husband, Bob, is retired and is a chronic alcohol abuser with a history of violence directed at his family. One morning, a neighbor sees a chair crash through the kitchen window and calls the police. The police find Gail unconscious on the kitchen floor and Jane bound and gagged on a mattress in the bedroom. Feces and urine are all over Jane's body. EMTs arriving at the scene find that the bed springs have broken Jane's skin. She also appears extremely malnourished and dehydrated.

Do you think John or Jane have been victims of elder abuse? Why or why not?

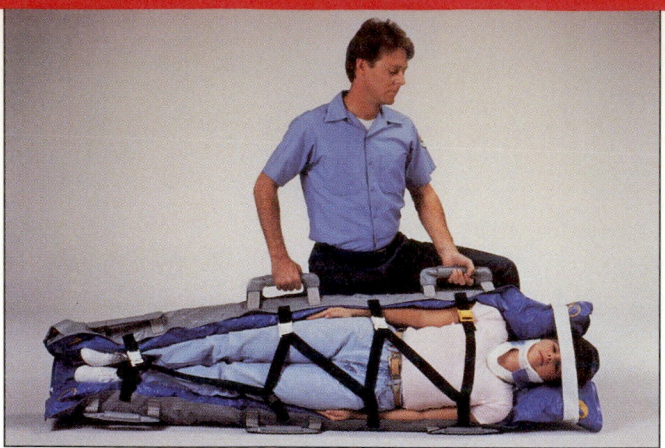

FIGURE 10-6 Vacuum mattresses that conform to body contours are a good choice for immobilizing the elderly.

and ability to keep the effects of even a simple injury localized. Your assessment of the patient's condition and stability must include past medical conditions, even if they are not currently acute or symptomatic. For example, suppose you respond to a call about a patient with a history of unstable angina who sustains a simple isolated fracture of the ankle. You must consider this patient to be highly unstable and provide prompt transport before the stress and simple trauma worsen the angina and patient instability occurs.

Falls and Trauma

A medical condition such as fainting, a cardiac rhythm disturbance, or a medication interaction may lead to a fall that causes injury to the patient. Whenever you assess an elderly patient who has fallen, you must find out why the fall occurred. Did a fainting episode cause the fall and injury, or did the patient trip on something or lose his or her balance? Again, history is important. Sometimes, a recent history of starting or stopping blood pressure medication is enough to cause a patient to become dizzy and fall. Before you assume that the patient tripped before falling, obtain a careful history and bystander account. Consider that the fall may have been caused by a medical condition, and look carefully for clues from the patient, bystanders, and the environment. Although the trauma that the patient sustains from the fall can be serious, you should also consider that the medical condition that caused the fall may be life threatening.

When you respond to a motor vehicle crash, be alert to the possibility that a medical emergency may have caused the accident, especially in single vehicle collisions with no apparent cause.

Even if a patient has no life-threatening medical condition, injuries can lead to a downward spiral of loss of strength, mobility, and weakness, resulting in immobility and an inability to conduct activities of daily living.

Because brain tissue shrinks with age, the elderly are more likely to sustain closed head injuries, such as subdural hematomas. As a result of bone loss from <u>osteoporosis</u>, a generalized bone disease that is common among postmenopausal women, elderly patients are also prone to fractures, especially in areas such as the hip. With age, the spine stiffens as a result of shrinkage of disk spaces, and vertebrae become brittle. Fracture of the spine and spinal cord injuries are more likely to occur.

Because of the amount of flexion that occurs in the spinal column, hip, or knee of elderly patients, use of conventional splints and backboards to immobilize the patient may be difficult or impossible unless a lot of padding is used. What is considered a normal anatomic position for children and adults is often very abnormal for some elderly trauma patients. You should try to determine the patient's baseline condition and what was normal for the patient before the accident. Trying to force a patient with pronounced joint flexion into "normal" anatomic position can be very painful for the patient and frustrating for you. Some devices, such as traction splints, simply do not work on patients with flexed hips and knees. Splinting devices, such as vacuum mattresses that conform to body contours, may be a better choice for immobilization than a conventional backboard (Figure 10-6).

Remember that when you treat an elderly trauma patient, you must assess the injuries and carefully look for the cause of the fall or crash.

Cardiovascular Emergencies

Syncope

You should always assume that <u>syncope</u>, or fainting, in the elderly is a life-threatening problem until proven otherwise. Syncope is caused by an interruption of blood flow to the brain. Syncope has many causes; some are serious and others are not. Either way, an elderly person who has a period of unconsciousness should be examined to determine the cause of the syncope. Table 10-2 shows some of the causes of syncope in an elderly patient.

Heart Attack

The classic symptoms of a heart attack are often not present in the elderly. As many as one-third of elderly patients have "silent" heart attacks in which the usual chest pain is not present. Table 10-3 shows signs and symptoms that are commonly noted in elderly patients who are experiencing a heart attack.

TABLE 10-2	Possible Causes of Syncope in an Elderly Patient
Cardiac Dysrhythmias/ Dysrhythmias/ Heart Attack	The heart is beating too fast or too slowly, the cardiac output drops, and blood flow to the brain is interrupted. A heart attack can also cause syncope.
Vascular and Volume	Medication interactions can cause venous pooling and <u>vasodilation</u>, a widening of the blood vessel, resulting in a drop in blood pressure and inadequate blood flow to the brain. Another cause can be a drop in blood volume because of hidden bleeding from a condition such as an aneurysm.
Neurologic	A transient ischemic attack or a "brain attack" can sometimes mimic syncope.

TABLE 10-3	Common Signs and Symptoms of Heart Attack in an Elderly Patient
Dyspnea	<u>Dyspnea</u>, the feeling of shortness of breath or difficulty in breathing, is a common complaint in the elderly and is most often associated with heart attack. It is often combined with other symptoms, such as nausea, weakness, and sweating. Chest pain associated with angina typically has an onset during periods of stress or exertion. In the elderly, chest pain is often not present, but exertional dyspnea is. As the disease progresses, dyspnea may have an onset without exertion. Dyspnea in the elderly is often the equivalent of chest pain in younger patients who are having angina or a heart attack. In addition, congestive heart failure and acute pulmonary edema may result from the "silent" heart attack.
A Weak Feeling	Weakness can be caused by many things. However, you should suspect a heart attack in a patient with a sudden onset of weakness. Weakness is often associated with sweating.
Syncope/Confusion/ Altered Mental Status	Syncope can have many causes, and in the elderly, none of these causes should be presumed to be minor. Major life-threatening causes of syncope are often cardiac in origin. Altered mental status is usually a signal of poor blood supply to the brain, often from cardiac dysrhythmia and heart attack.

The Acute Abdomen

A number of life-threatening abdominal catastrophes are common in elderly patients. Because of pain referral patterns and the possibility that the patient does not feel any pain, abdominal complaints in the elderly are notoriously difficult to assess. In the field, the one result of abdominal catastrophe is blood loss, which leads to shock and death. *Abdominal aortic aneurysm* (AAA) is one of the most rapidly fatal conditions. AAA tends to develop in individuals who have a history of hypertension and atherosclerosis.

Elderly patients are also more prone to abdominal problems because of the loss of collagen, which makes vessels and connective tissue weaker. The walls of the aorta weaken, and blood begins to leak into the layers of the vessel, causing the aorta to bulge like a bubble on a tire. If enough blood is lost into the vessel wall itself, shock occurs. If the wall bursts, it rapidly leads to fatal blood loss. When the problem is caught early, there is a chance to repair the vessel before rupture and fatal blood loss occur.

A patient with an abdominal aortic aneurysm most commonly reports abdominal pain radiating through to the back with occasional flank pain. If the AAA becomes large enough, it can be felt as a pulsating mass in the midline of the abdomen during physical examination. Occasionally, the AAA causes a decrease in blood flow to one of the iliac arteries, and the patient complains of some discomfort in the affected extremity. Assessment may also reveal diminished or absent pulses in the extremity. <u>Compensated shock</u> (early shock) and <u>decompensated shock</u> (late shock) as a result of blood loss are common occurrences. Because of a decrease in blood volume and decreased blood flow to the brain, the patient may experience syncope. You should treat the patient for shock and provide prompt transport to the hospital.

Another cause of abdominal pain and shock is gastrointestinal bleeding, which can occur for a variety of reasons and is usually heralded by the vomiting of blood or material that looks like coffee grounds. Bleeding in the lower digestive tract is usually manifested by black or tarry stools. A patient with gastrointestinal bleeding may experience weakness, dizziness, or syncope. Bleeding into the gastrointestinal system can be life threatening because of the potential for blood loss and shock.

Altered Mental Status

Because of our stereotypical perceptions about the elderly, we may expect them to forget names or not be able to remember events or learn new things. However, these types of changes in mental status are not part of the normal aging process. They may be part of a slow deterioration or a condition or disease of rapid onset, neither of which is normal. To determine the onset of this change in mental status, you must compare the patient's ability to function with that of the recent past. This will help to establish a baseline and give some perspective on the onset of the change. The two terms that are often used to describe a change in mental status are "delirium" and "dementia."

<u>Delirium</u> is a change in mental status that is marked by the inability to focus, think logically, and maintain attention. Acute anxiety may be present in addition to the other symptoms. Usually, memory remains mostly intact. Delirium is commonly marked by an acute or recent onset and is a "red flag" for some type of new health problem. Delirium may be caused by tumors, fever, or drug or alcohol intoxication or withdrawal. Delirium can be present from metabolic causes as well. Any time a patient has an acute onset of delirious behavior, you should rapidly assess the patient for the following three conditions:

- Hypoxia
- Hypovolemia
- Hypoglycemia

Any of these three conditions, if left unrecognized or untreated, may be rapidly fatal.

<u>Dementia</u> is the slow onset of progressive disorientation, shortened attention span, and loss of cognitive function. Dementia develops slowly over a period of years rather than a few days. Alzheimer's disease, brain attacks, or genetic factors may cause dementia. Dementia is usually considered irreversible and is an expected course of the pathophysiologic neurologic disease process. The patient's history and determination of function in the recent past are key factors in determining the baseline. Delirium is caused by emergent problems; dementia is not.

Advance Directives

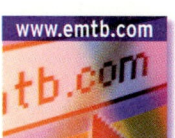

Many individuals today are making use of <u>advance directives</u>, specific legal papers that direct relatives and caregivers about what kind of medical treatment may be given to them if they cannot speak for themselves. An advance directive is also commonly called a living will. It can also take the form of "Do not resuscitate" (DNR) orders and health care proxies. DNR orders give you permission *not* to attempt resuscitation. However, for a DNR order to be valid, the patient's medical problems must be clearly stated, and the form must be signed by the patient or legal guardian and by one or more physicians. The form must be dated within the preceding 12 months. Even in the presence of a DNR order, you are still obligated to provide supportive measures, such as oxygen, pain relief, and comfort when you can.

A health care proxy is exercised by an individual who has been authorized by the patient to make medical decisions for the patient. Be sure to follow your service's protocol when faced with an advance directive.

Mentally competent adults and emancipated minors have the right to consent to or decline treatment, provided that they are competent to do so. The definition of competence is often hotly debated, but a person who is older than 18 years of age, alert, and not intoxicated and who understands the consequences of his or her decision is generally deemed competent. Unfortunately, patients who are unconscious or in a medical crisis are not able to inform medical personnel about their wishes to consent to or decline treatment. It is dangerous to take someone else's word for what the patient's wishes are; this is the reason that written advance directives have been developed.

Dealing with advance directives has become more common for EMS providers as more individuals are electing to use hospice services and spend their final days at home. Although advance directives may be in place, family members or caregivers who are present at the time of death or when the patient's condition worsens often become alarmed and call 9-1-1. Family members and caretakers may then become upset when you take resuscitative action and begin transportation to the hospital.

Another common situation is the transportation of patients from nursing facilities. Specific guidelines vary from state to state; however, you should consider the following general guidelines:

- Patients have the right to refuse treatment, including resuscitative efforts, provided that they are able to communicate their wishes.
- A DNR order is valid in a health care facility only if it is in the form of a written order by a physician.
- You should periodically review state and local protocols and legislation regarding advance directives.
- When you are in doubt or when there are no written orders, you should try to resuscitate the patient.

It is absolutely essential that every EMT-B becomes familiar with his or her state regulations regarding advance directives. Every service should also provide additional training on the actions you should take when presented with advance directives. When in doubt, your best course of action is to take resuscitative action that is appropriate to the situation and to practice sound medical treatment.

Elder Abuse

Reports and complaints of abuse, neglect, and other related problems among the nation's elderly are on the rise. The exact extent of elder abuse is not known for several reasons, including the following:

- Elder abuse is a problem that has been largely hidden from society.
- The definitions of abuse and neglect among the elderly vary.
- Victims of elder abuse are often hesitant to report the problem to law enforcement agencies or human and social welfare personnel.

In 1981, The House Select Committee on Aging concluded that 4% of the elderly nationwide, or more than 1.1 million individuals, were victims of some kind of abuse.

A parent who feels ashamed or guilty because he or she raised the abuser is often a typical victim of elder abuse. The abused individual may also feel traumatized by the situation or be afraid that the abuser will try to get back at him or her. In some areas of the country, there is a lack of formal reporting mechanisms, and some states lack statutory provisions that require that elder abuse be reported.

The physical and emotional signs of abuse, such as rape, spouse beating, or nutritional deprivation, are often overlooked or not accurately identified. Older women in particular are not likely to report incidents of sexual assault to law enforcement agencies. Patients with sensory deficits, senility, and other forms of altered mental status, such as drug-induced depression, may not be able to report abuse.

Elder abuse is defined as any action on the part of an elderly individual's family member, caretaker, or other associated person that takes advantage of the elderly individual's person, property, or emotional state; it is also called *granny battering* or *parent battering*.

The elderly individual who is likely to be abused is generally older than 65 years of age. Elder abuse occurs most often in women older than 75 years of age. The abused person is often frail with multiple chronic medical conditions, has dementia, and may suffer from an impaired sleep cycle, sleepwalking, and periods of shouting at others. The individual may be incontinent and in general is dependent on others for activities of daily living.

Abusers of the elderly are often products of child abuse themselves, and the abuse that is inflicted upon the elderly may be a retaliatory matter. As with cases of child and spousal abuse, if the family history indicates patterns of abuse or weak family ties, or if children have been ill treated or treated violently, the probability of elder abuse is greater. Because many elderly individuals live in a family environment and are typically women older than 75 years of age, you must try to find clues from the environment. The abuser is frequently the spouse or a middle-aged daughter-in-law who is caring for dependent children and dependent parents while perhaps holding full- or part-time employment. Most of these abusers are not trained in the particular care that the elderly require and have little relief time from the constant care demands of their own family, children, and spouse. Their lives are now complicated by the often less-than-flexible elderly individual they have to care for.

The abuser may also suffer from marked fatigue, be unemployed with financial difficulties, and be a substance abuser.

Abuse is not restricted to the home; environments such as nursing, convalescent, and continuing care centers are also sites where the elderly sustain physical, chemical, or pharmacologic harm. Often, care providers in these environments consider the elderly to represent management problems or categorize them as obstinate and undesirable patients. When called to the scene to treat an elderly patient who you suspect may have been abused, you may find that elder abuse can be gruesome, vulgar, barbaric, or worse than that inflicted upon children.

Assessment of Elder Abuse

While assessing the patient, you should try to obtain an explanation of what happened. You should suspect abuse when frank answers to questions about what caused the injury are concealed or avoided.

You must also suspect abuse when you are given unbelievable answers from anyone other than the patient, the possible abuser, or significant witnesses. Answers to questions you ask such as "Exactly where did this happen?," "Exactly what was the patient doing?," and "What time did it happen?" may provide valuable clues to whether the patient was abused. You should be suspicious if you think "Does this make sense?" or "Do I really believe this story?" while reviewing the patient's history. If you see burns, especially cigarette burns or physical marks that indicate that certain parts of the patient's body have been scalded systematically, you must also suspect abuse. As an EMT-B, you may be the first health care provider to observe possible abuse. You should try to find out information related to violent incidents when gathering the patient's medical history. Information that may be important in assessing possible abuse includes the following:

- Repeated visits to the emergency department or clinic
- A history of being "accident prone"
- Soft-tissue injuries
- Unbelievable or vague explanations of injuries
- Psychosomatic complaints
- Chronic pain
- Self-destructive behavior
- Eating and sleep disorders
- Depression or a lack of energy
- Substance and/or sexual abuse

You should remember that many patients suffering abuse are so afraid of retribution that they make false statements. An elderly patient who is being abused by family members may lie about the origin of abuse for fear of being removed from the home. In other cases of elder abuse, sensory deprivation or dementia may hinder adequate explanation.

Your assessment of the patient is important, not only to identify abuse that may not be reported by the patient, but also to uncover pathology. A physician may have to diagnose some abuse cases with X-rays or magnetic resonance imagery. You can observe other abuse, such as malnutrition, by visual examination; you can discover such abuse as swelling of an extremity by palpation.

In addition to the lifesaving care that you can provide the patient, your examination of the patient can help to reduce further trauma from abuse through its very identification. Repeated abuse can lead to a high risk of death. A preventive measure in reducing additional maltreatment of the patient is identification of the abuse by emergency medical providers. This may allow for referral and protective services of human, social, and public safety agencies (Table 10-4).

TABLE 10-4	Categories of Elder Abuse
Physical	• Assault
	• Neglect
	• Dietary
	• Poor maintenance of home
	• Poor personal care
Psychological	• Benign neglect
	• Verbal
	• Being treated as an infant
	• Deprivation of sensory stimulation
Financial	• Theft of valuables
	• Embezzlement

Signs of Physical Abuse

Signs of abuse may be quite obvious or subtle. Obvious signs include bruises; burns; head, chest, abdominal, or bone injuries; and sexual abuse injuries. Subtle signs include undernourishment or a failure to thrive. You must record and document your findings when you examine the patient.

Inflicted bruises are usually found on the buttocks and lower back, genitals and inner thighs, cheeks or earlobes, upper lip and inside the mouth, and neck. Pressure bruises caused by the human hand may be identified by oval grab marks, pinch marks, hand prints, linear marks, or bruises that encircle the trunk. Human bites are typically inflicted on the upper extremities. Human bites can cause lacerations, crushing, and infection.

You should also investigate multiple bruises in various states of healing by questioning the patient and reviewing the patient's activities of daily living.

Burns are a common form of abuse. Most of these burns are not examined in a medical setting. Typical abuse from burns are caused by contact with cigarettes, matches, heating devices, heated metal, forced immersion in hot liquids, chemicals, and electrical power sources.

Your assessment of a patient who has been burned should include attention to burns that may cause airway distress, especially facial burns, burned sputum, and singeing of facial and nasal hair.

As in all abuse cases, you should obtain a history of the injury, especially in burn cases. Pay special attention to the need for life support measures. Burns can lead to death in many elderly patients. Be sure to observe the patient's body for blisters, fresh burns, and imprints of items such as a hot poker or iron. Remove any jewelry from the patient's arm or hand to prevent constriction.

Injuries to the head from direct blows are generally a high cause of mortality in abused patients. Pay special attention to the ABCD in patients who have received a head injury.

Specific head injuries include blows, lacerations, and pulling of hair from the scalp. Because of the scalp's abundant blood supply, significant blood loss can occur. Blunt trauma, impalement injuries, and bullet wounds to the head can lead to subdural hematomas. Bleeding from the nose, wounds or burns of the lips and tongue, missing or loose teeth, broken bones in the face, and bruises in the corners of the mouth may indicate abuse.

Damage to the eyes is of particular concern in cases of elder abuse. Was there blunt or penetrating trauma? Were chemicals involved?

You should also inspect the patient's ears for indications of twisting, pulling, or pinching or evidence of frequent blows to the outer ears.

The chest is often an area of assault. Be sure to inspect the patient's chest for evidence of blunt or penetrating trauma. Blunt trauma may result from a hit with a baseball bat, a fist, or a hard bar of soap wrapped in a towel. Penetrating trauma may be evident from sharp instruments such as an ice pick, knife, or screwdriver. Elderly individuals may be restrained by the abuser with various tie devices that can result in rib fractures or internal damage to organs in the thoracic cage. You must immediately treat any impairment of breathing.

Injury to organs in the abdominal cavity are serious and may be life threatening. Blunt and penetrating trauma are the usual mechanisms of injury; however, poisoning or forced ingestion of caustic substances may be involved. Damage to the internal organs may be caused by blows from the back of a fist. Unrecognized abdominal injury can lead to death.

Be sure to examine the extremities for bruises or deformity, in addition to distal circulation. Ordinarily, fractures are not life threatening; however, multiple fractures to the femur or pelvis can lead to blood loss and death.

It may be difficult to see a failure to thrive in an elderly patient who has been abused. You should observe the patient's weight and try to determine whether the patient appears undernourished or has been unable to gain weight in the current environment. Does the patient have a ravenous appetite? Has medication been withheld? Is money being withheld, so the patient cannot buy food or medicine? You should also check for signs of neglect, such as evidence of a lack of hygiene, poor dental hygiene, poor temperature regulation or lack of reasonable amenities in the home.

You must regard injuries to the genitals or rectum with no reported trauma as evidence of sexual abuse in any patient. Elderly patients with altered mental status may never be able to report sexual abuse. In addition, many women do not report cases of sexual abuse because of shame and the pressure to forget. Sexually abused patients often have difficulty reporting the violence, so you must carefully scrutinize and review implausible explanations.

Renal injury may occur from blunt trauma to the flank or back, indicated by contusions, hematomas, or ecchymosis. Perforation of the ureter and bladder may result from penetrating trauma.

Lacerations, bruises, or injury to the genitalia, incontinence, and evidence of sexually transmitted disease or other infection must raise the question in your mind as to the cause.

prep kit

ready for review

Management of elderly patients can present you with many challenges that are not encountered with younger patients and confront you with a host of different problems that may be quite difficult and frustrating to solve. The health problems of the elderly are multifaceted, and frequent barriers to communication can be expected. In managing the elderly patient, things may not be packaged in their normal framework.

Although assessment of the elderly patient involves the same basic approach as with any other patient, you must take a more wary approach to the elderly patient. The injury or medical condition may be worse than is indicated by the existing signs and symptoms, and the injuries and conditions that are found will have a more profound effect than they would in a younger patient. You should also note that in addition to the critical needs that an underlying medical problem may cause, the elderly patient may be more unstable than a younger patient, thus having an increased possibility for sudden rapid deterioration.

The exact extent of elder abuse is not known because many patients do not report it. Victims of elder abuse are generally women older than 65 years of age. Abusers are often family members who must care for the elderly person in addition to caring for their own spouses and children. Elder abuse also occurs in nursing, convalescent, and continuing care centers. Elder abuse can be gruesome, vulgar, and barbaric, and is often worse than abuse inflicted on children. You must provide lifesaving care to the patient and also try to reduce additional abuse through identification of the problem. Identification of abuse by emergency medical providers can lead to referral and protective services of human, social, and public safety agencies.

Remember, the elderly patient you are caring for has made it to this age. Whether because of better medical care, genetics, or some other factor, the patient has survived. Growing old is not easy work, and neither is the emergency medical care of the elderly patient. You must be careful to obtain an accurate history of the patient, be patient, and communicate effectively. The duty that we owe to our elders and the sense of service provided to them is one of our more important callings.

vital vocabulary

www.emtb.com

advance directives Written documentation that specifies medical treatment for a competent patient should he or she become unable to make decisions.

aneurysm An abnormal blood-filled dilation of a blood vessel.

atherosclerosis A disease in which fatty material is deposited and accumulates in the innermost layer of medium- and large-sized arteries.

arteriosclerosis A disease that is characterized by hardening and thickening of the arterial walls.

cataract Clouding of the lens of the eye or its surrounding transparent membrane.

collagen A protein that is the chief component of connective tissue fibrils and bones.

compensated shock Early shock.

decompensated shock Late shock.

delirium A change in mental status marked by the inability to focus, think logically, and maintain attention.

dementia The slow onset of progressive disorientation, shortened attention span, and loss of cognitive function.

dyspnea Shortness of breath or difficulty breathing.

elder abuse Any action on the part of an elderly individual's family member, caretaker, or other associated person that takes advantage of the elderly individual's person, property, or emotional state; also called *granny battering* or *parent battering*.

hypoxia A dangerous condition in which the body tissues and cells do not have enough oxygen.

osteoporosis A generalized bone disease that is common among postmenopausal women in which there is a reduction in the amount of bone mass, leading to fractures after minimal trauma.

syncope Fainting caused by an interruption of blood flow to the brain.

vasodilation Widening of a blood vessel.

assessment in action

You and your partner are called to a private residence for a woman who had fallen. Upon arrival, you are met at the door by the patient, an 83-year-old woman. She states that she does not think she needs an ambulance but her neighbor, who was visiting at the time she fell, insisted on calling 9-1-1. You find out that the woman actually fell about an hour ago. She landed squarely on her buttocks.

You note that the patient is limping markedly, but your assessment reveals only minimal swelling and no obvious deformity. The patient is alert and oriented but appears very pale. She has a blood pressure of 88/70 mm Hg, a pulse of 58 beats/min, and respirations of 26 breaths/min.

As you and your partner lift the patient onto the stretcher, she cries out in pain, and you now note an obvious, significant deformity just below her right hip. Test results at the hospital reveal that she has a blood alcohol level of 0.282 and a fractured right hip.

1. Which of the patient's vital signs is within normal limits for her age group?
   A. Pulse
   B. Skin color
   C. Respirations
   D. Blood pressure

2. Assessment of a patient with a suspected fracture of the hip should **NOT** include an evaluation of the patient's:
   A. ability to bear weight or walk.
   B. ability to move the toes on the injured extremity.
   C. ability to feel sensations distal to the injury.
   D. skin color and distal pulses in the injured extremity.

3. Which of the following statements about fractures of the hip is true?
   A. Distal circulation is usually not affected.
   B. Swelling and deformity of the extremity are often absent.
   C. The patient may be able to stand and walk.
   D. Internal rotation of the affected foot is a common presentation.

4. Which of the following statements about alcohol intoxication in the elderly is true?
   A. Alcohol intoxication may alter pain sensation.
   B. An alcohol odor on the breath may be present but overlooked.
   C. Elderly patients from lower income socioeconomic groups are more likely to be alcoholics.
   D. Increased liver function in the elderly easily eliminates alcohol from the patient's system.

5. What is the most likely reason the EMT-Bs overlooked the possibility that the patient was intoxicated?
   A. The patient would have had flushed skin if she were intoxicated.
   B. The patient would have had a higher blood pressure if she were intoxicated.
   C. The patient would have shown obvious signs of alcohol use.
   D. The patient would have been vomiting if she were intoxicated.

prep kit 10

points to ponder

You respond to a call about an elderly man with severe abdominal pain. When you arrive, his wife lets you in and tells you that she called for you. She says that he has had pain for about three hours now. You find the man sitting at the kitchen table. He is wearing very thick glasses and asks who is there as you walk into the room. It is obvious that his vision is very poor. As you begin talking to him, you find out that he is also quite deaf. You must yell to him to communicate, and at that, he appears to hear only about one-third of what you are saying. He appears confused and disoriented, but you are not sure whether that is mental or because he cannot see or hear very well. He is complaining about pain in his feet. He says that he does have abdominal pain, but mostly it is his feet. His feet feel cold and are a little cyanotic, but both are about the same. His wife insists that he was having severe abdominal pain earlier. When you ask about medications, he produces a shoe box with about 20 pill bottles, 12 of which he says he takes at least once a week. You find yourself very frustrated with the lack of information you are able to obtain.

• How would you treat this man? Would you transport him? How else could you get more information? He is not refusing care, but it is unclear whether he needs it. On what would you base your decisions?

online outlook

In order to provide effective treatment to the growing number of elderly patients, all EMTs must have an increased understanding of geriatric care issues. Learn more about the health of geriatric Americans by completing Exercise 10 at www.emtb.com.

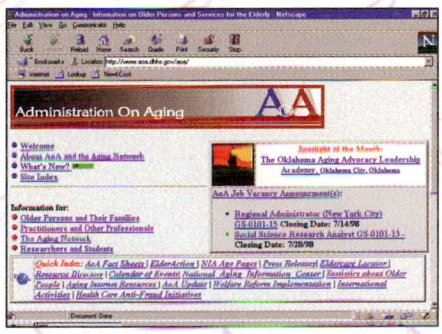

Medical Emergencies

Paul E. Pepe, MD, MPH, FACEP, FCCM

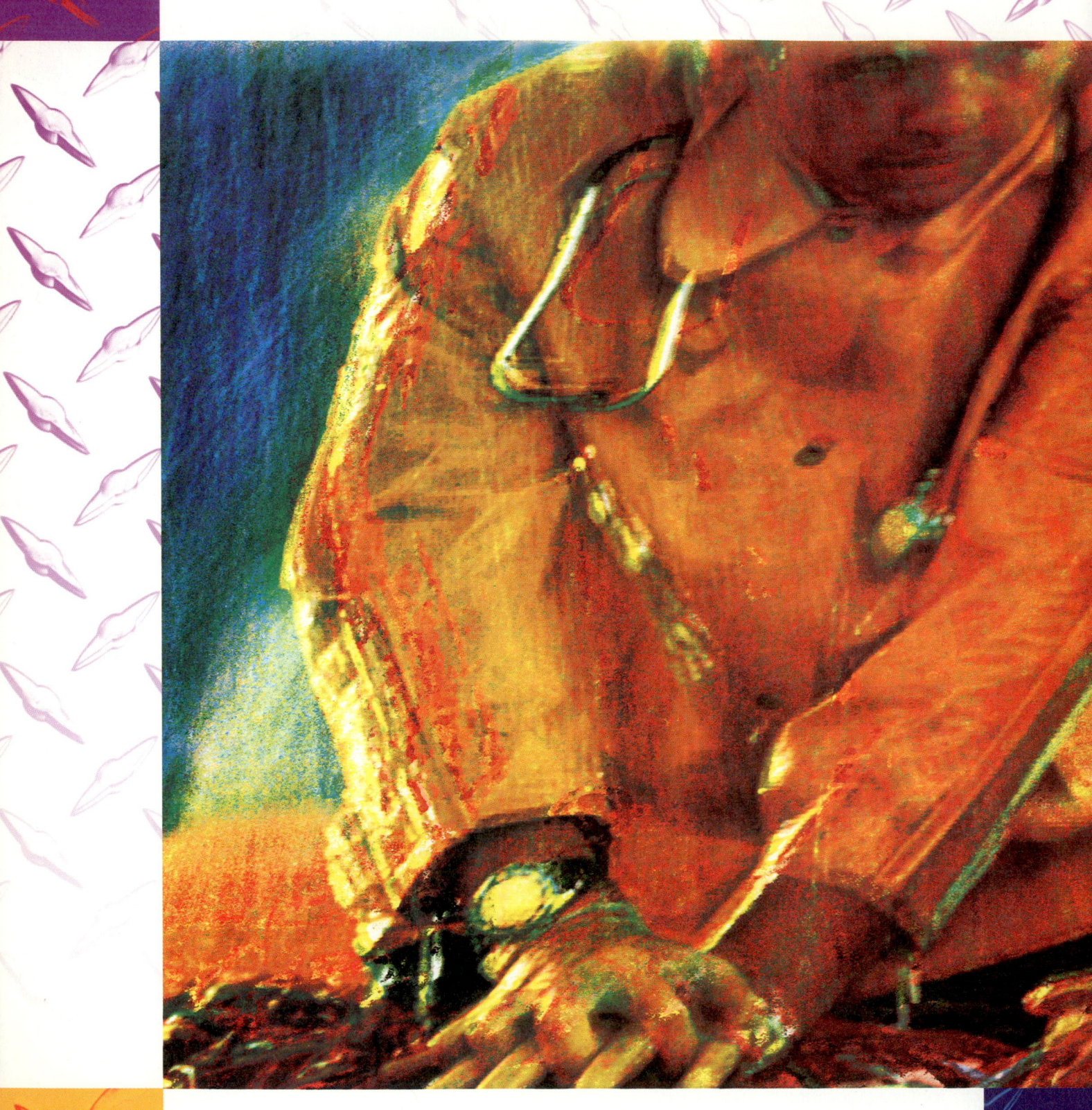

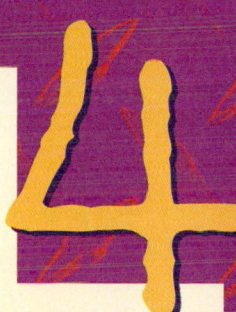

section 4

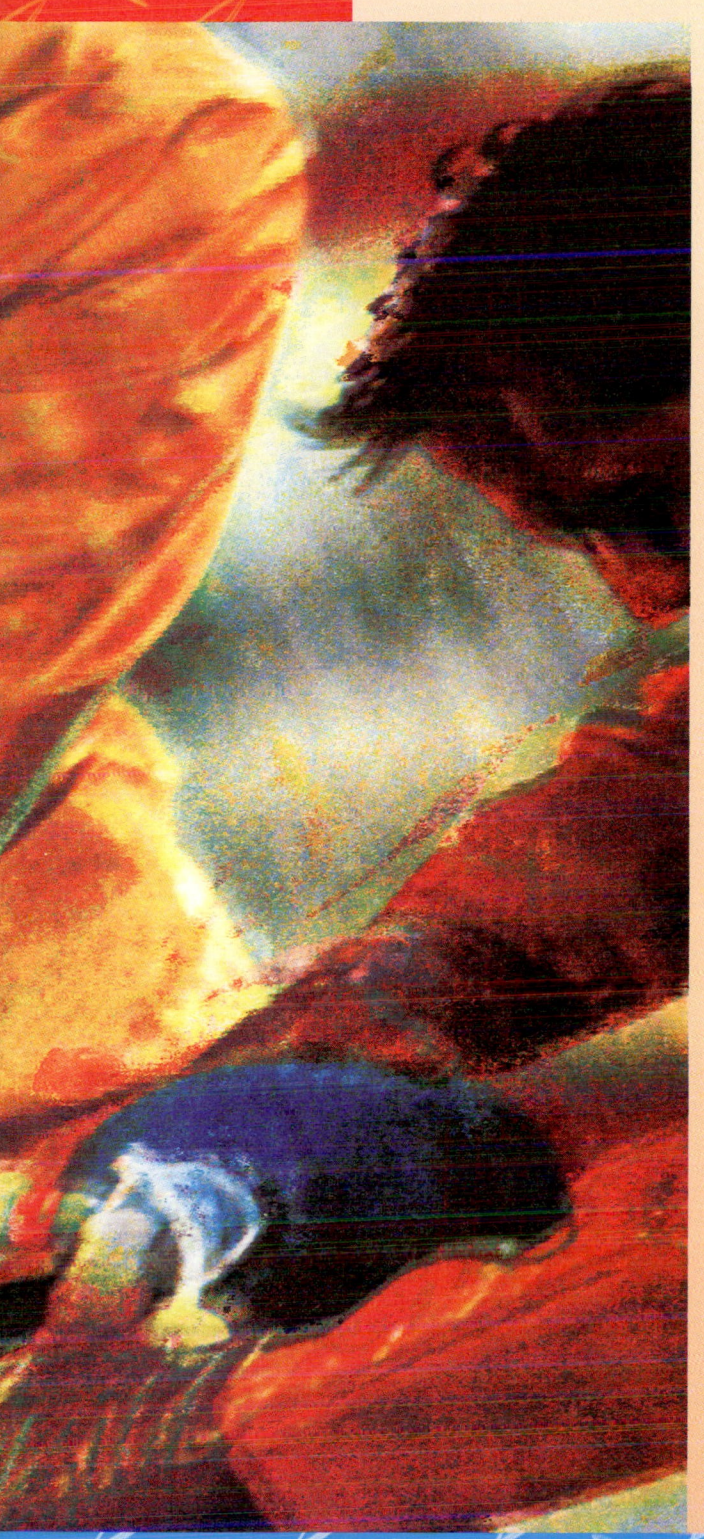

General Pharmacology

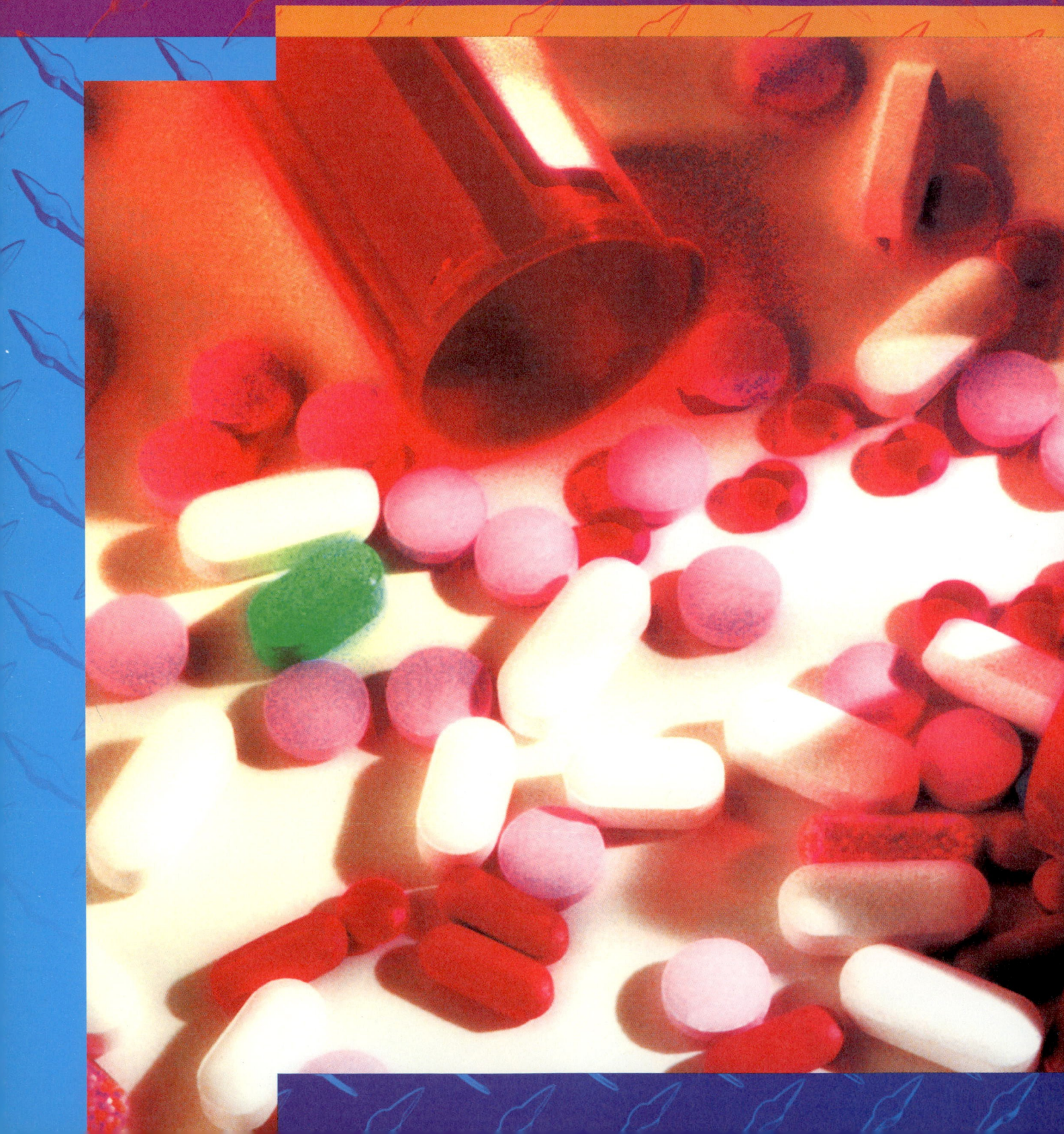

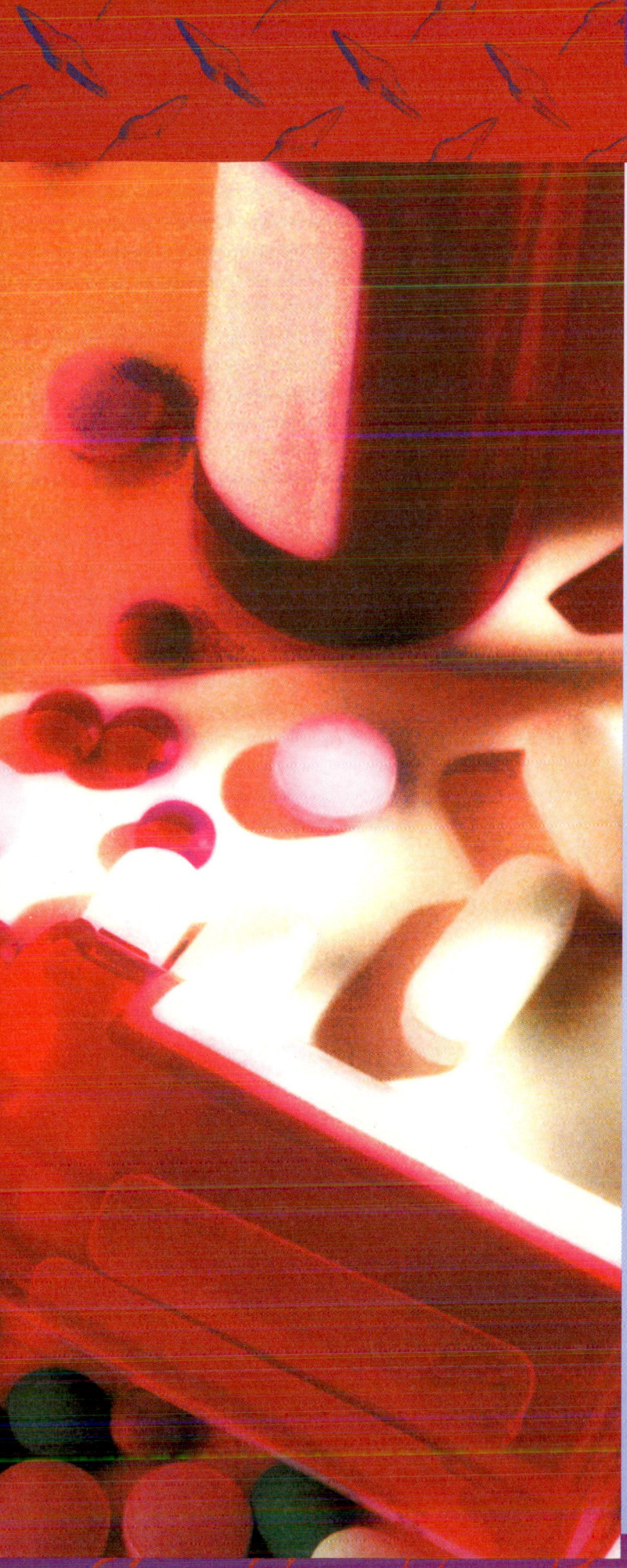

objectives

Cognitive

1. Identify which medications will be carried on the unit.

2. State the medications carried on the unit by the generic name.

3. Identify the medications with which the EMT-B may assist the patient with administering.

4. State the medications the EMT-B can assist the patient with by the generic name.

5. Discuss the forms in which medications may be found.

Affective

6. Explain the rationale for the administration of medications.

Psychomotor

7. Demonstrate general steps for assisting the patient with self-administration of medications.

8. Read the labels and inspect each type of medication.

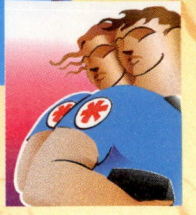

you are the emt

Rescue 6 please respond to 103 Claremont for a 38-year-old woman experiencing a severe allergic reaction after starting a new antibiotic. She reports she has an Epi-Pen to use for another allergy that her doctor said she could use in case of an emergency, but she is too dizzy to reach it . . . .

EMT-Bs can now assist patients with the administration of their medications, increasing the likelihood that you will encounter this type of call. This chapter will help to prepare you as it provides a baseline for understanding pharmacology and will help you to answer the following questions:

1. What medications can you assist patients in taking?
2. How does this task change your roles and responsibilities?

General Pharmacology

Administering medications is a serious business. Used appropriately, a medication may alleviate pain, ease suffering, and improve a patient's well-being. However, used inappropriately, medication may cause harm and even death. As an EMT-B, you will be responsible for administering certain drugs to patients and helping them to self-administer others. You will ask patients about their medications and drug allergies, and you will report this information to hospital personnel. To act without understanding how medications work is to place patients and yourself in danger.

This chapter describes the various forms of medications, the different ways in which they can be administered, and how they work. It then takes a close look at each of the six medications you may be called upon to administer or help patients to self-administer.

How Medications Work

Pharmacology is the study of the properties (characteristics) and effects of drugs and medications. Although these two terms are often used interchangeably, "drugs" may make some people think of narcotics or illegal substances. For this reason, you should try to use the word "medications," especially when interviewing patients and families. In general terms, a medication is a chemical substance that is used to treat or prevent disease or relieve pain.

The **dose** is the amount of the medication that is given. The dose depends on the patient's size or age;

adults and children will get different amounts of the same drug. It also depends on the desired action of the drug. The **action** is the therapeutic effect that a drug is expected to have on the body. For example, nitroglycerin relaxes the walls of the blood vessels and may dilate the arteries. This increases the blood flow, and thus the supply of oxygen, to the heart muscle. In this way, nitroglycerin relieves the squeezing or crushing pain that occurs with the cardiac condition called angina. Nitroglycerin is therefore indicated for chest pain associated with angina. **Indications** are the therapeutic uses for a particular medication.

There are times when you should not a give a patient medication, even if it is indicated for that person's condition. Such situations are called **contraindications**. A drug is contraindicated when it would either harm the patient or have no positive effect on the patient's condition. For example, giving activated charcoal is indicated when a patient has swallowed a poison. Generally, activated charcoal, premixed with water, is used to prevent the body from absorbing a poison. However, activated charcoal would be contraindicated if the patient were unconscious and could not swallow.

Side effects are any actions of a drug other than the desired ones. Side effects may occur even when a medication is administered properly. For example, giving epinephrine to a patient who is having an allergic reaction should dilate the bronchioles and decrease wheezing. However, two side effects of epinephrine are cardiac stimulation and constriction of the arteries, which may elevate the patient's heart rate and blood pressure. These side effects are predictable; others are not.

Medication Names

A medication may have many different names. A <u>trade name</u> is the brand name that a manufacturer gives to a drug, such as Tylenol or Lasix. As a proper noun, a trade name begins with a capital letter. Trade names are used in every aspect of our daily lives, not just in drugs. Well-known examples include Jell-O gelatin, Band-Aid adhesive bandages, and Hershey chocolate candy. A drug may have many different trade names, depending on how many companies manufacture it. Advil, Nuprin, and Motrin all are trade names for the same generic medication: ibuprofen.

The <u>generic name</u> of a drug (such as ibuprofen) is usually its original chemical name, which is not capitalized. Sometimes a drug is called by its generic name more often than by any of its trade names. For example, you may hear the term "nitroglycerin" used more often than the trade names Isordil and Nitrostat. All drugs that are licensed for use in the United States are listed by their generic names in the *United States Pharmacopoeia.*

Medications may be <u>prescription drugs</u> or <u>over-the-counter (OTC) drugs</u>. Prescription drugs are distributed to patients only by pharmacists according to a physician's order. OTC drugs may be purchased directly from a wholesale or retail source, such as a discount store or supermarket, without a prescription. In recent years, the number of prescription drugs that have become available OTC has increased dramatically. Therefore, many of the problems that are attributable to prescription drugs may become more common. You may also come into contact with patients who have taken "street" drugs such as heroin or cocaine. Although street drugs lack the pharmaceutical purity of OTC or prescribed drugs, they still are pharmacologically active and will cause an effect.

Routes of Administration

<u>Absorption</u> is the process by which medications travel through body tissues until they reach the bloodstream. There are nine routes of medication delivery into the body. All except intravenous injection involve absorption.

- <u>Intravenous (IV) injection</u>. "Intravenous" means "into the vein." Medications that need to enter the bloodstream immediately may be injected directly into a vein. This is the fastest way to deliver a chemical substance, but the IV route cannot be used for all chemicals. For example, aspirin, oxygen, or charcoal cannot be given by the IV route.

- <u>Oral</u>. Many medications are taken by mouth (<u>Per os</u>, or PO) and enter the bloodstream through the digestive system. This process often takes as much as 1 hour.

- <u>Sublingual (SL)</u>. "Sublingual" means "under the tongue." Medications that take the SL route, such as nitroglycerin tablets, are absorbed by the venous plexus under the tongue and enter the bloodstream through the oral mucous membranes within minutes. This route is not only faster, it protects medications from chemicals in the digestive system, such as acids that can weaken or inactivate them.

- <u>Intramuscular (IM) injection</u>. "Intramuscular" means "into the muscle." Usually, medications that are administered via IM injection are absorbed quickly, because muscles have a lot of blood vessels. Some types of medications, though, are designed for a slower, sustained release from the muscle. Many such medications have the prefix "depo" in their names, meaning that they form a depository in the muscle after being injected. However, not all medications can be administered intramuscularly. Intramuscular injections can cause damage to muscle tissue and result in uneven, unreliable absorption. This is especially true in people who are experiencing decreased tissue perfusion or shock.

- <u>Intraosseous (IO)</u>. "Intraosseous" means "into the bone." Medications that are delivered via this route reach the blood through the bone marrow. To get medication into the marrow requires drilling a needle through the bone cortex. Because this is painful, the IO route of delivery is used most often in patients who are unconscious as a result of cardiac arrest or extreme shock. Most commonly, the IO route is reserved for children who have less available (or difficult to access) IV sites.

- <u>Subcutaneous (SC) injection</u>. "Subcutaneous" means "beneath the skin." An SC injection is given into the tissue between the skin and the muscle. Because there is less blood here than in the muscles, medications that are delivered via this route are generally absorbed more slowly, and their effects last longer. An SC injection is a useful way to deliver medications that cannot be taken by mouth, as long as they do not irritate or damage the tissue. Commonly, a daily insulin shot is given this way to a patient with diabetes. Also, epinephrine can be given by this route.

- **Transcutaneous**. Transcutaneous means "through the skin." Some medications can be absorbed transcutaneously, such as "nicotine patches" in individuals who are trying to quit smoking. On occasion, a medication that comes in another form is administered transcutaneously to achieve a slower, longer-lasting effect. An example is an adhesive patch containing nitroglycerin.

- **Inhalation**. Some medications are inhaled into the lungs so that they can be absorbed into the blood more quickly. Others are inhaled because they actually work in the lungs. Generally, inhalation helps to minimize the effects of the medication in other body tissues. Such medications come in the form of aerosols, fine powders, or sprays.

- **Per rectum (PR)**. "Per rectum" means "by rectum." This route of delivery is frequently used with children because of easier administration and more reliable absorption. (Children often regurgitate some or all of a medication.) For similar reasons, many medications that are used for nausea and vomiting come in a rectal suppository form. Some medications to control seizures are administered PR when it is impossible to administer them intravenously.

Table 11-1 lists the words that are used for routes of medication delivery, along with their meanings

Dosage Forms

The form that a medication comes in usually dictates its route of delivery. For instance, a tablet or a spray cannot be delivered through a needle. The manufacturer chooses the form to ensure the proper route of the medication, the timing of its release into the bloodstream, and its effects on the target organs or body systems. As an EMT-B, you should be familiar with all of the following seven dosage forms.

Tablets and Capsules

Most medications that are given by mouth to adult patients are in tablet or capsule form (Figure 11-1). Capsules are gelatin shells filled with powdered or liquid medication. If the capsule contains liquid, the shell is sealed and usually soft. If the capsule contains powder, the shell can usually be pulled apart. Tablets often contain other materials that are mixed with the medication and compressed under high pressure.

Some tablets are designed to dissolve very quickly in small amounts of liquid so that they can be given sublingually and absorbed rapidly. An example is the sublingual nitroglycerin tablet used for chest pain by patients with cardiac conditions. These medications are especially useful in emergency situations. Generally, a

TABLE 11-1	Routes of Administration: Words and Their Meanings	
This Word . . .	**From These Latin Words . . .**	**Means**
Inhalation	*inhalatio* (drawing air into the lungs)	inhaling or breathing in
Intramuscular (IM)	*intra* (into) and *muscularis* (of the muscles)	into muscle
Intraosseous (IO)	*intra* (into) and *ossa* (bone)	into bone
Intravenous (IV)	*intra* (into) and *venosus* (of the veins)	into vein
Per)s (PO)	*per* (by) and *os* (mouth)	by mouth
Per Rectum (PR)	*per* (by) and *rectum* (rectum)	by rectum
Subcutaneous (SC)	*sub* (under) and *cutis* (skin)	under the skin
Sublingual (SL)	*sub* (under) and *lingua* (relating to the tongue)	under the tongue
Transcutaneous	*trans* (through) and *cutis* (skin)	through the skin

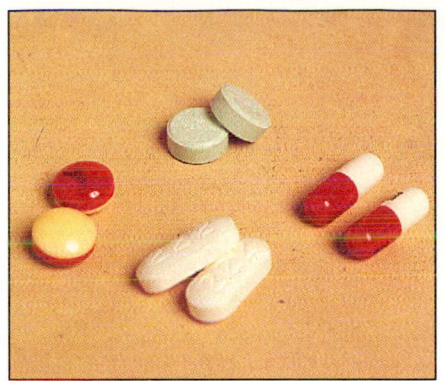

FIGURE 11-1 Tablets and capsules are typically taken by mouth and enter the bloodstream through the digestive system.

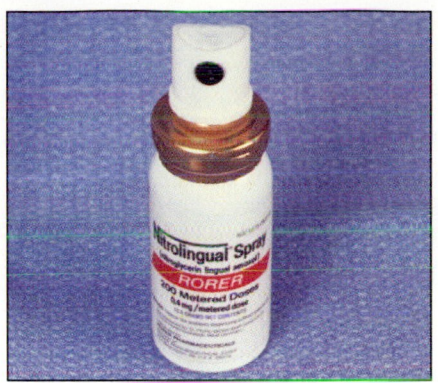

FIGURE 11-2 Nitroglycerin, which is prescribed for chest pain, is often given sublingually (SL) as a spray or a tablet.

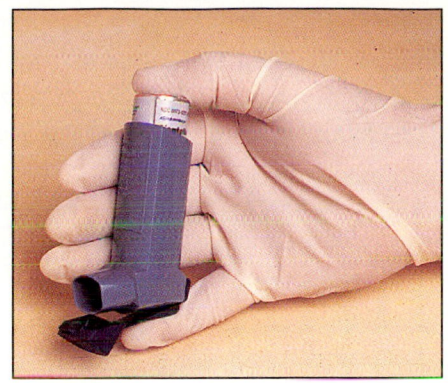

FIGURE 11-3 Some medications are inhaled into the lungs with a metered-dose inhaler so that they can be absorbed into the bloodstream more quickly.

medication that must be swallowed is less useful in an emergency, since the digestive tract provides a slower route of delivery. For example, an oral pain medication is less useful than an IV pain medication when pain relief is needed within minutes.

Solutions and Suspensions

A **solution** is a liquid mixture of one or more substances that cannot be separated by filtering or allowing the mixture to stand. Solutions can be given by almost any route. When given by mouth, solutions may be absorbed from the stomach fairly quickly because the drug is already dissolved. Solutions that irritate the stomach may be given rectally, applied topically to the skin, sprayed sublingually, or inhaled. For example, you may need to help in the sublingual delivery of a nitroglycerin spray (Figure 11-2). Many solutions can be given as an IV, IM, or SC injection. If a patient has a severe allergic reaction, you may help to administer a solution of epinephrine subcutaneously, using an autoinjector.

Many substances do not dissolve well in liquids. Some of these can be ground into fine particles and evenly distributed throughout a liquid by shaking or stirring. This type of mixture is called a **suspension**. An example is activated charcoal, which you may give to patients who have taken overdoses of certain drugs or ingested certain poisons.

Suspensions separate if they stand or are filtered. It is very important that you shake or swirl a suspension before administering it to ensure that the patient receives the right amount of medication. For example, if you are a parent, you may have had to shake a suspension of oral antibiotic before giving it to your child.

Suspensions usually are administered by mouth but sometimes are given rectally. Occasionally, suspensions are applied directly to the skin to treat skin problems. You may have used calamine lotion in this way. Injectable suspensions are given via IM or SC injection only. Certain hormone shots or vaccinations are given this way because of the suspended particles. They cannot be given via IV injection because the suspended particles do not remain dissolved.

Metered-Dose Inhalers

If liquids or solids are broken into small enough droplets or particles, they can be inhaled. A **metered-dose inhaler (MDI)** is a miniature spray canister, used to direct such substances through the mouth and into the lungs (Figure 11-3). An MDI delivers the same amount of medication each time it is used. Since an inhaled medication usually is a suspension, the MDI must be shaken hard before the medication is administered. MDIs are often used by patients with respiratory illnesses such as asthma or emphysema.

Topical Medications

Lotions, creams, and ointments all are **topical medications**, that is, they are applied to the surface of the skin and affect only that area. Ointments contain the least amount of water, lotions the most. You have probably

As an EMT-B, you should be familiar with the serum dosage forms.

noticed that OTC lotions are oilier than prescribed lotions. The smaller the amount of water in the preparation, the slower the rate of absorption of the medication. For example, hand lotions usually are absorbed faster than facial creams. Calamine lotion is an example of a medical lotion. Creams, in turn, are absorbed faster than ointments such as Neosporin first-aid ointment. Hydrocortisone cream to diminish skin itching is an example of a medical cream that can also be given in ointment form.

Transcutaneous Medications

Transdermal medications are designed to be absorbed through the skin, or transcutaneously. Medications such as nitroglycerin paste usually have properties or delivery systems that help to dilate the blood vessels in the skin and thus speed absorption into the bloodstream. In contrast to most topical medicines, which work directly on the application site, transdermal medications are usually intended for systemic (whole-body) effects. A note of caution: If you touch such a medication with your bare skin while administering it, you will absorb it just as readily as the patient will.

Newer delivery systems for transcutaneous medications include the adhesive patch. Patches attach to the skin and allow even absorption of a drug for many hours (Figure 11-4). Both prescription and OTC medications come in this form. Two common examples are nitroglycerin and nicotine.

Gels

A **gel** is a semi-liquid substance that is administered orally through capsules or plastic tubes. Gels usually have the consistency of paste or creams but are transparent (clear). "Gelatinous" means thick and sticky, like gelatin. Depending on your local medical directives, as an EMT-B, you may give oral glucose in gel form to a patient with diabetes (Figure 11-5).

Gases for Inhalation

Gaseous medications are neither solid nor liquid and most often are delivered in an operating room (OR). The medication that is most commonly used in gas form outside the OR is oxygen. You might not think of oxygen as a medication because it is all around us and we all use it. However, in its concentrated form, it is a potent medication that has systemic effects, that is, effects throughout the body (Figure 11-6). You will usually administer oxygen through a face mask or nasal cannula.

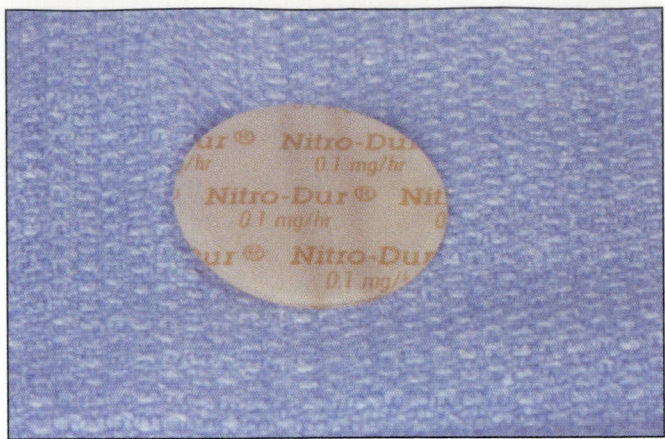

FIGURE 11-4 Some drugs are transcutaneous, or administered through the skin, such as the nitroglycerin patch shown.

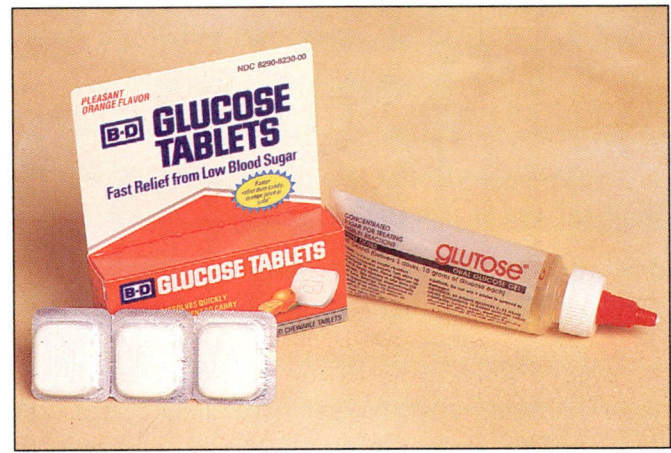

FIGURE 11-5 Oral glucose, used in diabetic emergencies, is available in both gel and tablet form.

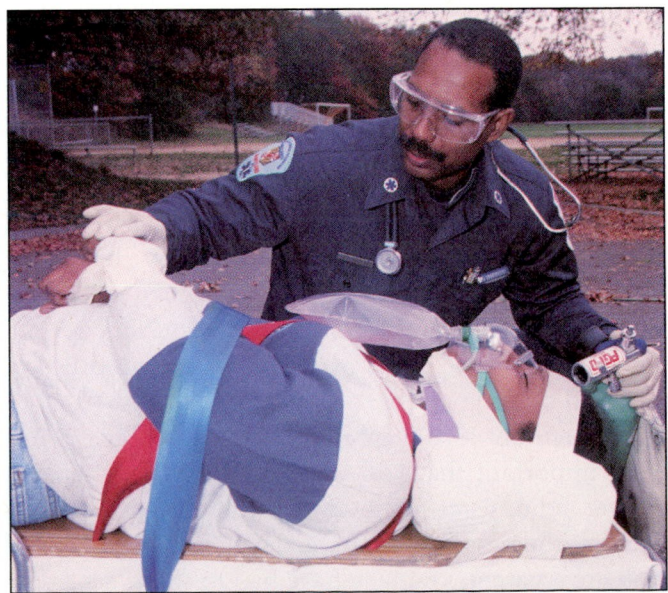

FIGURE 11-6 Oxygen is a potent medication that you will typically give through a nonrebreathing mask.

Medications Carried on the EMS Unit

The three medications that may be carried on the EMS unit are oxygen, oral glucose, and activated charcoal. Used wisely, each can be a powerful tool. Keep in mind, however, that you may deliver these medications only according to standing orders in a protocol (off-line medical control) or a direct order (on-line medical control).

Oxygen

All cells need <u>oxygen</u> to function properly. The heart and brain, especially, cannot function for long if oxygen levels go down, which is why oxygen was chosen as an on-board medication for EMS units.

If a patient is not breathing or is having trouble getting air into the lungs, you should administer supplemental oxygen. In general, you will be giving oxygen via a nonrebreathing mask at 10 to 15 L/min or via nasal cannula at 2 to 6 L/min. However, if the patient is not breathing, you must also provide artificial ventilations, so you will need to use the BVM device. Oxygen is usually delivered at 15 L/min with this technique.

Outside a hospital, the nonrebreathing mask (a mask containing a reservoir tube or bag) is the preferred method of giving oxygen to patients who are experiencing significant respiratory difficulties or shock. With a good mask-to-mouth seal, this mask can provide up to 95% inspired oxygen (Figure 11-7). With a nasal cannula, oxygen flows through two small, tubelike prongs that fit into the patient's nostrils. This device can provide up to 35% to 40% inspired oxygen if the flowmeter is set at 6 L/min. Settings that are higher than this do not provide much additional benefit and tend to dry the nasal mucosa.

Remember that, although oxygen itself does not burn, it allows other things to burn. If there is extra oxygen in the air, objects will burn more easily. So make sure there are no open flames, lit cigarettes, or sparks in the area in which you are administering oxygen. The

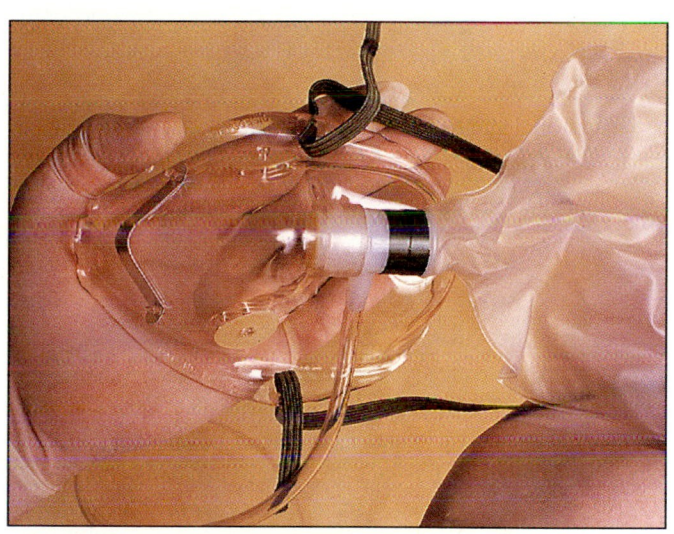

FIGURE 11-7 A nonrebreathing mask is the preferred method of giving oxygen, as it provides up to 95% inspired oxygen.

know these medications

Under the U.S. Department of Transportation's 1994 EMT-Basic National Standard Curriculum, an EMT-B is allowed to administer or help patients self-administer the following six medications.

You may be called upon to administer these medications:

- Oxygen
- Activated charcoal
- Oral glucose

You may help patients self-administer these medications:

- Epinephrine
- Metered-dose inhaler medications
- Nitroglycerin

However, you may administer or help to administer these medications *only* under the following conditions:

- A licensed physician gives you a direct order to administer a medication, and/or the local medical protocols under which you are working permit you to administer that medication. Some local protocols exclude one or more of the six medications listed above.

- The local medical protocols under which you are working include standing orders for the use of a medication in defined situations. It is imperative that you do *not* give or help patients take any other medications under any circumstances.

patient's clothing and blankets may be saturated with oxygen and can easily burst into flame if exposed to one of these triggers.

Activated Charcoal

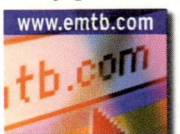

Many poisoning emergencies involve overdoses of drugs taken by mouth. Fortunately, many drugs adsorb activated charcoal, which keeps the drugs from being absorbed by the body. **Adsorption** means to bind to or stick to a surface. **Activated charcoal** is ground into a very fine powder to provide the greatest possible surface area for binding. You will probably carry a container with a premixed suspension of activated charcoal powder and water in the EMS unit, if allowed by local protocol (Figure 11-8).

The bond between drug and charcoal is not permanent. Because the drug may break free and be absorbed into the bloodstream if activated charcoal remains in the digestive system throughout a normal day, charcoal is frequently suspended with another medication called sorbitol (a complex sugar). This suspension has a laxative effect that causes the entire mixture, including the drug, to move quickly through the digestive system.

Activated charcoal is given by mouth. Although sorbitol sweetens the suspension, the black color of the

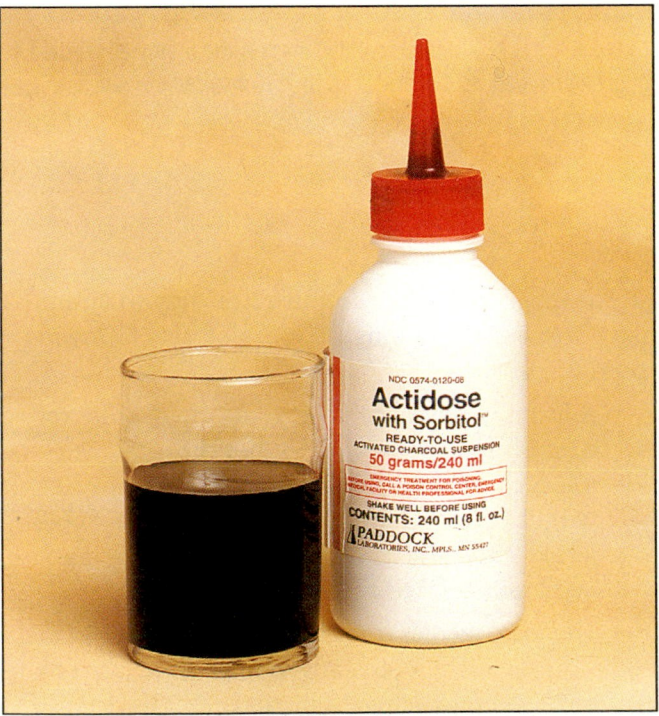

FIGURE 11-8 Activated charcoal is a suspension that is often used for patients who have taken a drug overdose or swallowed a poison.

The three medications that may be carried on the EMS unit are oxygen, oral glucose, and activated charcoal. Used wisely, each can be a powerful tool.

charcoal makes it look unappealing. For this reason, you should use a covered container and ask the patient to drink the fluid through a straw.

Oral Glucose

Glucose is a sugar that our cells use as fuel. Although some cells can use other sugars, brain cells must have glucose. If the level of glucose in the blood gets too low, a person can lose consciousness, have seizures, and ultimately die.

The medical term for an extremely low blood glucose level is **hypoglycemia**. Hypoglycemia can be caused by an excess of insulin, which is taken to control blood glucose levels. Patients with diabetes who use insulin regularly understand the effects of this medication on the body. If they ever inject more insulin than the body can use, hours later they may need to eat a candy bar or drink a sugared cola to try to counteract the insulin's action. The **oral glucose** that is carried in the EMS unit can counteract the effects of hypoglycemia in the same way as a candy bar or sweet drink, but faster. This is because common table sugar (sucrose) and fruit sugars (fructose) are complex sugars and must be split before they can be absorbed. Glucose is a simple sugar that is readily absorbed by the bloodstream.

Hospital personnel and paramedics can give glucose through an IV line. As an EMT-B, you can give glucose only by mouth. Glucose is available as a gel designed to be spread on the mucous membranes between the cheek and gum; however, absorption through this route is not as reliable as with injection. Because the patient may be conscious one moment and unconscious the next, you must be very careful when administering oral glucose. If the patient is unable to swallow well, you should not give glucose, as it might be accidentally inhaled into the lungs.

Assisted-Administration Medications

The three prescribed medications that you may help patients self-administer are epinephrine, metered-dose inhaler medications, and nitroglycerin. These medications, prescribed by doctors for self-administration by patients, have risks as well as benefits, and you must understand them.

Epinephrine

Epinephrine is the main hormone that controls the body's fight-or-flight response. It is released inside the body when there is sudden stress, such as during exercise or when the patient becomes suddenly scared. Because epinephrine is secreted by the adrenal glands, it is also known as adrenaline. Epinephrine has different effects on different body tissues and is used as a medication in several forms. Generally, epinephrine will increase heart rate and blood pressure and decrease the muscle tone of the bronchiole tree. Therefore, it can ease breathing problems caused by the bronchiole spasms that are common in asthma and allergic reactions. In a person who is close to anaphylactic shock as a result of an allergic reaction, epinephrine may also help to prevent a dramatic decrease in blood pressure.

Epinephrine has the following characteristics:

- Secreted naturally by adrenal glands
- Decreases muscle tone of bronchiole tree
- Dilates passages in lungs
- Constricts blood vessels
- Increases heart rate and blood pressure

Depending on the condition being treated, epinephrine can be delivered by MDI or by SC, IM, or IV injection. You may be allowed to assist with all but the last form of delivery.

Administering epinephrine by metered-dose inhaler. Asthma, also known as "reactive airway disease," can be a life-threatening condition. Therefore, some patients use epinephrine inhalers to relieve bronchial spasms quickly. The trade names of some of these inhalers include Primatene Mist, Bronitin Mist, Bronkaid Mist, and Medihaler-Epi. Since epinephrine tends to increase heart rate and blood pressure, most patients with asthma also use certain chemical cousins of epinephrine that produce fewer side effects. Metaproterenol (Alupent or Metaprel) and albuterol (Proventil or Ventolin) both work more on the bronchial spasms and less on the cardiovascular system.

Administering epinephrine by injection. Patients who know that they are allergic to insect stings often

caring for the elderly

Geriatric patients often take many medications. They might also save medications left over from prior medical conditions. Make every effort to identify which medications are current and what they are being used to treat. Ask family members to help distinguish current from outdated medications, or look at the expiration dates on the medication labels. Take either a list of the current medications or the drugs themselves with you to the emergency department.

Elderly patients can become confused about their drug regimen. Uncertainty as to whether or not they missed a dose may cause the patients to repeat the drug, possibly leading to an overdose. If you think an overdose has occurred, contact medical control.

Remember, medications can interact with each other, creating potentially harmful conditions for the patient. Even though a medication may be indicated for a special condition, it might be contraindicated in the presence of another drug. For example, if the patient is taking the heart medication propranolol (Inderal) and has an acute episode of shortness of breath, any asthma remedy might be rendered ineffective by the heart medication.

The new drug sildenafil (Viagra) can have potentially fatal drug interactions with common heart medications. Ask a patient who has prescribed nitroglycerin if he has used Viagra within the previous 24 hours. Report this to medical control.

While medications do help people to recover from acute conditions and adjust to chronic diseases, they can pose serious problems for the geriatric patient. You should distinguish current from prior medications, suspect accidental or intentional overdoses, and be prepared for potentially lethal drug interactions. Document all findings and inform medical control.

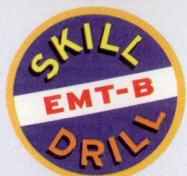

Administering an SC or IM Injection

Figure 11-9

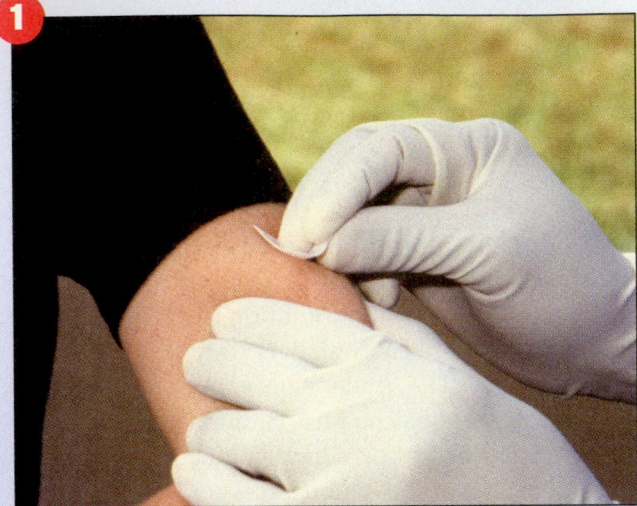

1 Before giving an injection, you should prepare the skin with an appropriate antiseptic.

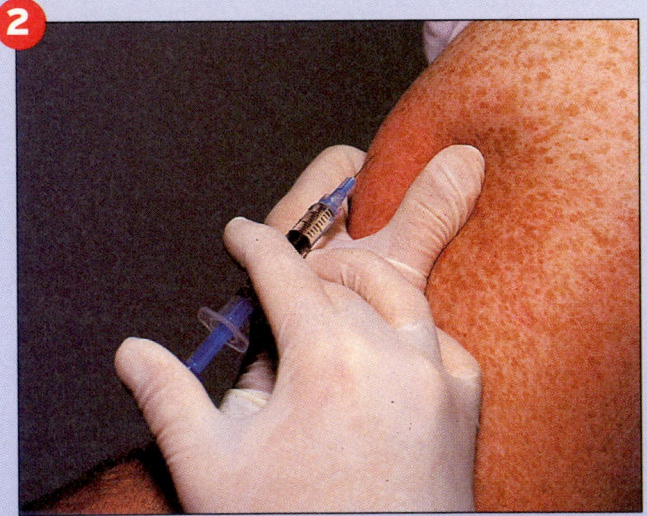

2 For an SC injection, you should pinch the skin while inserting the needle at a 45-degree angle.

carry epinephrine for SC or IM injections, just in case they are stung. In these individuals, insect venom causes the body to release histamine, which lowers blood pressure by relaxing the small blood vessels and allowing them to leak. The release of histamine may also cause wheezing from bronchial spasms and swelling of the airway tissues (edema), which make it difficult for the patient to breathe. Epinephrine acts as a specific antidote to histamine, countering both of these harmful effects. It constricts (or tightens) the blood vessels, allowing blood pressure to rise and reducing the swelling. In the lung's airways, it has the opposite effect; it dilates (or enlarges) these passages, so the flow of air is less restricted. You can also expect the patient's heart rate to increase after administration of epinephrine.

You may be trained to administer SC and IM injections of epinephrine, depending on local protocol. Remember that an SC injection puts the epinephrine into the tissue between the skin and the muscle. Therefore, it is usually helpful to pinch the skin lightly to lift it away from the muscle. A syringe used for SC injections has a short, thin needle, typically between 1/2″ and 5/8″ long. The syringe for IM use has a longer, thicker needle that is between 1 and 1 1/2″ long so that it can reach into the muscle.

Follow these steps for either an SC or an IM injection (Figure 11-9):

1. Sterilize the skin with the appropriate antiseptic.

2. Insert the needle into the skin (or muscle). Then draw the syringe's plunger back slightly before injecting the medication.

3. Check to see whether any blood seeps into the syringe. If it does, you have accidentally placed the needle in a small blood vessel and will need to withdraw the needle and start again using the same syringe (assuming that the skin remains sterilized).

4. If no blood returns when you pull back on the needle, push the plunger on the syringe to inject the medication.

5. Once the needle has been injected into the patient's skin, it becomes contaminated with potential viruses and other infectious agents from the patient. Appropriate disposal precautions must be taken.

Epinephrine may also be dispensed from an auto-injector, which automatically delivers a preset amount of the medication (Figure 11-10). This is the method that you will most likely use. Pressing the device into the skin activates the mechanism. Regardless of the

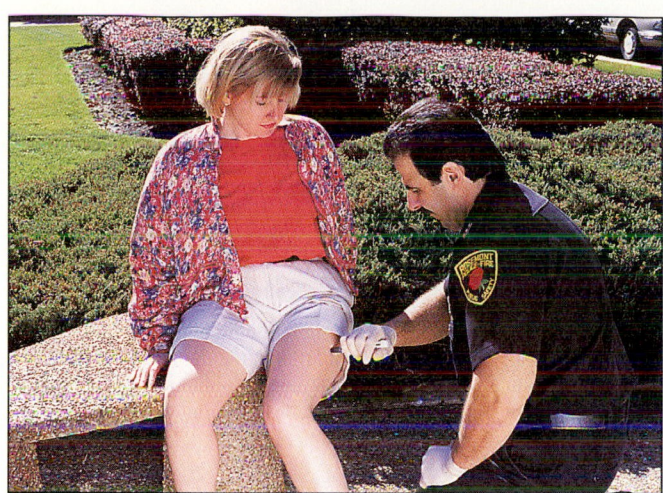

FIGURE 11-10 An Epi-Pen™ auto-injector may be used to administer a preset dose of epinephrine.

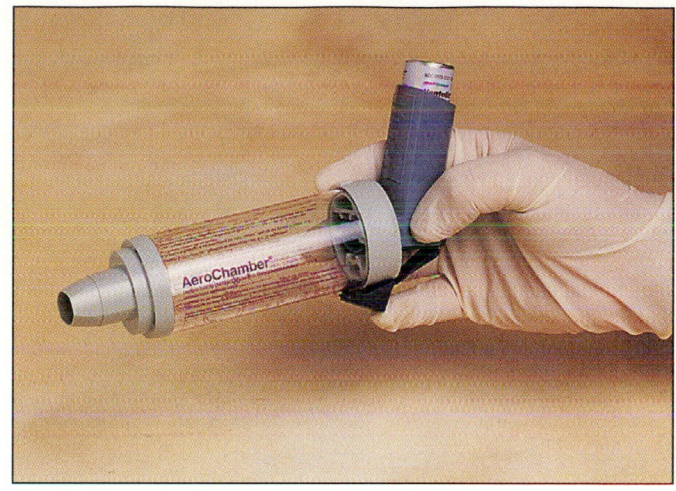

FIGURE 11-11 Some inhalers have spacer devices to better direct the medication spray.

method used, epinephrine causes a burning sensation where it is injected, and the patient's heart rate will increase after the injection.

Metered-Dose Inhaler Medications

Sometimes, a respiratory condition such as asthma is not severe enough to require the use of epinephrine. In such cases, patients may use one of the epinephrine cousins that is more narrowly focused on the lungs. These medications are delivered with a metered-dose inhaler. An MDI requires a great deal of coordination, something that may be in short supply when an individual is having trouble breathing. Patients must aim properly and spray just as they start to inhale. An adapter, which fits over the inhaler like a sleeve, can be used; however, most of the medication tends to end up on the roof of the patient's mouth. To avoid misdirecting the spray, many physicians prescribe "spacer" devices for use with the inhaler (Figure 11-11). The inhaler fits into an opening on one end of the spacer's chamber, and the mouthpiece fits on the other end. The patient sprays the prescribed dose into the chamber and then breathes in and out of the mouthpiece until the mist is completely inhaled.

If the patient does not have a spacer, you can quickly improvise by using the cardboard tube from a roll of paper towels or toilet paper. This is a reasonable alternative as long as you can do it in a minute or less. You may need to cut the tube to get a length of 4" to 6". Have the patient open his or her lips inside one end of the tube as you place the plastic adapter on the inhaler and hold the mouthpiece at the other end of the tube. Activate the spray by pressing the canister into the adapter just as the patient starts to inhale. If relief is not achieved, wait

about 3 minutes and repeat this sequence. Above all, it is important to ensure that the patient inhales all the medication in a single-sprayed dose.

Nitroglycerin

Many patients with cardiac conditions carry some form of fast-acting nitroglycerin to relieve the pain of angina. Nitroglycerin is the same substance as TNT (trinitro-toluene), which is why the term "nitro" is used both in medicine and the explosives business. Fortunately, the forms of nitroglycerin that you will use have been stabilized so that they are not explosive.

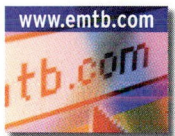

If you have ever run for a prolonged period of time, you probably remember that your muscles developed a painful, heavy, burning sensation. This is because the demand for oxygen to those muscles exceeded the supply. When heart muscle develops a similar pain, it is called angina pectoris. The cause is the same: not enough oxygen, in this case because of a blockage or narrowing in the blood vessels that supply the heart. Occasionally, the cause is a spasm in these blood vessels. Unlike the runner with sore legs, of course, the heart muscle cannot stop and rest until the pain goes away.

The purpose of **nitroglycerin** is to increase blood flow by relieving the spasms or causing the arteries to dilate. It does this by relaxing the muscular walls of the coronary arteries and veins. Nitroglycerin also relaxes veins throughout the body, so less blood is returned to the heart and the heart does not have to work as hard each time it contracts. In short, blood pressure is decreased. Because of this, however, it is important that you always take the patient's blood pressure before administering nitroglycerin. If the systolic blood pressure is less than 100 mm Hg, the nitroglycerin may have the harmful effect of lowering the blood flow to the heart's own blood vessels. Even a patient who has adequate blood pressure should sit or lie down with head elevated before taking this drug. If the patient is standing, he or she may faint when blood flow to the brain is reduced as the nitroglycerin starts to work. If a significant drop in the patient's blood pressure (15 to 20 mm Hg) occurs and the patient suddenly feels dizzy or sick, lay the patient down and raise the legs.

During a heart attack (myocardial infarction, or MI), a blood clot forms in a narrowed coronary artery, blocking the blood flow to a section of the heart muscle. If the blockage is not cleared in time (usually an hour or more), that section of the heart muscle will die. If nitroglycerin no longer brings relief to a person in whom it has previously worked, the person may be experiencing an MI instead of an angina attack. Therefore, it is important to know how much nitroglycerin a patient has needed in the past to relieve chest pain and how much has been taken during the current emergency. Always report this information to medical control. Remember, you cannot administer this medication without clearance from medical control or standing orders.

Nitroglycerin has the following effects:

- Relaxes the muscular walls of coronary arteries and veins
- Less blood is returned to the heart
- Decreases blood pressure
- Relaxes veins throughout the body
- Often causes a mild headache after administration

Administering nitroglycerin by tablet. Nitroglycerin is usually taken sublingually: The patient places a tiny tablet under the tongue, where it dissolves. The tablet should create a slight tingling or burning sensation. If the nitroglycerin has lost its usual "bite," it may have lost potency because of aging or improper storage. Be sure to check the expiration date on the bottle.

Sublingual nitroglycerin tablets should be stored in their original glass container with the cap screwed on tightly. Note that what looks like cotton in the container is actually rayon. If real cotton is placed in the container, it can absorb nitroglycerin, thus reducing the tablets' potency. Other medications placed in the container can likewise rob nitroglycerin of its power. If you notice any signs of improper storage, be sure to include that information in the patient's medical history.

Administering nitroglycerin by metered-dose spray. Some patients who take nitroglycerin use a metered-dose spray, which deposits medication on or under the tongue. Each spray is equivalent to one tablet. To ensure direct, proper dosing on the bottom of the tongue, do not use a spacer with the metered-dose canister when delivering nitroglycerin by this method.

Whether using the tablets or the metered-dose spray, you should wait 5 minutes for a response before repeating. Closely monitor the patient's vital signs, particularly the blood pressure.

General Steps to Administering Medication

As an EMT-B, you must be familiar with the five general steps of administering any medication to a patient:

1. **Obtain an order from medical control.**
   This order may be given to you directly, through on-line medical control via telephone or radio. Or it may be indirect, through protocols that contain standing orders for the administration of certain medications. For example, your system may use a protocol that describes how the medical director wants you to deal with a patient who is having respiratory difficulties. Part of this protocol may direct you to use a nonrebreathing mask to deliver oxygen to such a patient at 15 L/min. You may do this without calling on-line medical control if the patient meets the criteria of the protocol.

   But what if the same patient is also having chest pain "just like my other heart attack"? In that case, you may be able to apply the oxygen, but you will have to call medical control or follow standing orders before helping to administer the patient's nitroglycerin spray. Knowing and understanding the local protocols under which you will be working are absolutely essential.

   In addition to getting approval to administer a medication, you must verify the on-line order, which means that you should restate the name of the drug, the dose to be given, and the route of administration to medical control. Verifying the order will help to reduce the chance of a miscommunication leading to the administration of an inappropriate medication.

Next, you must reconfirm that the patient can tolerate the medication. For example, suppose that you have received and verified the order to give one sublingual nitroglycerin tablet to a patient with a cardiac condition. While you were getting the order, however, the patient began to sweat more and became less responsive. A repeat blood pressure is 80/60 mm Hg. Using your knowledge about nitroglycerin, you would decide not to give the medication. Instead, you would notify medical control of the changes in the patient's condition and seek further orders.

2. **Verify the proper medication and prescription.** You have received and confirmed the medication order and determined that the patient is still a candidate for the drug. You must now make sure that the drug you are about to deliver is really the one you asked for. Carefully read the label. If it is the patient's own prescription, the bottle may show the trade name or the generic name. If you have any questions at all, contact on-line medical control. Make sure that the medication is, indeed, the patient's own and does not belong to a friend or relative. You should never give a medication to a patient that has been prescribed for someone else. The only exception to this rule is if you are ordered to do so by medical control and you are sure that they understand that the medication does not belong to the patient.

3. **Verify the form, dose, and route of the medication.** You have confirmed your order and verified that the medication is the one you want to give. Now you must make sure that the form of the medication, the dose, and the route are all compatible with the order you received. For example, suppose that you are told to give the patient a sublingual nitroglycerin tablet. The patient's nitroglycerin tablet bottle is empty, but he has another bottle of nitroglycerin capsules. These are to be swallowed four times a day. The medication is the same, but the form, dose, and route of delivery are different from the order given. You may not substitute the capsules for the tablets without specific orders from medical control.

general steps to administering medication

1. Obtain an order from medical control.
2. Verify the proper medication and prescription.
3. Verify the form, dose, and route of the medication.
4. Check the expiration date and condition of the medication.
5. Reassess the vital signs, especially heart rate and blood pressure, at least every 5 minutes or as the patient's condition changes.
6. Document.

4. **Check the expiration date and condition of the medication.** The last step before administering a medication is to make sure it has not expired. Prescription and OTC drugs alike should have an expiration date on their labels. Check the date. If no date can be found, you should examine the drug with suspicion. In addition, if you find discoloration, cloudiness, or particles in a liquid medication, you should not use it. If a patient with asthma gives you an MDI and the expiration date on it is smudged, you should not use it.

5. **Reassess the vital signs, especially heart rate and blood pressure, at least every 5 minutes or as the patient's condition changes.**

6. **Document.** Remember the EMS rule: The work is not done until the paperwork is done. Once the medication has been delivered, you must document your actions and the patient's response. This includes the time you gave the medication as well as the name, dose, and route of administration. Did the patient improve, get worse, or not change at all? Were there any side effects? A second EMS rule says that "if you did not write it down, it did not happen." If your performance should ever be questioned, documentation is your best defense.

prep kit

ready for review

Medications come in seven different forms: tablets and capsules, solutions and suspensions, metered-dose inhalers, topical medications, transdermal medications, gels, and gases. They may be administered through nine different routes: intravenous, intramuscular, or subcutaneous injection; orally; sublingually; intraosseously; transcutaneously; by inhalation; and by rectum. In all but the intravenous injection route, the medication is absorbed into the bloodstream through various body tissues. These routes of administration often determine the speed with which the medication takes effect.

Three medications are typically carried on the EMS unit: oxygen, oral glucose, and activated charcoal. There are three additional medications that the EMT-B may help the patient self-administer: metered-dose inhaler medications, nitroglycerin, and epinephrine. Remember, though, that these may differ depending on local protocol. The administration of any drug requires approval by medical control, either through direct orders given on-line or standing orders that are part of the local protocols.

There are five steps to follow in administering medications, four of which occur before you give the drug: Obtain an order from medical control, verify the proper medication, verify the dose and route, and check the expiration date of the medication. The fifth step is to accurately document the patient's history, assessment, treatment, and response

vital vocabulary

www.emtb.com

absorption   The process by which medications travel through body tissues until they reach the bloodstream.

action   The effect of a drug on the body.

activated charcoal   Charcoal ground into a very fine powder that provides the greatest possible surface area for binding drugs that have been taken by mouth; it is carried on the EMS unit.

adsorption   To bind to or stick to a surface.

contraindication   Situations in which a drug should not be given because it would not help or may actually harm a patient.

dose   The amount of medication given on the basis of the patient's size and age.

epinephrine   Medication that increases heart rate and blood pressure but also eases breathing problems by decreasing muscle tone of the bronchiole tree; the EMT-B may be allowed to help the patient self-administer the medication.

gel   A semi-liquid substance that is administered orally through capsules or plastic tubes.

generic name   The original chemical name of a drug (in contrast to one of its "trade names").

hypoglycemia   An extremely low blood glucose level.

indication   A therapeutic use for a specific medication.

inhalation   Breathing into the lungs; a medication delivery route.

intramuscular (IM) injection   An injection into a muscle.

intraosseous (IO)   Into the bone; a medication delivery route.

intravenous (IV) injection   An injection directly into a vein.

metered-dose inhaler (MDI)   A miniature spray canister through which droplets or particles may be inhaled.

nitroglycerin   Medication that increases blood flow by relieving spasms or causing arteries to dilate; the EMT-B may be allowed to help the patient self-administer the medication.

oral   By mouth; a medication delivery route.

oral glucose   A simple sugar that is readily absorbed by the bloodstream; it is carried on the EMS unit.

over-the-counter (OTC) drugs   Drugs that may be purchased directly by a patient without a prescription.

oxygen   A gas that all cells need in order to metabolize; the heart and brain, especially, cannot function without oxygen.

per os   Through the mouth; a medication delivery route.

per rectum   Through the rectum; a medication delivery route.

pharmacology   The study of the properties and effects of medications.

prescription drugs   Drugs that are distributed to patients only by pharmacists according to a physician's order.

side effects   Any effects of a drug other than the desired ones.

solution   A liquid mixture that cannot be separated by filtering or allowing the mixture to stand.

sublingual (SL)   Under the tongue; a medication delivery route.

suspension   A mixture of ground particles that are distributed evenly throughout a liquid.

subcutaneous (SC) injection   An injection into the tissue between the skin and muscle.

topical medications   Lotions, creams, and ointments that are applied to the surface of the skin and affect only that area.

trade name   The brand name that a manufacturer gives a drug.

transcutaneous   Through the skin; a medication delivery route.

transdermal medications   Medications that are designed to be absorbed through the skin.

assessment in action

You are heading back to the station after a call when you and your partner are summoned to a local homeless shelter for a "sick man." At the scene, you are directed down a poorly lit hall to room 35, where you find an unkempt 51-year-old man lying on a vomit-encrusted bed. The patient says that he wants to go to the hospital but first wants you to find his medications. He has slurred speech, he can barely stand, and his breath odor suggests that he's been drinking. When questioned, the patient denies drinking for the last several days. After a quick search of the room, your partner finds a large, unmarked pill bottle that is about half filled with four or five different kinds of pills. As the patient struggles to put on his socks, he asks you to give him a pink pill and a big white pill from the bottle.

1. What should you do when the patient asks you to give him his medications?
   A. Give him the pink pill but not the white pill.
   B. Give him the white pill but not the pink pill.
   C. Give him both pills, and then prepare for transport.
   D. Contact medical control before you give him any medications.

2. The label on a prescription pill bottle identifies the proper dose of the medication. What is the definition of a dose of medication?
   A. The expected action of the medication
   B. How much of the medication should be taken
   C. How long the medication is supposed to work
   D. The reason the patient is taking the medication

3. Which of the following terms describes when a medication should **NOT** be used because it may be ineffective or possibly even harmful to the patient?
   A. Preparation
   B. Loading dosage
   C. Specific action
   D. Contraindication

4. Who would be liable if the patient suddenly became gravely ill after you helped him to take the medications in the unmarked bottle?
   A. You
   B. The patient
   C. Your medical director
   D. The emergency department physician

5. Which of the following statements about prescription medications is true?
   A. Prescription medications rarely have any side effects.
   B. A double dose of a medication makes it work twice as well.
   C. The route of administration for a medication does affect how it works.
   D. All prescription medications may have dangers associated with them.

points to ponder

Objectives 1-1.8, 1-5.31, 3-6.2, 4-1.8

You respond to a 34-year-old patient who is complaining of a diabetic problem. When you enter the apartment, you find it to be very messy and dirty. The smell is difficult to bear and is a mixture of urine, body odor, and something rotting. You find the patient on the couch and immediately notice large ulcers and dead tissue on her feet. The patient is less than alert but not unconscious and is able to communicate in slow, slurred speech. She confirms that she is diabetic and says that she has been taking her insulin. You ask to see it, and she tells you it is in a drawer in the kitchen. When you open the drawer, you find many medications, including insulin and syringes. While looking for the most recent insulin, you notice about 20 bottles, most empty, of different pain killers. All of these are dated within the last three months, and about half of them are prescribed by one physician; the others are from different physicians.

- Why might the patient have so many empty bottles of pain medication? Would you report this? If so, to whom? Was it appropriate to look at the other medications when you asked only about the insulin? Why or why not? Would this affect how you thought of the patient? Would this change how you treat the patient?

online outlook

A medication may have many different names, which may be a bit confusing for you at first. To learn more about trade names and generic names of medications, complete Exercise 11 at the www.emtb.com.

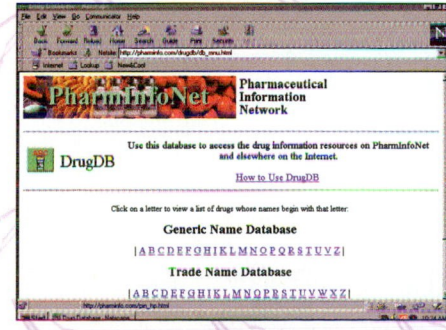

Respiratory Emergencies

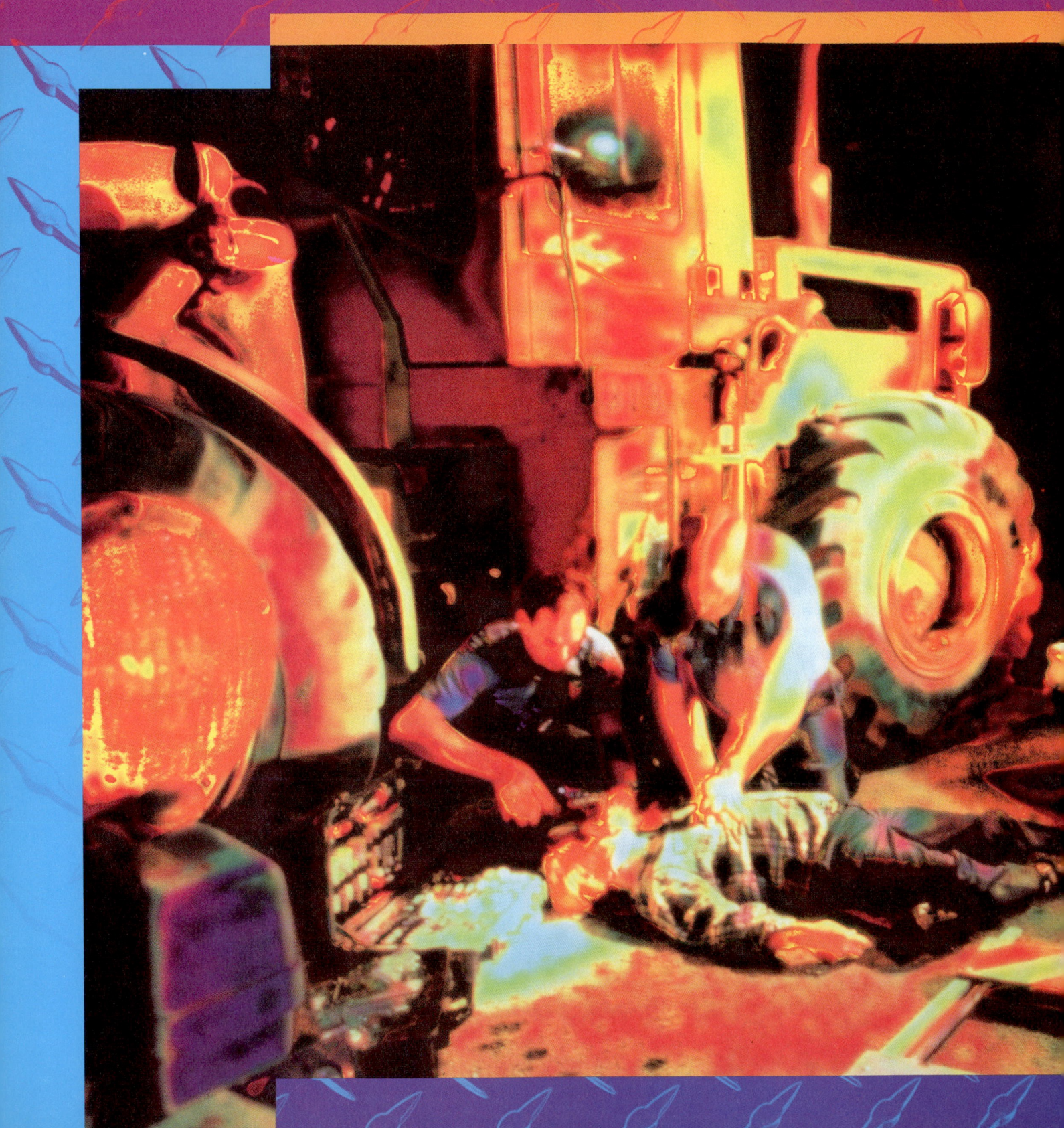

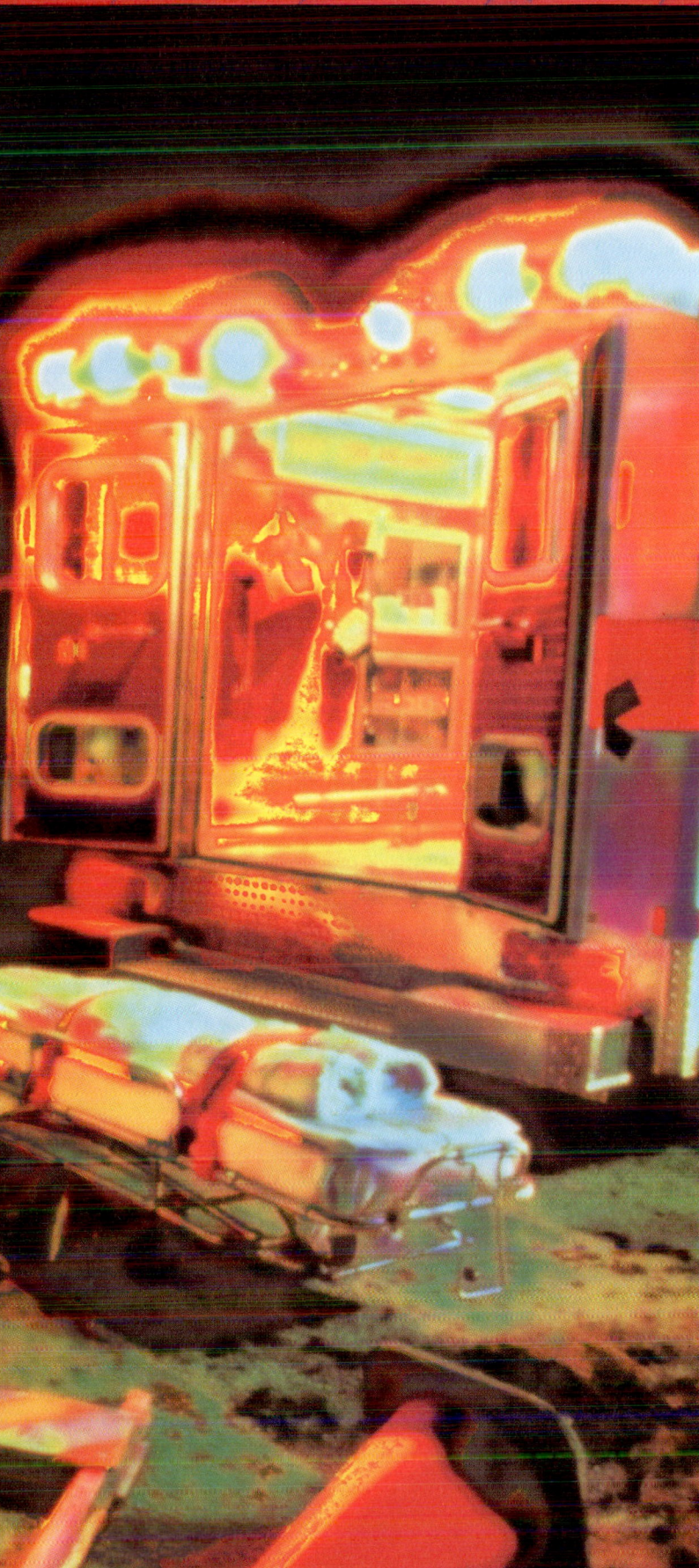

objectives

Cognitive

1. List the structure and function of the respiratory system.

2. State the signs and symptoms of a patient with breathing difficulty.

3. Describe the emergency medical care of the patient with breathing difficulty.

4. Recognize the need for medical direction to assist in the emergency medical care of the patient with breathing difficulty.

5. Describe the emergency medical care of the patient with breathing distress.

6. Establish the relationship between airway management and the patient with breathing difficulty.

7. List signs of adequate air exchange.

8. State the generic name, medication forms, dose, administration, action, indications, and contraindications for the prescribed inhaler.

9. Distinguish between the emergency medical care of the infant, child, and adult patient with breathing difficulty.

10. Differentiate between upper airway obstruction and lower airway disease in the infant and child patient.

Affective

11. Defend EMT-Basic treatment regimens for various respiratory emergencies.

12. Explain the rationale for administering an inhaler.

Psychomotor

13. Demonstrate the emergency medical care for breathing difficulty.

14. Perform the steps in facilitating the use of an inhaler.

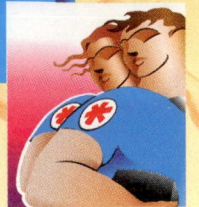

you are the emt

Rescue 6 please respond to the Altwood Apartments at 126th and Lexington for a man having shortness of breath. He is in Building C, apartment 9. Be advised that Engine 7 is already en route.

Calls for "breathing problems" are dispatched routinely every day. In fact, this is the most common reason people call 9-1-1. This chapter will prepare you to respond to many types of respiratory problems that you will encounter as an EMT-B and will help you to answer the following questions:

1. What type of respiratory emergencies should you expect to see as an EMT-B?

2. What is your role in caring for patients with this type of emergency?

Respiratory Emergencies

Dyspnea, the feeling of being short of breath, is a complaint that you will encounter often. It is a symptom of many different conditions, from the common cold and asthma to heart failure and pulmonary embolism. You may or may not be able to determine what is causing dyspnea in a particular patient; this can be difficult even for physicians in a hospital setting. Also, several different problems may contribute to a patient's dyspnea at the same time, including some that are serious or life threatening. Even without a definitive diagnosis, however, you may still be able to save a life.

This chapter begins with a basic explanation of how the lungs function. It then looks at common medical problems that can impede normal functioning and cause dyspnea, including acute pulmonary edema, chronic obstructive pulmonary disease, and asthma. You will learn the signs and symptoms of each condition. You should keep all these possible medical problems in mind as you take the patient's history and perform a physical assessment, a process that the chapter describes in detail. The information that you collect will help you to decide on the proper treatment, which differs according to the probable cause of the dyspnea.

Remember, the sensation of not getting enough air can be terrifying, regardless of its cause. As an EMT-B, you should be prepared to treat not just the symptom and the underlying problem, if you know it, but also the anxiety that it produces.

Anatomy and Function of the Lungs

The respiratory system consists of all the structures of the body that contribute to the breathing process. Important anatomic features include the upper and lower airways, the lungs, and the diaphragm (Figure 12-1). Air enters the trachea and moves along the bronchial tubes to the air spaces, called alveoli, where oxygen and carbon dioxide are exchanged.

The principal function of the lungs is respiration, which is the exchange of oxygen and carbon dioxide. The two processes that occur during respiration are inspiration, the act of breathing in or inhaling, and expiration, the act of breathing out or exhaling. During respiration, oxygen is provided to the blood, and carbon dioxide is removed from it. This exchange of gases takes place rapidly in normal lungs at the level of the alveoli. Alveoli are microscopic, thin-walled air sacs that lie against the pulmonary capillary vessels. Oxygen and carbon dioxide must be able to pass freely between the alveoli and the capillaries (Figure 12-2). Oxygen entering the alveoli from inhalation passes through tiny passages in the alveolar wall into the capillaries, which carry the oxygen back to the heart. The heart pumps the oxygen around the body. Carbon dioxide, which is produced by the body's cells, is brought back to the lungs by the blood that circulates through and around the alveolar air spaces. The carbon dioxide diffuses back into the alveoli and, in turn, travels back up the bronchial tree and out the upper airways during exhalation. Again, carbon dioxide is "exchanged" for oxygen,

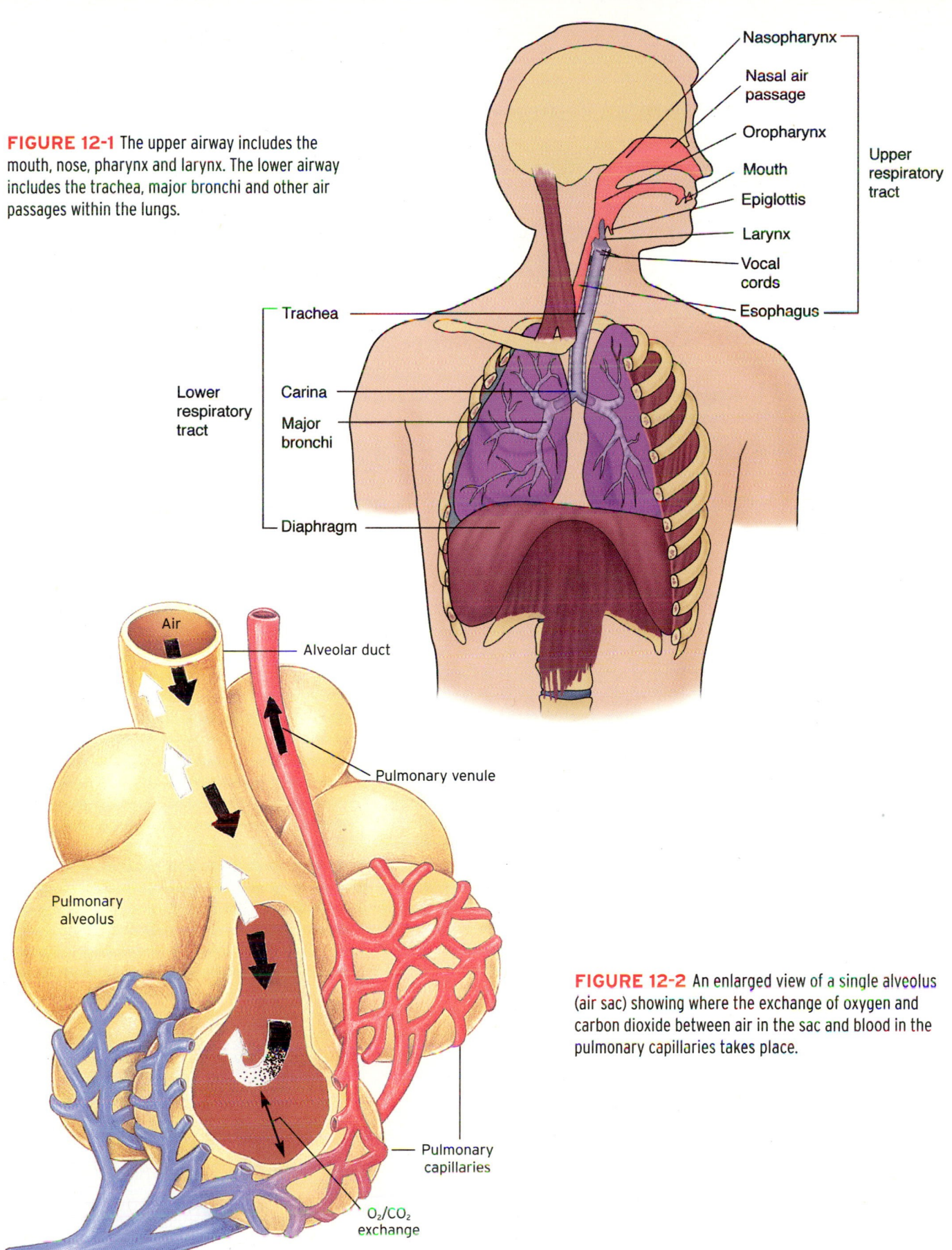

FIGURE 12-1 The upper airway includes the mouth, nose, pharynx and larynx. The lower airway includes the trachea, major bronchi and other air passages within the lungs.

Nasopharynx

Nasal air passage

Oropharynx

Mouth

Epiglottis

Larynx

Vocal cords

Esophagus

Upper respiratory tract

Trachea

Carina

Major bronchi

Diaphragm

Lower respiratory tract

Air

Alveolar duct

Pulmonary venule

Pulmonary alveolus

Pulmonary capillaries

FIGURE 12-2 An enlarged view of a single alveolus (air sac) showing where the exchange of oxygen and carbon dioxide between air in the sac and blood in the pulmonary capillaries takes place.

O_2/CO_2 exchange

Pulmonary arteriole

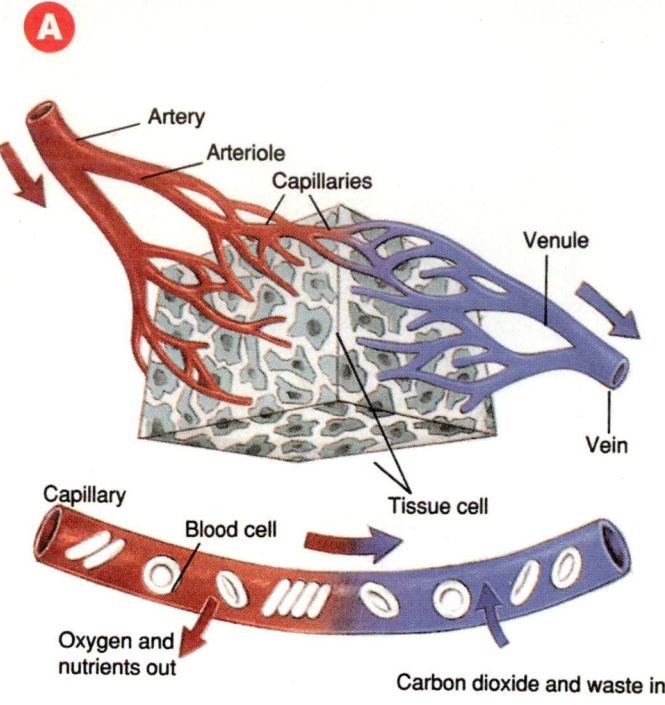

A

Artery
Arteriole
Capillaries
Venule
Vein
Capillary
Blood cell
Tissue cell
Oxygen and nutrients out
Carbon dioxide and waste in

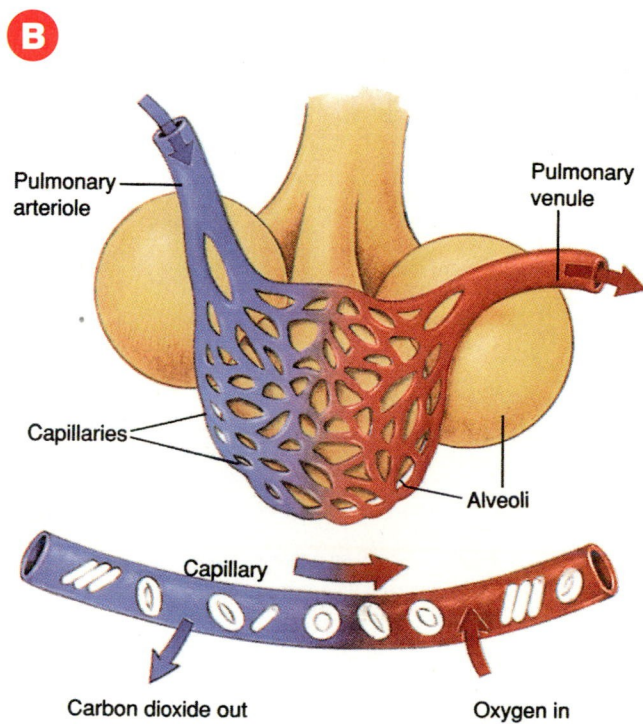

B

Pulmonary arteriole
Pulmonary venule
Capillaries
Alveoli
Capillary
Carbon dioxide out
Oxygen in

FIGURE 12-3 The exchange of oxygen and carbon dioxide in respiration. **A:** Oxygen passes from the blood through capillaries to tissue cells. Carbon dioxide passes from tissue cells through capillaries to the blood. **B:** In the lungs, oxygen is picked up by the blood and carbon dioxide is given off.

> Pulmonary edema is one of the most common causes of hospital admission in the United States. It is not uncommon for a patient to have repeated bouts.

which travels in exactly the opposite direction (during inhalation) (Figure 12-3).

In most disorders of the lung, one or more of the following situations exists:

- The pulmonary vessels are actually obstructed from absorbing oxygen or releasing carbon dioxide by fluid, infection, or collapsed air spaces.
- The alveoli are damaged and cannot transport gases properly across their own walls.
- The air passages are obstructed by muscle spasm, mucus, or weakened floppy airway walls.
- Blood flow to the lungs is obstructed by blood clots.
- The pleural space is filled with air or excess fluid, so the lung cannot properly expand.

All these conditions prevent the proper exchange of oxygen and carbon dioxide. In addition, the pulmonary blood vessels themselves may have abnormalities that interfere with blood flow and thus with the transfer of gases.

The brain stem senses the level of carbon dioxide in the arterial blood. The level of carbon dioxide bathing the brain stem is what stimulates a healthy person to breathe. If the level drops too low, the person automatically breathes at a slower rate and less deeply. As a result, less carbon dioxide is expired, allowing carbon dioxide levels in the blood to return to normal. If the level of carbon dioxide in the arterial blood rises above normal, the patient breathes more rapidly and more deeply. When more fresh air (containing no carbon dioxide) is brought into the alveoli, more carbon dioxide diffuses out of the bloodstream, thereby lowering the level.

The following are the characteristics of normal breathing:

- A normal rate and depth
- A regular pattern of inhalation and exhalation
- Good audible breath sounds on both sides of the chest
- A regular rise and fall movement on both sides of the chest
- Movement of the abdomen

The following are signs that a patient is not breathing normally:

- A rate of breathing that is slower than 8 breaths/min or faster than 24 breaths/min
- Muscle retractions above the clavicles, between the ribs, and below the rib cage, especially in children
- Pale or cyanotic skin
- Cool, damp (clammy) skin
- Shallow or irregular respirations
- Pursed lips
- Nasal flaring

The level of carbon dioxide in the arterial blood can rise for a number of reasons. The exhalation process may be impaired by various types of lung disease. Otherwise, the body may produce too much carbon dioxide, either temporarily or chronically, depending on the disease or abnormality.

If, over a period of years, arterial carbon dioxide levels rise slowly to an abnormally high level and remain there, the respiratory center in the brain, which senses carbon dioxide levels and controls breathing, may work less efficiently. The failure of this center to respond normally to a rise in arterial levels of carbon dioxide is called chronic carbon dioxide retention. If the condition is severe, respiration will stop unless there is a secondary drive to stimulate the respiratory center. Fortunately, a second stimulus does develop in patients with chronically high blood carbon dioxide levels, namely, a low level of oxygen in the blood. Low blood oxygen causes the respiratory center to respond and stimulate respiration. If the arterial level of oxygen is then raised, as happens when the patient is given additional oxygen, there is no longer any stimulus to breathe; both the high carbon dioxide and low oxygen drives are lost. Patients with chronic lung diseases frequently have a chronically high level of blood carbon dioxide. Therefore, giving too much oxygen to these patients may actually depress, or completely stop, the respirations. Individuals older than age 65 years are especially prone to problems with respiration, either from occult (not obvious) stroke, lung disease, cardiovascular disease, liver disease, or certain medications.

> Patients with chronic lung diseases frequently have a chronically high level of blood carbon dioxide.

Causes of Dyspnea

Dyspnea is shortness of breath or difficulty breathing. Many different medical problems may cause dyspnea. Be aware that if the problem is severe and the brain is deprived of oxygen, the patient may not be alert enough to complain of shortness of breath. More commonly, altered mental status is a sign of hypoxia of the brain.

Patients often develop breathing difficulty or hypoxia with the following medical conditions:

- Upper or lower airway infection
- Acute pulmonary edema
- Chronic obstructive pulmonary disease (COPD)
- Spontaneous pneumothorax
- Asthma or allergic reactions
- Pleural effusion
- Prolonged seizures
- Mechanical obstruction of the airway
- Pulmonary embolism
- Hyperventilation
- Severe pain, particularly chest pain

Upper or Lower Airway Infection

Infectious diseases causing dyspnea may affect all parts of the airway. Some cause mild discomfort. Others obstruct the airway to the point that patients require a full range of respiratory support. In general, the problem is always some form of obstruction, either to the flow of air in the major passages (colds, diphtheria, epiglottitis, and croup) or to the exchange of gases between the alveoli and the capillaries (pneumonia). Table 12-1 (see page 16) shows infectious diseases that are associated with some degree of dyspnea.

Acute Pulmonary Edema

Sometimes, the heart muscle is so injured after an acute myocardial infarction or other illness that it cannot circulate blood properly. In these cases, the left side of the heart cannot remove blood from the lung as fast as the right side delivers it. As a result, fluid builds up within the alveoli as well as in the lung tissue between the alveoli and the pulmonary capillaries. This accumulation of fluid, called pulmonary edema, can develop quickly after a major heart attack. By physically separating alveoli from pulmonary capillary vessels, the edema interferes with the exchange of

TABLE 12-1   Infectious Diseases Associated with Dyspnea

Disease	Characteristics	Disease	Characteristics
Common Cold	• Usually associated with swollen nasal mucous membranes and the production of fluid from the sinuses and nose. • Dyspnea is not severe; patients complain of "stuffiness" or difficulty breathing through the nose.	Epiglottitis	• A bacterial infection of the epiglottis that can produce severe swelling of the flap over the larynx. • In preschool and school-aged children especially, the epiglottis can swell to two to three times its normal size (Figure 12-4). • The airway may become completely obstructed, sometimes quite suddenly.
Diphtheria	• Although well controlled in the past decade, it is still highly contagious and serious when it occurs. • The disease causes the formation of a diphtheritic membrane lining the pharynx that is composed of debris, inflammatory cells, and mucus. This membrane can rapidly and severely obstruct the passage of air into the larynx.		
Pneumonia	• An acute bacterial or viral infection of the lung that damages and destroys lung tissue, usually associated with fever, cough, and production of sputum. • Fluid also accumulates in the surrounding normal lung tissue, separating the alveoli from their capillaries. (Sometimes, fluid can also accumulate in the pleural space.) • The lung's ability to exchange oxygen and carbon dioxide is impaired. • The breathing pattern in pneumonia does not indicate major airway obstruction, but the patient may experience tachypnea, an increase in the breathing rate, which is an attempt to compensate for the reduced amount of normal lung tissue and for the buildup of fluid.		

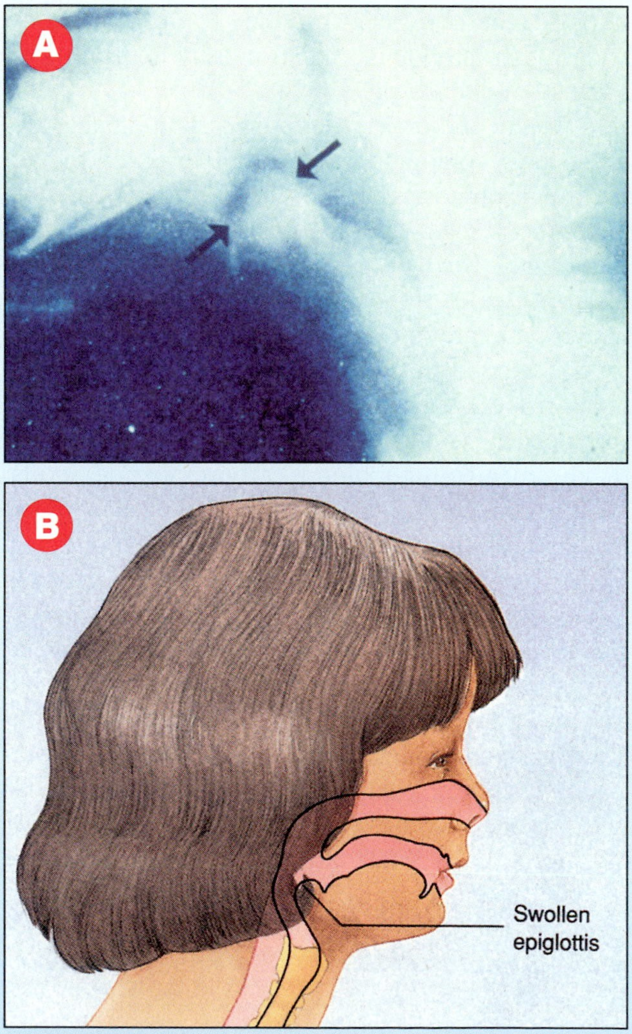

FIGURE 12-4 Acute epiglottitis. **A:** Epiglottitis is caused by a bacterial infection resulting in severe swelling of the epiglottis. **B:** The epiglottis is massively swollen and almost fully obstructs the airway.

Disease	Characteristics
	• <u>Stridor</u> (abnormal, high-pitched, rough barking inspiratory sounds) may be heard late in the development of airway obstruction.
	• Acute epiglottitis in the adult is characterized by a severe sore throat.
	• The disease is now much less common than it was 20 years ago because of a vaccine that can help to prevent most cases.
<u>Croup</u>	• An inflammation and swelling of the lining of the larynx, the narrowest point of the airway, typically seen in children between ages 6 months and 3 years (Figure 12-5).
	• The common signs of croup are stridor and a seal-bark cough, which signal a significant narrowing of the air passage of the larynx that may progress to significant obstruction.
	• Croup often responds well to the administration of humidified oxygen.

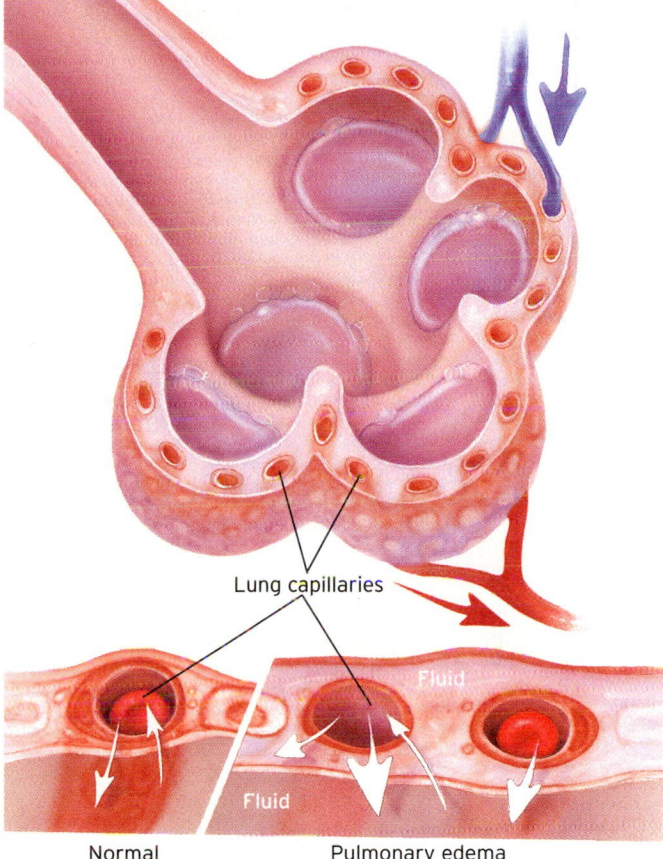

FIGURE 12-6 In pulmonary edema, fluid fills the alveoli and separate the capillaries from the alveolar wall, interfering with the exchange of oxygen and carbon dioxide.

Lung capillaries

Fluid

Normal   Fluid   Pulmonary edema

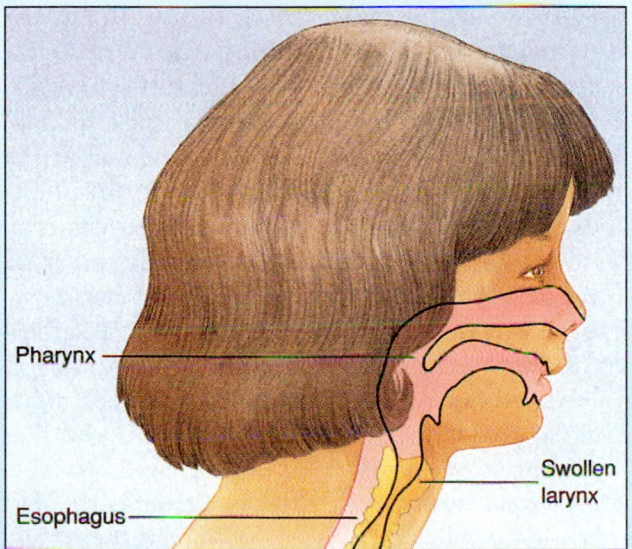

Pharynx

Swollen larynx

Esophagus

FIGURE 12-5 (below) Croup swells the lining of the larynx, which is the narrowest point in a child's airway.

carbon dioxide and oxygen (Figure 12-6). There is not enough room left in the lung for slow, deep breaths. The patient usually experiences dyspnea with rapid, shallow respirations. In the most severe instances, you will see a frothy pink sputum at the nose and mouth.

In most cases, patients have a longstanding history of chronic congestive heart failure that can be kept under control with medication. However, acute worsening may occur if the patient stops taking the medication, eats food that is too salty, or has a stressful illness, a new heart attack, or an abnormal heart rhythm. Pulmonary edema is one of the most common causes of hospital admission in the United States. It is not uncommon for a patient to have repeated bouts.

Some patients who have pulmonary edema do not have heart disease. Inhaling large amounts of smoke or toxic chemical fumes can produce pulmonary edema, as can traumatic injuries of the chest. In these cases, fluid collects in alveoli and lung tissue in response to damage to the tissues of the lung or the bronchi.

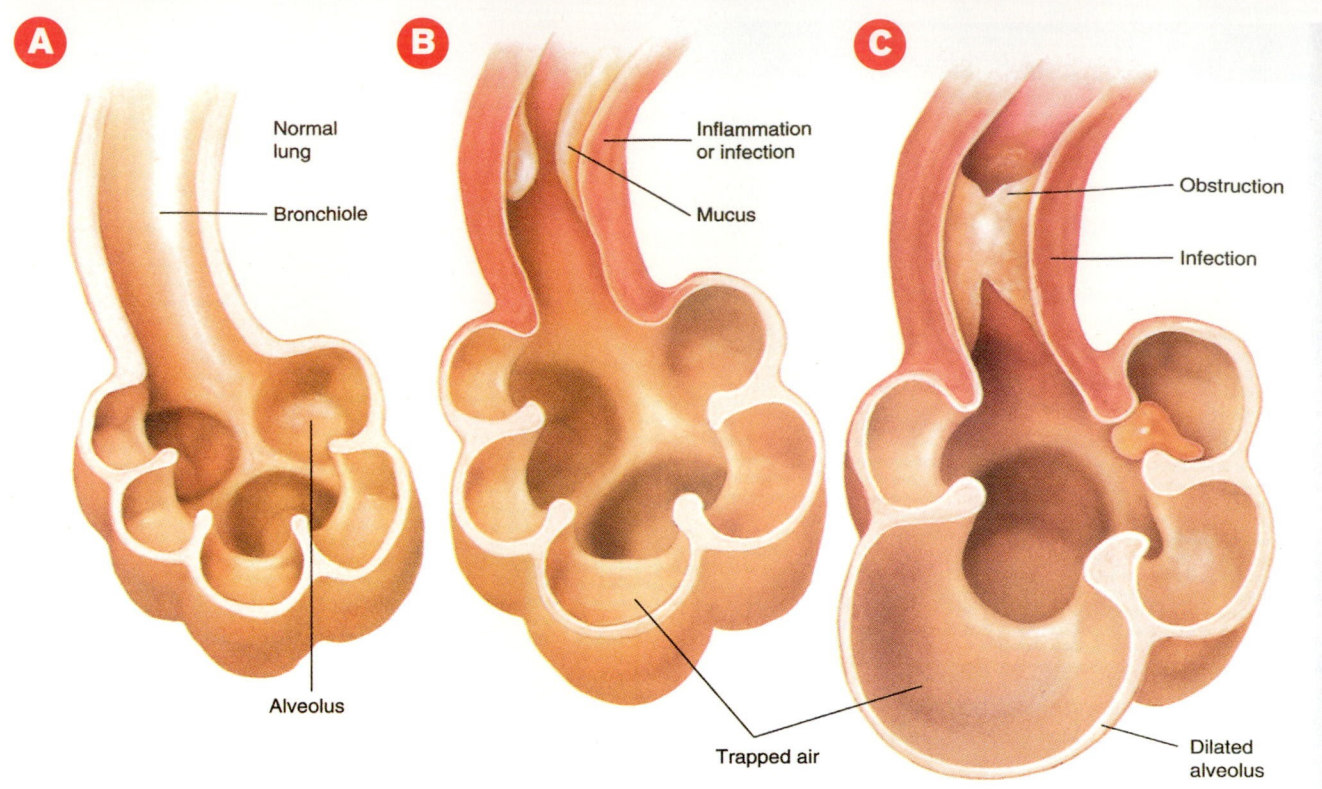

FIGURE 12-7 Repeated episodes of irritation and inflammation in the alveoli result in obstruction, scarring, and some dilation of the alveolar sac. **A:** Normal alveolus. **B:** Infection produces mucus and swelling. **C:** A mucus plug creates an obstruction and further dilation of the alveolus.

Chronic Obstructive Pulmonary Disease

<u>Chronic obstructive pulmonary disease (COPD)</u> is a common lung condition, affecting some 10% to 20% of the entire adult population in the United States. It is the end of a slow process, which over several years results in disruption of the airways, the alveoli, and the pulmonary blood vessels. The process itself may be a result of direct lung and airway damage from repeated infections or inhalation of toxic agents such as industrial gases, but most often, it results from cigarette smoking. Although it is well known that cigarettes are a direct cause of lung cancer, their role in the development of COPD is far more significant and less well publicized.

Tobacco smoke is itself a bronchial irritant and can create a chronic <u>bronchitis</u>, an ongoing irritation of the trachea and bronchi.

With bronchitis, excess mucus is constantly produced, obstructing small airways and alveoli. Protective cells and lung mechanisms that remove foreign particles are destroyed, further weakening the airways. Chronic oxygenation problems can also lead to right heart failure and fluid retention, such as edema in the leg. Pneumonia develops easily when the passages are persistently obstructed. Ultimately, repeated episodes of irritation and pneumonia cause scarring in the lung and some dilation of the obstructed alveoli, leading to COPD (Figure 12-7).

Another type of COPD is called <u>emphysema</u>. Emphysema is a loss of the elastic material around the air spaces as a result of chronic stretching of the alveoli when bronchitic airways obstruct easy expulsion of gases. Smoking can also directly destroy the elasticity of the lung tissue. Normally, lungs act like a spongy balloon that is inflated; once they are inflated, they will naturally recoil because of their elastic nature, expelling gas rapidly. However, when they are constantly obstructed or when the "balloon's" elasticity is diminished, air is no longer expelled rapidly, and the walls of the alveoli eventually fall apart, leaving large "holes" in the lung that resemble a large air pocket or cavity. This condition is called emphysema.

Most patients with COPD have elements of both chronic bronchitis and emphysema. Some patients will have more elements of one condition than the other; few patients will have only emphysema or bronchitis. Therefore, most patients with COPD will chronically produce sputum, have a chronic cough, and have difficulty expelling air from their lungs, with long expiration phases and wheezing.

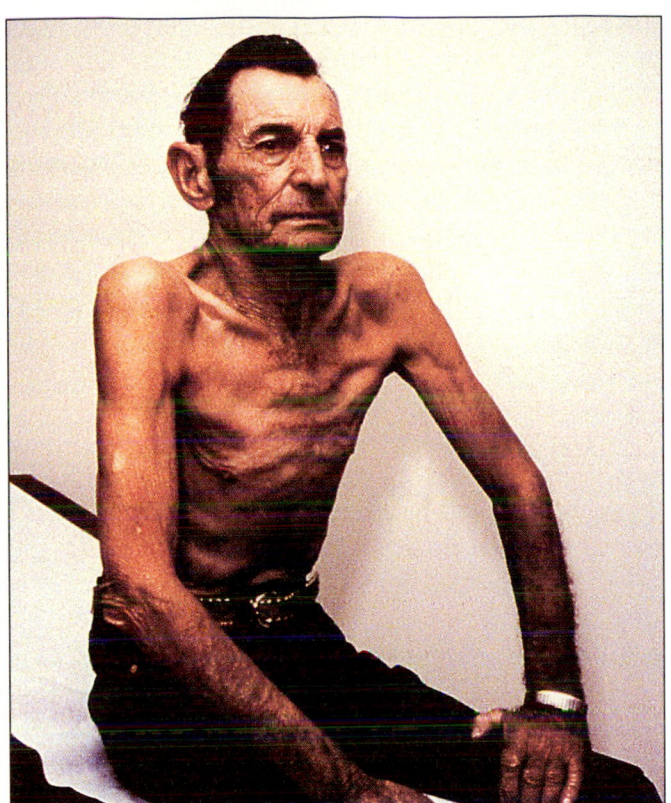

FIGURE 12-8 Typically, a patient with COPD has a barrel-shaped chest and uses accessory muscles and pursed lips for breathing. Notice, also, that the patient is sitting in the tripod position.

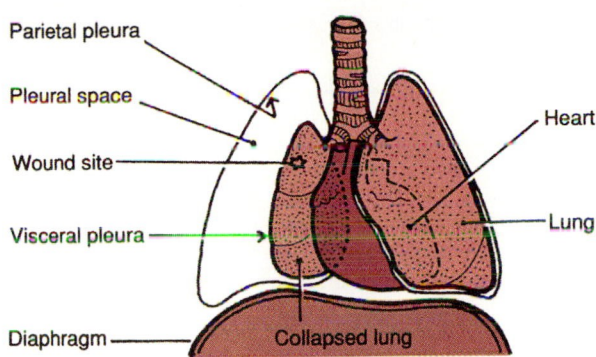

FIGURE 12-9 A pneumothorax occurs when air leaks into the pleural space from an opening in the chest wall or the surface of the lung. The lung collapses as air fills the pleural space and the two pleural surfaces are no longer in contact.

Patients with COPD cannot handle pulmonary infections well, because the existing airway damage makes them unable to cough up the mucus or sputum produced by the infection. The chronic airway obstruction makes it difficult to breathe deeply enough to clear the lungs. Gradually, the arterial oxygen level falls, and the carbon dioxide level rises. If a new infection of the lung occurs in a patient with COPD, the arterial oxygen level may fall rapidly. In a few patients, the carbon dioxide level may rise high enough to cause sleepiness. These patients require respiratory support and careful administration of oxygen.

Patients with COPD usually are older than age 50 years. They will always have a history of recurring lung problems and are almost always long-term cigarette smokers. Patients with COPD may complain of tightness in the chest and constant fatigue. Because air has been gradually and continuously trapped in their lungs in increasing amounts, their chests often have a barrel-like appearance (Figure 12-8). If you listen to the chest with a stethoscope, you will hear abnormal breath sounds. These may include **rales**, which are crackling, rattling sounds that are usually associated with fluid in the lungs but here are related to chronic scarring of small airways. **Rhonchi**, which are coarse gravelly

sounds, and high-pitched, whistling **wheezes**, which are expiratory sounds common to patients with asthma, may be heard as well. Because of large emphysematous air pockets and diminished airflow, sounds of breathing are frequently hard to hear and may be detected only high up on the posterior chest.

The patient with COPD usually presents with a long history of dyspnea with a sudden increase in shortness of breath. There is rarely a history of chest pain. More often, the patient will remember having had a recent "chest cold" with fever and either inability to cough up mucus or a sudden increase in sputum. If the patient is able to cough up sputum, it will be thick and is often green or yellow. The blood pressure of patients with COPD is normal; however, the pulse, is rapid and occasionally irregular. Pay particular attention to the respirations. They may be rapid, or they may be very slow, as in carbon dioxide retention.

Spontaneous Pneumothorax

Normally, the "vacuum" pressure in the pleural space keeps the lung inflated. When the surface of the lung is disrupted, however, air escapes into the pleural cavity, and the negative vacuum pressure is lost; the natural elasticity of the lung tissue causes the lung to collapse. The accumulation of air in the pleural space, which may be partial or complete, is called a **pneumothorax** (Figure 12-9). Pneumothorax is most often caused by trauma, but it can also be caused by some medical conditions without any injury. In these patients, the condition is called a "spontaneous" pneumothorax.

Spontaneous pneumothorax may occur in patients with certain chronic lung infections or in young people born with weak areas of the lung. Patients with emphysema and asthma are at high risk for spontaneous pneumothorax when a weakened portion of lung

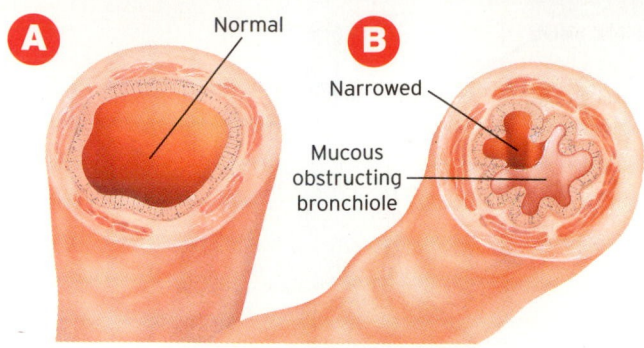

FIGURE 12-10 Asthma is an acute spasm of the bronchioles. **A:** Cross section of a normal bronchiole. **B:** The bronchiole in spasm; a mucus plug has formed and partially obstructed the bronchiole.

ruptures, often during coughing. A patient with a spontaneous pneumothorax becomes dyspneic (short of breath) and can complain of **pleuritic chest pain**, a sharp, stabbing pain on one side that is worse during breathing or with certain movement of the chest wall. By listening to the chest with the stethoscope, you can sometimes tell that breath sounds are absent or decreased on the affected side. However, altered breath sounds are very difficult to detect in a patient with severe emphysema. Spontaneous pneumothorax may be the cause of sudden dyspnea in a patient with underlying emphysema.

Asthma and Allergic Reactions

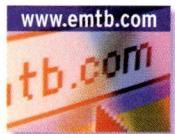

Asthma is an acute spasm of the smaller air passages called bronchioles, associated with excessive mucus production and sometimes with spasm of the bronchiolar muscles (Figure 12-10). It is a common but serious disease, affecting about 6 million Americans and killing some 4,000 to 5,000 Americans each year. Asthma produces a characteristic wheezing as patients attempt to exhale through partially obstructed air passages. These same air passages open easily during inspiration. In other words, when patients inhale, breathing appears relatively normal; the wheezing is heard only when they exhale. This wheezing may be so loud that you can hear it without a stethoscope. In other cases, the airways are so blocked that no air movement is heard. In severe cases, the actual work of exhaling is very tiring, and cyanosis and/or respiratory arrest may quickly develop, even within 60 minutes.

Asthma affects patients of all ages and is usually the result of an allergic reaction to an inhaled, ingested, or injected substance. Note that the substance itself is not the cause of the allergic reaction; rather, it is an exaggerated response of the body's immune system to that substance that causes the reaction. In some cases, however, there is no identifiable substance, or **allergen**, that triggers the body's immune system. Almost anything can be considered an allergen. An allergic response to certain foods or some other allergen may produce an acute asthma attack. Between attacks, patients may breathe normally. In its most severe form, an allergic reaction can produce anaphylaxis and even anaphylactic shock. This, in turn, may cause respiratory distress that is severe enough to result in coma and death. Asthma attacks may also be caused by severe emotional stress, exercise, or respiratory infections.

Most patients with asthma are familiar with their symptoms and know when an attack is imminent. Typically, they will have appropriate medication either with them or at home. You should listen carefully to what these patients tell you; they often know exactly what they need.

Asthma and anaphylactic reactions. Patients who do not have asthma may still have severe allergic reactions. The same allergens that may cause asthma attacks may cause anaphylaxis, a reaction characterized by airway swelling and dilation of blood vessels all over the body, which may lower blood pressure significantly. Anaphylaxis may be associated with widespread itching and an asthmalike condition. The airway may swell so much that breathing problems can progress from extreme difficulty in breathing to total airway obstruction in a matter of a few minutes. Most anaphylactic reactions occur within 30 minutes of exposure to the allergen, which can be anything from eating certain nuts to receiving a penicillin injection. For some patients, this may be the first time they had such a reaction to the substance. Therefore, they may not know what caused the swelling and allergic reaction. In other cases, the patient may know of the allergen but not be aware of exposure. In severe cases, epinephrine is the treatment of choice. Oxygen and antihistamines are also useful. As always, medical direction should guide appropriate therapy.

Hay fever. A much milder and more common allergy problem is hay fever. This is caused by an allergic reaction to pollen. In some areas of the country where pollen is present in the air throughout the year, hay fever is almost a universal illness. Generally, it does not produce major emergency problems. It does produce a number of difficulties in the upper respiratory tract, such as a stuffy or runny nose and sneezing.

Pleural Effusions

A **pleural effusion** is a collection of fluid outside the lung on one or both sides of the chest; in compressing the lung or lungs, it causes dyspnea (Figure 12-11). This

are sitting upright. Nothing will really relieve their symptoms, however, except removal of the fluid, which must be done by a physician in the hospital.

Mechanical Obstruction of the Airway

As an EMT-B, you should always be aware of the possibility that a patient with dyspnea may have a mechanical obstruction of the airway and be prepared to treat it quickly. In semiconscious and unconscious individuals, the obstruction may be the result of the position of the head, obstruction by the tongue, or aspiration of vomitus or a foreign object (Figure 12-12). Opening the airway with the head-tilt or chin-lift maneuver may solve the problem. You should perform this maneuver only after you have ruled out a head or neck injury. If simply opening the airway does not correct the breathing problem, you will have to search the upper airway for the obstruction.

Always consider upper airway obstruction from a foreign body first in patients who were eating just before becoming short of breath. The same is true of young children, especially crawling babies, who might have swallowed and choked on a small object.

Pulmonary Embolism

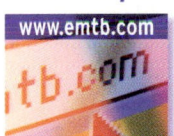

An **embolus** is anything in the circulatory system that moves from its point of origin to a distant site and lodges there, obstructing subsequent blood flow in that area. Beyond the point of obstruction, circulation can be completely cut off or at least markedly decreased, which can result in a serious, life-threatening condition. Emboli can be fragments of blood clots in an artery or vein that break off and travel through the bloodstream. They also can be foreign bodies that enter the circulation, such as a bullet or a bubble of air.

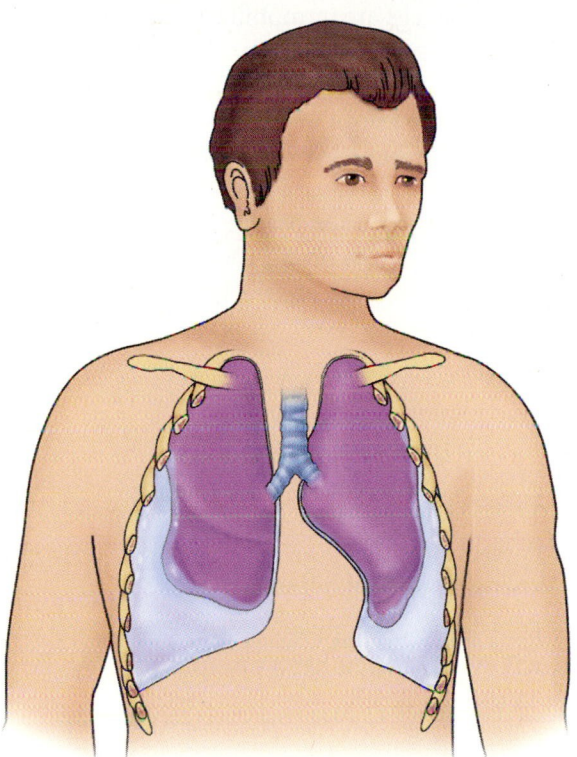

FIGURE 12-11 With a pleural effusion, fluid may accumulate in large volumes on one or both sides, compressing the lungs and causing dyspnea.

fluid may collect in large volumes in response to any irritation, infection, or cancer. Though it can build up gradually, over days or even weeks, patients often report that their dyspnea came on suddenly. Pleural effusions should be considered as a contributing diagnosis in any patient with lung cancer and shortness of breath.

When you listen with a stethoscope to the chest of a patient with dyspnea resulting from pleural effusions, you will hear decreased breath sounds over the region of the chest where fluid has moved the lung away from the chest wall. These patients frequently feel better if they

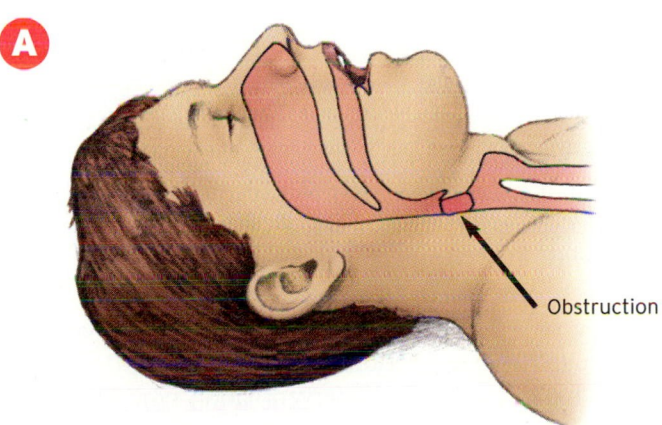

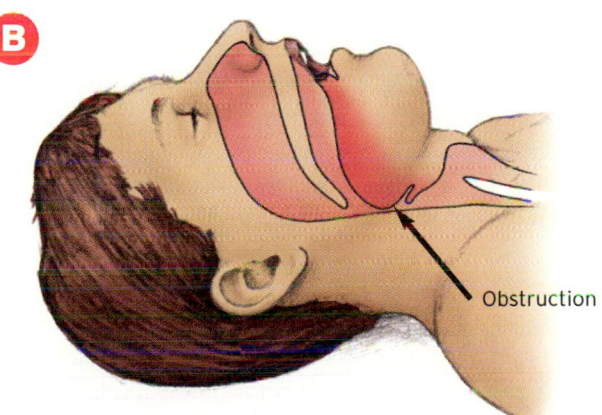

FIGURE 12-12 A. Foreign body obstruction occurs when an object, such as food, is lodged in the airway. **B.** Mechanical obstruction also occurs when the head is not properly positioned, causing the tongue to fall back into the throat.

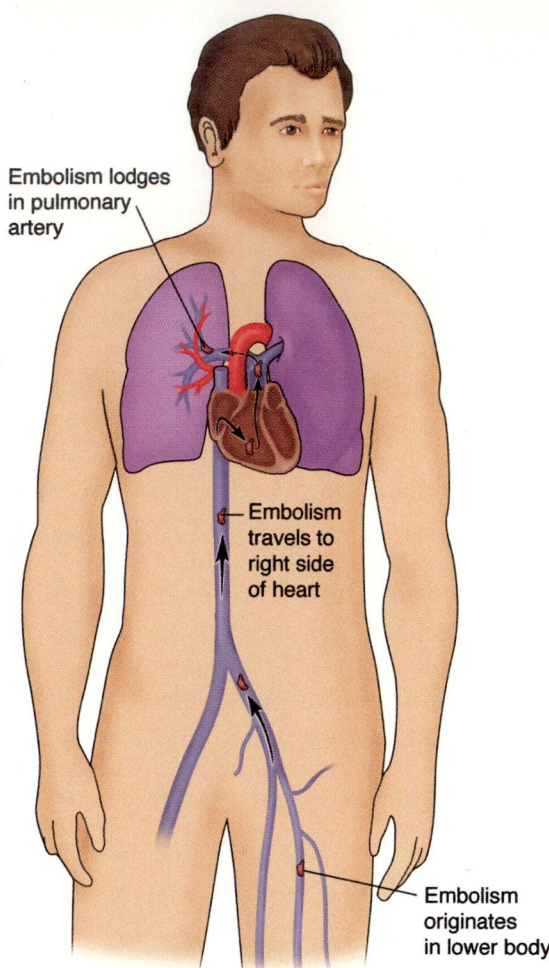

Embolism lodges
in pulmonary
artery

Embolism
travels to
right side
of heart

Embolism
originates
in lower body

FIGURE 12-13 A pulmonary embolus is a blood clot from the vein that breaks off, circulates through the venous system, and moves through the right side of the heart into the pulmonary artery. Here, it can become lodged and significantly obstruct blood flow.

A pulmonary embolism is the passage of a blood clot formed in a vein, usually in the legs or pelvis, that breaks off and circulates through the venous system. The large clot moves through the right side of the heart and into the pulmonary artery, where it becomes lodged, significantly decreasing or blocking blood flow (Figure 12-13). Even though the lung is actively involved in inhalation and exhalation of air, no exchange of oxygen or carbon dioxide takes place in the areas of blocked blood flow because there is no effective circulation. In this circumstance, the level of arterial carbon dioxide usually rises, and the oxygen level may drop enough to cause cyanosis. More important, they can inhibit circulation and cause significant dyspnea.

Pulmonary emboli may occur as a result of damage to the lining of vessels, a tendency for blood to clot unusually fast, or, most often, slow blood flow in a lower extremity. Slow blood flow in the legs is usually caused by bed rest, which can lead to the collapse of veins.

Patients whose legs are immobilized following a fracture or recent surgery are at risk for pulmonary emboli for days or weeks after the incident. Only rarely do pulmonary emboli occur in active, healthy individuals.

Although they are fairly common, pulmonary emboli are difficult to diagnose. They occur about 650,000 times a year in the United States. Ten percent are immediately fatal, but most often, the patient never notices them. Symptoms and signs, when they do occur, include the following:

- Dyspnea
- Acute pleuritic chest pain
- Hemoptysis (coughing up blood)
- Cyanosis
- Tachypnea
- Varying degrees of hypoxia

With a large enough embolus, complete, sudden obstruction of the right heart's output of blood flow can result in sudden death.

Hyperventilation Syndrome

When dyspnea occurs in a patient with no lung abnormalities, it is called hyperventilation syndrome. Hyperventilation is defined as overbreathing to the point that the level of arterial carbon dioxide falls below normal. This may be an indicator of major, life-threatening illness. For example, a patient with diabetes who has very high blood glucose levels, a patient poisoned with aspirin, or a patient with a severe infection is likely to hyperventilate. In these patients, rapid, deep breathing is the body's attempt to stay alive. The body is trying to compensate for *acidosis,* the buildup of excess acid in the blood or body tissues, resulting from the primary illness. Because carbon dioxide, mixed with water in the bloodstream, can add to the blood's acidity, lowering the level of carbon dioxide helps to compensate for the other acids.

Similarly, in an otherwise healthy person, blood acidity can be diminished by excessive breathing, because it "blows off" too much carbon dioxide. The result is a relative lack of acids. The resulting condition, *alkalosis,* is the buildup of excess base (lack of acids), in the body fluids.

Alkalosis is the cause of many of the symptoms associated with *hyperventilation syndrome,* including anxiety, dizziness, numbness, tingling of the hands and feet, and even a sense of dyspnea despite the rapid breathing. Although hyperventilation can be the response to illness and a buildup of acids, hyperventilation syndrome is not the same thing. Instead, this syndrome occurs in the absence of other physical problems. However, it is very common during psychological stress, affecting some 10%

of the population at one time or another. The respirations of an individual who is experiencing hyperventilation syndrome may be as high as more than 40 shallow breaths/min or as low as only 20 very deep breaths/min.

The decision whether hyperventilation is being caused by a life-threatening illness or a panic attack should not be made outside the hospital. All patients who are hyperventilating should be given supplemental oxygen and transported to the hospital, where physicians will make that medical decision.

Treatment of Dyspnea

When taking the initial vital signs of a person with dyspnea, you should pay particular attention to respirations. Always speak with assurance and assume a concerned, professional approach to reassure the patient, who is probably very frightened. You will usually administer oxygen. Take great care in monitoring the respirations as you do so. Reevaluate the respirations and the patient's response to oxygen repeatedly, at least every 5 minutes, until you reach the emergency department. In a person with a chronically high carbon dioxide level (e.g., certain patients with COPD), this is critical, because the supplemental oxygen may cause a rapid rise in the arterial oxygen level. This, in turn, may abolish the secondary respiratory oxygen drive and cause respiratory arrest.

Do *not* withhold oxygen for fear of depressing or stopping breathing in a patient with COPD who needs oxygen. Slowing of respirations after administration of oxygen does not necessarily mean that the patient no longer needs the oxygen; he or she may need it even more. If respirations slow and the patient becomes unconscious, you should assist breathing.

Approach to the Patient in Respiratory Distress

Your first questions are always the same: Is the patient conscious? Is he or she breathing? If not, you must take action. Assess the airway and give two quick breaths via mouth-to-mask or BVM device, whatever is required by local protocol. As you ventilate, you need to ask another series of questions, as follows:

1. **Is air going into the lungs?** Look for clues in the rise and fall of the chest, the respirations, and the heart rate.

2. **When you compress the BVM device, does the chest wall expand?**

3. **When you release the bag, does the chest go back down?** If not, something is wrong. Try to reposition the patient and insert an oral airway to keep the tongue from blocking the airway. Reposition the head. Reassess your hand position and face mask seal.

caring for the elderly

As we get older, normal aging processes alter the respiratory system and our ability to exchange oxygen and carbon dioxide. If the patient is a smoker, the disease processes of emphysema or chronic bronchitis can hasten or worsen these changes.

Several changes occur as we age. The chest wall, including the muscles and ribs, become less resilient. Additionally, the bronchi and bronchioles lose their muscle mass or tone, and the air sacs (alveoli) become stiffer and less able to recoil (relax and empty) in exhaling. If the chest wall, including muscles and ribs, is weaker or less flexible, the chest cavity cannot expand as easily, and the total amount of air that is allowed into the lungs will be reduced. With decreased recoil of the lungs, alveoli can become distended with air trapped inside. If you are required to ventilate the apneic (non-breathing) geriatric patient, you will notice that it is more difficult because of increased resistance of the chest and airways as well as reduced compliance of the lungs.

The geriatric patient is at an increased risk of pneumonia or a worsening of asthma or COPD if the airways have lost muscle mass or tone. Secretions might not be expelled from the airways, allowing pneumonia to develop.

The result of normal changes with aging is a reduction of the total amount of air the lungs can hold, air becoming trapped in overstretched alveoli, and increased resistance to air flow into and out of the lungs. Ultimately, all these changes cause a decreased oxygen/carbon dioxide exchange in the respiratory system with reduced oxygen delivery to the cells. Be sure to consider changes in aging that affect the respiratory system and provide adequate ventilation and oxygenation according to the patient's needs. The geriatric patient may need ventilatory support for conditions that, in the younger adult, are easily accommodated by the respiratory system.

Next, assess the rate at which you are assisting the patient's ventilations. You need to give breaths at roughly the same rate as the patient would if he or she were breathing spontaneously (e.g., 10 to 15/min). Rescuers often get excited and ventilate the patient too quickly. Breathing for the patient too rapidly can cause harm. With rapid squeezing of the bag, higher pressures force the air rapidly into the lungs. Higher pressures can fill the stomach, as well as the lungs, with air. If the air and fluid in the stomach come back up the esophagus, vomit may enter the lungs, which can cause a serious form of pneumonia. Adults should be given one breath every 5 seconds. School-aged children need a smaller breath every 3 seconds. Infants need a small breath every 3 seconds.

Finally, assess the pulse. If the patient has a pulse, continue to support respirations. Measure the pulse rate; if it is normal, chances are that the patient is receiving enough oxygen to support life. If the pulse rate is too fast (more than 100/min) or too slow (less than 60/min), the patient may not be getting enough oxygen. Recheck everything. Is the oxygen bottle hooked up to the mask? Is the oxygen turned on? Is the flow rate adequate (more than 10 L/min)? Is there a good face mask seal? Is the chest rising and falling with each breath? Is the airway blocked with vomit or the tongue?

Signs and symptoms. If the patient is breathing, you need to decide whether the breathing is normal. Table 12-2 lists the clues that will help you to decide if there is a breathing difficulty.

Focused history and physical examination. After you form your initial impression, ask the patient to describe the problem. Begin by asking an open-ended question: "What can you tell me about your breathing?" Pay close attention to OPQRST: when the problem began (onset), what makes the breathing difficulty worse (provocation), how the breathing feels (quality), and whether the discomfort moves (radiation). How much of a problem is the patient having (severity)? Is the problem continuous or intermittent (time)? If it is intermittent, how long does it last?

Find out what the patient has already done for the breathing problem. Does the patient use a prescribed inhaler? If so, when was it used last? How many doses have been taken? Does the patient use more than one inhaler? Find out whether the patient has any allergies or history of drug reactions.

Interventions. If the patient complains of breathing difficulty, you should administer supplemental oxygen. In general, you do not need to worry about giving too much oxygen. Put a nonrebreathing face mask on the patient and supply oxygen at a rate of 10 to 15 L/min (enough to maintain the reservoir bag) in a patient with severe diffi-

culty breathing. Then continue your assessment. Obtain a set of vital signs and document them.

As was stated previously, there is some concern about suppression of the "hypoxic" drive to breathe in some patients with COPD. Unless these patients are unresponsive, a more conservative approach is suggested. In patients who have longstanding COPD and probable carbon dioxide retention, administration of low-flow oxygen (2 L/min) is a good place to start, with adjustments to 3 L/min, then 4 L/min, and so on until symptoms have improved (for example, the patient has less dyspnea or a better mental status). When in doubt, err on the side of more oxygen, and monitor the patient closely.

Patients who call for help because of breathing difficulty are likely to have had the same trouble before. They probably have prescribed medications to use that are delivered by inhaler. If so, you may be able to help them use it. Consult medical control. Remember to report what the medication is, when the patient last took a puff, how many puffs were used at that time, and what the label states regarding dosage. If medical control permits, you may help the patient to self-administer the medication. Be certain that the inhaler belongs to the patient, it contains the correct medication, the expiration date has not passed, and the correct dose is being administered. Administer repeat doses of the medication if the maximum dose has not been exceeded and the patient is still experiencing shortness of breath.

If the patient does not have a prescribed inhaler, continue with the focused history and physical exam. Even patients who use their inhaler may continue to get worse. You need to reassess breathing frequently and be prepared to assist ventilations in severe cases. You must assist ventilation in a patient who is having an asthma attack, using slow, gentle breaths. Remember, the problem in asthma is getting the air out of the lungs, not into them. Resist the temptation to squeeze the bag hard and fast. Always assist with ventilations as a last resort, and then provide only about 10 to 12 shallow breaths/min.

Prescribed Inhalers

Some of the most common medications used for shortness of breath are called inhaled beta-agonists, which dilate breathing passages. Typical trade names are Proventil, Ventolin, Alupent, Metaprel, and Brethine. The generic name for Proventil and Ventolin is albuterol; for Alupent and Metaprel, it is metaproterenol; and for Brethine, it is terbutaline. The action of most of these medications is to relax the muscles that surround the bronchioles in the lungs, leading to enlargement (dilation) of the airways and easier passage of air. Common side effects of inhalers used for acute shortness of breath include increased pulse rate, nervousness, and muscle tremors.

TABLE 12-2 Signs and Symptoms of Respiratory Impairment

- **The patient complains of breathing difficulty.**

- **The patient appears anxious or restless.** This can happen if the brain is not getting enough oxygen for its needs. Check the vital signs.

- **The patient has low respirations.** If the respirations are less than 10 breaths/min., you may need to assist ventilations with a BVM device.

- **The patient's skin is blue.** The tongue, nailbeds, and inside the lips are good places to look for cyanosis. These all have a large collection of blood vessels and thin skin, making bluish blood easy to see.

- **The patient's breathing features wheezing, gurgling, snoring, stridor, or crowing.** Common causes of stridor include a foreign body obstruction and infection of the trachea.

- **The patient cannot speak more than few words between breaths.** Ask the patient something such as "How are you doing?" If the patient cannot speak at all, he or she probably has a breathing emergency that will need immediate attention.

- **The patient is using the accessory muscles in the neck to assist breathing.** If the patient is using only the diaphragm to breathe, suspect damage to the nerves that carry breathing commands to the chest muscles; the diaphragm may be getting the command to breathe, but because of spinal cord injury, the chest muscles may not.

- **The patient has an altered mental status associated with shallow or slow breathing.**

- **The patient is coughing excessively,** which might mean that the patient has anything from mild upper respiratory infection or hay fever to pneumonia, asthma, or heart failure.

- **The patient's breathing rhythm is irregular.** Because the brain controls breathing, an irregular breathing rhythm may signal a head injury. In this case, the patient will probably be unresponsive.

- **The patient is sitting up, leaning forward** with palms flat on the bed or the arms of the chair. This is called the tripod position, because the back and two arms are working together to support the upper body. This position allows the diaphragm the most room to function and helps the patient to use accessory muscles to assist breathing. It is usually a good idea to let the patient stay in the most comfortable position.

- **The chest has a barrel shape.** In certain chronic lung diseases, because air has been gradually and continuously trapped within the lung in increasing amounts, the distance from front to back gets longer, nearly equaling the side-to-side distance. A barrel chest may indicate a long history of breathing problems.

- **The conjunctivae are pale.** Perhaps the patient is short of breath because there are not enough red blood cells to carry oxygen to the tissues.

- **The patient has an increased pulse and respirations** (heart rate more than 100/min or respirations more than 20/min).

If the patient has a prescribed metered-dose inhaler, read the label carefully to make sure that the medication is to be used for shortness of breath and that it has, in fact, been prescribed by a physician (Figure 12-14). When in doubt, consult medical control.

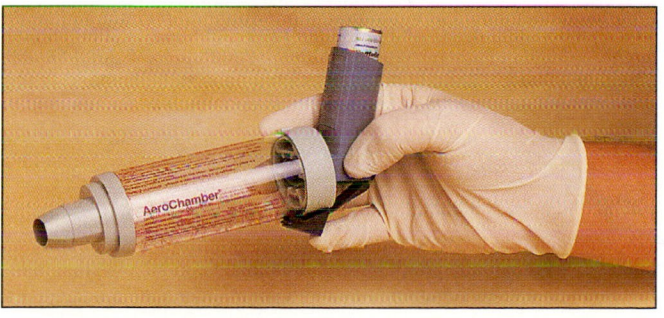

FIGURE 12-14 Some inhalers have spacer devices to better direct the medication spray.

Before helping a patient to self-administer any metered-dose inhaler medication, make sure that the medication is indicated, that is, the patient has signs and symptoms of shortness of breath. Finally, check that there are no contraindications for its use, such as the following:

- The patient is unable to help coordinate inhalation with depression of the trigger, perhaps because the patient is too confused.

- The inhaler is not prescribed for this patient.

- You did not obtain permission from medical control or local protocol.

- The patient had already met the maximum prescribed dose before your arrival.

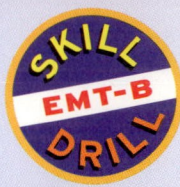

Administering a Metered-Dose Inhaler
Figure 12-15

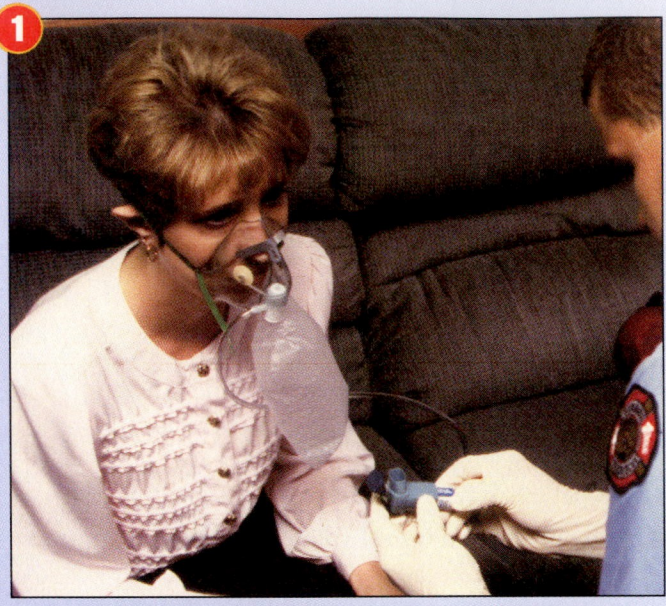

① After you have applied oxygen, check to ensure that you have the correct medication and that it has not expired.

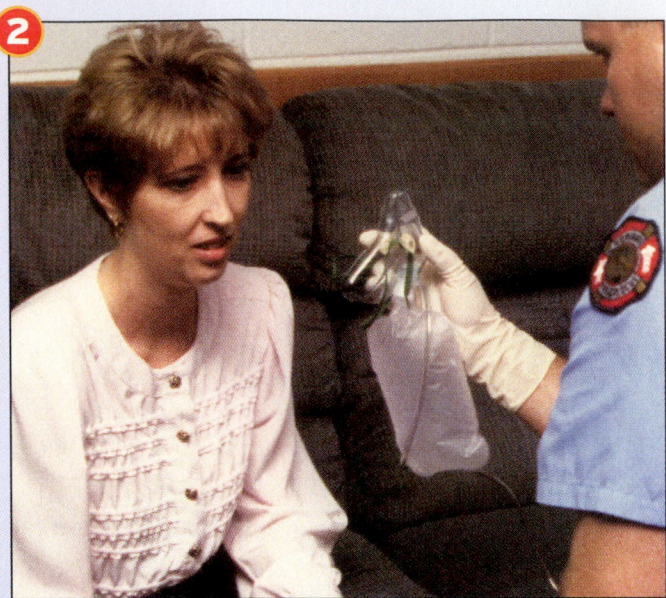

② Remove the oxygen mask, shake the inhaler vigorously, hand the patient the inhaler, and have the patient exhale deeply.

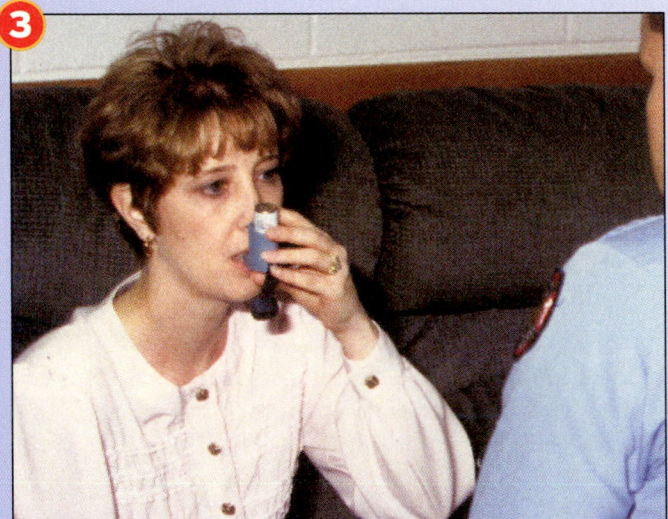

③ Have the patient depress the inhaler and inhale deeply. Advise the patient to hold his or her breath for as long as is comfortable.

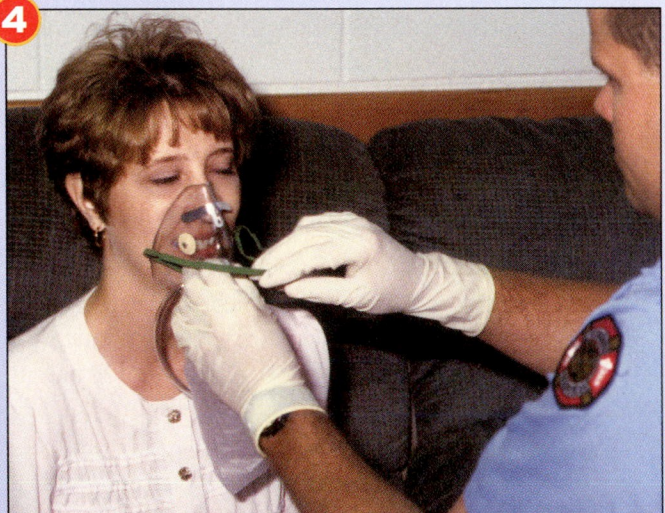

④ Reapply the oxygen, and allow the patient to breathe normally. Repeat with a second dose as instructed by medical control or local protocol.

Administration of metered-dose inhaler medication.
To help a patient self-administer medication from an inhaler, follow these steps:

1. **Obtain an order** from medical control or local protocol.

2. **Check that you have** the right medication, the right patient, and the right route.

3. **Make sure that the patient is alert** enough to use the inhaler.

4. **Check the expiration date** of the inhaler.

5. **Check to see whether the patient** has already taken any doses.

6. **Make sure the inhaler** is at room temperature or warmer.

7. **Shake the inhaler** vigorously several times.

8. **Stop administering** supplemental oxygen and remove any mask from the patient's face.

9. **Ask the patient** to exhale deeply and, before inhaling, to put his or her lips around the opening of the inhaler.

10. **If the patient has a spacer**, use it to allow more effective use of the medication.

11. **Have the patient** depress the hand-held inhaler as he or she begins to inhale deeply.

12. **Instruct the patient** to hold his or her breath for as long as is comfortable to help the body absorb the medication.

13. **Continue to administer** supplemental oxygen.

14. **Allow the patient** to breathe a few times, then repeat second dose per direction from medical control or local protocol.

Reassessment. You need to carefully watch patients with shortness of breath. About 5 minutes after the patient uses an inhaler, repeat the vital signs and perform a focused reassessment. Ask the patient whether the treatment made any difference. Look at the patient's chest to see whether the patient is still using accessory muscles to breathe. Listen to the patient's speech pattern. Keep in mind that the patient may get worse instead of better, and be prepared to provide assisted breathing with positive pressure ventilation.

After helping the patient with the inhaler treatment, transport the patient to the emergency department. While en route, continue to assess the patient's breathing. Try talking to calm and reassure the patient and continue to give supplemental oxygen.

At the hospital, report what you did for the patient, then document your assessment and actions.

The steps for the administration of metered-dose medication are reviewed in the Skill Drill "Administration of a metered-dose inhaler," (Figure 12-15).

caring for kids

Asthma is a common childhood illness. When assessing a pediatric patient, look for retraction of the skin above the sternum and between the ribs. Retractions are typically easier to see in children than in adults. Cyanosis is a late finding in children. Keep in mind that a cough may not be a symptom of a cold; it could signal pneumonia or asthma. Even if you do not hear much wheezing, the presence of a cough can indicate that some degree of reactive airway disease, or a frank asthma attack may be taking place.

The emergency care of a child with shortness of breath is the same as it is for an adult, including the use of supplemental oxygen. However, many small children will not tolerate (or may refuse to wear) a face mask. Rather than fighting with the child, hold the oxygen mask in front of the child's face or ask the parent to hold the mask (Figure 12-16). Many children with asthma also will have prescribed hand-held metered-dose inhalers. Use these inhalers just as you would with an adult.

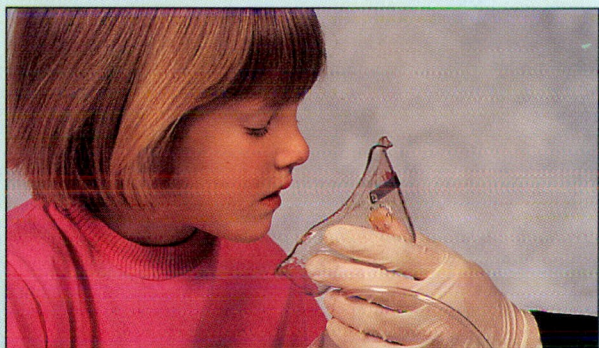

FIGURE 12-16 Because children may refuse to wear an oxygen mask, you may have to hold the mask in front of the child's face. If the child still refuses, enlist the parents' help.

Treatment of Specific Conditions

Infection of the upper or lower airway. Dyspnea associated with acute infections is quite common. Except for the patient with pneumonia, acute bronchitis, or epiglottitis, it is rarely serious. The acute congestion and stuffiness of a common cold hardly ever require emergency care. Indeed, most people with colds treat themselves with OTC medications. However, individuals

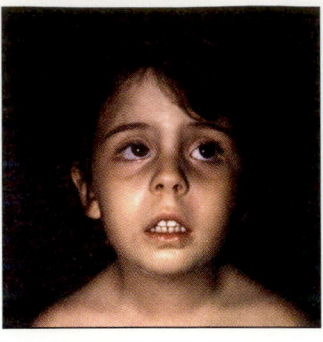
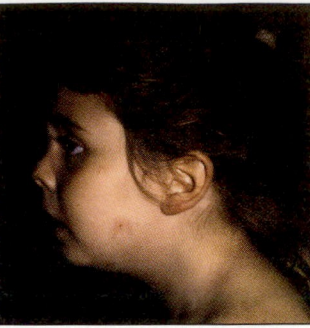

FIGURE 12-17 A child with epiglottis may be more comfortable sitting up and leaning forward.

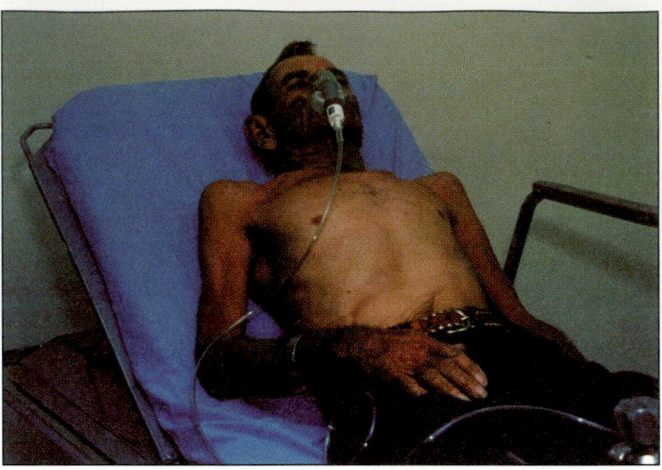

FIGURE 12-18 Transport a patient with COPD in an upright position if it is most comfortable. Ensure that you continue to give oxygen and reassess respirations en route.

with a common cold who have underlying problems such as asthma or heart failure may experience a worsening of their condition as a result of the additional stress of the infection. In addition, cold medications may also have stressful side effects, such as agitation, increased heart rate, and increased blood pressure.

For patients with upper airway infections and dyspnea, administer warm humidified oxygen. Do not attempt to suction the airway or place an oropharyngeal airway in a patient with suspected epiglottitis, because these maneuvers may cause complete airway obstruction. Transport the patient promptly to the hospital. Allow the patient to sit in the position that is most comfortable. For someone with epiglottitis, this is usually sitting upright and leaning forward, the "sniffing position" (Figure 12-17). To force a patient with epiglottitis to lie supine may cause upper airway obstruction that could result in death.

The dyspnea of pneumonia is caused not by upper airway obstruction but by the loss of effective lung volume and a need for more rapid air exchange. Here again, the problem will not be helped by the use of artificial airways but may improve with the administration of oxygen.

Acute pulmonary edema. Dyspnea caused by acute pulmonary edema may be associated with cardiac disease or direct lung damage. In either case, administer 100% oxygen, and, if necessary, carefully suction any secretions from the airway. Provide prompt transport to the emergency department. The best position for a conscious patient who has a myocardial infarction or direct lung injury is the one in which it is easiest to breathe. Usually, this is sitting up. Rarely will you need to use an artificial airway, because no upper airway obstruction problem exists. However, an unconscious patient with acute pulmonary edema may require full ventilatory support, including airway, positive pressure ventilation with oxygen, and suctioning.

Chronic obstructive pulmonary disease. Patients with COPD may be semiconscious or unconscious from **hypoxia**, a condition in which the body's cells and tis-

sues do not get enough oxygen, or from carbon dioxide retention. They may appear to be in respiratory distress and/or be cyanotic. They may have pursed lips and may be using accessory muscles to breathe, including those in the neck and shoulders.

Transport patients with COPD as promptly as possible to the emergency department, allowing them to sit upright if this is most comfortable (Figure 12-18). Patients with COPD often find breathing difficult when lying down.

Spontaneous pneumothorax. Patients with spontaneous pneumothorax may have severe respiratory distress, or they may have no distress at all and complain only of pleuritic chest pain. Provide supplemental oxygen at low levels, and provide prompt transport to the hospital. Like most dyspneic patients, those with spontaneous pneumothorax are usually more comfortable sitting up. Monitor the patient carefully, watching for any sudden deterioration in the respiratory status. Be ready to support the airway, assist respirations, and give full cardiopulmonary support if it becomes necessary.

Asthma or allergic reactions. Many lung problems are incorrectly labeled "asthma"; therefore, your assessment of the patient is critical. A patient who truly has asthma will have a history of repeated episodes of sudden shortness of breath, in which he or she had difficulty exhaling. Confirm whether the patient is able to breathe normally at other times. If possible, ask family members to describe the patient's asthma. Even if they only identify wheezing as a problem, be aware that some forms of heart failure, foreign body aspiration, or toxic fumes inhalation may cause wheezing.

As you assess the patient's vital signs, note that the pulse rate will be normal or elevated, the blood pressure may be slightly elevated, and respirations will be increased.

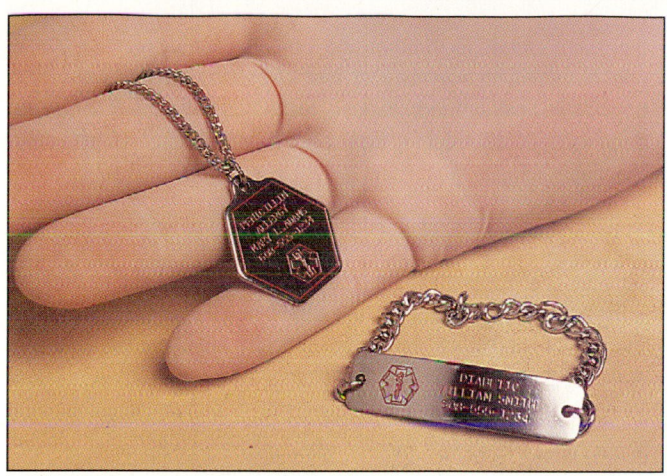

FIGURE 12-19 Some patients who are known to be severely allergic to bee stings, certain medications, or other substances often wear a medical identification tag.

Administer oxygen, and allow the patient to sit in an upright position, which makes breathing easier. Be reassuring; tension and anxiety make asthma attacks worse.

Ask questions about how and when the symptoms began, as reactions that follow a bee or wasp sting may progress rapidly to anaphylactic shock. A patient in anaphylactic shock may quickly become unconscious and require assisted ventilations and supplemental oxygen. If the patient is already unconscious upon your arrival, look for a medical identification tag that may provide a clue (Figure 12-19). Unconscious patients require prompt transport to the emergency department.

As you care for the patient, be prepared to suction large amounts of mucus from the mouth and to administer oxygen. If you do suction, do not withhold oxygen for more than 10 to 15 seconds. Allow some time for oxygenation between suction attempts. If the patient is unconscious, you may have to provide airway maintenance. Occasionally, CPR is required for an episode of anaphylaxis.

If the patient carries medication for an asthma attack or allergic reaction, you may help with its administration, as directed by local protocol. Keep in mind that epinephrine is a very potent agent with a number of significant side effects. Do not give it unless you are certain that the patient is having a severe asthma attack or severe allergic reaction and you know the history of the episode.

A prolonged asthma attack that is unrelieved by epinephrine may progress into a condition known as *status asthmaticus*. The patient is likely to be frightened, frantically trying to breathe, while using all the accessory muscles. Status asthmaticus is a true emergency, and the patient must be given oxygen and transported immediately to the emergency department.

The effort to breathe during an asthma attack is very tiring, and the patient may be exhausted by the time you arrive. An exhausted patient may have stopped feeling anxious or even struggling to breathe. This patient is not recovering; he or she is at a very critical stage and is likely to stop breathing. Aggressive airway management, oxygen administration, and prompt transport are essential in this situation.

Pleural effusions. Treatment of pleural effusions consists of removal of fluid collected outside the lung, which must be done by a physician in a hospital setting. However, you should provide oxygen and other routine support measures.

Obstruction of the upper airway. If the patient is a small child or someone who was eating just before dyspnea developed, you may assume that the problem is an inhaled or aspirated foreign body. If the patient is old enough to talk but cannot make any noise, upper airway obstruction is the likely cause.

The first thing to do is clear the upper airway. Then, whether or not you are successful, administer supplemental oxygen and transport the patient promptly to the emergency department.

Pulmonary embolism. Because a considerable amount of lung tissue may not be functioning, supplemental oxygen is mandatory in a patient with a pulmonary embolism. Place the patient in a comfortable position, usually sitting, and assist breathing as necessary. Hemoptysis, if present, is usually not severe, but any blood that has been coughed up should be cleared from the airway. You should expect an unusually rapid and possibly irregular heartbeat. Transport the patient to the emergency department promptly. Be aware that pulmonary emboli may cause cardiac arrest, requiring CPR.

Hyperventilation. When you respond to a patient who is hyperventilating, complete an initial assessment and history of the event. Is the patient having chest pain or coughing blood? Is there a history of cardiac problems or diabetes? You must always assume a serious underlying problem even if you suspect that the underlying problem is stress. Do not have the patient breathe into a paper bag, even though it is thought to be the traditional technique for managing hyperventilation syndrome. In theory, breathing into a paper bag causes the patient to rebreathe exhaled carbon dioxide, allowing the level of carbon dioxide in the blood to return to normal. In fact, if the patient is hyperventilating because of a serious medical problem, this maneuver could make things worse. A patient with underlying pulmonary disease who breathes into a bag may become severely hypoxic. Treatment should instead consist of reassuring the patient in a calm, professional manner; supplying supplemental oxygen; and providing prompt transport to the emergency department. Patients who hyperventilate need to be evaluated in the hospital setting.

prep kit

ready for review

Dyspnea is a common complaint that may be caused by numerous medical problems, including infections of the upper or lower airways, acute pulmonary edema, chronic obstructive pulmonary disease, spontaneous pneumothorax, asthma or allergic reactions, pleural effusions, mechanical obstruction of the airway, pulmonary embolism, and hyperventilation. Each of these lung disorders interferes in one way or another with the exchange of oxygen and carbon dioxide that takes place during respiration. This interference may be in the form of damage to the alveoli, separation of the alveoli from the pulmonary vessels by fluid or infection, obstruction of the air passages, or air or excess fluid in the pleural space. Patients with longstanding lung diseases often have chronically high levels of blood carbon dioxide; in some cases, giving too much oxygen to these patients may depress or stop respirations. However, judicious use of oxygen is always an important priority in patients with dyspnea.

Signs and symptoms of breathing difficulty include unusual breath sounds, including wheezing, stridor, rales, and rhonchi; nasal flaring; pursed lip breathing; cyanosis; inability to talk; use of accessory muscles to breathe; and sitting in the tripod position, which allows the diaphragm the most room to function.

In treating dyspnea, it is important to reassure the patient and provide supplemental oxygen. Remember to maintain the patient in a position that is comfortable for breathing, usually sitting upright. If the patient is not breathing, use a BVM device to assist breathing. If the patient is breathing with great difficulty, apply oxygen through a nonrebreathing face mask with the oxygen flow set at 10 to 15 L/min. Next, perform a focused history and physical exam, including vital signs. If the patient has a prescribed inhaler or epinephrine injector, consult medical control to assist with its use. Then transport the patient to the hospital, monitoring his or her condition on the way. Talking with the patient is a good way to monitor a breathing problem.

Remember, a patient who is breathing rapidly may be getting insufficient oxygen as a result of respiratory distress from a variety of problems, including pneumonia or a pulmonary embolism; trying to "blow off" more carbon dioxide to compensate for acidosis caused by a poison, a severe infection, or a high level of blood glucose; or having a stress reaction. In every case, prompt recognition of the problem, giving oxygen, and prompt transport are essential.

vital vocabulary

www.emtb.com

allergen   A substance that causes an allergic reaction.

asthma   A disease of the lungs in which muscle spasm in the small air passageways and the production of large amounts of mucus result in airway obstruction.

bronchitis   Irritation of the major lung passageways, from either infectious disease or irritants such as smoke.

carbon dioxide retention   A condition characterized by a chronically high blood level of carbon dioxide in which the respiratory center no longer responds to high blood levels of carbon dioxide.

chronic obstructive pulmonary disease (COPD)   A slow process of dilation and disruption of the airways and alveoli, caused by chronic bronchial obstruction.

common cold   Usually associated with swollen nasal mucous membranes and the production of fluid from the sinuses and nose.

croup   An infectious disease of the upper respiratory system that may cause partial airway obstruction and is characterized by a barking cough; usually seen in children.

diphtheria   An infectious disease in which a membrane lining the pharynx is formed that can severely obstruct passage of air into the larynx.

dyspnea   Shortness of breath or difficulty breathing.

embolus   A blood clot or other substance that has formed in a blood vessel or in the heart that breaks off and travels to another blood vessel, where it causes blockage.

emphysema   A disease of the lungs in which there is extreme dilation and eventual destruction of pulmonary alveoli with poor exchange of oxygen and carbon dioxide; it is one form of chronic obstructive pulmonary disease (COPD).

epiglottitis   An infectious disease in which the epiglottis becomes inflamed and enlarged and may cause upper airway obstruction.

hyperventilation   A lowering of blood carbon dioxide levels, usually through rapid or deep breathing.

hypoxia   A condition in which the body's cells and tissues do not have enough oxygen.

pleural effusion   A collection of fluid between the lung and chest wall that may compress the lung.

pleuritic chest pain   Sharp, stabbing pain in the chest that is worsened by a deep breath; often caused by inflammation or irritation of the pleura.

pneumonia   An infectious disease of the lung that damages and destroys lung tissue.

pneumothorax   A partial or complete accumulation of air in the pleural space.

pulmonary edema   A buildup of fluid in the lungs, usually as a result of congestive heart failure.

pulmonary embolism   The condition in which a blood clot breaks off from a large vein and travels to the blood vessels of the lung, causing obstruction of blood flow.

rales   Crackling, rattling breath sounds signaling fluid in the air spaces of the lungs.

rhonchi   Coarse breath sounds heard in patients with chronic mucus in the airways.

stridor   A harsh, high-pitched inspiratory sound, such as the sound often heard in acute laryngeal (upper airway) obstruction.

wheeze   A high-pitched, whistling breath sound, characteristically heard on expiration in patients with asthma or COPD.

12 prep kit

assessment in action

You receive a call for assistance from a local bookseller specializing in old and antique books. When you arrive, you find one of the customers, a 38-year-old man, seated in a hunched-over position in one of the back aisles. You notice immediately that the patient seems to be breathing very fast. As you begin to ask him questions, you find that he can speak only in short, 3- and 4-word bursts. He manages to tell you that he had been looking at old books for the last hour when his chest started to tighten up, possibly from the dust. The patient also tells you that he uses a Ventolin inhaler, but he left it in his car. The patient says that he smokes about two packs of cigarettes a week. Your partner obtains baseline vital signs. The patient has a blood pressure of 152/90 mm Hg, a regular pulse of 122 beats/min, and shallow respirations of 34 breaths/min.

1. Which of the following steps would be **LEAST** helpful in assessing this patient's respiratory status?
   A. Assessing the depth of the breaths
   B. Evaluating the use of accessory muscles
   C. Counting the number of breaths in a minute
   D. Compressing the rib cage for injuries or deformity

2. Another customer offers to let the patient use her inhaler when he states that he thinks he needs an inhaler. The most appropriate course of action would be to:
   A. thank the other customer and state that the patient needs his own inhaler.
   B. check for breath sounds, then let the patient use the other customer's inhaler.
   C. observe the patient as the other customer helps the patient use her inhaler.
   D. obtain another set of vital signs, then let the patient use the other customer's inhaler.

3. Which of the following statements about administering medication via an inhaler is **FALSE**?
   A. The medication in the inhaler does not expire.
   B. The inhaler should be shaken vigorously before each use.
   C. The inhaler should be used at room temperature or warmer.
   D. The medication in the inhaler relaxes the muscles that surround the bronchioles.

4. The patient finds an almost-empty inhaler in his briefcase and uses it. Which of the following would **NOT** be considered a side effect of using his inhaler?
   A. Nervousness
   B. Symptom relief
   C. Increased pulse
   D. Tremors or shaking

5. Which of the following facts from the patient's history is **LEAST** important as you assess the patient and plan his care?
   A. The patient is a 38-year-old man.
   B. The patient uses Ventolin to treat his asthma.
   C. The patient smokes two packs of cigarettes a week.
   D. The patient is currently taking antibiotics for a sinus infection.

points to ponder

Objectives 1-2.5, 1-2.6

You are returning from lunch when you hear the dispatch of another unit to a drowning at an apartment complex about half a block away from where you are. You "jump" the call and turn into the complex. You arrive at the pool as the rescuers hand out an 18-month-old child. The child is cyanotic and unresponsive. You find a pulse but no breathing. Your partner has a child about that same age and is shaken by this call. Just before transport, the child "crashes," losing its pulse also. Even with the best care you could provide, the child does not make it. Now you are back out on duty, your partner is barely functioning, and when you close your eyes, you can see the child and the look on your partner's face as you took control of the scene. There are about 6 hours left in your shift.

• Would you stay on duty? What would you do to help your partner? What would you do to help yourself?

online outlook

The term "chronic obstructive pulmonary disease" (COPD) comprises emphysema and chronic bronchitis. The number of lives that are claimed by chronic lung disease has increased sharply. In 1979, it accounted for about 50,000 deaths. In 1982, the number rose to 59,000, and by 1992, the number of deaths reached 86,974. To learn more about COPD, complete Exercise 12 at the www.emtb.com.

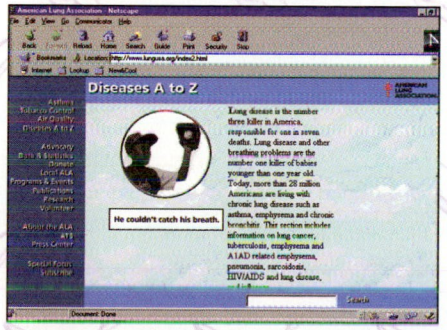

prep kit 12

Cardiovascular Emergencies

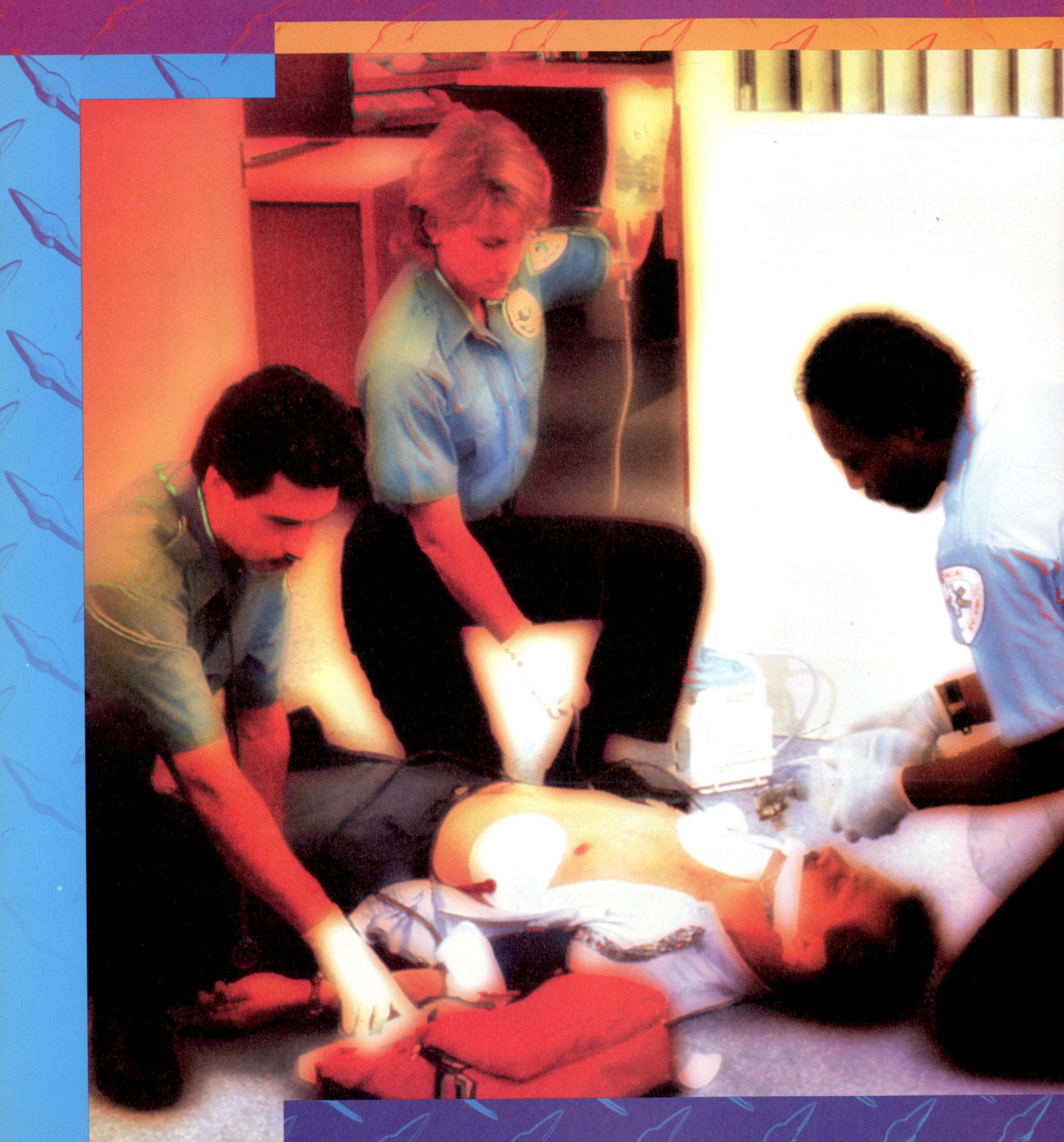

objectives

Cognitive

1. Describe the structure and function of the cardiovascular system.

2. Describe the emergency medical care of the patient experiencing chest pain/discomfort.

3. List the indications for automated external defibrillation (AED).

4. List the contraindications for automated external defibrillation.

5. Define the role of EMT-B in the emergency cardiac care system.

6. Explain the impact of age and weight on defibrillation.

7. Discuss the position of comfort for patients with various cardiac emergencies.

8. Establish the relationship between airway management and the patient with cardiovascular compromise.

9. Predict the relationship between the patient experiencing cardiovascular compromise and basic life support.

10. Discuss the fundamentals of early defibrillation.

11. Explain the rationale for early defibrillation.

12. Explain that not all chest pain patients result in cardiac arrest and do not need to be attached to an automated external defibrillator.

13. Explain the importance of prehospital ACLS intervention if it is available.

14. Explain the importance of urgent transport to a facility with Advanced Cardiac Life Support if it is not available in the prehospital setting.

15. Discuss the various types of automated external defibrillators.

16. Differentiate between the fully automated and the semi-automated defibrillator.

17. Discuss the procedures that must be taken into consideration for standard operations of the various types of automated external defibrillators.

18. State the reasons for assuring that the patient is pulseless and apneic when using the automated external defibrillator.

19. Discuss the circumstances which may result in inappropriate shocks.

20. Explain the considerations for interruption of CPR, when using the automated external defibrillator.

21. Discuss the advantages and disadvantages of automated external defibrillators.

22. Summarize the speed of operation of automated external defibrillation.

23. Discuss the use of remote defibrillation through adhesive pads.

24. Discuss the special considerations for rhythm monitoring.

25. List the steps in the operation of the automated external defibrillator.

26. Discuss the standard of care that should be used to provide care to a patient with persistent ventricular fibrillation and no available ACLS.

27. Discuss the standard of care that should be used to provide care to a patient with recurrent ventricular fibrillation and no available ACLS.

28. Differentiate between the single rescuer and multi-rescuer care with an automated external defibrillator.

29. Explain the reason for pulses not being checked between shocks with an automated external defibrillator.

30. Discuss the importance of coordinating ACLS trained providers with personnel using automated external defibrillators.

31. Discuss the importance of postresuscitation care.

32. List the components of postresuscitation care.

33. Explain the importance of frequent practice with the automated external defibrillator.

34. Discuss the need to complete the Automated Defibrillator: Operator's Shift Checklist.

(Continued)

objectives—cont'd.

35. Discuss the role of the American Heart Association (AHA) in the use of automated external defibrillation.

36. Explain the role medical direction plays in the use of automated external defibrillation.

37. State the reasons why a case review should be completed following the use of the automated external defibrillator.

38. Discuss the components that should be included in a case review.

39. Discuss the goal of quality improvement in automated external defibrillation.

40. Recognize the need for medical direction of protocols to assist in the emergency medical care of the patient with chest pain.

41. List the indications for the use of nitroglycerin.

42. State the contraindications and side effects for the use of nitroglycerin.

43. Define the function of all controls on an automated external defibrillator, and describe event documentation and battery defibrillator maintenance.

Affective

44. Defend the reasons for obtaining initial training in automated external defibrillation and the importance of continuing education.

45. Defend the reason for maintenance of automated external defibrillators.

46. Explain the rationale for administering nitroglycerin to a patient with chest pain or discomfort.

Psychomotor

47. Demonstrate the assessment and emergency medical care of a patient experiencing chest pain/discomfort.

48. Demonstrate the application and operation of the automated external defibrillator.

49. Demonstrate the maintenance of an automated external defibrillator.

50. Demonstrate the assessment and documentation of patient response to the automated external defibrillator.

51. Demonstrate the skills necessary to complete the Automated Defibrillator: Operator's Shift Checklist.

52. Perform the steps in facilitating the use of nitroglycerin for chest pain or discomfort.

53. Demonstrate the assessment and documentation of patient response to nitroglycerin.

54. Practice completing a prehospital care report for patients with cardiac emergencies.

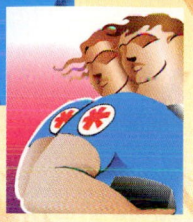

you are the emt

You are called to an apartment complex for a "man not feeling well." As you make your way down the hall, you can already hear someone crying, as well as a voice saying, "One and two and three and four and five and . . ." CPR is clearly in progress. This situation is a bit different from what you expected based on the call to 9-1-1.

Cardiac emergencies are one of the most common reasons EMS in requested. This chapter will provide you with the information necessary so that you can contribute to the reduction of mortality and morbidity associated with emergency cardiac care in the prehospital setting, and it will help you to answer the following questions.

1. What are the key factors in improving survivability for cardiac patients?
2. What is the role of an EMT-B in caring for a cardiac patient?

Cardiovascular Emergencies

Heart attacks and other cardiac emergencies affect millions of Americans each year, nearly 1 million persons dying from a cardiovascular problem annually. As a result, heart disease remains the leading cause of death. In fact, about one third of Americans will eventually die as a result of heart disease. Thus, many of your calls will involve some type of cardiac emergency.

This chapter begins with a brief description of the heart and how it works. It then discusses the relationship between chest pain and ischemic heart disease. It explains how to recognize and treat acute myocardial infarction (classic heart attack) and the complications of sudden death, cardiogenic shock, and congestive heart failure. The use of nitroglycerin is described. The last part of the chapter is devoted to the use and maintenance of the automated external defibrillator (AED).

Cardiac Structure and Function

The heart is a relatively simple organ with a simple job. It has to pump blood to supply oxygen-enriched red blood cells to the tissues of the body. The heart is divided down the middle into two sides (left and right) by a wall called the septum. Each side of the heart has an **atrium**, or upper chamber, and a **ventricle**, or lower chamber (Figure 13-1). Blood leaves each of the four

chambers of the heart through a one-way valve. These valves keep the blood moving through the circulatory system in the proper direction. The largest valve is the **aortic valve**, lying between the left ventricle and the aorta. The **aorta**, the body's main artery, receives the blood ejected from the left ventricle and delivers it to all the other arteries so that they can carry blood to the tissues of the body.

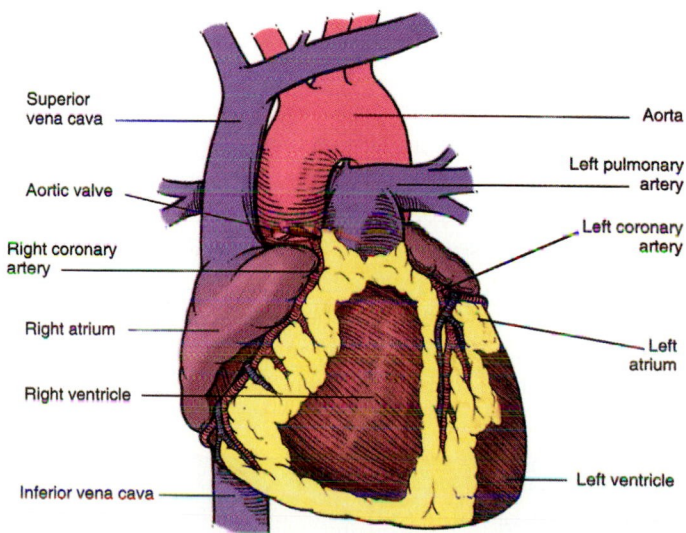

Superior vena cava	Aorta
Aortic valve	Left pulmonary artery
Right coronary artery	Left coronary artery
Right atrium	Left atrium
Right ventricle	Left ventricle
Inferior vena cava	

FIGURE 13-1 The heart is a four-chambered muscle that pumps blood to all parts of the body.

A

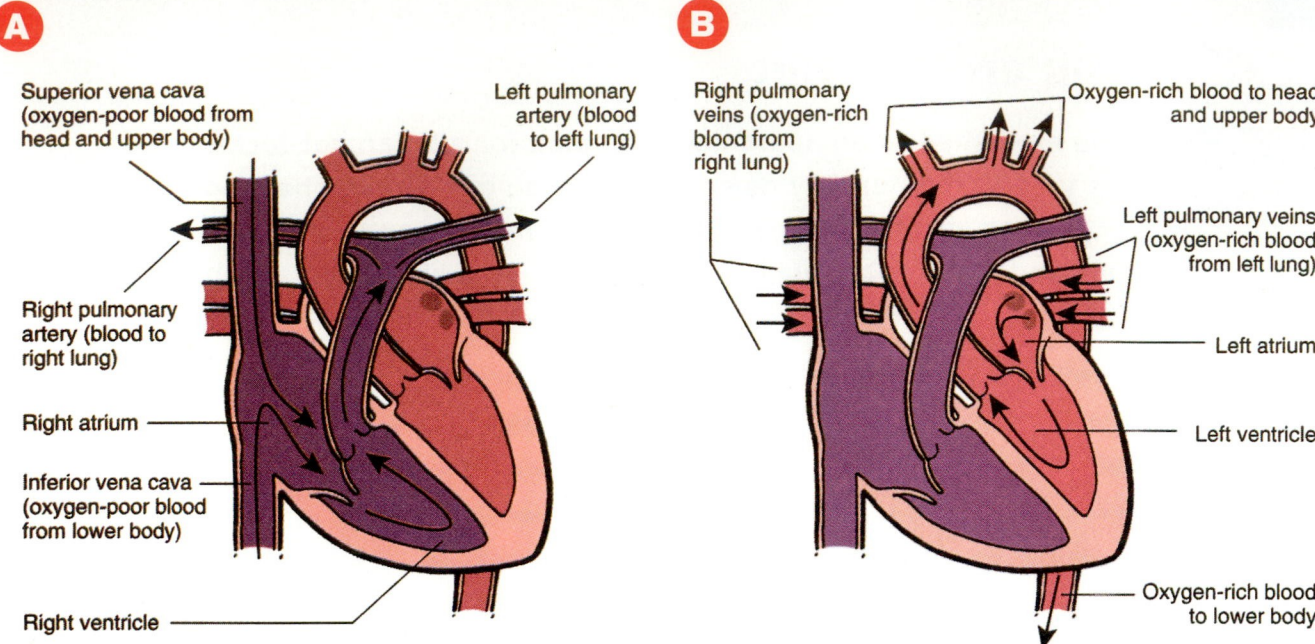

Superior vena cava (oxygen-poor blood from head and upper body)

Left pulmonary artery (blood to left lung)

Right pulmonary artery (blood to right lung)

Right atrium

Inferior vena cava (oxygen-poor blood from lower body)

Right ventricle

B

Right pulmonary veins (oxygen-rich blood from right lung)

Oxygen-rich blood to head and upper body

Left pulmonary veins (oxygen-rich blood from left lung)

Left atrium

Left ventricle

Oxygen-rich blood to lower body

FIGURE 13-2 A: The right side of the heart receives oxygen-poor blood from the veins. **B:** The left side of the heart receives oxygen-rich blood from the lungs through the pulmonary veins.

The right side of the heart receives oxygen-poor (deoxygenated) blood from the veins of the body (Figure 13-2). Blood enters into the right atrium from the vena cava, which then fills the right ventricle. After contraction of the right ventricle, blood flows into the pulmonary artery and the pulmonary circulation, where the blood is oxygenated. The left side of the heart receives oxygen-rich (oxygenated) blood from the lungs through the pulmonary veins. Blood enters into the atrium, then passes into the left ventricle. This side of the heart is more muscular than the other because it must pump blood into the aorta and all the other arteries of the body.

The heart contains more than muscle tissue. The heart's electrical system, which is distributed throughout the entire heart, controls heart rate and enables the atria and ventricles to work together (Figure 13-3). Normal electrical impulses begin in the sinus node, just above the atria. The impulses travel across both atria, causing them to contract. Between the atria and the ventricles, the impulses cross over a bridge of special electrical tissue called the atrioventricular (AV) node. Here the

signal is slowed down for about one tenth to two tenths of a second to allow blood time to pass from the atria to the ventricles. Then the impulses exit the AV node and spread throughout both ventricles, causing the ventricular muscle cells to contract.

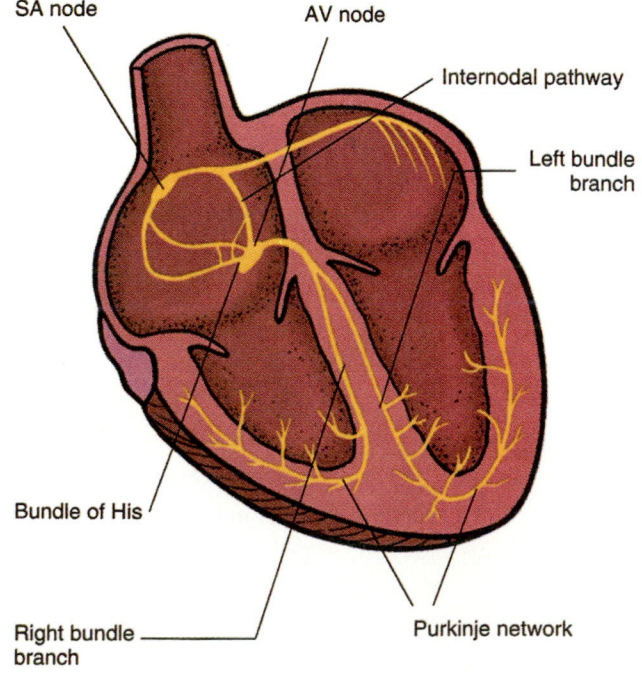

SA node

AV node

Internodal pathway

Left bundle branch

Bundle of His

Right bundle branch

Purkinje network

FIGURE 13-3 The electrical conduction system of the heart controls most aspects of heart rate and enables the four chambers to work together.

> About one third of Americans will eventually die as a result of heart disease.

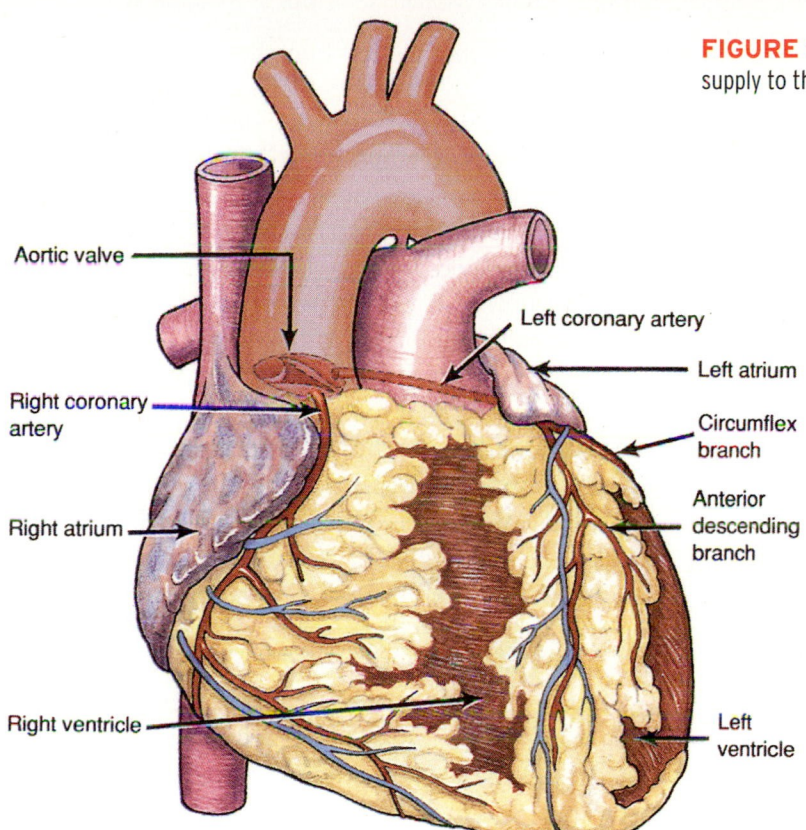

FIGURE 13-4 The coronary arteries carry the blood supply to the heart.

Aortic valve

Left coronary artery

Left atrium

Right coronary artery

Circumflex branch

Anterior descending branch

Right atrium

Right ventricle

Left ventricle

Circulation

To carry out its function of pumping blood, the **myocardium**, or heart muscle, must have a continuous supply of oxygen and nutrients. During periods of physical exertion or stress, the myocardium requires more oxygen, so the heart must increase its output of blood. In the normal heart, the increased need for blood is easily supplied by **dilation**, or widening, of the coronary arteries, which increases blood flow. The **coronary arteries** are the blood vessels that supply blood to the heart muscle. They start at the first part of the aorta, just above the aortic valve. The right coronary artery supplies blood to the right ventricle and, in most people, the bottom part, or inferior wall, of the left ventricle. The left coronary artery divides into two major branches, both of which supply the left ventricle (Figure 13-4).

Two major arteries branching from the upper aorta supply blood to the head and arms. The right and left carotid arteries supply the head and brain with blood. The subclavian arteries (under the clavicles) supply blood to the upper extremities. As the subclavian artery enters each arm, it becomes the brachial artery, the major vessel that supplies blood to each arm. Just below the elbow, the brachial artery divides into two major branches: the radial and ulnar arteries (Figure 13-5).

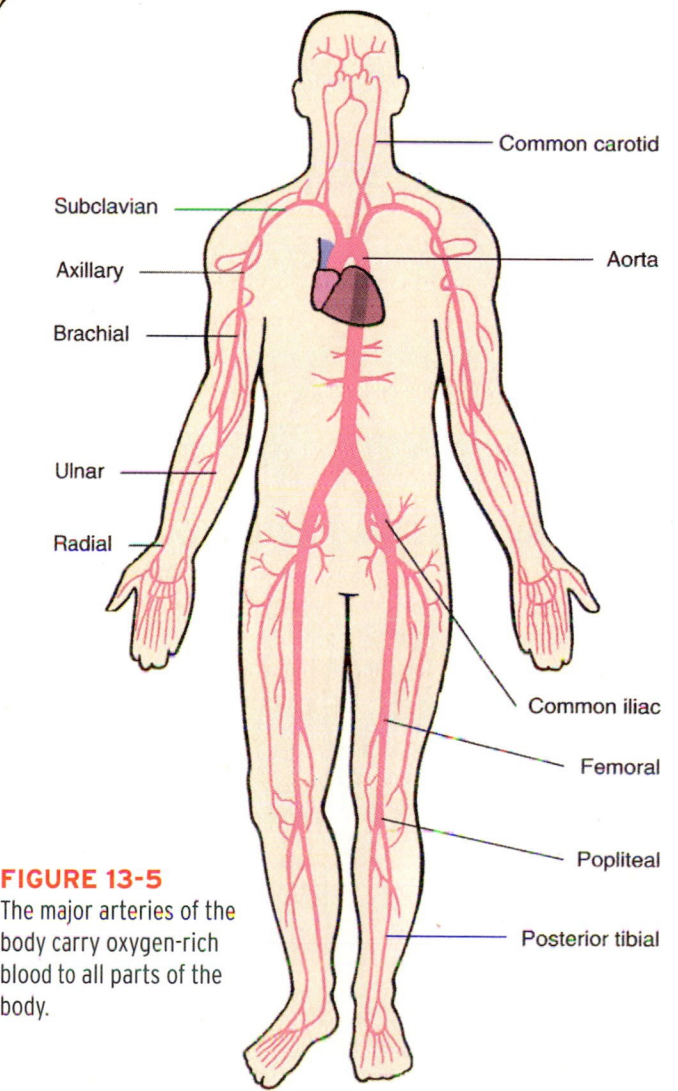

Common carotid

Subclavian

Axillary

Aorta

Brachial

Ulnar

Radial

Common iliac

Femoral

Popliteal

Posterior tibial

FIGURE 13-5 The major arteries of the body carry oxygen-rich blood to all parts of the body.

At the level of the navel, the aorta divides into two main branches called the right and left iliac arteries, which supply blood to the groin, pelvis, and legs. As the iliac arteries enter the legs through the groin, they become the right and left femoral arteries. At the level of the knee, the femoral artery divides into the **anterior** (front) and **posterior** (behind) tibial artery and the peroneal artery.

After blood travels through the arteries, it enters smaller and smaller vessels, called arterioles and capillaries. The capillaries are tiny blood vessels that connect arterioles to venules. Capillaries, which are found in all parts of the body, allow the exchange of nutrients and waste at the cellular level.

Venules are the smallest branches of veins. After traveling through the capillaries, blood enters the system of veins, starting with the venules, on its way back to the heart. The veins become larger and larger and eventually form the two large venae cavae: the upper vena cava and the lower vena cava. The **superior** (upper) vena cava carries blood from the head and arms back to the right atrium. The **inferior** (lower) vena cava carries blood from the abdomen, kidneys, and legs back to the right atrium. The superior and inferior venae cavae join at the right atrium of the heart, where blood is eventually returned into the pulmonary circulation for oxygenation (Figure 13-6).

Blood consists of several types of cells and fluid (Figure 13-7). *Red blood cells* are the most numerous and give the blood its color. Red blood cells carry oxygen to the body's tissues and then remove carbon dioxide. Larger *white blood cells* help to fight infection. *Platelets,* which help the blood clot, are much smaller than either red or white blood cells. *Plasma* is the fluid that the cells float in. It is a mixture of water, salts, nutrients, and proteins.

Blood pressure is the pressure of circulating blood against the walls of the arteries. Systolic blood pressure is the maximum pressure exerted by the left ventricle as it contracts. As the left ventricle relaxes, the arterial pressure falls. When the aortic valve closes, blood flow stops. The diastolic blood pressure is the pressure exerted against the walls of the arteries while the left ventricle is at rest. Remember that the top number in a blood pressure reading is the systolic pressure, and the bottom number is the diastolic or resting pressure.

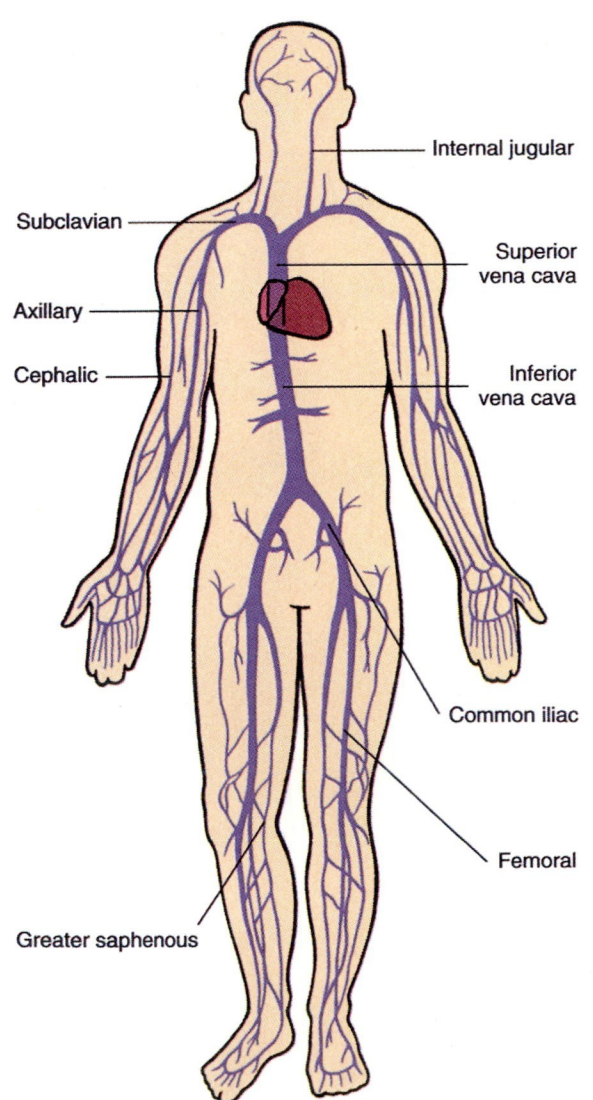

FIGURE 13-6 The veins carry blood from the body back to the heart, which pumps it through the lungs for oxygenation.

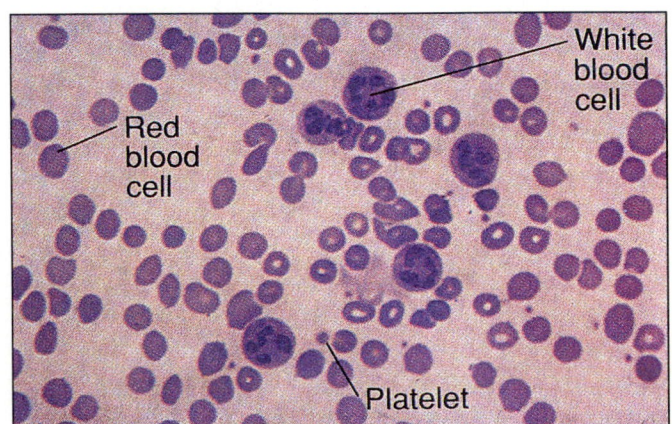

FIGURE 13-7 Blood consists of several types of cells and fluids, including red blood cells, white blood cells, and platelets.

pulsation

As the left ventricle contracts, it ejects a forceful wave of blood through the arteries. You can feel that wave in areas where the artery is near the surface of the skin. This wave is called the pulse. Common places to feel for a pulse include the following (Figure 13-8):

- The *carotid pulse* can be felt in the neck, two fingerbreadths on either side of the Adam's apple (thyroid cartilage).

- The *femoral pulse* can be felt in the groin, right at the crease dividing the lower abdomen from the leg.

- The *brachial pulse* can be felt on the inside of the elbow, right at the level of the crease. Pulsations also can be palpated on the inside of the arm between the elbow and armpit. This is the pulse that you listen to when you take blood pressure.

- The *radial pulse* can be felt on the thumb side of the wrist, about one finger width above the wrist crease.

- The *posterior tibial pulse* can be felt on the inside of the ankle, just posterior to the medial malleolus. The medial malleolus is the bony bump at the end of the tibia.

- The *dorsalis pedis pulse* can be felt at the top of the foot. This artery is not in the exact same place in all people. To find its pulse, place your hand across the top of the foot just below the ankle crease. Once you feel something that might be a pulse, use your fingertips to confirm that finding.

Practice feeling for these pulses on yourself and on friends and family members.

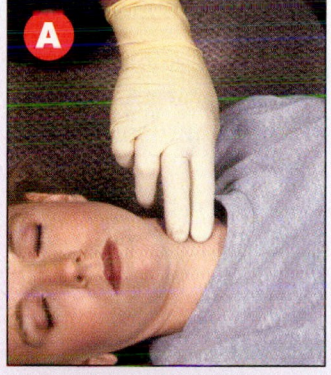
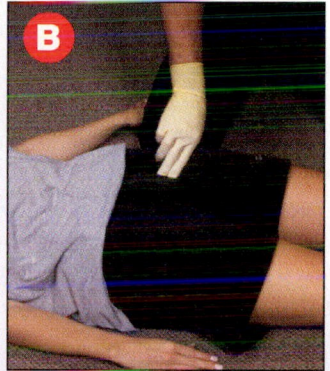
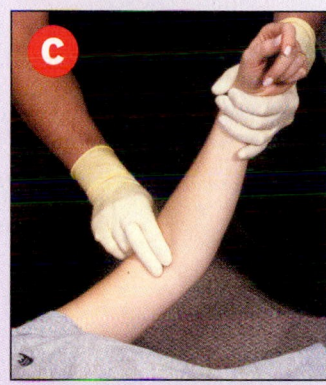
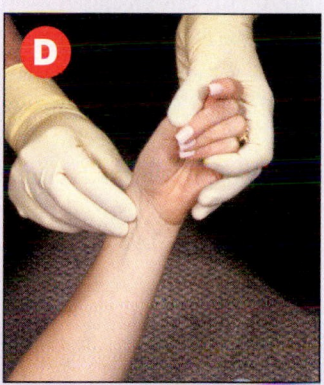
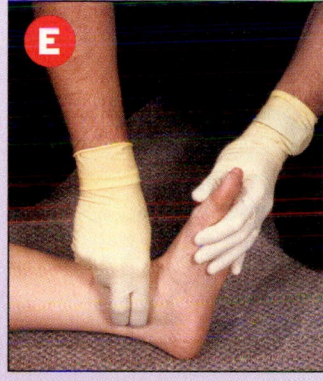
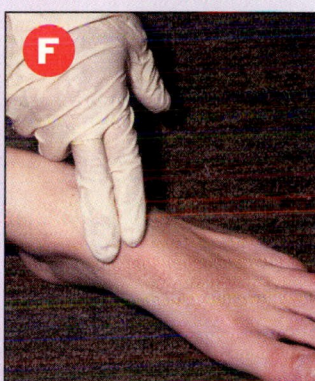

FIGURE 13-8 Common pulse points.
A: The carotid pulse is taken at the neck.
B: The femoral pulse is felt in the groin area.
C: The brachial pulse can be felt on the inside of the upper arm.
D: The radial pulse can be felt on the thumb side of the wrist.
E: The posterior tibial pulse can be felt on the inside of the ankle.
F: The dorsalis pedis pulse can be felt at the top of the foot.

Cardiac Compromise

Chest pain or discomfort that is related to the heart usually stems from a condition called <u>ischemia</u>, or insufficient oxygen. Because of a partial or complete blockage of blood flow through the coronary arteries, heart tissues fail to get enough oxygen and nutrients. The tissue soon begins to starve and, if blood flow is not restored, eventually dies. Ischemic heart disease, then, is disease involving a decrease in blood flow to one or more portions of the heart muscle.

Atherosclerosis

Most often, the low blood flow to heart tissue is caused by coronary artery atherosclerosis. <u>Atherosclerosis</u> is a disorder in which calcium and a fatty material called cholesterol build up and form a plaque inside the walls of blood vessels, obstructing flow and interfering with their ability to dilate or contract (Figure 13-9). Eventually, atherosclerosis can even cause complete <u>occlusion</u>, or blockage, of a coronary artery. Atherosclerosis usually involves other arteries of the body, as well.

The problem begins when the first deposit of cholesterol is laid down on the inside of an artery. This may happen during the teenage years. As a person ages, more of this fatty material is deposited; the <u>lumen</u>, or the inside diameter of the artery, narrows. As the cholesterol deposits grow, calcium deposits can form as well. The inner wall of the artery, which is normally smooth and elastic, becomes rough and brittle with these atherosclerotic plaques. Damage to the coronary arteries may become so extensive that they cannot accommodate increased blood flow at times of maximum need.

For reasons that are still not completely understood, a brittle plaque will sometimes develop a crack, exposing the inside of the atherosclerotic wall. Acting like a torn blood vessel, the ragged edge of the crack activates the blood-clotting system, just as it does when an injury has caused bleeding. In this situation, however, the resulting blood clot will partially or completely block the lumen of the artery. Tissues downstream from the blood clot will suffer from lack of oxygen (ischemia). If blood flow is resumed in a short time, the ischemic tissues will recover. However, if too much time goes by before blood flow is resumed, the tissues will die. This sequence of events is known as an <u>acute myocardial infarction (AMI)</u>, a classic heart attack. <u>Infarction</u> means the death of tissue (Figure 13-10). The same sequence may also cause the death of cells in other organs, such as the brain. In this case, the death of heart

muscle can lead to severe diminishment of the heart's ability to pump.

In the United States, coronary artery disease is the number one cause of death for both men and women. The peak incidence of heart disease occurs between ages 40 and 70 years, but it can also strike teens or individuals in their 90s. You must be alert to the possibility that, although less likely, a 26-year-old person with chest pain could actually be having a heart attack, especially if he or she has a higher than usual risk.

Factors that place a person at higher risk for a myocardial infarction are called risk factors. The major controllable factors are cigarette smoking, high blood pressure, elevated cholesterol levels, elevated blood sugar levels (diabetes), lack of exercise, and stress. The major risk factors that cannot be controlled are older age, family history of atherosclerotic coronary artery disease, and male gender.

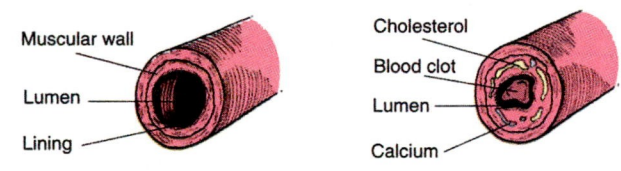

FIGURE 13-9 In atherosclerosis, calcium and cholesterol build up inside the walls of the blood vessels, causing an obstruction in blood flow to the heart.

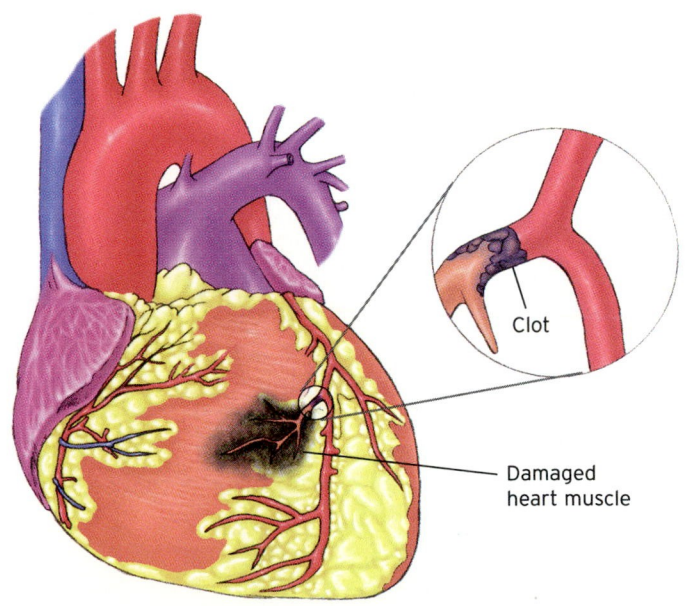

FIGURE 13-10 An acute myocardial infarction occurs when a blood clot prevents blood flow to an area of the heart muscle. If left untreated, this can result in death of heart tissue.

Angina Pectoris

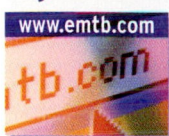

Chest pain does not always mean that a person is having an AMI. When, for a brief period of time, heart tissues are not getting enough oxygen, the pain is called **angina pectoris**, or angina. Although it can result from a spasm of the artery, angina is most often a symptom of atherosclerotic coronary artery disease. Angina occurs when the heart's need for oxygen exceeds its supply, usually during periods of physical or emotional stress when the heart is working hard. A large meal or sudden fear may also trigger an attack. When the demand for extra oxygen goes away (e.g., the person stops exercising), the pain typically goes away.

Angina pain is typically described as crushing, squeezing, or "like somebody standing on my chest." It is usually felt in the midchest, under the sternum. However, it can radiate to the jaw, the arms (frequently the left arm), the midback, or the epigastrium (the upper-middle region of the abdomen). The pain usually lasts from 3 to 8 minutes, rarely longer than 15 minutes. It may be associated with shortness of breath, nausea, or sweating. It disappears promptly with rest, supplemental oxygen, or nitroglycerin, all of which increase the supply of oxygen to the heart. Although angina pectoris is frightening, it does not mean that heart cells are dying, nor does it usually lead to death or permanent heart damage. It is, however, a warning that you and the patient should both take seriously. Even with angina, because oxygen supply to the heart is diminished, the electrical system can be compromised and the person is at risk for significant cardiac rhythm problems.

Keep in mind that it can be very difficult even for doctors in hospitals to distinguish between the pain of angina and the pain of heart attack. You must assume the worst-case scenario, but at the same time, reassure the patient that you will be taking good care of him or her.

Acute Myocardial Infarction

As we have seen, the pain of AMI signals the actual death of cells in the area of the heart where blood flow is obstructed. Once dead, the cells cannot be revived. Instead, they will eventually turn to scar tissue and become a burden to the beating heart. This is why fast action is so critical in treating a heart attack. The sooner the blockage can be cleared, the fewer the cells that may die. About 30 minutes after blood flow is cut off, some heart muscle cells begin to die. After about 2 hours, as many as half of the cells in the area can be dead; in most cases, after 4 to 6 hours, more than 90% of them will be dead. However, studies show that in many cases, opening the coronary artery with either "clot-busting" drugs or angioplasty (mechanical clearing of the artery) can prevent damage to the heart muscle if done within the first hour after the onset of symptoms. Therefore, immediate transport to the emergency department is essential.

AMI is more apt to occur in the larger, thick-walled left ventricle, which needs more blood and oxygen, than in the right ventricle. The left ventricle is larger because it has to send the blood much farther away, to the whole body, than the right ventricle, which has to send blood only to the lungs.

The Pain of Acute Myocardial Infarction

The pain of AMI differs from the pain of angina in three important ways:

- **It may or may not be caused by exertion** but can occur at any time, sometimes when a person is sitting quietly or even sleeping.
- **It does not resolve in a few minutes**; rather, it can last between 30 minutes and several hours.
- **It may or may not be relieved by rest** or nitroglycerin.

Note that not all patients who are having an AMI experience pain or recognize it when it does occur. In fact, about one third of patients never seek medical attention. This can be attributed, in part, to the fact that people are afraid of dying and do not wish to face the possibility that their symptoms may be serious. Middle-aged men, in particular, are likely to minimize their symptoms. However, a few patients, particularly elderly individuals or those with diabetes, do not experience any pain during an AMI. Others may feel only mild discomfort and call it "indigestion."

Therefore, when you are called to a scene where the chief complaint is chest pain, complete a thorough assessment, no matter what the patient says. Any complaint of chest discomfort in a person older than age 21 years is a serious matter. In fact, the best thing you can do is to assume the worst.

Consequences of Acute Myocardial Infarction

Acute myocardial infarction can have three serious consequences:

- Sudden death
- Cardiogenic shock
- Congestive heart failure

Sudden death. Approximately 40% of all patients with AMI never reach the hospital. Sudden death usually is the result of **cardiac arrest**, in which the heart fails to generate an effective blood flow. Although you cannot feel a pulse in someone experiencing cardiac arrest, the heart may still be twitching, though erratically. The heart is using up energy without pumping. Such an abnormality of heart rhythm is a ventricular arrhythmia, known as ventricular fibrillation.

A variety of other lethal and nonlethal arrhythmias may follow AMI, usually within the first hour. In most cases, it is premature ventricular contractions (PVCs), or extra beats in the damaged ventricle. PVCs by themselves are a harmless arrhythmia that is common among healthy, as well as sick, individuals. Other arrhythmias are much more dangerous (Figure 13-11). These include the following:

- **Tachycardia**: Rapid beating of the heart, 100 beats/min or more.

- **Bradycardia**: Unusually slow beating of the heart, 60 beats/min or less.

- **Ventricular tachycardia (VT)**: Rapid heart rhythm, usually at a rate of 150 to 200 beats/min. The electrical activity starts in the ventricle instead of the atrium. This rhythm usually does not allow adequate time between each beat for the left ventricle to fill with blood. Therefore, the patient's blood pressure may fall. He or she may also feel weak or lightheaded or may even become unresponsive. In some cases, the patient may develop worsening chest pain or chest pain that was not there before onset of the arrhythmia. A string of six or more rapid PVCs, back to back, can be called a "run of VT." Most cases of VT will be more sustained and may deteriorate into ventricular fibrillation.

- **Ventricular fibrillation**: Disorganized, ineffective quivering of the ventricles. No blood gets to the body, and the patient usually becomes unconscious within 10 seconds. The only way to treat this arrhythmia is to electrically defibrillate the heart. To **defibrillate** means to shock the heart with a specialized electrical current in an attempt to restore a normal rhythmic beat. Defibrillation is highly successful in terms of saving a life if begun within a minute or two. If a defibrillator is not immediately available, basic CPR must be initiated within the first few minutes, to buy a few more minutes for the defibrillator. Even if CPR is begun right at the time of collapse, chances of survival diminish each minute until defibrillation is accomplished.

If uncorrected, unstable ventricular tachycardia or ventricular fibrillation will eventually lead to **asystole**, the absence of all heart electrical activity. Without CPR, this will occur within 10 to 15 minutes. Because it reflects a long period of ischemia, nearly all patients you find in asystole will die.

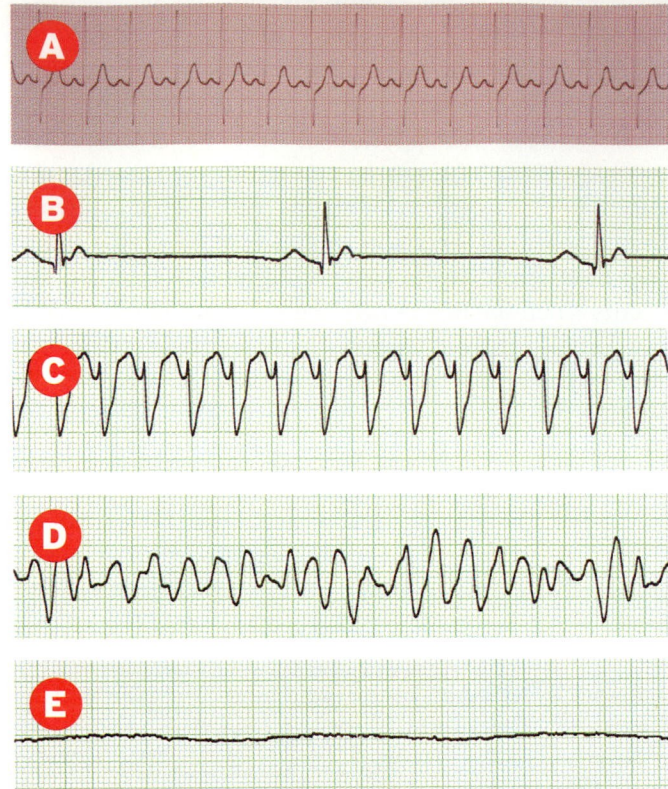

FIGURE 13-11 Common heart arrhythmias **A:** Sinus tachycardia **B:** Bradycardia **C:** Ventricular tachycardia (VT) **D:** Ventricular fibrillation (VF) **E:** Asystole

Cardiogenic shock. Shock is a simple concept but one that few people without medical training really understand. For that reason, Chapter 25 is devoted to a discussion of shock. The discussion of shock in this chapter is limited to that associated with cardiac problems.

For an EMT-B, shock is also a critical concept. Shock is present when body tissues do not get enough oxygen, causing body organs to malfunction. In **cardiogenic shock**, often caused by a heart attack, the problem is that the heart lacks enough power to force the proper volume of blood through the circulatory system. Cardiogenic shock can occur immediately or as late as 24 hours after the onset of the AMI. The various signs and symptoms of cardiogenic shock are produced by the improper functioning of the body's organs. The challenge for you is to recognize shock in its early stages, when treatment is much more successful.

Congestive heart failure. Failure of the heart occurs when the ventricular heart muscle is so damaged that it can no longer keep up with the return flow of blood from the atria. **Congestive heart failure (CHF)** can occur any time after a myocardial infarction, heart valve damage, or longstanding high blood pressure, but it usually happens between the first few hours and the first few days after an acute myocardial infarction.

more about shock

Signs and symptoms.

- One of the first signs of shock is *anxiety or restlessness* as the brain becomes relatively starved for oxygen. The patient may complain of *"air hunger."* Think of the possibility of shock when the patient is yelling, "I can't breathe." Obviously, the patient can breathe, because he or she can talk. However, the patient's brain is sensing that it is not getting enough oxygen.
- As the shock continues, the body tries to send blood to the most important organs, such as the brain and heart, and away from less important organs, such as the skin. Therefore, you may see *pale, clammy skin* in patients with shock.
- As the shock gets worse, the body will attempt to compensate by increasing the amount of blood pumped through the heart. Therefore, the *pulse rate will be higher than normal.* In severe shock the heart rate will usually, but not always, be greater than 120 beats/min.
- Shock can also be characterized by rapid and shallow breathing, nausea and vomiting, and a decrease in body temperature.
- Finally, as the heart and other organs begin to malfunction, the *blood pressure will fall below normal.* A systolic blood pressure less than 90 mm Hg is easy to recognize, but it is a late finding that indicates severe shock. Do not assume that shock is not present just because the blood pressure is normal.

Treatment of patients with shock. Take the following steps when treating patients with signs and symptoms of shock:

1. Position the patient comfortably. Most patients with heart failure will be more comfortable in semi-Fowler's position; however, those with low blood pressure may not tolerate a semi-upright position. These patients may be more comfortable and be more alert in a supine position.
2. Administer oxygen.
3. Assist ventilations as necessary.
4. Provide prompt transport to the emergency department.

more about CHF

Signs and symptoms.

Watch for the following signs and symptoms in a patient you suspect has CHF:

- The patient finds it easier to breathe when sitting up. When the patient is lying down, more blood is returned to the right ventricle and to the lungs, causing further pulmonary congestion.
- Often, the patient is mildly or severely agitated.
- Chest pain may or may not be present.
- The patient often has greatly distended neck veins that do not collapse even when the patient is sitting.
- The patient may have swollen limbs from pedal edema.
- The patient generally will have a high blood pressure, rapid heart rate, and rapid respirations.
- The patient will usually be using accessory breathing muscles of the neck and ribs, reflecting the additional hard work of breathing.
- The fluid surrounding small airways may produce rales, best heard by listening to either side of the patient's chest, about midway down the back. In severe congestive heart failure, these soft sounds can be heard even at the top of the lung.

Once congestive heart failure develops, it can be treated but not cured. Regular use of medications may reduce the severity of the symptoms and allow patients to resume normal activities. However, these patients often become ill again and are frequently admitted to the hospital. Approximately half of them will be dead within 5 years of the onset of symptoms.

Treatment of CHF. Basically, you should treat the patient with congestive heart failure the same way as the patient with chest pain:

1. Take the vital signs, monitor heart rhythm, and give oxygen by nonrebreathing face mask with an oxygen flow of 10 to 15 L/min.
2. Allow the patient to remain sitting in an upright position with the legs down.
3. Be reassuring; many patients with CHF are quite anxious because they cannot breathe.
4. Patients who have had problems with CHF before will usually have specific medications for its treatment. Gather these medications and take them along to the hospital.
5. Nitroglycerin may be of value if the patient's blood pressure is adequate. If the patient has prescribed nitroglycerin, and medical control advises you to do so, you can attempt to administer it sublingually.
6. Prompt transport to the emergency department is essential.

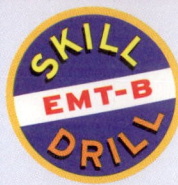

Treating a Conscious Patient with Chest Pain
Figure 13-12

1

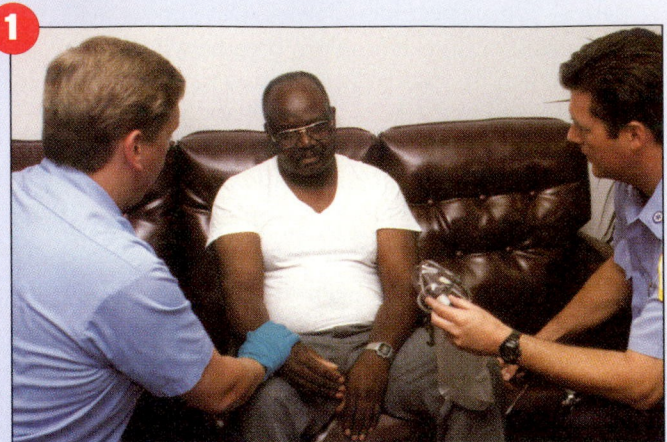

Reassure the patient as you perform the initial assessment and apply oxygen. Ask about the patient's discomfort using OPQRST.

2

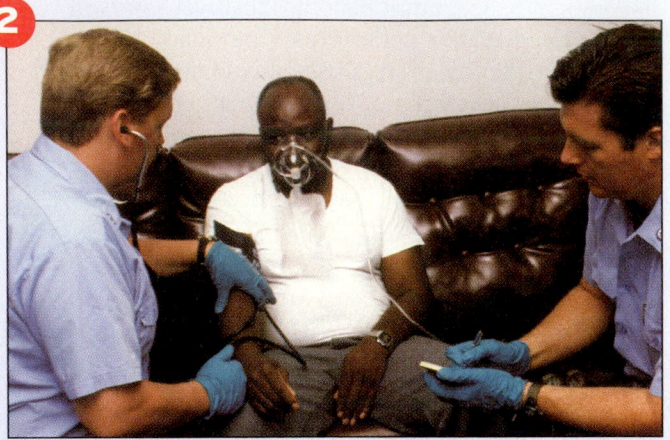

Place the patient in a comfortable position. Measure and record the baseline vital signs.

3

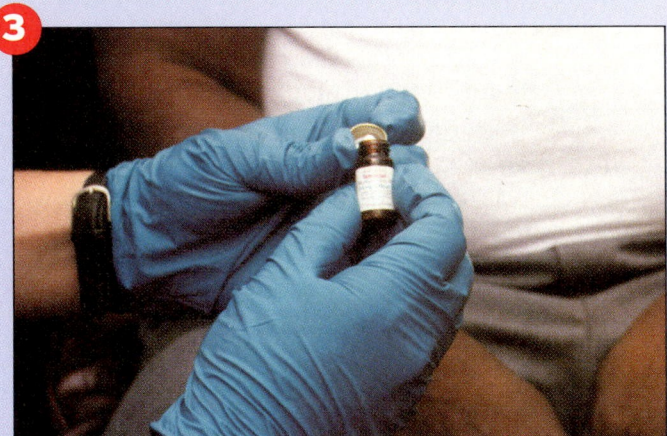

Check medication and expiration date.

4

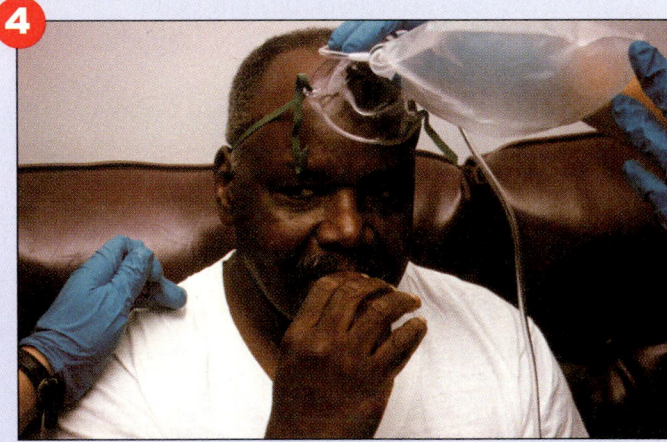

Help to administer nitroglycerin.

5

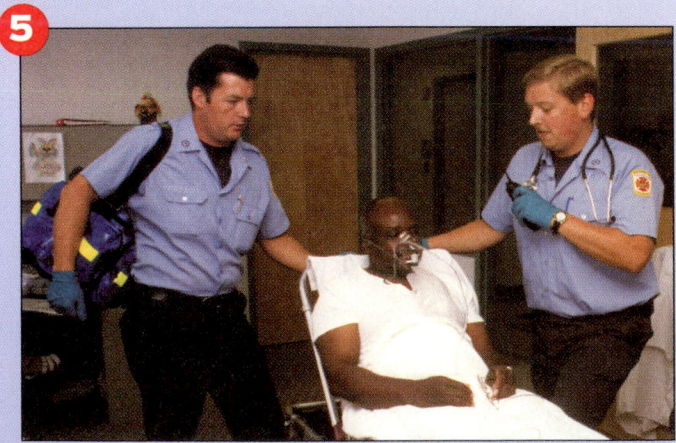

Prepare to transport the patient. Report to medical control.

Just as the pumping function of the left ventricle can be damaged by coronary artery disease, it can also be damaged by diseased heart valves or chronic hypertension. In any of these cases, when the muscle can no longer contract effectively, the heart tries other ways to maintain an adequate cardiac output. Two specific changes in heart function occur: The heart rate increases, and the left ventricle enlarges in an effort to increase the amount of blood pumped each minute.

When these adaptations can no longer make up for the decreased heart function, congestive heart failure eventually develops. It is called "congestive" heart failure because the lungs become congested with fluid once the heart fails to pump the blood effectively. Blood tends to back up in the pulmonary veins, increasing the pressure in the capillaries of the lungs. When the pressure in the capillaries exceeds a certain level, fluid (mostly water) passes through the walls of the capillary vessels and into the alveoli. This condition is called pulmonary edema. It may occur suddenly, as in AMI, or slowly over months, as in chronic congestive heart failure. Sometimes pulmonary edema, in which the patient has pink, frothy sputum and severe dyspnea, is the first sign of AMI.

Fluid also collects elsewhere in the body, usually in the feet and legs. This is called **pedal edema**. The swelling causes relatively few symptoms other than discomfort. However, chronic pedal edema may indicate underlying heart disease even in the absence of pain or other symptoms.

Recognizing and Treating Acute Myocardial Infarction

A patient with an acute myocardial infarction may show any of the following signs and symptoms:

- Sudden onset of weakness, nausea, and sweating without an obvious cause
- Chest pain/discomfort that is often crushing or squeezing and that does not change with each breath
- Pain in the lower jaw, arms, or neck
- Sudden arrhythmia with **syncope** (fainting)
- Pulmonary edema
- Sudden death

Physical Findings of AMI and Cardiac Compromise

The physical findings of AMI vary, depending on the extent and severity of heart muscle damage. The following are the most common:

- **Pulse.** Generally, the pulse rate increases as a normal response to pain, stress, fear, or actual injury to the myocardium. Because arrhythmias are common in AMI, you may feel an irregularity of the pulse.
- **Blood pressure.** Blood pressure may fall as a result of diminished cardiac output and diminished capability of the left ventricle to pump. However, most patients with AMI will have a normal or, most likely, elevated blood pressure.
- **Respiration.** Respirations are usually normal unless the patient has congestive heart failure. In that case, respirations may become rapid and difficult.
- **General appearance.** The patient often appears frightened. There may be nausea, vomiting, and a cold sweat. The skin is often ashen gray because of poor cardiac output and the loss of skin **perfusion**, or blood flow through the tissue. Occasionally, the skin will have a bluish tint, called cyanosis; this is the result of poor oxygenation of the circulating blood. With acute congestive heart failure, you may see swollen neck veins that do not collapse when the patient sits up.
- **Mental state.** Patients with AMI sometimes experience an almost overwhelming feeling of impending doom. If a patient tells you, "I think I am going to die," pay attention.

Approach to the Patient with Chest Pain

All patient assessments begin by determining whether or not the patient is responsive. If the patient is not responsive and weighs at least 55 lb, you must decide whether or not, on the basis of your local protocols, to use the automated external defibrillator (AED) and begin CPR. If the patient weighs less than 55 lb (usually patients younger than age 8 years), use of the AED is not advised. Generally, the AED should be applied if the patient is pulseless and appears to be a candidate for CPR. If the patient is responsive, a series of steps must be taken. Specifically, take the following steps when you are treating a conscious patient who complains of chest discomfort (Figure 13-12):

1. **Reassure the patient** and perform the initial assessment. After confirming consciousness and the chief complaint of chest pain, reassure the patient as you apply oxygen. Act professionally; be calm. Speak to the patient in a normal voice that is neither too loud nor too soft. Let the patient know that trained individuals, including yourself, are present to provide care and that he or she will soon be taken to the hospital. Remember, some patients may act carefree, while others may be demanding.

However, most are still frightened. Your professional attitude may be the single most important factor in winning the patient's cooperation and helping him or her through this event. Patients often have a good idea about what is happening, so do not lie and offer false reassurance. If asked, "Am I having a heart attack?" you can say, "I do not know for sure, but in case you are, we are taking care of you. We are helping you now by giving oxygen, and we will be taking you to the hospital. You are in good hands."

2. **Measure and record the patient's vital signs.** As your partner obtains the history, you should take vital signs, including pulse, blood pressure, and the rate and depth of breathing. You must obtain readings for both systolic and diastolic blood pressures. Note the exact time that the baseline vital signs are measured. Vital signs should be reassessed at least every 5 minutes or as significant changes in the patient's condition occur. It is essential to monitor the patient with an AMI closely, because sudden cardiac arrest is always a risk. If cardiac arrest occurs, you must be ready to begin automated defibrillation or CPR immediately. If an AED is immediately available, use it; if not, do CPR until the AED is available.

3. **Position the patient.** If you suspect AMI, place the patient in a comfortable position, usually sitting up and well supported. Make sure the patient has no difficulty breathing and has no airway obstruction. Try not to allow the patient to exert himself or herself, strain, or walk. If necessary, lift the patient, using care.

4. **Apply oxygen,** if not already done. Unless the patient has severe difficulty breathing, giving oxygen by nasal cannula at 2 to 3 L/min is a reasonable course of action. *However, some protocols call for use of a nonrebreathing mask in all cases to ensure adequate oxygenation.* If the patient is having severe difficulty breathing or shows signs of shock, apply a nonrebreathing mask at 10 to 15 L/min.

5. **Obtain a focused history and physical exam.** Take a brief history from the patient. Friends or family members who are present often have helpful information. Ask them the following questions:
   - Has the patient ever had a heart attack before?
   - Has the patient been told about having previous heart problems?
   - Are there any risk factors for coronary artery disease?

You can use the ABCDEF approach, as follows, to find additional information:

- **A**ge
- **B**lood pressure problems
- **C**igarette smoking history
- **D**iabetes
- **E**levated blood lipids (cholesterol, triglycerides)
- **F**amily history of heart disease

In terms of the physical exam, check the skin color, temperature, and feel of the skin. Is it cool, moist? How do the mucous membranes look? Are they pink, ashen, or bluish? Are the lung sounds clear? Are the neck veins distended?

6. **Ask specific questions** about the patient's chest discomfort. Use the OPQRST mnemonic to determine the type of pain, as follows:
   - **Onset.** Determine what time the discomfort that motivated the call for help began.
   - **Provocation.** Ask what makes the pain or discomfort worse. Is it positional? Does a deep breath or pressing on the chest over the painful spot make it worse? Is the pain steady?
   - **Quality.** Ask what type of pain it is. Let the patient use his or her own words to describe what is happening. Try to avoid supplying the patient with only one option. Do not ask "Does it feel like an elephant is sitting on your chest?" Instead, say "Tell me what the pain feels like." If the patient cannot answer an open-ended question, then provide a list of alternatives. "There are lots of different kinds of pain. Is your pain more like a heaviness, pressure, burning, tearing, dull ache, stabbing, or needlelike pain?"
   - **Radiation.** Ask whether the pain travels to another part of the body.
   - **Severity.** Ask the patient to rate the pain on a simple scale. Often, a scale ranging from 0 to 10 is used, in which 0 represents no pain at all and 10 represents the worst pain imaginable. Do not use the patient's answer to determine whether the pain has a serious cause. Do use it to check whether the pain is getting better or worse; after supplying oxygen or doing something else for the problem, ask the patient to rate the pain again.
   - **Time.** Find out how long the pain lasts when it is present and whether it has been intermittent or continuous.

In addition, ask whether the patient has had the same pain before. If so, ask "Do you take any medications for the pain?" and "Do you have any of the medication with you?" If the patient has had a heart attack or angina before, ask whether this is the same type of pain.

7. **Administer prescribed nitroglycerin.** Nitroglycerin works in most patients within 5 minutes to relieve the pain of angina. Most patients who have been prescribed nitroglycerin carry a supply with them. Trade names of nitroglycerin include Nitrostat and others. Patients take one dose of nitroglycerin under the tongue whenever they have an episode of angina that does not immediately go away with rest. If the pain is still present after 5 minutes, patients are typically instructed by their doctors to take a second dose. If the second dose does not work, most patients are told to take a third dose and then call for EMS. If the patient has not taken all three doses, you can help to administer the medication, if you are allowed to do so by local protocol.

Nitroglycerin comes in several forms: as a small white pill, placed sublingually (under the tongue); as a spray, also taken sublingually; or as a skin patch applied to the chest (Figure 13-13). In any form, the effect is the same. Nitroglycerin relaxes the muscle of blood vessel walls, dilates coronary arteries, increases blood flow and the supply of oxygen to the heart muscle, and decreases the workload of the heart. Nitroglycerin also dilates blood vessels in other parts of the body and can sometimes cause low blood pressure and/or a severe headache. As a result, it also can cause pulse rate increases, usually to make up for any fallen blood pressure. For this reason, you should take the patient's blood pressure within 5 minutes after each dose. If the systolic blood pressure is less than 100 mm Hg, do not give any more medication. Other contraindications to nitroglycerin include the presence of head injury, age younger than 15 years, or maximum prescribed dose already given in the past hour (usually three doses).

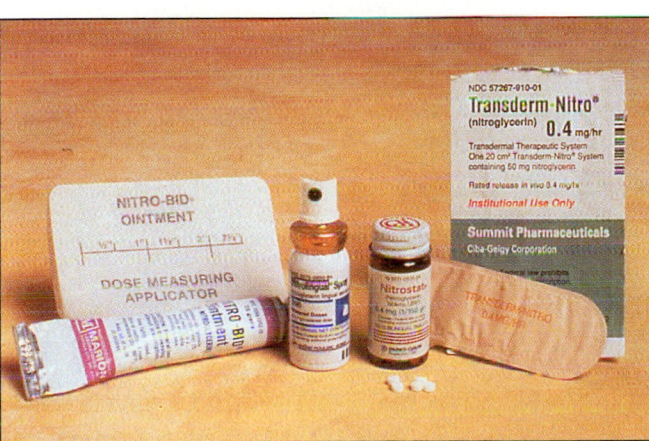

FIGURE 13-13 Nitroglycerin used to treat AMI comes in many forms, including paste, spray, tablets, and skin patches.

If the patient does not have prescribed nitroglycerin, continue with your focused assessment and prepare to transport. Be sure that this process does not consume too much time. Do not delay transport to assist with administration of nitroglycerin. The drug can be given en route. To safely assist the patient with nitroglycerin, you will need to do the following:

- Obtain an order from medical direction either on-line or by prescribed protocol.

- Perform a focused assessment for patients with cardiac problems.

- Measure the patient's blood pressure. Continue with administration of nitroglycerin only if the systolic blood pressure is greater than 100 mm Hg.

- Contact medical control if you have no standing orders.

- Check that you have the right medication, the right patient, and the right delivery route.

- Check the expiration date of the nitroglycerin.

- Question the patient about the last dose he or she took and its effects. Make sure that the patient understands the route of administration.

- When you give a patient nitroglycerin, you should be prepared to have the patient lie down to prevent fainting if the nitroglycerin substantially lowers the patient's blood pressure (the patient gets dizzy or feels faint).

- Ask the patient to lift his or her tongue. Place the tablet or spray the dose underneath the tongue (while wearing gloves), or have the patient do so.

- Have the patient keep his or her mouth closed with the tablet under the tongue until it is dissolved and absorbed. Caution the patient against swallowing the tablet.

- Recheck blood pressure within 2 minutes.

- Record each activity and the time of application.

- Perform continued reassessment.

After giving nitroglycerin, reassess the patient and note the response to the medication. If the chest pain persists and the patient still has a systolic blood pressure greater than 100 mm Hg, then repeat the dose in 3 to 5 minutes as authorized by your medical control. In general, a maximum of three doses of nitroglycerin are given for any one episode of chest pain.

8. **Transport the patient.** Early, prompt transport to the emergency department is critical so that newer treatments, such as clot-busting drugs or angioplasty, can be initiated. To be most effective, these treatments must be started as soon as possible after the onset of the attack. Therefore, alert the emergency department about the status of your patient and your estimated time of arrival. Describe the patient's condition to the emergency department staff on arrival, and leave a copy of the ambulance report form for the patient's hospital records.

9. **Report to medical control.** Report to the hospital by radio or cellular telephone while en route. Give the patient's history, vital signs, repeat vital signs, medications being taken, and the treatment you are giving. Follow the instructions of your medical control physician.

Heart Operations and Pacemakers

Over the last 20 years, hundreds of thousands of open heart operations were performed to bypass damaged segments of coronary arteries in the heart. In the coronary artery bypass graft (CABG) operation, a blood vessel from the chest or leg is sewn directly from the aorta to a coronary artery beyond the point of the obstruction. Other patients may have had a procedure called percutaneous transluminal coronary angioplasty (PTCA), which aims to dilate, rather than bypass, the coronary artery. In this procedure, usually called an angioplasty or balloon angioplasty, a tiny balloon is attached to the end of a long, thin tube. The tube is introduced through the skin into a large vein, usually in the groin, and then threaded into the narrowed coronary artery, with radiographs serving as a guide. Once the balloon is in position inside the coronary artery, it is inflated. The balloon is then deflated, and the tube is removed from the body. Sometimes, a metal mesh called a stent is placed inside the artery either instead of or after the balloon. The stent is left in place permanently to help keep the artery from narrowing again.

You will almost certainly have a patient with previous AMI or angina who has had one of these procedures. Patients who have had a bypass graft will have a long surgical scar on their chest from the operation (Figure 13-14). Patients who have had an angioplasty or coronary artery stent usually will not. However, newer "keyhole" surgical techniques may not produce a large scar. You should not assume that a patient who has a small scar has not had bypass surgery. Chest pain in a patient who has had any of these procedures should be treated the same as chest pain in patients who have not had any heart surgery. In any event, chest pain in a

patient who has undergone either procedure is treated exactly the same as chest pain in a patient who has not. Carry out all the described tasks, and transport the patient promptly to the emergency department of the hospital. If CPR is required, perform it in the usual way, regardless of the scar on the patient's chest. Likewise, if indicated, an AED should be administered as well.

Many people with heart disease in the United States have cardiac pacemakers to maintain a regular cardiac rhythm and rate. Pacemakers are inserted when the electrical control system of the heart is so damaged that it cannot function properly. These battery-powered devices deliver an electrical impulse through wires that are in direct contact with the myocardium. The generating unit is generally placed under a heavy muscle or a fold of skin; it typically resembles a small silver dollar under the skin in the left upper chest (Figure 13-15).

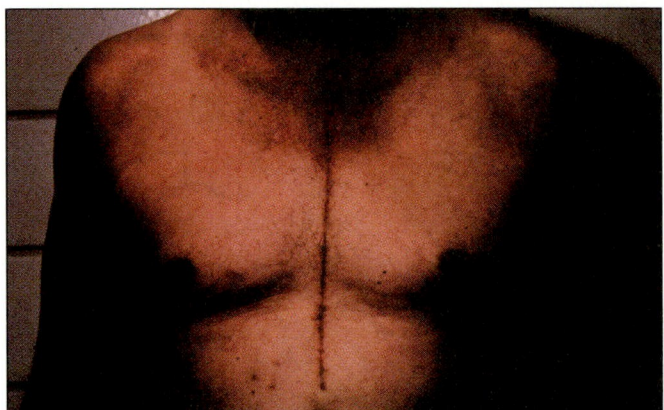

FIGURE 13-14 The surgical scar on the patient's chest implies a previous coronary artery bypass graft (CABG) surgery.

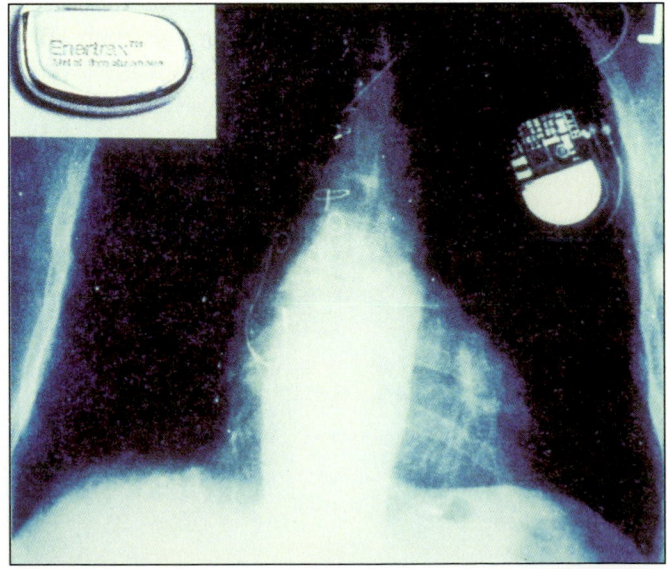

FIGURE 13-15 A pacemaker, which is typically inserted under the skin in the left upper chest, delivers an electrical impulse to regulate heartbeat.

caring for kids

Heart problems in childhood are uncommon and usually congenital, meaning that the patient was born with the problem. In general, your approach to these patients should be the same as that for an adult. You should attempt to reassure the patient. If possible, administer oxygen. If the patient will not wear a face mask, have the parent hold the oxygen in front of the child's face.

Cardiac arrest in younger children is less common than in older children and is usually caused by a breathing problem. The energy levels of the electrical shock delivered by most AEDs are too high for children who are younger than 8 years or weigh less than 55 lb; therefore, do not use an AED on children who fall into either of these categories. Teenagers, who may occasionally have a cardiac arrest related to a heart problem, may benefit from external defibrillation.

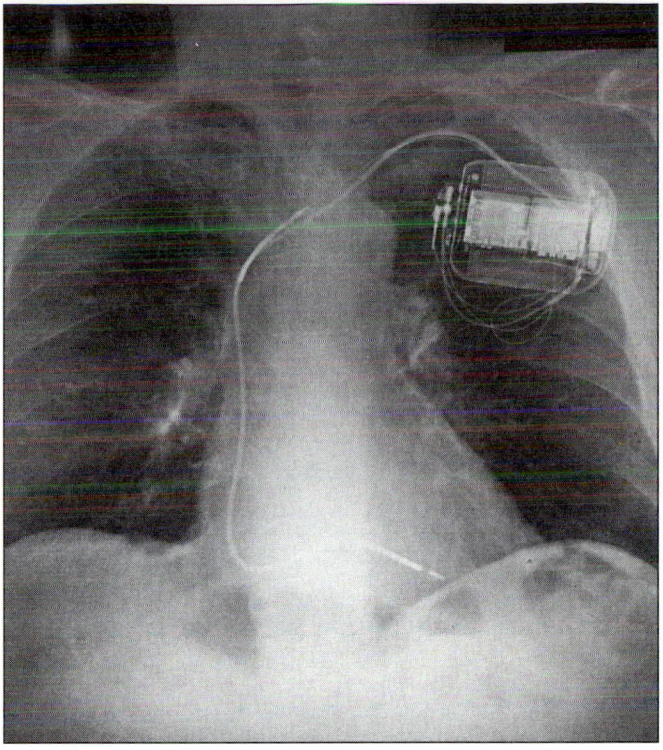

FIGURE 13-16 An AICD is attached directly to the heart and continuously monitors heart rhythm, delivering shocks as needed. The electricity from the AICD is so low that it has no effect on rescuers.

Normally, you do not need to be concerned about problems with pacemakers. Thanks to modern technology, an implanted unit will not require replacement or a battery charge for years. Wires are well protected and rarely broken. In the past, pacemakers sometimes malfunctioned when a patient got too close to an electrical radiation source, such as a microwave oven, but this is no longer the case. Every patient with a pacemaker still should be aware of the precautions, if any, that must be taken to maintain its proper functioning.

If a pacemaker does not function properly, as when the battery wears out, the patient may experience syncope, dizziness, or weakness because of an excessively slow heart rate. The pulse ordinarily will be less than 60 beats/min because the heart is beating without the stimulus of the pacemaker and without the regulation of its own electrical system, which may be damaged. In these circumstances, the heart tends to assume a fixed slow rate that is not fast enough to allow the patient to function normally. A patient with a malfunctioning pacemaker should be promptly transported to the emergency department; repair of the problem may require an operation. When an AED is used, the patches should not be placed directly over the pacemaker. This will ensure a better flow of electricity through the patient's body.

Automatic Implantable Cardiac Defibrillators

More and more patients who survive ventricular fibrillation cardiac arrests have a small automatic implantable cardiac defibrillator (AICD) implanted. Some patients who are at particularly high risk for a cardiac arrest have them as well. These devices are attached directly to the heart and can prolong the lives of certain patients. They continuously monitor the heart rhythm, delivering shocks as needed (Figure 13-16). Regardless of whether a patient having an AMI has an AICD, he or she should be treated like all other AMI patients; treatment should include performing CPR and using an AED if the patient goes into cardiac arrest. Generally, the electricity from an AICD is so low that it will have no effect on rescuers and therefore should not be of concern to you.

Many people with heart disease in the United States have cardiac pacemakers to maintain a regular cardiac rhythm and rate.

Automated External Defibrillation

In the late 1970s and early 1980s, scientists developed a small computer that could analyze electrical signals from the heart and determine when ventricular fibrillation was taking place. This development, along with improved battery technology, made possible the automated portable defibrillator, which can automatically administer an electrical shock to the heart when needed.

AED machines come in two basic forms (Figure 13-17). The automated defibrillator needs an operator to perform just two tasks: applying the pads and turning the machine on. The semi-automated defibrillator requires some operator interaction. All semi-automated defibrillators have two buttons: one that turns the machine on and one that delivers the electrical shock. Most automated defibrillators use a computer voice synthesizer to advise the EMT which steps to take on the basis of the AED's analysis. Some models have a third button that tells the computer to analyze the heart's electrical rhythm; other models start doing this as soon as they are turned on. In the United States, the vast majority of the AEDs are semi-automated.

The computer inside the AED is specially programmed to recognize rhythms that require defibrillation to correct, most commonly ventricular fibrillation. The current programs are extremely accurate. It would be extremely rare for them to recommend a shock when a shock would not be called for, and they rarely fail to recommend one when it would be helpful. Therefore, if the AED recommends a shock, you can believe that it is indicated.

When an error does occur, it is usually the operator's fault. The most common error is not having a charged battery. To avoid this problem, many defibrillator companies have built smarter machines that will warn the operator that the battery is unlikely to work. However, some of the older models do not have this feature. You should check the AED daily and exercise the battery as often as the manufacturer recommends.

Another error occurs when the AED is applied to a patient who is moving. The computer may be unable to tell the difference between electrical signals from the heart and electrical signals from the arms and chest muscles that are moving. The way to avoid this error is to apply the AED only to pulseless, unresponsive patients and to stay clear of the patient (do not touch the patient) during analysis and shock.

A third error can occur when the AED is applied to a responsive patient with a rapid heart rate. Most computers identify a regular rhythm faster than 150 or 180 beats/min as ventricular tachycardia, which should be shocked. Sometimes, though, a patient has another heart rhythm that should not be shocked but that is fast enough to confuse the computer. Again, to avoid this problem, you should apply the AED only to unresponsive patients with no pulse.

Automated external defibrillation offers the EMT-B a number of advantages. First, of course, the machine is fast, and it delivers the most important treatment for the patient in ventricular fibrillation: an electrical shock. It can be delivered within 1 minute of the EMT's arrival at the patient's side. Second, you will find that using an AED is easier than performing CPR. ALS

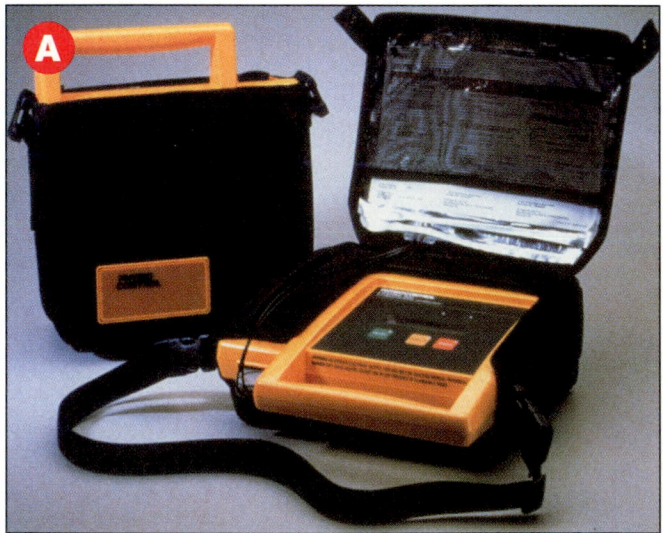
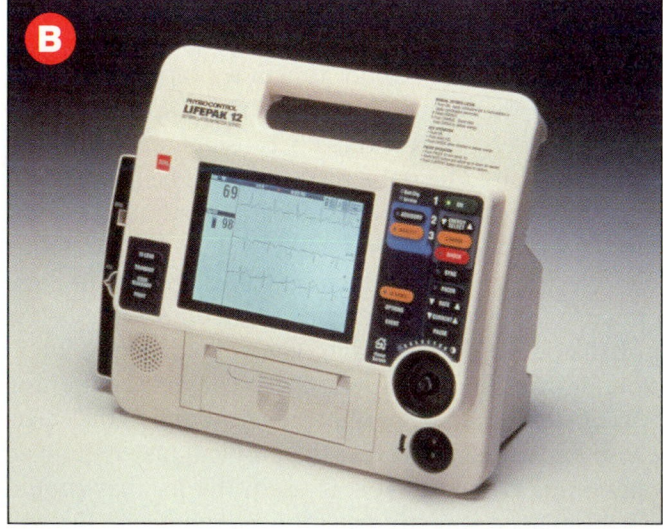

FIGURE 13-17 AEDs come in two forms. **A:** Automated. **B:** Semiautomated.

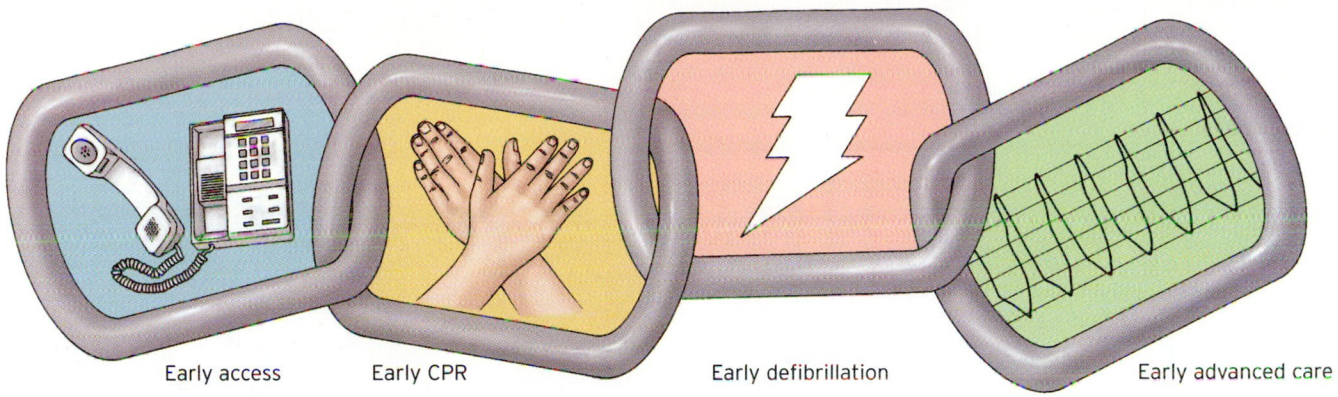

Early access   Early CPR   Early defibrillation   Early advanced care

FIGURE 13-18 The four links of the American Heart Association's chain of survival.

> You should check the AED daily and exercise the battery as often as the manufacturer recommends.

The four main links in the chain of survival are as follows (Figure 13-18):

- Recognition of early warning signs and immediate activation of EMS

- Immediate CPR

- Early defibrillation

- Early advanced care, such as on-scene intubation, and certain intravenous medications followed by expert follow-up care in the hospital

providers do not have to be on the scene to provide this definitive care.

Current AEDs offer two other advantages. The shock can be given through remote, adhesive defibrillator pads, which are safer for you than paddles. Also, the pad area is larger than paddles, which means that the transmission of electricity is more efficient. Usually, there are pictures on the pads to remind you where they go on the patient's chest.

Not all patients in cardiac arrest require an electrical shock. Although all patients in cardiac arrest should be analyzed with an AED, some do not have shockable rhythms (eg, pulseless electrical activity and asystole). Asystole (flatline) indicates that no electrical activity remains. Pulseless electrical activity usually refers to a state of cardiac arrest despite an organized electrical complex.

Rationale for Early Defibrillation

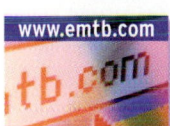

Few patients who experience sudden cardiac arrest outside of a hospital survive unless a rapid sequence of events takes place. The chain of survival is a way of describing the ideal sequence of events that can take place when such an arrest occurs.

If any one of the links in the chain is absent, the patient is more likely to die. For example, few patients benefit from defibrillation when more than 10 minutes elapse before administration of the first shock or if CPR is not performed in the first 2 to 3 minutes. If all links in the chain are strong, the patient has the best possible chance of survival.

CPR helps patients in cardiac arrest because it prolongs the period of time during which defibrillation can be effective. Rapid defibrillation has successfully resuscitated many patients with cardiac arrest from ventricular fibrillation. However, defibrillation works best if it takes place within 2 minutes of the onset of the cardiac arrest. To try to achieve better survival rates among cardiac arrest victims, many communities are exploring the idea that nontraditional first responders should be trained to administer early defibrillation. These responders would include police officers, security personnel, lifeguards, maintenance workers, and flight attendants. As an EMT-B, you should support these efforts to shorten the time interval until defibrillation. Remember, seconds really do matter when the patient is in cardiac arrest.

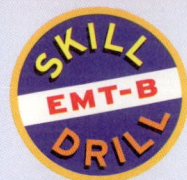

Performing AED and CPR

Figure 13-19

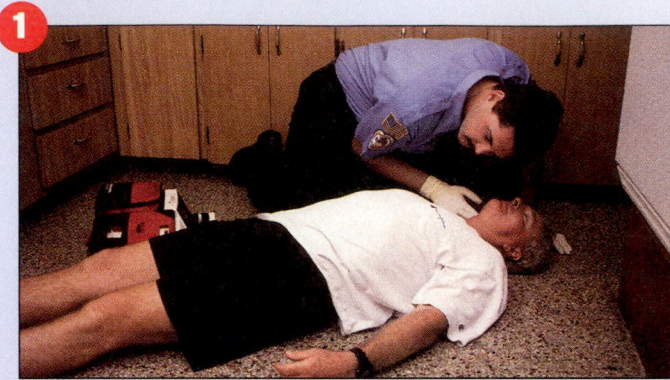

1 Perform an initial assessment, checking for breathing and pulselessness. If the patient is unresponsive and not breathing (or taking gasping breaths), one person should prepare to apply the AED. The other person should begin CPR.

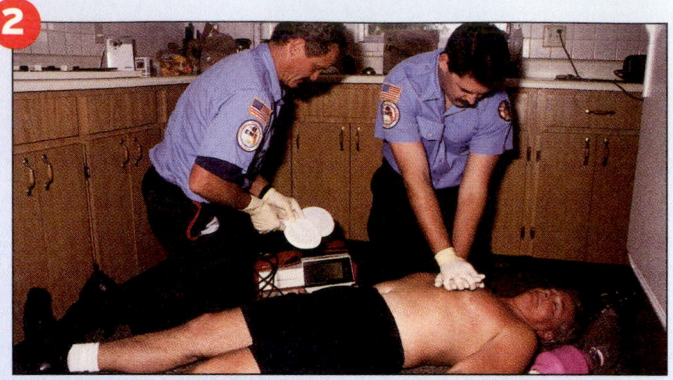

2 As your partner performs CPR, prepare to apply the AED pads.

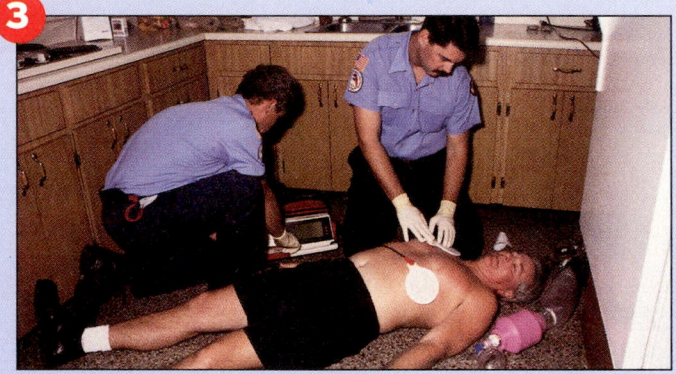

3 Stop CPR. Apply the AED pads; one just right of the sternum and below the clavicle, the other on the left side of the chest, 2" to 3" below the armpit.

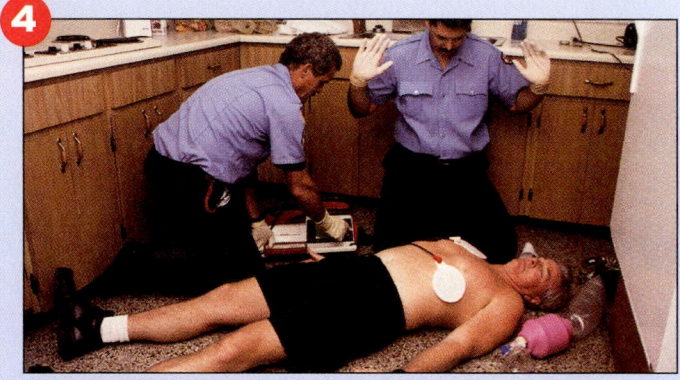

4 Say "Clear the patient," and push the analyze button, if there is one. If the machine advises shock, push the shock button. Repeat this sequence up to three times.

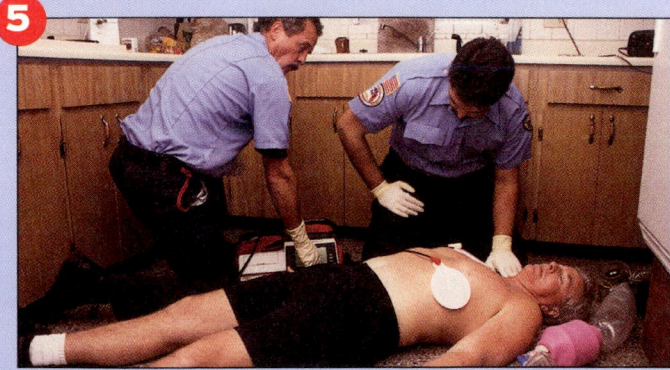

5 Check for a pulse. If the pulse has resumed, check for the patient's breathing.

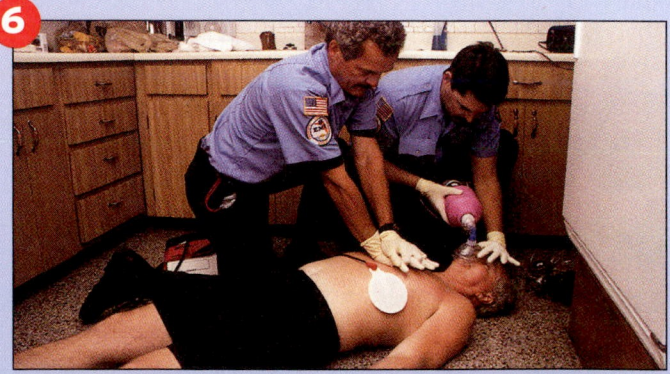

6 If the patient has no pulse, resume CPR for 1 minute, then stop CPR. Check for pulse, and if absent, then push the analyze button again. If needed, repeat one cycle of three stacked shocks, then prepare the patient for transport and report to medical control.

Integrating the AED and CPR

Since most cardiac arrests occur in the home, a bystander at the scene may already have started CPR before you arrive. For this reason, you must know how to work the AED into the CPR sequence. Remember that the AED is not very complex; it may not be able to distinguish other movements from ventricular fibrillation. Therefore, do *not* touch the patient while the AED is analyzing the heart rhythm and delivering shocks. Stop CPR, and let the AED do its job. CPR may be stopped for up to 90 seconds if three shocks are necessary. This is entirely proper; defibrillation is more important than CPR when ventricular fibrillation is present.

Prepare with BSI techniques while you are en route to the scene. Upon arrival at the scene, make sure that the scene is safe for you and your partner to enter. Ask any bystanders or first responders who are performing CPR to stop so that you can apply the AED and defibrillate the patient. Take the following steps if allowed by your local protocols (Figure 13-19):

1. Arrive on scene and perform your initial assessment. Assess responsiveness. If the patient is responsive, do not apply the AED.

2. Stop CPR if it is in progress.

3. Verify pulselessness and apnea. Check for breathing and a pulse even if the patient appears to be breathing.

4. If the patient is unresponsive and not breathing or is breathing agonally (slow, gasping breaths), give two quick breaths using a pocket mask or other quick airway adjunct.

5. Have your partner resume CPR.

6. If there is no pulse and an AED is close at hand, use the AED.

7. Remove clothing from the patient's chest area. Apply the pads to the chest: one just to the right of the breastbone (sternum) just below the collarbone (clavicle), the other on the left chest with the top of the pad 2" to 3" below the armpit. Ensure that the pads are attached to the wires leading up to the AED (and that they are attached to the AED in some models).

8. Turn on the machine and begin your narrative, if the machine has a tape recorder.

9. Stop CPR.

10. State aloud, "Clear the patient," and ensure that no one is touching the patient.

11. Push the analyze button, if there is one.

12. Wait for the computer in the AED to determine whether a shockable rhythm is present.

13. If a shock is not needed, go to step 18 (CPR only). If a shock is advised, make sure that no one is touching the patient. When the area is clear, push the shock button (in a semi-automated device).

14. After the shock is given, most AEDs will automatically reanalyze the rhythm; if not, push the analyze button again.

15. If the machine advises a shock, deliver a second shock.

16. Reanalyze the rhythm.

17. If the machine advises a shock, deliver a third shock.

18. Check for a pulse to see whether the patient now has a heart rhythm.

19. If the patient has a pulse, check the patient's breathing.

20. If the patient is breathing adequately, give the patient oxygen via nonrebreathing mask and transport. If the patient is not breathing adequately, use necessary airway adjuncts and proper positioning of the head and jaw to ensure an open airway. Provide artificial ventilations with high-concentration oxygen and transport.

21. If the patient has no pulse, perform 1 minute of CPR.

22. After 1 minute of CPR, make sure no one is touching the patient. Push the analyze button again (as applicable).

23. If necessary, repeat one cycle of up to three stacked shocks.

24. Transport and check with medical control.

25. Continue to support breathing until the patient begins to breathe normally.

If, after any rhythm analysis, the AED advises no shock, check the patient's pulse. If the patient has a pulse, check the patient's breathing. If the patient is breathing adequately, give high-concentration oxygen via nonrebreathing mask and transport. If the patient is not breathing adequately, provide artificial ventilations with high-concentration oxygen via a BVM device or oxygen-powered device, and transport. Ensure that appropriate airway techniques are used at all times.

If the patient has no pulse, resume CPR for 1 minute, then have the AED reanalyze the heart rhythm. If the AED advises shock, deliver up to two sets of three stacked shocks. Separate each set of three shocks with 1 minute of CPR.

If the AED advises no shock and the patient has no pulse, resume CPR for 1 minute, then stop and reanalyze the heart rhythm for a third time. If the AED advises shock, deliver up to two sets of three stacked shocks with 1 minute of CPR between the two sets. If the AED still advises no shock, check with medical control, resume CPR, and transport.

If you are the only rescuer at the scene and you have an AED, take the following steps:

1. Perform an initial assessment. Assess responsiveness. If the patient is responsive, do not apply the AED.

2. Verify that the patient has no pulse and is not breathing (or is breathing with inadequate gasping breaths).

3. If the patient is not breathing or is gasping, give two quick breaths using a pocket mask or other quick airway adjunct.

4. Remove clothing from the patient's chest area. Apply one pad just to the right of the breastbone (sternum), just below the collarbone (clavicle), and the other on the left chest with the top of the pad 2" to 3" below the armpit.

5. Turn on the defibrillator power.

6. Push the analyze button, if there is one.

7. Deliver up to three shocks, if indicated.

8. Follow your local protocol. If the AED indicates no need for shocks, provide CPR.

If another person is available who knows CPR, ask for help. You will perform the steps in the same order. The only difference is that the other person can continue CPR while you are getting the AED out and hooked up to the patient.

After AED Shocks

The care of the patient after the AED delivers its shock depends on your location and EMS system; therefore, you should follow your local protocols. After the AED protocol is completed, the patient is likely to have had one of the following occur:

- Regained a pulse

- No pulse, and the AED indicates that no shock advised

- No pulse, and the AED indicates that a shock is advised

If you got to the patient quickly and the patient started breathing on his or her own, administer oxygen by nonrebreathing face mask with the oxygen flow set to 10 to 15 L/min. Check the patient's pulse, using the carotid artery, if possible. If the patient has a pulse but is not breathing adequately, assist ventilations, using a BVM device with high-flow oxygen. Prepare for transport, keeping the AED attached to the patient. Recheck the pulse frequently, at least every 30 seconds. In applicable devices, push the analyze button on the AED if the pulse is lost. Commonly, patients who are successfully defibrillated by AED will develop a normal heart rhythm for a while. However, since the heart still is not receiving optimal amounts of oxygen, ventricular fibrillation will often recur.

Patients who fail to regain a pulse on the scene of the cardiac arrest usually do not do well. What you do with these patients will, again, depend on your EMS system. Whether you should transport the patient or wait for ALS to arrive should be in the local protocols established by medical direction. If paramedics or another advanced life support service is responding to the scene, the best option usually is to stay where you are and continue the sequence of shocks and CPR. Administering CPR while patients are being moved or transported is usually not effective. Patients' best chance of survival is if they are resuscitated where they are found, unless the location is unsafe.

If an advanced life support service is not responding to the scene and your local protocols agree, you should begin transport when one of the following occurs:

- The patient regains a pulse.

- Six shocks are delivered.

- The machine gives three consecutive messages (separated by one minute of CPR) that no shock is advised.

If you must transport a patient while performing CPR, you need a plan for managing the patient in the ambulance. Ideally, you will have two EMT-Bs in the patient compartment while a third drives. After six shocks on the scene, prepare for transport. You may deliver additional shocks at the scene or en route with the approval of medical control. Keep in mind that AEDs cannot analyze rhythm while the vehicle is in motion. Nor is it as safe to defibrillate in a moving ambulance. Therefore, you should come to a complete stop if more shocks are ordered. Be sure to memorize the protocol of your EMS service so that you will know how to manage patients in this situation.

Cardiac Arrest During Transport

If you are traveling to the hospital with an unconscious patient, check the pulse at least every 30 seconds. If a pulse is not present, take the following steps:

1. Stop the vehicle.

2. If the AED is not immediately ready, perform CPR until it is ready.

3. Analyze the rhythm.

4. Deliver the shock, if indicated.

5. Continue resuscitation according to your local protocol.

If you are en route with a conscious patient who is having chest pain and who becomes unconscious, take the following steps:

1. Check for a pulse.

2. Stop the vehicle.

3. If the AED is not immediately ready, perform CPR until it is ready.

4. Analyze the rhythm.

5. Deliver up to three shocks, if indicated.

6. Continue resuscitation according to your local protocol. If a "no shock" message is given and no pulse is present, you should start or resume CPR, then transport. If the AED advises you to shock, give up to two sets of three stacked shocks and continue to transport the patient.

Coordination with ALS

The time to defibrillation is critical to survival after cardiac arrest. As an EMT-B equipped with an AED, you

AED operational tips

- One EMT-B operates the defibrillator while another does CPR.

- Defibrillation comes first. Do not hook up oxygen or do anything else that delays analysis of rhythm or defibrillation.

- Be familiar with the AED device used by your EMS system.

- Avoid all contact with the patient during analysis of the rhythm.

- State, "Clear the patient" before shocking. Another popular phrase is "I'm clear, you're clear, we're all clear" before delivering shocks.

- In applicable models of AEDs, check the batteries at the beginning of your shift; carry an extra charged battery with your AED.

- Do not use an AED for cardiac arrest in children younger than age 8 years (i.e., those who weigh less than 55 lb).

- Unless indicated otherwise by local protocol, you do not need to perform pulse checks during rhythm analysis; typically, there will be no pulse check between stacked shocks 1 and 2 and stacked shocks 2 and 3.

- Continued airway maintenance and artificial ventilation are of prime importance.

have the one tool that the dying patient in ventricular fibrillation needs most. Furthermore, it is very hard to hurt someone with an AED. Therefore, if you have an AED available, do not wait for the paramedics to arrive to administer a shock. Waiting might seem like a good idea. It is not. It is throwing away the patient's best chance for survival.

If the patient is unresponsive and does not have a pulse, apply the AED and push the analyze button (if there is one) as quickly as you can. Notify the ALS personnel as soon as possible after you recognize a cardiac arrest, but do not delay defibrillation. After the paramedics arrive at the scene, you should interact with them according to your local protocols.

AUTOMATED EXTERNAL DEFIBRILLATOR
Daily/Shift Inspection Checklist

Serial # _____   Date _____   Time _____

Model # _____   Inspected by _____

Item	Pass	Fail
Exterior/Cables:		
Nothing stored on top of unit		
Carry case intact and clean		
Exterior/LCD screen clean and undamaged		
Cables/connectors clean and undamaged		
Cables securely attached to unit		
Batteries:		
Unit charger is plugged in and operational (if applicable)		
Fully charged battery in unit		
Fully charged spare battery		
Spare battery charger plugged in and operational (if applicable)		
Valid expiration date on both batteries		
Supplies:		
Two sets of electrodes		
Electrodes in sealed packages with valid expiration dates		
Razor		
Hand towel		
Alcohol wipes		
Memory/voice recording device—module, card, microcassette		
Manual override—module, key (if applicable)		
Printer paper (if applicable)		
Operation:		
Unit self-test per manufacturer's recommendation/instructions		
Display (if applicable)		
Visual indicators		
Verbal prompts		
Printer (if applicable)		
Attach AED to simulator/tester:		
Recognizes shockable rhythm		
Charges to correct energy level within manufacturer's specifications		
Delivers charge		
Recognizes nonshockable rhythm		
Manual override system in working order (if applicable)		

Signature:

FIGURE 13-20 A sample daily checklist for the AED.

Safety Considerations

As the operator of the AED, you are responsible for making sure that the electricity injures no one, including yourself. As long as you place the pads in the correct position and make sure no one is touching the patient, you should be safe. Do not defibrillate a patient whose chest is under water. While there is some danger to you if you are also in the water, there is another problem. Electricity follows the path of least resistance; instead of traveling between the pads and through the patient's heart, it will diffuse into the water. Therefore, the heart will not receive enough electricity to cause defibrillation. You can defibrillate a soaking wet patient, but try first to dry the patient's chest. Do not defibrillate someone who is touching metal that others are touching, and carefully remove a nitroglycerin patch from a patient's chest before defibrillation to prevent ignition of the patch.

AED Maintenance

One of your primary missions as an EMT-B is to deliver an electrical shock to a patient in ventricular fibrillation. To accomplish this mission, you need to have a *working* defibrillator. You must become familiar with the maintenance procedures required for the brand of AED your service uses. Read the operator's manual (Figure 13-20). If your defibrillator does not work on the scene, someone will want to know what went wrong. That person may be your system's administrator, your medical director, the local newspaper reporter, or the family's attorney. You will be asked to show proof that you maintained the defibrillator properly.

The main legal risk in using the AED is failing to deliver a shock when one was needed. The most common reason for this failure is that the battery did not work, usually because it was not properly maintained. Another problem is operator error. This means not pushing the analyze or shock buttons when the machine advises you to do so or failing to apply the AED to a patient in cardiac arrest. Of course, the AED is like any other manufactured item. It can fail, although this is rare. Ideally, you will encounter any such failure while doing routine maintenance, not while caring for a patient in cardiac arrest. Check your equipment, including your AED, at the beginning of each shift. Ask the manufacturer for a checklist of items that should be checked daily, weekly, or less often.

If you do have an AED failure while caring for a patient, you must report that problem to the manufacturer and to the U.S. Food and Drug Administration (FDA). Be sure to follow your EMS procedures for notifying these organizations.

Medical Direction

Defibrillation of the heart is a medical procedure. While AEDs have made the process of delivering electricity much simpler, there is still a benefit in having a physician's help. The medical director of your service should help to teach you how to use the AED, attending some or all of the training sessions. At the very least, he or she should approve the written protocol that you will follow in caring for patients in cardiac arrest. In most states, successful completion of AED training in an EMT-B course is not permitted without approval by state laws, rules, and local medical direction authority.

There should be a review of each incident in which the AED is used. After returning from the hospital or the scene, sit down with the rest of the team and go over what happened. What went particularly well? What could have gone better? Decide what you will do differently the next time. This discussion will help all members of the team to learn from the incident. Review such events by using the written report, any voice-ECG tape recorder, and the device's solid-state memory modules and magnetic tape recordings, if applicable.

caring for the elderly

Like the other body systems, the cardiovascular system undergoes changes as we get older. The heart, like other major organs, will show the effects of aging. As the heart's muscle mass and tone decrease, the amount of blood pumped out of the heart per beat is decreased. The residual (reserve) capacity of the heart is also reduced; therefore, when the vital organs of the body need additional blood flow, the heart cannot meet the need. When blood flow to the tissues is decreased, the organs suffer. If blood flow to the brain is inadequate, the patient may complain of weakness, fatigue, or dizziness and may develop syncope (fainting). If the patient fatigues during your assessment, allowing the patient to rest may allow better tissue perfusion, since the physical demands on the heart will be reduced.

The power to the heart muscle can fail. The heart runs on electricity and has its own electrical system. Under normal conditions, electrical impulses travel throughout the heart resulting in the contraction of the heart muscle and the pumping of blood from the heart's chambers. With aging, the electrical system can deteriorate, causing the heart's contraction to weaken or, if blood flow to the heart muscle is affected, extra beats to form. With a decreased strength of contraction, the heartbeat is weaker and blood flow to the tissues is reduced. If extra beats are allowed to form, the patient's heart rhythm will be irregular. While some irregular heart rhythms are acceptable, others can be potentially lethal.

The arteries are also affected by aging. Arteriosclerosis (hardening of the arteries) can develop, affecting perfusion of the tissues. There is an increased chance of heart attack or stroke from decreased blood flow or plaque formation (arteriosclerosis) in the narrowed arteries.

Patients with diabetes can experience reduced circulation to the hands and feet; this makes peripheral pulses harder to detect. It also puts the hands and feet at particular risk for developing infection or ulcerations.

In some older patients, particularly diabetics, chest pain is absent, and the clinical picture can be confused with other, noncardiac conditions.

The cardiovascular system is affected by aging. You should be aware of the changes, seeking to determine what is normal versus what is chronic for the patient as opposed to what is an acute condition. Sometimes, the weakening of the heart muscle, the deterioration of its electrical system, and the hardening of the arteries make the task of assessing and caring for the elderly patient more difficult.

There should also be a review of the incident by your service's medical director or quality improvement officer. Quality improvement involves both individuals using AEDs and the responsible EMS system managers. This review should focus on speed of defibrillation, that is, the interval between the moment the call for help was received in the primary public safety answering point (PSAP) and the moment the first shock was delivered. A typical standard used states that, at a minimum, your service should deliver the first shock to the patient within 8 minutes in more than 90% of cases, preferably sooner. If you have reached this benchmark, you should continue to work to improve your record. Few systems will achieve the ultimate goal: shocking 100% of patients within 1 minute of the call. However, all systems can try. Mandatory continuing education with skill competency review is generally required for EMS providers, with a continuing competency skill review every 3 to 6 months for the EMT-B. Most systems allow 90 days between practice drills to reassess competency in AED use.

> Quality improvement involves both individuals using AEDs and the responsible EMS system managers.

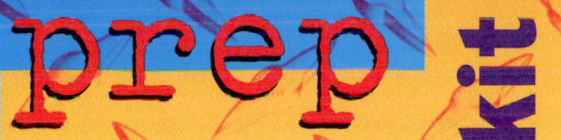

ready for review

The heart is divided down the middle into two sides, right and left, each with an upper chamber called the atrium and a lower chamber called the ventricle. The largest of the four heart valves that keep blood moving through the circulatory system in the proper direction is the aortic valve, which lies between the left ventricle and the aorta, the body's main artery. The heart's electrical system controls heart rate and guarantees that the atria and ventricles work together.

During periods of exertion or stress, the myocardium requires more oxygen. This is supplied by dilation of the coronary arteries, which increases blood flow. Common places to feel for a pulse include the carotid, femoral, brachial, radial, ulnar, posterior tibial, and dorsalis pedis arteries.

Low blood flow is usually caused by coronary artery atherosclerosis, a disease in which cholesterol plaques build up inside blood vessels, eventually occluding them. Occasionally, a brittle plaque will crack, causing a blood clot to form. Heart tissue downstream suffers from a lack of oxygen and, within 30 minutes, will begin to die. This is called an acute myocardial infarction (AMI), or heart attack. Heart tissues that are not getting enough oxygen but are not yet dying can cause pain called angina. The pain of AMI is different from the pain of angina in that it can come at any time, not just with exertion; it lasts up to several hours, rather than just a few moments; and it is not relieved by rest or nitroglycerin. In addition to crushing chest pain, signs of AMI include sudden onset of weakness, nausea, and sweating; sudden arrhythmia; pulmonary edema; and even sudden death.

Heart attacks can have three serious consequences. One is sudden death, usually the result of cardiac arrest caused by abnormal heart rhythms called arrhythmias. These include tachycardia, bradycardia, ventricular tachycardia, and, most commonly, ventricular fibrillation. The second consequence is cardiogenic shock, in which body organs, starved for oxygen, malfunction; symptoms include restlessness; anxiety; pale, clammy skin; pulse rate higher than normal; and blood pressure lower than normal. Patients with these symptoms should receive oxygen, assisted ventilations as needed, and immediate transport.

The third consequence of AMI is congestive heart failure, in which damaged heart muscle can no longer contract effectively enough to pump blood through the system. The lungs become congested with fluid, breathing becomes difficult, the heart rate increases, and the left ventricle enlarges. Signs include swollen limbs from pedal edema, high blood pressure, rapid heart rate and respirations, rales, and sometimes the pink sputum and dyspnea of pulmonary edema. Treat a patient with CHF as you would a patient with chest pain. Monitor the heart rhythm, give oxygen via nonrebreathing face mask, allow the patient to remain sitting up, and transport promptly.

In treating patients with chest pain, take a medical history, following the OPQRST mnemonic to understand the pain; measure and record vital signs; put the patient in a comfortable position, usually sitting up; administer prescribed nitroglycerin and oxygen; and transport the patient, reporting to medical control as you do. If a patient is not responsive and weighs at least 55 lb, you must decide whether to use the automated external defibrillator (AED); if the patient weighs less than 55 lb, you may have to begin CPR directly.

The fully automated AED needs an operator to perform two tasks: apply the pads to the patient's chest and turn the machine on; the semi-automated models also require the operator to press a button to analyze the heart's electrical rhythm and/or deliver the shock. The computer inside the AED recognizes rhythms that require shocking and will not mislead you. The three most common errors in using certain AEDs are failure to keep a charged battery in the machine, applying the AED to a patient who is moving, and applying the AED to a responsive patient with a rapid heart rate. Do not touch the patient while the AED is analyzing the heart rhythm or delivering shocks. In integrating use of the AED and CPR, you should perform CPR only after giving up to three successful shocks, if these are all needed. If you still cannot get a pulse, follow local protocol. If advanced life support service is responding to the scene, stay where you are and continue the sequence of shocks and CPR. Do not wait for ALS to arrive to begin defibrillation. If ALS is not responding, begin transport after six shocks or after the machine gives three consecutive messages that no shock is advised. If an unconscious patient has a pulse but loses it during transport, you must stop the vehicle, start CPR if the defibrillator is not ready, then apply the AED; if a conscious patient becomes unconscious, do the same thing, delivering up to three shocks if necessary, then continue to transport.

At a minimum, your service should try to deliver the first shock to a patient within 8 minutes of the call for help in 90% of cases, preferably sooner.

The chain of survival, which is the sequence of events that must happen for a patient with cardiac arrest to have the best chance of survival, includes recognition of early warning signs and immediate activation of EMS, immediate CPR by bystanders, early defibrillation, and early advanced care. Seconds count at every stage.

prep kit

vital vocabulary

www.emtb.com

acute myocardial infarction (AMI) Heart attack; death of the heart muscle following obstruction of blood flow to it. Acute in this context means "new" or "happening right now."

angina pectoris Transient (short-lived) chest discomfort caused by partial or temporary blockage of blood flow to the heart muscle.

anterior A directional term meaning "front."

aorta The main artery, which receives blood from the left ventricle and delivers it to all the other arteries that carry blood to the tissues of the body.

aortic valve A structure that lies between the left ventricle and the aorta. It keeps blood from flowing back into the left ventricle after the left ventricle ejects its blood into the aorta. It is one of four heart valves that ensure that blood flows in only one direction.

arrhythmia An irregular or abnormal heart rhythm.

atherosclerosis A disorder in which cholesterol and calcium build up inside the walls of blood vessels, eventually leading to partial or complete blockage of blood flow.

asystole Complete absence of heart electrical activity.

atrium One of two (right and left) upper chambers of the heart. The right atrium receives blood from the vena cava and delivers it to the right ventricle, which, in turn, pumps blood into the blood vessels of the lungs. The left atrium receives blood from pulmonary veins and delivers it to the left ventricle.

bradycardia Slow heart rate, less than 60 beats/min.

cardiac arrest A state in which the heart fails to generate an effective and detectable blood flow; pulses are not palpable in cardiac arrest, even if muscular and electrical activity continues in the heart.

cardiogenic shock A state in which not enough oxygen is delivered to the tissues of the body, caused by low output of blood from the heart. It can be a severe complication of a large acute myocardial infarction, as well as other conditions.

congestive heart failure (CHF) A disorder in which the heart loses part of its ability to effectively pump blood, usually as a result of damage to the heart muscle and usually resulting in a backup of fluid into the lungs.

coronary artery A blood vessel that carries blood and nutrients to the heart muscle.

defibrillate To shock a fibrillating (chaotically beating) heart with specialized electrical current in an attempt to restore a normal rhythmic beat.

dilation Widening of a tubular structure such as a coronary artery.

fibrillation Completely disorganized, ineffective twitching of the heart muscle.

infarction Death of a body tissue, usually caused by interruption of its blood supply.

inferior A directional term meaning "below" or "at the bottom."

ischemia A lack of oxygen that deprives tissues of necessary nutrients, resulting from partial or complete blockage of blood flow; ischemia implies that the problem is still potentially reversible and that permanent injury has not yet occurred.

lumen The inside diameter of an artery or other hollow structure.

myocardium Heart muscle.

occlusion Blockage, usually of a tubular structure such as a blood vessel.

pedal edema Swelling of the feet and ankles caused by collection of fluid in the tissues.

perfusion The flowing of blood through body tissues and vessels.

posterior A directional term meaning "behind" or "rear."

superior A directional term meaning "above" or "on top."

syncope Fainting spell or transient loss of consciousness.

tachycardia Rapid heart rhythm, more than 100 beats/min.

ventricle One of two (right and left) lower chambers of the heart. As the main pumping chamber of the heart, the left ventricle receives blood from the left atrium (upper chamber) and delivers blood to the aorta, which, in turn, delivers it to the rest of the body.

ventricular fibrillation Disorganized, ineffective twitching of the ventricles, resulting in no blood flow and a state of cardiac arrest.

ventricular tachycardia Rapid heart rhythm in which the electrical impulse begins in the ventricle (instead of the atrium), which may result in inadequate blood flow and eventually deteriorate into cardiac arrest.

assessment in action

You have just cleared a call at the hospital when dispatch sends you to a private residence for a "man with chest pain." You are met at the door by a tiny, elderly woman. The woman leads you to the bedroom where her husband is lying in bed. As the wife begins introducing her husband, he clutches his chest and falls over. You and your partner roll the patient over and quickly slide him to the floor. Your partner then opens the patient's airway while you run for the AED.

1. Your partner determines that the patient is not breathing, but when he attempts to ventilate, the breaths do not go in. Your partner should immediately:
   A. perform 1 minute of CPR and then attempt to ventilate again.
   B. reposition the patient to open the airway and then attempt to ventilate again.
   C. give five quick back blows, followed by five abdominal thrusts.
   D. give five abdominal thrusts and then attempt to ventilate again.

2. You arrive with the AED just as your partner has secured the patient's airway. You should now:
   A. give five more abdominal thrusts.
   B. prepare to defibrillate as soon as possible.
   C. perform 2 minutes of CPR and then defibrillate.
   D. perform 5 minutes of CPR and then defibrillate.

3. The AED electrodes do not stay attached to the patient, despite several attempts to attach them. The patient's chest is dry, and he has little hair, so the problem most likely is that:
   A. there is too much adhesive on the electrodes.
   B. the patient weighs too much.
   C. the adhesive on the electrodes is dried out.
   D. the electrodes are too complicated for you to work.

4. The AED is finally applied correctly and advises a shock. After one shock is delivered, the AED reanalyzes the heart rhythm and now prompts that "no shock is advised." You should immediately:
   A. reassess the patient's airway, breathing, and circulation.
   B. perform CPR at a ratio of 15 compressions, followed by two breaths.
   C. give five quick abdominal thrusts and then check the airway again.
   D. provide rescue breathing at a rate of one breath every 5 seconds.

5. En route, the AED begins to display a "low battery/change battery now" message. If you were to attempt to defibrillate without changing the battery, what is most likely to happen?
   A. Large, blistered burn marks would appear under the pads.
   B. There would be inadequate or no current delivery to the heart.
   C. An excessively large shock would be delivered to the heart.
   D. The probability of a first shock conversion in increased.

prep kit 13

points to ponder

Objectives 4-3.3, 4-3.5, 4-3.8, 4-3.38, 4-3.44

You are first on scene at a cardiac arrest involving a 65-year-old woman. You have initiated CPR while your partner is setting up the AED. Another squad arrives, and one of the older members takes over breaths without saying anything to you. You immediately start counting out loud and on three, the other member gives a breath. You pause long enough for the air to go in and mention that it is suppose to be after the fifth compression. The other member laughs and says, "This ain't no book. Out here, we breathe when it's convenient."

- How would you deal with this person both during patient care and afterward?

online outlook

In an average lifetime, the heart beats more than two and a half billion times, without ever pausing to rest. Like a pumping machine, the heart provides the power that is needed for life. To learn more about the heart and cardiovascular system, complete Exercise 13 at www.emtb.com.

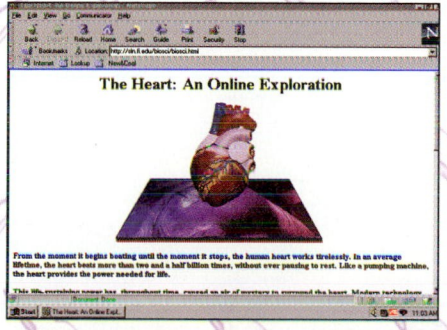

Neurologic Emergencies

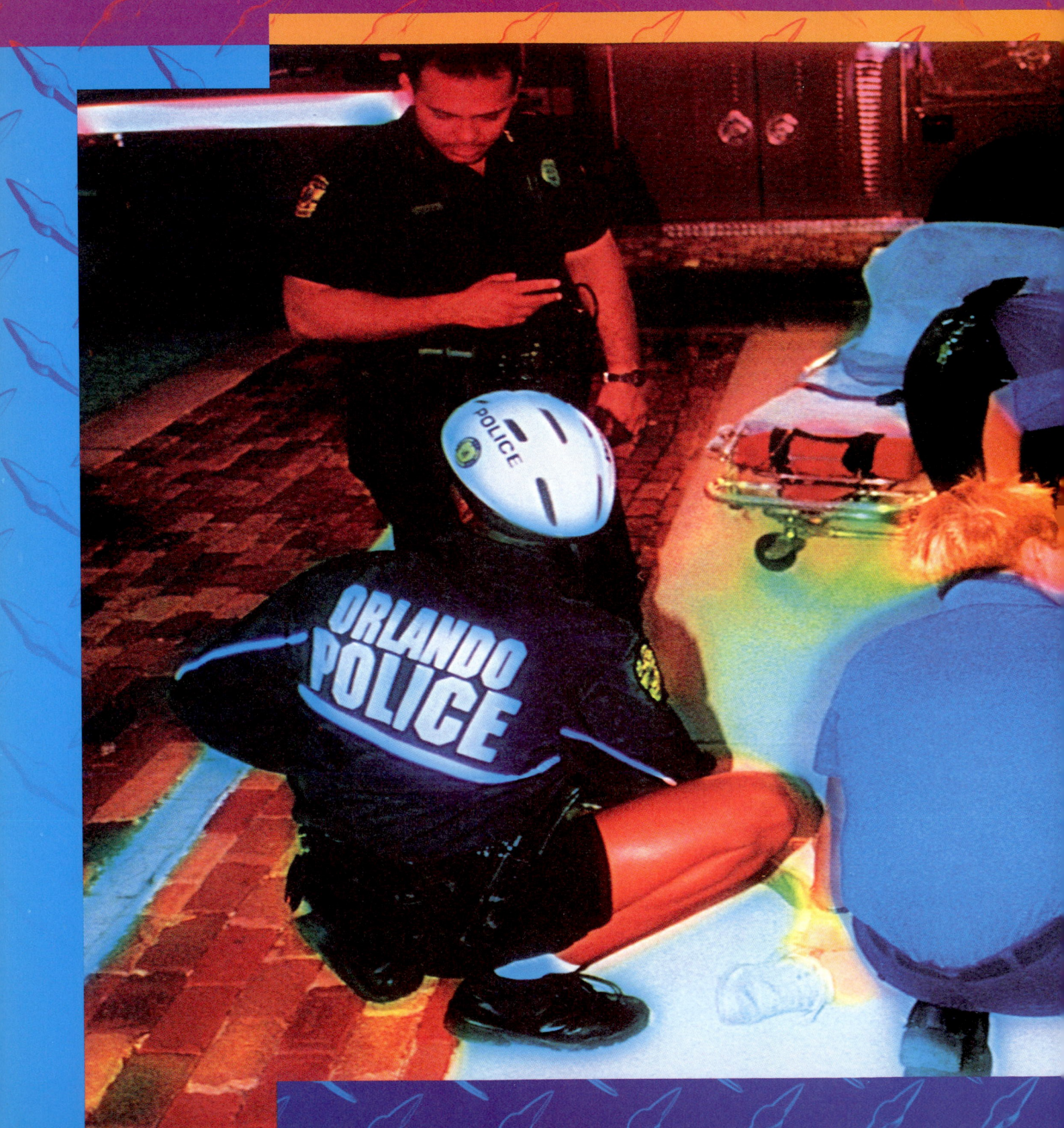

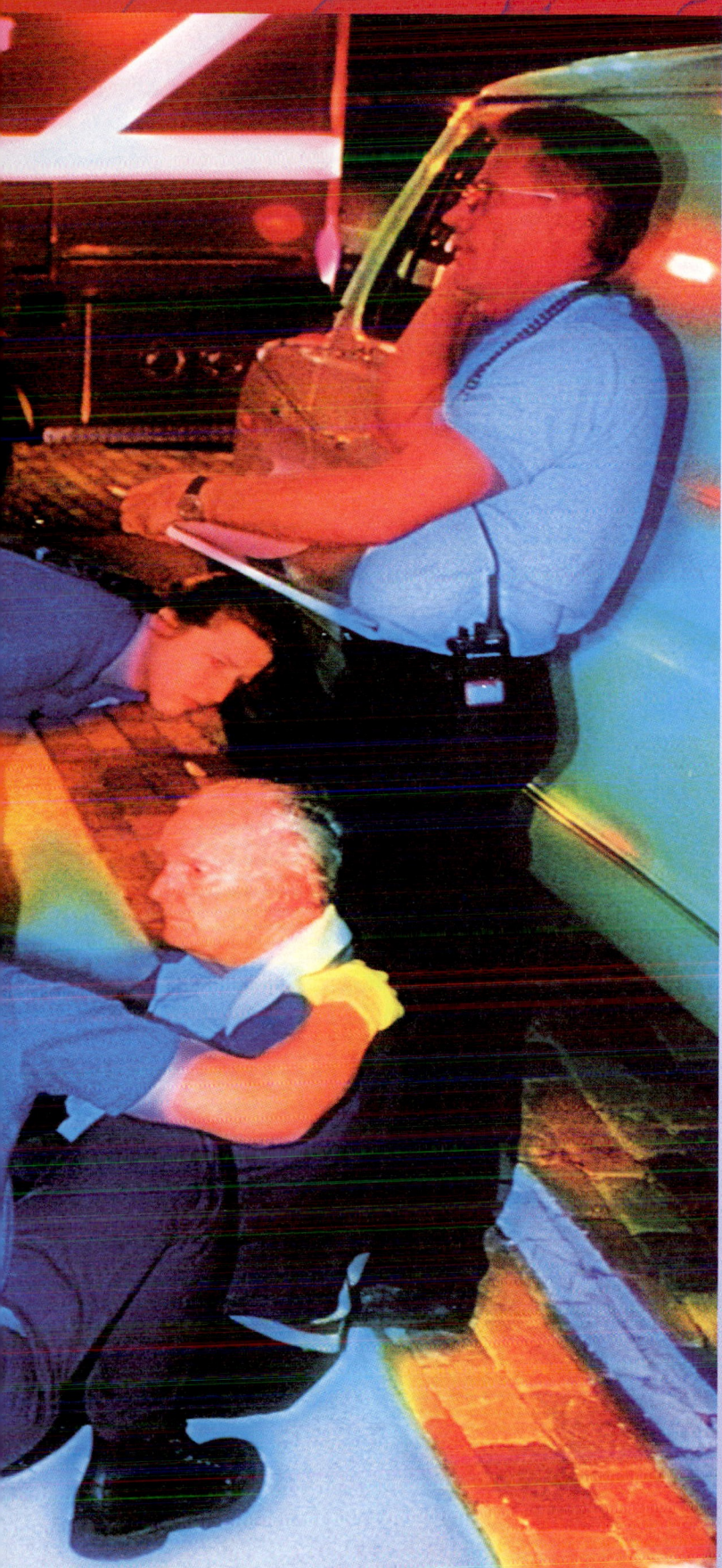

objectives*

Cognitive

1. Describe the causes of stroke, including the two major types of stroke and the three conditions that cause blockages.

2. Describe the sequence of events that occur during a stroke.

3. Obtain and interpret the key vital signs in the stroke patient, including the time of onset of the symptoms.

4. State the reason stroke must be treated within the first 3 to 6 hours.

5. Identify the signs and symptoms of stroke.

6. Describe the significance of a transient ischemic attack (TIA).

7. Define seizure, including the two major types of seizure.

8. Describe the parts of a seizure.

9. List possible causes of seizure.

10. Explain the importance of recognizing seizures.

11. Describe characteristics of the postseizure state.

12. Define altered mental status.

13. List possible causes of altered mental status.

Affective

14. Explain the importance of tolerance and patience when caring for a patient who has had a stroke, seizure, or who has altered mental status.

Psychomotor

15. Demonstrate the steps in the emergency medical care for the patient who has had a stroke.

16. Demonstrate testing for aphasia, facial weakness, and motor weakness.

17. Demonstrate the steps in the emergency medical care for the patient who has had a seizure.

18. Demonstrate the steps in the emergency medical care for the patient who has altered mental status.

* These are non-curriculum objectives.

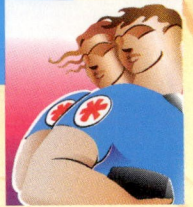

you are the emt

Squad 14 respond to 9th and Linder Drive and see the man who was picked up for strange behavior by the police officer on the scene.

The list of reasons that an individual may display so-called strange behavior is long and varied. The condition *altered mental status* refers to changes in a person's behavior. Calls in response to changes in behavior represent some of the most challenging cases you will encounter. This chapter will help to equip you with knowledge and skills so that you can provide high-quality care for patients who are experiencing neurologic emergencies and will help you to answer the following questions:

1. How can your care make a difference for patients with neurologic emergencies?

2. Is prompt transport using lights and sirens indicated for every patient who is experiencing a neurologic emergency?

Neurologic Emergencies

Stroke is the third most common cause of death in the United States, after heart disease and cancer. In the past few years, there has been a revolution in the treatment of stroke. For the most part, emergency treatment had not previously been available for patients with stroke, who typically faced years of painful rehabilitation or lifelong paralysis. Now, emergency physicians, neurologists, and neurosurgeons can help some patients with acute stroke to avoid the most devastating consequences of this disease, assuming that they get to the hospital in time.

Seizures and altered mental status also occur when there is a disorder in the brain. Seizures may occur as a result of a recent or old head injury, a brain tumor, a metabolic problem, or simply a genetic disposition. Your ability to recognize when a seizure has occurred or is occurring is critical for the patient, as it helps to direct appropriate treatment.

Altered mental status is a common presentation in patients with a wide variety of medical problems. Though it is tempting, you should not make assumptions about the cause of altered mental status. Causes range from alcohol intoxication to stroke. Obviously, treatment varies widely as well. Patients with altered mental status present a particular challenge in that they may be difficult to handle and frustrating to treat at times. Your professionalism is paramount in these situations.

The chapter opens with a description of the structure and function of the brain and what goes wrong in the most common causes of brain disorder, including stroke, seizure, and altered mental status. It then discusses the signs and symptoms of each condition. You will learn how to approach and assess a patient with a brain disorder and why prompt transport to an appropriate medical facility is so important. The chapter then describes key assessment strategies for stroke, seizure, and altered mental status. Appropriate management of each is then discussed.

Brain Structure and Function

The brain is the body's computer. It controls breathing, speech, and all other body functions. All your thoughts, memories, wants, needs, and desires reside in the brain. Different parts of the brain do different things. For example, some receive input from the senses, including sight, hearing, taste, smell, and touch; others control the muscles and movement, while others control the formation of speech.

The brain is divided into three major parts: the brain stem, the cerebellum, and the largest part, the cerebrum (Figure 14-1). The brain stem controls the most basic functions of the body, such as breathing, blood pressure, swallowing, and pupil constriction. Just behind the brain stem, the cerebellum controls muscle and body coordination. It is responsible for coordinating complex tasks that involve many muscles, such as standing on one foot without falling, walking, writing, picking up a coin, or playing the piano.

The cerebrum, located above the cerebellum, is divided down the middle into the right and left cerebral hemispheres. Each hemisphere controls activities on the opposite side of the body and the same side of the face. The front part of the cerebrum controls emotion and thought, and the middle part controls touch and move-

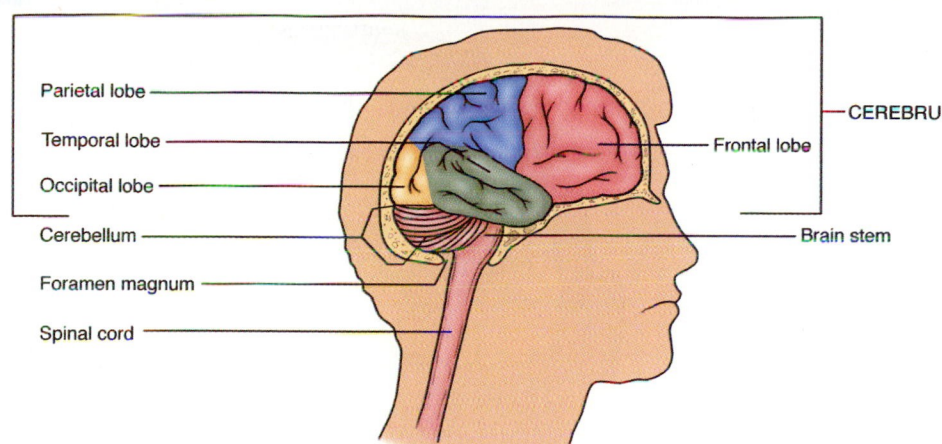

FIGURE 14-1 The brain lies well protected within the skull. Its major parts are the cerebrum, the cerebellum, and the brain stem.

ment. The back part of the cerebrum processes sight. In most people, speech is controlled on the left side of the brain near the middle of the cerebrum.

All the messages traveling to and from the brain travel along nerves. Twelve cranial nerves run directly from the brain to various parts of the head, such as the eyes, ears, nose, and face. All the rest of the nerves join in the spinal cord and exit the brain through a large hole in the base of the skull called the foramen magnum (Figure 14-2). At each vertebra in the neck and back, two nerves, called spinal nerves, branch out from the spinal cord and carry signals to and from the body.

Common Causes of Brain Disorder

Stroke is a common cause of brain disorder that is potentially treatable. Other brain disorders include coma, infection, and tumor. Although these specific problems are not covered here, the seizures or altered mental status that often accompany them are discussed. The information in this section will help you better understand, communicate with, and care for patients who have experienced some type of brain disorder.

Stroke

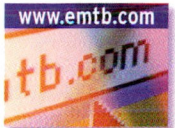

A <u>cerebrovascular accident (CVA)</u> is an interruption of blood flow to the brain that results in the loss of brain function. <u>Stroke</u> is the loss of brain function that results from a CVA and occurs when part of the blood flow to the brain is suddenly cut off. Lacking oxygen, brain cells stop working and begin to die; these dead cells are called <u>infarcted cells</u>. Medical science currently has little to offer these cells once they are dead. However, it may take several hours or more for cell death to occur, even when it appears that severe disability will occur. Also, in some cases, a trickle of blood may still be getting

through to the affected area of the brain. This blood may supply enough oxygen to keep a larger group of brain cells, called <u>ischemic cells</u>, alive but not enough to let the cells work properly and perform their given jobs. For example, if ischemic cells are responsible for controlling the left arm, the patient will not be able to move that arm. If normal blood flow is restored to that area of the brain in time, the patient will regain use of the arm.

New therapies, such as "clot busters," have been shown to reverse symptoms and thus abort the stroke, if given within 2 to 3 hours. These therapies may not

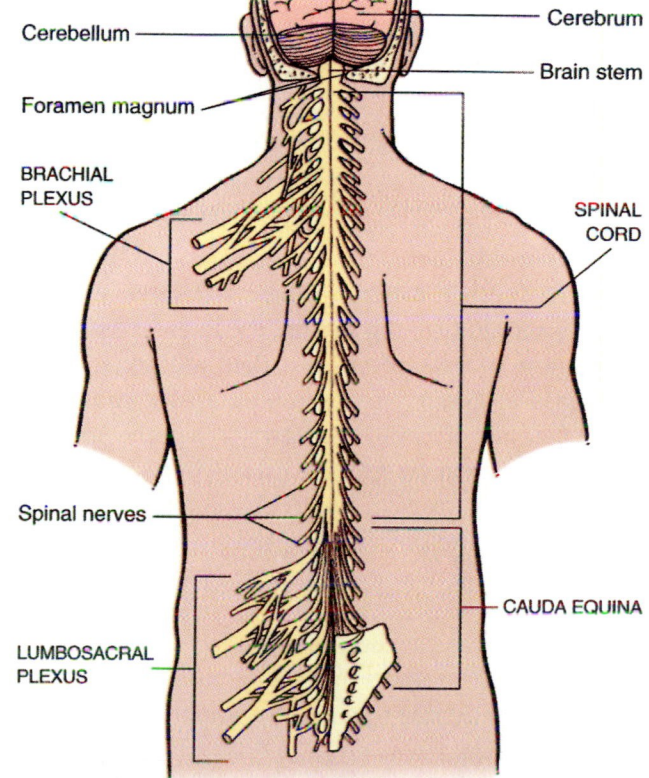

FIGURE 14-2 The spinal cord is the continuation of the brain stem. It exits the skull at the foramen magnum and extends down to the level of the second lumbar vertebra.

work for all patients, and they cannot be given to patients with bleeding-type strokes. Nevertheless, until the potential for definitive treatment is ruled out at the hospital, you should proceed under the assumption that the area of the brain can still be saved. The sooner the treatment is begun, the better for the patient.

Interruption of cerebral blood flow may result from <u>thrombosis</u>, clotting of the cerebral arteries; <u>arterial rupture</u>, rupture of a cerebral artery; or <u>cerebral embolism</u>, obstruction of a cerebral artery caused by a clot that was formed elsewhere and traveled to the brain.

There are two main types of stroke: hemorrhagic (usually from arterial rupture) and ischemic (from embolism or thrombosis). Their symptoms are the same, although the events taking place inside the brain are different.

Hemorrhagic stroke. A <u>hemorrhagic stroke</u> occurs as a result of bleeding inside the brain. The free blood then forms a clot, which squeezes the brain tissue next to it. When that tissue is squeezed hard enough, oxygenated blood cannot get into the area, and the surrounding cells begin to die.

Certain types of patients are at higher risk of hemorrhagic stroke. The patients who are at highest risk are those who have very high or long-term elevated blood pressure that is not treated. After many years of high pressure, the blood vessels in the brain weaken. Eventually, one of the vessels may rupture, and blood will spurt out of the hole and into the brain. Proper treatment of high blood pressure can help to prevent this long-term damage to the blood vessels.

Some individuals may have been born with weaknesses, called *aneurysms*, in the arteries' walls. Many of these individuals have a sudden onset of "bad headache." When a hemorrhagic stroke occurs in an otherwise healthy young person, the likely cause is often a weakness in a blood vessel called a *berry aneurysm*. This type of aneurysm resembles a tiny balloon (or berry) that juts out from the artery. When the aneurysm is overstretched and ruptures, blood spurts into an area around the coverings of the brain called the subarachnoid space. Therefore, these types of strokes are called subarachnoid hemorrhages. Again, patients with this type of stroke experience a sudden severe headache, typically described as the worst headache they have ever had. If the patient seeks medical attention immediately, surgeons may be able to repair the aneurysm.

Ischemic stroke. When blood flow to a particular part of the brain is cut off by a blockage inside a blood vessel, the result is an <u>ischemic stroke</u>. This can occur with thrombosis or with embolism that blocks blood flow. As with coronary artery disease, atherosclerosis in the

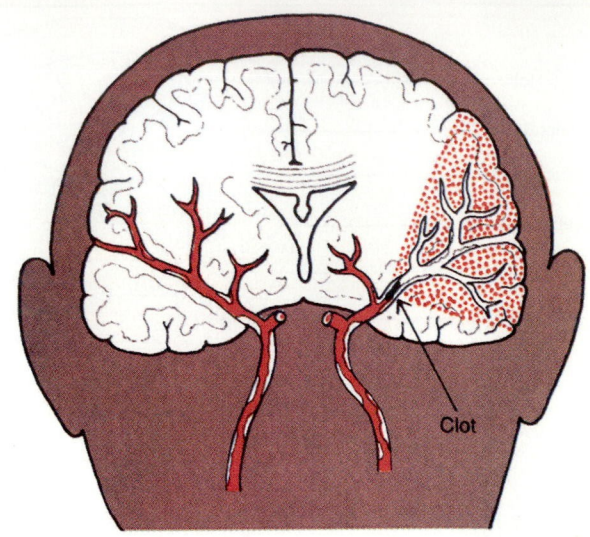

FIGURE 14-3 Atherosclerosis can damage the wall of a cerebral artery, producing narrowing and a clot. When the vessel is narrowed or completely blocked, blood flow to that part of the brain may be blocked, and the cells begin to die.

blood vessels is usually the cause. <u>Atherosclerosis</u> is a disorder in which calcium and a fatty material called cholesterol build up, forming a plaque inside the walls of blood vessels. This plaque obstructs blood flow, interfering with the vessel's ability to dilate. Eventually, atherosclerosis can cause complete occlusion (blockage) of an artery (Figure 14-3). In other cases, an atherosclerotic plaque in the carotid artery in the neck will rupture. A blood clot will form over the crack in the plaque, sometimes growing big enough to completely block all blood flow through that artery. Deprived of oxygen, parts of the brain supplied by the artery will stop working. Patients with such ischemic strokes will have dramatic symptoms, including loss of movement on the opposite side of the body.

Even if the blockage in the carotid artery is not complete, smaller pieces of the clot may embolize (break off and be carried by the blood flow) deep into the brain. There, a piece of clot will lodge in a branch blood vessel. This cerebral embolism then blocks blood flow (Figure 14-4). Depending on the location of the lodged clot, the patient may experience anything from no symptoms at all to being completely unable to move one side of the body.

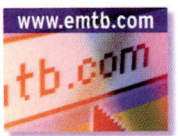

Transient ischemic attack. In some patients, normal processes in the body will break up a blood clot in the brain. When that happens quickly, blood flow is restored to the affected area, and the patient will regain use of the affected body part. When stroke symptoms go away on their own in less than 24 hours, the event is called a <u>transient ischemic attack (TIA)</u>. Some patients call these mini-strokes.

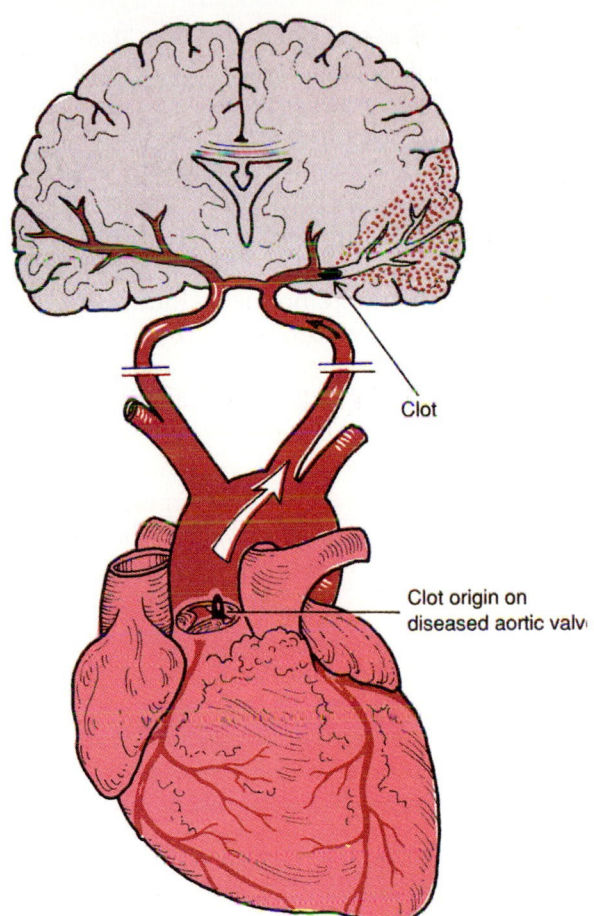

FIGURE 14-4 An embolus, a blood clot usually formed on a diseased heart valve, can travel through the body's vascular system, lodge in a cerebral artery, and cause a stroke.

Clot

Clot origin on diseased aortic valve

TABLE 14-1	Common Causes of Seizures
Type	**Cause**
Epileptic	Congenital in origin
Structural	Tumor (benign or cancerous) Infection (brain abscess) Scar from injury
Metabolic	Abnormal blood chemistry Hypoglycemia Poisoning Drug overdose Sudden withdrawal from alcohol, drugs
Febrile	Sudden high fever

Although most patients with TIAs do well, every TIA is an emergency. It may be a warning sign that a larger, permanent stroke is about to occur. For this reason, all patients with a new TIA should be evaluated by a physician to determine whether preventive action can be taken.

Seizures

A **seizure** is typically characterized by unconsciousness and a generalized severe twitching of all of the body's muscles that lasts several minutes or longer. This type of seizure is often called a **generalized seizure** or *grand mal seizure*. In other cases, the seizure may simply be characterized by a brief lapse of attention in which the patient seems to just stare and does not seem to respond to anyone. This type of seizure, called an **absence** (ob-sáhnz) **seizure** or *petit mal seizure,* typically occurs in young children.

Characteristics of seizures. Some seizures occur on only one side of the body. Others begin on one side and gradually progress to a generalized seizure that affects the entire body. Most individuals with lifelong or chronic seizures tolerate these events reasonably well without complications, but in some situations, seizures may signal life-threatening conditions.

Most seizures last 3 to 5 minutes and are followed by a lengthy period (5 to 30 minutes or more) of what is called a **postictal state**, in which the patient remains unconscious and unresponsive. Gradually, the patient begins to awaken unless some other severe abnormality causes the seizure. In contrast, a petit mal seizure can last for just a fraction of minute, after which the patient fully recovers immediately with only a brief lapse of memory of the event.

Seizures that recur every few minutes are referred to as **status epilepticus**, also known as status seizures. For obvious reasons, recurring seizures should be considered serious situations in which patients need immediate medical care.

Causes of seizures. Some seizure disorders, such as epilepsy, are congenital, which means that the patient was born with the condition. Other types of seizures may be due to high fevers, structural problems in the brain, or metabolic or chemical problems in the body (Table 14-1). Epileptic seizures can usually be controlled with medications such as phenytoin (Dilantin), phenobarbital, or carbamazepine (Tegretol). Patients with epilepsy will often have seizures if they stop taking their medications or if they do not take an adequate dose.

Seizures may also be caused by an area of abnormality in the brain, such as a benign or cancerous tumor, an infection (brain abscess), or a scar from some type of injury. These seizures are said to have a *structural* cause; in other cases, the seizures are *metabolic*. With the latter, seizures can be caused by abnormal levels of certain blood chemicals (eg, extremely low sodium levels), hypoglycemia (low blood glucose), poisons, drug overdoses, or sudden withdrawal from routine and heavy alcohol or sedative drug usage or even from prescribed medications. Dilantin, a drug that is used to control seizures, can cause seizures itself if the person takes too much.

Seizures can also result from sudden high fevers, particularly in children. Such convulsions, known as **febrile seizures**, are usually very unnerving for parents to observe but are generally well tolerated by the child. Nevertheless, you must transport a child who has had a febrile seizure, as this condition needs to be evaluated in the hospital. The fact that a second seizure may occur is very worrisome, and if it occurs, the patient requires rapid hospital evaluation to identify possible causes, such as serious infection within the brain or tissues covering the brain.

The importance of recognizing seizures. Regardless of the type of seizure, it is extremely important for you to recognize when a seizure is occurring or whether one has already occurred. You must also determine whether this episode differs from any previous ones. For example, if the previous seizure occurred on only one side of the body and this seizure occurs over the entire body, some additional or new problem may be involved. In addition to recognizing that seizure activity has occurred and/or that something different may now be occurring, you must also recognize the postictal state as well as the complications of seizures.

Because most seizures involve a vigorous twitching of the muscles, they use lots of oxygen. This excessive demand consumes oxygen that was being delivered by the circulation to the vital functions of the body. It is similar to a situation in which you exercise vigorously without giving your body a chance to rest. As a result, there is a buildup of acids in the bloodstream, and the patient will turn cyanotic (bluish lips, tongue, and skin in Caucasians) from the lack of oxygen. Often, the seizures themselves prevent the patient from breathing normally, making the problem worse.

Recognizing seizure activity also means looking at other problems associated with the seizure. For example, the patient may have fallen during the seizure episode and injured some part of the body; head injury is the most serious possibility. Patients having a generalized seizure may become incontinent, meaning that they may lose bowel and bladder control. Therefore, one clue that unresponsive or confused patients may have had a seizure is to find that they urinated into their clothing. Although incontinence is possible with other medical conditions, sudden incontinence is very likely a sign that a seizure has occurred.

The postictal state. Once a seizure has stopped, the patient's muscles relax, becoming almost flaccid, or floppy, and the breathing becomes labored (fast and deep) in an attempt to compensate for the buildup of acids in the bloodstream. By breathing faster and more deeply, the body can balance the acidity in the bloodstream. With a normal circulation and liver function, the acids clear away within minutes, and the patient will begin to breathe more normally. Intuitively, the longer and harder the convulsions are, the longer it will take for this imbalance to correct itself. Likewise, longer and more severe seizures will result in longer postictal unresponsiveness and confusion.

In some situations, the postictal state may be characterized by **hemiparesis**, or weakness on one side of the body, resembling a stroke. Unlike the typical stroke, hemiparesis soon resolves itself. Most commonly, the postictal state is characterized by lethargy and confusion to the point that the patient may be combative and appear angry. You must be prepared for these circumstances, both in your approach to scene control and in your treatment of the patient's symptoms. If the patient's condition does not improve, you should consider other possible underlying problems, including hypoglycemia or infection.

Altered Mental Status

Aside from stroke and seizures, the most common type of neurologic emergency that you will encounter is altered mental status. Simply put, altered mental status means that the patient is not thinking clearly or is incapable of being aroused. In some instances, patients will be unconscious; in others, they may be alert but confused (Figure 14-5). The range of problems is wide, and the causes are many, including common problems such as **hypoglycemia** (low blood glucose), hypoxemia, intoxication, drug overdose, unrecognized head injury, brain infection, body temperature abnormalities, and uncommon conditions such as brain tumors, glandular abnormalities, and chronic poisonings.

Hypoglycemia. The clinical picture of patients with altered mental status due to hypoglycemia is very complex. Patients can have signs and symptoms that mimic stroke and seizures. Because both oxygen and glucose are needed for brain function, hypoglycemia can mimic low-oxygen conditions in the brain such as those associated with stroke. In these instances, the patient may have hemiparesis, similar to what occurs as a result of a stroke. The principal difference, however, is that a patient who has had a stroke may be alert and attempting to communicate normally, whereas a patient with hypoglycemia almost always has an altered or decreased level of consciousness (Figure 14-6).

Patients with hypoglycemia commonly, but not always, take medications that lower blood glucose levels.

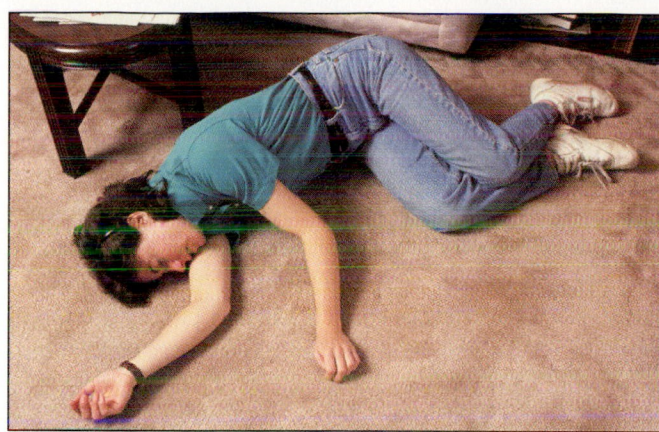

FIGURE 14-5 A patient with altered mental status can be unconscious in some instances; in others, the patient may be alert but confused.

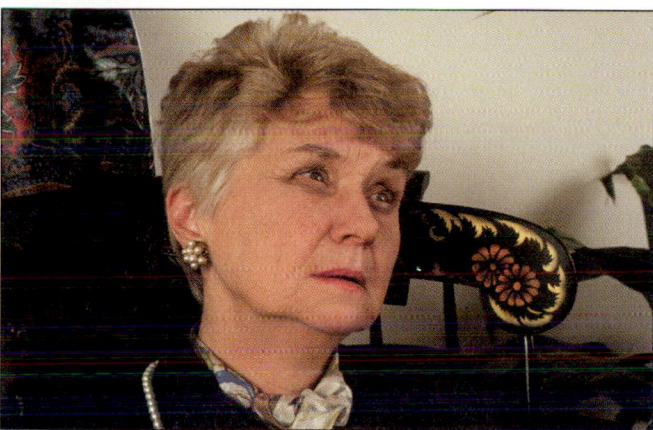

FIGURE 14-6 During your assessment of a patient with an altered or decreased level of consciousness, consider the possibility of hypoglycemia.

Thus, if the patient appears to have signs and symptoms of stroke and an altered mental status, you should report your findings to medical control and treat the patient accordingly. Check for and report medications, but remember that not all patients who have diabetes take insulin or other medications to lower blood glucose. Remember, also, that patients with a decreased level of consciousness should not be given anything by mouth. Again, local protocols should guide your actions.

Patients with hypoglycemia can also experience seizures, and you may arrive at the scene to find a patient in a postictal state: confused and disoriented or unresponsive. The mental status of a patient who has had a typical seizure is likely to improve; however, in a patient with hypoglycemia, the mental status is not likely to improve, even after several minutes. Therefore, you should consider the possibility of hypoglycemia in a patient who has had a seizure.

Likewise, you should consider hypoglycemia in a patient who has altered mental status after an injury such as a motor vehicle crash, even when there is an accompanying head injury. As with any other patient, you should look for medical identification bracelets or medications that might confirm your suspicions.

Other causes of altered mental status. Altered mental status can occur as a result of hypoglycemia, but there are many other possibilities as well, including unrecognized head injury with internal bleeding or severe alcohol intoxication. Your consideration of other possibilities becomes important because a patient with altered mental status may be combative and refuse treatment and transport. You should be prepared for difficult patient encounters and follow local protocols for dealing with these situations, recognizing the potential for serious underlying problems.

In most cases, a patient who appears intoxicated most likely is just that; however, you must consider these other problems as well. Individuals with chronic alcoholism can have abnormalities in liver function and in their blood-clotting and immune systems, which can predispose them to intracranial bleeding, brain and bloodstream infections, and hypoglycemia, along with many other problems.

Psychological problems and complications from medications are also possible causes of altered mental status. A person who appears to have a psychological problem may also have an underlying medical condition such as alcohol withdrawal syndrome or abnormal blood chemistry.

Infections are another possible cause, particularly those involving the brain or bloodstream. Infections in these areas are obviously life threatening and need immediate attention. Patients may not demonstrate typical signs of infection, such as fever, particularly if they are very young or very old or have impaired immune systems.

Altered mental status can also be caused by drug overdose or poisonings; therefore, you should monitor patients closely for accompanying cardiac and breathing problems. Likewise, altered mental status can be caused by abnormalities in blood chemistry, which can lead to heart and breathing problems as well.

Thus, the presentation of altered mental status varies widely from simple confusion to coma. No matter what the cause, you should consider altered mental status to be an emergency that requires immediate attention even when it appears that the culprit may simply be alcohol intoxication or a minor car crash or fall.

Signs and Symptoms of Brain Disorder

Many different disorders can cause brain or other neurologic symptoms, which can affect level of consciousness, speech, and voluntary muscle control. As a general rule, if the brain problem is caused primarily by disorders in the heart and lungs, the entire brain will be affected. For example, without any blood flow (cardiac arrest), the patient will go into a coma and can have permanent brain damage within minutes, even if CPR is begun soon thereafter. However, if the primary problem is in the brain, such as a poor blood supply to the middle part of the left cerebral hemisphere, the patient may not be able to move some parts of the right side of the body. This might be the right arm, the right leg, or the facial muscles on the lower part of the right side of the face. Low oxygen levels in the bloodstream, due to lung disease, for example, will affect the entire brain, causing anxiety, restlessness, and confusion.

Stroke

Left hemisphere problems. If the left cerebral hemisphere has been affected, the patient may have a speech disorder called <u>aphasia</u>, an inability to produce or understand speech. Speech problems can vary widely. Patients may have trouble understanding speech but can speak clearly. This condition is called receptive aphasia. You can detect this problem by asking the patient a question such as "What day is today?" In response, the patient with aphasia may say, "Green." The speech is clear, but it does not make sense. Other patients will be able to understand the question but cannot produce the right sounds in order to answer. Only grunts or other incomprehensible sounds emerge. These patients have expressive aphasia.

Right hemisphere problems. If the right cerebral hemisphere of the brain is not getting enough blood, patients will have trouble moving the muscles on the left side of the body. Usually, they will understand language and be able to speak, but their words may be slurred and hard to understand. This problem is called <u>dysarthria</u>.

Interestingly, patients with right hemisphere strokes may be completely oblivious to their problem. If you ask these patients to lift their left arm and they cannot, they will lift their right arm instead. They seem to have forgotten that the left arm even exists. This symptom is called neglect. Patients with a problem affecting the back part of the cerebrum may neglect certain parts of their vision. Generally, this is hard to detect in the field, but you should be aware of the possibility. Try to sit or stand on the patient's good side, since he or she may be unable to see things on the "bad" side.

The problem of neglect causes many patients who have had large strokes to delay seeking help. Strokes are not painful. Therefore, a patient may be unaware that there is a problem until a family member or friend points out that some part of the patient's body is not working correctly.

Bleeding in the brain. Patients who have bleeding in their brain may have very high blood pressure. Sometimes, this is the cause of the bleeding, but many times it is a response to the bleeding: The brain is raising the blood pressure in an attempt to force more oxygen into its injured parts. High blood pressure in stroke patients should not be treated in the field. Quite often, blood pressure will return to normal or may drop significantly on its own.

Other Conditions

The following three conditions may simulate stroke:

- Hypoglycemia
- A postictal state
- Subdural or epidural bleeding (a blood clot near the skull that presses on the brain)

Because both oxygen and glucose are needed for brain metabolism, a patient with hypoglycemia may look like a patient who is having a stroke. You should find out whether the patient has diabetes and takes insulin or a glucose-lowering medication.

A patient in the postictal state may look like a patient who is having a stroke. However, in most cases, a patient having a seizure will recover rapidly, within the next few minutes.

Subdural and epidural bleeding usually occur as a result of trauma (Figure 14-7). The dura is a leathery covering over the brain, next to the skull. A fracture near the temples may cause an artery to bleed on top of the dura and the resulting clot presses on the brain. Onset is usually very rapid after injury. In other cases, the veins just below the dura may be torn and bleed (a subdural bleed). Onset occurs more slowly, sometimes over a period of several days.

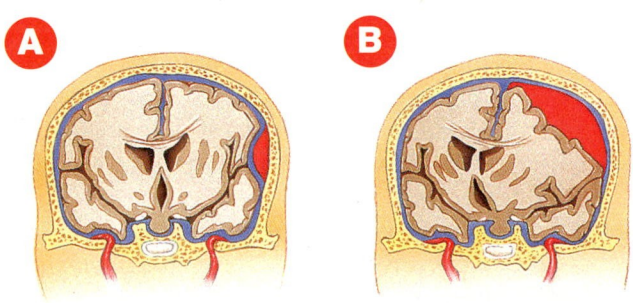

FIGURE 14-7 Trauma to the head can result in intracranial bleeding. **A:** Bleeding outside the dura and under the skull is epidural. **B:** Bleeding beneath the dura but outside the brain is subdural.

The onset of strokelike signs and symptoms may be subtle; the original injury may not even be remembered. Patients with chronic alcoholism or bleeding problems are at most risk and should be considered for aggressive care in the hospital if stroke symptoms are present.

Assessing the Patient

Stroke

When you are called to assist a patient with a possible stroke, you should first determine whether the patient is responsive and breathing. Friends and family members may think that the patient has had a stroke when he or she has really had a cardiac arrest.

Initial assessment. Upon arrival, you should check and care for immediate problems with the patient's ABCD. If the patient is responsive and breathing, obtain a history. Also try to speak with relatives or friends who may have seen what happened (Figure 14-8). Make a special effort to determine when the patient last appeared to be normal. This will tell physicians in the emergency department whether it is safe to begin certain treatments that must be given in the first hours after onset. Since you may be the only person on the emergency medical team with the opportunity to speak with bystanders, you may be the only one who can make this

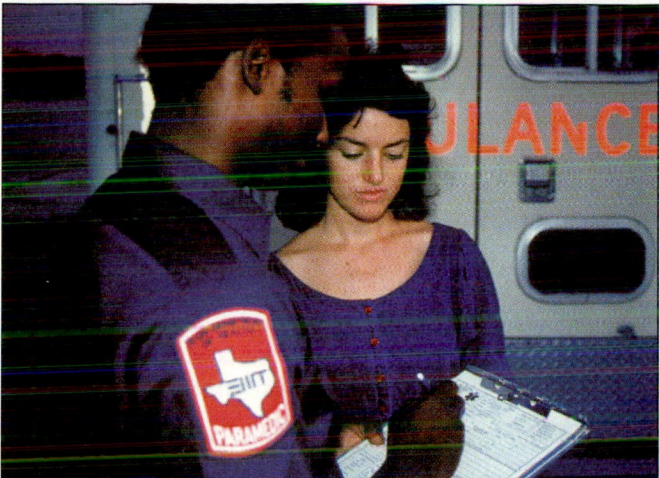

FIGURE 14-8 Try to speak with family members or bystanders who may have seen what happened. They may also be able to tell you when the patient last appeared "normal."

critical determination. Many times, you will be able to find out only that the patient was normal when he or she went to sleep the night before. Note that in such cases, the time the patient was last seen to be normal was at bedtime, not when the patient awoke with symptoms. Take the phone numbers of witnesses and family members to the hospital. Also collect or list all medications the patient has taken.

Although a stroke patient may appear to be unconscious and unable to speak, the patient may still be able

caring for the elderly

Over time, the brain will gradually deteriorate and shrink as a part of the normal aging process. This can increase the risk of head injury from minor forces, since the brain can bounce off the inside of the skull. A reduced brain mass can also reduce the patient's mental status and capacity. A smaller brain can impair memory function, and with lapses in short-term memory, the geriatric patient can ask the same or similar questions repeatedly.

When you are called to care for an elderly patient with an altered mental status, consider the possibility of a stroke or transient ischemic attack (TIA). At the scene of a motor vehicle crash involving an elderly driver, consider a stroke or TIA as the precipitating factor in the crash. Be alert for an altered mental state or unusual pupil responses in low light (ie, constricted or unequal pupils in dim light).

Beware of headache. Although elderly patients do get tension headaches, they are far less common in the elderly population. You should consider any headache as potentially serious.

As with the general population, the elderly can also sustain seizures. Remember that seizures are not necessarily due to epilepsy. You should consider and assess for the possibility of a drug overdose, stroke, head injury, or central nervous system infection. Status epilepticus in an elderly patient can have harmful effects such as hypoxia, irregular heart rhythm, hypotension, elevated body temperatures, low blood glucose, and, if the patient vomits, aspiration.

Remember that the elderly patient is at higher risk for central nervous system illnesses and injuries, including brain injury, TIA, stroke, and seizures. Do not be surprised to find a serious head injury from what you might consider a simple bump on the head.

to hear and understand what is taking place. Be careful what you say, avoiding all unnecessary or inappropriate remarks. Try to communicate with the patient by looking for indications that the patient can understand you, such as a glance, gaze, motion or pressure of the hand, efforts to speak, or nodding the head. Establishing effective communication can help you to calm the patient and lessen the fear that accompanies an inability to communicate (Figure 14-9).

As you perform the initial assessment, give supplemental oxygen using a nasal cannula or nonrebreathing mask, whichever local protocol prefers. Then begin your focused assessment, including vital signs. If necessary, provide assisted ventilation, protect the airway, and suction to prevent aspiration. Remember to check for any history of diabetes, seizure, or recent head injury.

Focused history and physical exam. As soon as possible, perform a neurologic exam as part of your focused physical exam. You should perform at least three key physical tests on patients you suspect of having had a stroke: tests of speech, facial movement, and arm movement. If any one of the three is positive (abnormal), the patient may be having a new stroke (Table 14-2).

To test speech, simply ask the patient to repeat a simple phrase such as "The sky is blue in Cincinnati." If the patient does this correctly, you know that he or she both understands and can produce speech. If the patient cannot repeat the phrase, the problem may be with either function: understanding speech or producing it.

To test facial movement, ask the patient to show his or her teeth (or gums, if there are no teeth). Watch to see that both sides of the face around the mouth move equally. If only one side is moving well, then you know that something is wrong with the control of the muscles on the other side.

To test arm movement, ask the patient to hold both arms in front of his or her body, palms up toward the

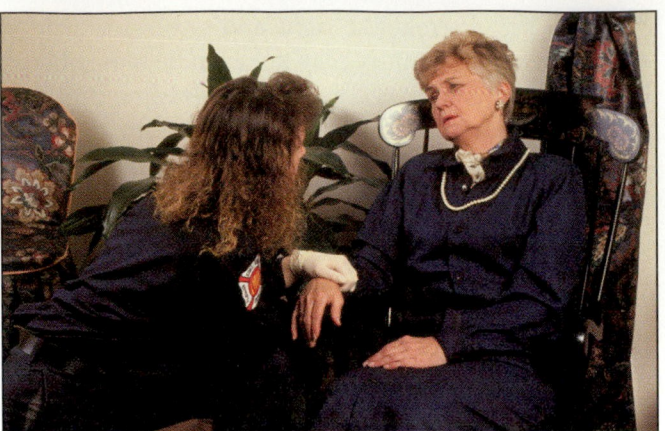

FIGURE 14-9 Make a special effort to establish communication with a patient who may have had a stroke. Look for indications that the patient understands you, such as a glance, gaze, squeeze of the hand, efforts to speak, or nodding the head.

sky, with eyes closed and without moving. Over the next 10 seconds, watch the patient's hands. If you see one side drift down toward the ground, then you know that side is weak. If both arms stay up and do not move, then you know that both sides of the brain are working.

If both arms fall to the ground, you have not really learned anything. Perhaps the patient did not understand your instructions. Try the arm test again, but this time move the patient's arms into position yourself. Another possibility to consider is that the patient is having a problem other than stroke. This is likely to be the answer if both sides of the brain are working improperly.

Transport considerations. After you have performed the neurologic exam, prepare the patient for transport. You want to spend as little time on the scene as possible. Remember, stroke is an emergency. There may be treatment available for the patient at the hospital. Place the patient in a comfortable position, usually on one side, with the paralyzed side down and well protected with

TABLE 14-2	Key Neurologic Tests for Assessing Stroke	
Test	**Normal**	**Abnormal**
Facial Droop (Ask patient to show teeth or smile.)	Both sides of face move equally well.	One side of face does not move as well as the other.
Arm Drift (Ask patient to close eyes and hold both arms out with palms up.)	Both arms move the same, or both arms do not move.	One arm does not move, or one arm drifts down compared with the other side.
Speech (Ask patient to say, "The sky is blue in Cincinnati.")	Patient uses correct words with no slurring.	Patient slurs words, uses inappropriate words, or is unable to speak.

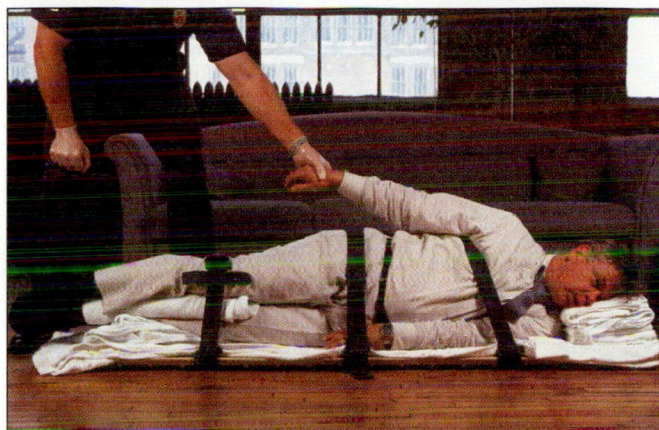

FIGURE 14-10 A patient who has had a stroke should be positioned with the paralyzed side down and well protected with padding. Elevate the head about 6".

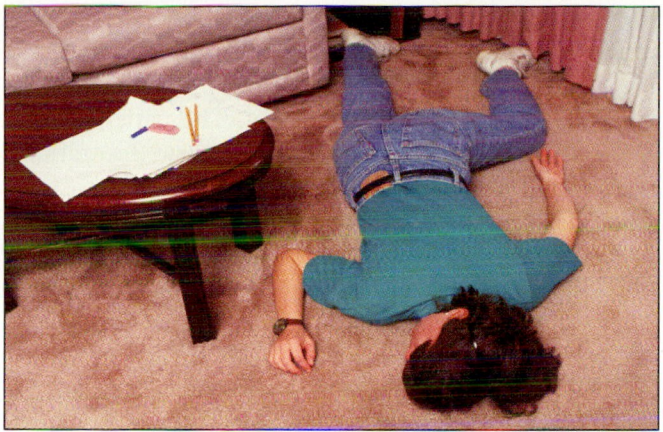

FIGURE 14-11 A patient who has had a seizure may be found in the postictal state when you arrive. If this is the case, be sure to ask family members or bystanders to verify that a seizure has occurred and how the seizure developed.

padding (Figure 14-10). The patient's head should be elevated about 6". Continue giving oxygen while en route.

After you begin transport, you should relay the information you have learned to the receiving hospital. Be sure to include the time that the patient was last seen to be normal, the findings of your neurologic examination, and the time you anticipate arriving at the hospital. This information will help the emergency department to conduct triage. After you arrive at the hospital, give a verbal report to the staff at the bedside. Then write a complete report detailing your findings and interventions.

Seizures

You are typically called to care for a patient who has had a seizure because someone actually witnessed the seizure. However, you may also be called to see an unresponsive patient when the patient is found in a postictal state (Figure 14-11). In other situations, you may be called to care for a patient who is having seizures and find that the patient actually has some other medical problem, such as cardiac arrest or some psychological problem. Therefore, thorough assessment is key because the information gathered at the scene may be extremely important to the hospital staff who must soon care for the patient.

In most instances, you will arrive sometime after the seizure has occurred, as it only lasts a few minutes. By the time someone recognizes the problem, calls for help, and receives a response, the patient should be in a postictal state. Thus, you must gather as much information from family or bystanders as possible to verify that a seizure has occurred and to obtain a description of the way the seizure developed.

Initial assessment. As with any other situation, you should focus on ABCD upon arrival. The patient may have been eating or chewing gum at the time of the seizure, and so there may be a foreign body obstruction. Bystanders may have tried to put objects in a patient's mouth "to help them breathe better," even though this practice is ill advised. Breathing and circulation should be confirmed as normal or treated as necessary. Again, in the immediate postictal state following a major seizure, you should anticipate rapid, deep respirations and an accompanying fast heart rate due to the stress of the severe convulsions. However, both respirations and heart rate should begin to slow to normal rates after several minutes. If not, you might suspect problems beyond the seizure alone.

Focused history and physical exam. You should obtain a SAMPLE history, including whether the patient has a history of seizures. If so, it is important to find out how the patient's seizures typically occur and whether this episode differs in some way from previous episodes. You should also ask what medications the patient has been taking. If the patient takes Dilantin and phenobarbital, he or she most likely has chronic problems. You might find that the patient ran out of medication or stopped taking medication for a while.

If the patient has no previous history of convulsions and now has a sudden focal (not generalized) seizure, a serious condition, such as brain tumor, intracranial bleeding, or serious infection should be suspected. Assessment is also the time to determine whether the patient takes medications that lower blood glucose such as insulin or oral hypoglycemic agents. In other situations, you may want to inquire about drug use or exposure to poisons.

As you document the physical signs of seizure, observe for recurrent seizures. If they occur, note whether the seizure starts at a focal part of the body (eg, one arm or one leg) and then progresses to the rest of the body. Otherwise, you should check for signs of incontinence. Most important, evaluate the patient's mental status, and monitor it every several minutes to verify progressive improvement. The patient should be checked for injuries, including head lacerations, shoulder dislocations, bitten tongue, and occasional extremity fractures. Also assess for weakness or loss of sensation on one side of the body, and reassess for improvement in such findings.

Altered Mental Status

Although the presentation of altered mental status is relatively straightforward, you should attempt to categorize the severity of the problem and look for accompanying or underlying conditions as you assess the patient. Use the AVPU scale to classify severity.

During your assessment, you should also consider other underlying medical conditions; the most important are those that are easily reversible. Therefore, you should consider hypoxemia and hypoglycemia as possible causes. Monitor these patients closely for depressed respirations that might need assisted ventilation. Likewise, a patient with a decreased level of consciousness may not be able to protect the airway; therefore, you should make sure that basic airway maneuvers are followed and suctioning available, particularly in those patients at the P or U level on the AVPU scale (Figure 14-12). Prompt transport is necessary, with close monitoring of vital signs en route.

Coordination with ALS

Most patients who have had a stroke or a seizure do not need advanced life support procedures in the field. However, if paramedics are available, you should

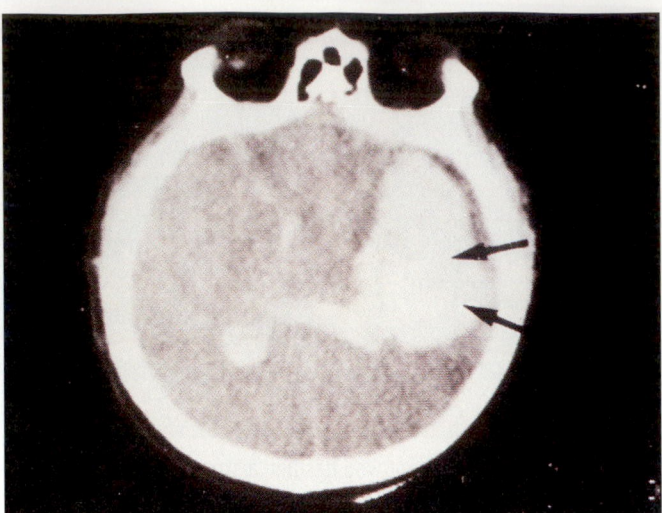

FIGURE 14-13 A CT scan of a ruptured cerebral aneurysm. The light area represents hemorrhage into the brain tissue (arrows).

request their assistance if the patient is unresponsive or has any signs of airway compromise, particularly if the patient takes insulin or glucose-lowering medication.

Emergency Medical Care

Stroke

In most patients with suspected stroke, physicians in the emergency department need to determine whether there is bleeding in the brain. If there is no bleeding, the patient may be a candidate for medication to help break up the blood clot or to help brain cells survive the reduced amount of oxygen. The only reliable way to tell whether there is bleeding is with a special type of X-ray test called computed tomography (CT). Blood is usually easy to see on the CT scan (Figure 14-13).

Most hospitals have only one CT scanner. The technician who knows how to run the machine may not be in the hospital in the middle of the night. That is why it is important that you recognize the signs and symptoms of stroke. If the emergency department staff knows that you are transporting a patient with a possible stroke, they may be able to call in the technician before you even arrive, or they may decide to delay a CT scan on another patient who has a less critical problem.

Keep in mind that most treatments for stroke must be started as soon as possible after the onset of the event (Table 14-3). Few, if any, current treatments do any good if they are started more than 3 to 6 hours after the stroke begins. Even if 3 hours have passed, prompt action on your part is essential. Newer therapy is under development that may be more flexible.

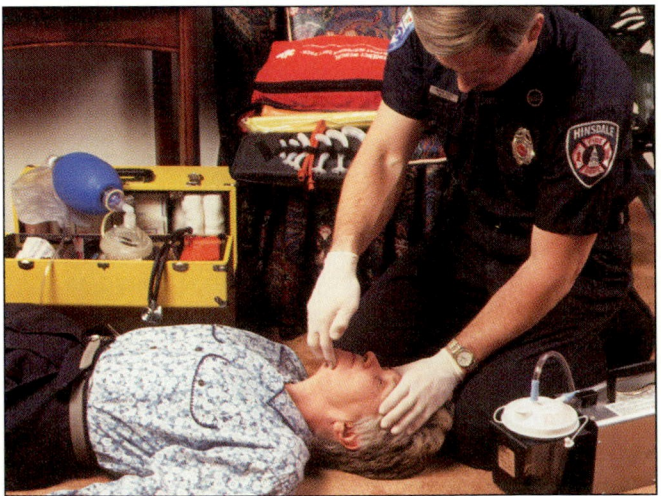

FIGURE 14-12 Securing and maintaining the airway in a patient who is unconscious is critical; also be sure to have suction readily available in the event that the patient vomits.

TABLE 14-3   Tips on Patient Care

- Patients who experience a TIA may have most of the same signs and symptoms as patients with a stroke. These signs and symptoms can last from minutes up to 24 hours. Therefore, the signs of stroke that you note on arrival may gradually disappear. Patients who appear to have had a TIA should be transported for further evaluation.

- Place the patient's affected or paralyzed extremity in a secure and safe position during patient movement and transport.

- Some patients who have had a stroke may be unable to communicate, but they can often understand what is being said around them. Be aware of this possibility.

- New therapies for stroke must be used shortly after the start of symptoms. Minimize time on the scene and notify the receiving hospital as soon as possible.

Seizures

In most situations, patients who have had a seizure require definitive evaluation and treatment in the hospital. Even a patient who has a history of chronic epilepsy that is controlled with medications may have an occasional seizure, commonly referred to as a breakthrough seizure. These patients should also be taken to the hospital for observation. At the hospital, blood levels of seizure medications are checked to ensure that patients are receiving the correct dose. Clearly, patients who have just had their first seizure or those with chronic seizures who have had an episode that is "different" require immediate examination to rule out life-threatening conditions. Unless the patient has a well-established history of seizures and is completely alert and oriented, supplemental oxygen is strongly advised, not only to provide extra oxygen but also to prevent the possibility of a recurrent seizure if there is a hypoxic component to the source of the convulsion.

Depending on local protocols, you should assess and treat the patient for possible hypoglycemia (diabetic with altered mental status who takes insulin or oral agents that lower blood glucose levels). If a severe injury has occurred, provide spinal immobilization, as well as any other splinting that may be needed. With recurrent seizures, protect the patient from further injury and apply appropriate airway procedures once the seizure ceases.

If you are treating a child who is having a febrile seizure, you should attempt to lower the child's temperature by removing his or her clothing and spraying/wiping the child with tepid water, particularly about the head and neck, and then fanning the moistened areas.

If the patient has been exposed to a toxin or poison, you should remove the source if possible. Suction should be readily available in case a patient with a decreased level of consciousness begins to vomit.

In all instances, you should be patient and tolerant with these patients, as many of them are likely to be confused and occasionally frightened. Many patients who experience seizures are frustrated with their condition and may refuse transport. Kindness and professional behavior are required to help convince the patient that transport is necessary for definitive care.

caring for kids

Children can have altered mental status caused by strokes, seizures, and other brain emergencies. However, children who have subarachnoid hemorrhages may not have a berry aneurysm; instead, they may have a congenital problem with the blood vessels in the brain. Children who have sickle-cell anemia are at particularly high risk for ischemic stroke. Treat stroke in children the same way that you do in adults.

As was mentioned earlier in this chapter, seizures can result from sudden high fevers, particularly in children. Remember that although febrile seizures are generally well tolerated by children, you must transport these patients to the hospital. The possibility of a second seizure makes transport mandatory so that if other problems develop, the child is in the hospital and can receive immediate definitive care.

If you suspect that a patient with altered mental status has hypoglycemia and you have the ability to test for it, you should do so and treat the patient according to local protocols. Also these patients require close monitoring, particularly of the airway, en route to the hospital.

prep kit

ready for review

The cerebrum, the largest part of the brain, is divided into right and left hemispheres, each controlling the opposite side of the body. Different parts of the brain control different functions: The front part of the cerebrum controls emotion and thought; the middle controls touch and movement; the back part of the cerebrum receives sight. In most people, speech is controlled on the left side of the brain, near the middle of the cerebrum.

Many different disorders can cause brain or other neurologic symptoms. As a general rule, if the problem is primarily in the brain, only part of the brain will be affected. If the problem is in the heart or lungs, the whole brain will be affected. Stroke is an important brain disorder because it is common and potentially treatable. Seizures and altered mental status are also common, and you must learn to recognize the signs and symptoms of each. Other brain diseases include coma, infections, and tumors.

Strokes occur when part of the blood flow to the brain is suddenly cut off; within minutes, brain cells begin to die of lack of oxygen. Signs and symptoms of stroke include receptive or expressive aphasia, dysarthria, muscle weakness or numbness on one side, facial droop, and sometimes high blood pressure. You should always do at least three neurologic tests on patients you suspect of having a stroke: testing speech, facial movement, and arm movement. In a transient ischemic attack (TIA), normal body processes break up the blood clot, restoring blood flow and ending symptoms in less than 24 hours. However, patients with TIA are at high risk for a permanent stroke. Because current treatments must be administered within 3 to 6 hours (and preferably within 2 hours) of the onset of symptoms to be most effective, you should provide prompt transport. Also, always notify the hospital as soon as possible that you are bringing in a possible stroke patient, so that staff there can prepare to test and treat the patient without delay.

Seizures are characterized by unconsciousness and generalized twitching of all or part of the body. There are types of seizures that you should learn to recognize: generalized, absence, and febrile convulsions. Most seizures last between 3 and 5 minutes and are followed by a postictal state in which the patient may be unresponsive, have labored breathing, and have hemiparesis and may have urinated on himself or herself. It is important for you to recognize the signs and symptoms of seizures so that you can provide emergency department staff with information as you transport the patient.

Altered mental status is also a common neurologic problem that you will encounter as an EMT-B. Signs and symptoms vary widely, as do the causes for this condition. Among the most common causes are hypoglycemia, intoxication, drug overdose, and poisoning. As you assess the patient with altered mental status, do not always assume intoxication; hypoglycemia is just as likely a cause. Prompt transport with close monitoring of vital signs en route is indicated.

vital vocabulary

www.emtb.com

absence seizure Seizure that may be characterized by a brief lapse of attention in which the patient may stare and does not respond. Also known as *petit mal seizure*.

aphasia The inability to understand or produce speech.

arterial rupture Rupture of a cerebral artery that may contribute to interruption of cerebral blood flow.

atherosclerosis A disorder in which cholesterol and calcium build up inside the walls of blood vessels, forming plaque, which eventually leads to partial or complete blockage of blood flow. An atherosclerotic plaque can also become a site where blood clots can form, break off, and embolize elsewhere in the circulation.

cerebral embolism Obstruction of a cerebral artery caused by a clot that was formed elsewhere in the body and traveled to the brain.

cerebrovascular accident (CVA) The interruption of blood flow to the brain that results in the loss of brain function.

dysarthria The inability to pronounce speech clearly, often due to loss of the nerves or brain cells that control the small muscles in the larynx.

febrile seizures Convulsions that result from sudden high fevers, particularly in children.

generalized seizure Seizure characterized by severe twitching of all the body's muscles that may last several minutes or more; also known as a grand mal seizure.

hemiparesis Weakness on one side of the body.

hemorrhagic stroke One of the two main types of stroke; occurs as a result of bleeding inside the brain.

hypoglycemia A condition characterized by low blood glucose.

infarcted cells Cells in the brain that die as a result of loss of blood flow to the brain.

ischemic cells Cells in the brain that receive enough blood after a cerebrovascular accident to stay alive but not to function properly.

ischemic stroke One of the two main types of stroke; occurs when blood flow to a particular part of the brain is cut off by a blockage (eg, a clot) inside a blood vessel.

postictal state Period following a seizure that lasts between 5 and 30 minutes, characterized by labored respirations and some degree of altered mental status.

seizure Generalized, uncoordinated muscular activity associated with loss of consciousness; a convulsion.

status epilepticus A condition in which seizures recur every few minutes.

stroke A loss of brain function in certain brain cells because they suddenly do not get enough oxygen. Usually caused by obstruction of the blood vessels in the brain that feed oxygen to those brain cells.

thrombosis Clotting of the cerebral arteries that may result in the interruption of cerebral blood flow and subsequent stroke.

transient ischemic attack (TIA) A disorder of the brain in which brain cells temporarily stop working because of insufficient oxygen, causing strokelike symptoms that resolve completely within 24 hours of onset.

assessment in action

A man on a corner flags you down as your partner slows your rig to stop at a red light. You see a small crowd standing around someone who is sitting propped against a street vendor's espresso stand. You find a 77-year-old woman with an obvious facial droop on the left side. According to her friend, the patient suddenly slumped to the ground and actually seemed unable to speak. The friend states that the facial droop developed soon after the patient slumped to the ground and that the patient then lost the ability to control her left arm. Assessment reveals that the patient is alert and able to respond to commands, although she cannot speak coherently. Her left arm is limp, but the skin color and capillary refill are both normal. The friend tells you that she sees the patient regularly and that the patient has been in excellent health, although she knows that the patient had surgery about a year ago to "clean the junk out of the arteries in her neck." Vital signs reveal a blood pressure of 188/92 mm Hg, a pulse of 104 beats/min, and quiet respirations of 28 breaths/min.

1. Your first step in caring for this patient should be to:
   A. ask the patient to try to stand on her own.
   B. obtain a blood pressure to check for hypertension.
   C. contact a family member to obtain permission to treat the patient.
   D. ensure that her airway is open and give her supplemental oxygen.

2. Although the patient keeps trying to answer your questions, she is unable to do so and is now becoming obviously agitated. At this point, you should:
   A. ignore her and ask the friend for information.
   B. firmly advise the patient to "get with the program-now."
   C. stop asking questions and try to calm the patient.
   D. step away and leave the patient alone until she quiets down.

3. What potentially life-threatening condition is associated with the patient's facial droop?
   A. Serious depression
   B. Impending heart attack
   C. Possible airway compromise
   D. Increasing respirations and hyperventilation

4. You are back at the hospital about an hour later, and your partner looks in to see how the patient is doing. He states that she has begun to speak again and has also regained partial use of her left arm. This improvement has most likely occurred because she may have:
   A. had hypothermia.
   B. had a transient ischemic attack.
   C. had a cerebrovascular accident.
   D. pretended to be ill to gain attention.

5. Which of the following interventions most likely contributed to the patient's rather quick neurologic turnaround?
   A. Giving high-flow supplemental oxygen
   B. Keeping the patient agitated
   C. Obtaining prompt vital signs
   D. Providing prompt transport to the hospital

points to ponder

Objectives 4-6.3, 4-6.10, 4-6.15, 4-8.1, 4-8.7, 4-8.8, 4-8.11

You arrive at an auto-pedestrian accident involving two children and a middle-aged patient. The two children were crossing the street and one was struck by the car. Your partner goes to the one who was struck and yells that she is bad. You check the other girl and she is uninjured. You ask some bystanders to stay with her and go check on the driver. The driver appears to be unconscious and is bleeding freely from a forehead laceration. As you establish responsiveness, it is obvious that the driver is drunk. The driver complains of neck pain and, when coherent, is quite abusive and won't stay still.

- Explain your treatment of the driver, including how you would keep him or her still.

online outlook

Different parts of the brain do different things. For example, some parts receive input from the senses, including sight, hearing, taste, smell, and touch; others control the muscles and movement; and still others control the formation of speech. To see many pictures of the brain and learn more about its function centers, complete Exercise 14 at www.emtb.com.

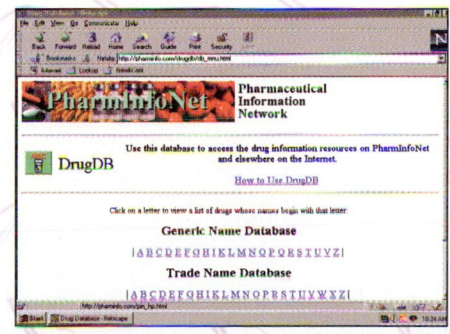

Communicable Diseases

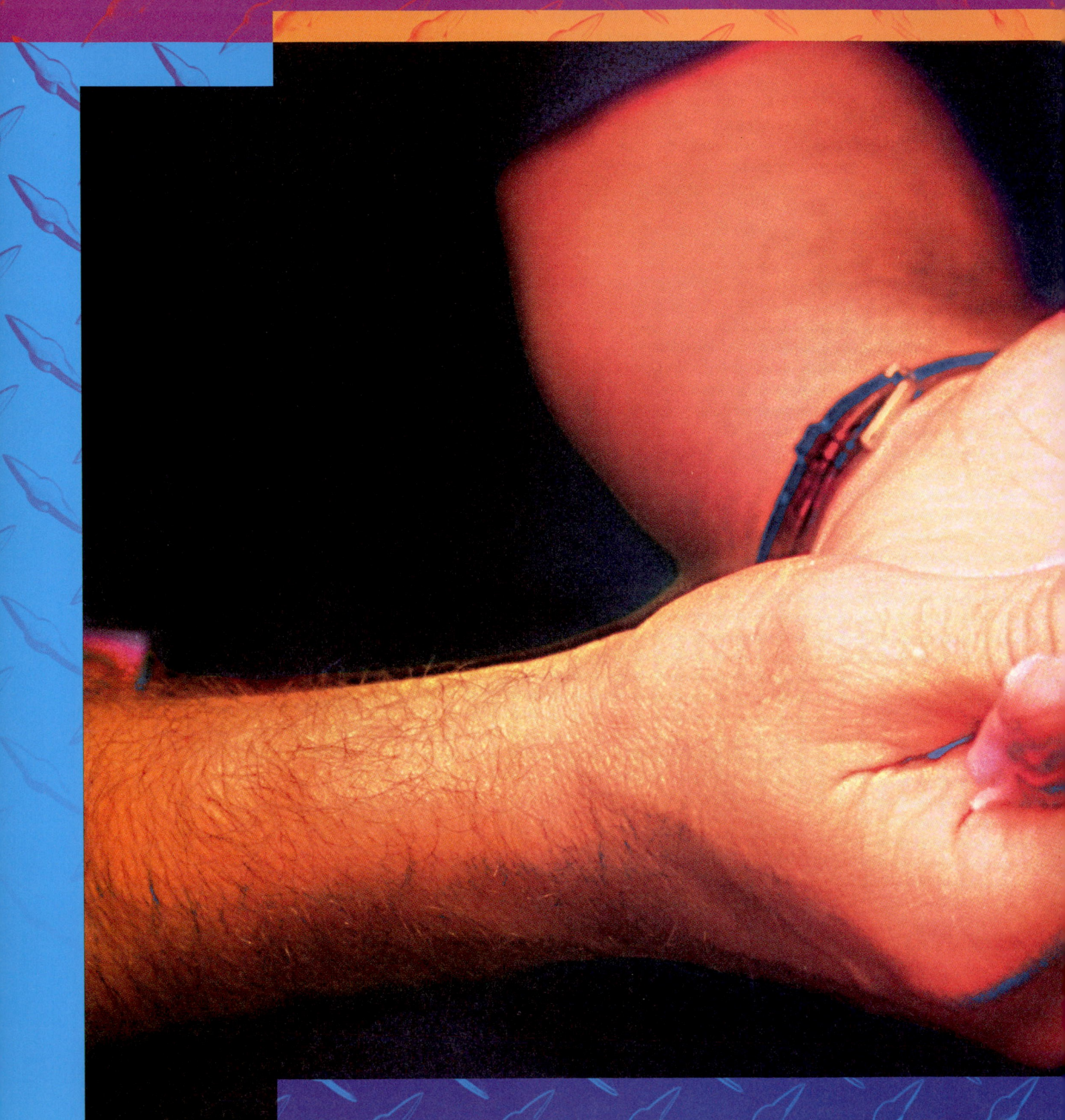

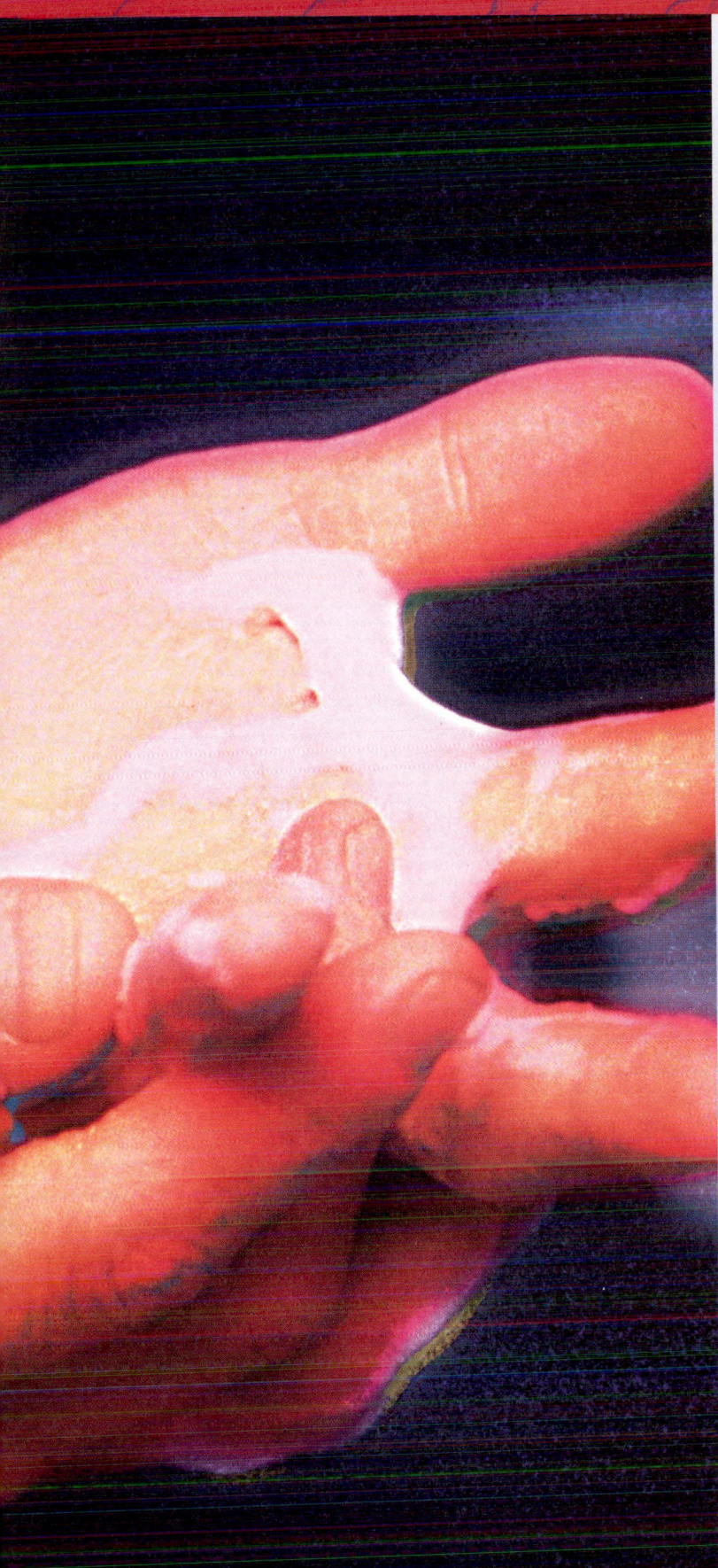

objectives

Cognitive

1. Describe the various ways by which communicable diseases can be transmitted from one person to another.

2. Identify how the following diseases are transmitted and discuss the steps to take to prevent and/or deal with an exposure to each: hepatitis, meningitis, tuberculosis, HIV/AIDS.

3. List the mechanisms of disease transmission.

4. Identify possible occupational diseases and methods of risk assessment.

5. Discuss the importance of obtaining a patient's history and assessment findings to identify possible communicable diseases.

6. Define the term "universal precautions" and describe when it is appropriate to use such measures.

7. Identify appropriate task-specific personal protective equipment (PPE).

8. Identify the role of a testing and immunization program in protecting the EMT from communicable diseases.

9. Identify the benefits of an exposure control plan.

10. List the components of postexposure management and reporting.

Affective

11. Explain the duty to care for patients with communicable diseases.

Psychomotor

None

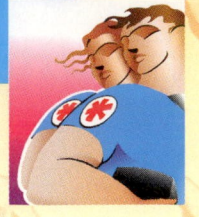

Communicable Diseases

Each handful of earth, each cup of water is home to hundreds of thousands of germs, including bacteria, fungi, protozoa, and viruses. However, humans are so well adapted to their environment that the vast majority of germs we encounter every day are basically harmless to us. On the other hand, many germs can become equally well adapted to the environment of the human body. Most of the time, such germs live quietly in the bowel, on the skin, or elsewhere in our bodies, doing no damage. Many such bacteria, such as those that produce vitamin K in humans, are beneficial. Indeed, it is in their best interests to cause their human hosts no harm. However, other germs can become temporary invaders, causing an acute infection and then either dying or becoming dormant. Fortunately, there are far more harmless colonizers than there are harmful invaders.

As an EMT-B, you will be called upon to treat and transport patients with a variety of communicable or infectious diseases. Most of these diseases are much harder to catch than is commonly believed. In addition, there are many immunizations, protective techniques, and devices that can minimize the health care provider's risk of infection. When these protective measures are used, the risk of the health care provider contracting a serious communicable disease is negligible. This chapter briefly discusses these precautionary measures. It describes the various ways in which diseases are spread from one person to the next, focusing on four diseases that are of special concern to the EMT: hepatitis, HIV infection, meningitis, and tuberculosis. You will learn how to prevent and handle exposure to each of these.

Routes of Transmission

While all infections result from an abnormal invasion of body spaces and tissues by germs, different germs use different means of attack. We refer to these as the mechanisms of transmission. **Transmission** is the way an infectious agent is spread. There are four basic mechanisms: direct transmission, vehicle-borne, vector-borne, and airborne (Table 15-1). In this context, "vehicle" means an inanimate object, while "vector" means a living object.

Because health care workers are exposed to so many different kinds of infections, the Centers for Disease Control and Prevention (CDC) developed a set of **universal precautions** for health care workers to use in treating patients. These protective measures are designed to prevent workers from coming into direct contact with germs carried by patients. **Direct contact** is the exposure or transmission of a communicable disease from one person to another. Gonorrhea is transmitted by direct contact, usually sexual. **Exposure** is contact with blood, body fluids, tissues, or airborne droplets by direct or indirect contact. **Indirect contact** is exposure or transmission of a disease from one person to another by contact with a contaminated object. Common colds are probably spread in this way, but gonorrhea is not. The goal of universal precautions is to interrupt the transmission of germs by decreasing the chance that you will come into contact with them. Universal precautions are not universal in the sense that they will help to protect you against all infectious diseases. Instead, the word "universal" is meant to remind you to apply precautions in all situations in which you

TABLE 15-1 Mechanisms of Transmission of Infectious Diseases

In this table (Data taken from Benenson AS (ed): *Control of Communicable Diseases in Man*, 15th edition, Washington, DC, American Public Health Association, 1990), the routes of transmission and some examples are outlined. Remember, while some germs frequently cause disease after transmission, transmission to a susceptible host is much more likely to cause asymptomatic infection and colonization.

Route	Descriptions	Source	Examples	
Direct	Contact, directly either with the person or with droplets sprayed (eg, by sneezing, coughing contact)	Ordinary contact	Measles, mumps, chickenpox, bacterial meningitis, influenza, diphtheria, herpes simplex	Universal Precautions
		Sexual contact	Syphilis, gonorrhea, HIV infection, hepatitis B, herpes simplex	
Indirect **Vehicle-Borne**	Spread by inanimate objects (eg, food, needles, clothing, transfused blood)	Food or water	Hepatitis A, B, C, salmonella, *Shigella*, poliomyelitis	
		Blood	HIV infection	
		Other	Measles, tetanus	
Vector-Borne Mechanical	Simple carriage by insects. The vector simply carries the germs.	Houseflies	*Shigella*	
Biological	Transmission by insect in which the germ lives and grows	Ticks	Lyme disease, Rocky Mountain spotted fever	
		Mosquitoes	Malaria, equine encephalitis	
Airborne Droplet nuclei	Residues after partial evaporation of droplets. Germs may remain viable, and the droplets may remain suspended for long periods		*Mycobacterium tuberculosis*, chickenpox	Airborne Disease Precautions
Dust	Small particles of dust from the soil may carry fungal spores and remain airborne for long times.		*Histoplasma, Coccidioides, Mycobacterium-avium intracellular*	

infectious, contagious, or communicable

Many people confuse the terms "infectious" and "contagious." In fact, all contagious diseases are infectious, but only some infectious diseases are contagious. For example, pneumonia caused by the pneumococcus bacteria is an *infectious* process, but it is not *contagious*. In other words, it will not be transmitted from one person to another. However, other infectious agents, such as the hepatitis B virus, are contagious because they can be transmitted from one person to another. An **infection** is an abnormal invasion of a host or host tissue by organisms such as bacteria, viruses, or parasites. A pathogen is a microorganism that is capable of causing disease in a host. A **host** is simply the organism or individual that is invaded. An **infectious disease**, then, is a disease that is caused by an infection. For example, Lyme disease is an infectious disease, caused by the Borrelia burgdorferi bacterium, which lives in deer ticks. However, Lyme disease is not contagious. Again, a **contagious** or **communicable disease** can be transmitted from one person to another. The only way to get Lyme disease is to be bitten by a deer tick.

TABLE 15-2   Parts of an Exposure Control Plan

Determination of Exposure	• Determines who is at risk for ongoing contact with blood and other body fluids • Creates a list of tasks that pose a risk for contact blood or other body fluids • Includes personal protective equipment (PPE) required by OSHA
Education and Training	• Explains why a qualified individual is required to answer questions about communicable diseases and infection control, rather than relying on packaged training materials • Includes availability of an instructor able to train EMTs regarding blood-borne and airborne pathogens, such as hepatitis B and C, HIV, syphilis, and tuberculosis. • Ensures that the instructor provides appropriate education, which is the best means for correcting many myths surrounding these issues
Hepatitis B Vaccine Program	• Spells out the vaccine offered, its safety and efficacy, record keeping, and tracking • Addresses the need for postvaccine antibody titers to identify individuals who do not respond to the initial three-dose vaccination series
Personal Protective Equipment (PPE)	• Lists the PPE offered and why it was selected • Lists how much equipment is available and where to obtain additional PPE • States when each type of PPE is to be used for each risk procedure
Cleaning and Disinfection Practices	• Describes how to care for and maintain vehicles and equipment • Identifies where and when cleaning should be performed, how it is to be done, what PPE is to be used, and what cleaning solution is to be used • Addresses medical waste collection, storage, and disposal
Tuberculin Skin Testing/Fit Testing	• Addresses how often employees should undergo Mantoux skin testing • Addresses how often fit testing should be done to determine the proper size mask to protect the EMT from tuberculosis • Addresses all issues dealing with HEPA respirator masks
Postexposure Management	• Identifies who to notify when exposure may have occurred, forms to be filled out, where to go for treatment, and what treatment is to be given
Compliance Monitoring	• Addresses how the service or department evaluates employee compliance with each aspect of the plan • Ensures that employees understand what they are to do and why it is important • States that noncompliance should be documented • Indicates what disciplinary action should be taken in the face of continued noncompliance
Record Keeping	• Outlines all records that will be kept, how confidentiality will be maintained, and how records can be assessed and by whom

have direct patient contact. It is impossible to tell whether an individual is free from a communicable disease in all situations, even if he or she appears healthy. Therefore, you should always take precautions.

You can also reduce your risk of exposure by following **body substance isolation (BSI)** techniques. BSI is the preferred infection control concept for fire and EMS personnel and is based on the assumption that all body fluids are potentially infectious. BSI differs from universal precautions in that in using universal precautions, you assume that blood and certain body fluids pose a risk for transmission of hepatitis B and HIV. In 1988, the CDC removed many body fluids, such as sweat, tears, saliva, urine, feces, vomitus, nasal secretions, and sputum, from the risk category unless these fluids contain visible blood. However, in the dark, you may not be able to see any blood. Therefore, EMS follows the BSI concept rather than relying on universal precautions.

Another way to reduce risk of exposure is by following your department's **exposure control plan**, which is a comprehensive plan that incorporates CDC guidelines, OSHA regulations, NFPA Infection Control Standard 1581, and other applicable state and local regulations (Table 15-2).

Even if germs do reach you, they may not infect you. For example, you may be *immune*, or resistant, to those particular germs. Immunity is a major factor in determining which hosts become ill from which germs. One way to gain immunity from many diseases today is to be immunized, or vaccinated, against them. Vaccinations have almost eliminated some childhood diseases, such as measles and polio.

Another way in which the body becomes immune to a disease is to recover from an infection from that germ (Table 15-3). Afterward, the body recognizes and repels that germ when it shows up again. Once experienced, many common infections provide lifelong immunity.

TABLE 15-3 Immunity to Infectious Diseases			
Type of Immunity	**Characteristics**	**Examples**	**Comments**
Lifelong	The illness will not recur	Measles Mumps Polio Rubella Hepatitis A Hepatitis B	Infection or vaccination provides long-term immunity to new infection. A live vaccine is required for measles only.
Partial	The person who has recovered from a first infection is unlikely to get a new infection from another person but may develop illness from germs that lie dormant from the initial infection.	Chickenpox Tuberculosis	Infection provides lifelong immunity to the patient from acquiring a new infection, but the original illness may recur, or it may recur in a different way. In the case of chickenpox, which is caused by the herpes zoster virus, an infection may recur years later in the form of shingles.
None	Exposure confers no protection from reinfection. The infection may wear down the patient's resistance.	Gonorrhea Syphilis HIV infection	No vaccine is available. Repeated infections are common. For example, there is effective immediate treatment for gonorrhea, and the germs may be eradicated; however, reinfection is likely if the high-risk practices (eg, unprotected sex) continue. For syphilis and HIV infection, the lack of immunity allows the germs to continue to cause damage within the host.

For example, a person who contracts and becomes infected with the hepatitis A virus may be ill for several weeks but, because an immunity has been built up, will not have to worry about getting the illness again. Sometimes, however, the immunity is only partial. Partial immunity protects against new infections. But germs that remain in the body from the first illness may still be able to cause the same disease again when the body is stressed or has some impairment in its immune system. For example, tuberculosis can cause a mild, unnoticeable infection before the body builds up a partial immunity. If the infection is never treated, the infection may be reactivated when immunity is weakened; however, such individuals are protected against a new infection from another person.

Humans seem unable to mount an effective immune response to some infections, such as **HIV infection**, which is infection with the human immunodeficiency virus (HIV) that can progress to acquired immunodeficiency syndrome (AIDS).

As an EMT-B, you can reduce your risk of infection in the following ways:

1. **Make sure you have all immunizations** recommended by OSHA, including the following:
   - Measles (necessary only if you have never had measles)
   - Rubella (German measles) (necessary only if you have never had rubella)
   - Mumps (necessary only if you have never had mumps)
   - Tetanus-diphtheria boosters (every 10 years)
   - Hepatitis B (required by OSHA)

   Although hepatitis A immunization is not required by OSHA, you may wish to be vaccinated as a preventive measure. Hepatitis A vaccination is not necessary if you have had hepatitis A in the past. All these vaccines are effective and rarely cause side effects. Many communities require you to show proof that you are up to date with their immunizations.

2. **Always follow BSI techniques**, which include the following:
   - Although intact skin is generally an excellent seal against the environment, breaks in the skin and exposure to the mucous membranes are a potential route for transmission of serious infections such as HIV and hepatitis B. Wear gloves, mask, and goggles if you have reason to think that you may be exposed to direct contact with blood or splashes of blood or other body fluids, especially if you have a break in

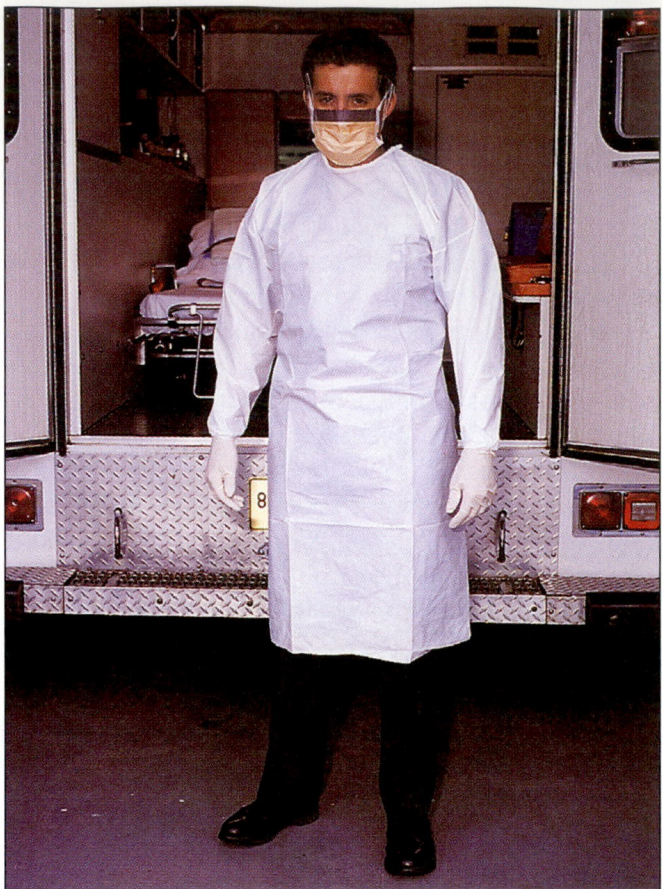

FIGURE 15-1 Gloves, a mask with shield or mask with goggles, and gown (optional) are necessary protection when you believe that the risk of direct exposure to blood or splashes of blood or other body fluids is possible.

your own skin (Figure 15-1). It does little good to put these items on after the contact has occurred. Make sure you have no unprotected breaks in your skin or on other parts of your body, such as on your arms. Blood can soak through your clothing and come into contact with these breaks. You may wish to use lotions to keep your skin supple and intact. If a patient appears to have a cough or a fever and/or a rash, use a disposable mask. Masks not only prevent your inhaling droplets in the air; they also keep you from carrying germs on your hand to your nose and mouth.

- Always use protective artificial ventilation devices instead of performing direct mouth-to-mouth resuscitation (with no protective devices) (Figure 15-2).

- Always wash after contact with a patient. The longer the germs remain with you, the better are their odds of getting through your barriers (Figure 15-3). Although soap and

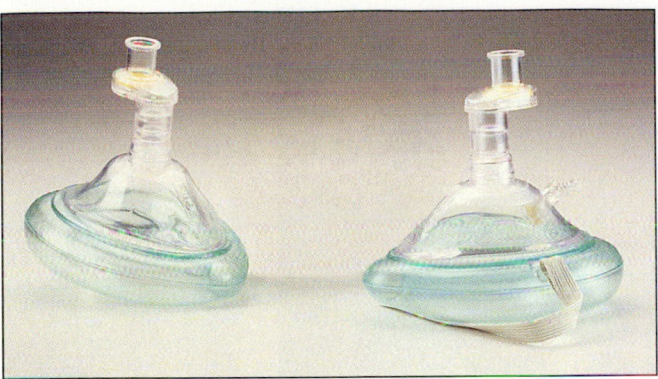

FIGURE 15-2 Barrier devices such as a pocket mask are necessary in providing artificial ventilations.

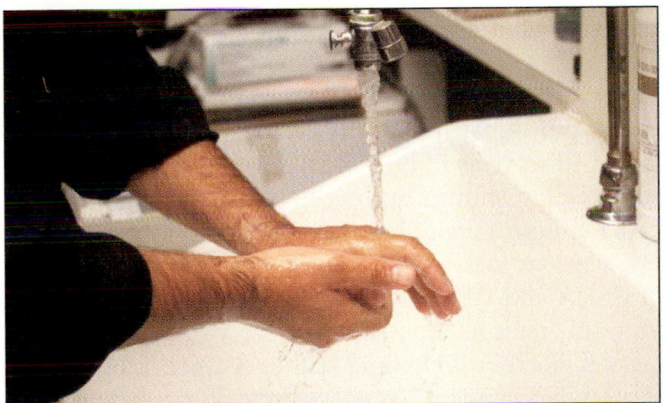
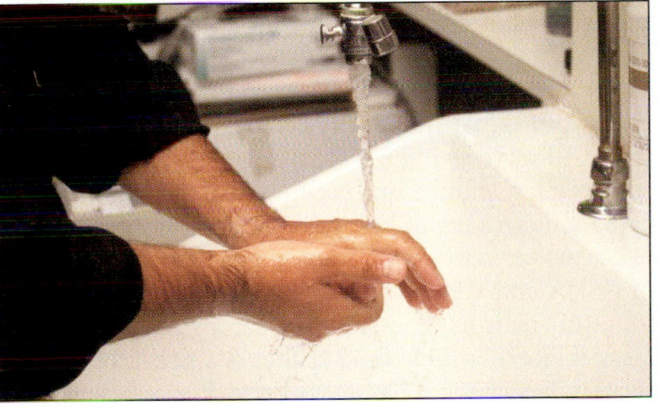

FIGURE 15-3 The single most important measure for self-protection against contagious disease is thorough handwashing.

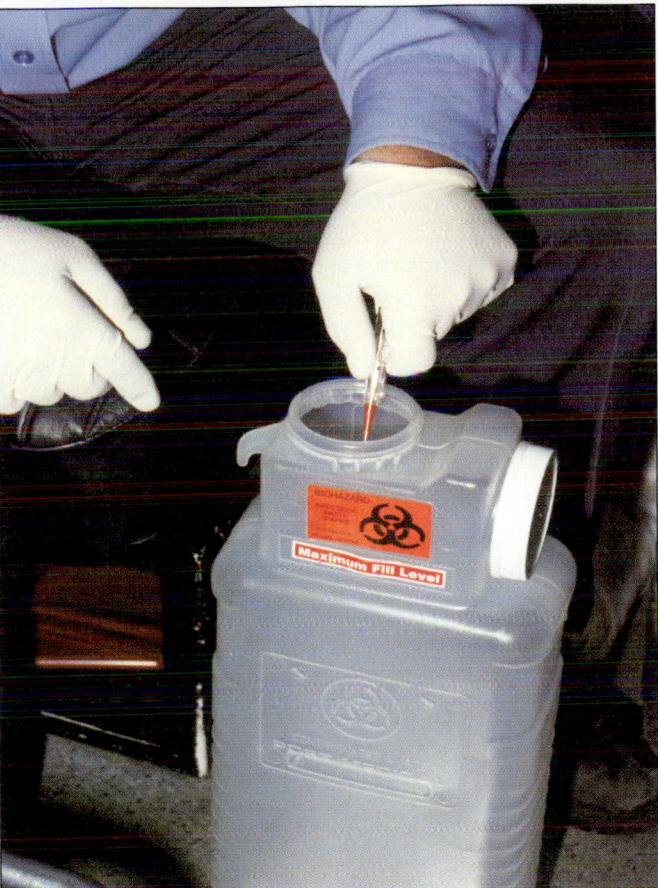

FIGURE 15-4 The proper disposal of sharps in a closed, rigid, marked container.

water are not protective in all cases, in certain cases they can be an excellent protection against further transmission from your skin to others.

3. **Be careful when handling needles,** scalpels, and other sharp items. The spread of HIV and hepatitis in the health care setting can usually be traced to careless handling of "sharps."

   - Do not recap needles. Even the most careful individuals miss occasionally.
   - Dispose of all sharp items that have been in contact with human secretions in closed, rigid containers (Figure 15-4).

   Remember, germs that cause no symptoms in one person may cause serious illness in another.

Duty to Care

You cannot deny care to a patient who you suspect has a communicable disease, even if you believe that the patient poses a risk to your safety. To deny care to such a patient is considered to be abandonment, which is legally and ethically a serious matter that can result in both civil and criminal actions against you. It can also be considered a breach of duty (a situation in which the EMT-B does not act within an expected and reasonable standard of care). In addition to breach of duty, if the following factors are present, you may be considered negligent in your duties:

- Duty (acting reasonably in a way that a person with similar training would act)
- Damages (physically or psychologically harming a patient)
- Cause (reasonable cause and effect—having a duty and abusing it and harming another individual)

Denying care to a patient who you suspect has a communicable disease can also be considered discrimination according to the Americans with Disabilities Act (ADA), especially when a public department or agency such as EMS is involved.

You must understand the disease process and the factors necessary to put you at risk because your response to them sometimes has legal consequences.

Risk Reduction and Prevention

Employer Responsibilities

Your employer cannot guarantee a 100% risk-free environment. Taking the risk of exposure to or acquisition of a communicable disease is a part of your job. You have a right to know about diseases that may pose a risk to you. Remember, though, that your risk for infection is not high; however, OSHA regulations, especially for private and federal agencies, require that all employees be offered a workplace environment that *reduces* the risk for exposure. Note that in some states that have their own OSHA plans, state and municipal employees must also be covered.

In addition to OSHA guidelines, other national guidelines and standards, including those from CDC and NFPA Infection Control Standard 1581, address reducing the risk for exposure to bloodborne **pathogens** and airborne diseases. The standards set by these agencies set a standard of care for all fire and EMS personnel and apply whether you are a full-time paid employee or a volunteer.

Personal Protective Equipment

Personal protective equipment (PPE) is equipment that blocks entry of an organism into the body. OSHA requires that the following PPE be made available to you:

- Vinyl and latex gloves
- Heavy-duty gloves for cleaning
- Protective eyewear
- Masks (including a HEPA respirator)
- Cover gowns
- Devices for respiratory assistance

The proper PPE for each task is selected according to the way in which a communicable disease is transmitted. For example, transmission of an airborne disease can be blocked by a mask. Blood spatter into the eye can be prevented by wearing eye protection.

Gloves are the most common type of PPE. Vinyl and latex gloves provide equal protection. You should evaluate each situation and choose the glove that works best. (Some individuals are allergic to latex. If you suspect that you are allergic, consult your supervisor for options.) Vinyl gloves may be best for routine procedures, and latex gloves may be best for invasive procedures. You must use heavy-duty rubber gloves for all cleaning and disinfecting procedures (Figure 15-5). Never use vinyl or latex gloves for cleaning.

Wear protective eyewear whenever there is a possibility that blood or another body fluid will splatter into your eyes. If you wear prescription eyeglasses, you can

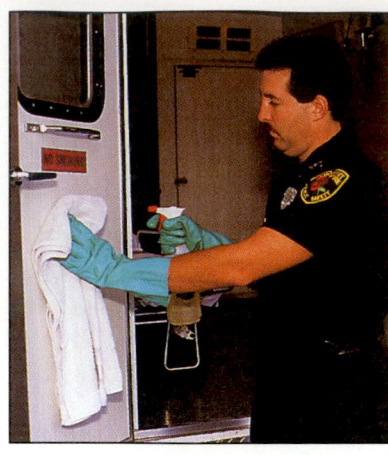

FIGURE 15-5
Heavy-duty rubber gloves must be used for cleaning and disinfecting procedures.

add removable side shields to your glasses while you are on duty.

Because some cover gowns are not practical in the field, your department will decide whether your uniform will serve as PPE. If so, the department's exposure control plan should outline how and where contaminated uniforms are to be laundered.

The use of masks is a complex issue, especially in light of OSHA and CDC requirements regarding protection from tuberculosis. You should wear a standard surgical mask if blood or body fluid spatter is a possibility. If you suspect that a patient has an airborne disease, you should place a surgical mask on the patient. However, if you suspect that the patient has tuberculosis, place a surgical mask on the patient and a HEPA respirator on yourself. Do not place a HEPA respirator on the patient; it is unnecessary and uncomfortable. A simple surgical mask will reduce the risk of transmission of germs from the patient into the air. Use of a HEPA respirator should comply with OSHA standards, which state that facial hair, such as long sideburns or a mustache, will prevent a proper fit.

Although there are no documented cases of disease transmission to rescuers as a result of performing unprotected mouth-to-mouth resuscitation on a patient with an infection, you should use a barrier or BVM device. Mouth-to-mouth resuscitation is rarely necessary in a work situation. Reusable BVM devices must be properly cleaned after the routine for high-level disinfection.

The recommendations for PPE use should be followed; however, OSHA recognizes that there are times when these procedures cannot be performed. There is an "exception" statement in the OSHA regulation that states that when you believe that taking the time to use PPE will delay delivery of care to the patient or will pose a risk to your personal safety, you may choose not to use PPE. Risk to personal safety refers to the likelihood of being attacked by a person or an animal, not to concern over acquiring a communicable disease. If you choose not to use PPE, you will have to justify this action, as an inquiry will follow.

Some Diseases of Special Concern

HIV Infection

Exposure to the HIV virus that causes AIDS is the most feared infection risk for EMTs. It is this prospect that led to the development of universal precautions and BSI. There is no vaccine to protect against HIV, and despite great progress in drug treatments, AIDS is still fatal. Fortunately, it is not easily transmitted in your work setting. For example, it is far less contagious than hepatitis B. HIV is a potential hazard only when deposited on a mucous membrane or directly into the bloodstream. Therefore, assuming that there is no sexual contact with a patient, your real risk of infection is limited to exposure to an infected patient's blood. Exposure can take place in the following ways:

- The patient's blood is splashed or sprayed into your eyes, nose, or mouth or into an open sore or cut, however tiny; even a microscopic opening in the skin is an invitation to a virus.

- You have blood from the infected patient on your hands and then touch your own eyes, nose, mouth, or an open sore or cut.

- A needle used to inject the patient breaks your skin. The risk to you from a single injection, even with a hollow-bore needle, is small, probably less than 1 in 1,000. However, this is by far the most dangerous form of exposure.

- Broken glass at a motor vehicle accident or other incident may penetrate your glove (and skin), which may have already been covered with blood from an infected patient.

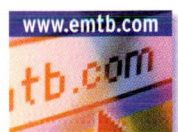

Many patients who are infected with HIV do not show any symptoms. This is why the government requires health care workers to wear certain types of gloves any time they are likely to come into contact with secretions or blood from any patient. You should always put on the proper type of gloves before leaving the ambulance to care for a patient. In addition, you must take great care in handling and disposing of needles and scalpels so that others are not inadvertently exposed to them. Finally, you should cover any open wounds that you have whenever you are on the job.

If you have any reason to think that a patient's blood or secretions may have entered your system, especially through inoculation of a patient's blood, you should seek medical advice as soon as possible. If you know that the patient is infected with HIV, your physician may suggest immediate treatment to try to keep the infection from establishing itself in you. However, if the patient seems an unlikely candidate for HIV infection, your physician may recommend that both you and the patient be tested before you undergo therapy. As scientists learn more about HIV, testing and treatment recommendations change. So it is important that you immediately see your doctor (or your program's designated physician) every time you are potentially exposed to a communicable disease.

Hepatitis

The term **hepatitis** refers to an inflammation (and often infection) of the liver. Hepatitis causes fever, loss of appetite, jaundice, and fatigue. It can be caused by a number of different viruses and toxins. There is no sure way to tell which patients with hepatitis have a contagious form of the disease and which do not. Table 15-4 on the next page shows the characteristics of different types of hepatitis, from which you can assess your risk of exposure. Hepatitis A can be transmitted only from a patient who has an acute infection, while hepatitis B and hepatitis C can also be transmitted from chronic carriers who have no signs of illness. A **carrier** is a person (or animal) in whom an infectious organism has taken up permanent residence and who may or may not cause any active disease. Carriers may never know that they harbor the organism; however, they can infect other individuals.

Hepatitis A is transmitted orally via oral/fecal contamination. This means that, generally, you must eat or drink something that is contaminated with the virus. **Contamination** is the presence of an infectious organism on or in an object. The organisms that cause hepatitis B and C are transmitted through vehicles other than food or water. For example, these organisms may enter the body through a transfusion or needlestick with infected blood, which puts health care workers at high risk for contracting hepatitis B, the more contagious and virulent form. **Virulence** is the strength or ability of a pathogen to produce disease. Hepatitis B is far more contagious than HIV. For this reason, vaccination with hepatitis B vaccine is highly recommended for EMTs. Unfortunately, not everyone who is vaccinated develops immediate immunity to the virus. Sometimes, but not always, an additional dose will provide immunity. You should be tested after vaccination to determine your immune status.

> You cannot deny care to a patient who you suspect has a communicable disease.

If you are stuck with a needle or injured in some other way while caring for a patient who might have hepatitis, see your physician immediately.

Meningitis

Meningitis is an inflammation of the meningeal coverings of the brain. Patients with meningitis will have signs and symptoms such as fever, headache, stiff neck, and altered mental status. It is an uncommon but very frightening infectious disease. Meningitis can be caused by viruses or bacteria, most of which are not contagious. However, one form, meningococcus meningitis, is highly contagious. The meningococcal bacterium colonizes the human nose and throat and only rarely causes an acute infection. When it does, it can be lethal. Patients with this kind of infection often have red blotches on their skin; however, many patient with forms of meningitis that are not contagious also have red blotches.

Because only laboratory tests can sort out the different forms of meningitis, you should use universal precautions and follow BSI techniques with any patient who is suspected of having meningitis. Gloves and a mask will go a long way to prevent the patient's secretions from getting into your nose and mouth. Again, the risk of infection is small, even if the organism is transmitted. For this reason, vaccines, which are available for most types of meningococcus, are rarely used. There are no effective treatments for the disease.

After treating a patient with meningitis, you should contact your employer health representative to make arrangements for counseling.

Tuberculosis

Most patients who are infected with *Mycobacterium tuberculosis* (the tubercle bacillus) are well most of the time. If the disease involves the bone or kidneys, the patient is only slightly contagious. In the United States, however,

TABLE 15-4   Characteristics of Hepatitis

Type	Route of Infection	Incubation Period (time before clinical signs and **symptoms** appear but infection may still be transmitted)	Acute Disease (when patient usually appears sick)
Viral (infectious)			
Hepatitis A	Fecal-oral, infected food	2 to 6 weeks	Early symptoms of all viral hepatitis include loss of appetite, vomiting, fever, fatigue, sore throat, cough, and muscle and joint pain. Several weeks later, jaundice (yellow eyes and skin) and right upper quadrant abdominal pain develop.
Hepatitis B	Blood, saliva, urine sexual contact, breast milk	4 to 12 weeks	
Hepatitis C	Blood, sexual contact	2 to 10 weeks	
Hepatitis D	Blood, sexual contact	4 to 12 weeks	
Toxin-Induced			
Medication, Drugs, Alcohol	Inhalation, skin exposure, oral ingestion, exposure or IV administration	Within hour to days following exposure	Severity of disease depends on amount of agent absorbed and duration of exposure.

tuberculosis is a chronic bacterial disease that usually strikes the lungs. Disease that occurs shortly after infection is called primary tuberculosis. Except in infants, this infection is not usually serious. After the primary infection, the tubercle bacillus is rendered dormant by the patient's immune system. However, even after decades of lying dormant, this germ can reactivate. Reactive tuberculosis is common and can be much more difficult to treat, especially because an increasing number of tuberculosis strains have grown resistant to most antibiotics.

Although tuberculosis is often hard to distinguish from other diseases, patients who pose the highest risk almost invariably have a cough. Therefore, for your safety, you should consider respiratory tuberculosis to be the only contagious form, as it is the only one that is spread by airborne transmission. The droplets that are produced by coughing are not the real problem. The real problem is the droplet nuclei, which are what remains of droplets after excess water has evaporated. These particles are tiny enough to be totally invisible and can remain suspended in the air for a long time. In fact, as long as they are shielded from ultraviolet light, they can remain alive for decades. So you may be at risk by simply entering a closed room that the patient actually left long ago. Particles of that size of droplet nuclei are not stopped by routine surgical masks. Inhaled, they are carried directly to the alveoli of the lungs, where the bacteria may begin to grow.

Why is tuberculosis not more common than it is? After all, absolute protection from infection with the tubercle bacillus does not exist. Everyone who breathes is at risk. And the vaccine for tuberculosis, called BCG, is only rarely used in the United States. Under normal circumstances, however, the mechanism of transmission used by M. tuberculosis is not very efficient. Infected air is easily diluted with uninfected air. And M. tuberculosis is one of those germs that typically causes no illness in a new host. In fact, many patients with tuberculosis do not even transmit the infection to family members. In crowded environments with poor ventilation, however, the disease spreads relatively easily.

Chronic Infection (patient may no longer have signs of the relevant illness)	Vaccine Available?	Treatment	Comments
Chronic condition does not exist.	Yes	None	Mild illness; approximately 2% of patients die. After acute infection, patient has life-long immunity.
Chronic infection affects up to 10% of patients; up to 90% of newborns who have the disease.	Yes	Yes, but poor	Up to 30% of patients may become chronic carriers. Patients are asymptomatic and without signs of liver disease, but they may infect others. Approximately 1% to 2% of patients die.
Chronic infection affects 90% of patients.	No	Yes, but poor	Cirrhosis of the liver develops in 50% of patients with chronic hepatitis C; chronic infection increases the risk of cancer of the liver.
Chronic infection is very common.	No	None	Occurs only in patients with active hepatitis B infection. Fulminant disease may develop in 20% of patients.
Some chemicals may initiate an inflammatory response that continues to cause liver damage long after the chemical is out of the body.	No	Stop exposure. In patients with overdose of acetaminophen, certain drugs may subdue liver injury if given early enough.	This type of hepatitis is not contagious. Patients with toxin-induced hepatitis may have liver damage, such as jaundice. Not every exposure to a toxin will cause liver damage.

If you are exposed to a patient who is found to have pulmonary tuberculosis, you will be given a tuberculin skin (Mantoux) test. This simple skin test determines whether a person has been infected with *M. tuberculosis.* A positive result means that infection has occurred; it does *not* mean that the person has active tuberculosis. It takes at least 6 weeks for the bacteria to show up in the laboratory test. So if you have the test within a few weeks of the exposure and results are positive, this means that you had already acquired the infection from somebody else. You will probably never identify the source. Most transmissions occur silently. This is why health care workers have tuberculin skin tests regularly. If the infection is found before the individual becomes ill, preventive therapy is almost 100% effective. Usually, a daily dose of isoniazid (INH) will cure the patient.

Other Diseases of Concern

Syphilis. Although syphilis is commonly thought of as a sexually transmitted disease, it is also a blood-borne disease. There is a small risk for transmission through a contaminated needlestick injury or direct blood-to-blood contact.

caring for the elderly

Everyone has defenses against getting sick, but the aging process can pose a threat to our natural defense mechanisms against invading microorganisms. Our physical defenses weaken or are eliminated as we age. The skin's thinning and loss of supportive collagen, along with a reduction in the number of blood vessels, can allow bacteria or viruses to enter the body with minimal resistance. The respiratory system cannot trap and eliminate bacteria or viruses in the airways as it once did. Finally, the gastrointestinal system allows an easier entry for bacteria or viruses through the intestines. Not only do our physical barriers to entry weaken, but our immune system deteriorates, and invading organisms are not as easily identified as abnormal. Infectious agents can take hold in the elderly patient much more easily because of reduced defenses.

When transporting the senior citizen, protect the patient from the environment, since extremes in heat or cold can further reduce the body's defenses. If you have a cold or the flu, use respiratory precautions, including a face mask for yourself so that the patient does not get exposed to the viruses. If your patient has a cold or the flu, protect yourself. However, remember that your defense system is probably much stronger than that of the patient.

Whooping cough. Whooping cough, also called pertussis, is an airborne disease caused by bacteria that mostly affects children younger than age 6 years. Signs and symptoms include fever and a "whoop" sound that occurs when the patient tries to inhale after a coughing attack.

The best way to prevent exposure is to try to place a mask on the patient. If the patient will not wear a mask, place one on yourself.

Newly recognized diseases. Newly recognized diseases, such as those caused by Hantavirus or enteropathogenic *Escherichia coli,* are being reported. These diseases are not transmitted from person to person. They are not communicable diseases and do not pose a risk to you during patient care.

Multiple antibiotic-resistant organisms have recently been the subject of media scrutiny. These organisms should be viewed as no more or less contagious than other less resistant organisms of the same type. The same precautions apply.

General Postexposure Management

In many instances, you will not know that a patient has an airborne or blood-borne disease, and you could be exposed without knowing it. The Ryan White Law requires that the hospital notify your department's <u>designated officer</u>, the individual in the department who is charged with the responsibility of managing exposures and infection control issues, within 48 hours of the time the hospital identifies the patient's disease (Figure 15-6). In the event of possible exposure, there should be a protocol in place to obtain information from your local hospital or other medical resource. You should be screened and given information about the necessity of medical follow-up. Treatment depends on the disease. Your designated officer will assist you with the necessary information.

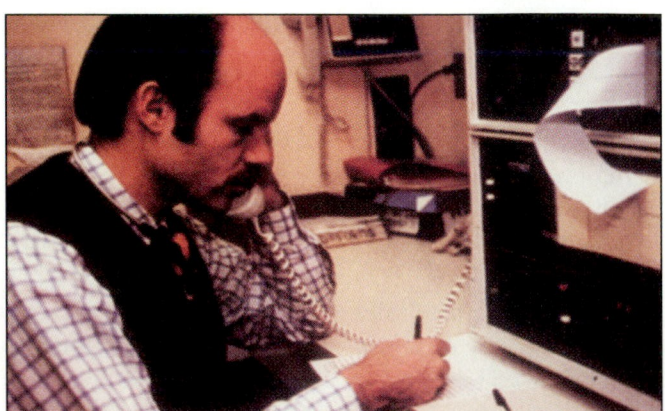

FIGURE 15-6 The Ryan White Law requires that the hospital notify your designated officer within 48 hours of the time the hospital identifies the patient's disease.

If you experience a needlestick injury or some other unprotected exposure to blood, you must notify your department's designated officer as soon as possible and complete an incident report. The designated officer can contact the hospital for information; the hospital has 48 hours to report back to the designated officer. Depending on your state laws and whether it is possible, patient testing should be done, followed by baseline testing on you.

Because there are many diseases for which there are no outward signs of infection, your protection lies in the use of PPE and/or prompt reporting of exposure. Be familiar with the postexposure protocols outlined in your department's exposure control plan.

Establishing an Infection Control Routine

Infection control, procedures to reduce infection in patients and health care personnel, should be an important part of your daily routine. Take the following steps in dealing with potential exposure situations:

1. **En route to the scene**, make sure that all equipment is out and available.

2. **Upon arrival**, make sure the scene is safe to enter, then do a quick visual assessment of the patient, noting whether any blood is present.

3. **Select the proper PPE** according to the tasks you are likely to perform. *Remember that good hand-washing is always necessary.*

4. **Change gloves and wash hands** between patients, especially if there is a great deal of blood at the scene; however, do not delay treatment for use of PPE if it puts patients at risk. Remove gloves and other gear after contact with the patient, unless you are in the patient compartment.

5. **Limit the number of people** who are involved in patient care if there are multiple injuries and a great deal of blood at the scene.

6. **If you or your partner is exposed** while providing care, try to relieve one another as soon as possible so that you can seek care. Make sure to call the designated officer and report the incident. This will also help to maintain confidentiality.

Be sure to routinely clean the ambulance after each run and on a daily basis. Cleaning is an essential part of the prevention and control of communicable diseases and will remove surface organisms that may remain in the unit.

You should clean your unit rather quickly so that it can be returned to service. Address the high-contact areas, including surfaces that were in direct contact with the patient's blood or body fluids or surfaces that you touched while caring for the patient after having contact with the patient's blood or body fluids.

Whenever possible, cleaning should be done at the hospital. If you clean the unit back at the station, make sure you have a designated area with good ventilation and a floor drain.

Bag any medical waste and dispose of it at the hospital whenever possible. Any contaminated equipment that is left with the patient at the hospital should be cleaned by hospital staff or bagged for transport and cleaning at the station.

You can use a bleach and water solution at a 1:10 dilution to clean the unit. A hospital-approved disinfectant that is effective against *M. tuberculosis* can also be used. Use the cleaning solution in a bucket or pistol-handled spray container. Do not use alcohol or aerosol spray products to clean the unit.

Remove contaminated linen, and place it into an appropriate bag for handling. Each hospital may have a different system for handling contaminated linen; you should learn hospital protocols (Figure 15-7).

Learn the regulations defining medical waste in your area. The disposal of infectious waste, such as needles, sharps, and heavily soiled dressings, may vary from hospital to hospital and from state to state.

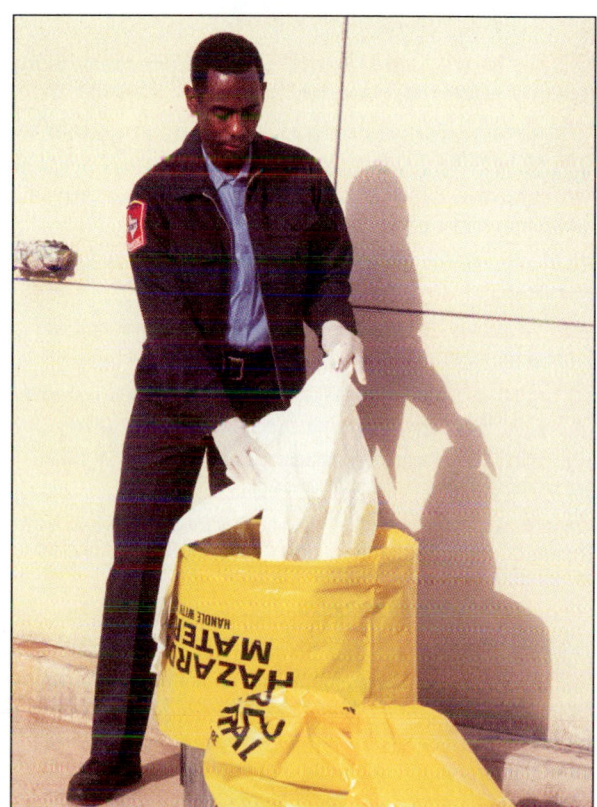

FIGURE 15-7 Contaminated linen should be bagged appropriately and disposed according to your local hospital protocols.

prep kit

ready for review

nfectious diseases can be transmitted in one of four ways: direct transmission, vehicle-borne, vector-borne, and airborne. Even if you are exposed to an infectious disease, your risk of becoming ill is small. Whether or not an acute infection occurs depends on several factors, including the amount and type of the infectious organism and your resistance to that infection. Most germs colonize the human body without causing any disease at all.

You can take several steps to protect yourself against exposure to infectious diseases, including keeping up to date with recommended vaccinations, using universal precautions and following BSI techniques at all times, and handling all needles and other sharp objects with great care. Sharp items should be disposed of in closed, rigid containers. Because it is often impossible to tell which patients have infectious diseases, you should avoid direct contact with the blood and body fluids of all patients. Use special caution if you have any open sores or cuts, no matter how small. If you think you may have been exposed to an infectious disease, see your physician (or your employer's designated physician) immediately.

The four infectious diseases of special concern are HIV infection, hepatitis B, meningitis, and tuberculosis. Of these, only meningitis and tuberculosis are transmitted through the air. The tubercle bacillus can remain dormant for decades without causing disease. Because medical therapy is almost always effective if you have not already become ill, you should get a tuberculosis test on a regular basis. Hepatitis B is by far the most common threat to health care workers. It is highly contagious and usually transmitted by needle-stick. Vaccination with hepatitis B vaccine is highly recommended. Meningitis is very rare; your risk of disease, even if you acquire this infection, is very small. Using a mask and gloves will go a long way to protect you against meningitis.

You should know what to do if you are exposed to an airborne or blood-borne disease. Your department's designated officer will be able to help you follow the protocol set up in your area.

Infection control should be an important part of your daily routine. Be sure to follow the proper steps when dealing with potential exposure situations.

Your ambulance should be cleaned after each run and on a daily basis. Know hospital protocols for laundering contaminated linens and disposal of infectious waste.

vital vocabulary

www.emtb.com

body substance isolation (BSI) An infection control concept and practice that assumes that all body fluids are potentially infectious.

carrier An animal or person who may transmit an infectious disease but does not display any symptoms of it.

communicable disease Any disease that can be spread from person to person, or from animal to person.

contagious An infectious disease that is capable of being transmitted from one person to another.

contamination The presence of infective organisms on or in objects such as dressings, water, food, needles, wounds, or a patient's body.

designated officer The individual in the department who is charged with the responsibility of managing exposures and infection control issues.

direct contact Exposure or transmission of a communicable disease from one person to another by physical touching.

exposure A situation in which a person has had contact with blood, body fluids, tissues, or airborne particles in a manner that suggests that disease transmission may occur.

exposure control plan A comprehensive plan that helps employees to reduce their risk of exposure to or acquisition of communicable diseases.

hepatitis An infection of the liver, usually caused by a virus, that causes fever, loss of appetite, jaundice, fatigue, and altered liver function.

HIV infection Infection with the human immunodeficiency virus (HIV) that can progress to acquired immunodeficiency syndrome (AIDS).

host The organism or individual that is attacked by the infecting agent; the host is infected by the agent.

indirect contact Exposure or transmission of disease from one person to another by contact with a contaminated object.

infection The abnormal invasion of a host or host tissue by organisms such as bacteria, viruses, or parasites, with or without signs or symptoms of disease.

infection control Procedures to reduce transmission of infection among patients and health care personnel.

infectious disease A disease that is caused by infection, in contrast to one caused by faulty genes, metabolic or hormonal disturbances, emotional trauma, or another cause.

meningitis An inflammation of the meningeal coverings of the brain; it is usually caused by a virus or a bacterium.

pathogen A microorganism that is capable of causing disease in a susceptible host.

personal protective equipment (PPE) Protective equipment that OSHA requires to be made available to the EMT.

transmission The way in which an infectious agent is spread: contact, airborne, by vehicles, or by vectors.

tuberculosis A chronic bacterial disease, caused by *Mycobacterium tuberculosis*, that usually affects the lungs but can also affect other organs such as the brain or kidneys.

universal precautions Protective measures that have traditionally been developed by the Centers for Disease Control and Prevention for use in dealing with objects, blood, body fluids, or other potential exposure risks of communicable disease.

virulence The strength or ability of a pathogen to produce disease.

assessment in action

Dispatch sends you to the Fun Time Daycare Center for a "sick child." On arrival, you find a lethargic 2-year-old boy in the sick room. A staff person tells you that the child has not been feeling well for several days but was still allowed to come to day care. Today, shortly after arriving, the boy became even more ill, and the parents were called but could not be located. Because they could not find the mother and the boy seemed to be getting sicker, the day care center staff decided to call 9-1-1.

On examination, you find that the child has a faint rash under his arms as well as over his abdomen and groin. A closer look reveals that the rash appears to consist of tiny blisters. He has a blood pressure of 96/64 mm Hg, a pulse of 130/min, and respirations of 36/min. Because you cannot do much for the patient in the field, you try to make him as comfortable as possible and transport him to the emergency department. The hospital is less than 5 minutes away, so your partner's radio report is short. He states only that you are transporting a sick child and then lists the vital signs.

Shortly after you and your partner return to quarters, the hospital staff calls to notify you that the child has chickenpox. They are unhappy that the information about the blisterlike rash was omitted from the radio report. Your partner is unhappy because he has never had chickenpox.

1. Chickenpox is transmitted through:
   A. the respiratory system only.
   B. contact with the dry, scabbed-over lesions.
   C. contact with the fluid drainage from the lesions.
   D. either the respiratory system or contact with fluid drainage.

2. Which of the following statements about the risk of contracting chickenpox is **FALSE**?
   A. It is very easy to contract chickenpox.
   B. It is very difficult to contract chickenpox.
   C. Chickenpox is considered communicable until the rash dries and scabs over.
   D. Chickenpox is considered communicable up to 5 days before the rash appears.

3. The rash associated with chickenpox most often first appears on the:
   A. face and scalp only.
   B. scalp and groin and under the armpits.
   C. palms of the hands and soles of the feet.
   D. trunk and then is distributed evenly across the body.

4. Because the EMT-Bs did not take protective measures, the most appropriate course of action at this time would be to:
   A. complete the appropriate exposure paperwork and report the incident to the shift supervisor.
   B. report the unprotected exposure to the ED physician and complete the appropriate exposure paperwork.
   C. report the unprotected exposure to the ED physician and to the shift supervisor.
   D. shower and change uniforms after the call and then report the incident to the shift supervisor.

5. Which of the following statements about the exposed EMT-B's risk of contracting chickenpox is true?
   A. He should be considered highly infectious, immediately isolated from patients and co-workers, and then sent home.
   B. He will almost certainly contract chickenpox, since there is no effective immunization.
   C. He should be considered infectious and should be isolated from co-workers from the tenth to the twenty-first day after exposure.
   D. He will not contract chickenpox despite never having had it, because once you reach adulthood, you develop a natural immunity.

points to ponder

Objectives 7-1.1, 7-1.8, 7-1.11, 7-1.13, 7-1.14, 1-1.4, 1-2.8, 1-2.9, 1-2.10, 1-2.11, 1-2.12, 1-2.13

Today you are assigned to transfers. Your third transfer of the morning is to take a 54-year-old, terminally ill patient from a hospital to an extended care facility. The hospital staff informs you that the patient has infectious tuberculosis, hands you a surgical mask, and tells you in what room to find the patient. You double-check your chart, and there is no indication that this patient may be infectious. Your ambulance is equipped for standard street care. You have four more transfers before you are scheduled to return to base.

- Would you accept this patient? If so, what actions and precautions would you take? If not, how would you justify it?

online outlook

BSI is an infection control concept and practice that assumes that all body fluids are potentially infectious. EMS follows the BSI concept rather than relying on universal precautions (UP). To learn more about UP and BSI, complete Exercise 15 at www.emtb.com.

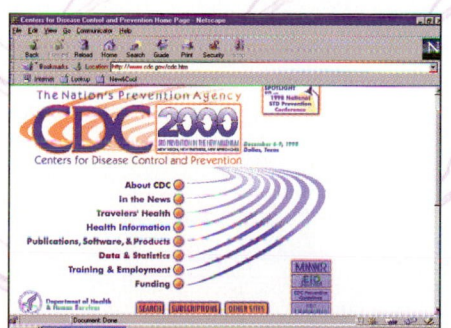

prep kit 15

The Acute Abdomen

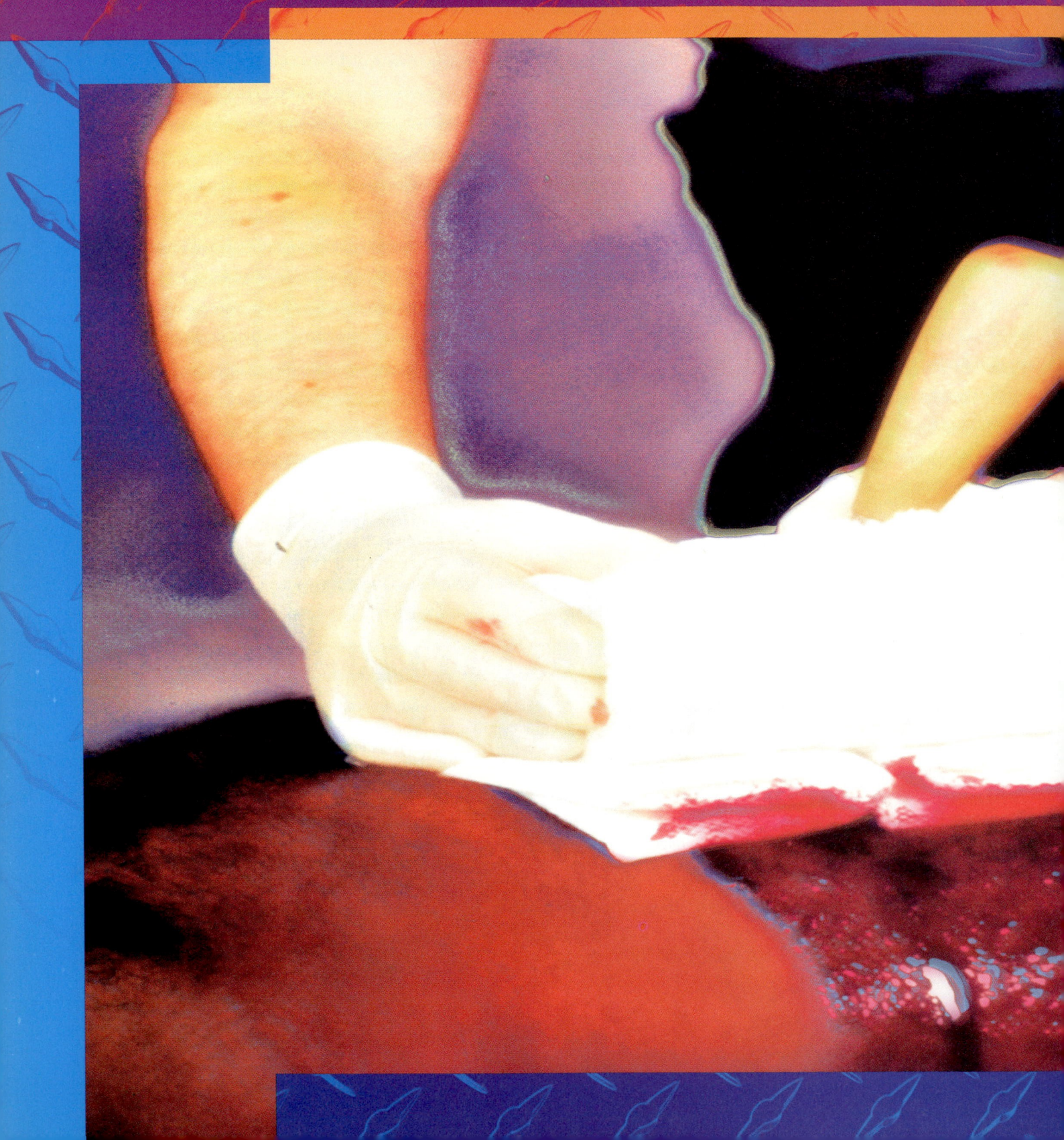

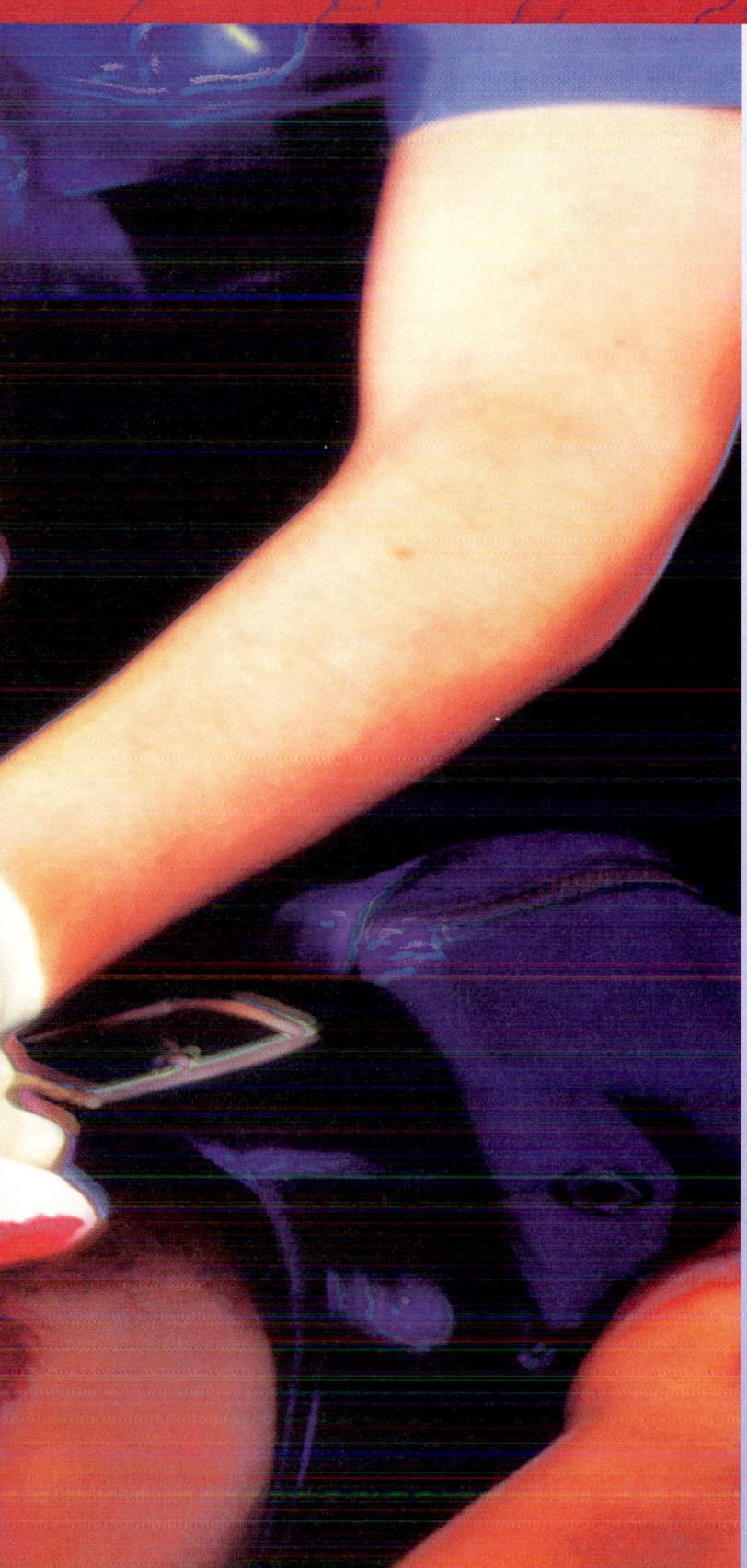

objectives*

Cognitive

1. Define the term "acute abdomen."

2. Identify the signs and symptoms of the acute abdomen and the necessity for immediate transport of patients with these symptoms.

3. Define the concept of "referred pain."

4. Describe the areas of pain or referred pain seen with the common causes of the acute abdomen.

5. Explain that pain in the abdomen can arise from other body systems.

Affective

None

Psychomotor

6. Perform a rapid gentle assessment of the abdomen.

* These are non-curriculum objectives.

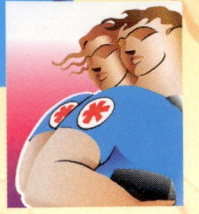

you are the emt

Rescue 6 please respond to a house at 847 Cook Road. The mother of a 12-year-old girl reports that her daughter has a severe stomach ache.

Information that is given to dispatch is often not complete. A call that sounds as minor as a stomach ache might turn out to be quite serious. This chapter will help you to understand the wide and varied problems associated with "an acute abdomen" and will help you to answer the following questions:

1. Under what circumstances is it appropriate not to transport a patient with abdominal pain?

2. Are there significant differences between male and female patients who have chief complaints of abdominal pain? Between different age groups? If so, what are they?

The Acute Abdomen

Abdominal pain is a common complaint, but the cause is often difficult to identify, even for a physician. As an EMT-B, you do not need to determine the exact cause of acute abdominal pain. You simply need to be able to recognize a life-threatening problem and act swiftly in response. Remember, the patient is in pain and is probably anxious, requiring all your skills of rapid assessment and emotional support.

This chapter begins by explaining the physiology of the abdomen. It then describes the signs and symptoms of the acute abdomen and explains how to examine the abdomen. Next, it discusses the different causes of the acute abdomen and appropriate emergency medical care.

The Physiology of the Abdomen

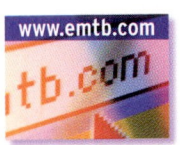

Acute abdomen is a medical term referring to the sudden onset of abdominal pain, that indicates an irritation of the **peritoneum**, the thin membrane that lines the entire abdominal cavity. This condition, called **peritonitis**, can be caused by an infection, a penetrating abdominal wound, a blunt injury severe enough to damage abdominal organs, and many diseases. In all cases, the major symptom is the same: severe pain. The major clinical signs are abdominal tenderness and distention.

Anatomically, the peritoneum is not one membrane, but two. The *parietal peritoneum* lines the walls of the abdominal cavity; the *visceral peritoneum* covers the surface of each of the organs in the abdominal cavity.

Two different types of nerves supply these two areas of the peritoneum. The parietal peritoneum is supplied by the same nerves from the spinal cord that supply the skin of the abdomen; it can therefore perceive much the same sensations: pain, touch, pressure, heat, and cold. These sensory nerves can easily identify and localize a point of irritation. In contrast, the visceral peritoneum is supplied by the autonomic nervous system. These nerves are far less able to localize sensation. The visceral peritoneum is stimulated when distention or contraction of the hollow abdominal organs activates the stretch receptors. This sensation is usually interpreted as **colic**, a severe, intermittent cramping pain. Other painful sensations that occur because of an irritated visceral peritoneum may be perceived at a distant point on the surface of the body, such as the back or shoulder. This phenomenon is called **referred pain**.

Referred pain is the result of connections between the body's two separate nervous systems. The spinal cord supplies sensory nerves to the skin and muscles; these nerves are called the somatic nervous system. The autonomic nervous system controls the abdominal organs and the blood vessels. The nerves connecting these two systems cause the stimulation of the autonomic nerves to be perceived as stimulation of the spinal sensory nerves. For example, *acute cholecystitis* (inflammation of the gallbladder) may cause pain in the right shoulder, because the autonomic nerves serving the gallbladder lie near the spinal cord at the same anatomic level as the spinal sensory nerves that supply the skin of the shoulder (Figure 16-1).

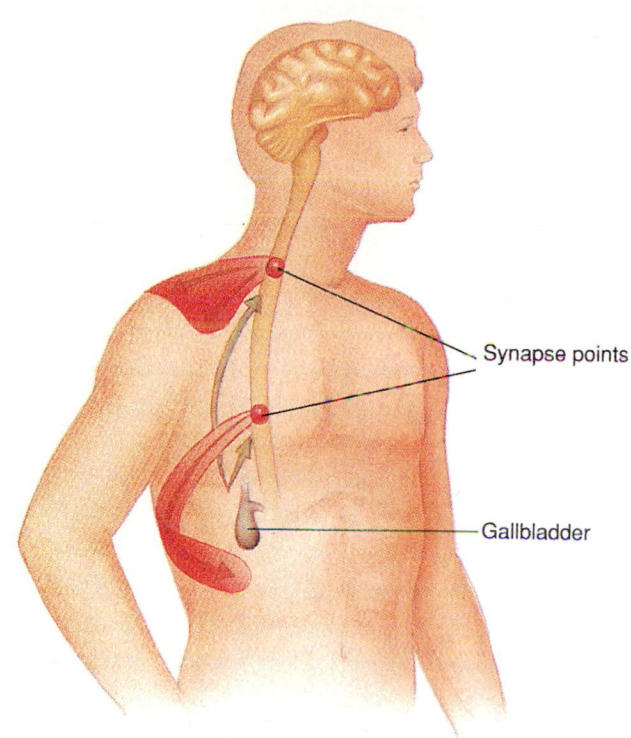

FIGURE 16-1 Acute cholecystitis causes referred pain in the shoulder as well as abdominal pain.

An acute abdomen is characterized by abdominal pain and tenderness.

Signs and Symptoms of Acute Abdomen

Peritonitis typically causes **ileus**, or paralysis of the muscular contractions that normally propel material through the intestine. The retained gas and feces, in turn, cause abdominal distention. In the presence of such paralysis, nothing that is eaten can pass normally out of the stomach or through the bowel. The only way the stomach can empty itself, then, is by **emesis**, or vomiting. For this reason, peritonitis is almost always associated with nausea and vomiting, usually in that order. These complaints do not point to a particular cause, since they can accompany almost every type of gastrointestinal disease or injury.

Similarly, **anorexia**, loss of hunger or appetite, is a nonspecific symptom. It, too, is an almost universal complaint in gastrointestinal and abdominal disease or injury. In fact, if a patient does not have anorexia, the situation may not be as serious as it otherwise appears.

Peritonitis is associated with a loss of body fluid into the abdominal cavity. The loss of fluid usually results from abnormal shifts of fluid from the bloodstream into body tissues. This decreases the volume of circulating blood and may eventually cause *hypovolemic shock*. This problem can be compounded by massive internal or external bleeding, resulting in severely inadequate perfusion. The patient may have normal vital signs or, if the peritonitis has progressed farther, may have tachycardia and hypotension. When peritonitis is accompanied by hemorrhage, the signs of shock are much more apparent.

Fever may or may not be present, depending on the cause of the peritonitis. Patients with *diverticulitis* (an inflammation of small pockets in the colon) or cholecystitis may have a substantial elevation in temperature. However, patients with acute appendicitis may have a normal temperature until the appendix ruptures and an abscess starts to form.

As we have seen, an acute abdomen is characterized by abdominal pain and tenderness. The pain may be sharply localized or diffuse and will vary in its severity. Localized pain gives a clue to the problem organ or area causing it. Tenderness may be minimal or so great that the patient will not allow you to touch the abdomen.

Another sign of the acute abdomen is tenseness of the abdominal muscles over the irritated area. In some instances, the muscles of the abdominal wall become rigid in an involuntary effort to protect the abdomen from further irritation. This boardlike muscle spasm, called **guarding**, can be seen with major problems such as a perforated peptic ulcer or pancreatitis. In some situations, patients are comfortable only when lying in one particular position, which tends to relax muscles adjacent to the inflamed organ and thus lessen the pain. Therefore, the position of the patient may provide an important clue. For example, a patient with appendicitis may draw up the right knee. A patient with pancreatitis may lie curled up on one side.

To gauge the degree of distention, simply look at the patient's abdomen. Distention begins shortly after muscular contractions of the bowel have ceased. Pulse and blood pressure may undergo significant change or none at all. These findings usually reflect the severity of the process, its duration, and the amount of fluid lost into the abdomen.

Remember, the patient with peritonitis usually has abdominal pain, even when lying quietly. The patient can be quiet but have difficulty breathing and may take rapid, shallow breaths because of the pain. Usually, you will find tenderness on palpation of the abdomen or when the patient moves. The degree of pain and tenderness is usually related directly to the severity of peritoneal inflammation.

The following is a checklist of common signs and symptoms of irritation or inflammation of the peritoneum that you can use to determine whether a patient has an acute abdomen:

- Local or diffuse abdominal pain and/or tenderness
- A quiet patient who is guarding the abdomen (in shock)
- Rapid breathing with shallow breaths
- Referred (distant) pain
- Anorexia, nausea, vomiting
- Tense, often distended, abdomen
- Sudden constipation or bloody diarrhea
- Tachycardia
- Hypotension
- Fever
- Rebound tenderness (hurts less when direct pressure is applied, but very painful when pressure is released)

Use the following steps to examine the abdomen quickly:

1. Explain to the patient what you are about to do.

2. Place the patient supine with the legs drawn up and flexed at the knees to relax the abdominal muscles.

3. Determine whether the patient is restless or quiet; whether motion causes pain; or whether any characteristic position, distention, or obvious abnormality is present.

4. Palpate the abdomen gently to determine whether it is tense (guarded) or soft (Figure 16-2).

5. Determine whether the patient can relax the abdominal wall on command.

6. Determine whether the abdomen is tender when palpated.

Although such an examination will yield much information, it should not be prolonged. The physician will do a much more detailed examination in the hospital.

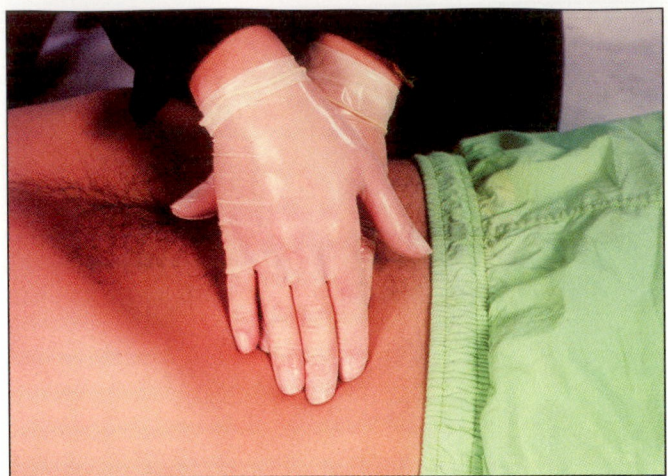

FIGURE 16-2 Check tenderness or rigidity by gently palpating the abdomen.

Remember to be very gentle when palpating the abdomen. Occasionally, an organ within the abdomen will be enlarged and very fragile, and rough palpation could cause further damage.

Causes of Abdominal Pain

Gastrointestinal and Urinary Tract

The abdominal cavity contains the solid and hollow organs that make up the gastrointestinal, genital, and urinary systems (Figure 16-3). Many of these organs, such as the bowel, are covered by visceral peritoneum; parietal peritoneum covers the inside aspect of the abdominal wall that forms the abdominal cavity. The entire abdominal cavity normally contains a very small amount of peritoneal fluid to bathe the organs. Any condition that allows pus, blood, feces, urine, gastric juice, intestinal contents, bile, pancreatic juice, amniotic fluid, or other foreign material to lie within or adjacent to this cavity can cause an acute abdomen. Technically, organs such as kidneys, ovaries, and other genitourinary structures are *retroperitoneal* (behind the peritoneum) (Figure 16-4). However, because they lie next to the peritoneum, problems in these organs can lead to an acute abdomen. Therefore, nearly every kind of abdominal problem can cause an acute abdomen.

Among the common diseases that produce signs of an acute abdomen are acute appendicitis, perforated gastric ulcer, cholecystitis, and diverticulitis. The more common emergency problems, with most common locations of direct and referred pain, are listed in Table 16-1.

Because the parietal peritoneum is richly supplied with very sensitive nerves, disease or inflammation of

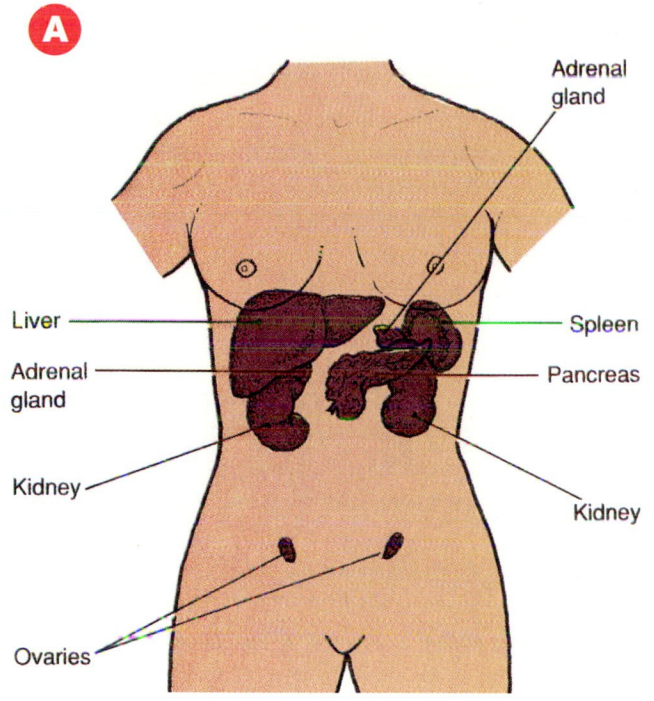

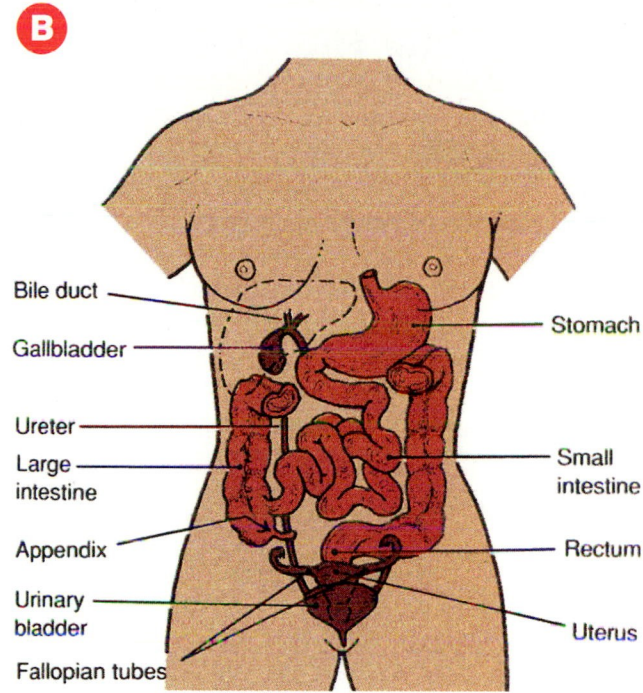

FIGURE 16-3 The solid and hollow organs of the abdomen. **A:** Solid organs include the liver, adrenal gland, spleen, pancreas, kidneys, and ovaries (in women). **B:** Hollow organs include the gallbladder, stomach, small and large intestine, and bladder.

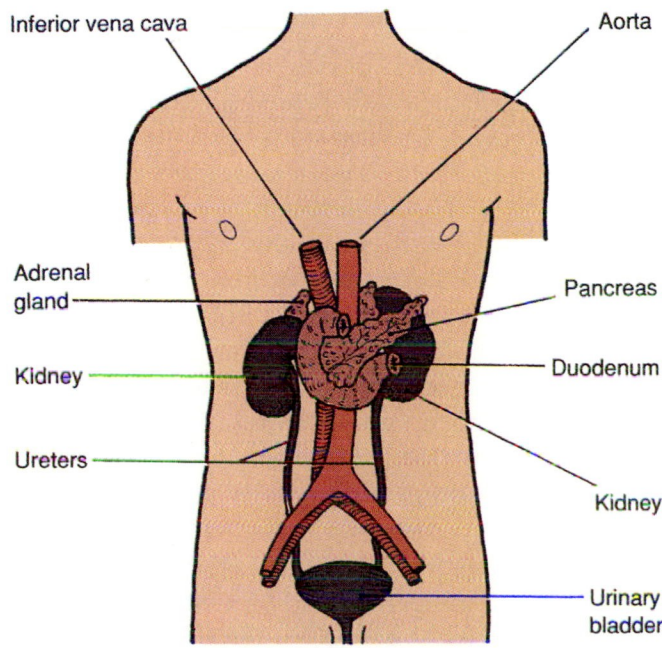

FIGURE 16-4 The major organs of the retroperitoneal space include the kidneys, ovaries, and other genitourinary structures.

TABLE 16-1	Common Abdominal Conditions
Condition	**Localization of Pain**
Appendicitis	Around navel (referred); right lower quadrant (direct)
Cholecystitis	Right shoulder (referred); right upper quadrant (direct)
Duodenal ulcer	Upper midabdomen or upper back
Diverticulitis	Left lower quadrant
Aortic Aneurysm (ruptured or dissecting)	Low back and right lower quadrant
Cystitis (inflammation of the bladder)	Lower midabdomen (retropubic)
Kidney Infection	Costovertebral angle
Kidney Stone	Right or left flanks, radiating to genitalia (referred)
Pelvic Inflammation (in women)	Both lower quadrants
Pancreatitis	Upper abdomen (both quadrants); back

caring for the elderly

The elderly patient is just as susceptible to the acute abdomen as the younger adult is. However, their signs and symptoms might be different. Because of altered pain sensation, the geriatric patient with an acute abdomen may not feel any discomfort or may describe the discomfort as mild, even in severe conditions.

Because the elderly patient has decreased body temperature regulation and response, the patient with an acute abdomen, including peritonitis, may not have a fever. However, if a fever is present, it can be minimal.

Because of the elderly patient's response to the acute abdomen, a delay in identifying the condition and seeking medical attention is possible, putting the patient at risk for complications. You should ask about the patient's medical history, especially the history of recent illness, to identify a potential illness. Ask about abdominal discomfort, when the patient last had a bowel movement, whether she or he was constipated or had diarrhea, when the patient last ate, and whether she or he vomited. Ruling out appendicitis, bowel obstruction, or ruptured bowel can hasten proper treatment and recovery.

organs that lie behind or beneath the abdominal cavity can also cause the signs of peritonitis. These signs and symptoms are similar to those produced by actual inflammation within the abdominal cavity. Pancreatitis, for example, can produce a severe reaction that is hard to distinguish from a perforated ulcer. Kidney stones that cause colic of the ureter are frequently associated with ileus. Infections of the urinary tract may also cause peritoneal irritation.

Uterus and Ovaries

Gynecologic problems are a common cause of acute abdominal pain. Always consider that a woman with lower abdominal pain and tenderness may have a problem related to her ovaries, fallopian tubes, or uterus.

Abdominal pains may also be related to the normal menstrual cycle. A common lower abdominal pain, often confused with appendicitis but fairly short lived, is called *mittelschmerz*. It is associated with the release of an egg from the ovary, characteristically occurring in the middle of the menstrual cycle, between menstrual periods. Mittelschmerz may also be associated with lower abdominal tenderness. Some women experience painful cramps at the time of their menstrual periods. In some, the discomfort may be crippling and the menstrual flow severe.

A common cause of an acute abdomen in women is *pelvic inflammatory disease (PID)*, an infection of the fallopian tubes and the surrounding tissues of the pelvis. With PID, acute pain and tenderness in the lower abdomen may be intense and accompanied by a high fever. If you suspect PID, promptly transport the patient to the emergency department for treatment.

Between 1% and 2% of all pregnancies are ectopic. The term *ectopic pregnancy* means that a fertilized egg has come to lie in an area outside the uterus, usually in a fallopian tube. A fallopian tube is simply not large enough to support the growth of a fetus and placenta for more than about 6 to 8 weeks. When the tube ruptures, it produces massive internal hemorrhage and abrupt abdominal pain. In this situation, the acute abdomen may be associated with the onset of hypovolemic shock. This combination mandates immediate transport to the hospital.

Other Organ Systems

The aorta lies immediately behind the peritoneum on the spinal column. In older individuals, the wall of the aorta sometimes develops weak areas that swell to form an **aneurysm**. The development of an aneurysm is rarely associated with symptoms because it occurs slowly, but if the aneurysm ruptures, massive hemorrhage may occur and, with it, the signs of acute peritoneal irritation. The patient may also experience severe back pain, because the peritoneum can, at times, be rapidly stripped away from the wall of the main abdominal cavity by the hemorrhage. Pain can also be associated with the pressure of blood on the back itself. In such instances, bleeding usually leads to profound shock. Again, the association of acute abdominal signs and symptoms with shock requires prompt transportation. Because this is a fragile situation with a large, leaking artery, avoid unnecessary or vigorous palpation of the abdomen. Remember to handle the patient gently during transport.

Pneumonia, especially in the lower parts of the lung, may cause both ileus pain and abdominal pain. In this instance, the problem lies in an adjacent body cavity, but the intense inflammatory response can affect the abdomen. Treat and transport this patient as you would any patient with abdominal pain.

A <u>hernia</u> is a protrusion of an organ or tissue through a hole in the body wall covering its normal site. Virtually every organ or tissue in the body will herniate through its covering membranes in certain circumstances. Hernias can occur as a result of the following:

- A congenital defect, as around the umbilicus
- A surgical wound that has failed to heal properly
- Some natural weakness in an area such as in the groin

Hernias always produce a mass or lump that the patient will be aware of. At times, the mass will disappear back into the body cavity in which it belongs. In this case, the hernia is said to be *reducible*. If the mass cannot be pushed back within the body, it is said to be *incarcerated*.

Reducible hernias pose little risk to the patient; some individuals live with them for years. When a hernia is incarcerated, however, its contents may become seriously compressed by the surrounding tissue, eventually compromising the blood supply. This situation, called <u>strangulation</u>, is a serious medical emergency. Immediate surgery is required to remove any dead tissue and repair the hernia.

The following signs and symptoms indicate a serious hernia problem:

- The existence of the hernia itself
- A clear statement that a mass that was reducible can no longer be pushed back inside the body
- Pain at the hernia site
- Tenderness when the hernia is palpated
- Red or blue skin discoloration over the hernia

Any of these signs and symptoms, other than the hernia itself, is cause for prompt transport to the emergency department.

Emergency Medical Care

The signs and symptoms of an acute abdomen signal a serious medical or surgical emergency. Ensure that you provide prompt, gentle transport for the patient; do not delay transport. Carry out the following steps as quickly as possible before transport.

1. **Do not attempt to diagnose the cause** of the acute abdomen.

2. **Clear and maintain the airway.**

3. **Anticipate vomiting.**

4. **Give oxygen.**

5. **Do not give the patient anything by mouth.** Food or fluid will only aggravate many of the symptoms, since intestinal paralysis will prevent it from passing out of the stomach. The presence of food in the stomach will make any emergency surgery more dangerous.

6. **Do not administer any sedative or analgesic agent** unless instructed to by medical control. Medications may mask the physical findings, thus delaying a diagnosis in the hospital. Medications can also increase the risk of aspiration (inhalation) of stomach contents into the lungs if the patient continues to vomit.

7. **Document all pertinent information:** Onset, Provocation, Quality, Radiation, Severity, Time and treatment (OPQRST). Note the presence of abdominal tenderness, distention, or guarding.

8. **Anticipate the development of hypovolemic shock.** Treat the patient for shock when it is evident.

9. **Make the patient as comfortable** as possible for transport. Conserve body heat with blankets, as needed.

10. **Monitor vital signs;** these may change quickly.

prep kit

ready to review

The acute abdomen is a medical emergency, requiring prompt but gentle transport. The pain, tenderness, and abdominal distention associated with acute abdomen are signs of peritonitis, which may be caused by any condition that allows pus, blood, feces, urine, gastric juice, intestinal contents, bile, pancreatic juice, amniotic fluid, or other foreign material to lie within or adjacent to the peritoneum. In addition to abdominal disease or injury, problems in the gastrointestinal, genital, and urinary systems may also cause peritonitis. Appendicitis, perforated gastric ulcer, cholecystitis, and diverticulitis are common causes of an acute abdomen. A strangulated hernia is another.

Signs and symptoms of acute abdomen include pain, nausea, vomiting, and a tense, distended abdomen. Pain is common directly over the inflamed area of the peritoneum, or it may be referred to another part of the body. Referred pain occurs because of the connections between the two different nervous systems supplying the parietal peritoneum and the visceral peritoneum.

Your first priorities are to assess airway, breathing, and circulation and then apply oxygen. Next, obtain a pertinent medical history: When did the symptoms begin? How have they changed over time? Where exactly is the pain? What does it feel like? How long does it last and how intense is it? Has there been a loss of fluid volume as a result of vomiting or diarrhea? Take vital signs and gently palpate the abdomen. The presence of abdominal tenderness will confirm the need to transport the patient to the emergency department in an urgent manner.

Do not give the patient with an acute abdomen anything by mouth. In all likelihood, the bowel is paralyzed, making it impossible for food to pass out of the stomach. Unless instructed to by medical control, do not give medication, as this may mask the symptoms.

vital vocabulary

www.emtb.com

acute abdomen A condition of sudden onset of pain within the abdomen, demanding immediate medical or surgical treatment.

aneurysm A swelling or enlargement of a part of an artery, resulting from weakening of the arterial wall.

anorexia Lack or loss of appetite for food.

colic Acute cramping abdominal pain.

emesis Vomiting.

guarding Involuntary muscle contractions of the abdominal wall, an effort to protect the inflamed abdomen.

hernia The protrusion of a loop of an organ or tissue through an abnormal body opening.

ileus Paralysis of the bowel, arising from any one of several causes.

peritoneum The membrane lining the abdominal cavity (parietal peritoneum) and covering the abdominal organs (visceral peritoneum).

peritonitis Inflammation of the peritoneum.

referred pain Pain felt in an area of the body other than the area where the cause of pain is located.

strangulation Complete obstruction of blood circulation in a given organ as a result of compression or entrapment, a situation causing death of tissue.

assessment in action

You and your partner are dispatched to a small apartment complex on the west side of town for a "man with belly pain." On arrival, you find a 39-year-old man in a small apartment that is furnished only with a couch with no legs, a TV, and a mattress. Beer cans, empty pizza boxes, and alcohol bottles litter the floor.

The patient is very pale and appears unsteady on his feet as he makes his way back to the couch after letting you and your partner in the door. He tells you that his stomach has been bothering him for about a week but that 2 days ago, it "really got worse." He then says that when he awoke this morning, it hurt to get out of bed. In fact, the only reason he got out of bed was to throw up. In response to your questions, he tells you that the vomit appeared "brownish-blackish" and had a bad odor. He denies any recent injury.

Assessment reveals that he has cool, quite moist skin and that his radial pulse is so fast that you can barely feel it. His abdomen feels firm and is tender to even the slightest touch. He has a blood pressure of 102/68 mm Hg, a pulse of 136 beats/min, and respirations of 32 breaths/min.

1. Of the following, which condition is the most potentially life threatening for this patient?
   A. Shock
   B. Intoxication
   C. Dehydration
   D. Malnutrition

2. What is the significance of the patient's description of the emesis?
   A. It confirms that the patient has abused alcohol.
   B. It confirms that the patient has bleeding hemorrhoids.
   C. It suggests that the patient is vomiting well-digested food.
   D. It suggests that the patient is vomiting partially digested blood.

3. Treatment at this time should consist of administering high-flow supplemental oxygen and:
   A. elevating the patient's head and shoulders.
   B. placing the patient in the recovery position.
   C. placing the patient supine with his knees flexed.
   D. placing the patient in Trendelenburg's position.

4. On the basis of the available information, which of the following statements best describes the patient's condition?
   A. The patient is in shock associated with gastrointestinal bleeding.
   B. The patient has a ruptured liver as a result of chronic alcohol abuse.
   C. The patient has a head injury from a fall that was caused by intoxication.
   D. The patient's condition is a result of acute alcohol withdrawal syndrome.

5. Which of the following statements best describes alcohol abuse and this patient's signs and symptoms?
   A. Long-term alcohol abuse usually affects only a single body system.
   B. Gastrointestinal bleeding is most often associated with a single episode of alcohol abuse.
   C. The patient's apparent alcohol abuse and his symptoms are not related.
   D. Chronic alcohol abusers are more likely to experience gastrointestinal bleeding than are individuals with no history of alcohol abuse.

points to ponder

Objectives 3-4.1, 3-4.2, 3-4.5, 4-9.1, 4-9.3

You respond to the local high school to find a 15-year-old girl with severe lower abdominal pain. History reveals that she normally has significant pain with menstruation and that she is experiencing vaginal bleeding currently but that it is "more red" than normal. She has not had a period for two months and thought she might be pregnant, so she went to "a guy that her friend knows and had that fixed a few days ago." This "guy" was not a physician, just a friend of a friend. She does not want to go to the hospital because her parents may find out what she has done.

• Would you advise her to go to the hospital? Why or why not? How would you encourage her to go to the hospital if you thought it was important?

online outlook

A hernia is a protrusion of an organ or tissue through a hole in the body wall covering its normal site. Virtually every organ or tissue in the body will herniate through its covering membranes in certain circumstances. Learn about the surgical repair of a hernia by completing Exercise 16 at www.emtb.com.

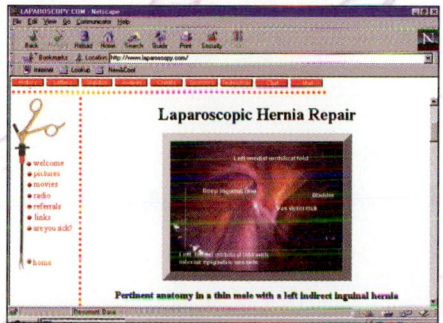

prep kit 16

Diabetic Emergencies

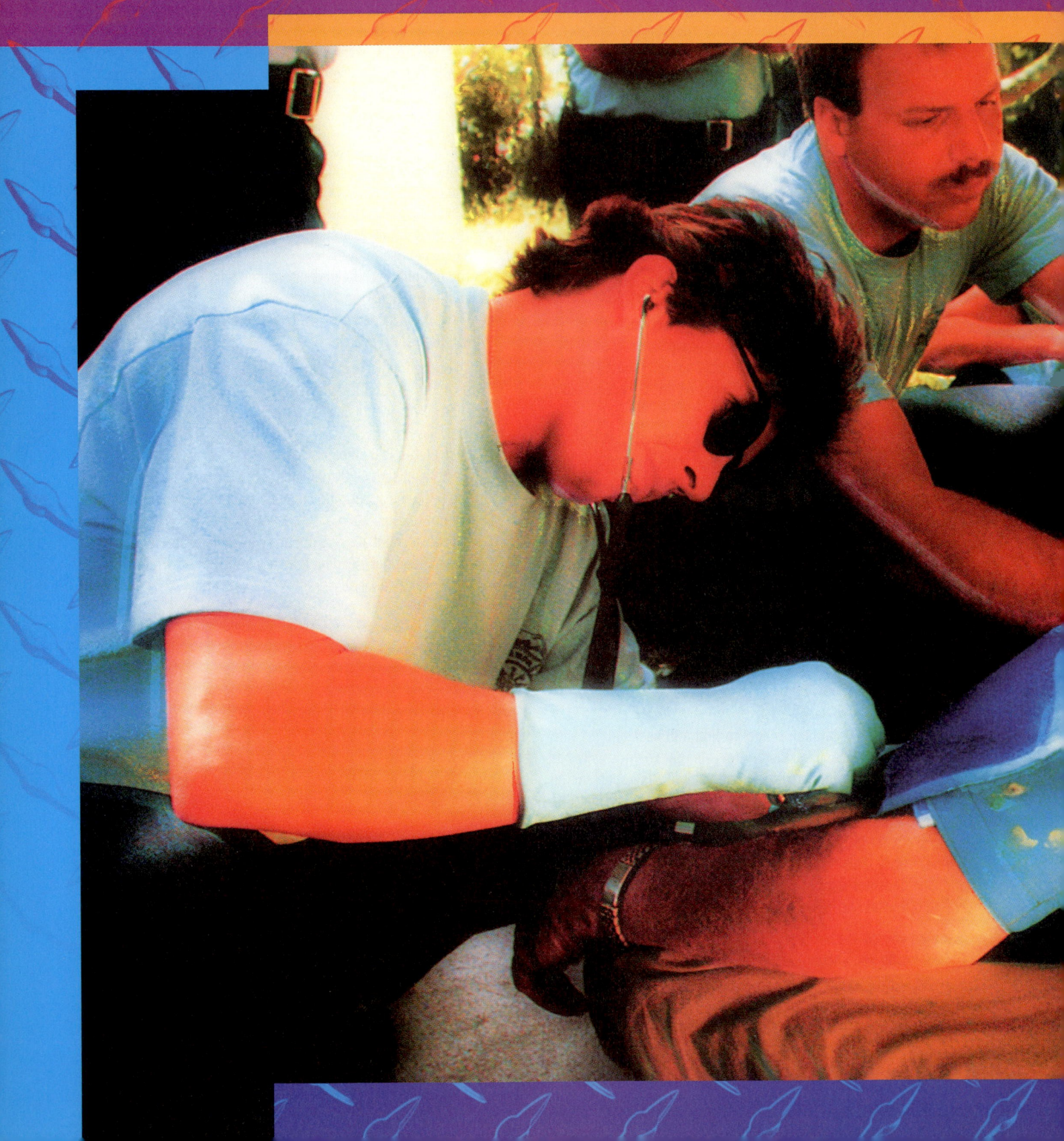

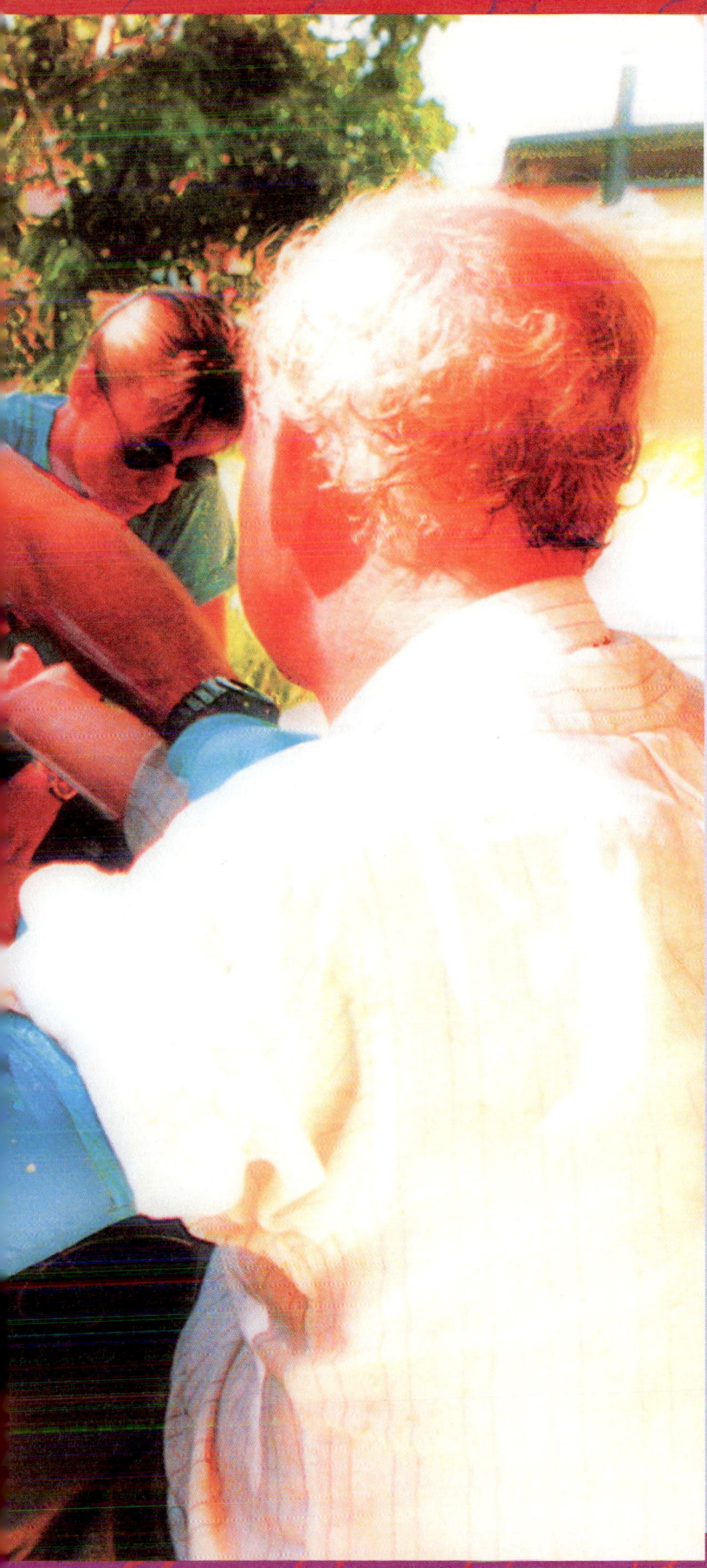

objectives

Cognitive

1. Identify the patient taking diabetic medications with altered mental status and the implications of a history of diabetes.

2. State the steps in the emergency medical care of the patient taking diabetic medicine with an altered mental status and a history of diabetes.

3. Establish the relationship between airway management and the patient with altered mental status.

4. State the generic and trade names, medication forms, dose, administration, action, and contraindications for oral glucose.

5. Evaluate the need for medical direction in the emergency medical care of the diabetic patient.

Affective

6. Explain the rationale for administering oral glucose.

Psychomotor

7. Demonstrate the steps in the emergency medical care for the patient taking diabetic medicine with an altered mental status and a history of diabetes.

8. Demonstrate the steps in the administration of oral glucose.

9. Demonstrate the assessment and documentation of patient response to oral glucose.

10. Demonstrate how to complete a prehospital care report for patients with diabetic emergencies.

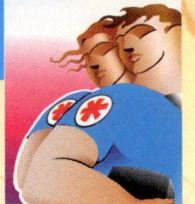

you are the emt

Rescue 6 please respond to Wally's Convenience Store at 188 Central Street . . . a young boy has just called in reporting what appears to be an intoxicated man who just fell down in the parking lot . . .

While the patient may, in fact, be intoxicated, there are other possible explanations for his appearance—diabetes, for example. This chapter will provide you with the background information you will need to care for a patient experiencing a diabetic emergency and will help you to answer the following questions:

1. How does the prehospital care for a patient with high blood glucose differ from that for a patient with low blood glucose?

2. How do patients with insulin-dependent diabetes mellitus differ from those with non-insulin-dependent diabetes mellitus?

Diabetic Emergencies

Diabetes is a very common disease, affecting about 6% of the population. It is a metabolic disorder in which the hormone that is needed to regulate blood glucose levels is missing or ineffective. Without treatment, blood glucose levels become too high and can cause coma and death. If properly treated, most people with diabetes can live a relatively normal life. However, diabetes can have many severe complications that affect the length and quality of life, including blindness, cardiovascular disease, and kidney failure. Also, treatment to lower high blood glucose levels can overshoot and cause a life-threatening state of hypoglycemia (low blood glucose). Therefore, as an EMT-B, you need to know the signs and symptoms of a blood glucose level that is either too high or too low so that you can administer the proper lifesaving treatment.

This chapter explains the two types of diabetes and how they are controlled, including the role of glucose and insulin. You will learn how to distinguish between diabetic coma and insulin shock, which often resemble each other. The chapter discusses how to identify and treat diabetic emergencies in the prehospital setting. Complications, such as seizures, altered mental status, and heart attack are also briefly discussed, as are the emergency medical care for each, in addition to the relationship of diabetes and an altered mental status to airway management.

Diabetes

Defining Diabetes

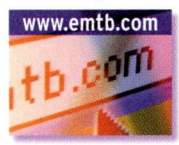

Literally, the word "diabetes" means "a passer through; a siphon." Medically, the term refers to a metabolic disorder in which the body's ability to metabolize simple carbohydrates (blood glucose) is impaired. It is characterized by the passage of large quantities of urine containing glucose, significant thirst, and deterioration of body functions. **Glucose**, or dextrose, is one of the basic sugars in the body and, along with oxygen, is the primary fuel for cellular metabolism.

The central problem in diabetes is the lack or ineffective action of **insulin**, a hormone that is normally produced by the pancreas that enables the cells to metabolize glucose. A **hormone** is a chemical substance produced by a gland that has special regulatory effects on other body organs and tissues. Without insulin, cells begin to "starve" because insulin is needed, like a key, to let glucose into the cells.

The full name of diabetes is **diabetes mellitus**, which means "sweet diabetes." This refers to the presence of sugar (glucose) in the urine. Diabetes mellitus is considered a metabolic disorder in which the body cannot metabolize glucose, usually because of the lack of insulin; the result is a wasting of glucose in the urine. *Diabetes insipidus,* a rare condition, also involves excessive urination, but here the missing hormone is one that regulates urinary fluid reabsorption. In this book, the term "diabetes" always refers to diabetes mellitus.

Left untreated, diabetes leads to a wasting of body tissues and death. Even with medical care, some patients with particularly aggressive forms of diabetes will die relatively young from one or more complications of the disease. Most patients with diabetes, however, can live out a normal life span. But they must be willing to adjust their lives to the demands of the disease, especially their eating habits and activities.

Types of Diabetes

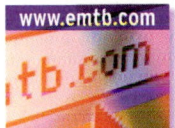

Diabetes is a disease with two distinct onset patterns. It may become evident when the patient is a child, or it may develop in later life, usually when the patient is middle-aged.

In **type I diabetes**, or *insulin-dependent diabetes,* most patients do not produce insulin at all. They need daily injections of supplemental, synthetic insulin throughout their lives to control blood glucose. Since this is the type of diabetes that strikes children, it used to be called "juvenile diabetes." However, it can, in some cases, develop in later life as well. Patients with type I diabetes are more likely to have metabolic problems and organ damage, such as blindness, heart disease, kidney failure, and nerve disorders.

In **type II diabetes**, or *non-insulin-dependent diabetes,* which usually appears later in life, patients produce inadequate amounts of insulin. In other cases, they may produce a fairly normal amount but the insulin does not function effectively. Although some patients with non-insulin-dependent diabetes may require some supplemental insulin, most can be treated with diet and non-insulin-type oral medications (hypoglycemic agents), such as chlorpropamide (Diabinase), tolbutamide (Orinase), and glyburide (Micronase). These medications stimulate the pancreas to produce more insulin and thus lower blood glucose. In some cases, these drugs can lead to hypoglycemia, particularly when patient activity and exercise levels are too vigorous or excessive. Patients with **hypoglycemia** have an abnormally low level of blood glucose. Non-insulin-dependent diabetes used to be called adult- (maturity) onset diabetes. Again, some patients with non-insulin-dependent diabetes may, in fact, be dependent on insulin.

The two types of diabetes are equally serious, although non-insulin-dependent diabetes is easier to regulate. Both can affect many tissues and functions other than the glucose-regulating mechanism. Both require lifelong medical management. Diabetes is considered to be an autoimmune problem, in which the body becomes allergic to its own tissues and literally destroys them. The severity of diabetes relates to the amount of insulin-producing tissue that is damaged or destroyed, as well as the time of life when the process started.

The Role of Glucose and Insulin

Glucose is the major source of energy for the body, and all cells need it to function properly. Some cells will not function at all without glucose. A constant supply of glucose is as important as oxygen to the brain. Without glucose, or with very low levels, brain cells rapidly suffer permanent damage. With the exception of the brain, insulin is needed to allow glucose to enter individual body cells to fuel their functioning. For this reason, insulin is said to be a "cellular key" (Figure 17-1).

Without insulin, glucose from food remains in the blood and gradually rises to extremely high levels. This condition is called **hyperglycemia**. Once the blood glucose levels reach 200 mg/dL or more, or twice the

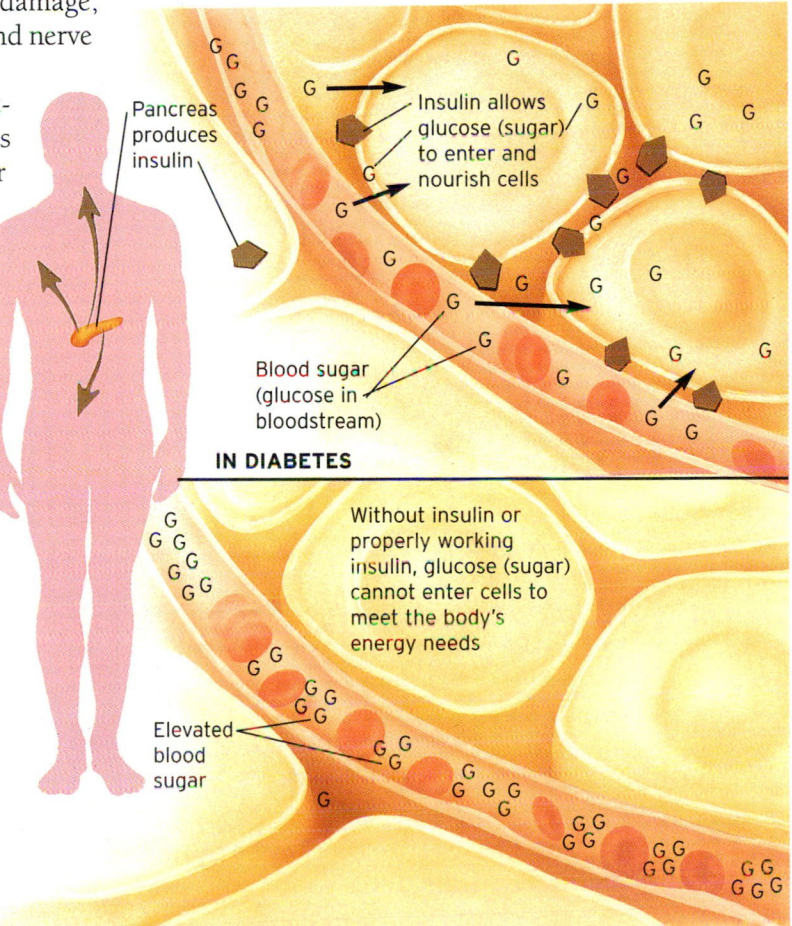

FIGURE 17-1 Diabetes is defined as a lack of or ineffective action of insulin. Without insulin, cells begin to "starve" because insulin is needed to allow glucose to enter and nourish the cells.

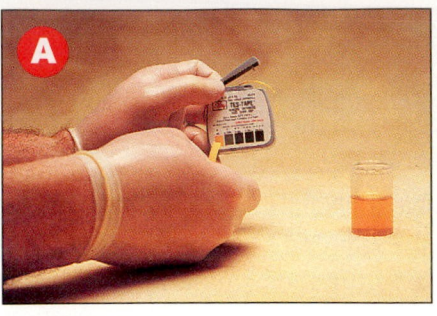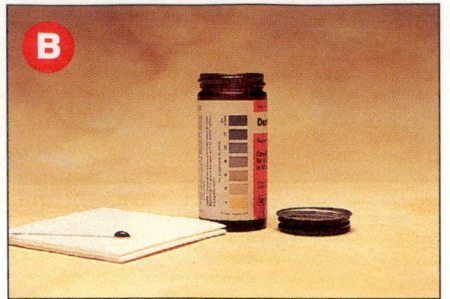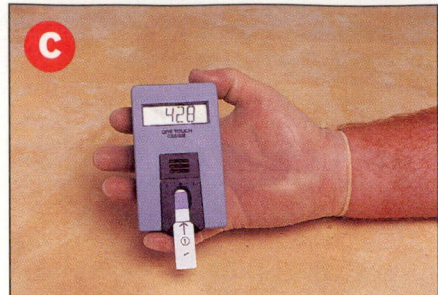

FIGURE 17-2 A: Urine testing kit. **B:** Glucose test strips for blood analysis. **C:** Blood glucose self-monitoring kit.

usual amount (normally 80 to 120 mg/dL), excess glucose is excreted by the kidney. This process requires a large amount of water. The loss of water in such large amounts causes the classic symptoms of uncontrolled diabetes, the "3 Ps":

- **Polyuria**, frequent and plentiful urination
- **Polydipsia**, frequent drinking of liquid to satisfy continuous thirst (secondary to the loss of so much body water)
- **Polyphagia**, excessive eating as a result of cellular "hunger"; seen only occasionally

Without glucose to supply energy for cells, the body must turn to other fuel sources. The most abundant is fat. Unfortunately, when fat is used as an immediate energy source, chemicals called *ketones* and *fatty acids* are formed as waste products and are hard for the body to excrete. As they accumulate in blood and tissue, certain ketones can produce a dangerous condition called **acidosis**. The form of acidosis seen in uncontrolled diabetes is called **diabetic ketoacidosis**, in which an accumulation of certain acids occurs when insulin is not available in the body. Signs and symptoms of diabetic ketoacidosis include vomiting, abdominal pain, and a type of deep, rapid breathing called *Kussmaul respirations*. When the acid levels in the body become too high, individual cells will cease to function. If the patient is not given proper fluid and insulin to reverse fat metabolism and restore use of glucose as a source of energy, ketoacidosis will progress to unconsciousness, diabetic coma, and eventually death.

As we have seen, diabetes mellitus is treatable; however, treatment must be tailored for the individual patient. The trick is to balance constantly the patient's need for glucose with the available supply of insulin by testing either the blood or the urine. In the past, most patients tested their urine daily for the presence of glucose and acetone. *Acetone* is one type of ketone, indicating the presence of ketones in the blood, but its absence does not mean that there are no ketones in the blood. Many patients now measure the level of glucose in the blood instead, using a *blood glucose self-monitoring*

unit. This is a much simpler and more accurate procedure: A drop of blood from the fingertip is placed on a thin strip of chemically treated paper. The paper turns color and is compared with a color chart, which matches colors with approximate blood glucose readings. The readings are in milligrams per deciliter of blood; remember that the normal blood glucose level is between 80 and 120 mg/dL. Patients can also buy devices for pricking the fingertip with a fine needle, standard tables for reading the strips, or a more elaborate unit that automatically analyzes the test strip and provides a digital readout of the blood glucose level (Figure 17-2).

Diabetic Coma and Insulin Shock

Two different conditions can lead to a diabetic emergency: diabetic coma (high blood glucose, or extreme hyperglycemia) or insulin shock (low blood glucose, or hypoglycemia) (Figure 17-3). The signs and symptoms of the two conditions can be quite similar (Table 17-1). For example, staggering and an intoxicated appearance to complete unresponsiveness are signs and symptoms of

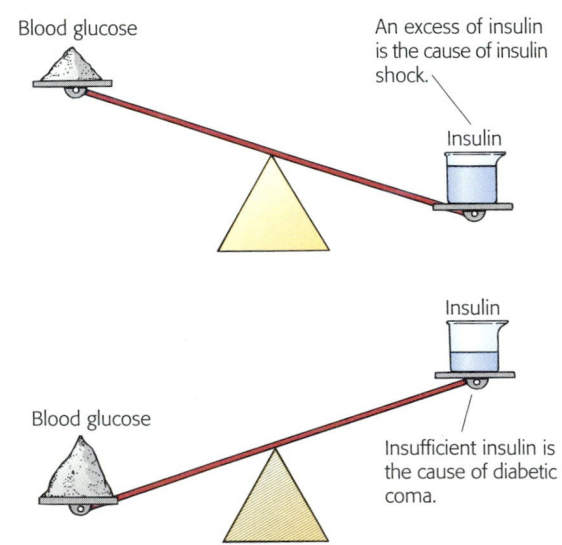

FIGURE 17-3 The two most common diabetic emergencies, diabetic coma and insulin shock, develop when the patient has either too much or too little glucose in the blood, respectively.

TABLE 17-1   Characteristics of Diabetic Emergencies

	Diabetic Coma	Insulin Shock
History		
Food intake	Excessive	Insufficient
Insulin dosage	Insufficient	Excessive
Onset	Gradual	Rapid, within minutes
Skin	Warm and dry	Pale and moist
Infection	Common	Uncommon
Gastrointestinal Tract		
Thirst	Intense	Absent
Hunger	Absent	Intense
Vomiting	Common	Uncommon
Respiratory System		
Breathing	Air hunger	Normal or rapid
Odor of breath	Sweet, fruity	Normal
Cardiovascular System		
Blood pressure	Low	Normal
Pulse	Rapid, weak	Normal or rapid and full
Nervous System		
Headache	Absent	Present
Consciousness	Restless merging to coma	Irritability, confusion, seizure, or coma
Urine		
Sugar	Present	Absent
Acetone	Present	Absent
Treatment		
Response	Gradual, within 6 to 12 hours following medication and fluid	Immediately after glucose

both. Note that your assessment of these potential emergencies should not prevent you from providing prompt care and transport as detailed in this chapter. However, in such urgent emergencies, the earlier clues are gathered, the better for the patient. With specific information about the type of emergency, you can help the hospital to prepare prompt, definitive care for the patient.

Diabetic coma. Diabetic coma is a state of unconsciousness resulting from several problems, including ketoacidosis, dehydration because of excessive urination, and hyperglycemia. Too much blood glucose by itself does not always cause diabetic coma, but on some occasions, it can lead to it.

Diabetic coma occurs in the patient who is not under medical treatment, who takes insufficient insulin, who markedly overeats, or who is undergoing some sort of stress, such as an infection, illness, overexertion, fatigue, or drinking alcohol. Usually, ketoacidosis develops over a period of time lasting from hours to days. The patient may ultimately be found comatose with the following physical signs:

- Air hunger, as indicated by Kussmaul respirations
- Dehydration, as indicated by dry, warm skin and sunken eyes
- A sweet or fruity (acetone) odor on the breath, caused by the unusual waste products in the blood (ketones)
- A rapid, weak ("thready") pulse
- A normal or slightly low blood pressure
- Varying degrees of unresponsiveness

Insulin shock. In insulin shock, the problem is hypoglycemia, insufficient glucose in the blood. When insulin levels remain high, glucose is rapidly taken out of the blood to fuel the cells. If glucose levels get too low, there may be an insufficient amount to supply the brain. If blood glucose remains low, unconsciousness and permanent brain damage can quickly follow.

Insulin shock occurs when the patient has done one of the following:

- Taken too much insulin
- Taken a regular dose of insulin but has not eaten enough food
- Had an unusual amount of activity or vigorous exercise and used up all available glucose

Insulin shock may also occur after the patient vomits a meal on a day when he or she took a regular dose of insulin. At times, insulin shock may occur with no identifiable predisposing factor.

Children who have diabetes may pose a particular management problem. First, their high levels of activity mean that they can use up circulating glucose more quickly than adults do, even after a normal insulin injection. Second, they do not always eat correctly and on schedule. As a result, insulin shock can develop more often and more severely in children than in adult patients.

Insulin shock develops much more quickly than diabetic coma. In some instances, it can occur in a matter of minutes. Hypoglycemia can be associated with the following signs and symptoms:

- Normal or rapid, deep sighing respirations
- Pale, moist (clammy) skin
- Diaphoresis (sweating)
- Dizziness, headache
- Rapid, bounding pulse
- Normal or slightly elevated blood pressure
- Aggressive, confused, lethargic, or unusual behavior
- Anxious or combative behavior
- Hunger
- Fainting, seizure, or coma
- Weakness on one side of the body (may mimic stroke)

Both diabetic coma and insulin shock produce unconsciousness and, in some instances, death. But they call for very different treatment. Diabetic coma is a complex metabolic condition that usually develops over time and involves all the tissues of the body. Correcting this condition may take many hours in a

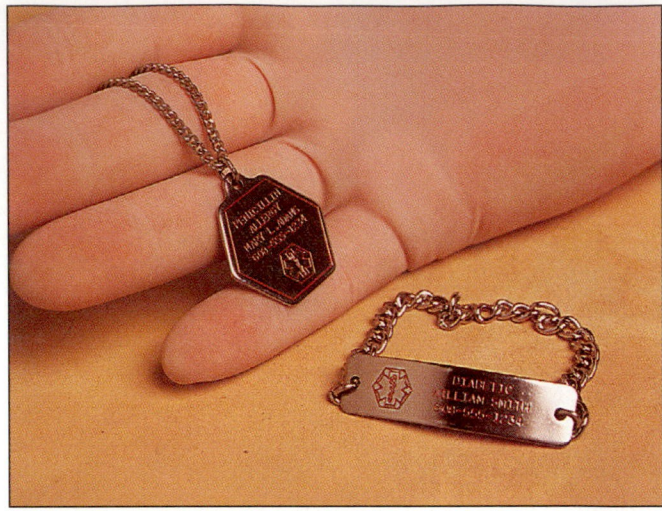

FIGURE 17-4 Some patients with diabetes will have a medical identification bracelet or necklace.

well-controlled hospital setting. Insulin shock, however, is an acute condition that can develop rapidly. A patient with diabetes who has taken his or her standard insulin dose and missed lunch may be in insulin shock before dinner. The condition is just as quickly reversed by giving the patient glucose. Without that glucose, however, the patient will suffer permanent brain damage. Minutes count.

Most individuals with diabetes understand and manage their disease well. Still, emergencies occur. In addition to diabetic coma and insulin shock, patients with diabetes may have "silent," or painless, heart attacks, a possibility that you should always consider. Their only symptom may be "not feeling so well."

Diabetes and the alcoholic. Occasionally, patients in insulin shock or a diabetic coma are thought to be intoxicated, especially if their condition has caused a motor vehicle crash or other incident. Confined by police in a "drunk tank," a patient with diabetes is at high risk of dying. In such situations, an emergency medical identification bracelet, necklace, or card may help to save the patient's life (Figure 17-4). Often, only a blood glucose test performed at the scene or in the emergency department will identify the real problem. In some EMS systems, you will be trained and allowed to perform the blood glucose test at the scene. Otherwise, you must always suspect hypoglycemia in any patient with altered mental status.

Certainly, diabetes and alcoholism can coexist in a patient. But you must be alert to the similarity in symptoms of acute alcohol intoxication and diabetic emergencies. Likewise, hypoglycemia and a head injury can coexist, and you must appreciate the potential even when the head injury is obvious.

Emergency Medical Care

You should ask the following questions of any ill patient who you know has diabetes:

- Do you take insulin or any pills that lower your blood sugar?

- Have you taken your usual dose of insulin (or pills) today?

- Have you eaten normally today?

- Have you had any illness, unusual amount of activity, or stress today?

If the patient has eaten but has not taken insulin, it is more likely that diabetic ketoacidosis is developing. If the patient has taken insulin but has not eaten, the problem is more likely to be insulin shock. A patient with diabetes will often know what is wrong. If the patient is not thinking or speaking clearly (or is unconscious), ask a family member the same questions.

The first step in caring for the patient is to perform an initial assessment to verify that the airway is open. If the patient is not breathing or is having difficulty breathing, open the airway and assist ventilations. Continue to monitor the airway as you provide care. Perform the focused assessment and detailed physical exam while your partner obtains the baseline vital signs and SAMPLE history.

When assessing a patient who you suspect might have diabetes, check to see whether he or she has an emergency medical identification symbol: a wallet card, necklace, or bracelet. Any one of the three will help you to determine whether the patient has diabetes. Or ask the patient or family if the patient has diabetes. Remember, however, that just because a person has diabetes does not mean that the diabetes is causing the current problem. He or she might be having a heart attack, stroke, or other medical emergency. For this reason, you must always do a full, careful assessment, paying attention to ABCD.

Inform medical control that you are at the scene of a diabetic emergency. At this point, ask the patient or family about the patient's last meal and insulin dose.

In the past, EMTs were often advised to place oral glucose gel or glucose tablets under the tongue or in the mouth of the unconscious patient. Very little sugar is actually absorbed in this manner. The risk of choking or aspirating liquid into the lungs probably outweighs the benefits of providing such small amounts of glucose. Therefore, although glucose is very important to give to patients with diabetes with altered mental status, *you should not attempt to give anything by mouth to an unconscious patient,* even if you suspect insulin shock. These patients need IV glucose, which you are not authorized

to give. Your responsibility is to provide prompt transport to the hospital, where the proper care can be given.

What if no one else is present, but you know that the unconscious patient has diabetes? Then you must use your knowledge of the signs and symptoms to decide whether the problem is diabetic coma or insulin shock. Remember, however, this assessment should not prevent you from providing prompt treatment and transport. The primary visible difference will be the patient's breathing: deep, sighing respirations in diabetic coma and normal or rapid respirations in insulin shock. However, the patient with diabetes who is unconscious and having convulsions is more likely to be in insulin shock, and deep sighing respirations may occur after a seizure.

Keep in mind that any unconscious patient may have undiagnosed diabetes. In patients with an altered mental status, you may be able to determine this in the field, if you have the proper equipment to test for blood glucose. Without this critical knowledge, treat this patient as you would any other unconscious individual. Provide full life support, particularly airway management, and prompt transport. At the emergency department, the diabetes and its complication can quickly be diagnosed.

Giving Oral Glucose

Oral glucose is a commercially available gel that dissolves when placed in the mouth. One toothpaste-type tube of gel equals one dose (Figure 17-5). Trade names for the gel include Glutose and Insta-Glucose. Glucose gel, which acts to increase blood glucose levels, should be given to any patient with a decreased level of consciousness who has diabetes that is controlled by medication. The only contraindications to glucose are an inability to swallow or unconsciousness, since aspiration (inhalation of the substance) can occur. Oral glucose itself has no side effects if it is administered properly; however, the risk of aspiration in a patient who is unable to gag can be dangerous. A conscious patient (even if confused) who does not really

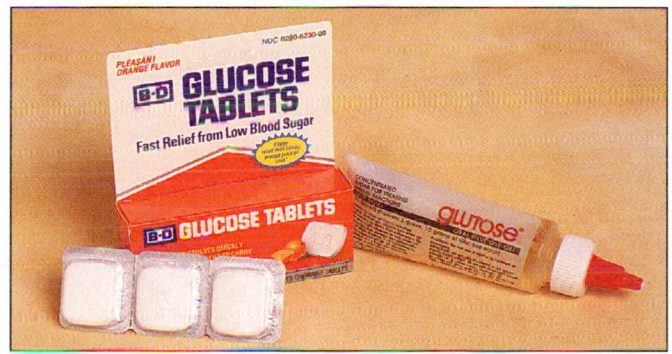

FIGURE 17-5 Oral glucose is commercially available in gel and tablet form. One tube of gel equals one dose.

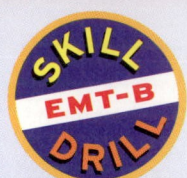

Administering Glucose

Figure 17-6

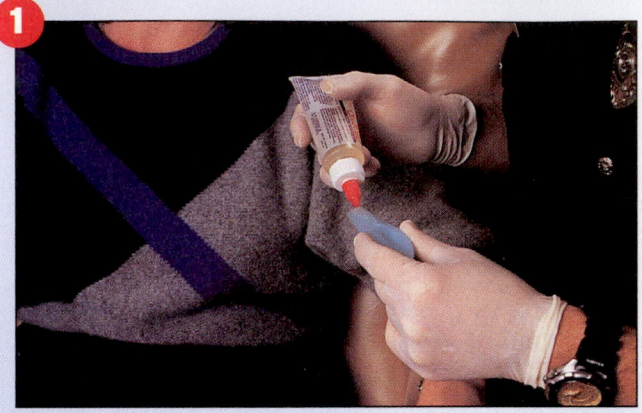

Squeeze the entire tube of oral glucose onto the bottom third of the tongue depressor or bite stick.

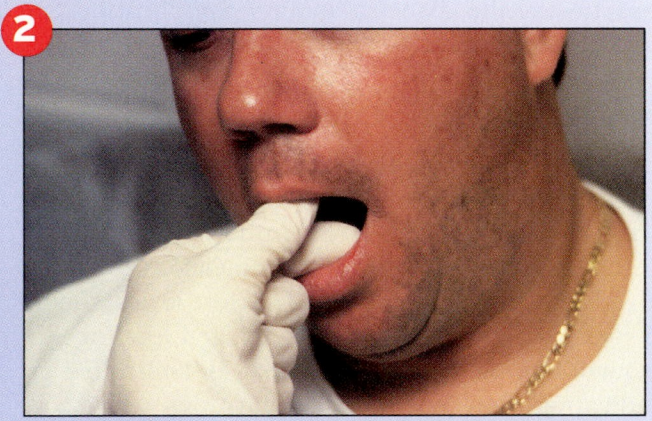

Open the patient's mouth using the cross-finger technique.

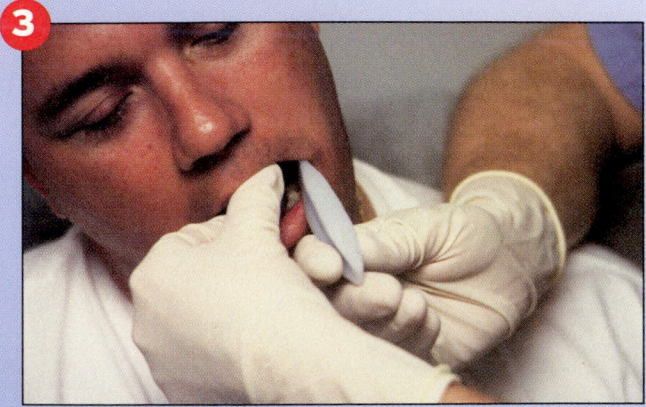

Place the tongue depressor or bite stick on the mucous membrane between the cheek and gum, with the gel side next to the cheek.

EMT-B safety

Managing problems related to diabetes and altered mental status poses very little risk to you, because exposure to body fluids is generally very limited. However, some patients can become confused and even aggressive at times. Follow BSI techniques, as you would with any other patient. Always use gloves, and wash your hands carefully after obtaining and checking a blood sample or if you perform airway techniques.

need glucose will not be harmed by it. Therefore, do not hesitate to give it under these circumstances.

As always, be sure to wear gloves before placing anything into a patient's mouth. After you have confirmed that the patient is conscious and able to swallow, squeeze the entire tube onto the bottom third of a tongue depressor and place the tongue depressor on the mucous membranes between the cheek and gum, with the gel side next to the cheek (Figure 17-6). Once the gel is dissolved, *or* if the patient loses consciousness or has a seizure, you should remove the tongue depressor.

Reassess the patient regularly after giving glucose, even if you see rapid improvement in the patient's condition. Watch for airway problems, sudden loss of consciousness, or seizures. Provide prompt transport to the hospital; do not delay transport just to give additional oral glucose.

A patient in insulin shock (rapid onset of coma, hypoglycemia) needs sugar immediately, and a patient in diabetic coma (acidosis, dehydration, hyperglycemia) needs insulin, complex IV fluid treatment, and probably other medications. These patients need prompt transport to the hospital for appropriate medical care.

For the conscious patient in insulin shock, medical protocols usually recommend sugar cubes, granulated sugar, maple syrup, honey, candy, fruit juice (sweetened with granulated sugar if available), oral glucose gel, or sweetened soft drinks. These will usually reverse the reaction within several minutes. Do not be afraid to give too much sugar. The problem often will not be solved with just a sip of juice. An entire candy bar or a full glass of sweetened juice is often needed. Do not give sugar-free drinks that are sweetened with saccharin or other synthetic sweetening compounds, as they will have little or no effect. Remember that even if the patient responds after receiving glucose, he or she may still need additional treatment. Therefore, you must transport the patient to the hospital as soon as possible.

caring for the elderly

You might encounter an elderly patient who has undiagnosed diabetes. These patients report that they have not been feeling well for a while but have not seen a physician. A patient with undiagnosed diabetes or one who is in denial or ignores the advice of his or her physician may call 9-1-1 when the signs and symptoms become annoying. Nonhealing wounds, blindness, and renal failure, and other complications are associated with poorly controlled or uncontrolled diabetes. As an EMT-B, you might be the first to recognize and suggest medical treatment to an elderly patient who might otherwise ignore his or her condition. It is important that you recognize the signs and symptoms of diabetes. As you obtain a SAMPLE history, also ask the patient whether he or she has noticed an increase in the number of ants in the bathroom, especially around the toilet. Ants like sugar, and excess sugar is excreted in the urine. An infestation of ants around the toilet could indicate sugar excreted in the urine and hence elevated blood glucose and the possibility of diabetes.

When there is any doubt about whether a conscious patient with diabetes is going into insulin shock or diabetic coma, most protocols will err on the side of giving glucose, even though the patient may have diabetic ketoacidosis. Untreated insulin shock will result in unconsciousness and can quickly cause significant brain damage or death. Compared with the patient in diabetic ketoacidosis, the patient in insulin shock is in a far more critical condition and far more likely to experience permanent problems. Furthermore, the amount of sugar that is typically given to such a patient is very unlikely to make a patient in diabetic ketoacidosis significantly worse. When in doubt, consult medical control.

Complications of Diabetes

Diabetes is a systemic disease affecting all tissues of the body, especially the kidneys, eyes, small arteries, and peripheral nerves. Therefore, you are likely to be called to treat patients with a variety of complications of diabetes, such as heart disease, visual disturbances, renal failure, stroke, and ulcers or infections of the feet or toes. With the exception of heart attack and stroke, most of these will not be acute emergencies. Considering that diabetes is a major risk factor for cardiovascular disease, individuals with diabetes should always be suspected of having a potential for heart attack, particularly older

patients, even when they do not present with classic symptoms such as chest pain.

Seizures

Although seizures are rarely life threatening, you should consider them very serious, even in patients with a history of chronic seizures, Seizures, which may be brief or prolonged, are caused by fever, infections, poisoning, hypoglycemia, trauma, or decreased levels of oxygen. They can also be idiopathic (of unknown cause) in children. Although brief seizures are not harmful, they may indicate a more dangerous and potentially life-threatening underlying condition. Because seizures can be caused by head injury, consider trauma as a cause. In the patient with diabetes, you should also consider hypoglycemia.

Emergency medical care of seizures includes ensuring that the airway is clear and placing the patient on his or her side if there is no possibility of cervical spine trauma. Do not attempt to place anything in the patient's mouth (eg, a bite stick or oral airway). Be sure to have suctioning equipment ready in case the patient vomits. Provide artificial ventilation if the patient is cyanotic or appears to be breathing inadequately, and provide prompt transport.

Altered Mental Status

Although altered mental status is often caused by complications of diabetes, it may also be caused by a variety of conditions, including poisoning, part of the postseizure state, infection, head injury, and decreased levels of oxygen.

Begin emergency medical care of altered mental status by ensuring that the airway is clear. Be prepared to provide artificial ventilation and suctioning in case the patient vomits, and provide prompt transport.

Relationship to Airway Management

Patients with altered mental status, particularly those who are difficult to awaken, are at risk for losing their gag reflex. When the gag reflex is not working, patients cannot reject foreign materials in their mouth (including vomit), and their tongues will often relax and obstruct the airway. Therefore, you must carefully monitor the airway in patients with hypoglycemia, diabetic coma, or a diabetic complication such as stroke or seizure. Place the patient in a lateral recumbent position, and make sure suction is readily available.

prep kit

ready for review

Diabetes is a metabolic disorder caused by the lack of insulin, a hormone that enables glucose to enter the cells, where it can be used for energy. Diabetes is typically characterized by excessive urination and resulting thirst, along with deterioration of body tissues. There are two types of diabetes. Type I diabetes, or insulin-dependent diabetes, usually starts in childhood and requires daily insulin to control blood glucose. Type II diabetes, or non-insulin-dependent diabetes, usually develops in middle age and often can be controlled with diet and oral medications. Both are serious systemic diseases, especially affecting the kidneys, eyes, small arteries, and peripheral nerves.

Patients with diabetes have chronic complications that place them at risk for other diseases such as heart attack, stroke, and infections. Most often, however, you will be called upon to treat the acute complications of blood glucose imbalance. These include hyperglycemia (excess blood glucose) and hypoglycemia (not enough blood glucose). Symptoms of hypoglycemia classically include confusion, rapid respirations, pale, moist skin, diaphoresis, dizziness, fainting, and even coma and seizures. This condition, called insulin shock, is rapidly reversible with the administration of glucose or sugar. Without treatment, however, permanent brain damage and death can occur. Hyperglycemia is usually associated with dehydration and ketoacidosis. It can result in diabetic coma, marked by rapid (often deep) respirations; warm, dry skin; a weak pulse; and a fruity breath odor. Hyperglycemia must be treated in the hospital with insulin and IV fluids.

Since either too much or too little blood glucose can result in altered mental status, you must perform a thorough history and patient assessment. When you cannot determine the nature of the problem, it is best to treat the patient for hypoglycemia. Be prepared to give oral glucose to a conscious patient who is confused or has a slightly decreased level of consciousness; however, do not give oral glucose to a patient who is unconscious or otherwise unable to swallow properly or protect his or her own airway. Remember, in all cases, providing basic life support and prompt transport is your primary responsibility.

vital vocabulary

acidosis   A pathologic condition resulting from the accumulation of acids in the body.

diabetes mellitus   A metabolic disorder in which the ability to metabolize carbohydrates (sugars) is impaired, usually because of a lack of insulin.

diabetic coma   Unconsciousness caused by dehydration, very high blood glucose, and acidosis in diabetes.

diabetic ketoacidosis   A form of acidosis in uncontrolled diabetes in which an accumulation of certain acids occurs when insulin is not available in the body.

glucose   One of the basic sugars; it is the primary fuel, along with oxygen, for cellular metabolism.

hormone   One of several chemical substances that regulate the activity of body organs and tissues; produced by a gland.

hyperglycemia   Abnormally increased glucose level in the blood.

hypoglycemia   Abnormally decreased glucose level in the blood.

insulin   A hormone produced by the pancreas that enables sugar in the blood to enter the cells of the body; used in synthetic form to treat and control diabetes mellitus.

www.emtb.com

insulin shock   Unconsciousness or altered mental status in a patient with diabetes caused by significant hypoglycemia; usually the result of excessive exercise and activity or failure to eat after a routine dose of insulin.

polydipsia   Excessive thirst persisting for long periods of time despite reasonable fluid intake; often the result of excessive urination; in patients with diabetes, the excessive urination is caused by the wasting of glucose in the urine when blood levels are high.

polyphagia   Excessive eating; in diabetes, the inability to use glucose properly can cause a sense of hunger.

polyuria   The passage of an unusually large volume of urine in a given period; in diabetes, this can result from wasting of glucose in the urine.

type I diabetes   The type of diabetic disease that usually starts in childhood and requires insulin for proper treatment and control; also known as insulin-dependent diabetes.

type II diabetes   The type of diabetic disease that usually starts in later life and often can be controlled through diet and oral medications; also known as non-insulin-dependent diabetes.

assessment in action

A college student returns to her apartment and finds her boyfriend lying on the sofa unconscious and unresponsive. She immediately calls 9-1-1. When you arrive, you find a 21-year-old man dressed in jogging gear. The patient is unresponsive to any stimuli and is breathing quickly with no apparent airway problems. As you check for a pulse, you notice that his skin is cool and clammy. The woman tells you that the patient was "fine" a couple of hours ago when she left. She states that he said he was not feeling well at breakfast and promised to eat something later. She also states that the patient has no known allergies and does not take any medicine except for a daily dose of insulin. Finally, she tells you that he began jogging a few weeks ago to try to get back into shape. While you have been asking questions, your partner has obtained baseline vital signs. The patient has a blood pressure of 88/54 mm Hg, a rapid, regular pulse of 128 beats/min, and respirations of 28 breaths/min.

1. Your protocol allows you to test the patient's blood using a Dexi-stick test. On the basis of the rapid onset of symptoms and the history provided by the patient's girlfriend, you expect the patient's blood glucose level to be:

   A. very low.
   B. within normal limits.
   C. very high.
   D. too high to measure.

2. A patient who has hypoglycemia in association with diabetes is **NOT** likely to:

   A. appear intoxicated.
   B. appear anxious or combative.
   C. report severe, crushing chest pain.
   D. have slurred or incomprehensible speech.

3. Why is the administration of oral glucose not indicated in this situation?

   A. The patient is younger than age 25 years.
   B. The patient was recently exercising heavily.
   C. The patient is unconscious and unresponsive.
   D. An acute onset of symptoms developed.

4. What is the proper way to administer oral glucose to a patient with diabetes?

   A. Place the gel between the cheek and the gum.
   B. Forcefully squirt the gel directly down into the throat.
   C. Spread the gel as far back on the tongue as possible.
   D. Squirt the gel deep in the throat on either side of the tongue.

5. Oral glucose is likely to take effect in:

   A. a few minutes.
   B. about 1 hour.
   C. more than 2 hours.
   D. about 12 hours.

points to ponder

Objectives 4-4.1, 4-4.2, 4-4.10, 4-6.3, 4-6.7, 4-6.10

It is 8:30 A.M., and you are called to a construction site for an unconscious employee. The coworkers are yelling at the patient and tell you that he was slurring his speech and staggering around for about an hour, then complained of feeling nauseated, went into the bathroom, and passed out. His breath smells sweet like alcohol. The patient is not wearing a medical information tag, and nobody knows much about him. The foreman is saying that the company won't pay for an ambulance to take a drunk to sober up.

- How would you deal with this situation? What other problems, besides alcohol intoxication, may present the same signs and symptoms? How would you tell them apart? Would you transport this patient?

online outlook

There is a wealth of information about diabetes on the World Wide Web. Explore some of these Internet resources by completing Exercise 17 at www.emtb.com.

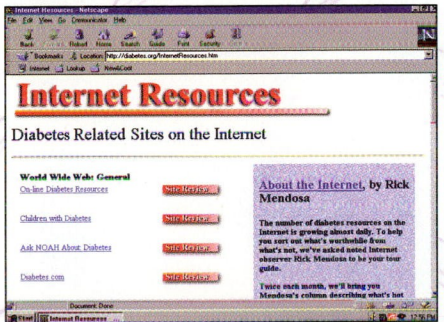

Allergic Reactions and Envenomations

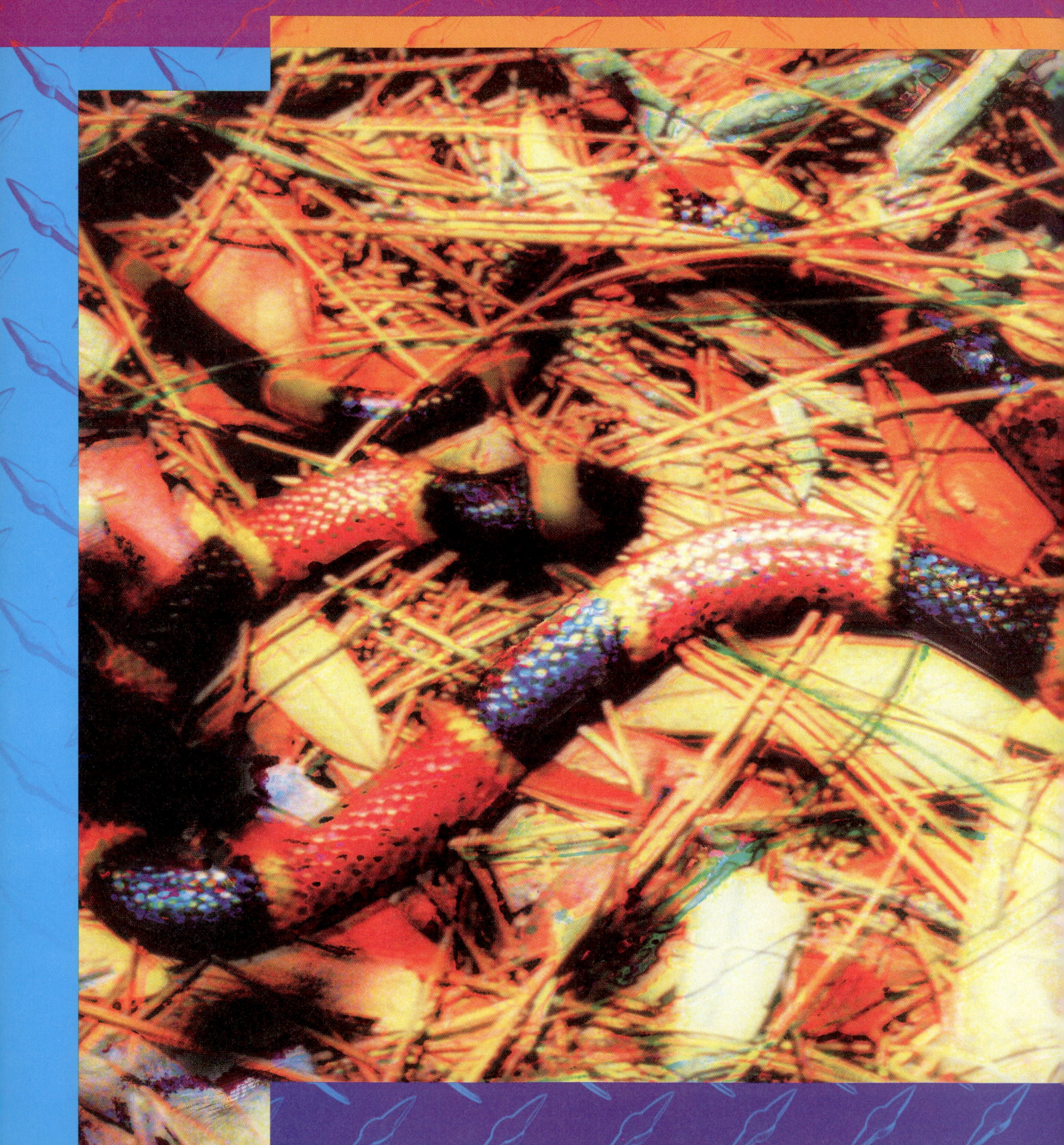

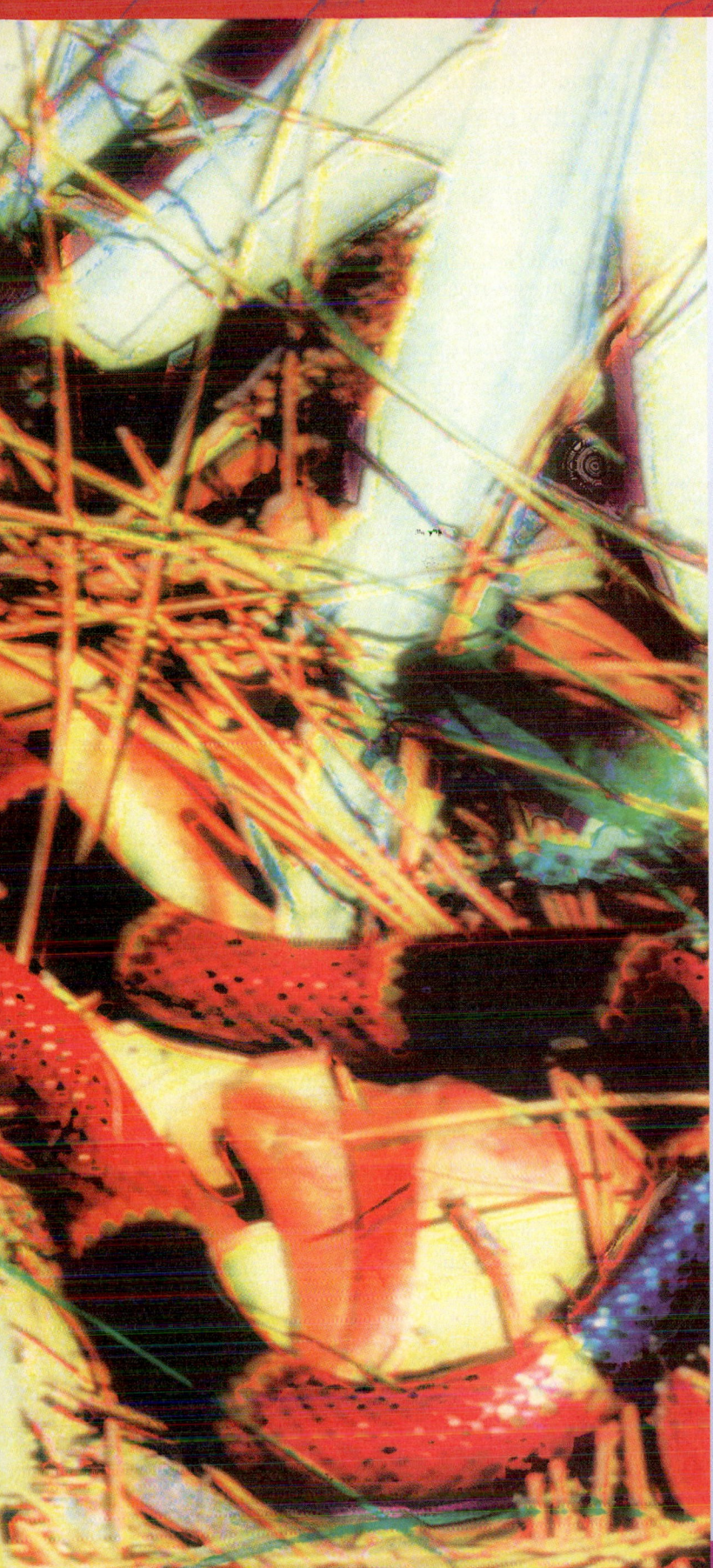

objectives

Cognitive

1. Recognize the patient experiencing an allergic reaction.

2. Describe the emergency medical care of the patient with an allergic reaction.

3. Establish the relationship between the patient with an allergic reaction and airway management.

4. Describe the mechanisms of allergic response and the implications for airway management.

5. State the generic and trade names, medication forms, dose, administration, action, and contraindications for the epinephrine auto-injector.

6. Evaluate the need for medical direction in the emergency medical care of the patient with an allergic reaction.

7. Differentiate between the general category of those patients having an allergic reaction, and those patients having an allergic reaction and requiring immediate medical care, including immediate use of an epinephrine auto-injector.

Affective

8. Explain the rationale for administering epinephrine using an auto-injector.

Psychomotor

9. Demonstrate the emergency medical care of the patient experiencing an allergic reaction.

10. Demonstrate the use of an epinephrine auto-injector.

11. Demonstrate the assessment and documentation of patient response to an epinephrine injection.

12. Demonstrate proper disposal of equipment.

13. Demonstrate completing a prehospital care report for patients with allergic emergencies.

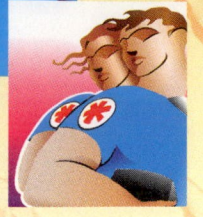

you are the emt

Rescue 6 please respond to 813 Dogwood Lane for a 7-year-old boy who is experiencing hives and difficulty breathing . . . his mother reports that he is severely allergic to eggs and he has just consumed more than ten cookies containing eggs . . .

Few calls will have the intensity of responding to an acute allergic reaction. This chapter will prepare you for responding to these frequent yet harrowing calls and will help you answer the following questions:

1. Why is prehospital care for allergic reactions based on assessment findings rather than on the diagnoses?

2. Is definitive treatment of acute allergic reactions really "time sensitive"?

Allergic Reactions and Envenomations

Every year, at least 1,000 Americans die from acute allergic reactions. In dealing with allergy-related emergencies, you must be aware of the possibility of acute airway obstruction and cardiovascular collapse and be prepared to treat these life-threatening complications. You must also be able to distinguish between the body's usual response to a sting or bite and an allergic reaction, which may require epinephrine. Your ability to recognize and manage the many signs and symptoms of allergic reactions may be the only thing standing between a patient and imminent death.

This chapter begins by describing the five categories of stimuli that may provoke allergic reactions. It then goes into considerable detail about insect stings and the typical reactions to them that occur among people who are, and those who are not, allergic to bees, wasps, yellow jackets, and hornets. You will learn what to look for in assessing patients who may be having an allergic reaction and how to care for them, including administration of epinephrine. The chapter then describes specific bites from poisonous spiders and snakes, ticks, dogs, humans, and marine animals.

Allergic Reactions

Contrary to what many people think, an **allergic reaction**, an exaggerated immune response to any substance, is not caused directly by an outside stimulus, such as a bite or sting. Rather, it is a reaction by the body's immune system, which releases chemicals to combat the stimulus. Among these chemicals are **histamines** and **leukotrienes**. An allergic reaction may be mild and local, involving hives, itching, or tenderness, or it may be severe and systemic, resulting in shock and respiratory failure.

Anaphylaxis is an extreme allergic reaction that is not always life threatening, but it typically involves multiple organ systems. In severe cases, anaphylaxis can rapidly result in death. Two of the most common signs of anaphylaxis are **wheezing**, a high-pitched, whistling breath sound usually resulting from blockage of the airway and heard on expiration, and widespread urticaria, or hives. **Urticaria** consists of small areas of generalized itching or burning that appear as multiple, small, raised areas on the skin (Figure 18-1).

Given the right person and the right circumstances, almost any substance can trigger the body's immune system and cause an allergic reaction: animal bites, food, latex gloves, or even semen can be an **allergen**. The most common allergens, however, fall into the following five general categories:

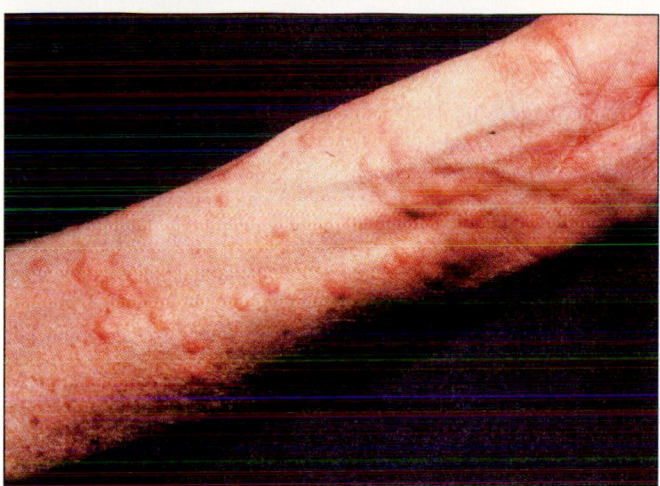

FIGURE 18-1 Urticaria, or hives, may appear following a sting and is characterized by multiple, small, raised areas on the skin. Urticaria may be one of the warning signs of impending anaphylactic reaction.

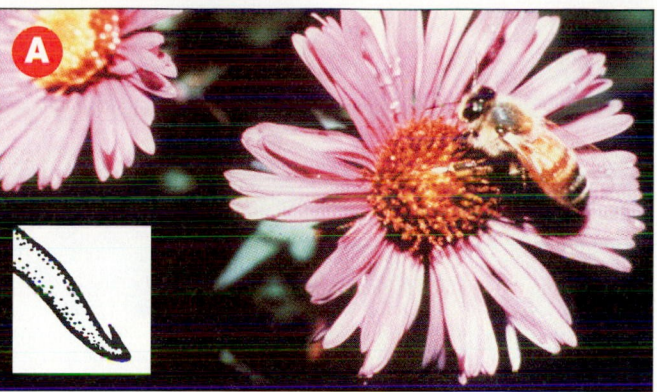

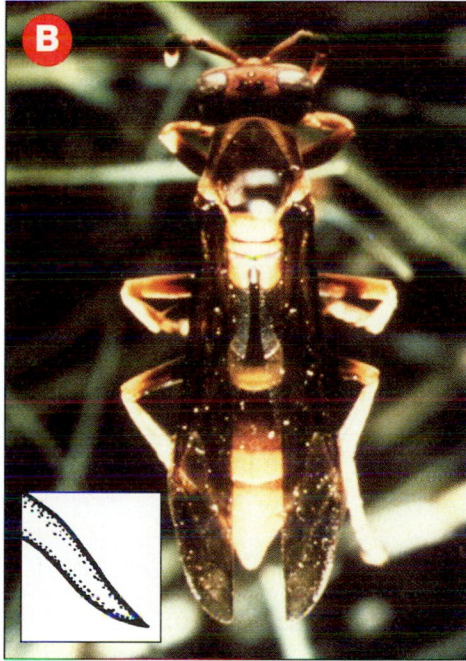

FIGURE 18-2 Most stinging insects inject venom through a small, hollow spine that projects from the abdomen. **A:** The stinger of the honeybee is barbed and cannot be withdrawn once the bee has stung someone. **B:** The wasp's is unbarbed, meaning that it can inflict multiple stings.

- **Insect bites and stings.** When an insect bites you and injects the bite with its venom, the act is called <u>envenomation</u> or, more commonly, a sting. The sting of a honeybee, wasp, ant, yellow jacket, or hornet may cause a severe reaction with the swiftness of an injected medication. The reaction may be local, causing swelling and itchiness in the surrounding tissue, or it may be systemic, involving the entire body. Such a total body reaction would be considered an anaphylactic reaction.

- **Medications.** Injection of drugs such as penicillin may cause an immediate (within 30 minutes) and severe allergic reaction. However, reactions to oral medications, such as oral penicillin, may be slower in onset (more than 30 minutes) but equally severe. The fact that a person has taken a medication once without experiencing an allergic reaction is no guarantee that he or she will not have an allergic reaction to it the next time around.

- **Plants.** Individuals who inhale dusts, pollens, or other plant materials to which they are sensitive may experience a rapid and severe allergic reaction.

- **Food.** Eating certain foods, such as shellfish or nuts, may result in a relatively slow (more than 30 minutes) reaction that still can be quite severe. The person may be unaware of the exposure or inciting agent.

- **Chemicals.** Certain chemicals, makeup, soap, latex, and various other substances can cause severe allergic reactions.

Insect Stings

There are more than 100,000 species of bees, wasps, and hornets. Deaths from anaphylactic reactions to stinging insects far outnumber deaths from snake bites. The stinging organ of most bees, wasps, yellow jackets, and hornets is a small hollow spine projecting from the abdomen (Figure 18-2). Venom can be injected through this spine directly into the skin. The stinger of the honeybee is barbed, so the bee cannot withdraw it. Therefore, the bee leaves a part of its abdomen embedded with the stinger and dies shortly after flying away. Wasps and hornets have no such handicap; they can sting repeatedly. Since these insects usually fly away after stinging, it is often impossible to identify which species was responsible for the injury.

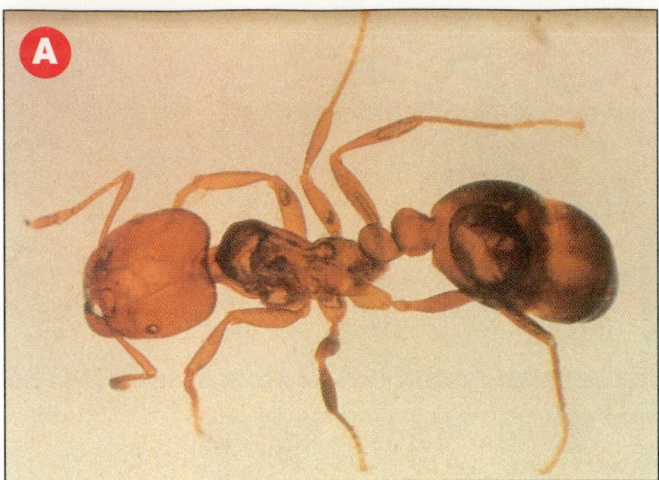

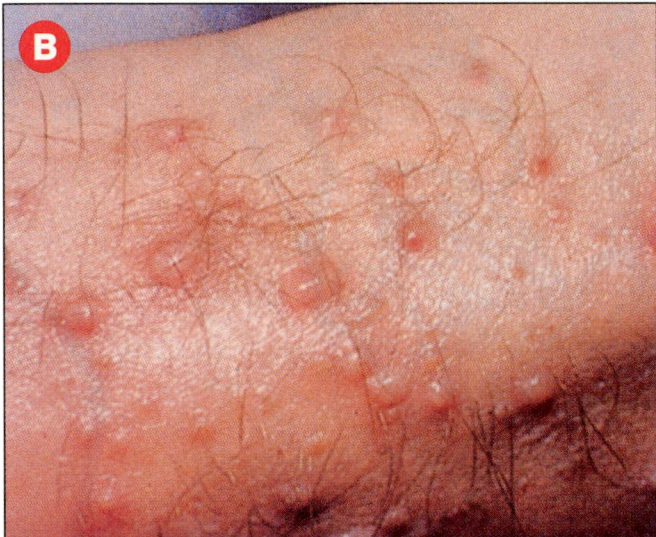

FIGURE 18-3 A: Fire ants inject an irritating toxin at multiple sites. **B:** Fire ant bites are generally found on the feet and the legs and appear as multiple small raised pustules.

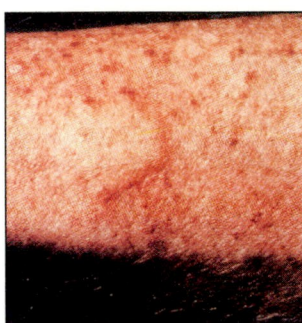

FIGURE 18-4 A wheal is a whitish, firm elevation of the skin that occurs after an insect sting or bite.

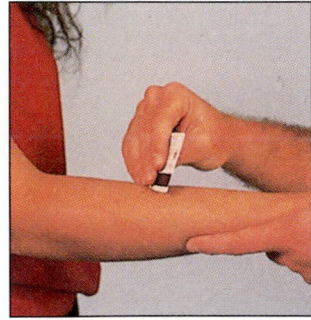

FIGURE 18-5 To remove the stinger of a honeybee, gently scrape the skin with the edge of a sharp, stiff object such as a credit card.

Some ants, especially the fire ant (Formicoidea), also strike repeatedly, often injecting a particularly irritating <u>toxin</u>, or poison, at the bite sites. It is not uncommon for a patient to sustain multiple ant bites, usually on the feet and legs, within a very short period of time (Figure 18-3).

Signs and symptoms of insect stings or bites include sudden pain, swelling, localized heat, and redness in light-skinned individuals, usually at the site of injury. There may be itching and sometimes a <u>wheal</u>, which is a raised, swollen, well-defined area on the skin (Figure 18-4). There is no specific treatment for these injuries, although applying ice sometimes makes them less irritating. The swelling associated with an insect bite may be dramatic and sometimes frightening to patients. However, these local manifestations are usually not serious.

Because the stinger of the honeybee remains in the wound, it can continue to inject venom for up to 20 minutes after the bee has flown away. In caring for a patient who has been stung by a honeybee, you should gently attempt to remove the stinger and attached muscle by scraping the skin with the edge of a sharp, stiff object such as a credit card (Figure 18-5). Generally, you should not use tweezers or forceps, as squeezing may cause the stinger to inject still more venom into the bite wound. Gently wash the area with soap and water or a mild antiseptic. Try to remove any jewelry from the area before swelling begins. Position the injection site slightly below the level of the heart and apply ice or cold packs to the area, but not directly on the skin, to help relieve pain and slow the absorption of the toxin. Be alert for vomiting or any signs of shock or allergic reaction, and do not give the patient anything by mouth. Place the patient in the shock position and give oxygen if needed. Monitor the patient's vital signs and be prepared to provide further support as needed.

Anaphylactic Reaction to Stings

Approximately 5% of all people are allergic to the venom of the bee, hornet, yellow jacket, or wasp. This type of allergy, which accounts for about 200 deaths per year, can cause very severe reactions, including anaphylaxis. Patients may experience generalized itching and burning, widespread urticaria, wheals, swelling about the lips and tongue, bronchospasm and wheezing, chest tightness and coughing, dyspnea, anxiety, abdominal cramps, and hypotension. Occasionally, respiratory failure occurs.

If untreated, such an anaphylactic reaction can proceed rapidly to death. In fact, more than two thirds of patients who die from anaphylaxis do so within the first half hour, so speed on your part is essential.

Patient Assessment

Allergic symptoms are almost as varied as allergens themselves. Your assessment of the patient experiencing an allergic reaction should include evaluations of the respiratory system, circulatory system, mental status, and the skin (Table 18-1).

Wheezing occurs because excessive fluid and mucus are secreted into the bronchial passages, and muscles around these passages tighten in reaction to the allergen. Exhalation, normally the passive, relaxed part of breathing, becomes harder as the patient tries to cough up the secretions or move air past the constricted airways. The fluid in the air passages and the constricted bronchi together produce the wheezing sound. Breathing rapidly becomes more difficult, and the patient may even stop breathing. Prolonged respiratory difficulty can cause a rapid heartbeat (tachycardia), shock, and even death. Stridor, a harsh, high-pitched inspiratory sound, occurs when swelling in the upper airway (near the vocal cords and throat) closes off the airway and can eventually lead to total obstruction.

Remember, the presence of hypoperfusion (shock) or respiratory distress indicates that the patient is having a severe enough allergic reaction to lead to death.

Emergency Medical Care

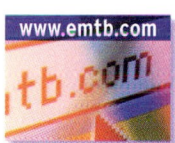
www.emtb.com

If the patient seems to be having an allergic reaction, you should give oxygen as you complete the initial assessment. Perform a focused history and physical examination. Find out whether the patient has a history of allergies, what the patient was exposed to, and how the patient was exposed. Determine what the effects of the exposure have been and how they have progressed. Find out what interventions have been completed. Next, obtain baseline vital signs and a SAMPLE history. Inform medical control about the patient's condition, then find out whether the patient has any prescribed, preloaded medications for allergic reactions. If necessary, be prepared to use standard airway procedures and positive pressure ventilation according to the principles identified in Chapters 7 and 39.

If the patient appears to be having a severe allergic (or anaphylactic) reaction, you should administer BLS at once and provide prompt transport to the hospital. You may wish to request ALS backup if you work in a tiered response system. In addition to providing oxygen, you should be prepared to maintain an airway or give CPR. Placing ice over the injury site has been thought to slow

TABLE 18-1   Common Signs and Symptoms of Allergic Reaction

Respiratory System

- Sneezing or an itchy, runny nose (initially)
- Tightness in the chest or throat
- Irritating, persistent dry cough
- Hoarseness
- Respirations that become rapid, labored, or noisy
- Wheezing and/or stridor

Circulatory System

- Decrease in blood pressure as the blood vessels dilate
- Increase in pulse rate (initially)
- Pale skin and dizziness, as the vascular system fails
- Loss of consciousness and coma

Skin

- Flushing, itching, or burning skin; especially common over the face and upper chest
- Urticaria over large areas of the body, both internally and externally
- Swelling, especially of the face, neck, hands, feet, and/or tongue
- Swelling and cyanosis or pallor around the lips
- Warm, tingling feeling in the face, mouth, chest, feet, and hands

Other Findings

- Anxiety, a sense of impending doom
- Abdominal cramps
- Headache
- Itchy, watery eyes
- Decreasing mental status

absorption of the toxin and diminish swelling, but ice packs placed directly on the skin may freeze it and cause more damage. Like any other attempt to reduce swelling with ice, you should be careful not to overdo the icing. In some areas, you may be allowed to assist the patient with epinephrine.

Whether made by the body (adrenaline) or by a drug manufacturer, epinephrine works rapidly to raise the pulse rate and blood pressure by constricting the blood

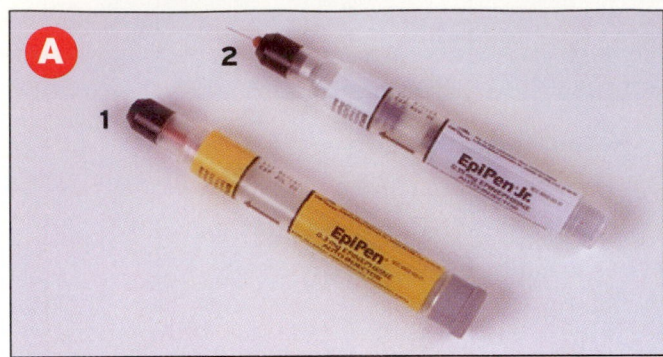

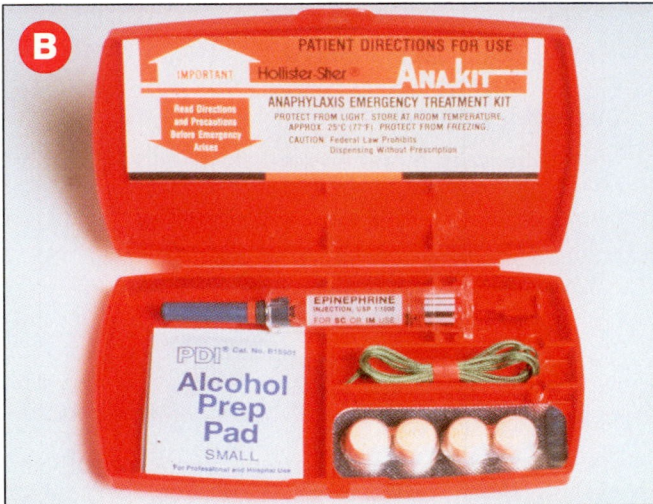

FIGURE 18-6 Patients who experience severe allergic reactions often carry their own epinephrine, which comes commercially as a predosed auto-injector. **A:** EpiPen (1-unfired, 2-fired). **B:** AnaKit.

1. **Receive a direct order from medical control** or follow local protocols or standing orders.

2. **Follow BSI techniques.**

3. **Make sure the medication has been prescribed** specifically for that patient. If it has not, do not give the medication, inform medical control, and provide immediate transport.

4. **Make sure the medication is not discolored** or expired.

You are now ready to give the medication, using the following steps:

1. **Remove the safety cap** from the auto-injector and, if possible, wipe the patient's thigh with alcohol or some other antiseptic. However, do not delay administration of the drug.

2. **Place the tip of the auto-injector** against the lateral part of the patient's thigh, midway between the waist and the knee.

3. **Push the injector firmly** against the thigh until the injector activates, about 5 to 10 seconds. This action will help prevent the kick that the spring-loaded syringe can cause when the needle is pulled from the injection site too soon. Hold the injector in place until the medication is injected.

4. **Remove the injector** from the patient's thigh and dispose of it in the proper biohazard container.

5. **Record the time and dose** of injection on your run sheet.

6. **Reassess and record** the patient's vital signs 2 minutes after using the auto-injector.

vessels. Epinephrine also inhibits the allergic reaction and dilates the bronchioles. All bee sting kits should contain a prepared syringe of epinephrine, ready for injection, along with instructions for its use. Your EMS service may or may not allow you to help patients self-administer epinephrine to combat allergic reactions or anaphylaxis. In some places, the medical director may authorize you to carry an epinephrine auto-injector (EpiPen). If the patient is known to be allergic, he or she might carry a commercial bee sting kit (Ana-Kit) that contains epinephrine (Figure 18-6). The adult system delivers 0.3 mg of epinephrine via an automatic needle and syringe system; the infant/child system delivers 0.15 mg.

Other bee sting kits contain some oral or IV *antihistamines,* agents that block the effect of histamine. These work relatively slowly, within several minutes to 1 hour. Because epinephrine can have an effect within 1 minute, it is the primary way to save the life of someone having a severe anaphylactic reaction.

If the patient is able to use the auto-injector on his or her own, your role is limited to helping. To use, or help the patient use, the auto-injector, you must take the following steps (Figure 18-7):

In some areas of the country, EMT-Bs can inject epinephrine for anaphylaxis. Follow your local protocols or medical direction, but generally you will inject 0.33 to 0.5 mL of 1/1,000 epinephrine solution to an adult weighing more than 50 kg intramuscularly or subcutaneously at intervals of 5 to 15 minutes, as needed. Doses for children vary, ranging from 0.1 to 0.33 mL, depending on the patient's weight. Be aware that the medication may cause significant tachycardia as well as increased anxiety or nervousness. Complete the emergency care outlined for this patient above, and provide prompt transport, closely monitoring vital signs frequently. Remember that all patients with suspected anaphylaxis should be given high-flow, high-concentration oxygen.

Because epinephrine constricts blood vessels, it may cause the patient's blood pressure to rise significantly. Other side effects include tachycardia, pallor, dizziness, chest pain, headache, nausea, and vomiting. All these effects may cause the patient to feel anxious or excited.

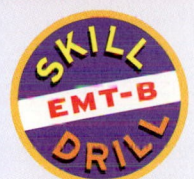

Using an Auto-Injector

Figure 18-7

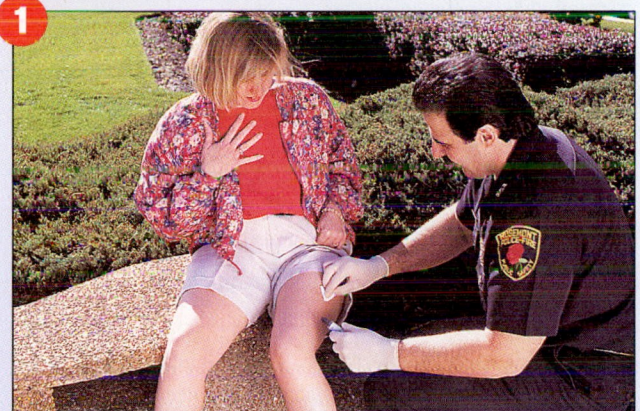

1 Prepare the patient's thigh by quickly wiping it with antiseptic.

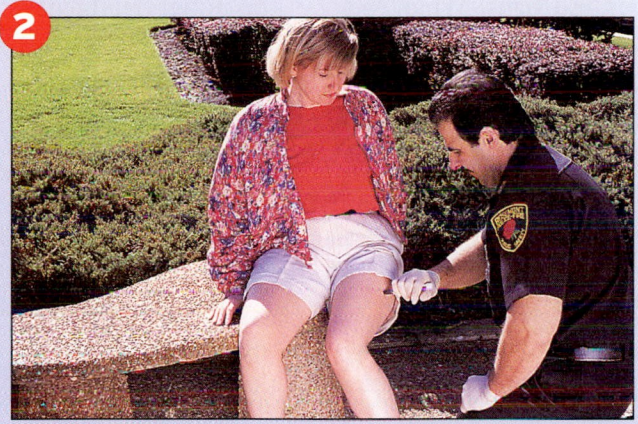

2 Place the tip of the auto-injector against the lateral aspect of the patient's thigh.

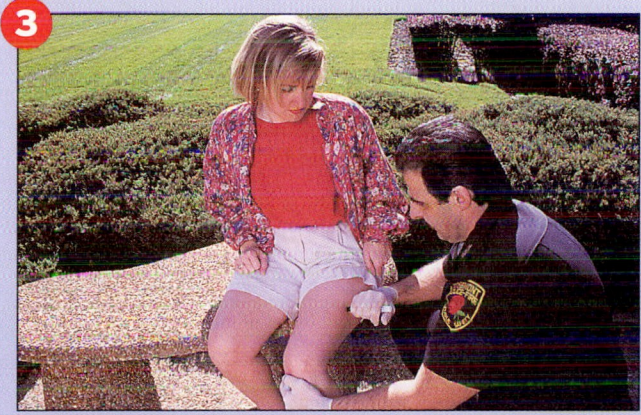

3 Push the auto-injector firmly against the thigh until the injector activates. Hold the injector in place until all the medication is injected.

These side effects are worth the trade-off when epinephrine is used in a life-threatening situation. However, if the patient has no signs of respiratory distress or shock after contact with a substance that causes an allergic reaction, continue with the focused assessment. Note that patients who are not wheezing, or who have no signs of respiratory compromise or hypotension, should not be given epinephrine.

Whether or not your emergency treatment includes epinephrine, you should always provide prompt transport for any patient who may be having an allergic reaction or has experienced a poisonous envenomation or bite. Continue to reassess the patient's vital signs en route; remember that signs and symptoms may change rapidly. You may need to give more than one injection of epinephrine if you note that the patient has decreasing mental status, increased breathing difficulty, or a decreasing blood pressure. Be sure to consult medical control first. Current auto-injectors give only one dose, and a patient who needs more than one dose will need to have more than one injector. As with any patient you are transporting, be prepared to treat for shock, begin BLS measures, or use the automated external defibrillator if necessary.

If the patient's condition improves, provide supportive care, including giving the patient oxygen during transport.

Specific Bites and Envenomations

Spider Bites

Spiders are both numerous and widespread in the United States. Many species of spiders bite. However, only two, the female black widow spider and the brown recluse spider, are able to deliver serious, even life-threatening bites. When you care for a patient who has had some type of bite, be alert to the possibility that the spider may still be in the area, although it is not likely. Remember that your safety is of paramount importance.

Black widow spider. The female black widow spider (*Latrodectus*) is fairly large as far as spiders go, measuring approximately 2" long with its legs extended. It is usually black and has a distinctive, bright red-orange marking in the shape of an hourglass on its abdomen (Figure 18-8). The female is larger and more toxic than the male. Black widow spiders are found in

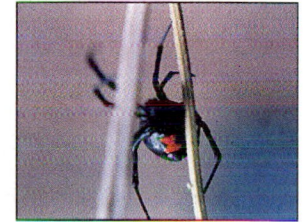

FIGURE 18-8
Black widow spiders are distinguished by their glossy black color and bright orange hourglass marking on the abdomen.

every state except Alaska. They prefer dry, dim places around buildings, in woodpiles, and among debris.

The bite of the black widow spider is sometimes overlooked. If the site becomes numb right away, the patient may not even recall being bit. However, most black widow spider bites cause localized pain and symptoms, including agonizing muscle spasms. In some cases, a bite on the abdomen causes muscle spasms so severe that the patient may be thought to have an acute abdomen, possibly peritonitis. The main danger with this type of bite, however, comes from the fact that the black widow's venom is poisonous to nerve tissues (neurotoxic). Other systemic symptoms include dizziness, sweating, nausea, vomiting, and skin rashes. Tightness in the chest and difficulty breathing develop within 24 hours, as well as severe cramps, with boardlike rigidity of the abdominal muscles. Generally, these signs and symptoms subside over 48 hours.

If necessary, a physician can administer a specific **antivenin**, a serum containing antibodies that counteract the venom, but because of a high incidence of side effects, its use is reserved for very severe bites, for the aged or very feeble, and for children younger than age 5 years. The severe muscle spasms are usually treated in the hospital with IV benzodiazepines such as diazepam (Valium) or lorazepam (Ativan). In general, emergency treatment for a black widow spider bite consists of BLS for the patient in respiratory distress. Much more often, the patient will merely require relief from pain. Transport the patient to the emergency department as soon as possible for treatment of both pain and muscle rigidity. If possible, bring the spider along.

Brown recluse spider. The brown recluse spider (*Loxosceles*) is dull brown in color and, at 1", somewhat smaller than the black widow (Figure 18-9). The short-haired body has a violin-shaped mark, brown to yellow in color, on its back. Although it lives mostly in the southern and central parts of the country, the brown recluse may be found throughout the continental United States. The spider takes its name from the fact that it tends to live in dark areas: in corners of old, unused buildings, under rocks, and in woodpiles. In cooler areas, it moves indoors to closets, drawers, cellars, and old piles of clothing.

In contrast to the venom of the black widow spider, the venom of the brown recluse spider is not neurotoxic but cytotoxic; that is, it causes severe local tissue damage. Typically, the bite is not painful at first but becomes so within hours. The area becomes swollen and tender, developing a pale, mottled, cyanotic center and possibly a small blister (Figure 18-10). Over the next

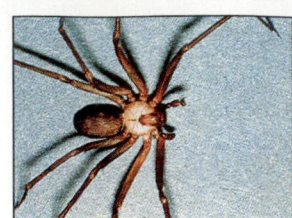

FIGURE 18-9
Brown recluse spiders are dull brown and have a dark, violin-shaped mark on the back.

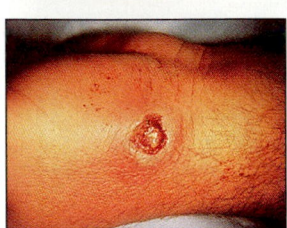

FIGURE 18-10
The bite of a brown recluse spider is characterized by swelling, tenderness, and a pale, mottled cyanotic center. There may also be a small blister on the bite.

several days, a scab of dead skin, fat, and debris will form and dig down into the skin, producing a large ulcer that may not heal unless treated promptly. Transport patients with such symptoms as soon as possible.

Brown recluse spider bites rarely cause systemic symptoms and signs. When they do, the initial treatment is BLS and transportation to the emergency department. Again, it is helpful if you can identify the spider and bring it to the hospital along with the patient.

Snake Bites

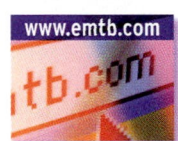

Snake bites are a worldwide problem of some significance. More than 300,000 injuries from snake bites occur annually, including 30,000 to 40,000 deaths. The greatest number of the fatalities occur in Southeast Asia and India (25,000 to 30,000) and in South America (3,000 to 4,000). In the United States, 40,000 to 50,000 snake bites are reported annually, about 7,000 of them caused by poisonous snakes. However, snake bite fatalities in the United States are extremely rare, about 15 a year for the entire country.

Of the approximately 115 different species of snakes in the United States, only 19 are venomous. These include the rattlesnake (*Crotalus*), the copperhead, the cottonmouth, or water moccasin (*Agkistrodon pisci-vorus*), and the coral snakes (*Micrurus* and *Micruroides*) (Figure 18-11). At least one of these poisonous species is found in every state except Alaska, Hawaii, and Maine. As a general rule, these creatures are timid. They usually do not bite unless provoked, angered, or accidentally injured, as when they are stepped on. There are a few exceptions to these rules. Cottonmouths are often rather aggressive, and very little provocation is needed to annoy a rattlesnake. Coral snakes, by contrast, are very shy and usually bite only when they are being handled.

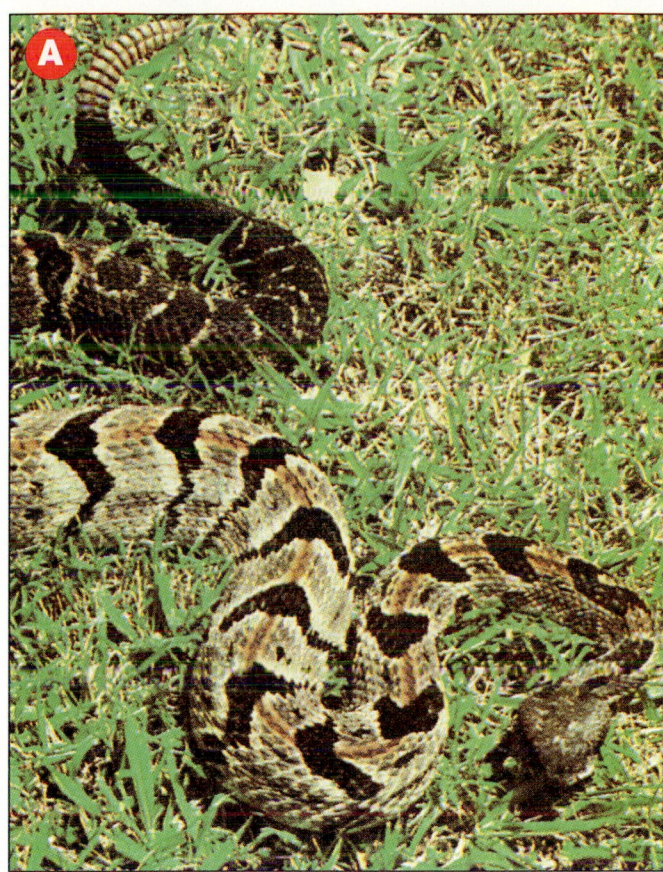

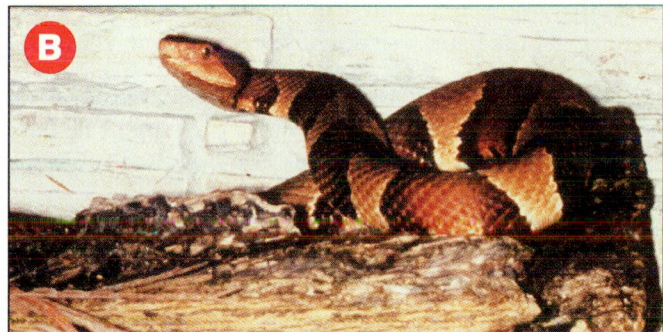

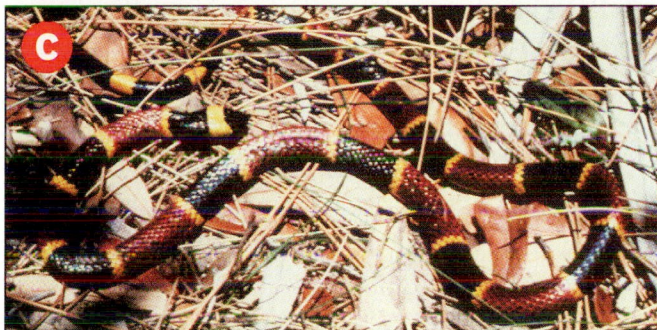

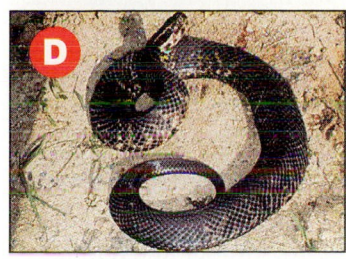

FIGURE 18-11
A: Rattlesnake.
B: Copperhead.
C: Coral snake.
D: Cottonmouth.

Most snake bites occur between April and October, when the animals are active, and tend to involve young men who have been drinking alcohol. Texas reports the largest number of bites. Other states with a major concentration of snake bites are Louisiana, Georgia, Oklahoma, North Carolina, Arkansas, West Virginia, and Mississippi. If you work in one of these areas, you should be thoroughly familiar with the emergency handling of snake bites. Remember, almost any time you are caring for a patient with a snake bite, another snake could come along and create a second victim: you. Therefore, use extreme caution on these calls, and be sure to wear the proper protective equipment for the area.

In general, only a third of snake bites result in significant local or systemic injuries. Often, envenomation does not occur because the snake has recently struck another animal and exhausted its supply of venom.

With the exception of the coral snake, poisonous snakes native to the United States all have hollow fangs in the roof of the mouth that inject the poison from two sacs at the back of the head. The classic appearance of the poisonous snake bite, therefore, is two small puncture wounds, usually about 1/2" apart, with discoloration, swelling, and pain surrounding them (Figure 18-12). Nonpoisonous snakes can also bite, usually leaving a horseshoe of tooth marks. However, some poisonous snakes have teeth as well as fangs, making it impossible to say which kind is responsible for a given set of tooth marks. On the other hand, fang marks are a clear indication of a poisonous snake bite.

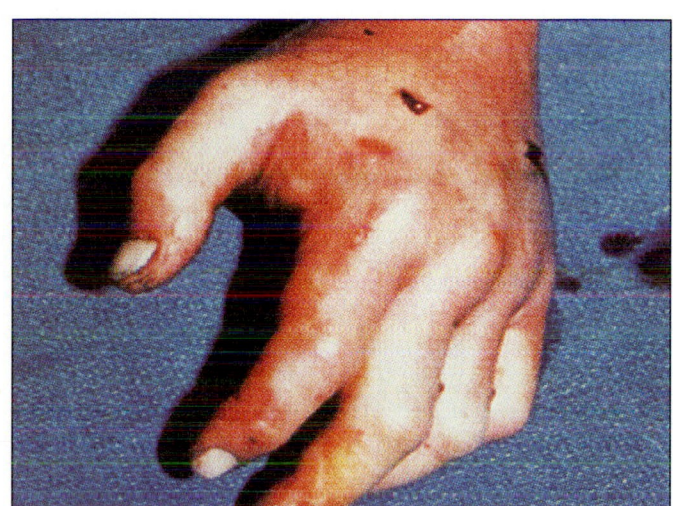

FIGURE 18-12 A snake bite wound from a poisonous snake has characteristic markings: two small puncture wounds about 1/2" apart, discoloration, and swelling.

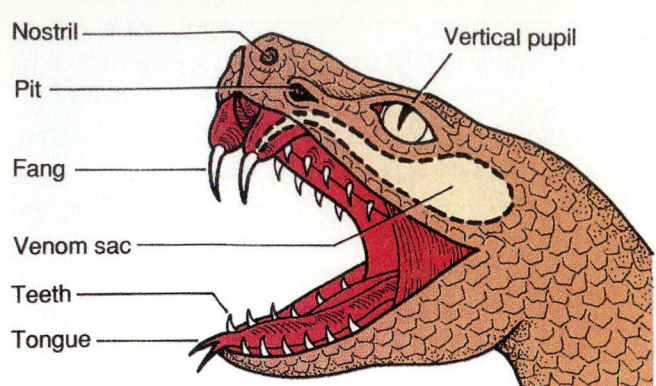

FIGURE 18-13 Pit vipers have small, heat-sensing organs (pits) located in front of their eyes that allow them to strike at warm targets, even in the dark.

Pit vipers. Rattlesnakes, copperheads, and cottonmouths are all pit vipers, with triangular-shaped, flat heads (Figure 18-13). They take their name from the small pits located just behind each nostril and in front of each eye. The pit is a heat-sensing organ that allows the snake to strike accurately at any warm target, especially in the dark when it cannot see through its vertical, slit-like pupils.

The fangs of the pit viper normally lie flat against the roof of the mouth and are hinged to swing back and forth as the mouth opens. When the snake is striking, the mouth opens wide and the fangs extend; in this way, the fangs penetrate whatever the mouth strikes. The fangs are actually special hollow teeth that act much like hypodermic needles. They are connected to a sac containing a reservoir of venom, which in turn is attached to a poison gland. The gland itself is a specially adapted salivary gland, which produces powerful enzymes that digest and destroy tissue. The primary purpose of the venom is to kill small animals and to start the digestive process prior to their being eaten.

The most common form of pit viper is the rattlesnake. Several different species of rattlesnake can be identified by the rattle on the tail. The rattle is actually numerous layers of dried skin that were shed but failed to fall off, coming to rest against a small knob on the end of the tail. Rattlesnakes have many patterns of color, often with a diamond pattern. They can grow to 6′ or more in length.

Copperheads are smaller than rattlesnakes, usually 2′ to 3′ long, with a reddish coppery color crossed with brown or red bands. These snakes typically inhabit woodpiles and abandoned dwellings, often close to areas of habitation. Although they account for most of the venomous snake bites in the eastern United States, copperhead bites are almost never fatal; however, note that the venom can destroy extremities.

Cottonmouths grow to about 4′ in length. Also called water moccasins, these snakes are olive or brown, with black cross-bands and a yellow undersurface. They are water snakes, with a particularly aggressive pattern of behavior. Although fatalities from these snake bites are rare, tissue destruction from the venom may be severe.

The signs of envenomation by a pit viper are severe burning pain at the site of the injury, followed by swelling and a bluish discoloration (ecchymosis) in light-skinned individuals that signals bleeding under the skin. These signs are evident within 5 to 10 minutes after the bite has occurred and spread over the next 36 hours. In addition to destroying tissues locally, the venom of the pit viper can also interfere with the body's clotting mechanism and cause bleeding at various distant sites. Other systemic signs, which may or may not occur, include weakness, sweating, fainting, and shock. If the patient has no local signs an hour after being bitten, it is safe to assume that envenomation did not take place. If swelling has occurred, you should mark its edges on the skin. This will allow physicians to assess what has happened, and when it happened, with greater accuracy.

Occasionally, a patient bitten by a snake will faint from fright. The patient will usually regain consciousness promptly when placed in a supine position. Do not confuse a fainting spell with shock. If shock occurs, it will happen much later.

In treating a snake bite from a pit viper, follow these steps to get the patient to the hospital in a timely fashion:

1. Calm the patient; assure him or her that poisonous snake bites are rarely fatal. Have the patient lie flat, face up, and explain that staying quiet will slow the spread of any venom through the system.

2. Locate the bite area; clean it gently with soap and water or a mild antiseptic. **Do not apply ice to the area.**

3. If the bite occurred on an arm or leg, splint the extremity to decrease movement.

4. Be alert for vomiting, which may be a sign of anxiety rather than the toxin itself.

5. Do not give anything by mouth, especially alcohol.

6. If, as rarely happens, the patient was bitten on the trunk, keep him or her supine and quiet and transport as quickly as possible.

7. Monitor the patient's vital signs and mark the skin with a pen over the area that is swollen, proximal to the swelling, to note whether swelling is spreading.

8. If there are any signs of shock, place the patient in the shock position and give oxygen.

9. If the snake has been killed, as is often the case, be sure to bring it with you so that physicians can identify it and administer the proper antivenin.

10. Notify the hospital that you are bringing in a snake bite patient; if possible, describe the snake.

11. Transport the patient promptly to the hospital.

If the patient shows no sign of envenomation, provide BLS as needed, place a sterile dressing over the suspected bite area, and immobilize the injury site. All patients with suspected snake bite should be taken to the emergency department, whether they show signs of envenomation or not. Treat the wound as you would any deep puncture wound to prevent infection.

If you work in an area where poisonous snakes are known to live, you should know the local medical protocol for handling snake bites. You should also know the address of the nearest facility where antivenin is available. This may be a nearby zoo, the local or public state health department, or a local community hospital.

Coral snakes. The coral snake is a small reptile with a series of bright red, yellow, and black bands completely encircling the body. Many harmless snakes have similar coloring, but only the coral snake has red and yellow bands next to one another, as this helpful rhyme suggests: "Red on yellow will kill a fellow; red on black, venom will lack."

A rare creature that lives primarily in Florida and in the desert Southwest, the coral snake is a relative of the cobra. It has tiny fangs and injects the venom with its teeth by a chewing motion, leaving behind one or more puncture or scratchlike wounds. Because of its small mouth and teeth and limited jaw expansion, the coral snake usually bites its victims on a small part of the body, such as a finger or toe.

Coral snake venom is a powerful toxin that causes paralysis of the nervous system. Within a few hours of being bitten, a patient will exhibit bizarre behavior, followed by progressive paralysis of eye movements and respiration. Often, there are limited or no local symptoms.

Successful treatment, either emergency or long term, depends on positive identification of the snake and support of respiration. Antivenin is available, but most hospitals do not stock it. Therefore, you should notify the hospital of the need for it as soon as possible. The steps for emergency care of a coral snake bite are as follows:

1. Immediately quiet and reassure the patient.

2. Flush the area of the bite with 1 to 2 quarts of warm, soapy water to wash away any poison left on the surface of the skin. **Do not apply ice to the region.**

3. Splint the extremity to minimize movement and the spread of venom at the site.

4. Check the patient's vital signs and continue to monitor them.

5. Keep the patient warm and elevate the lower extremities to help prevent shock.

6. Give supplemental oxygen if needed.

7. Transport the patient promptly to the emergency department, giving advance notice that the patient has been bitten by a coral snake.

8. Give the patient nothing by mouth.

Scorpion Stings

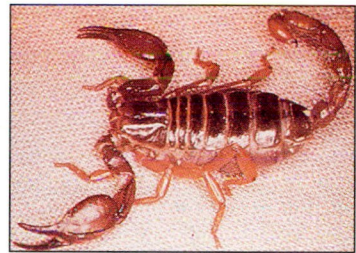

FIGURE 18-14 The sting of a scorpion is more painful than it is dangerous, causing localized swelling and discoloration.

Scorpions are eight-legged arachnids from the biological group Arachnida with a venom gland and a stinger at the end of their tail (Figure 18-14). Scorpions are rare; they live primarily in the southwestern United States and in deserts. With one exception, a scorpion's sting is usually very painful but not dangerous, causing localized swelling and discoloration. The exception is the *Centruroides sculpturatus*. Although it is found naturally in Arizona and New Mexico, as well as parts of Texas, California, and Nevada, it may be kept as a pet by anyone. The venom of this particular species may produce a severe systemic reaction that brings about circulatory collapse, severe muscle contractions, excessive salivation, hypertension, convulsions, and cardiac failure. Antivenin is available but must be administered by a physician. If you are called to care for a patient with a suspected sting from *Centruroides sculpturatus*, you should notify medical control as soon as possible. Administer all the elements of BLS and transport the patient to the emergency department as rapidly as possible.

Tick Bites

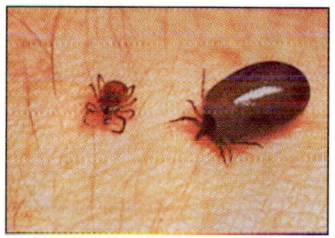

FIGURE 18-15 Ticks typically attach themselves directly to the skin.

Found most often on brush, shrubs, trees, sand dunes, or other animals, ticks are tiny insects that usually attach themselves directly to the skin (Figure 18-15). Only a fraction of an inch long, they can easily be mistaken for a freckle, especially since their bite is not painful. Indeed, the danger with a tick bite is not from the bite itself, but from the infecting

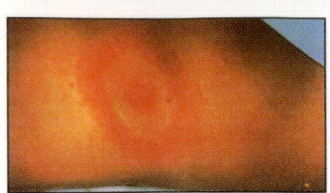

FIGURE 18-16
The rash associated with Lyme disease has a characteristic "bull's eye" pattern.

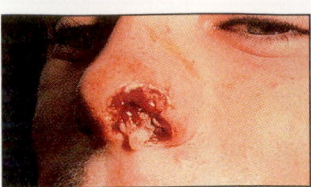

FIGURE 18-17
Dog bite wounds should be examined at the hospital, as these wounds are heavily contaminated with virulent bacteria.

organisms that the tick carries. Ticks commonly carry two infectious diseases: Rocky Mountain spotted fever and Lyme disease. Both are spread through the tick's saliva, which is injected into the skin when the tick attaches itself.

Rocky Mountain spotted fever, which is not limited to the Rocky Mountains, occurs within 7 to 10 days after a bite by an infected tick. Its symptoms include nausea, vomiting, headache, weakness, paralysis, and possibly cardiorespiratory collapse.

Lyme disease has received extensive publicity. It is, after AIDS, the second most rapidly growing infectious disease in the United States. Originally seen only in Connecticut, Lyme disease has now been reported in 35 states. It occurs most commonly in the Northeast, the Great Lake States, and the Pacific Northwest; New York State reports the largest number of cases. The first symptom, a rash that may spread to several parts of the body, begins about 3 days after the bite of an infected tick. The rash may eventually resemble a target bull's-eye pattern in one third of patients (Figure 18-16). After a few more days or weeks, painful swelling of the joints, particularly the knees, occurs. Lyme disease may be confused with rheumatoid arthritis and, like that disease, may result in permanent disability. However, if it is recognized and treated promptly with antibiotics, the patient may recover completely.

Tick bites occur most commonly during the summer months, when people are out in the woods wearing little protective clothing. Transmission of the infection from tick to person takes at least 12 hours, so if you are called on to remove a tick, you should proceed carefully and slowly. Do not attempt to suffocate the tick with gasoline or Vaseline or burn it with a lighted match; you will only burn the patient. Instead, using a fine tweezers, grasp the tick by the body and pull it straight out of the skin. This method will usually remove the whole tick. Even if part of the tick is left embedded in the skin, the part containing the infecting organisms has been removed. Once the tick is removed, paint the area with disinfectant and save the tick in a glass jar or other container so that it can be identified. Do not handle the tick with your fingers. Provide any necessary supportive emergency care, and transport the patient to the hospital.

Remind the patient that the symptoms of Rocky Mountain spotted fever and Lyme disease do not occur for several days after a bite, and advise him or her to see a physician within the next day or two.

Dog Bites and Rabies

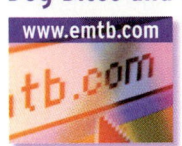

Most people who are bitten by dogs do not report the incident to a physician, believing that dog bites are not serious. They can be very serious, however. A dog's mouth is heavily contaminated with virulent bacteria. You should consider all dog bites as contaminated and potentially infected wounds that may require antibiotics, tetanus prophylaxis, and suturing (Figure 18-17). Occasionally, dog bites result in mangled, complex wounds that require surgical repair. For these reasons, all dog bites should be treated by a physician. Place a dry, sterile dressing over the wound, and promptly transport the patient to the emergency department. If an arm or leg was injured, splint that extremity. Often, the patient will be extremely upset and frightened, a situation that calls for calm reassurance on your part.

A major concern with dog bites is the spread of *rabies,* an acute, fatal viral infection of the central nervous system that can affect all warm-blooded animals. Although rabies is extremely rare today, particularly with widespread inoculation of pets, it still exists. Stray dogs that have not been inoculated can be carriers of the disease, as can squirrels, bats, foxes, skunks, and raccoons. The virus is in the saliva of a **rabid**, or infected, animal and is transmitted through biting or licking an open wound. Infection can be prevented in a person who has been bitten by such an animal only by a series of special vaccine injections, a painful procedure that must be begun soon after the bite. Since animals that have rabies do not always show it immediately in their behavior, a person's only chance to avoid the vaccine is to find the animal and turn it over to the health department for observation and/or testing. Unless the animal is a pet and has a rabies tag indicating that it has been inoculated, you should let an animal control officer capture and transport it.

Children, particularly young ones, may be seriously injured or even killed by dogs. These dogs are not always vicious or rabid; sometimes, the child had unknowingly provoked the animal. However, you must assume that it may turn and attack you as well. Therefore, you generally should not enter the scene until the animal has been secured by either the police or an animal control officer. Then you may carry out the necessary emergency care and transport the child to the emergency department.

Human Bites

More so than even the dog's, the human mouth contains an exceptionally wide range of virulent bacteria and viruses. For this reason, you should regard any human bite that has penetrated the skin as a very serious injury. Similarly, any laceration caused by a human tooth can result in a serious, spreading infection (Figure 18-18). Remember this if

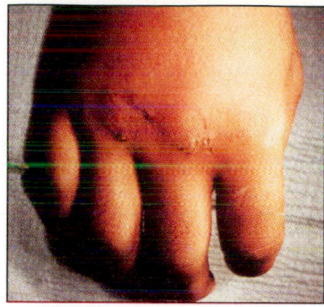

FIGURE 18-18
Human bites can result in serious, spreading infection. Thus, patients must be evaluated at the hospital.

you have occasion to treat someone who has been punched in the mouth: The person who delivered the punch may also need treatment.

The emergency treatment for human bites consists of the following steps:

1. Promptly immobilize the area with a splint or bandage.
2. Apply a dry, sterile dressing.
3. Provide transport to the emergency department for surgical cleansing of the wound and antibiotic therapy.

Injuries from Marine Animals

Coelenterates, including the fire coral, Portuguese man-of-war, sea wasp, sea nettles, true jellyfish, sea anemones, true coral, and soft coral, are responsible for more envenomations than any other marine animals (Figure 18-19). The stinging cells of the coelenterate are called nematocysts, and large animals may discharge hundreds of thousands of them. Envenomation causes very painful, reddish lesions in light-skinned individuals extending in a line from the site of the sting. Systemic symptoms include headache, dizziness, muscle cramps, and fainting.

To treat a sting from the tentacles of a jellyfish, a Portuguese man-of-war, various anemones, corals, or hydras, remove the patient from the water and pour any type of alcohol on the affected area. Unlike fresh water, alcohol will inactivate the nematocysts. Do not try to manipulate the remaining tentacles; this will only cause further discharge of the nematocysts. Remove the tentacles by scraping them off with the edge of a sharp, stiff object such as a credit card. Persistent pain may respond to immersion of the area in hot water (110° to 115°F, 43° to 46°C) for 30 minutes. On very rare occasions, a patient may have a systemic allergic reaction to the sting of one of these animals. Treat such a patient for anaphylactic shock. Give BLS, and provide immediate transport to the hospital.

TABLE 18-2	Common Marine Envenomations

Dogfish
Dragon fish
Fire coral
Hydroids
Jellyfish
Lionfish
Marine snail
Portuguese
   man-of-war
Ratfish
Scorpion fish
Sea anemone
Sea urchins
Starfish
Stingray
Stonefish
Tiger fish
Toadfish
Weever fish

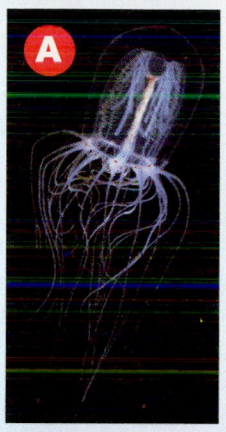
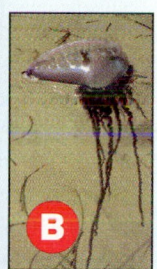
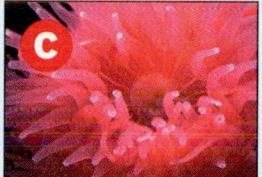

FIGURE 18-19
A: Portuguese man-of-war.
B: Jellyfish. **C:** Sea anemone.

Toxins from the spines of urchins, stingrays, and certain spiny fish such as the lionfish, scorpion fish, or stonefish are heat sensitive (Table 18-2). Therefore, the best treatment for such injuries is to immobilize the affected area and soak it in hot water for 30 minutes. This will often provide dramatic relief from local pain. However, the patient still needs to be transported to the emergency department, since he or she could develop an allergic reaction or infection, including tetanus.

If you work near the ocean, you should be familiar with the marine life in your area. The emergency treatment of common coelenterate envenomations consists of the following steps:

1. **Limit further discharge** of nematocysts by avoiding fresh water, wet sand, showers, or careless manipulation of the tentacles. Keep the patient calm, and reduce motion of the affected extremity.
2. **Inactivate the nematocysts** by applying alcohol. (Although isopropyl or rubbing alcohol is recommended, virtually any type of alcohol, including high proof liquor or cologne, is effective.)
3. **Remove the remaining tentacles** by scraping them off with the edge of a sharp, stiff object such as a credit card. Do not use your ungloved hand to remove the tentacles, because self-envenomation will occur. Persistent pain may respond to immersion in hot water (110° to 115°F, 43° to 46°C) for 30 minutes.
4. **Provide transport** to the emergency department.

prep kit

ready for review

An allergic reaction is a response to chemicals the body itself releases in order to combat certain stimuli, called allergens. Allergic reactions occur most often in response to five categories of stimuli: insect bites and stings, medications, food, plants, and chemicals. The reaction may be mild and local, involving itching, redness, and tenderness; or severe and systemic, including shock and respiratory failure. Anaphylaxis is a life-threatening allergic reaction mounted by multiple organ systems, which must be treated with epinephrine. Wheezing and skin wheals can be signs of anaphylaxis. People who know that they are allergic to bee, hornet, yellow jacket, or wasp venom often carry a bee sting kit that contains epinephrine in an auto-injector. You may help to administer this medication in this form with authorization from medical control. All patients with suspected anaphylaxis require oxygen.

In assessing a person who may be having an allergic reaction, you should check for flushing, itching, and swelling skin, hives, wheezing and stridor, a persistent cough, a decrease in blood pressure, a weak pulse, dizziness, abdominal cramps, and headache.

Poisonous spiders include the black widow spider and the brown recluse spider. Poisonous snakes include pit vipers and coral snakes. A person who has been bitten by a pit viper needs prompt transport; clean the bite area and keep the patient quiet to slow the spread of venom. Notify the hospital as soon as possible if a patient has been bitten by a coral snake, as its venom can cause paralysis of the nervous system, and most hospitals do not have appropriate antivenin on hand.

Patients who have been bitten by ticks may be infected with Rocky Mountain spotted fever or Lyme disease and should see a doctor within a day or two. Remove the tick using a tweezers, and save it for identification.

Dog and human bites can both lead to serious infection and must be treated by a physician. Dogs can carry rabies, a fatal viral infection present in their saliva. Painful vaccine treatment is necessary to prevent rabies in a person who has been bitten by a dog that cannot be captured or identified. Do not try to rescue a child who is being attacked by a dog without the help of police or animal control officers.

Remember that a hundred times more people die every year from allergic reactions to food, bee stings, or medications than from the bites of venomous snakes or marine animals. Many venomous snake bites may be treated with antivenin. Many marine envenomations may benefit from submersion in hot water to deactivate the heat-sensitive toxins. Such treatment may be started in the field at the request of medical control.

Always provide prompt transport to the hospital for any patient who is having an allergic reaction or has been bitten by a poisonous insect or animal. Remember that signs and symptoms can deteriorate rapidly. Carefully monitor the patient's vital signs en route, especially for airway compromise.

vital vocabulary

allergen A substance that causes an allergic reaction.

allergic reaction The body's immune response to an internal or surface agent.

anaphylaxis An extreme, life-threatening systemic allergic reaction that may include shock and respiratory failure.

antivenin A substance that is produced to counteract the effect of venom from an animal or insect.

envenomation The act of injecting venom.

epinephrine A substance produced by the body (adrenaline) and a drug produced by pharmaceutical companies to increase pulse and blood pressure; the drug of choice for an anaphylactic reaction.

histamine A substance produced by the body that is responsible for many of the symptoms of anaphylaxis.

leukotrienes Chemical substances made by the body that contribute to anaphylaxis.

www.emtb.com

rabid An adjective describing an animal that is infected with rabies.

stridor A harsh, high-pitched respiratory sound, generally heard during inspiration, that is caused by partial blockage and/or narrowing of the upper airway.

toxin A poison or harmful substance.

urticaria Small spots of generalized itching and/or burning that appear as multiple raised areas on the skin; hives.

wheal A raised, swollen area on the skin resulting from an insect bite or allergic reaction.

wheezing A high-pitched, whistling breath sound, usually caused by a partial airway blockage and characteristically heard on expiration.

assessment in action

A local middle-school class is on a nature hike when the teacher suddenly hears screaming. A 14-year-old girl is waving her arms frantically as a swarm of yellow jackets buzz around her.

The girl is stung several times and drops to the ground. The teacher sees that the girl has been stung and remembers that the girl had problems in the past with bee stings and carries some kind of medicine for bee stings. The teacher uses her cell phone to call 9-1-1. Your unit is dispatched to the call.

On arrival, you find the girl seated against a rock. She has six obvious stings, two of them on her face. The sting areas are red and swollen, and the girl says that they itch "a lot." Initial assessment reveals that the patient is breathing loudly and her skin is warm, pink, and moist. The patient has a blood pressure of 104/66 mm Hg, a regular pulse of 142 beats/min, and fast, shallow respirations of 40 breaths/min.

1. On the basis of your initial assessment, you would report to medical control that the patient is:
   A. having a life-threatening allergic reaction and needs immediate transport.
   B. in anaphylactic shock and needs a PASG applied.
   C. in severe respiratory distress and needs help in administering epinephrine.
   D. not in acute distress but needs prompt transport.

2. Because this patient has known allergies to bee stings, you should expect that she would carry:
   A. oral antibiotics.
   B. an oral insulin kit.
   C. a Proventil inhaler.
   D. an epinephrine auto-injector.

3. The patient suddenly collapses as you are trying to find the EpiPen in her backpack. Under normal circumstances, what would you do before administering epinephrine?
   A. Elevate her head.
   B. Contact medical control.
   C. Recheck her blood pressure.
   D. Place her in a sitting position.

4. Which of the following items is **NOT** considered a common cause of allergic reactions?
   A. Nuts
   B. Seafood
   C. Cola drinks
   D. Medications

5. What is the proper site for injecting the EpiPen?
   A. Dorsal aspect of the foot
   B. Midabdomen, just above the umbilicus
   C. Lateral thigh, between the waist and knee
   D. Middle of the neck, just above the shoulder

points to ponder

Objectives 4-5.1, 4-5.2, 4-5.3, 4-5.4, 4-5.6, 4-5.7, 4-5.8

You respond to a call to find a 24-year-old unconscious patient. Her face is quite cyanotic and swollen, and she appears to have a rash over most of her body. There is some respiratory effort, but there does not appear to be any air exchange. You contact the hospital and get a new physician, whom you do not recognize. The physician denies your request to administer epinephrine. By now, your partner has obtained vitals; they are blood pressure of 60/20 mm Hg, pulse of 140 beats/min, and no respirations. Your second request for epinephrine is denied. The hospital is 15 minutes away.

• How would you deal with this situation? Would you spend more time trying to convince the physician? What would your treatment include besides epinephrine?

online outlook

Given the right person, almost any substance can trigger the body's immune system and cause an allergic reaction. To learn more about common allergens, complete Exercise 18 at www.emtb.com.

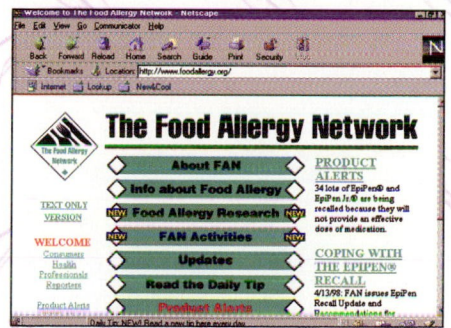

Substance Abuse
and Poisoning

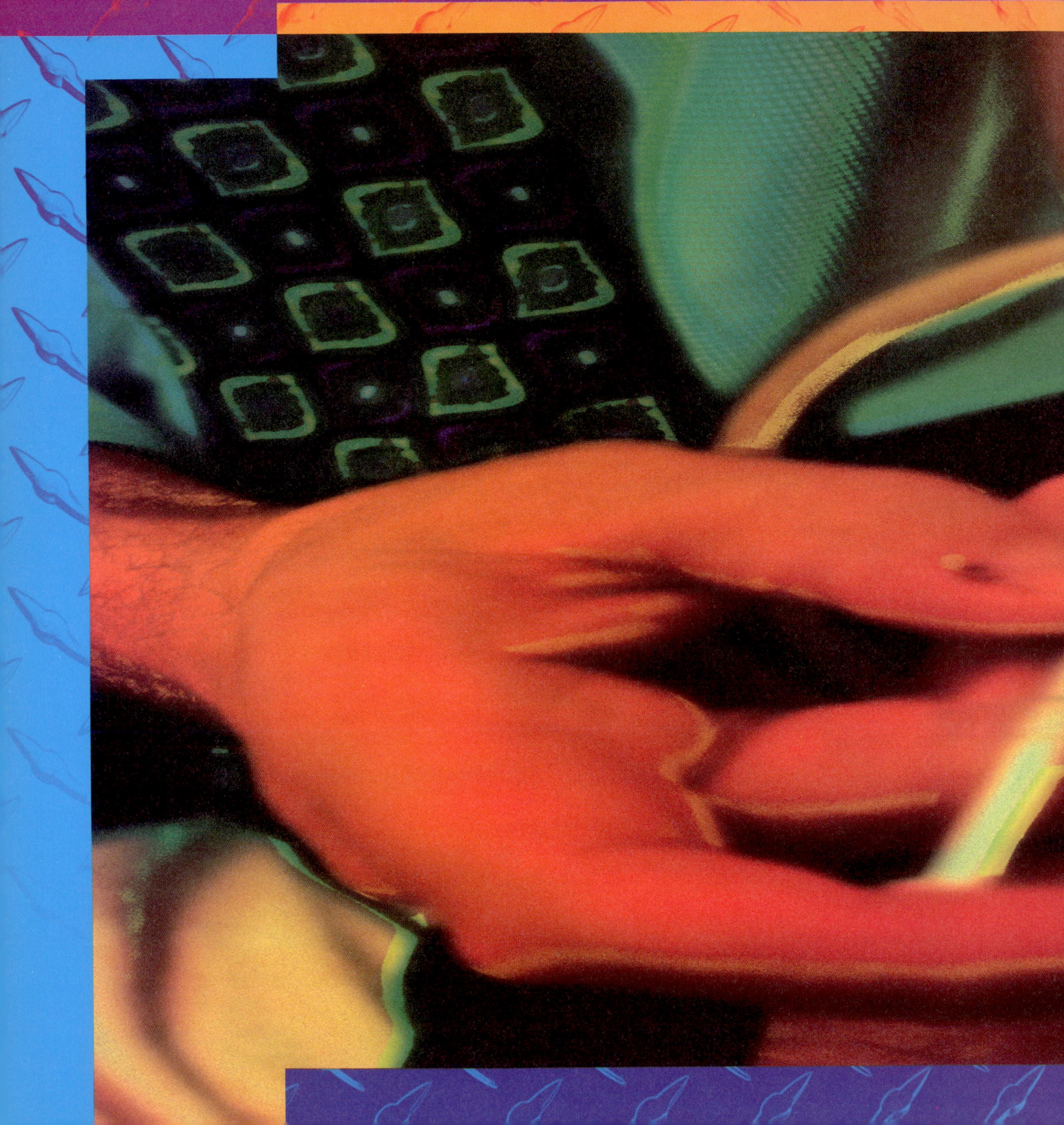

objectives

Cognitive

1. List various ways that poisons enter the body.

2. List signs and symptoms associated with poisoning.

3. Discuss the emergency medical care for the patient with possible overdose.

4. Describe the steps in the emergency medical care for the patient with suspected poisoning.

5. Establish the relationship between the patient suffering from poisoning or overdose and airway management.

6. State the generic and trade names, indications, contraindications, medication form, dose, administration, actions, side effects, and reassessment strategies for activated charcoal.

7. Recognize the need for medical direction in caring for the patient with poisoning or overdose.

Affective

8. Explain the rationale for administering activated charcoal.

9. Explain the rationale for contacting medical direction early in the prehospital management of the poisoning or overdose patient.

Psychomotor

10. Demonstrate the steps in the emergency medical care for the patient with possible overdose.

11. Demonstrate the steps in the emergency medical care for the patient with suspected poisoning.

12. Perform the necessary steps required to provide a patient with activated charcoal.

13. Demonstrate the assessment and documentation of patient response.

14. Demonstrate proper disposal of the equipment for the administration of activated charcoal.

15. Demonstrate completing a prehospital care report for patients with a poisoning/overdose emergency.

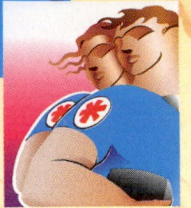

you are the emt

Rescue 6 please respond to Johnson Middle School for a possible overdose.

Whether you work on a volunteer squad in a small town or for a service in a big city, you will be called to treat patients who have abused drugs or other substances. This chapter will help you to understand the increasing problem of substance abuse in addition to what happens when a patient has been poisoned. It will also help you to answer the following questions:

1. Why is the problem with street drugs perceived as only a "big city" problem?
2. What are the main differences between legal and illegal drugs?

Substance Abuse and Poisoning

Every day, each of us comes into contact with things that are potentially poisonous. This is not surprising when you consider that almost any substance may be a poison in certain circumstances. Different doses can turn even a remedy into a poison. Consider aspirin. When taken in recommended doses, it is a safe and effective analgesic. Too much aspirin, however, can result in death.

Acute poisoning affects some 5 million children and adults each year. Chronic poisoning, often caused by abuse of drugs and other substances, including tobacco, is much more common. Fortunately, deaths from poisoning are fairly rare. Poisoning death rates for children have decreased steadily since the 1960s, when safety caps were introduced for drug bottles and containers. Poisoning deaths in adults, though, have been rising, the majority the result of drug abuse.

In this chapter, the term "poisoned" includes both acute and chronic poisonings. As an EMT-B, you must recognize that patients with either type of problem may have a variety of injuries. Although you cannot stop a chronic substance abuse problem, you may be able to prevent death from the acute effects of the poison.

This chapter discusses how to identify the patient who has been poisoned and how to gather clues about the poison. It describes the different ways in which poison is introduced into the body. It then discusses the signs, symptoms, and treatment of specific poisons, including opioids and sedatives. Food poisoning and plant poisoning are also discussed.

Identifying the Patient and the Poison

A **poison** is any substance whose chemical action can damage body structures or impair body function. A poison can be introduced into the body through a variety of means. Poisons act by changing the normal metabolism of cells or by actually destroying them. Poisons may act acutely, as in an overdose of heroin, or chronically, as in years of alcohol or other substance abuse. **Substance abuse** is the knowing misuse of any substance to produce a desired effect (eg, cocaine intoxication).

Your primary responsibility to the patient who has been poisoned is to recognize that a poisoning has occurred. Keep in mind that very small amounts of some poisons can cause considerable damage or death. If you have even the slightest suspicion that a patient has taken a poisonous substance, you should notify medical control and begin emergency treatment at once.

Symptoms and signs of poisoning vary according to the specific agent, as shown in Table 19-1. Some poisons cause the pulse to speed up, while others cause it to slow down; some cause the pupils to dilate, while others cause the pupils to constrict. If respiration is depressed or difficult, cyanosis may occur. Some chemical compounds will irritate or burn the skin or mucous membranes, resulting in burning or blistering. The presence of such injuries at the mouth strongly suggests the ingestion of a poison, such as lye. If possible, consider asking the patient the following questions:

- What substance did you take?
- When did you take it (or become exposed to it)?

TABLE 19-1	Toxidromes: Typical Signs and Symptoms of Specific Drug Overdose
Opioid	Hypoventilation/respiratory arrest Pinpoint pupils (miosis) Sedation/coma Hypotension
Sympathomimetics	Hypertension Tachycardia Dilated pupils (mydriasis) Agitation/seizures Hyperthermia
Sedative-Hypnotics	Slurred speech Sedation/coma Hypoventilation Hypotension
Anticholinergics	Tachycardia Hyperthermia Hypertension Dilated pupils (mydriasis) Dry skin and mucous membranes Sedation/agitation/seizures/ coma/delirium Decreased bowel sounds
Cholinergics	Excess defecation/urination Muscle fasciculations Pinpoint pupils (miosis) Excess lacrimation/ salivation Airway compromise Nausea/vomiting

poison control centers

There are several hundred poison centers in the United States. The phone number of your local poison control center is typically found on the inside cover of your local phone book. Staff at every center have access to information about virtually all of the commonly used drugs, chemicals, and substances that could possibly be poisonous. They know the appropriate emergency treatment for each, including the antidote, if there is one. An **antidote** is a substance that will counteract the effects of a particular poison.

If you believe that a patient has been poisoned, you should immediately provide medical control with all relevant information: when the poisoning occurred; a description of the suspected poison, including the amount involved; and the patient's size, weight, and age. If necessary, medical control can contact the regional poison center and relay specific instructions back to you.

A medical toxicologist is a physician who specializes in caring for patients who have been poisoned. About 100 of these specialists work in special hospitals called Medical Toxicology Treatment Centers, located throughout the United States. At times, your medical control may divert a patient who meets certain poisoning criteria to one of these centers instead of to the closest hospital.

You and your medical control should know the telephone number of your regional poison control center and have it available in case you come upon an unexpected case of poisoning.

- How much did you ingest?
- What actions have been taken?
- How much do you weigh?

Try to determine the nature of the poison. Objects at the scene may provide clues: an overturned bottle, a needle or syringe, scattered pills, chemicals, even an overturned or damaged plant. The remains of any nearby food or drink may also be important. Place any suspicious material in a plastic bag, and take it to the hospital, along with any containers you find.

Containers can provide critical information. In addition to the name and concentration of the drug, a pill bottle label may list specific ingredients, the number of pills that were originally in the bottle, and the name of the manufacturer and the dose that was prescribed. This information can help emergency department physicians to determine how much has been ingested and what specific treatment may be required. For certain food poisonings, a food container that lists the name and location of the maker or the vendor may be of equal importance in saving the life of the patient and possibly other people.

If the patient vomits, collect the material, called **vomitus**, in a separate plastic bag so that it can be analyzed at the hospital. After providing emergency care, collecting and bagging suspicious materials and vomitus may be the most important thing you can do for the patient.

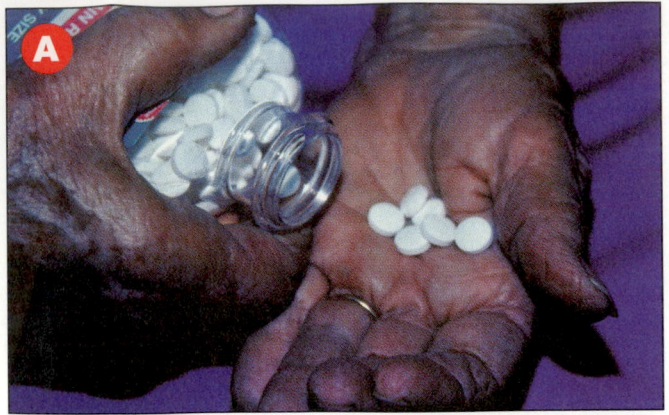

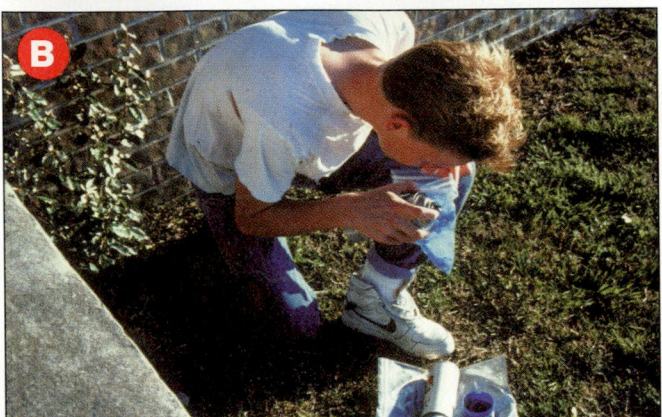

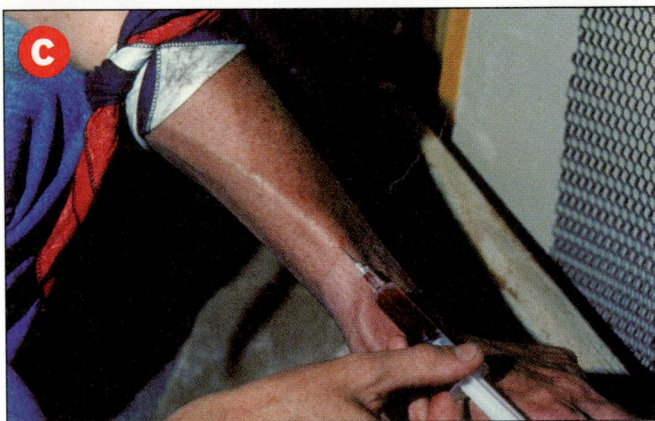

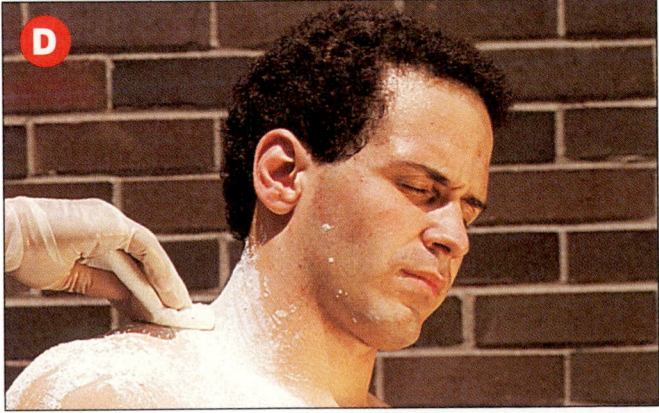

FIGURE 19-1 There are four routes by which a poison can enter the body. **A:** Ingestion. **B:** Inhalation. **C:** Injection. **D:** Absorption (surface contact)

How Poisons Get Into the Body

Emergency care for the patient who has been poisoned may include a range of actions from reassuring an anxious parent to instituting CPR. Most often, it will not include administering a specific antidote, because most poisons do not have one. Therefore, in general, the most important treatment for poisoning is diluting and/or physically removing the poisonous agent. How you do this depends on how the poison gets into the patient's body in the first place. Essentially, the four avenues to consider are as follows (Figure 19-1):

- Ingestion
- Inhalation
- Injection
- Surface contact (absorption)

Injection often can be the most worrisome avenue of poisoning. You can administer oxygen to a patient who has inhaled a poison, and you can give activated charcoal to one who has ingested a poison. You can flood the skin with water and wash out the eyes. However, it is difficult to remove or dilute injected poisons, a feature that makes these cases especially urgent. On the other hand, all routes of poisoning can be deadly, and each should be thought of as being equally serious.

Always consult medical control before you proceed with the treatment of any poisoning victim.

Ingested Poisons

Approximately 80% of all poisoning is by mouth, that is, by **ingestion**. Ingested poisons include liquids, household cleaners, contaminated food, plants, and, in the majority of cases, drugs. Ingested poisoning is usually accidental in children and, except for contaminated food, deliberate in adults. Plant poisonings are common among children, who like to explore and often bite the leaves of various bushes or shrubs.

Your goal as an EMT-B is to rapidly remove as much of the poison as possible from the gastrointestinal tract. For most poisoning victims, this emergency treatment is sufficient.

In the past, syrup of ipecac was used to cause vomiting, but today it is recommended in only a few situations in which the risk of losing consciousness is clearly ruled out. Because syrup of ipecac induces vomiting, individuals who have ingested substances that may cause diminished alertness over time might vomit and inhale the vomit into the lungs as they lose consciousness. As a result, syrup of ipecac is usually not carried on ambulances. Today, many EMS systems allow you to carry activated charcoal on your unit. Activated charcoal comes as a suspension that binds to the poison in the stomach and carries it out of the system. Therefore, it is both more effective and safer than syrup of ipecac. Because activated charcoal is an inky, messy fluid, you may have to do some coaxing to get a child to drink it; try to give it in a covered cup with a straw (Figure 19-2). Remember, you should never force this (or any other) liquid into a patient's mouth.

Although every poison will result in a specific set of symptoms and signs, you should always assess the airway, breathing, and circulation of every patient who has been poisoned. Many patients have died as a result of problems with ABCD that might have been managed easily. Be prepared to provide aggressive ventilatory support and CPR to a patient who has ingested an opiate, sedative, or barbiturate, each of which can cause depression of the central nervous system (CNS) and slow breathing. Make sure you use a barrier device when providing CPR. Again, whenever poisoning is involved, you should provide prompt transport to the emergency department. The patient may need IV support and other treatments that can be given only in the hospital. If you work in a tiered system, ALS backup also may be a good idea, as they often carry and can administer additional medications and therapies.

Inhaled Poisons

Patients who have inhaled poison, including natural gas, certain pesticides, carbon monoxide, chlorine, or other gases, should be moved into fresh air immediately (Figure 19-3). Depending on how long they were exposed, they may require supplemental oxygen and basic life support. Always use a self-contained breathing apparatus (SCBA) to protect yourself from poisonous fumes. Remember that once patients are removed from the toxic environment, they are not toxic to you. However, make certain that only trained rescuers remove the patient from the poisonous environment.

Some inhaled poisons, such as carbon monoxide, are odorless and produce severe hypoxia without damaging or even irritating the lungs. Others, such as chlorine, are very irritating and cause airway obstruction and pulmonary edema. The patient may report the following signs and symptoms: burning eyes, sore throat, cough, chest pain, hoarseness, wheezing, respiratory distress, dizziness, confusion, headache, or stridor in severe cases. The patient may also have seizures or an altered mental status. Some inhaled agents cause progressive lung damage, even after the patient is removed from direct exposure; the damage may not be evident for a

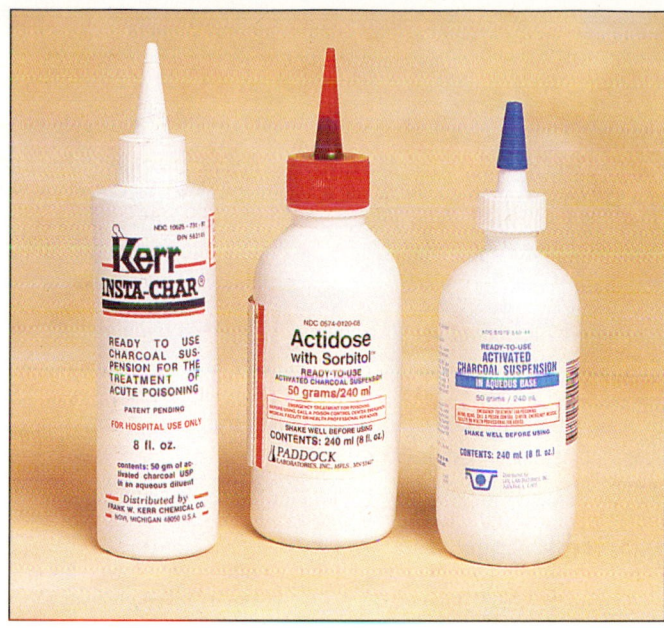

FIGURE 19-2 Activated charcoal comes as a premixed suspension that you should give, if local protocol allows, in a covered cup with a straw.

few hours. Meanwhile, it may take 2 or 3 days or more of intensive care to reestablish normal lung function. For this reason, all patients who have inhaled poison require immediate transport to an emergency department. Be prepared to use supplemental oxygen via nonrebreathing mask and/or ventilatory support with a BVM device, if necessary, and then continue BLS measures. Make sure a suctioning unit is available in case the patient vomits. As with other poisonings, it is helpful to bring containers, bottles, and labels when you transport the patient to the hospital.

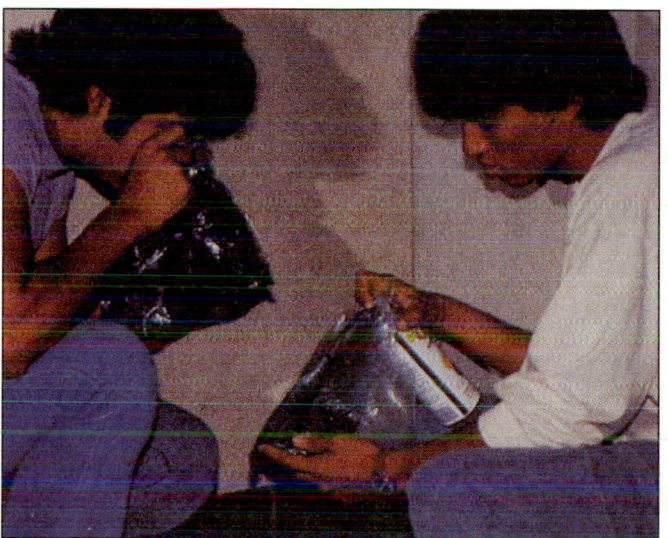

FIGURE 19-3 Patients who have inhaled poisons need supplemental oxygen and prompt transport to the emergency department.

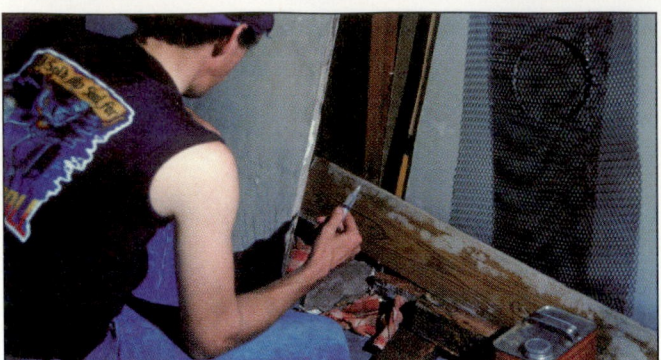

FIGURE 19-4 Injected poisons are impossible to dilute or remove from the body; therefore, prompt transport to the emergency department is critical.

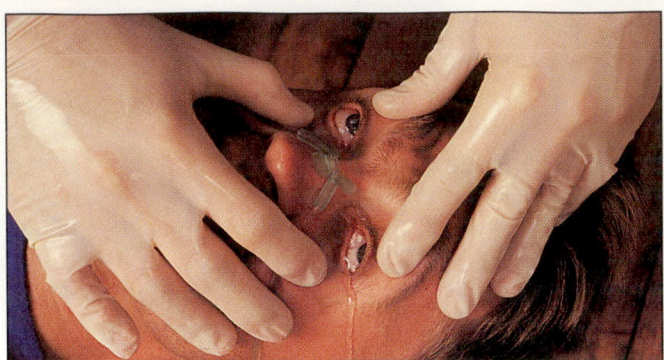

FIGURE 19-5 If chemical agents are in the patient's eyes, irrigate the eyes quickly and thoroughly, ensuring that the irrigation fluid runs from the bridge of the nose outward.

Injected Poisons

Poisoning by injection is almost always the result of a deliberate drug overdose, such as heroin or cocaine (Figure 19-4). Contrary to the thinking of television detectives, the only other parties who are likely to have injected a patient with poison are insects and animals.

Signs and symptoms of poisoning by injection can have a multitude of presentations, including weakness, dizziness, fever, chills, easy excitability, or unresponsiveness.

In general, injected poisons are impossible to dilute or remove, as they are usually absorbed quickly into the body or cause intense local tissue destruction. If you suspect that rapid absorption has occurred, monitor the patient's airway, provide high-flow oxygen, and be alert for nausea and vomiting. Remove rings, watches, and bracelets from areas around the injection site if swelling occurs. Prompt transport to the emergency department is essential. Bring all containers, bottles, and labels with the patient to the hospital.

Surface Contact (Absorbed) Poisons

Many corrosive substances will damage the skin, mucous membranes, or eyes, causing chemical burns, tell-tale rashes, or lesions. Acids, alkalis, and some petroleum (hydrocarbon) products are very destructive. Signs and symptoms of absorbed poisoning include a history of exposure, liquid or powder on a patient's skin, burns, itching, irritation, redness of the skin in light-skinned individuals, or typical odors of the substance.

Emergency treatment for a typical contact poisoning includes the following two steps:

1. Avoid contaminating yourself or others.
2. Remove the irritating or corrosive substance from the patient as rapidly as possible.

Remove all clothing that has been contaminated with poisons or irritating substances, thoroughly dust off any dry chemicals, flush the skin with running water, then wash the skin with soap and water. When a large amount of material has been spilled on a patient, flooding the affected part for at least 20 minutes may be the fastest and most effective treatment. If the patient has a chemical agent in the eyes, you should irrigate them quickly and thoroughly, at least 5 to 10 minutes for acid substances and 15 to 20 minutes for alkalis. As you irrigate the eyes, make sure that the fluid runs from the bridge of the nose outward (Figure 19-5).

Many chemical burns occur in industrial settings, where showers and specific protocols for handling surface burns are available. If you are called to such a scene, trained people usually will be there to assist you. Do not spend time trying to neutralize substances on the skin with additional chemicals. This may actually be more harmful. Instead, wash the substance off immediately with lots of water.

The only time you should not irrigate the contact area with water is when a poison reacts violently with water, such as contamination with phosphorus or elemental sodium. These substances ignite when they come into contact with water. Instead, brush the chemical off the patient, remove contaminated clothing, and apply a dry dressing to the burn area. Be sure to wear gloves and the proper protective clothing.

Provide prompt transport to the emergency department for definitive care. En route, continue irrigation and provide oxygen if possible.

> The most important treatment for poisoning is diluting and/or physically removing the poisonous agent.

Emergency Medical Care

External decontamination is important. Remove tablets or fragments from the patient's mouth, wash or brush poison from the patient's skin, and monitor the patient's breathing. Treatment focuses on support: assessing and maintaining the ABCD.

In some cases, you will give activated charcoal to patients who have ingested poison, if approved by medical control or local protocol. Charcoal is not indicated for patients who have ingested an acid, alkali, or petroleum product; who have a decreased level of consciousness; or who are unable to swallow.

Remember that activated charcoal adsorbs, or sticks to, many commonly ingested poisons, preventing the toxin from being absorbed into the body by the stomach or intestines. If local protocol permits, you will likely carry plastic bottles of premixed suspension, each containing up to 50 g of activated charcoal. Some common trade names for the suspension form are InstaChar, Actidose, and LiquiChar. The usual dosage for an adult or child is 1 g of activated charcoal per kilogram of body weight. The usual adult dose is 25 to 50 g, and the usual pediatric dose is 12.5 to 25 g.

Before you give a patient charcoal, obtain approval from medical control. Next, shake the bottle vigorously to mix the suspension. The medication looks like mud, so it is best to cover the outside of the container so that the fluid is not visible, and ask the patient to drink with a straw. You might need to persuade the patient to drink it, particularly if the patient is a child, but never force it. If the patient takes a long time to drink the mixture, you will have to shake the container frequently to keep the medication mixed. Be sure to record the time when you administered the activated charcoal.

The major side effect of ingesting activated charcoal is black stools. If the patient has ingested a poison that causes nausea, he or she may vomit after taking activated charcoal, and the dosage will have to be repeated. As you reassess the patient, be prepared for vomiting, nausea, and possible airway problems.

Specific Poisons

Over time, a person who routinely misuses a substance needs increasing amounts of it to achieve the same result. This is called developing a **tolerance** to the substance. Increasing tolerance can lead to addiction. A person with an **addiction** has an overwhelming desire or need to continue using the agent, at whatever cost, with a tendency to increase the dosage. This does not happen only with the classic drugs of abuse, such as cocaine. Almost any substance can be abused, including laxatives, nasal decongestants, vitamins, and food.

The importance of BSI techniques in caring for victims of drug abuse cannot be stressed enough. Known drug abusers have a fairly high incidence of serious and undiagnosed infections, including AIDS and hepatitis. These patients may bite, spit, hit, or otherwise injure you, causing you to come into contact with their blood and other body fluids. Always be sure to wear appropriate protective equipment. A calm, professional approach can defuse frightening situations, but keep your safety and that of your team uppermost in mind. Expect the unexpected and remember: The drug user, not the drug, can pose the greatest threat.

Alcohol

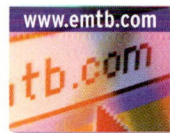 The most commonly abused drug in the United States is alcohol (Figure 19-6). It affects people from all walks of life and kills more than 200,000 of them each year. More than 50% of all traffic fatalities or injuries, 67% of murders, and 33% of suicides are related to alcohol, which impairs the capacity to think and function rationally. Alcoholism is one of the greatest national health problems, along with heart disease, cancer, and stroke.

Alcohol is a powerful CNS depressant. It is both a **sedative**, a substance that decreases activity and excitement, and a **hypnotic**, meaning that it induces sleep. In general, alcohol dulls the sense of awareness, slows reflexes, and reduces reaction time. It may also cause aggressive and inappropriate behavior and lack of coordination. However, a person who appears intoxicated may have other medical problems as well. Look for signs of head trauma, toxic reactions, or uncontrolled diabetes. Severe acute alcohol ingestion may cause hypoglycemia, which may contribute to the symptoms. At the very least, you should assume that all intoxicated patients are experiencing a drug overdose and require thorough examination by a physician. In most states, such patients cannot legally refuse transport.

If a patient exhibits signs of serious CNS depression, you must provide respiratory support. This may be

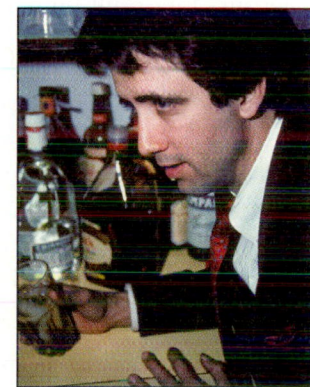

FIGURE 19-6 Alcohol intoxication often causes altered mental status, slowed reflexes, and impaired reaction time.

difficult, however, because depression of the respiratory system can also cause **emesis**, or vomiting. The vomiting may be very forceful or even bloody (**hematemesis**), since large amounts of alcohol irritate the stomach. Internal bleeding should also be considered if the patient appears to be in shock (hypoperfusion), as blood might not clot effectively in a patient who has a prolonged history of alcohol abuse.

A patient in alcohol withdrawal may experience frightening hallucinations or **delirium tremens (DTs)**, a syndrome characterized by restlessness, fever, sweating, disorientation, agitation, and even convulsions. These conditions may develop if patients no longer have their daily source of alcohol. Alcoholic hallucinations come and go. A patient with an otherwise fairly clear mental state may see fantastic shapes or figures or hear odd voices. Such auditory and visual hallucinations often precede DTs, which are a much more severe complication.

DTs may develop 1 to 7 days after a person stops drinking or when consumption levels are decreased suddenly. Again, patients may experience one or more of the following signs and symptoms:

- Agitation and restlessness
- Fever
- Sweating
- Confusion and/or disorientation
- Delusions and/or hallucinations
- Seizures

Provide prompt transport for these patients after you have completed your assessment and given necessary care. A person who is experiencing hallucinations or DTs is extremely ill. Should seizures develop, treat them as you would any other seizure. The patient should not be restrained, although you must protect him or her from self-injury. Give the patient oxygen, and watch carefully for vomiting. Hypovolemia may develop from sweating, fluid loss, insufficient fluid intake, or vomiting associated with DTs. If you see signs of hypovolemic shock, elevate the patient's feet slightly, clear the airway, and turn the head to one side to minimize the chance of aspiration during transport. These patients may not respond appropriately to suggestions or conversation; they are often confused and frightened. Therefore, your approach should be calm and relaxed. Reassure the patient and provide emotional support.

Opioids

The pain relievers called *opioid analgesics* are named for the opium in poppy seeds, the origin of heroin, codeine, and morphine. On the list of frequently abused drugs,

TABLE 19-2	Common Opoid Drugs

Butorphanol (Stadol)
Codeine
Fentanyl derivatives ("China White")
Heroin
Hydrocodone (Hycodan)
Hydromorphone (Dilaudid)
Meperidine (Demerol)
Methadone (Dolophine)
Morphine
Oxycodone (Percodan)
Pentazocine (Talwin)
Propoxyphene (Darvon)

they have been joined by a number of synthetic opioids, with origins in the laboratory. These include meperidine (Demerol), hydromorphone (Dilaudid), propoxyphene (Darvon), oxycodone (Percocet), hydrocodone (Vicodin), and methadone (Table 19-2). Most of these drugs have legitimate medical uses. With the exception of heroin, which is illegal in the United States, many addicts may have started using any of the opioids with an appropriate medical prescription.

These agents are CNS depressants and can cause severe respiratory depression. Administered intravenously, however, they produce a characteristic "high" or "kick." Tolerance develops rapidly, so some users may require massive doses to experience the same high. In general, emergency medical problems related to opioids are caused by respiratory depression, including a decreased volume of inspired air and decreased respirations. Patients typically appear sedated and cyanotic and have pinpoint pupils.

Treatment includes supporting the airway and breathing. You may try to arouse patients by talking loudly to them or shaking them gently. Always give supplemental oxygen, and be prepared for vomiting. Many home remedies are believed to reverse the respiratory depression associated with heroin overdose, including applying ice to the groin or forcing milk into the mouth. *None of these work, and they frequently complicate the clinical picture.* Nevertheless, you should be aware that a patient's friends may have attempted inappropriate methods of resuscitation. The only effective antidote to reverse the symptoms and signs of opioid overdose are certain so-called narcotic antagonists such as naloxone (Narcan). Patients will respond within 2 minutes to naloxone when it is given intravenously. Naloxone is usually administered by paramedics on-scene or, more often, by physicians at the emergency department.

TABLE 19-3   Examples of Sedative-Hypnotic Drugs

Barbiturates	Benzodiazepines	Others
Amobarbital	Alprazolam (Xanax)	Carisoprodol (Soma)
Butabarbital	Chlordiazepoxide (Librium)	Chloral hydrate ("Mickey Finn")
Pentobarbital	Diazepam (Valium)	Cyclobenzaprine (Flexeril)
Phenobarbital	Flunitrazepam (Rohypnol)	Ethchlorvynol (Placidyl)
Secobarbital	Lorazepam (Ativan)	Ethyl alcohol (drinking alcohol)
	Oxazepam (Serax)	Glutethimide (Doriden)
	Temazepam (Restoril)	Hydrocarbon inhalants
		Isopropyl alcohol (rubbing alcohol)
		Meprobamate (Equagesic)

Sedative-Hypnotic Drugs

Barbiturates and benzodiazepines have been a part of legitimate medicine for a long time. They are easy to obtain and relatively cheap. People sometimes solicit prescriptions from several physicians for the same or a variety of sedative-hypnotics. These drugs are CNS depressants and alter level of consciousness, with effects similar to those of alcohol so that the patient may appear drowsy, peaceful, or intoxicated (Table 19-3). By themselves, they do not relieve pain, nor do they produce a specific high, although users often take alcohol or an opioid at the same time to boost their effects.

In general, these agents are taken by mouth. Occasionally, however, contents of capsules are suspended or dissolved in water and injected to produce a rather sudden state of ease and contentment. Unfortunately, use of IV sedative-hypnotic drugs quickly induces tolerance, so an individual requires increasingly larger doses. As a result, you are less likely to be called upon to treat an acute overdose in someone who chronically abuses these drugs. However, you may be called to a scene of an attempted suicide in which the patient has taken large quantities of these drugs. In these situations, patients will have marked respiratory depression and may even be in a coma.

Sedative-hypnotic drugs may also be given to people unknowingly as a "knock-out" drink, or "Mickey Finn." More recently, drugs such as Rohypnol have been abused as a "date rape drug," causing the unwary individual to become sedated and even unconscious. The individual later begins to awaken, confused and unable to remember what happened.

In general, your treatment of patients who have overdosed with sedative-hypnotics and have respiratory depression is to provide airway clearance, ventilatory assistance, and prompt transport. Give supplemental oxygen, and be ready to assist ventilation. You may attempt to stimulate the person by speaking loudly or gently shaking him or her; remember to watch for vomiting.

A specific antidote is available for acute benzodiazepine overdose. It is called flumazenil and is given intravenously. Although it will reverse the sedation and respiratory depression of the benzodiazepine sedative-hypnotics, it will have no effect on the signs and symptoms of overdose from ethyl alcohol or barbiturates. Almost always, flumazenil is administered in the hospital after a physician's assessment.

As multi-drug use becomes more common, you may find it increasingly difficult to determine what agents the patients have taken. Your best approach is to treat any obvious injuries or illnesses, keeping in mind that drug use may complicate the picture and make full life support necessary. Focus on ABCD, especially the possibility of airway problems (relaxation of the tongue, causing obstruction), vomiting, respiratory depression, and, in severe cases, cardiac arrest.

Abused Inhalants

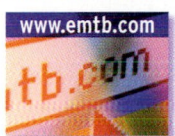 Many abused inhalants produce several of the same CNS effects as other sedative-hypnotics, but these agents are inhaled instead of ingested or injected. Some of the more common agents include acetone, toluene, xylene, and hexane, which are found in glues, cleaning compounds, paint thinners, and lacquers. Similarly, gasoline and various halogenated hydrocarbons, such as Freon, used as propellants in aerosol sprays, are also abused as inhalants. None of these inhalants is a medication. Since these are products that can be bought in hardware stores, they are commonly abused by teenagers seeking an alcohol-like high.

Always use special care in dealing with a patient who may have used inhalants. Their effects range from mild drowsiness to coma, but unlike most other sedative-hypnotics, these agents may often cause seizures. Also, halogenated hydrocarbon solvents can make the heart supersensitive to the patient's own adrenaline, putting the patient at high risk for sudden cardiac death from ventricular fibrillation; even the action of walking may release enough adrenaline to cause a fatal ventricular arrhythmia. You must try to keep such patients from struggling with you or exerting themselves. Give supplemental oxygen, and use a stretcher to move the patient. Prompt transport to the hospital is essential; monitor vital signs en route.

Sympathomimetics

Sympathomimetics are CNS stimulants that frequently cause hypertension, tachycardia, and dilated pupils. A **stimulant** is any agent that produces an excited state. Amphetamine and methamphetamine ("ice") are commonly taken by mouth. They are also injected by abusers in many cases. They typically are taken to make the user "feel good," improve task performance, suppress appetite, or prevent sleepiness. They may just as easily produce irritability, anxiety, lack of concentration, or seizures. Other common examples include phentermine and Benzedrine. Caffeine, theophylline, and phenylpropanolamine (a nasal decongestant) are all mild sympathomimetics. So-called "designer drugs," such as Ecstasy and Eve, are also frequently abused in certain areas of the country.

Sympathomimetic drugs are frequently called "uppers" (Table 19-4). Someone using one of these agents may display disorganized behavior, restlessness, and sometimes anxiety or great fear. Paranoia and delusions are common with sympathomimetic abuse.

Cocaine, also called coke, crack, crystal, snow, freebase, rock, gold dust, blow, and lady, may be taken in a number of different ways. Classically, it is inhaled into the nose and absorbed through the nasal mucosa, damaging tissue, causing nosebleeds, and ultimately destroying the nasal septum. It can also be injected intravenously or subcutaneously (skin-popping). Cocaine can be absorbed through all mucous membranes and even across the skin. In any form, the immediate effects of a given dose last less than an hour.

Another method of abusing cocaine is by smoking it. Crack is pure cocaine. It melts at 93°F (34°C) and vaporizes at a slightly higher temperature. Therefore, crack is easily smoked. In this form, it reaches the capillary network of the lungs and can be absorbed into the body in seconds. The immediate outflow of blood from the heart speeds the drug to the brain, so its effect is felt at once. Smoked crack produces the most rapid means of absorption and therefore the most potent effect.

Cocaine is one of the most addicting substances known, more so than heroin or nicotine. Its immediate effects include excitement and euphoria. Acute cocaine overdose is a genuine emergency, as patients are at high risk for seizures and cardiac arrhythmias. Chronic cocaine abuse may cause hallucinations; patients with "cocaine bugs" think that bugs are crawling out of their skin.

In caring for patients who have been poisoned with any of the sympathomimetics, be aware that their severe agitation can lead to tachycardia and hypertension. Patients may also be paranoid, putting you and other health care providers in danger. Law enforcement officers should be at the scene to restrain the patient, if necessary. Do not leave the patient unattended and unmonitored during transport.

All of these patients need to get to the emergency department promptly because of their risk of seizures, cardiac arrhythmias, and stroke. You may see blood pressures as high as 250/150 mm Hg. Give supplemental oxygen, and be ready to provide suctioning. If the patient is already having a seizure, you must protect him or her against self-injury.

TABLE 19-4	Street Names for Amphetamines
Adam	MDA
Bennies	Psychodrine
DOM	Speed
Ecstasy	STP
Eve	Uppers
Fen-phen	
Golden eagle	
Ice	

Marijuana

The flowering hemp plant *Cannabis sativa,* called marijuana, is abused throughout the world. It has been estimated that as many as 20 million people use marijuana daily in the United States. Inhaling marijuana smoke from a cigarette or pipe produces euphoria, relaxation, and drowsiness. It also impairs short-term memory and the capacity to do complex thinking and work. In some people, the euphoria progresses to depression and confusion. An altered perception of time is common, and anxiety and panic can occur. With very high doses, patients experience hallucinations.

A person who has been using marijuana rarely needs transport to the hospital. Exceptions may include someone who is hallucinating, very anxious, or paranoid. However, you should be aware that marijuana is often used as a vehicle to get other drugs into the body. For example, it may be covered with crack or PCP, also known as "angel dust."

Hallucinogens

Hallucinogens alter an individual's sense of perception (Table 19-5). The classic hallucinogen is lysergic acid diethylamide (LSD). Abuse of another hallucinogen, phencyclidine (PCP, "angel dust") is relatively uncommon among young adults. PCP is a dissociative anesthetic that is easily synthesized and highly potent. Its effectiveness by oral, nasal, pulmonary, and IV routes makes it easy to add to other street drugs. PCP is dangerous, as it causes severe behavioral changes in which individuals often inflict injury to themselves.

All these agents cause visual hallucinations, intensify both vision and hearing, and generally separate the user from reality. The user, of course, expects that the altered sensory state will be pleasurable. Often, however, it can be terrifying. At some point, you are bound to encounter patients who are having a "bad trip." They will usually be hypertensive, tachycardic, anxious, and probably paranoid.

Many of the hallucinogens have sympathomimetic properties. Indeed, your care for a patient who is having a bad reaction to a hallucinogenic agent is the same as that for a patient on a sympathomimetic. Use a calm,

TABLE 19-5	Commonly Abused Hallucinogens

Bufotenine (toad skin)
Dimethyltryptamine (DMT)
Jimsonweed
Lysergic acid diethylamide (LSD)
Marijuana
Mescaline
Morning glory
Nutmeg
Phencyclidine hydrochloride (PCP)
Psilocybin (mushroom)

professional manner, and provide emotional support. Do not use restraints unless you or the patient is in danger of injury and then always within the guidelines specified by local authorities. These patients may suddenly experience hallucinations or odd perceptions, so you must watch them carefully throughout transport. Never leave a patient who has taken a hallucinogen unattended and unmonitored.

Anticholinergic Agents

The classic picture of a person who has taken too much of an anticholinergic medication is "hot as a hare, blind as a bat, dry as a bone, red as a beet, and mad as a hatter." These are drugs that have properties that, among other effects, block the parasympathetic nerves. Common medications with a significant anticholinergic effect include atropine, diphenhydramine (Benadryl), jimsonweed, and certain cyclic antidepressants. With the exception of jimsonweed, these medications usually are not abused drugs but may be taken as an intentional overdose. You will find that it is often difficult to distinguish between an anticholinergic overdose and a sympathomimetic overdose. In both groups of patients, patients may be agitated and tachycardic and have dilated pupils. Once a pure anticholinergic poisoning has been diagnosed, the patient may be treated with physostigmine intravenously by staff in the emergency department, depending on the severity of the situation.

As newer, safer antidepressants such as fluoxetine (Prozac) and sertraline (Zoloft) crowd the market, you can expect to see fewer overdoses of cyclic antidepressants such as amitriptyline (Elavil) and imipramine (Tofranil). In addition to its anticholinergic effects, a cyclic antidepressant overdose may cause more serious, indeed life-threatening, effects. This is because the medication may block the electrical conduction system in the heart, leading to lethal cardiac arrhythmias. Patients with acute cyclic antidepressant overdose must be transported immediately to the emergency department; they may go from appearing "normal" to seizure and death within 30 minutes. The seizures and cardiac arrhythmias caused by a severe cyclic antidepressant overdose are best treated in the hospital with IV sodium bicarbonate. If you work in a tiered system, you should consider calling for ALS backup when you are en route to the scene.

Cholinergic Agents

The "nerve gases" designed for chemical warfare are cholinergic agents. These agents overstimulate normal body functions that are controlled by parasympathetic nerves, such as salivation, mucous secretion, urination, crying, and heart rate. Obviously, you are unlikely to run across these. However, you may well be called to care for patients who have been exposed to one of the organophosphate insecticides or certain wild mushrooms, which are also cholinergic agents. The signs and symptoms of cholinergic drug poisoning are easy to remember because of the mnemonic DUMBELS:

- **D**efecation
- **U**rination
- **M**iosis (contraction of the pupils)
- **B**ronchorrhea (discharge of mucus from the lungs)
- **E**mesis
- **L**acrimation (tearing)
- **S**alivation

Alternatively, you can use the mnemonic SLUDGE:

- **S**alivation
- **L**acrimation
- **U**rination
- **D**efecation
- **G**I irritation
- **E**ye constriction

In poisonings, patients will have excessive amounts of these normal functions and body secretions. In addition, patients may have either bradycardia or tachycardia.

The most important consideration in caring for a patient who has been exposed to an organophosphate insecticide or some other cholinergic agent is to avoid exposure yourself. Because such agents may cling to a patient's clothing and skin, decontamination may take priority over immediate transport to the emergency department. At the hospital, the anticholinergic drug atropine can be used to dry up the patient's secretions. In the meantime, your priority after decontamination is to decrease the secretions in the mouth and trachea that threaten to suffocate the patient and provide airway support. Depending on your local EMS protocol, this can be treated as a HazMat situation.

Miscellaneous Drugs

While not as common as it was 30 years ago, aspirin poisoning remains a potentially lethal condition. Ingesting too many aspirin tablets, either acutely or chronically, may result in nausea, vomiting, hyperventilation, and ringing in the ears. Patients with this problem are frequently anxious, confused, tachypneic, and in danger of having seizures. They should be transported quickly to the hospital.

Overdosing with *acetaminophen* is also very common, probably because acetaminophen is available in so many different preparations, such as Tylenol. The good news is that acetaminophen is generally not very toxic. A healthy patient could ingest 140 mg of acetaminophen for every kilogram of body weight without serious adverse effects. The bad news is that the symptoms of an overdose generally do not appear until it is too late. For example, massive liver failure may not be apparent for a full week. And patients may not provide the information necessary for a correct diagnosis. For this reason, gathering information at the scene is very important. By finding an empty acetaminophen bottle, you may save a patient's life. If given early enough (before liver failure occurs), a specific antidote may prevent liver damage.

Be extremely careful in dealing with a child who has unintentionally ingested a poisonous substance. Although such incidents usually do not lead to death, family members may be distraught, and your professional attitude will help to ease the tension. Remember, however, that a single swallow of some substances can kill a child (Table 19-6).

Some alcohols, including methyl alcohol and ethylene glycol, are even more toxic than ethyl alcohol (drinking alcohol). Although they may be used as a substitute by the chronic alcoholic who is unable to obtain ethyl alcohol, they are more often taken by someone attempting suicide. In either case, immediate transport to the emergency department is essential. Methyl alcohol is found in

TABLE 19-6   Fatal Injested Poisons
Benzocaine
Calcium channel blockers (verapamil, nifedipine, diltiazem)
Camphor
Chloroquine
Cyclic antidepressants (amitriptyline (Elavil), imipramine (Tofranil), nortriptyline (Pamelor))
Hydrocarbon solvents
Lomotil
Methanol/ethylene glycol
Methylsalicylate (oil of wintergreen)
Phenothiazines (Thorazine)
Quinine
Theophylline
Visine®

caring for the elderly

In an accidental overdose or poisoning, the elderly patient may have become confused about his or her drug regimen. He or she may have forgotten that the medication had been taken, repeating the dose a number of times. Or the patient could have forgotten the doctor's instructions to discard leftover medication and might have taken both the current and the older drug, resulting in an increase in effects or an unwanted drug interaction.

The elderly patient may also intentionally overdose in an attempt to commit suicide. Geriatric patients have been known to ingest common household chemicals such as insecticides, acetaminophen, aspirin, or caustic substances in an attempt to end their lives. Be alert for any indication of an intentional overdose or poisoning, even though the patient might deny an attempted suicide.

In considering any poisoning, remember the basics. Because of the aging process, the routes of administration in the elderly patient pose significant changes in the way the poison is absorbed into the body. In the senior citizen, damage to the stomach could be more severe, since increased gastric acids can alter absorption of the poison. Additionally, decreased gastric mobility slows absorption by delaying emptying of the stomach and, in the event of caustic substance ingestion, increases injury to the stomach.

If a senior citizen inhales a poison, even in tiny quantities, lung damage can be severe. Consider the decreased lung capacity and ability to exchange oxygen and carbon dioxide in the elderly patient's lungs. Pulmonary function could be worsened to potentially fatal levels with the inhalation of minute amounts of poison.

For poisons that are absorbed by or injected into the skin, reduced circulation to the skin can decrease or delay absorption into the body. Watch for an increased reaction or irritation at the skin site.

In the geriatric patient, the liver may not be able to metabolize the poison as effectively, or the kidneys may not be able to excrete the poison as quickly. In either case, the drug or poison remains in the body for a longer period of time, causing additional tissue damage. When a medication is not metabolized or excreted as quickly as before, the drug could accumulate to toxic levels and, ultimately, become fatal.

dry gas products and Sterno; ethylene glycol is found in some antifreeze products. Both cause a "drunken" feeling. Left untreated, both will also cause severe tachypnea, blindness (methyl alcohol), renal failure (ethylene glycol), and eventually death. Even ethyl alcohol (typical drinking alcohol) can stop a patient's breathing if taken in too high a dose or too fast, particularly in children.

Food Poisoning

The term "ptomaine poisoning" was coined in 1870 to indicate poisoning by a class of chemicals found in rotting food. It is still used today in many news accounts of food poisoning. This is unfortunate, because the term is misleading. Food poisoning is almost always caused by eating food that is contaminated by bacteria. The food may appear perfectly good, with little or no decay or odor to suggest danger.

There are two main types of food poisoning. In one, the organism itself causes disease; in the other, the organism produces toxins that cause disease (Table 19-7). A **toxin** is a poison or harmful substance produced by bacteria, animals, or plants.

One organism that produces direct effects of food poisoning is the *Salmonella* bacterium. The condition called salmonellosis is characterized by severe gastrointestinal symptoms within 72 hours of ingestion, including nausea, vomiting, abdominal pain, and diarrhea. In addition, patients suffering from salmonellosis may be systemically ill with fever and generalized weakness. Some people are carriers of certain bacteria; although they may not become ill themselves, they may transmit diseases,

TABLE 19-7	Common Sources of Food Poisoning
Bacillus cereus	Giardia lamblia
Campylobacter	Rotavirus
Clostridium botulinum toxin	Salmonella
	Shigella
Clostridium perfringens	Staphylococcus toxin
Cryptosporidium	Vibrio parahaemolyticus
Enterococcus	Yersinia enterocolitica
Escherichia coli	

particularly if they work in the food services industry. Usually, proper cooking kills bacteria, and proper cleanliness in the kitchen prevents the contamination of uncooked foods.

The more common cause of food poisoning is the ingestion of powerful toxins produced by bacteria, often in leftovers. The bacterium *Staphylococcus,* a common culprit, is quick to grow and produce toxins in foods that have been prepared in advance and kept too long, even in the refrigerator. Foods prepared with mayonnaise, when left unrefrigerated, are a common vehicle for the development of staphylococcal toxins. Usually, staphylococcal food poisoning results in sudden gastrointestinal symptoms, including nausea, vomiting, and diarrhea. Although time frames may vary from individual to individual, usually these symptoms may start within 2 to 3 hours after ingestion or as long as 8 to 12 hours after ingestion.

The most severe form of toxin ingestion is botulism. This often-fatal disease usually results from eating improperly canned food, in which the spores of *Clostridium* bacteria have grown and produced a toxin. The symptoms of botulism are neurologic: blurring of vision, weakness, and difficulty in speaking and breathing. Symptoms may develop as long as 4 days after ingestion or as early as the first 24 hours.

In general, you should not try to determine the specific cause of acute gastrointestinal problems. After all, severe vomiting may be a sign of a self-limiting food poisoning, a bowel obstruction requiring surgery, or another poison, such as copper, arsenic, zinc, cadmium, scombrotoxin (fish poison), or Clitocybe or Inocybe mushrooms. Instead, you should gather as much history as possible from the patient, and transport him or her promptly to the hospital. When two or more individuals in one group have the same illness, you should bring along some of the suspected food. In advanced cases of botulism, you may have to assist respirations and give basic life support.

Plant Poisoning

Several thousand cases of poisoning from plants occur each year, some severe. Many household plants are poisonous if ingested, as they may be by children who like to nibble leaves (Table 19-8). Some poisonous plants cause local irritation of the skin; others can affect the circulatory system, the gastrointestinal tract, or the central nervous system. It is impossible for you to memorize every plant and poison, let alone their effects (Figure 19-7). You can and should do the following:

1. Assess the patient's vital signs and airway.
2. Notify the regional poison center for assistance in identifying the plant.
3. Take the plant to the emergency department.
4. Provide prompt transport.

Irritation of the skin and/or mucous membranes is a problem with the common houseplant called dieffenbachia, which resembles "elephant ears." When chewed, a single leaf may irritate the lining of the upper airway enough to cause difficulty in swallowing, breathing, and speaking. In rare circumstances, the airway may be completely obstructed. For this reason, dieffenbachia has been called "dumb cane." Emergency medical treatment of dieffenbachia poisoning includes maintaining an open airway, giving oxygen, and transporting the patient as promptly as possible to the hospital for respiratory support. You should continue to assess the patient for airway difficulties throughout transport. If necessary, provide positive pressure ventilation.

TABLE 19-8 Common Toxic Plants	
Scientific Name	**Common Name**
Abrus precatorius	Jequirity bean/ rosary pea
Cicuta species	Water hemlock/ wild carrot
Colchicum autumnalel	Autumn crocus
Conium maculatum	Poison hemlock
Convallaria majalis	Lily of the valley
Datura species	Jimsonweed/stinkweed
Dieffenbachia	Dumbcane
Digitalis purpurea	Foxglove
Nerium oleander	Oleander/rose laurel
Nicotiana glauca	Tree tobacco
Phoradendron	Mistletoe
Phytolacca americana	Pokeweed
Rhododendron	Rhododendron/azaleas
Ricinus communis	Castor bean
Solarium nigrum	Nightshade
Zygadenus species	Death camas

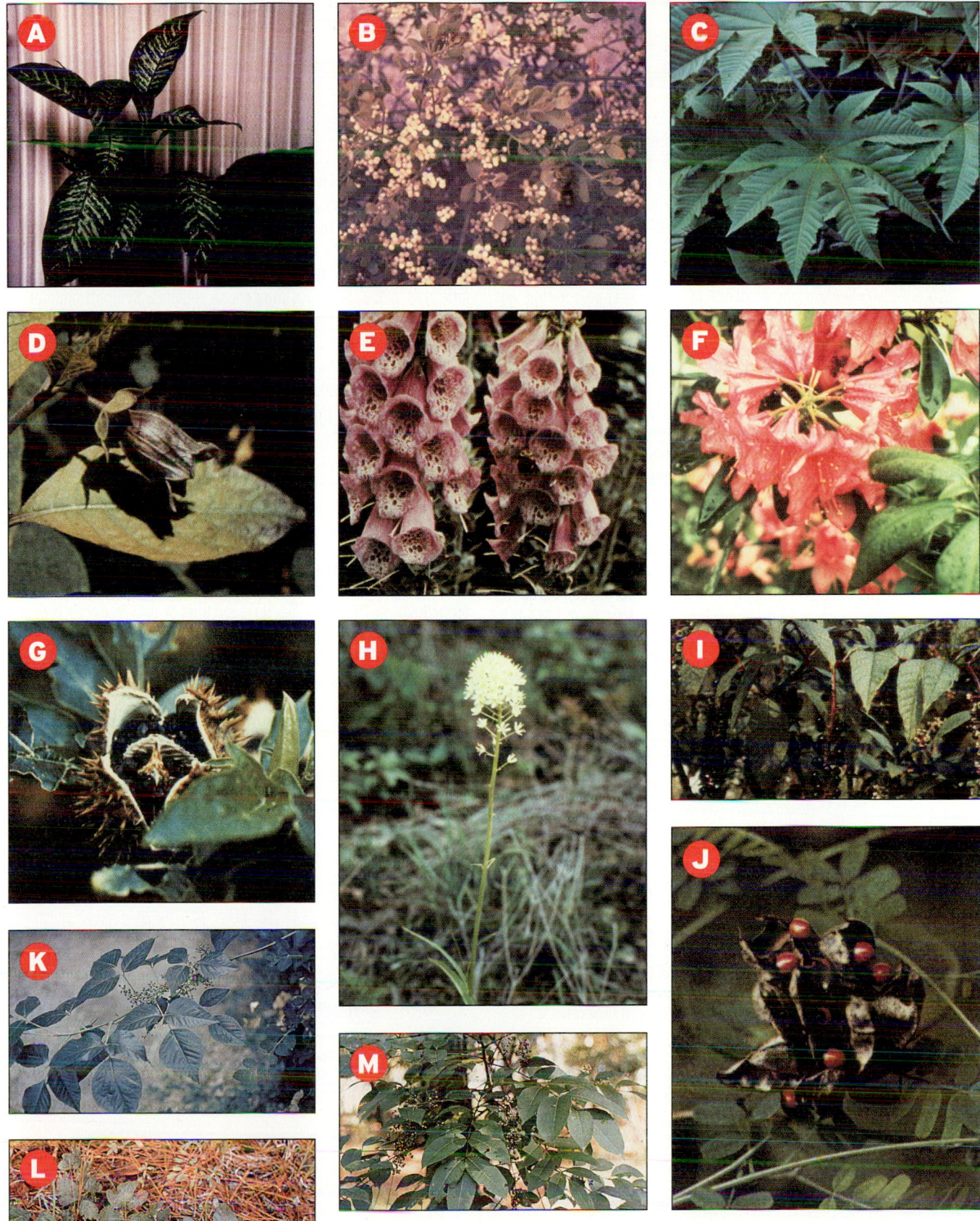

FIGURE 19-7 The toxins in these common poisonous plants are often ingested or absorbed through the skin. **A:** Dieffenbachia. **B:** Mistletoe. **C:** Castor bean. **D:** Nightshade. **E:** Foxglove. **F:** Rhododendron. **G:** Jimson weed. **H:** Death camus. **I:** Pokeweed. **J:** Rosary pea. **K:** Poison ivy. **L:** Poison oak. **M:** Poison sumac.

prep kit

ready for review

Poisons act acutely or chronically to destroy or impair body cells. If you believe a patient may have taken a poisonous substance, you should notify medical control and begin emergency treatment at once. This may include administration of an antidote, usually at the hospital, if an antidote exists. It also entails collecting any evidence of the type of poison that was used and bringing it to the hospital; diluting and physically removing the poisonous agent; providing respiratory support; and transporting the patient promptly to the hospital.

A poison can be introduced into the body in one of four ways: ingestion, inhalation, injection, or surface contact (absorption). Approximately 80% of all poisoning is by ingestion, including plants, contaminated food, and most drugs. In general, activated charcoal should be used in these patients. In the case of surface contact poisons, be sure to avoid contaminating yourself. You should then remove all contaminated substances and clothing from the patient, and flood the affected part. Move patients who have inhaled poison into the fresh air; be prepared to use supplemental oxygen via nonrebreathing mask and/or ventilatory support via BVM device. BLS may be needed for some patients, especially those who have injected poison, which is almost always a deliberate act.

People who abuse a substance can develop a tolerance to it, which may lead to addiction. Always use BSI techniques in caring for victims of drug abuse. In addition to alcohol and marijuana, commonly abused drugs fall into seven categories: opioid analgesics, sedative-hypnotics, inhalants, sympathomimetics, hallucinogens, anticholinergics, and cholinergics. Like alcohol, drugs in the first three categories depress the CNS and can cause respiratory depression. You must support the airway in such cases and be prepared for the patient to vomit. Take special care with patients who have used inhalants, since the drugs may cause seizures. Sympathomimetics, including cocaine, stimulate the CNS, causing hypertension, tachycardia, seizures, and dilated pupils. These patients may be paranoid, as may patients who have taken hallucinogens. Anticholinergic medications, often taken in suicide attempts, can cause a person to become hot, dry, blind, red-faced, and mentally unbalanced. An overdose of cyclic antidepressants can lead to cardiac arrhythmias. The symptoms of cholinergic medications, which include organophosphate insecticides, can be remembered by the mnemonic DUMBELS or SLUDGE, for excessive defecation, urination, miosis, bronchorrhea, emesis, lacrimation, and salivation.

Two main types of food poisoning cause gastrointestinal symptoms. In one type, bacteria in the food directly cause disease, such as salmonellosis; in the other, bacteria such as *Staphylococcus* produce powerful toxins, often in leftover food. The most severe form of toxin ingestion is botulism, which can first produce neurologic symptoms as late as 4 days after ingestion. Plant poisoning can affect the circulatory system, the gastrointestinal system, or the central nervous system. Some plants, such as the dieffenbachia, irritate the skin or mucous membranes, and even sometimes cause obstruction of the airway.

vital vocabulary

www.emtb.com

addiction A state characterized by an overwhelming obsession or physical need to continue the use of a drug or agent.

antidote A substance that is used to neutralize or counteract a poison.

delirium tremens (DTs) The clinical withdrawal syndrome seen in alcoholics who are deprived of ethyl alcohol; characterized by restlessness, fever, sweating, disorientation, agitation, and convulsions; in some cases, there is risk of death when untreated.

emesis Vomiting.

hallucinogen An agent that produces false perceptions in any one of the five senses.

hematemesis Vomiting blood.

hypnotic A sleep-inducing effect or agent.

ingestion Swallowing; taking a substance by mouth.

opioids Any drug or agent with actions similar to morphine.

poison A substance whose chemical action could damage structures or impair function when introduced into the body.

sedative A substance that decreases activity and excitement.

stimulant Any agent that produces an excited state.

substance abuse The knowing misuse of any substance to produce some desired effect.

tolerance The need for increasing amounts of a drug to obtain the same effect.

toxin A poison or harmful substance produced by bacteria, animals, or plants.

vomitus Vomited material.

assessment in action

A jogger who is just finishing his morning run through the park encounters a young woman who is crying and shaking a young man lying next to her on a blanket. She keeps repeating, "Please wake up, oh, please wake up!" The jogger tells her he will call for help and runs to his car to use his cell phone to call 9-1-1.

When you arrive several minutes later, you find a 24-year-old man who is unresponsive to any stimuli. He has slow, shallow respirations of 6 breaths/min. His pulse is almost too weak to feel. Because the patient is unable to answer questions, his girlfriend tries to answer them. She states that they live together in a nearby apartment and started using heroin about 4 months ago. What started as off-and-on weekend snorting has quickly progressed to regular IV use.

1. The patient has a blood pressure of 88/64 mm Hg, a pulse of 66 beats/min, and respirations of 8 breaths/min? Your next step should be to:
   A. carefully observe the patient.
   B. contact medical control for orders.
   C. quickly perform five abdominal thrusts.
   D. assist ventilations and give high-flow oxygen.

2. Because of the patient's history of IV drug abuse, you would suspect that he is at high risk for all of the following **EXCEPT**:
   A. HIV.
   B. AIDS.
   C. cancer.
   D. hepatitis.

3. The young woman pulls a small plastic bag from her purse and asks you to identify what is inside. The appropriate course of action would be to:
   A. focus on patient care.
   B. examine the contents of the bag.
   C. counsel her about substance abuse.
   D. identify the substance before continuing to treat the patient.

4. As you move the patient onto the stretcher and strap him in, he goes into respiratory arrest. What should you do?
   A. Begin immediate cardiopulmonary resuscitation.
   B. Apply a cervical collar and continue to strap him in.
   C. Open the patient's airway and give two rescue breaths.
   D. Provide prompt transport, and start writing your report.

5. The patient's respirations are now 4 to 5 breaths/min. At this point, the **LEAST** appropriate intervention would be to:
   A. prepare the suction unit.
   B. give oxygen via nasal cannula at 2 L/min.
   C. periodically reassess the patient's vital signs.
   D. monitor the patient's level of consciousness.

points to ponder

Objectives 1-1.8, 4-6.3, 4-6.5, 4-6.7, 4-6.9

You are called to provide medical support to a police SWAT team when they bust a local drug house. The entry goes well, and no one is injured. You are called into the house for a patient who reportedly had a seizure just a few moments ago. The patient appears to be unconscious. As you approach, you notice that the patient is heavily tattooed and has significant tracks on his arms from IV drug use. From the description provided by witnesses and the patient's response to painful stimulus, you question whether the patient actually had a seizure.

- How would you treat this patient? Would you attempt to prove that the patient is faking the seizure?

online outlook

The National Clearinghouse for Alcohol and Drug Information is a comprehensive source of information on drug abuse and its health consequences. Learn more from this web site by completing Exercise 19 at www.emtb.com.

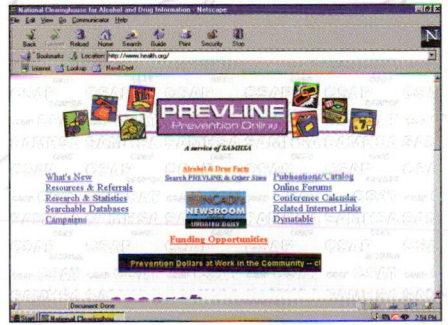

Environmental Emergencies

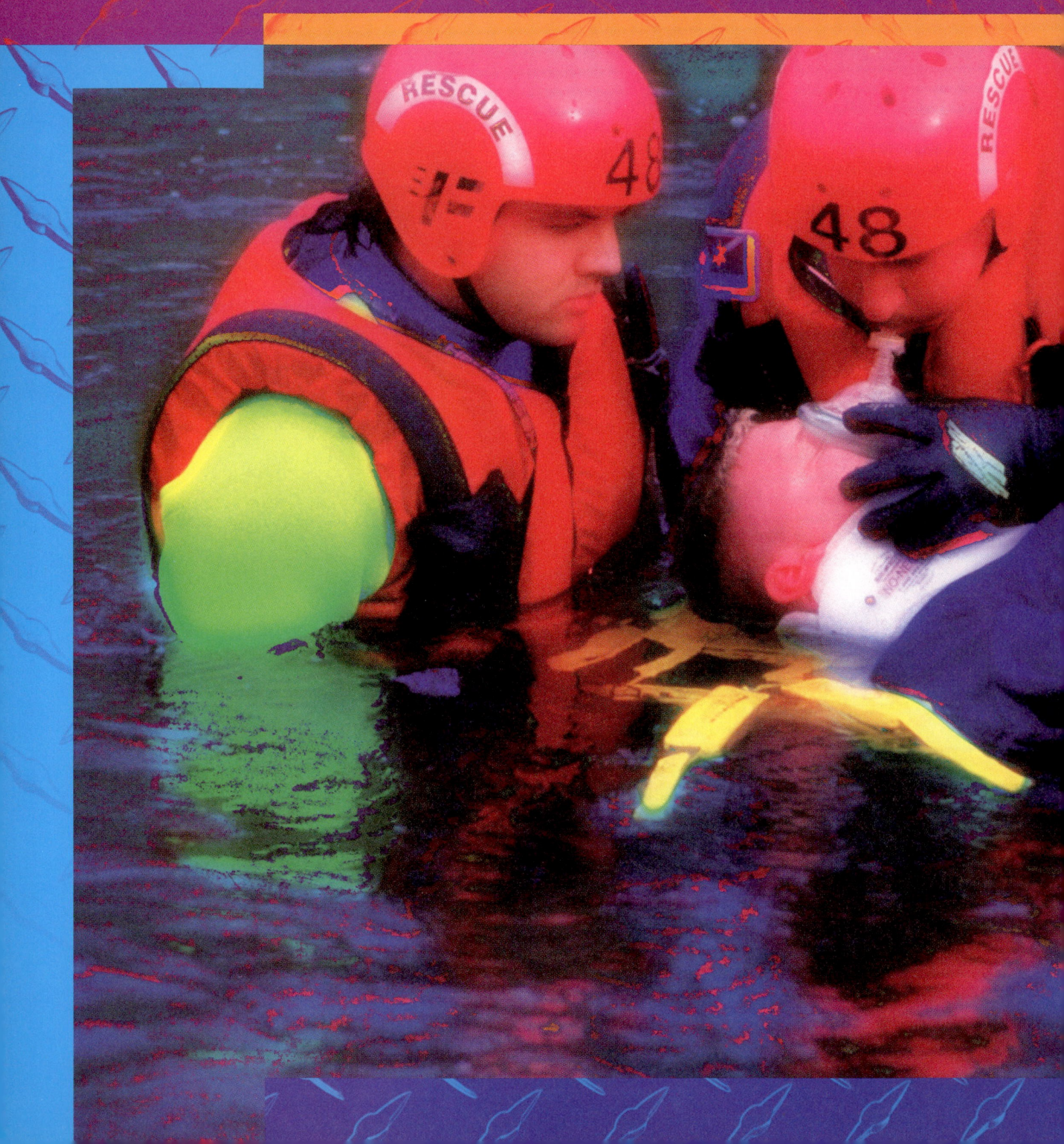

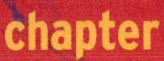

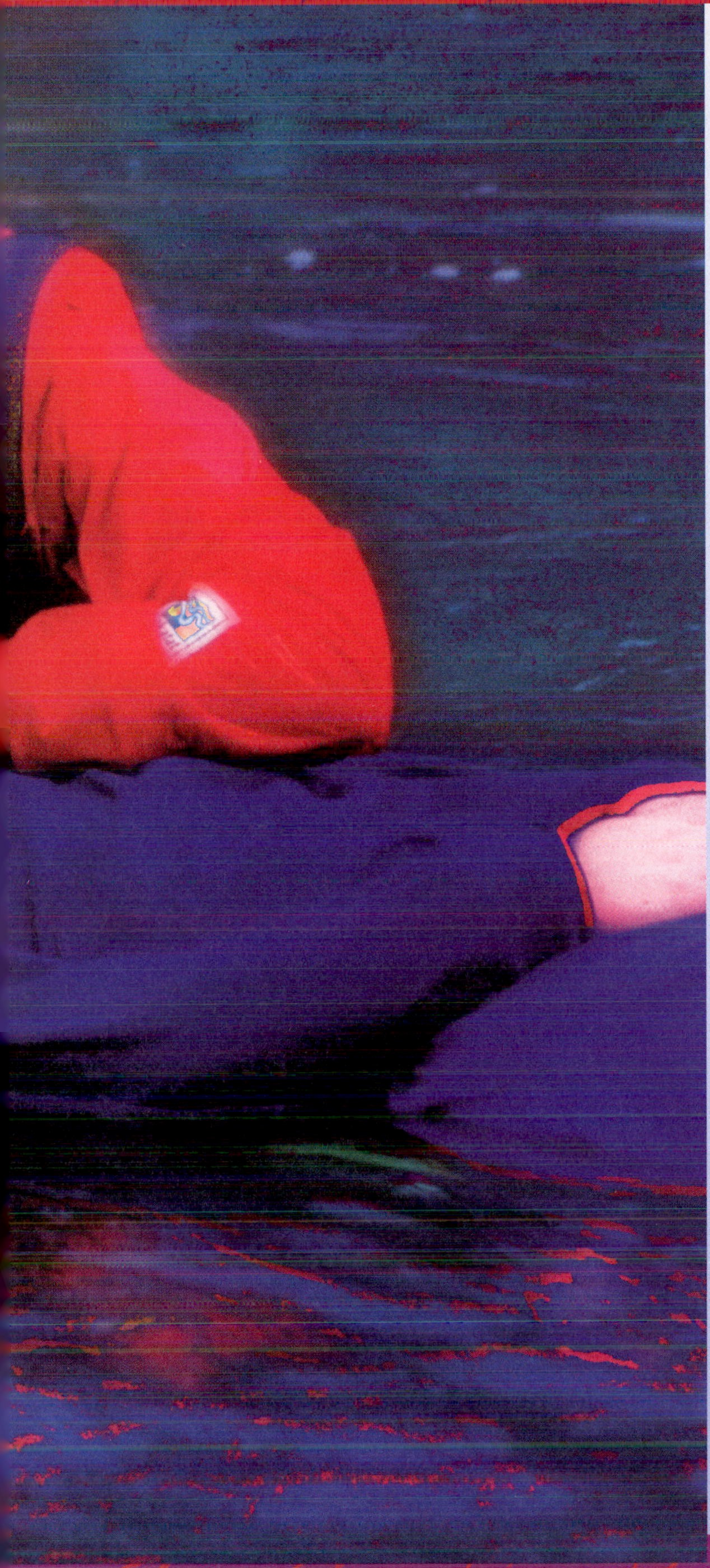

objectives

Cognitive

1. Describe the various ways that the body loses heat.
2. List the signs and symptoms of exposure to cold.
3. Explain the steps in providing emergency medical care to a patient exposed to cold.
4. List the signs and symptoms of exposure to heat.
5. Explain the steps in providing emergency care to a patient exposed to heat.
6. Recognize the signs and symptoms of water-related emergencies.
7. Describe the complications of near drowning.
8. Discuss the emergency medical care of bites and stings.*

Affective

None

Psychomotor

9. Demonstrate the assessment and emergency medical care of a patient with exposure to cold.
10. Demonstrate the assessment and emergency medical care of a patient with exposure to heat.
11. Demonstrate the assessment and emergency medical care of a near-drowning patient.
12. Demonstrate completing a prehospital care report for patients with environmental emergencies.

* Note that emergency medical care of bites and stings was covered in chapter 18.

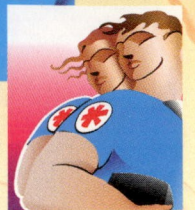

you are the emt

Rescue 6 please respond to Highway 7 and Arrow Lake for a child through the ice. Air temperature is 15°F.

You may be called frequently to care for patients experiencing heat- or cold-related problems, depending on your location. In all cold weather emergencies, you must be prepared to treat cardiac arrest as a result of hypothermia. This chapter will prepare you to care for these often-challenging situations. It will also help you to answer the following questions:

1. How do acute and chronic hypothermia events differ?
2. How does active rewarming differ from passive rewarming?

Environmental Emergencies

Heat and cold can both overwhelm the body's mechanisms for regulating temperature, including sweating and radiation of body heat into the atmosphere. A variety of medical emergencies can result from exposure to heat or cold, particularly in children, the elderly, people with chronic illnesses, and young adults who overexert themselves. There is also a range of medical emergencies that arise from water recreation, and these can sometimes be complicated by the cold. These emergencies include localized injuries and systemic illnesses. As an EMT-B, you can save lives by recognizing and responding properly to these emergencies, most of which require prompt treatment in the hospital.

This chapter describes how the body regulates core temperature and the ways in which body heat is lost to the environment. It then discusses the various forms of heat-, cold-, and water-related emergencies, including how to diagnose and treat hypothermia, hyperthermia, and diving injuries.

Cold Exposure

Normal body temperature must be maintained within a very narrow range for the body's chemistry to work efficiently. If the body, or any part of it, is exposed to cold environments, these mechanisms may be overwhelmed. Cold exposure may cause injury to individual parts of the body, such as the feet, hands, ears, or nose, or to the body as a whole. When the entire body temperature falls, the condition is called <u>hypothermia</u>.

Because heat always travels from a warmer place to a cooler place, the body will tend to lose heat to the environment. The body can lose heat in the following five ways:

- <u>Conduction</u> is the direct transfer of heat from a part of the body to a colder object, as when a warm hand touches cold metal or ice or is immersed in water with a temperature of less than 98°F (37°C). Heat passes directly from the body to the colder object.

- <u>Convection</u> occurs when heat is transferred to circulating air, as when cool air moves across the body surface. A person standing outside in windy winter weather, wearing lightweight clothing, is losing heat to the environment mostly by convection.

- <u>Evaporation</u> is the conversion of any liquid to a gas, a process that requires energy, or heat. Evaporation is the natural mechanism by which sweating cools the body. This is why swimmers coming out of the water feel a sensation of cold as the water evaporates from their skin. Individuals who exercise vigorously in a cool environment may sweat and feel warm at first, but later, as their sweat evaporates, they can become exceedingly cool.

- <u>Radiation</u> is the loss of body heat directly into still air in a colder environment. Because heat always travels from a warm object to a cooler one, a person standing in a cold room will lose heat by radiation.

- **Respiration.** Body heat is lost during normal breathing, as warm air in the lungs is exhaled into the atmosphere and cooler air is inhaled.

The rate and amount of heat loss by the body can be modified in three ways:

1. **Increase heat production.** One way for the body to increase its heat production is to increase the rate of metabolism of its cells, as occurs in shivering.

2. **Move to an area where heat loss is decreased.** The most obvious way to decrease heat loss from radiation and convection is to move out of a cold environment and seek shelter from wind. Just covering the head will minimize radiation heat loss by up to 70%.

3. **Wear insulated clothing, which helps to decrease heat loss in several ways.** Insulators, such as specific materials or dry, still air, do not conduct heat. Thus, layers of clothing that trap air provide good insulation, as do wool, down, and synthetic fabrics that have small pockets of trapped air. Protective clothing also traps perspiration and prevents evaporation. Sweating without evaporation will not result in cooling.

Hypothermia

Hypothermia literally means "low temperature." It is diagnosed when the **core temperature** of the body— the temperature of the heart, lungs, and vital organs —falls below 95°F (35°C). The body can usually tolerate a drop in core temperature of a few degrees. However, below this critical point, the body loses the ability to regulate its temperature and to generate body heat. Progressive loss of body heat then begins.

To protect itself against heat loss, the body normally constricts blood vessels in the skin; this results in the characteristic appearance of blue lips and/or fingertips. As a secondary precaution against heat loss, the body tends to create additional heat by shivering, which is the active moving of many muscles to generate heat. As cold exposure worsens and these mechanisms are over-whelmed, many body functions begin to slow down. Eventually, the functioning of key organs such as the heart begins to slow. Untreated, this can lead to death.

Hypothermia can develop either quickly, as when someone is immersed in cold water, or more gradually, as when a lost person is exposed to the cold environment for several hours or more. The temperature does not have to be below freezing for hypothermia to occur. In winter, homeless people and those whose homes lack heating may develop hypothermia at higher temperatures. Even in summer, swimmers who remain in the water for a long time are at risk of hypothermia. Like all heat and cold injuries, hypothermia is more common among elderly and ill individuals, who are less able to adjust to temperature extremes. Hypothermia is also common among the very young, who are unable to put on clothes to protect themselves against the cold. Infants and children are small, with a relatively large surface area, and have less body fat than do adults. Also, because of their small muscle mass, children may not be able to shiver as effectively as adults, and infants do not shiver at all.

Patients with injuries or illness, such as burns, shock, head injury, stroke, generalized infection, injuries to the spinal cord, diabetes, and hypoglycemia, are more prone to hypothermia, as are patients who have taken certain drugs or poisons.

Signs and symptoms. Signs and symptoms of hypothermia generally become progressively more severe as the core temperature falls. Hypothermia generally progresses through four general stages, as shown in Table 20-1. Although there is no clear distinction among the stages, the different signs and symptoms of each will help you estimate the severity of the problem. When you assess a patient in the field, you should be able to distinguish between mild and severe hypothermia.

To assess the patient's general temperature, place the back of your hand between the patient's clothing and

TABLE 20-1	Characteristics of Systemic Hypothermia			
Core Temperature	**93° to 95°F** (34° to 35°C)	**89° to 92°F** (32° to 33°C)	**80° to 88°F** (27° to 31°C)	**<80°F** (<27°C)
Signs and Symptoms	Shivering, foot stamping	Loss of coordination, muscle stiffness	Coma	Apparent death
Cardiorespiratory Response	Constricted blood vessels, rapid breathing	Slowing respirations, slow pulse	Weak pulse, arrhythmias, very slow respirations	Cardiac arrest
Level of Consciousness	Withdrawn	Confused, lethargic, sleepy	Unresponsive	Unresponsive

abdomen (Figure 20-1). If the abdomen feels cool, the patient is likely experiencing a generalized cold emergency. If you work in a cold environment, you may carry a hypothermia thermometer, which registers lower body temperatures (Figure 20-2). Note that regular thermometers will not register the temperature of a patient who has significant hypothermia. Mild hypothermia occurs when the core temperature is between 90° and 95°F (32° and 35°C). The patient is usually alert and shivering in an attempt to generate more heat through muscular activity. The patient may jump up and down and stamp his or her feet. Pulse rate and respirations are usually rapid. The skin in light-skinned individuals can be red, but may eventually appear pale, then cyanotic. As was noted previously, individuals in a cold environment may have blue lips or fingertips because of the body's constriction of blood vessels at the skin to retain heat.

More severe hypothermia occurs when the core temperature is less than 90°F (32°C). Shivering stops, and muscular activity decreases. At first, small, fine muscle activity such as coordinated finger motion ceases. Eventually, as the temperature falls further, all muscle activity stops.

As the core temperature drops toward 85°F (29°C), the patient becomes lethargic, usually losing interest in continuing to fight the cold. The level of consciousness decreases, and the patient may try to remove his or her own clothes. Poor coordination and memory loss follow, along with reduced or complete loss of sensation to touch, mood changes, and impaired judgment. The patient becomes less communicative, experiences joint or muscle stiffness, and has trouble speaking. The muscles eventually become rigid, and the patient begins to appear stiff or rigid.

If the temperature continues to fall to 80°F (27°C), vital signs slow; the pulse becomes weaker, and respirations slow to shallow or become absent. Cardiac arrhythmias may occur as the blood pressure decreases or disappears.

At a core temperature less than 80°F (27°C), all cardiorespiratory activity may cease, pupillary reaction is slow, and the patient may appear dead.

Never assume that a cold, pulseless patient is dead. Patients may survive even severe hypothermia, if proper emergency measures are carried out.

Emergency medical care. Even mild degrees of hypothermia can have serious consequences and complications. These include cardiac arrhythmia and blood-clotting abnormalities. Therefore, all patients with hypothermia require immediate transport for evaluation and treatment. Management of hypothermia in the field, regardless of the severity of the exposure, consists of

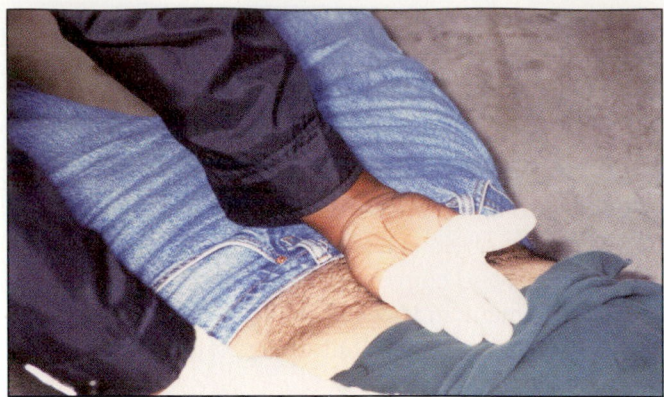

FIGURE 20-1 To assess a patient's temperature, pull back your glove and place the back of your hand on the patient's skin.

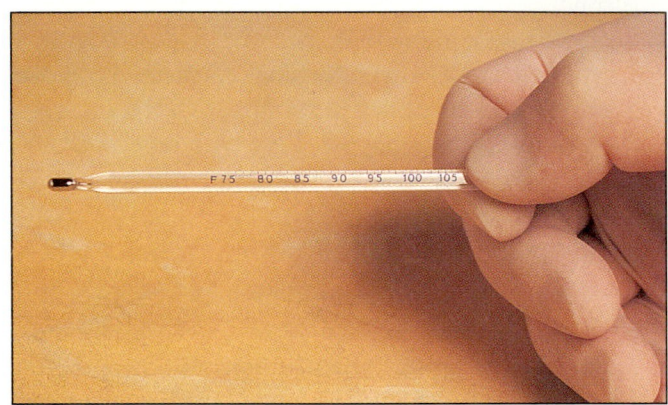

FIGURE 20-2 A special hypothermia thermometer registers temperatures well below that of a regular thermometer. It must be inserted in the rectum for an accurate reading.

stabilizing the vital functions and preventing further heat loss.

In most cases, you should move the patient from the cold environment to prevent further heat loss. To prevent further damage to the feet, do not allow the patient to walk. Remove any wet clothing, and cover the patient with a dry blanket. Always make sure to handle the patient gently so that you will not cause any pain or further injury to the skin. Do not massage the extremities. Do not allow the patient to eat, to use any stimulants, such as coffee, tea, or cola, or to smoke or chew tobacco.

You can give the patient warm, humidified oxygen if you have not already done so as part of the initial assessment. Next, assess the patient's pulse for 30 to 45 seconds, especially before considering CPR (Figure 20-3). Begin passive rewarming, which includes wrapping the patient in blankets and turning up the heat in the patient compartment of the ambulance.

If the patient is alert and responds appropriately, the hypothermia is mild, and you can begin active rewarming, which includes wrapping the patient in blankets

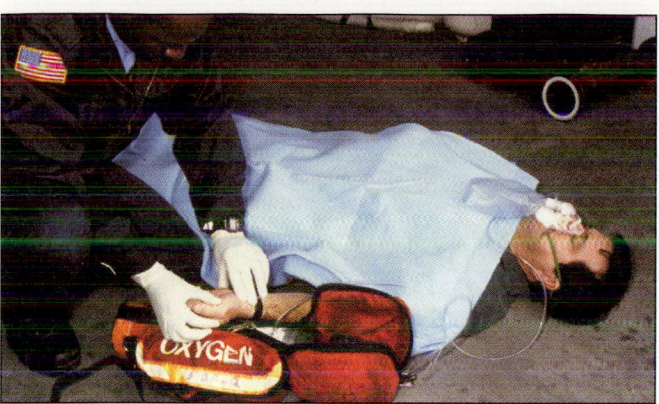

FIGURE 20-3 Cover the patient with a dry blanket, give oxygen, and assess the pulse before considering CPR.

and applying heat packs or hot water bottles to the groin, axillary, and cervical regions. Turn the heat up high in the patient compartment of the ambulance.

You must try to minimize further loss of body heat, especially when you cannot get to a hospital quickly. However, when the patient has moderate or severe hypothermia, you should never try to rewarm the patient actively (placing heat on or into the body). Rewarming too quickly may cause a fatal cardiac arrhythmia that requires defibrillation; for this reason, rewarming should be done in the hospital. Again, your goal is to prevent further heat loss. Remove the patient immediately from the cold environment. Place the patient in the ambulance, and warm it to a temperature of about 70°F (21.1°C). If you cannot get the patient out of the cold immediately, move him or her out of the wind and away from contact with any object that will conduct heat from the body. Place a protective cover on the patient, and remember that most heat is lost around the head and neck.

If the patient is alert and shivering, you may assume that the hypothermia is relatively mild. If possible, you can give warm fluids by mouth in this case, assuming that the patient can swallow without a problem. Remove all wet clothing, and cover the patient with a blanket. Notify the hospital of the patient's condition so that staff can prepare to start rewarming as soon as you arrive. When the patient is not shivering and is lethargic, moderate or severe hypothermia is probably present. A special low-temperature thermometer is required to take this patient's temperature, generally done through the rectum. A patient with a more severe form of hypothermia will have a core temperature of less than 90°F (32°C).

If you cannot feel a radial pulse, gently palpate for a carotid pulse and wait for 30 to 45 seconds before you decide that there is none.

Physicians disagree about the wisdom of performing

BLS (ie, CPR) on a patient with hypothermia who appears to be pulseless. Such a patient actually may be in a kind of "metabolic ice box," having achieved a metabolic balance that BLS may upset. Even a pulse rate of one or two beats per minute indicates cardiac activity, and cardiac activity may spontaneously recover once the core is warmed. However, there is evidence that when correctly done, BLS will increase blood flow to the critical parts of the body. For this reason, some authorities recommend starting BLS on a patient with hypothermia and no pulse. The American Heart Association recommends that CPR be started if the patient has no detectable pulse or breathing. Again, for a patient with hypothermia, this may require a prolonged pulse check. You can perform ventilation with warm, humidified oxygen. Remove wet clothing, and protect the patient from the cold and wind with blankets in a warmer environment.

If you are in an area where hypothermia is a common problem, you should have prearranged protocols for dealing with this situation. In all cases, consult medical control before proceeding with BLS.

Management of Cold Exposure in a Sick or Injured Person

All patients who are severely injured are at risk for hypothermia. Keep this in mind when you are evaluating a patient with multiple injuries.

A sick or injured person who has been trapped in a cold environment may develop hypothermia or may already have problems related to cold exposure. Such a person is more susceptible than a healthy person to cold injury. Take the following steps promptly to prevent further cold injury:

1. **Remove wet clothing** and keep the patient dry.
2. **Prevent conduction heat loss.** Move the patient away from any wet or cold surfaces, such as a car frame.
3. **Insulate all exposed body parts,** especially the head, by wrapping them in a blanket or any other available dry, bulky material.
4. **Prevent convection heat** loss by erecting a wind barrier around the patient.
5. **Remove the patient** from the cold environment as promptly as possible.

Regardless of the nature or severity of the cold injury, remember that even an unresponsive patient may be able to hear you. Some patients have told of hearing themselves pronounced dead by someone who had forgotten the old saying: "No one is dead unless he is warm and dead." If you carry an AED, you should consider defibrillation if the patient is in ventricular fibrillation (a shockable heart rhythm). Although this heart rhythm is unlikely in patients with hypothermia, it can develop in patients who are rewarmed too rapidly.

Local Cold Injuries

Most injuries from cold are confined to exposed parts of the body. The extremities, particularly the feet, and the exposed ears, nose, and face, are especially vulnerable to cold injury. When exposed parts of the body become very cold but not frozen, the condition is called frostnip, chilblains, or immersion foot (trench foot). When the parts become frozen, the injury is called <u>frostbite</u> (Figure 20-4).

You should try to find out the duration of the exposure, the temperature to which the body part was exposed, and the wind velocity during exposure. These are important factors in determining the severity of a local cold injury. You should also investigate a number of underlying factors:

- Exposure to wet conditions
- Inadequate insulation from cold or wind
- Restricted circulation from tight clothing or shoes or circulatory disease
- Fatigue
- Poor nutrition
- Alcohol or drug abuse
- Hypothermia
- Diabetes
- Cardiovascular disease
- Older age

In hypothermia, blood is shunted away from the extremities in an attempt to maintain the core temperature. This shunting of blood increases the risk of local cold injury to the extremities, ears, nose, and face. Thus, the patient with hypothermia should also be assessed for frostbite or other local cold injury. The reverse is also true. You must remember that both local and systemic cold exposure problems can occur in the same patient.

Frostnip and immersion foot. After prolonged exposure to the cold, the skin may be freezing while the deeper tissues are unaffected. This condition, which often affects the ears, nose, and fingers, is called frostnip. Because frostnip is usually not painful, the patient often is unaware that a cold injury has occurred. Immersion foot, also called trench foot, occurs after prolonged exposure to cold water. It is particularly common in hikers or hunters who stand for a long time

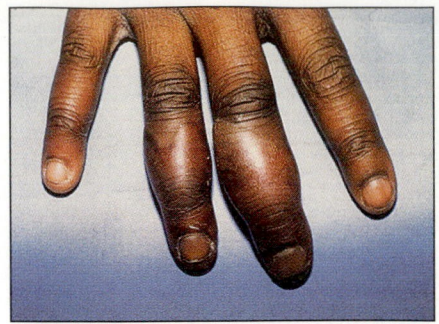
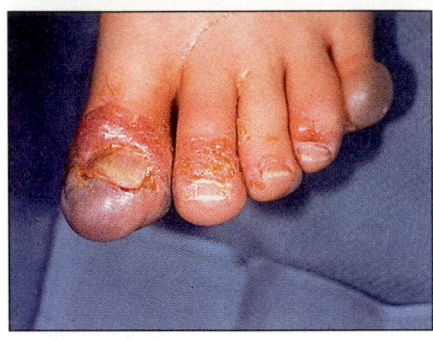
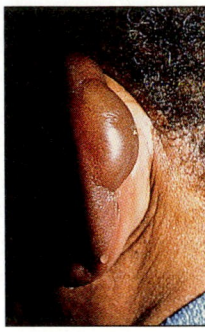

FIGURE 20-4 The extremities and the ears, nose, and face are particularly susceptible to frostbite.

in a river or lake. With both frostnip and immersion foot, the skin is pale (blanched) and cold to the touch; normal color does not return after palpation of the skin. In some cases, the skin of the foot will be wrinkled, but it can also remain soft. The patient complains of loss of feeling and sensation in the injured area.

As in all other hypothermia cases, the emergency treatment of these less severe local cold injuries consists of removing the patient from the cold, wet environment, but also rewarming the affected part. With frostnip, contact with a warm object may be all that is needed; you can use your hands, your breath, or the patient's own body. During rewarming, the affected part will often tingle and become red in light-skinned individuals. With immersion foot, remove wet shoes, boots, and socks, and rewarm the foot gradually, protecting it from further cold exposure.

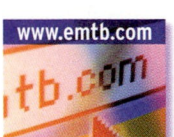

Frostbite. Frostbite is the most serious local cold injury, because the tissues are actually frozen. Freezing permanently damages cells, although the exact mechanism by which damage occurs is not known. The presence of ice crystals within the cells may cause physical damage. The change in the water content in the cells may also cause changes in the concentration of critical electrolytes, producing permanent changes in the chemistry of the cell. When the ice thaws, further chemical changes occur in the cell,

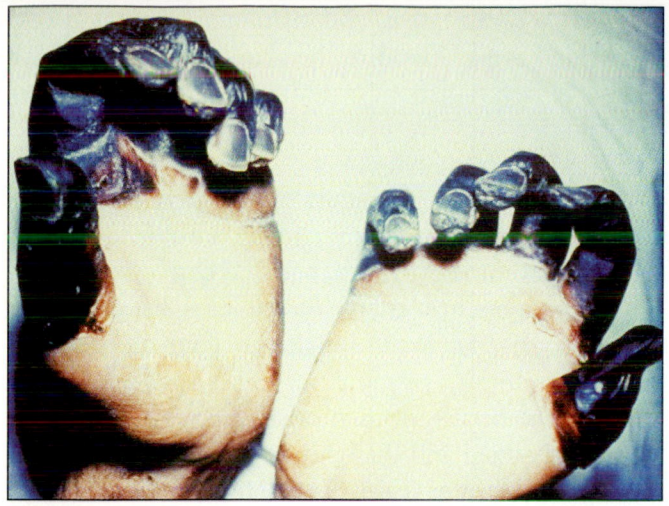

FIGURE 20-5 Gangrene, or permanent cell death, can occur when tissue is frozen and certain chemical changes occur in the cells.

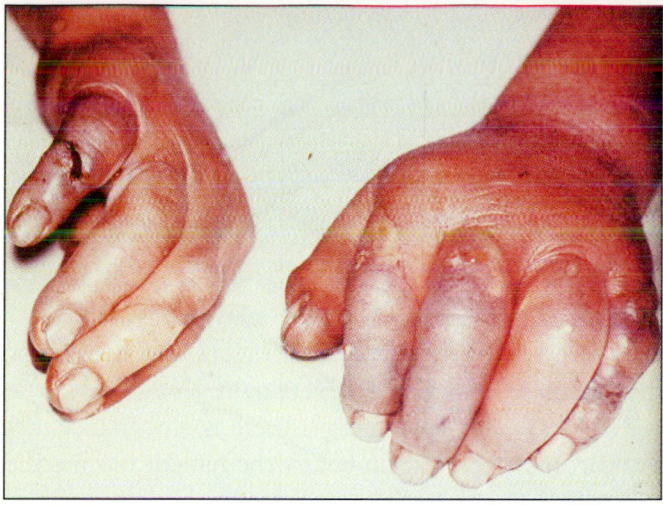

FIGURE 20-6 Frostbitten parts are often identified as hard and firm to touch.

causing permanent damage or cell death, called *gangrene* (Figure 20-5). If gangrene occurs, the dead tissue must be surgically removed, sometimes by amputation. Following less severe damage, the exposed part will become inflamed, tender to touch, and unable to tolerate exposure to cold.

Frostbite can be identified by the hard, frozen feel of the affected tissues. Most frostbitten parts are hard and waxy (Figure 20-6). The injured part feels firm to frozen as you gently touch it. Blisters and swelling may be present. In light-skinned individuals with a deep injury that has thawed or partially thawed, the skin may appear red with purple and white, or it may be mottled and cyanotic.

As with a burn, the depth of skin damage will vary. With superficial frostbite, only the skin is frozen; with deep frostbite, the deeper tissues are frozen as well. You may not be able to tell superficial from deep frostbite in the field. Even an experienced surgeon in a hospital setting may not be able to tell until several days have gone by.

Emergency medical care of local cold injury. The emergency treatment of local cold injuries in the field should include the following steps:

1. **Remove the patient** from further exposure to the cold.
2. **Handle the injured part gently,** and protect it from further injury.
3. **Administer oxygen,** if this was not already done as part of the initial assessment.
4. **Remove any wet or restricting clothing** over the injured part.

With an early or superficial injury, such as frostnip or immersion foot, splint the extremity and cover it loosely with a dry, sterile dressing. Never rub injured tissues with anything; rubbing just causes further damage. Do not reexpose the injury to cold.

With a late or deep cold injury, such as frostbite, be sure to remove any jewelry from the injured part and cover the injury loosely with a dry, sterile dressing. Do not break blisters or rub or massage the area. Do not apply heat or rewarm the part. Unlike frostnip and trenchfoot, rewarming of the frostbitten extremity is best accomplished under controlled circumstances in the emergency department. You can cause a great deal of further injury to fragile tissues by attempting to rewarm a frostbitten part. Never apply something warm or hot, such as the exhaust from the ambulance engine or, even worse, an open flame. Do not allow the patient to stand or walk on a frostbitten foot.

Evaluate the patient's general condition for the signs or symptoms of systemic hypothermia. Support the vital functions as necessary, and transport the patient promptly to the hospital.

If prompt hospital care is not available and medical control instructs you to institute rewarming in the field, use a warm-water bath. Immerse the frostbitten part in water with a temperature between 100° and 112°F (38° and 44.5°C). Check the water temperature with a thermometer before immersing the limb, and recheck it frequently during the rewarming process. The water temperature should never exceed 112°F (44.5°C). Stir the water continuously. Keep the frostbitten part in the water until it feels warm and sensation has returned to

As with so many hazards, you cannot help others if you do not practice self-protection.

the skin. Dress the area with dry, sterile dressings, placing them also between injured fingers or toes. Expect the patient to complain of severe pain.

Never attempt rewarming if there is any chance that the part may freeze again before the patient reaches the hospital. Some of the most severe consequences of frostbite, including gangrene and amputation, have occurred when parts were thawed and then refrozen.

Cover the frostbitten part with soft, padded, sterile cotton dressings. If blisters have formed, do not break them. Remember, you cannot accurately predict the outcome of a case of frostbite early in its course. Even body parts that appear gangrenous may recover following proper emergency and hospital treatment.

Cold Exposure and You

As an EMT-B, you are also at risk for hypothermia if you work in a cold environment. If cold weather search-and-rescue operations are a possibility in your assigned areas, you should receive survival training and precautionary tips. You should be thoroughly familiar with local conditions. Be aware of existing and potential weather conditions, and stay on top of changes that are forecast for the area. Make sure proper clothing is available, and wear it whenever appropriate. Your vehicle, too, must be properly equipped and maintained for a cold environment. As with so many hazards, you cannot help others if you do not practice self-protection. Never allow yourself to become a casualty!

Heat Exposure

Normal body temperature is 98.6°F (37°C). Complicated regulatory mechanisms keep this internal temperature constant, regardless of the **ambient temperature**, the temperature of the surrounding environment. In a hot environment or during vigorous physical activity, when the body itself produces excess heat, the body will try to rid itself of the excess heat. There are several ways of doing this. The two most efficient are sweating (and

evaporation of the sweat) and dilation of skin blood vessels, which brings blood to the skin surface to increase the rate of heat radiation. In addition, of course, the person who becomes overheated can remove clothing and try to find a cooler environment.

Ordinarily, the heat-regulating mechanisms of the body work very well, and individuals are able to tolerate significant temperature changes. When the body is exposed to more heat energy than it loses, hyperthermia results. **Hyperthermia** is a high core temperature, usually 101°F (38.3°C) or more.

When the body's mechanisms to decrease body heat are overwhelmed and the body is unable to tolerate the excessive heat, illness develops. High air temperature can reduce the body's ability to lose heat by radiation; high humidity reduces the ability to lose heat through evaporation. Another contributing factor is vigorous exercise, during which the body can lose more than 1 L of sweat an hour, causing loss of fluid and electrolytes. Illness from heat exposure can take the following three forms:

- Heat cramps
- Heat exhaustion
- Heatstroke

All three forms of heat illness may be present in the same patient, since untreated heat exhaustion may progress to heatstroke. Heatstroke is a life-threatening emergency.

Children; the elderly; patients with heart disease, COPD, diabetes, dehydration, and obesity; and those with limited mobility are at greatest risk for heat illnesses. The elderly, newborns, and infants exhibit poor thermoregulation. Newborns and infants often wear too much clothing. Alcohol and certain drugs, including medications that dehydrate the body or decrease the ability of the body to sweat, also make a person more susceptible to heat illnesses. When you are treating someone for a heat illness, always obtain a drug and medication history.

Heat Cramps

Heat cramps are painful muscle spasms that occur after vigorous exercise. They do not occur only when it is hot outdoors. They may be seen in factory workers and even well-conditioned athletes. The exact cause of heat cramps is not well understood. We know that sweat produced during strenuous exercise, particularly in a warm environment, causes a change in the body's electrolyte, or salt, balance. The result may be a loss of essential electrolytes from the cells. Dehydration may also play a role in the development of muscle cramps. Large amounts of water can be lost from the body as a result of excessive sweating. This loss of water may affect muscles that are being stressed and cause them to go into spasm.

Heat cramps usually occur in the leg or abdominal muscles. When the abdominal muscles are involved, the pain and muscle spasm may be so severe that the patient appears to have an acute abdominal problem. If a patient with a sudden onset of abdominal cramps has been exercising vigorously in a hot environment, you should suspect heat cramps.

Take the following steps to treat heat cramps in the field (Figure 20-7):

1. **Remove the patient** from the hot environment. Loosen any tight clothing.

2. **Rest the cramping muscles.** Have the patient sit or lie down until the cramps subside.

3. **Replace fluids by mouth.** Use water or a diluted (half-strength) balanced electrolyte solution, such as Gatorade. In most cases, plain water is the most useful. Do not give salt tablets or solutions that have a high salt concentration. The patient already has an adequate amount of electrolytes circulating; they are just not distributed properly. With adequate rest and fluid replacement, the body will adjust the distribution of electrolytes, and the cramps will disappear.

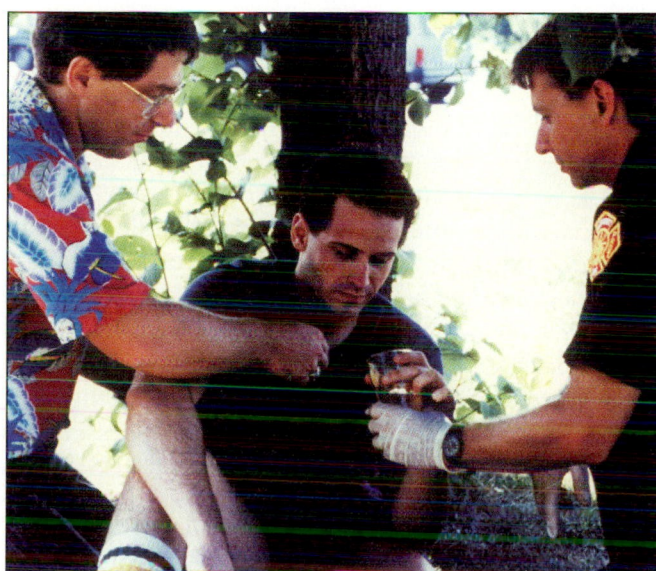

FIGURE 20-7 A patient with heat cramps should be moved to a cool environment as you begin your assessment and treatment.

If, after these measures, the cramps do not go away, transport the patient to the hospital.

Once the cramps are gone, the patient may resume activity. For example, an athlete can return to play once the heat cramps have disappeared. However, heavy sweating may cause the cramps to recur. Hydration by drinking lots of water is the best preventive and treatment strategy.

Heat Exhaustion

Heat exhaustion, also called *heat prostration* or *heat collapse,* is the most common serious illness caused by heat. It is the result of the body's losing so much water and so many electrolytes through very heavy sweating that hypovolemia (fluid depletion) occurs. For sweating to be an effective cooling mechanism, the sweat must be able to evaporate from the body. Otherwise, the body will continue to produce sweat, with further loss of body water. People standing in the hot sun and particularly those wearing several layers of clothing, such as football fans or parade watchers, may sweat profusely but experience little body cooling. High humidity will also decrease the amount of evaporation that can occur. Individuals working or exerting themselves in poorly ventilated areas are unable to release heat through convection. Thus, people who work or exercise vigorously and those who wear heavy clothing in a warm, humid, or poorly ventilated environment are particularly prone to heat exhaustion.

The signs and symptoms of heat exhaustion and those of associated hypovolemia are as follows:

- Onset while working hard or exercising in a hot, humid, or poorly ventilated environment and sweating heavily

- Onset, even at rest, in the elderly and infant age groups in hot, humid, and poorly ventilated environments or extended time in hot, humid environments

- Cold, clammy skin with ashen pallor

- Dry tongue and thirst

- Dizziness, weakness, or faintness, with accompanying nausea or headache

- Normal vital signs, although the pulse is often rapid and the diastolic blood pressure may be low

- Normal or slightly elevated body temperature on rare occasions, as high as 104°F (40°C)

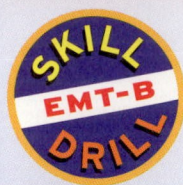

Treating for Heat Exhaustion

Figure 20-8

1

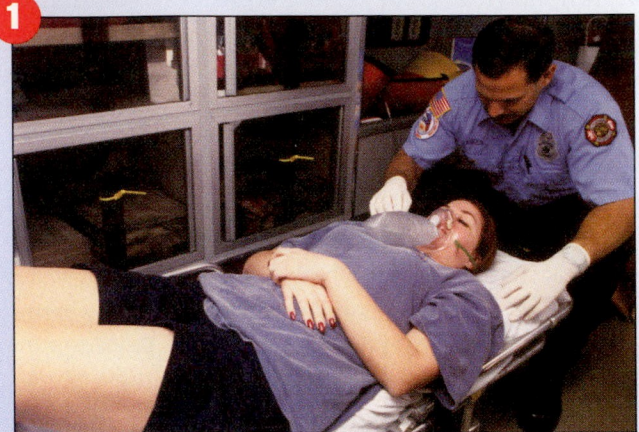

Remove a patient with heat exhaustion from the hot environment to the back of the ambulance. Place the patient in a supine position, give oxygen, and elevate the legs.

2

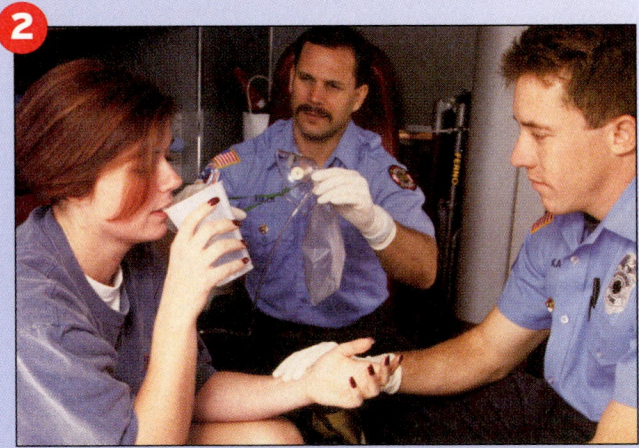

If the patient is fully alert, give him or her water to drink.

3

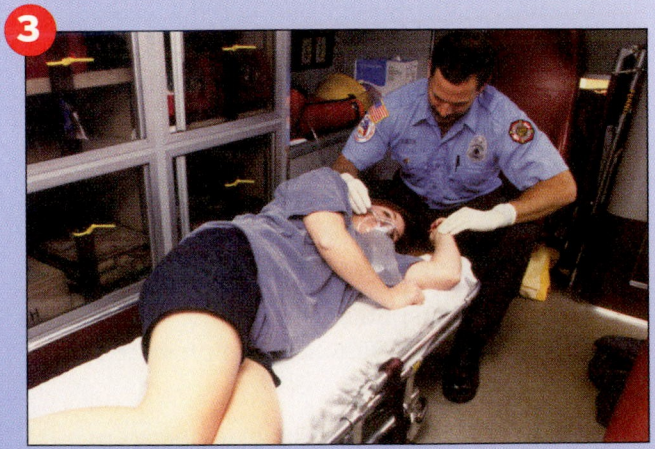

If the patient feels nauseated, transport on his or her side.

Treat the patient for mild hypovolemic shock. Remove the patient promptly from the hot environment and place him or her into the back of the air-conditioned ambulance. Give the patient oxygen if this was not already done as part of the initial assessment. Loosen any tight clothing, and remove any excessive layers of clothing particularly around the head and neck (Figure 20-8). Encourage the patient to lie down and elevate the legs. Fan the patient to cool him or her. If the patient is fully alert, you should encourage him or her to slowly drink up to a liter of water, as long as nausea does not develop. Never force fluids by mouth on a patient who is not fully alert, because the patient could aspirate the fluid into the lungs.

In most cases, these measures will reverse the symptoms, causing the patient to feel better within 30 minutes. But you should prepare to transport the patient to the hospital for more aggressive treatment, such as IV fluid therapy and close monitoring, especially in the following circumstances:

- The symptoms do not clear up promptly.
- The level of consciousness decreases.
- The temperature remains elevated.
- The person is very young, elderly, or has any underlying medical condition, such as diabetes, cardiovascular disease, or other worrisome condition.

You can transport the patient on his or her side if you think the patient may be nauseated and ready to vomit, but make certain that the patient is secured.

Heatstroke

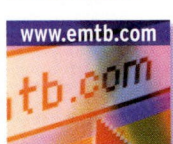

www.emtb.com

Heatstroke, the least common but most serious illness caused by heat exposure, occurs when the body is subjected to more heat than it can handle and normal mechanisms for getting rid of the excess heat are overwhelmed. The body temperature then rises rapidly to the level at which tissues are destroyed. Untreated heatstroke always results in death.

Heatstroke can develop in patients during vigorous physical activity or when they are outdoors or in a closed, poorly ventilated, humid space. It also occurs during heat waves among individuals (particularly the elderly) who live in buildings with no air conditioning or with poor ventilation. It may also develop in children who are left unattended in a locked car on a hot day.

Many patients with heatstroke have hot, dry, flushed skin because their sweating mechanism has been overwhelmed. However, early in the course of heatstroke, the skin may be moist or wet. Keep in mind that a patient can have heatstroke even if he or she is still sweating. The body temperature rises rapidly in patients with heatstroke. It may rise to 106°F (41°C) or more. As the body core temperature rises, the patient's level of consciousness falls.

Often, the first sign of heatstroke is a change in behavior. However, the patient then becomes unresponsive very quickly. The pulse is usually rapid and strong at first, but as the patient becomes increasingly unresponsive, the pulse becomes weaker and the blood pressure falls.

Recovery from heatstroke depends on the speed with which treatment is administered, so you must be able to identify this patient quickly. Emergency treatment has one object: Get the body temperature down by any means available. Take the following steps when treating a patient with heatstroke:

1. **Move the patient** out of the hot environment and into the ambulance.

2. **Set the air conditioning** to maximum cooling.

3. **Remove the patient's clothing.**

4. **Give the patient oxygen** if this was not done as part of the initial assessment.

5. **Apply cool packs** to the patient's neck, groin, and armpits (Figure 20-9).

6. **Cover the patient** with wet towels or sheets, or spray the patient with cool water and fan him or her to quickly evaporate the dampness on the skin.

7. **Aggressively and repeatedly fan** the patient with or without dampening the skin.

8. **Provide immediate transport** to the hospital.

9. **Notify the hospital** as soon as possible so that the staff can prepare to treat the patient immediately on arrival.

caring for the elderly

As we age, our bodies can lose their ability to respond to the environment. Older adults undergo changes in their ability to compensate for low or high ambient temperatures. For example, if the ambient temperature rises from 85 to 94°F (29.5° to 34.5°C), the older adult may not recognize the change or be able to compensate for it. Therefore, unless the person is accustomed to the heat, heatstroke can develop relatively quickly.

Shivering, a common effect of hypothermia, is the body's attempt to maintain heat. However, because of a decrease in muscle mass or tone, the hypothermic elderly patient may not shiver. Further, a decrease in muscle mass and body fat means that there is less insulation and protection from the cold. Because of the body's altered response to heat loss and its ability to gain heat, the health care provider might not suspect or report hypothermia. In caring for the geriatric patient in cold climates, be sure to protect the patient against unwanted heat loss. Cover all exposed areas with loose-fitting blankets. Pay particular attention to protecting the patient's head, since heat loss from the head is substantial.

Because of reduced circulation to the skin, heat loss via conduction, convection, and radiation is significantly lower. Additionally, the aging process alters the patient's ability to perspire; therefore, heat loss through evaporation is reduced. Since the elderly patient cannot disperse heat effectively, classic heatstroke can develop rapidly. Typically, the older adult will not go through an initial stage of heat exhaustion. During the summer, you should be acutely aware of the potential for heatstroke and factors that can predispose a patient to heat illness. Factors that increase the possibility of heatstroke include medications, diabetes, alcohol abuse, malnutrition, Parkinsonism, hyperthyroidism, and obesity.

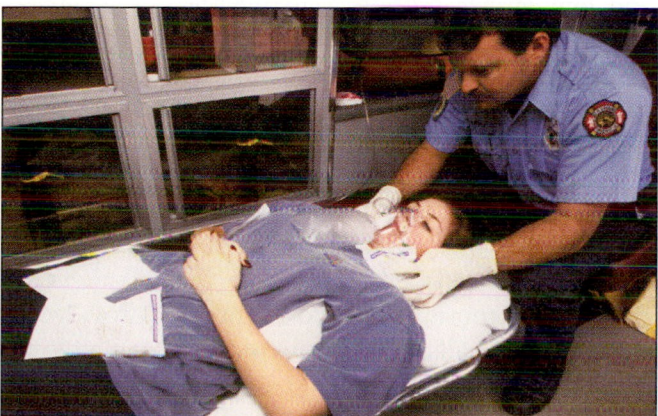

FIGURE 20-9 As part of treatment of heatstroke, give oxygen and place cool packs about the patient's neck, groin, and armpits.

Drowning and Near Drowning

Drowning is death from suffocation after submersion in water; near drowning is defined as survival, at least temporarily, after suffocation in water. Drowning is often the last in a cycle of events caused by panic in the water (Figure 20-10). It can happen to anyone who is submerged in water for even a short period of time. Struggling toward the surface or the shore, the person becomes fatigued or exhausted, which leads him or her to sink even deeper. However, drowning also occurs in mop buckets, puddles, bathtubs, and other places where the individual is not completely submerged. Small children can drown in only a few inches of water if unattended.

Inhaling very small amounts of either fresh or salt water can severely irritate the larynx, sending the muscles of the larynx and the vocal cords into spasm, called laryngospasm. The average person experiences this to a mild degree when a bit of a drink is inhaled and the patient coughs and seems to be choking for a few seconds. This is the body's attempt at self-preservation, since laryngospasm prevents more water from entering the lungs. But this can be too much of a good thing in severe cases such as water submersion, since the patient's lungs cannot be ventilated when significant laryngospasm is present. Instead, progressive hypoxia occurs until the patient becomes unconscious. At this point, the spasm relaxes, making rescue breathing possible. Of course, if the patient has not already been removed from the water, the patient may now inhale deeply, and more water may enter the lungs. In 85% to 90% of cases, significant amounts of water enter the lungs of the drowning victim.

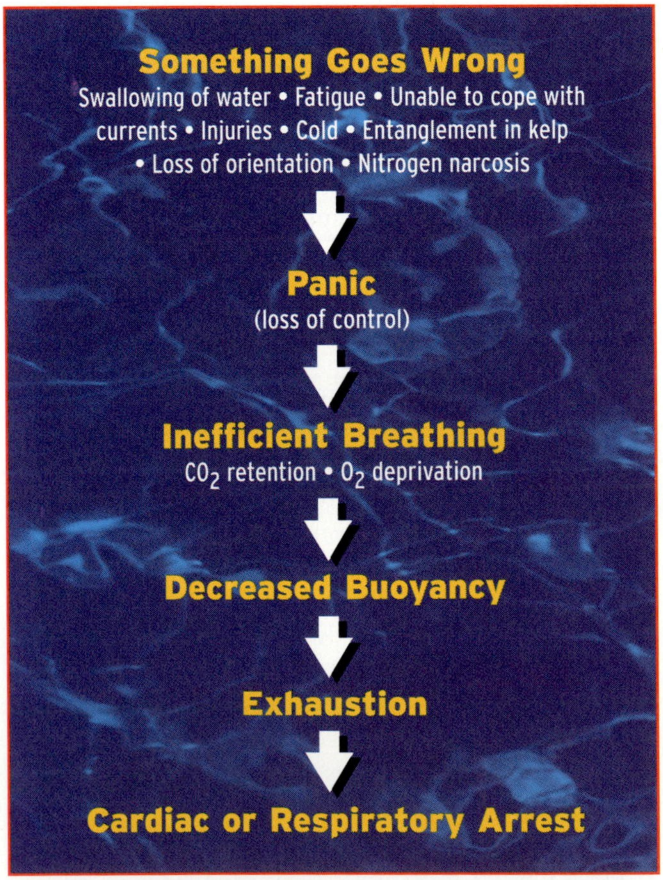

Emergency Medical Care

Treatment begins with rescue and removal from the water. When necessary, artificial ventilation should begin as soon as possible, even before the victim is removed from the water. At the same time, you must take care to stabilize and protect the patient's spine when a long fall or dive has occurred (or if this is a possibility when no information is provided). Associated cervical spine injuries are possible, especially in diving mishaps. In most cases, you will use mouth-to-mouth ventilation with the head in a neutral position, opening the airway with the jaw-thrust or chin-lift maneuver. If the patient does not have a possible spinal injury, you can turn the patient quickly to the left side to allow draining from the upper airway. Note that water will not drain from the lungs. If there is evidence of upper airway obstruction by foreign matter, remove the obstruction manually or, if available, by suction. If necessary, use abdominal thrusts, followed by assisted ventilations. Administer oxygen if this was not done as part of the initial assessment, either by mask for patients who are breathing spontaneously or via BVM device for those requiring assisted ventilation.

Check for a pulse immediately after the patient emerges from the water. It may be difficult to find a pulse because of constriction of the peripheral blood vessels and low cardiac output. Nevertheless, if the pulse is unmeasurable, start CPR if the patient is unresponsive.

Even if resuscitation in the field appears completely successful, you must always transport near-drowning patients to the hospital. Inhalation of any amount of fluid can lead to delayed complications lasting for days or weeks.

Make sure that the patient is kept warm, especially after cold water immersion. Make sure blankets and protection from the environment are provided as needed. If ventilation equipment is not available but oxygen is, you can breathe the oxygen in yourself and give mouth-to-mask ventilation until rescue equipment arrives. In this method, your expired air will have a higher percentage of oxygen.

Something Goes Wrong
Swallowing of water • Fatigue • Unable to cope with currents • Injuries • Cold • Entanglement in kelp • Loss of orientation • Nitrogen narcosis

⬇

Panic
(loss of control)

⬇

Inefficient Breathing
CO_2 retention • O_2 deprivation

⬇

Decreased Buoyancy

⬇

Exhaustion

⬇

Cardiac or Respiratory Arrest

FIGURE 20-10 Panic in the water often precedes drowning.

EMT-B safety

You must ensure the safety of rescue personnel before a water rescue can begin. If the patient is conscious and still in the water, you should perform a water rescue. An old saying sums up the basic rule of water rescue: "Reach, throw and row, and *only then* go" (Figure 20-11). First, try to reach for the patient. If that does not work, then throw the patient a rope, a life preserver, or any floatable object that is available. For example, an inflated spare tire, rim and all, will float well enough to support two people in the water. Do not attempt a swimming rescue unless you are trained and experienced in the proper techniques. Even then, you should always wear a helmet and a personal flotation device (Figure 20-12). Too many well-meaning individuals have themselves become victims while attempting a swimming rescue. In cold climates or cold water locations, rapid hypothermia is a concern as well for rescuers. Be prepared for this potential event.

If you work in a recreation area near lakes, rivers, or the ocean, you must have a prearranged plan for water rescue. This plan should include access to and cooperation with local personnel who are trained and skilled in water rescue; these personnel should help to develop the protocol for water rescue. Because the success of any water rescue depends on how rapidly the patient is removed from the water and ventilated, make sure you always have immediate access to personal flotation devices and other rescue equipment.

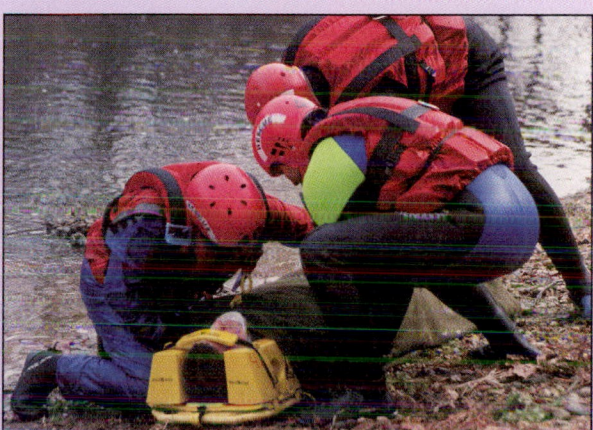

FIGURE 20-12 When performing a water rescue, you must wear proper personal protective equipment, including a personal flotation device.

Basic Rules of Water Rescue

Reach

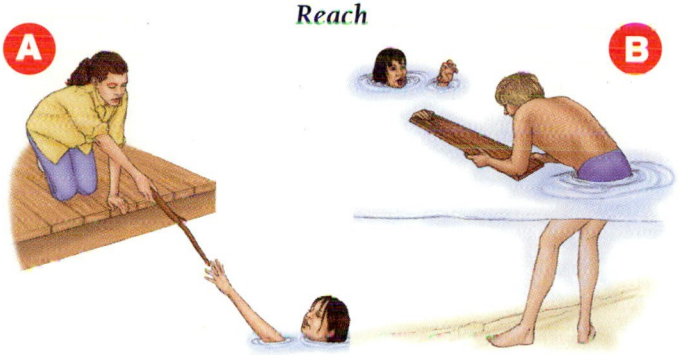

Throw and Tow

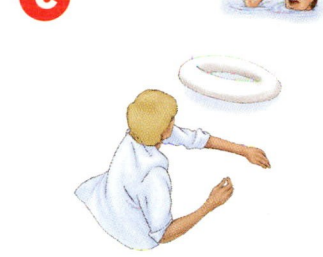

Row

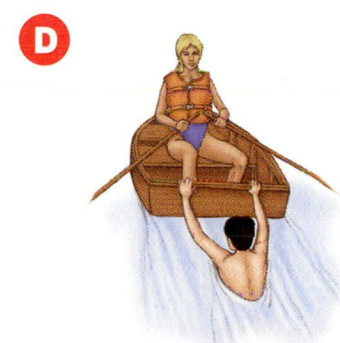

Only then Go

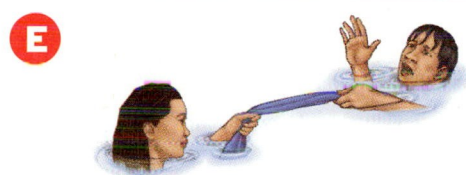

FIGURE 20-11
A: Reach the person from shore.
B: If you cannot reach the person from shore, wade closer.
C: If an object that floats is available, throw it to the person.
D: Use a boat if one is available.
E: If you must swim to the person, use a towel or board for him or her to hold onto. Do not let the person grab you.

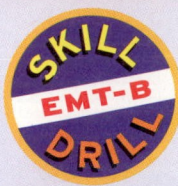

Stabilizing a Suspected Neck Injury

Figure 20-13

1

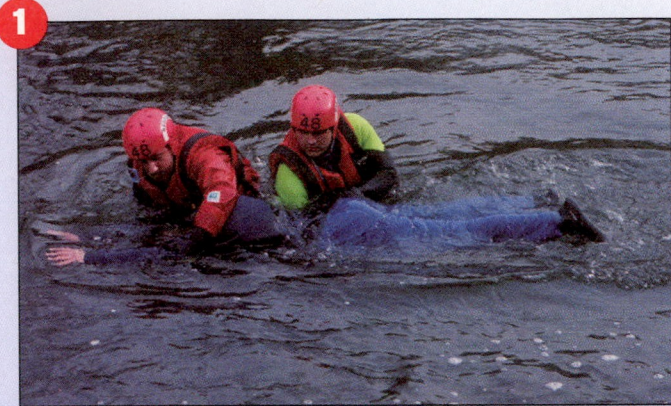

Turn the patient to a supine position by rotating the entire upper half of the body as a single unit.

2

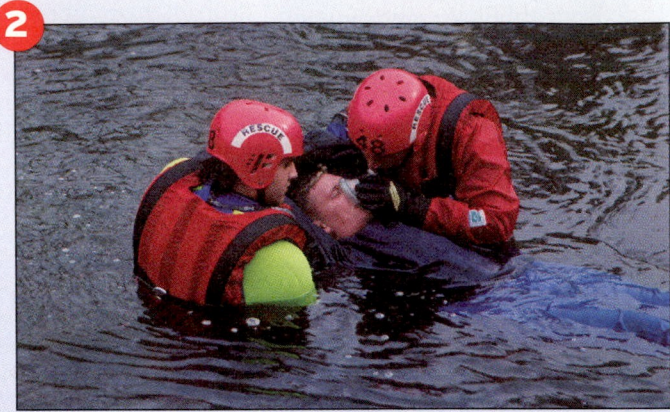

As soon as the patient is turned, begin artificial ventilation using the mouth-to-mouth method or a pocket mask.

3

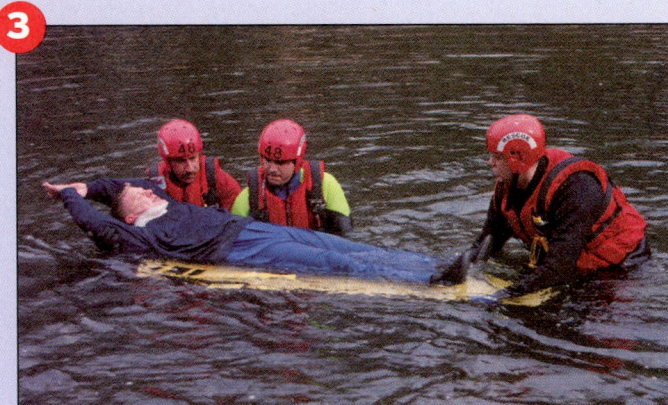

Float a buoyant spine board under the patient as you continue to provide artificial ventilation.

4

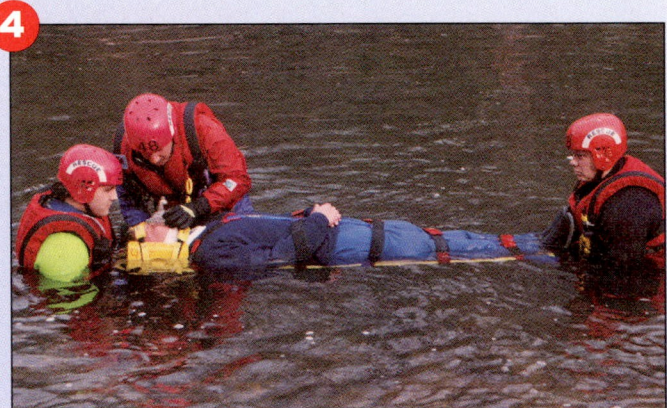

Secure the patient to the spine board.

5

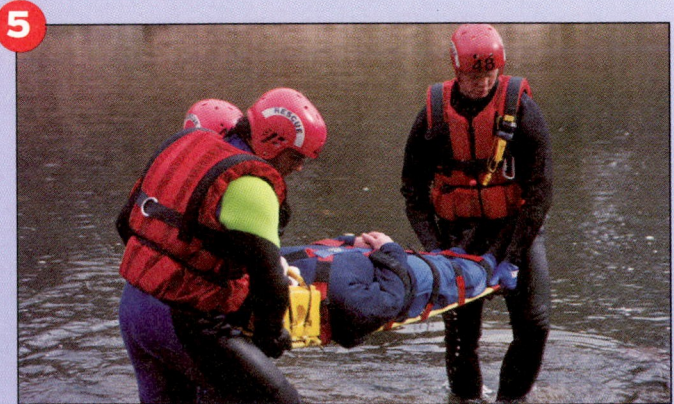

Remove the patient from the water.

6

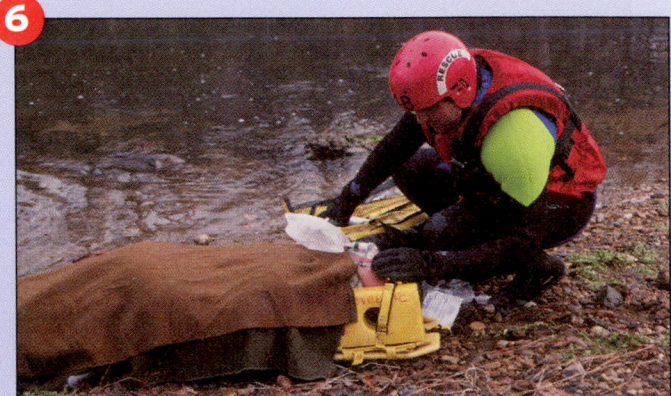

Once the patient is out of the water, cover him or her with a blanket. If the patient is breathing, apply oxygen. If the patient is not breathing and has no pulse, begin CPR.

Spinal Injuries in Submersion Incidents

Submersion incidents may be complicated by spinal fractures and spinal cord injuries. You must assume that spinal injury exists with the following conditions:

- The submersion has resulted from a diving mishap or long fall.
- The patient is unconscious, and no information is available to rule out the possibility of a mechanism causing neck injury.
- The patient is conscious but complains of weakness, paralysis, or numbness in the arms or legs.
- You suspect the possibility of spinal injury despite what witnesses say.

Most spinal injuries in diving incidents affect the cervical spine. When spinal injury is suspected, the neck must be protected from further injury. This means that you will have to stabilize the suspected injury while the patient is still in the water. In this situation, you should perform the following steps (Figure 20-13):

1. **Turn the patient supine.** Two rescuers are usually required to turn the patient safely, although in some cases one rescuer will suffice. Always rotate the entire upper half of the patient's body as a single unit. Twisting only the head, for example, may aggravate any injury to the cervical spine.

2. **Restore the airway and begin ventilation.** Immediate ventilation is the primary treatment of all drowning and near-drowning patients. As soon as the patient is face up in the water, apply the mouth-to-mouth method or, if it is available, an airway adjunct. Have the other rescuer support the head and trunk as a unit while you open the airway and begin artificial ventilation.

3. **Float a buoyant spine board under the patient.** Secure the head and trunk to the board to eliminate motion of the cervical spine. Do not remove the patient from the water until this is done.

4. **Remove the patient from the water on the board,** and if there is no pulse, begin CPR. Effective cardiac compression or CPR is extremely difficult to perform when the patient is still in the water.

Remember, always prevent further heat loss by keeping the patient warm with blankets. Give the patient high-flow oxygen and/or continue CPR en route if necessary.

Recovery Techniques

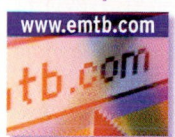

On occasion, you may be called to the scene of a drowning and find that the patient is not floating or visible in the water. An organized rescue effort in these circumstances calls for personnel who are experienced with recovery techniques and equipment, including snorkel, mask, and scuba gear. <u>Scuba (self-contained underwater breathing apparatus) gear</u> is a system that delivers air to the mouth and lungs at atmospheric pressures that increase with the depth of the dive.

As a last resort, when standard procedures for recovery are unsuccessful, you may have to use a grappling iron or large hook to drag the bottom for the victim. Although the hook could seriously wound the patient, it may be the only effective way to bring him or her to the surface for resuscitation efforts.

Resuscitation Efforts

You should *never* give up on resuscitating a cold-water drowning victim. When a person is submerged in water that is colder than body temperature, heat will be conducted from the body to the water. The resulting hypothermia can protect vital organs from the lack of oxygen. In addition, exposure to cold water will occasionally activate certain primitive reflexes, which may preserve basic body functions for prolonged periods. In one case, a $2^{1}/_{2}$-year-old girl recovered after being submerged in cold water for at least 66 minutes. Continue full resuscitation efforts until the patient recovers or is pronounced dead by a physician.

Also, whenever a person dives or jumps into very cold water, the <u>diving reflex</u>, slowing of the heart rate caused by submersion in cold water, may cause immediate <u>bradycardia</u>, a slow heart rhythm. Loss of consciousness and drowning may follow. However, the person may be able to survive for an extended period of time under water, thanks to a lowering of the metabolic rate associated with hypothermia. For this reason, you should continue full resuscitation efforts no matter how long the patient has been submerged.

> You should never give up on resuscitating a cold-water drowning victim.

Diving Problems

Most serious water-related injuries are associated with dives, with or without scuba gear. Some of these problems are related to the nature of the dive; others result from panic. Panic is not restricted to the person who is frightened by water. It can happen even to the experienced diver or swimmer.

There are more than 3,000,000 scuba sport divers in the United States, approximately 200,000 new divers being trained annually. Medical problems relating to scuba diving techniques and equipment are becoming increasingly common. These problems are separated into three phases of the dive: descent, bottom, and ascent.

Descent Problems

Descent problems are usually due to the sudden increase in pressure on the body as the person dives deeper into the water. Some body cavities cannot adjust to the increased external pressure of the water; the result is severe pain. The usual areas affected are the lungs, the sinus cavities, the middle ear, the teeth, and the area of the face surrounded by the diving mask. Usually, the pain caused by these "squeeze problems" forces the diver to return to the surface to equalize the pressures, and the problem clears up by itself. A diver who continues to complain of pain, particularly in the ear, after returning to the surface should be transported to the hospital.

A person with a perforated tympanic membrane (ruptured eardrum) may develop a special problem while diving. If cold water enters the middle ear through a ruptured eardrum, the diver may lose his or her balance and orientation. The diver may then shoot to the surface and run into ascent problems.

> Panic is not restricted to the person who is frightened by water. It can happen even to the experienced diver or swimmer.

Problems at the Bottom

Problems related to the bottom of the dive are rarely seen. They include inadequate mixing of oxygen and carbon dioxide in the air the diver breathes and accidental feeding of poisonous carbon monoxide into the breathing apparatus. Both are the result of faulty connections in the diving gear. These situations can cause drowning or rapid ascent; they require emergency resuscitation and transport of the patient.

Ascent Problems

Most of the serious injuries associated with diving are related to ascending from the bottom and are referred to as *ascent problems*. These emergencies usually require aggressive resuscitation. Two particularly dangerous medical emergencies are *air embolism* and *decompression sickness* (also called "the bends").

Air embolism. The most dangerous, and most common, emergency in scuba diving is <u>air embolism</u>, a condition caused by a bubble of air in the blood vessels. Air embolism may occur on a dive as shallow as 6 feet. The problem starts when the diver holds his or her breath during a rapid ascent. The air pressure in the lungs remains at a high level while the external pressure on the chest decreases. As a result, the air inside the lungs expands rapidly, causing the alveoli in the lungs to rupture. The air released from this rupture can cause the following injuries:

- Air may enter the pleural space and compress the lungs (a pneumothorax).

- Air may enter the mediastinum (the space within the thorax that contains the heart and great vessels), causing a condition called *pneumomediastinum*.

- Air may enter the bloodstream and create bubbles of air in the vessels called *air emboli*.

Pneumothorax and pneumomediastinum both result in pain and severe dyspnea. An air embolus will act as a plug and prevent the normal flow of blood and oxygen to a specific part of the body. The brain and spinal cord are the organs most severely affected by air embolism because they require a constant supply of oxygen.

The following are potential signs and symptoms of air embolism:

- Blotching (mottling of the skin)

- Froth (often pink or bloody) at the nose and mouth

- Severe pain in muscles, joints, or abdomen

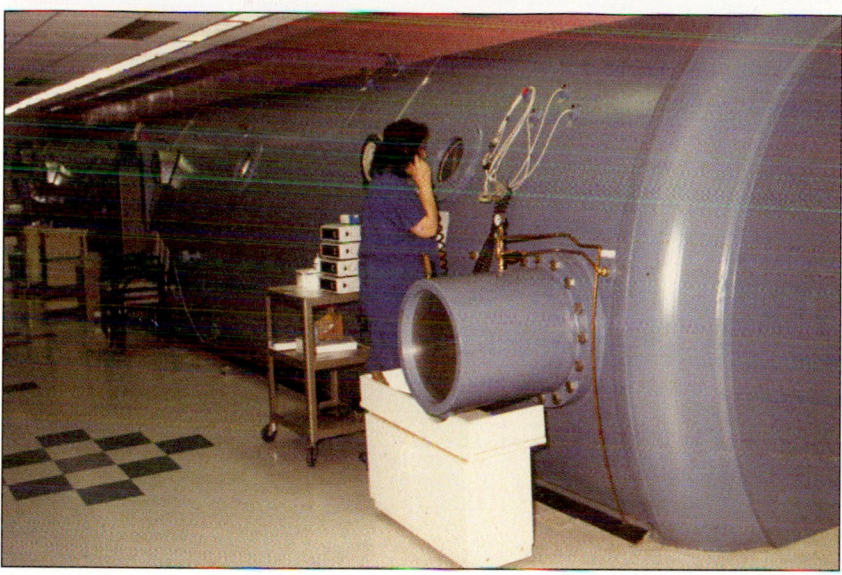

FIGURE 20-14 A hyperbaric chamber is usually a small room pressurized to more than atmospheric pressure used in the treatment of decompression sickness.

- Dyspnea and/or chest pain
- Dizziness, nausea, and vomiting
- Dysphasia (difficulty speaking)
- Difficulty with vision
- Paralysis and/or coma
- Irregular pulse and even cardiac arrest

Decompression sickness. <u>Decompression sickness</u>, commonly called <u>the bends</u>, occurs when bubbles of gas, especially nitrogen, obstruct the blood vessels. This condition also results from too rapid an ascent from a dive, although the exact mechanism of injury is unknown. During the dive, nitrogen that is being breathed dissolves in the blood and tissues because it is under pressure. When the diver ascends, the external pressure is decreased, and the dissolved nitrogen forms small bubbles within those tissues. These bubbles can lead to problems similar to those that occur in air embolism (blockage of tiny blood vessels, depriving parts of the body of their normal blood supply), but severe pain in certain tissues or spaces in the body is the most common problem.

The most striking symptom is abdominal and/or joint pain so severe that the patient literally doubles up or "bends." Dive tables and computers are available to show the proper rate of ascent from a dive, including the number and length of pauses that a diver should make on the way up. However, even divers who stay within these limits can suffer the bends.

Even after a "safe dive," decompression sickness can occur from driving a car up a mountain or flying in an unpressurized airplane that climbs too rapidly to a great

height. However, the risk of this diminishes after 24 to 48 hours. The problem is exactly the same as ascent from a deep dive: a sudden decrease of external pressure on the body and release of dissolved nitrogen from the blood that forms bubbles of nitrogen gas within the blood vessels.

You may find it difficult to distinguish between air embolism and decompression sickness. As a general rule, air embolism occurs immediately on return to the surface, whereas the symptoms of decompression sickness may not occur for several hours. The emergency treatment is the same for both. It consists of BLS followed by recompression in a <u>hyperbaric chamber</u>, a chamber, usually a small room that is pressurized to more than atmospheric pressure (Figure 20-14). Recompression treatment allows the bubbles of gas to dissolve into the blood and equalizes the pressures inside and outside the lungs. Once these pressures are equalized, gradual decompression can be accomplished under controlled conditions to prevent the bubbles from reforming.

In treating patients who are suspected of having air embolism or decompression sickness, you should follow these accepted treatment steps:

1. Remove the patient from the water. Try to keep the patient calm.

2. Begin BLS and administer oxygen.

3. Place the patient in a left lateral recumbent position with the head down.

4. Provide prompt transport to the nearest recompression facility for treatment.

Injury from decompression sickness is usually reversible with proper treatment. However, if the bubbles block critical blood vessels that supply the brain or spinal cord, permanent central nervous system injury may result. Therefore, the key in emergency management of these serious ascent problems is to recognize that an emergency exists and treat them as soon as possible. Begin BLS, administer oxygen, and arrange for recompression as rapidly as possible.

Other Water Hazards

You must pay close attention to the body temperature of a person who is rescued from cold water. Treat hypothermia caused by immersion in cold water the same way you treat hypothermia caused by cold exposure. Prevent further heat loss from contact with the ground, stretcher, or air, and transport the patient promptly.

A person swimming in shallow water may suffer from **breath-holding syncope**, a loss of consciousness caused by a decreased stimulus for breathing. This happens to swimmers who breathe in and out rapidly and deeply before entering the water in an effort to expand their capacity to stay underwater. While increasing the oxygen level, this hyperventilation lowers the carbon dioxide level. Because an elevated level of carbon dioxide in the blood is the strongest stimulus for breathing, the swimmer may not feel the need to breathe even after using up all the oxygen in his or her lungs. The emergency treatment for a breath-holding syncope is the same as that for a drowning or near drowning.

Injuries caused by boat propellers, sharp rocks, water skis, or dangerous marine life may be complicated by immersion in cold water. In these cases, remove the patient from the water, taking care to protect the spine, and give BLS as needed. Apply dressings and splints if indicated, and monitor the patient closely for any signs of immersion or cold injury.

You should be aware that a child who is involved in a drowning or near drowning may be the victim of child abuse. Although it may be difficult to prove, such incidents should be handled according to the rules set up for suspected child abuse.

Prevention

Appropriate precautions can prevent most immersion incidents. Each year, many small children drown in residential pools. All pools should be surrounded by a fence that is at least 6′ high, with slats no farther apart than 3″ and self-closing, self-locking gates. The most common problem is lack of adult supervision, even when attention is not given for a few seconds. Half of all teenage and adult drownings are associated with the use of alcohol. As a health care professional, you should be involved in public education efforts to make people aware of the hazards of swimming pools and water recreation.

prep kit

ready to review

Cold illness can be either a local or a systemic problem. Local cold injuries include frostbite, frostnip, and immersion foot. Frostbite is the most serious because tissues actually freeze with this injury. All patients with a local cold injury should be removed from the cold and protected from further exposure. You can rewarm frostnipped parts, including immersion foot, with your warm hands or breath. On the other hand, you can cause further damage to a frost-bitten part by attempting to rewarm it in the field. If this is necessary because you cannot transport the patient to the hospital, immerse the part in water at a temperature between 100° and 112°F (38° and 44.5°C).

Patients who are exposed to the cold can also become hypothermic. The key to treating such patients is to stabilize vital functions and prevent further heat loss. Do not attempt to rewarm patients who have moderate to severe hypothermia, because they are prone to developing arrhythmias unless handled very carefully. Even if you cannot find a pulse, do not consider a patient dead until he or she is "warm and dead." Local protocol will dictate whether or not such patients receive CPR or defibrillation in the field.

The body's regulatory mechanisms normally maintain body temperature within a very narrow range around 98.6°F (37°C). The body can increase its core temperature by increasing its metabolism, for example, by shivering. In general, however, body temperature is regulated by losing heat to the atmosphere. This can occur via five mechanisms: conduction, convection, evaporation, radiation, and respiration. Of these, evaporation, convection, and radiation are the most important. The very young and the very old, as well as patients with certain diseases and medication regimens, are at increased risk of heat or cold injuries because their regulatory mechanisms are not as efficient as those of other patients.

Heat illness can take three forms: heat cramps, heat exhaustion, and heatstroke. Heat cramps are painful muscle spasms that occur with vigorous exercise. They usually go away if you remove the patient from the hot environment, rest the affected muscles, and replace lost fluids (drinking lots of water).

Heat exhaustion, a more systemic illness, is essentially a form of hypovolemic shock. It occurs when the body loses so much water and so many electrolytes that it becomes dehydrated. Patients with heat exhaustion may be cold and clammy, weak or faint, confused, and have a headache. As with other patients in shock, the pulse is often rapid. Body temperature can be high, and the patient may or may not still be sweating. Treatment includes removing the patient, if feasible, from the heat and treating for mild hypovolemic shock, usually with oral fluids. More often, IV fluids will be necessary.

Heat exhaustion can progress to heatstroke. This is a life-threatening emergency, usually fatal if untreated. Patients with heatstroke may or may not still be sweating, but they will usually be dry and will have high body temperatures. Changes in mental status can include coma. Rapid lowering of the body temperature in the field can save the life of a patient with heatstroke. Fanning dampened skin and placement of cold packs around the neck, armpits, and groin are key.

Drowning and near-drowning incidents can occur even in areas that are not associated with water recreation. The first rule in caring for victims of such incidents is to be sure not to become a victim yourself. Take care to protect the spine when removing patients from the water, since spinal cord injuries, especially cervical spine injuries, are often involved in drownings. Be aware of the possibility of hypothermia, especially in cold water immersions.

While some injuries associated with scuba diving are immediately apparent, others may show up hours later. Most significant injuries occur during ascent. Patients with air embolism or decompression sickness may have pain, paralysis, or altered mental status. Be prepared to transport such patients to a recompression facility with a hyperbaric chamber.

20

prep kit

prep kit

vital vocabulary

air embolism A condition caused by air bubbles in the blood vessels.

ambient temperature The temperature of the surrounding environment.

bradycardia Slow heart rate, less than 60 beats/min.

breath-holding syncope Loss of consciousness caused by a decreased breathing stimulus.

conduction The loss of heat by direct contact (eg, when a body part comes into contact with a colder object).

convection The loss of body heat caused by air movement (eg, breeze blowing across the body).

core temperature The temperature of the central part of the body (eg, the heart, lungs, and vital organs).

decompression sickness (the bends) A condition seen in divers in which gas, especially nitrogen, forms bubbles in blood vessels, obstructing the vessels.

diving reflex Slowing of the heart rate caused by sudden submersion in cold water.

drowning Death from suffocation by submersion in water.

electrolytes Certain salts and other chemicals that are dissolved in body fluids and cells.

evaporation Conversion of water from a liquid to a gas.

frostbite Damage to tissues as the result of exposure to cold; frozen body parts.

www.emtb.com

heat cramps Painful muscle spasms usually associated with vigorous activity in a hot environment.

heat exhaustion A form of heat injury in which the body loses significant amounts of fluid and electrolytes from heavy sweating, which results in dizziness, nausea, confusion, collapse, and severe weakness; also called heat prostration or heat collapse.

heatstroke A life-threatening condition caused by exposure to excessive natural or artificial heat, marked by warm, dry skin; severely altered mental status; and often irreversible coma.

hyperbaric chamber A chamber, usually a small room, pressurized to more than atmospheric pressure.

hyperthermia A condition in which the internal body temperature rises to 101°F (38.3°C) or more.

hypothermia A condition in which the internal body temperature falls below 95°F (35°C) after exposure to a cold environment.

laryngospasm A severe constriction of the larynx and vocal cords.

near drowning Survival, at least temporarily, after suffocation in water.

radiation The direct loss of body heat to a colder air environment.

SCUBA (self-contained underwater breathing apparatus) A system that delivers air to the mouth and lungs at various atmospheric pressures, increasing with the depth of the dive.

online outlook

Hypothermia can develop either quickly, as when someone is immersed in cold water, or more gradually, as when a lost hunter is exposed to the cold environment for several hours or more. To learn more about preventing and treating hypothermia, complete Exercise 20 at www.emtb.com.

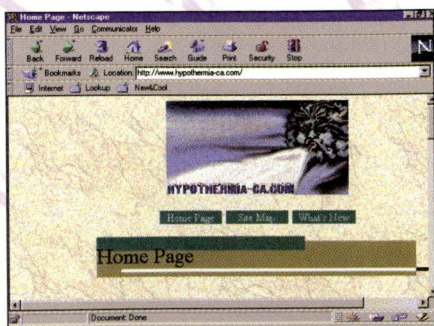

points to ponder

Objectives 1-3.3, 1-3.4, 4-7.1, 4-7.4, 4-7.5

You are at the park with a friend when you hear a yell for help. You turn to find a small group of people standing around someone who is lying on the ground. You identify yourself and take control of the scene. The patient is middle aged and, for religious reasons, is dressed in many layers of clothing, including a covering over the head. You find out that the people are on vacation from Alaska and have been here about a week. The weather is unusually hot, with temperatures over 100°F (38°C). The patient feels very hot, and what skin you can see is quite red. You suggest removing some of the patient's clothing, and the patient refuses. You move the patient to the shade and offer some water to drink. The patient again refuses to remove any clothing. The patient suddenly loses consciousness. EMS has not been activated and is approximately 15 minutes away.

- How would you treat this person? Would you remove some of the patient's clothing? Why or why not?

assessment in action

It is a hot, humid day in mid-August, and inside the North End Welding shop, the temperature is more than 120°F. Usually, the employees work for only 50 minutes between breaks. However, one welder is trying to catch up on a difficult job, so he skipped two consecutive breaks and collapsed suddenly. You arrive to find a 23-year-old man sitting on the floor against a wall. The patient reports that he feels weak and dizzy and as though someone had "punched him in the gut." A co-worker who saw the event reports that after he called 9-1-1, he checked on the patient and found that the patient could scarcely respond. The patient states that he has been battling the flu for the last couple of days and has had several episodes of vomiting and diarrhea. Because of that, he has had little to eat or drink.

Assessment reveals that the patient has cool, moist skin, a blood pressure of 118/68 mm Hg, a pulse of 126 beats/min, and respirations of 24 breaths/min.

1. The patient's severe muscle cramps have most likely developed because his:
   A. pulse rate is higher than normal.
   B. systolic blood pressure is extremely low.
   C. respirations are too fast and shallow for his metabolic needs.
   D. electrolytes have been depleted because of the vomiting, diarrhea, and sweating.

2. Your first step in caring for this patient should be to:
   A. listen to his breath sounds.
   B. move him to a cooler environment.
   C. give supplemental oxygen via nasal cannula.
   D. continue to ask him about his medical history.

3. The high temperature in the welding shop has reduced the patient's ability to:
   A. breathe normally.
   B. lose heat from sweating.
   C. exchange oxygen for carbon dioxide.
   D. exchange carbon dioxide for oxygen.

4. Once you have moved the patient to the ambulance, you decide to cool him with ice packs. Which of the following locations would be the **LEAST** effective for placing the ice packs?
   A. Neck
   B. Groin
   C. Armpits
   D. Forehead

5. The patient states that he cannot afford to take the time off to go to the hospital and that he really would like to return to work. At this point, you should:
   A. suggest that the patient drive himself home and go to bed.
   B. summon law enforcement and force him to go to the hospital.
   C. encourage the patient to go to the hospital for a complete evaluation.
   D. help the patient out of the ambulance and let him return to work.

prep kit

20

Behavioral Emergencies

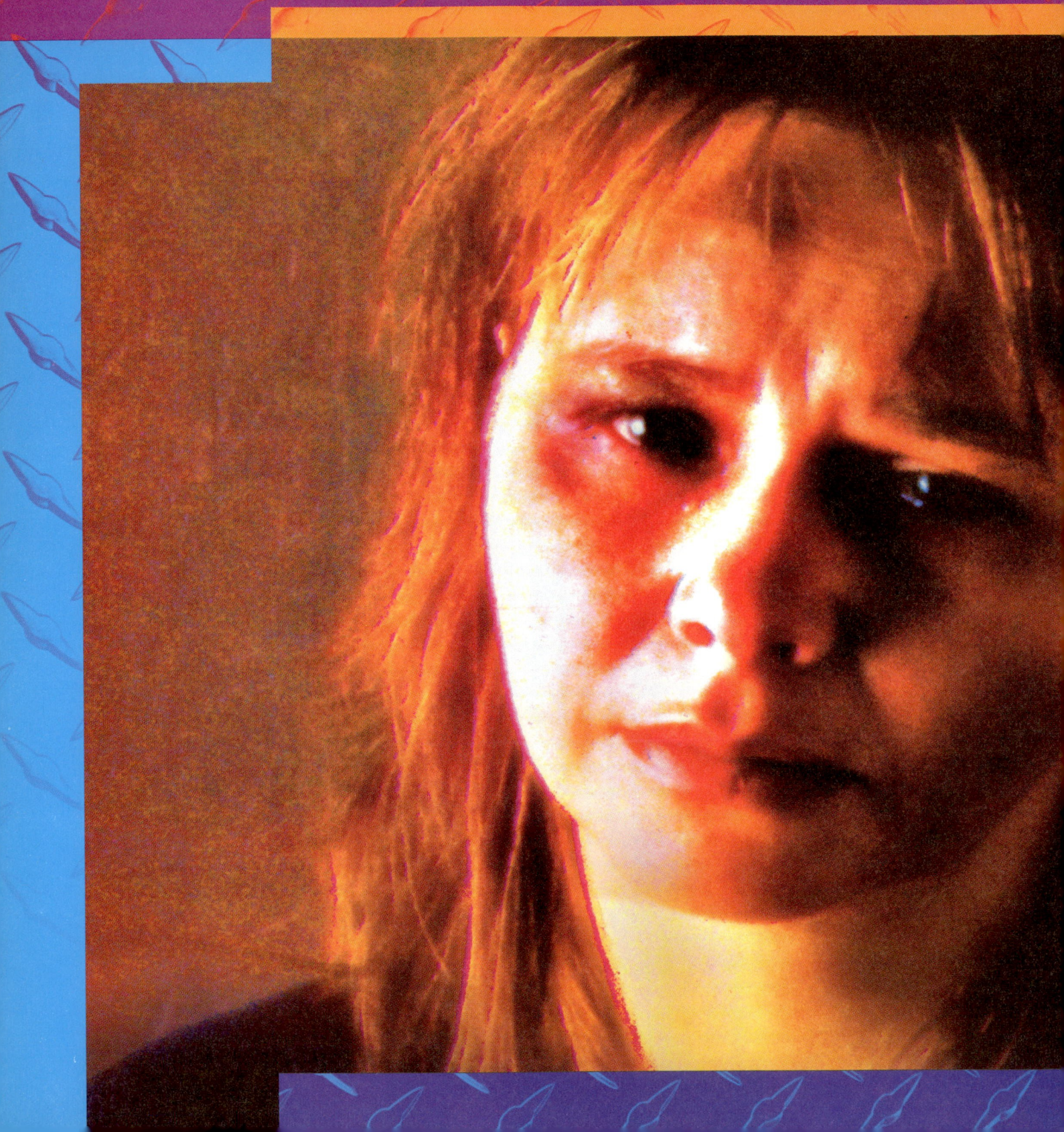

objectives

Cognitive

1. Define behavioral emergencies.

2. Discuss the general factors that may cause an alteration in a patient's behavior.

3. State the various reasons for psychological crises.

4. Discuss the characteristics of an individual's behavior which suggest that the patient is at risk for suicide.

5. Discuss special medicolegal considerations for managing behavioral emergencies.

6. Discuss the special considerations for assessing a patient with behavioral problems.

7. Discuss the general principles of an individual's behavior which suggest that the patient is at risk for violence.

8. Discuss methods to calm behavioral emergency patients.

Affective

9. Explain the rationale for learning how to modify your behavior toward the patient with a behavioral emergency.

Psychomotor

10. Demonstrate the assessment and emergency medical care of the patient experiencing a behavioral emergency.

11. Demonstrate various techniques to safely restrain a patient with a behavioral problem.

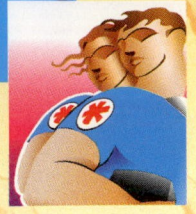

Behavioral emergencies are often stressful for the EMT-Bs because of the increased risk of danger to the patient, the bystanders, and to themselves. This chapter will prepare you for responding to these emergencies and will help you answer the following questions:

1. What is your role in responding to a behavioral emergency in which violence may be involved?

2. What are the advantages and disadvantages of having law enforcement officials at the scene of the behavioral emergency?

Behavioral Emergencies

As an EMT-B, you can expect to deal often with patients undergoing a psychological or behavioral crisis. The crisis may be due to the emergency situation, mental illness, mind-altering substances, stress, or many other causes. This chapter discusses various kinds of behavioral emergencies, including those involving overdoses, violent behavior, and mental illness. You will learn how to assess a person who exhibits signs and symptoms of a behavioral emergency and what kind of emergency care may be required in these situations. The chapter also covers legal concerns in dealing with disturbed patients. Finally, it describes how to identify and manage the potentially violent patient, including the use of restraints.

Myth and Reality

Everyone has mental illness problems at some point in life, some more severe than others. Perfectly healthy people may have some of the symptoms and signs of mental illness from time to time. Therefore, you should not jump to the conclusion that you are mentally disturbed when you behave in certain ways that are discussed in this chapter. For that matter, you also should not jump to this conclusion about a patient in any given situation.

The most common misconception about mental illness is that if you are feeling "bad" or "depressed," you must be "sick." That is simply untrue. There are many perfectly justifiable reasons for feeling depressed, including divorce, loss of a job, and the death of a relative or friend. For the teenager who just broke up with his girlfriend of 12 months, it is altogether normal to withdraw from ordinary activities and to feel "blue." This is a normal reaction to a crisis situation. However, when a person finds that Monday morning blues last until Friday, week after week, he or she may indeed have a behavioral problem.

Many people believe that all individuals with mental health disorders are dangerous, violent, or otherwise unmanageable. This is untrue. Only a small percentage of those with mental health problems fall into these categories. As an EMT-B, however, you may be exposed to a higher proportion of violent patients. After all, you are seeing people who are, by definition, considered to be having an emergency; otherwise, you probably would not be seeing them. You are there because family members or friends felt unable to manage the patient by themselves. This may be a result of the use or abuse of drugs or alcohol. It may be that the patient has a long history of mental illness and is reacting to a particularly stressful event.

While you cannot determine what has caused a person's behavioral problem, you may be able to predict that the person will become violent. The ability to predict violence is an important assessment tool for the EMT-B.

Defining Behavioral Emergencies

Behavior is what you can see of a person's response to the environment, his or her actions. Sometimes, it is obvious what a person is responding to: A person is punched, and he or she runs away or bursts into tears or hits back. Sometimes, it is less clear, as when someone is depressed for very complex reasons.

Most of the time, individuals respond to the environment in reasonable ways. Over the years, they have learned to adapt to a variety of situations in daily life, including stresses and strains. This is called *adjustment*. There are times, however, when the stress is so great that the normal ways of adjusting do not work. When this happens, a person's behavior is likely to change, even if only temporarily. The new behavior may not be appropriate, or normal.

The definition of a **behavioral crisis** or emergency is any reaction to events that interferes with the **activities of daily living (ADL)** or has become unacceptable to the patient, family, or community. For example, when someone experiences an interruption of the daily routine, such as washing, dressing, and eating, chances are his or her behavior has become a problem. For that person, at that time, a behavioral emergency may exist. If the interruption of daily routine tends to recur on a regular basis, the behavior is also considered a *mental health problem*. It is then a pattern, rather than an isolated incident.

For example, a person who suffers a panic attack after having a heart attack is not necessarily mentally ill. Likewise, you would expect a person who is fired from a job to have some sort of reaction, often sadness and depression. These behavioral problems are short-term and isolated events. However, the person who reacts with a fit of rage, attacking people and property or going on a "bender" for a week, has gone beyond what society considers appropriate or normal behavior. That person is clearly undergoing a behavioral emergency. Usually, if an abnormal or disturbing pattern of behavior lasts for at least a month, it is regarded as a matter of concern from a mental health standpoint. For example, chronic **depression**, a persistent feeling of sadness and despair, may be a symptom of a mental or physical disorder. This type of long-term problem would be labeled a mental health disorder.

A person who is no longer able to respond appropriately to the environment may be having what is called a psychological or psychiatric emergency. When a psychiatric emergency arises, the patient may show agitation or violence or become a threat to himself, herself, or others. This is more serious than a more typical behavioral emergency that causes inappropriate behavior such as interference with ADL or intolerable actions. An immediate threat to the person involved or to others in the immediate area, including family, friends, bystanders, and EMTs should be considered a psychiatric emergency. For example, a person might respond to the death of a spouse by attempting suicide. On the other hand, although this is a major life disruption, it does not have to involve violence or harm to an individual. Disruption can take many forms; not all involve violence nor are they all psychiatric emergencies.

The Magnitude of Mental Health Problems

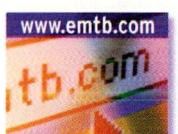

According to the National Institutes of Mental Health, at one time or another, one in five Americans has some type of **mental disorder**, an illness with psychological or behavioral symptoms that may result in an impairment in functioning. It can be caused by a social, psychological, genetic, physical, chemical, or biologic disturbance.

Pathology: Causes of Behavioral Emergencies

Although sudden grief, emotional conflicts, and other psychological problems can cause behavioral emergencies, sudden illness, recent trauma, drug or alcohol intoxication, and diseases of the brain, such as Alzheimer's disease, can produce abnormal behavior as well. Likewise, altered mental status can arise from low blood glucose, lack of oxygen, inadequate blood flow to the brain, and excessive heat or cold. As an EMT-B, you are not responsible for diagnosing the underlying cause of a behavioral or psychiatric emergency. However, you should know the two basic categories of diagnosis a physician will use: organic (physical) and functional (psychological).

Organic brain syndrome is a temporary or permanent dysfunction of the brain caused by a disturbance in the physical or physiologic functioning of brain tissue, such as the disturbances listed above. That is, something has gone wrong in the way the organ itself is working. For example, low blood glucose could cause organic brain syndrome. A **functional disorder** is one in which the abnormal operation of an organ cannot be traced to an obvious change in the actual structure, or physiology, of the organ. Something has gone wrong, but the root cause cannot be identified as the working of the organ itself. Schizophrenia is a good example of a functional disorder.

These two types of disorders can look very much alike. An **altered mental status**, or a change in the way a person thinks or behaves, is one indicator of central nervous system diseases. A patient displaying bizarre behavior may turn out to have an acute medical illness that is the cause, or a partial cause, of the behavior. Recognizing this possibility may allow you to save a life.

Safe Approach to a Behavioral Emergency

All the regular EMT skills—assessment, providing care, patient approach, history taking, and patient communication—are used in behavioral emergencies. However,

TABLE 21-1   Safety Guidelines for Behavioral Emergencies

- **Be prepared to spend extra time.** It may take longer to assess, listen to, and prepare the patient for transport.

- **Have a definite plan of action.** Decide who will do what. If restraint is needed, how will it be accomplished?

- **Identify yourself calmly.** Try to gain the patient's confidence. If you begin shouting, the patient is likely to shout louder or become more excited. A low, calm voice is often a quieting influence.

- **Be direct.** State your intentions and what you expect of the patient.

- **Assess the scene.** If the patient is armed or has potentially harmful objects in his or her possession, have these removed by law enforcement personnel before you provide care.

- **Stay with the patient.** *Do not let the patient leave the area, and do not leave yourself unless law enforcement personnel can stay with the patient.* Otherwise, the patient may go to another room and obtain weapons, lock himself or herself in the bathroom, or take pills.

- **Encourage purposeful movement:** Help the patient to get dressed and gather appropriate belongings to take to the hospital.

- **Express interest in the patient's story.** Let the patient tell you what happened or what is going on now in his or her own words. However, do not play along with auditory or visual disturbances.

- **Do not get too close to the patient;** everyone needs personal space. Furthermore, you want to be sure you can move quickly if the patient becomes violent or tries to run away. Do not physically talk down to or directly confront the patient. A squatting, 45° angle approach is usually not confrontational but may hinder your movements. Do not allow the patient to get between you and the exit.

- **Avoid fighting with the patient.** You do not want to get into a power struggle. Remember, the patient is not responding to you in a normal manner; he or she may be wrestling with internal forces over which neither of you has control. You and others may be stimulating these inner forces without knowing it. If you can respond with understanding to the feeling that the patient is expressing, whether this is anger or fear or desperation, you may be able to gain his or her cooperation. If it is necessary to use force, be sure you have adequate help and move toward the patient quietly and with assured firmness.

- **Be honest and reassuring.** If the patient asks whether he or she has to go to the hospital, the answer should be, "Yes, that is where you can receive medical help."

- **Do not judge.** You may see behavior that you dislike. Set those feelings aside and concentrate on providing emergency medical care.

---

other management techniques also come into play. There is not room in this chapter for a full discussion of these techniques, but you should follow general guidelines to ensure your safety at the scene of a behavioral emergency (Table 21-1).

Assessing a Behavioral Emergency

In evaluating a situation that is considered a behavioral emergency, the first things to consider are your safety and how the patient is responding to the environment (Table 21-2). Is the situation unduly dangerous to you and your partner? Do you need immediate law enforcement backup? Does the patient's behavior seem typical or normal in the circumstances? For example, a patient who has just been assaulted has good reason to be fear-

ful of other people, including you. On the other hand, if you ask a person, "Do you know where you are?" and he or she replies, "The planet Venus" (and does not seem to be joking), you may conclude that the person is disoriented, regardless of the cause.

A behavioral crisis puts tremendous stress on a person's coping mechanisms, including natural abilities and training. The person is actually incapable of responding reasonably to the demands of the environment. This state may be temporary, as in an acute illness, or longer-lived, as in a complex, chronic mental illness. In either case, the patient's perception of reality may be compromised or distorted.

Sometimes a patient in a behavioral or psychiatric emergency will not respond at all to your questions. In those cases, you may be able to tell quite a lot about the patient's emotional state from facial expressions, pulse, and respirations. Tears, sweating, and blushing may be significant indicators of state of mind. Also, make sure

TABLE 21-2 Questions to Ask in Evaluating a Behavioral Crisis

- How does the patient relate to you?
- Does the patient answer your questions appropriately?
- Is the patient withdrawn or detached?
- Is the patient hostile or friendly? Too friendly?
- Does the patient understand why you are there?
- How is the patient dressed? Is the dress appropriate for the time of year and occasion? Are the clothes clean or dirty?
- Are the patient's movements coordinated or jerky and awkward? Does he or she appear to be agitated?
- Are the patient's movements purposeful? Are the movements helping to accomplish a task, such as sitting down and putting on a pair of shoes, or do they appear to be aimless, such as rocking back and forth on the chair?
- Has the patient harmed himself or herself? Is there damage to the surroundings?
- Does the patient appear relaxed or stiff and guarded?
- What are the patient's facial expressions? Are they bland and flat or expressive? Does the patient show joy, fear, or anger as appropriate? To what degree?
- Are the patient's vocabulary and expressions what you would expect under the circumstances? Are they in line with the patient's social and educational background?
- Is the patient easily distracted?
- Are the patient's responses to what is going on around him or her appropriate?
- Is the patient's memory intact? Check orientation to time, place, person: Do you know what day/month/year it is? Do you know where you are? Do you know who I am?
- Is the patient alert and able to talk logically and coherently?
- What is the patient's mood? Does he or she seem agitated, elated, abnormally depressed?
- Does the patient appear fearful or worried?
- Does the patient express disordered thoughts, delusions, or hallucinations? That is, does he or she appear to be seeing, hearing, or responding to people or situations that are not present?

that you look at the patient's eyes; a patient who has a blank gaze or rapidly moving eyes may be experiencing CNS depression or some type of extra stress (Figure 21-1).

In trying to determine the reason for the patient's state, you should consider three major areas possible contributors:

- Is the patient's central nervous system functioning properly? For example, the patient may be experiencing diabetic problems, particularly hypoglycemia. He or she may have been poisoned or may be responding to a physical trauma of some sort. Any of these situations could cause the patient to behave in an unusual or irrational fashion.

- Are hallucinogens or other drugs or alcohol a factor? Does the patient see strange things? Is everything distorted? Do you smell alcohol on the patient's breath?

- Are **psychogenic** circumstances, symptoms, or illness (caused by mental rather than physical factors) involved? These might include the death of a loved one, severe depression, a history of mental illness, threats of suicide, or some other major interruption of ADL.

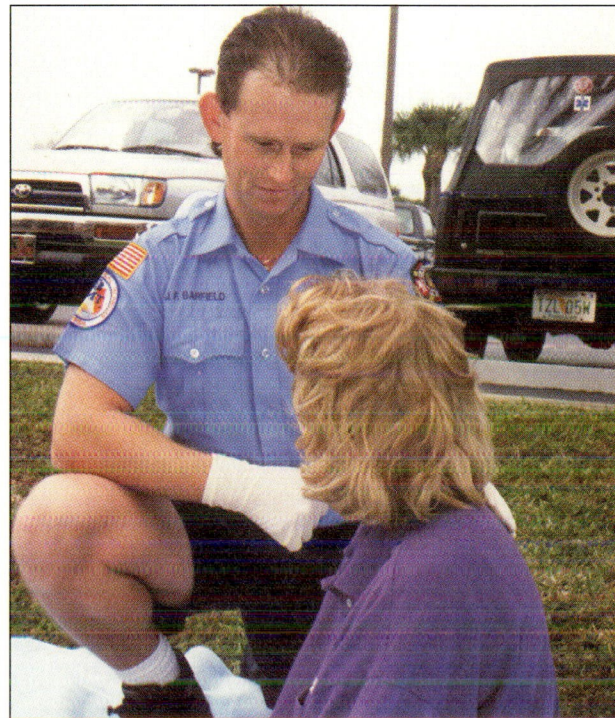

FIGURE 21-1 Making eye contact with a patient can provide useful clues about a patient's emotional state.

Family, friends, and observers may be of great help in answering these questions. Together with your observations and interaction with the patient, they should provide enough data for you to assess the situation. This assessment has two primary goals: recognizing major threats to life, and reducing the stress of the situation as much as possible.

Suicide

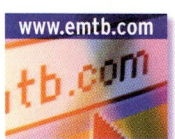 The single most significant factor that contributes to suicide is depression. Any time you encounter an emotionally depressed patient, you must consider the possibility of suicide. Risk factors for suicide are listed in Table 21-3.

It is a common misconception that people who threaten suicide never commit it. This is not correct. Suicide is a cry for help. Threatening suicide is an indication that someone is in a crisis he or she cannot handle. Immediate intervention is necessary.

Whether or not the patient has any of these risk factors, you must be alert to the following warning signs:

- Does the patient have an air of tearfulness, sadness, deep despair, or hopelessness that suggests depression?

- Does the patient avoid eye contact, speak slowly or haltingly, and project a sense of vacancy, as if he or she really isn't there?

- Does the patient seem unable to talk about the future? Ask the patient whether he or she has any vacation plans. Suicidal people consider the future so uninteresting that they do not think about it;

people who are seriously depressed consider the future so distant that they may not be able to think about it at all.

- Is there any suggestion of suicide? Even vague suggestions should not be taken lightly, even if presented as a joke. If you think that suicide is a possibility, do not hesitate to bring the subject up. You will not "give the patient ideas" if you ask directly, "Are you considering suicide?"

- Does the patient have any specific plans relating to death? Has the patient recently prepared a will? Given away significant possessions or advised close friends what he or she would like done with them? Arranged for a funeral service? These are critical warning signs.

Consider also the following additional risk factors for suicide:

- Are there any unsafe objects in the patient's hands or nearby (eg, a sharp knife, glass, poisons, a gun)?

- Is the environment unsafe (eg, an open window in a high-rise building, a patient standing on a bridge or precipice)?

- Is there evidence of self-destructive behavior (eg, partially cut wrists, large alcohol or drug intake)?

- Is there an imminent threat to the patient or others?

- Is there an underlying medical problem?

Remember, the suicidal patient may be homicidal as well. Do not jeopardize your life or the lives of your fellow EMT-Bs. If you have reason to believe that you are in danger, you must obtain police intervention. In the meantime, try not to frighten the patient or make him or her suspicious.

TABLE 21-3 Risk Factors for Suicide	
• Depression, any age	• Chronic debilitating illness or recent diagnosis of serious illness
• Previous suicide attempt (80% of successful suicides were preceded by at least one attempt.)	• Financial setback, loss of job, police arrest, imprisonment, or some sort of social embarrassment
• Current expression of wanting to commit suicide or sense of hopelessness	• Substance abuse, particularly with increasing usage
• Family history of suicide	• Children of an alcoholic parent
• Age older than 40 years, particularly for single, widowed, divorced, alcoholic, or depressed individuals (Men in this category who are older than age 55 years have an especially high risk.)	• Severe mental illness
	• Anniversary of death of loved one, job loss, marriage, etc.
• Recent loss of spouse, significant other, family member, or support system	• Unusual gathering or new acquisition of things that can cause death, such as purchase of a gun, a large volume of pills, or increased use of alcohol
• Holidays	

Medicolegal Considerations

The medical and legal aspects of emergency medical care become more complicated when the patient is undergoing a behavioral or psychiatric emergency. Nevertheless, legal problems are greatly reduced with the emotionally disturbed patient who consents to care. Gaining that patient's confidence is therefore a critical task for the EMT-B.

Mental incapacity can take many forms: unconsciousness (as a result of hypoxia, alcohol, or drugs), temporary but severe stress, or depression. Once you have determined that a patient has impaired mental

> When a patient is not mentally competent to grant consent for emergency medical care, the law assumes that there is implied consent.

capacity, you must decide whether he or she requires immediate emergency medical care. A patient who is mentally unstable may resist your attempts to render care. Nevertheless, you must *not* leave this patient alone. Doing so may expose you to civil action for abandonment or negligence. In such situations, you should

caring for the elderly

As the population ages, you will begin to see more patients in the over-65 age group. In responding to an increasing number of geriatric patients, you will probably notice some behavioral or mental health problems, including depression, dementia, and delirium. These mental status changes can affect your ability to thoroughly assess and treat the ill or injured geriatric patient. Understanding the causes of altered behavior in the elderly patient will help you in patient care.

Depression is one of the more common mental status problems that you will see in the older population. While a lot of attention has been paid to depression in younger adults, the media has not given much credence to the older adult's mental health challenges. As an EMT, you can recognize a problem and perhaps prevent a suicide in the depressed elderly person.

Depression has a number of causes, some organic, some psychological, and some cultural. Organic causes of depression include an emotional response to a major illness such as cancer or dementia. Further, medications can induce a feeling of depression, especially when interacting with other prescription drugs. Finally, changes in the endocrine system, such as menopause, can elicit depression.

With all the possible causes of depression, an older adult can feel helpless and hopeless. The depressed person can be either argumentative or placid. He or she might trivialize complaints, not wanting to be of a bother to anyone. Someone who sees no way out of his or her situation may turn to suicide. Be alert for a suicide gesture or ideation, even though it may not be obvious.

While depression can create behavioral problems in the elderly patient, dementia is another cause of abnormal behavior. The most common cause of dementia is primary progressive dementia, also known as Alzheimer's dementia. It is estimated that 10% of the population older than age 65 years and 50% of the population older than age 85 years have Alzheimer's dementia. Currently, there is no cure for Alzheimer's, and once it has been diagnosed, the patient's life expectancy can range from 7 to 20 years.

During the progression of the disease, the patient can develop openly hostile behavior, kicking, yelling, pinching, and hitting you, your partner, or the patient's caregiver. You might need to contain the violent patient, but do so gently and only to the point at which the violent behavior stops.

Other causes of altered behavior include diabetic emergencies, heat- and cold-related illnesses, poisoning or overdose, strokes or TIAs, and infection. It is interesting to note that, while the mechanism is not understood, urinary tract infection or constipation can alter an elderly person's behavior.

As the EMT responding to a call for help, you should accept the possibility of depression in the elderly patient. Do not discount the patient's feelings or devalue his or her emotions. Be alert for a suicide gesture, and pay attention to any statements about death. To get the patient's cooperation, you can elicit his or her help in providing care for the acute illness or injury. A smile and a touch can go a long way in alleviating fear in all of your patients, especially the elderly.

request that law enforcement personnel handle the patient. Another reason for seeking law enforcement support is for the patient who resists treatment; such a patient will often threaten EMT-Bs and others.

Consent

When a patient is not mentally competent to grant consent for emergency medical care, the law assumes that there is implied consent. For example, the consent of an unconscious patient is implied if life or health is at risk. The law refers to this as the emergency doctrine: consent is implied because of the necessity for immediate emergency treatment. In a situation that is not immediately life threatening, emergency medical care or transportation may be delayed until the proper consent is obtained.

In cases involving psychiatric emergencies, however, the matter is not always clear-cut. Does a life-threatening emergency exist or not? If you are not sure, you should request the assistance of law enforcement personnel.

Limited Legal Authority

As an EMT-B, you have limited legal authority to require or force a patient to undergo emergency medical care when no life-threatening emergency exists. Patients have the right to refuse care. However, most states have legal statutes regarding the emergency care of mentally ill and drug-impaired individuals. These statutory provisions permit law enforcement personnel to place such a person in protective custody so that emergency care can be rendered. You should be familiar with your local and state laws regarding these situations.

The typical provision states that "any police officer who has reasonable cause to believe that a person is mentally ill and dangerous to himself, herself, or others or gravely disabled…may take such person into custody and take or cause such person to be taken to a general hospital for emergency examination…" Again, since these provisions vary, you should become familiar with those in your state.

The general rule of law is that a competent adult has the right to refuse treatment, even if lifesaving care is involved. In psychiatric cases, however, a court of law would probably consider your actions in providing lifesaving care to be appropriate, particularly if you have a reasonable belief that the patient would harm himself, herself, or others without your intervention.

Restraint

Ordinarily, restraint of a person must be ordered by a physician, a court order, or a law enforcement officer.

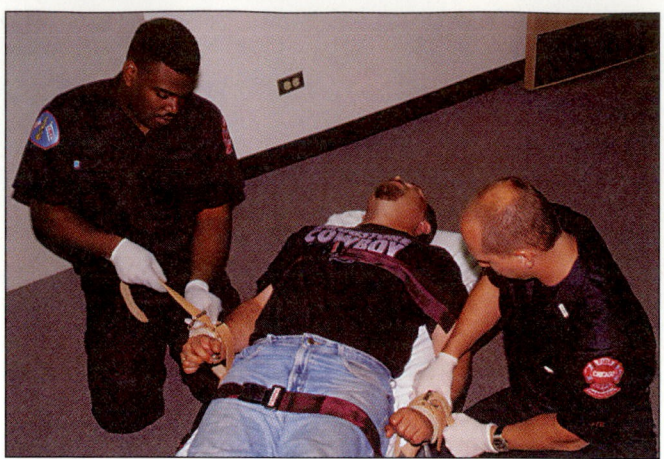

FIGURE 21-2 You may use restraints to prevent a patient from causing injury to himself or herself.

If you restrain a person without authority in a nonemergency situation, you expose yourself to a possible lawsuit, as well as to personal danger. Legal actions against the EMT can involve charges of assault, battery, false imprisonment, and violation of civil rights. You may use restraints only to protect yourself or others from bodily harm or to prevent the patient from causing injury to himself or herself (Figure 21-2). In either case, you may use only reasonable force as necessary to control the patient, something that different courts may define differently. For this reason, you should always consult medical control and contact law enforcement for help before restraining a patient.

In fact, you probably should always involve law enforcement personnel if you are called to assist a patient in a severe behavioral or psychiatric crisis. They will provide physical backup in managing the patient as well as the necessary witness and legal authority to restrain the patient. A patient who is restrained by law enforcement personnel is in their custody.

Always try to transport a disturbed patient without restraints if possible. Once the decision has been made to restrain a patient, however, you should carry it out quickly. Be aware of BSI considerations. If the patient is spitting, place a surgical mask over his or her mouth.

Make sure you have adequate help to safely restrain a patient. At least four people should be present to carry out the restraint, each being responsible for one extremity. Before you begin, discuss the plan of action. As you prepare to restrain the patient, stay outside the patient's range of motion.

In subduing a disturbed patient, use the minimum force necessary. You should avoid acts or physical force that may cause injury to the patient. The level of force will vary, depending on the following factors:

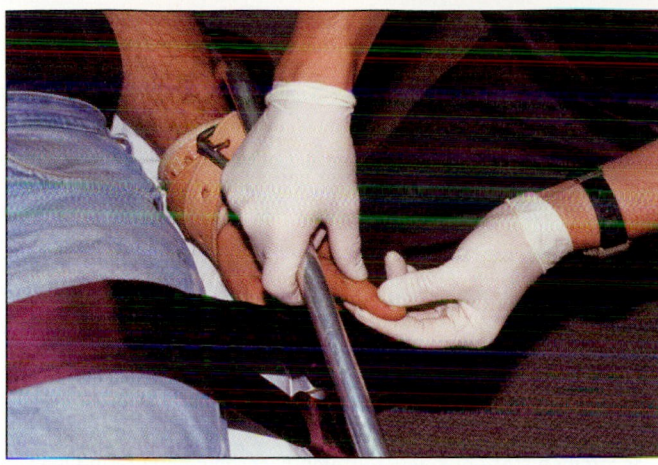

FIGURE 21-3 Assess circulation frequently while the patient is restrained.

- The degree of force that is necessary to keep the patient from injuring him or herself, or others

- A patient's gender, size, strength, and mental status

- The type of abnormal behavior the patient is exhibiting. You should use only restraint devices that have been approved by your state's health department for this purpose; soft, wide leather or cloth restraints are preferred to police-type handcuffs.

Acting at the same time, the police officers should secure the patient's extremities with approved equipment. Somebody, preferably you or your partner, should continue to talk to the patient throughout the process. Remember to treat the patient with dignity and respect at all times. Also, monitor the patient for vomiting, airway obstruction, and cardiovascular stability, since the patient cannot fend for himself or herself. Drug or alcohol intoxication may cause violent behavior but then lead to such physical problems as well. To enhance your protection of the patient, you might place the patient face down on a stretcher and secure the patient with multiple straps. However, assess the airway and circulation frequently while the patient is restrained (Figure 21-3). Document the reason for the restraint and the technique that was used. Be especially careful if a combative patient suddenly becomes calm and cooperative. This is the time not to relax but to secure the situation. The patient may suddenly become combative again and injure someone. Keep in mind that you may use reasonable force to defend yourself against an attack by an emotionally disturbed patient. It is extremely helpful to have (and document) witnesses in attendance even during transport to protect against false accusations. EMTs have been accused of sexual misconduct or other physical abuse in such circumstances.

The Potentially Violent Patient

Violent patients make up only a small percentage of those undergoing a behavioral or psychiatric crisis. However, the potential for violence by such a patient is always an important consideration for the EMT-B.

Use the following list of risk factors to assess the level of danger:

- **Past history.** Has the patient previously exhibited hostile, overly aggressive or violent behavior? Ask individuals at the scene, or request this information from law enforcement personnel or family.

- **Posture.** How is the patient sitting or standing? Is the patient tense, rigid, or sitting on the edge of his or her seat? Such physical tension is often a warning signal of impending hostility.

- **The scene.** Is the patient holding or near potentially lethal objects such as a knife, gun, glass, poker, or bat (or near a window or glass door)?

- **Vocal activity.** What kind of speech is the patient using? Loud, obscene, erratic, and bizarre speech patterns usually indicate emotional distress. Someone using quiet, ordered speech is not as likely to strike out as someone who is yelling and screaming.

- **Physical activity.** The motor activity of a person undergoing a psychiatric crisis may be the most telling factor of all. The patient who has tense muscles, clenched fists, or glaring eyes; is pacing; cannot sit still; or is fiercely protecting personal space requires careful watching. Agitation may predict a quick escalation to violence.

Other factors to consider in assessing a patient's potential for violence include the following:

- Poor impulse control

- A history of truancy, fighting, and uncontrollable temper

- Low socioeconomic status, unstable family structure, or inability to keep a steady job

- Tattoos, especially those with gang identification or statements such as "Born to Kill" or "Born to Lose"

- Substance abuse

- Depression, which accounts for 20% of violent attacks

- Functional disorder. (If the patient says that voices are telling him or her to kill, believe it.)

prep kit

ready for review

Behavioral emergencies can present the EMT-B with great difficulties in patient management. Your major responsibility in these situations is to defuse potentially life-threatening incidents and reduce the impact of the stressful condition without exposing yourself to unnecessary risks. While only a small percentage of individuals with mental health disorders are dangerous to themselves or others, you may be exposed to a higher proportion of violent individuals in your daily activities. There are a number of warning signs of violence, including a past history of hostile behavior, rigidity, loud and erratic speech patterns, agitation, and depression.

A behavioral emergency is any reaction to events that interferes with activities of daily living. A person who is no longer able to respond appropriately to the environment may be having a more serious psychiatric emergency. Not all behavioral emergencies involve a mental health problem, however. Some emergencies are a temporary response to a traumatic event.

Underlying causes of behavioral emergencies fall into two categories: organic brain syndrome and functional disorders.

Assessing a person who may be having a behavioral crisis involves observing the person, talking with the person, and talking with friends, family members, and witnesses to the person's behavior. You are looking for indications that the person's thoughts, feelings, and reactions are inappropriate for the circumstances.

Consider contributing factors in three areas: central nervous system functioning, drug or alcohol use, and psychogenic circumstances such as the death of a loved one or other major interruption of normal life.

The threat of suicide requires immediate intervention. Depression is the most significant risk factor for suicide. Others include personal or family history of suicide attempts, chronic debilitating illness, financial setback, and severe mental illness.

As an EMT-B, you have limited legal authority to require a patient to undergo emergency medical care in the absence of a life-threatening emergency. However, most states have provisions allowing law enforcement personnel to place mentally impaired persons in custody so that such care can be provided. You should always involve law enforcement personnel any time you are called to assist a patient in a severe behavioral or psychiatric crisis. Always consult medical control and contact law enforcement for help before restraining a patient. If restraints are required, use the minimum force necessary. Assess the airway and circulation frequently while the patient is restrained.

In providing emergency medical care for a patient having a behavioral emergency, be direct, honest, and calm; have a definite plan of action; stay with the patient at all times, but don't get too close; express interest in the patient's story, but do not judge his or her behavior. Always treat such patients with respect.

vital vocabulary

www.emtb.com

activities of daily living (ADL) The basic activities a person usually accomplishes during a normal day, such as eating, dressing, and washing.

altered mental status A change in the way a person thinks and behaves that signals disease in the central nervous system.

behavior How a person functions or acts.

behavioral crisis The point at which a person's reactions to events interfere with activities of daily living; a behavioral crisis becomes a psychiatric emergency when it causes a major life interruption, such as attempted suicide.

depression A persistent mood of sadness, despair, and discouragement; depression may be a symptom of many different mental and physical disorders, or it may be a disorder on its own.

functional disorder A disorder in which there is no known physiologic reason for the abnormal functioning of an organ or organ system.

mental disorder An illness with psychological or behavioral symptoms and/or impairment in functioning, caused by a social, psychological, genetic, physical, chemical, or biologic disturbance.

organic brain syndrome Temporary or permanent dysfunction of the brain, caused by a disturbance in the physical or physiologic functioning of brain tissue.

psychogenic A symptom or illness that is caused by mental factors as opposed to physical ones.

assessment in action

The off-going crew has barely finished giving their report when dispatch sends you to a duplex on 28th Street for an "unknown medical emergency." On arrival, you find an unkempt 57-year-old man lying on the couch in a well-furnished living room. He slowly awakens when you speak to him but still seems drowsy as you begin to ask questions. The woman who meets you at the door is apparently his soon-to-be ex-wife. She states that she and the patient have been fighting, and she leaves in a huff. Afterward, the patient tells you that he lost his job 2 months ago and has been unable to find work. He admits that he has probably been drinking too much, and now his wife is telling him that she wants a divorce. He yells, "I can't take anymore. Enough is enough!"

1. Your response to this situation need **NOT** include:
   A. an attempt to keep the patient as calm as possible.
   B. a scene size-up to evaluate for possible threats or hazards.
   C. an assessment of the patient as the situation and the patient allow.
   D. understanding and encouraging words to the patient to make a decision about his desire to commit suicide.

2. Which of the following is **LEAST** likely to be a factor in this patient's decision to attempt suicide?
   A. Job status
   B. Alcohol use
   C. Marital situation
   D. Living conditions

3. Which of the following approaches would be the **LEAST** effective in calming a patient during a behavioral emergency?
   A. Involving trusted family members and friends
   B. Responding honestly to the patient's questions
   C. Reminding the patient that you are there to help
   D. Keeping your scene time to the absolute minimum

4. In assessing the patient's potential for violence, which of the following factors concerns you the most?
   A. The patient is talking to you while he is lying on the couch.
   B. The patient yells at you when you ask him about the comment he made.
   C. A family member at the scene reports that the patient has no history of violence.
   D. The patient has a medium physical build and does not appear to have a weapon.

5. What would allow you to transport the patient immediately and against his will if you believed that this patient was a danger to himself?
   A. A court order
   B. Implied consent
   C. Informed consent
   D. The presence of law enforcement

points to ponder

Object. 1-2.7, 1-1.3, 1-1.4, 1-3.11, 1-3.12, 4-8.1, 4-8.5, 4-8.7, 4-8.8, 4-8.9

You respond to an address that you have been to several times before, where you find a woman who has once again been beaten up. She is scared and bruised and may have broken ribs. Her children are scared and crying and hide when you enter. You clean up some of the woman's scrapes and apply cold packs to her face. She has once again refused transport to the hospital. While you are treating her, the door opens. Her husband has returned. He is holding a knife and threatening you, your partner, and his wife.

- What is your first concern? What precautions should you have taken? How would you deal with this situation?

online outlook

Any time you encounter an emotionally depressed patient, you must consider the possibility of suicide. To learn more about suicide and suicide prevention, complete Exercise 21 at the www.emtb.com.

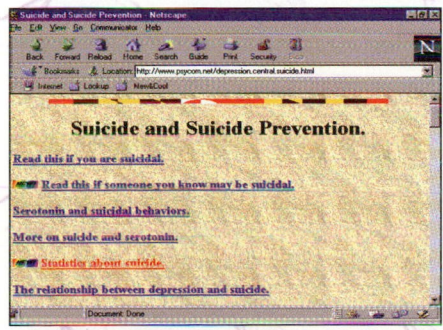

prep kit 21

Obstetrics and Gynecological Emergencies

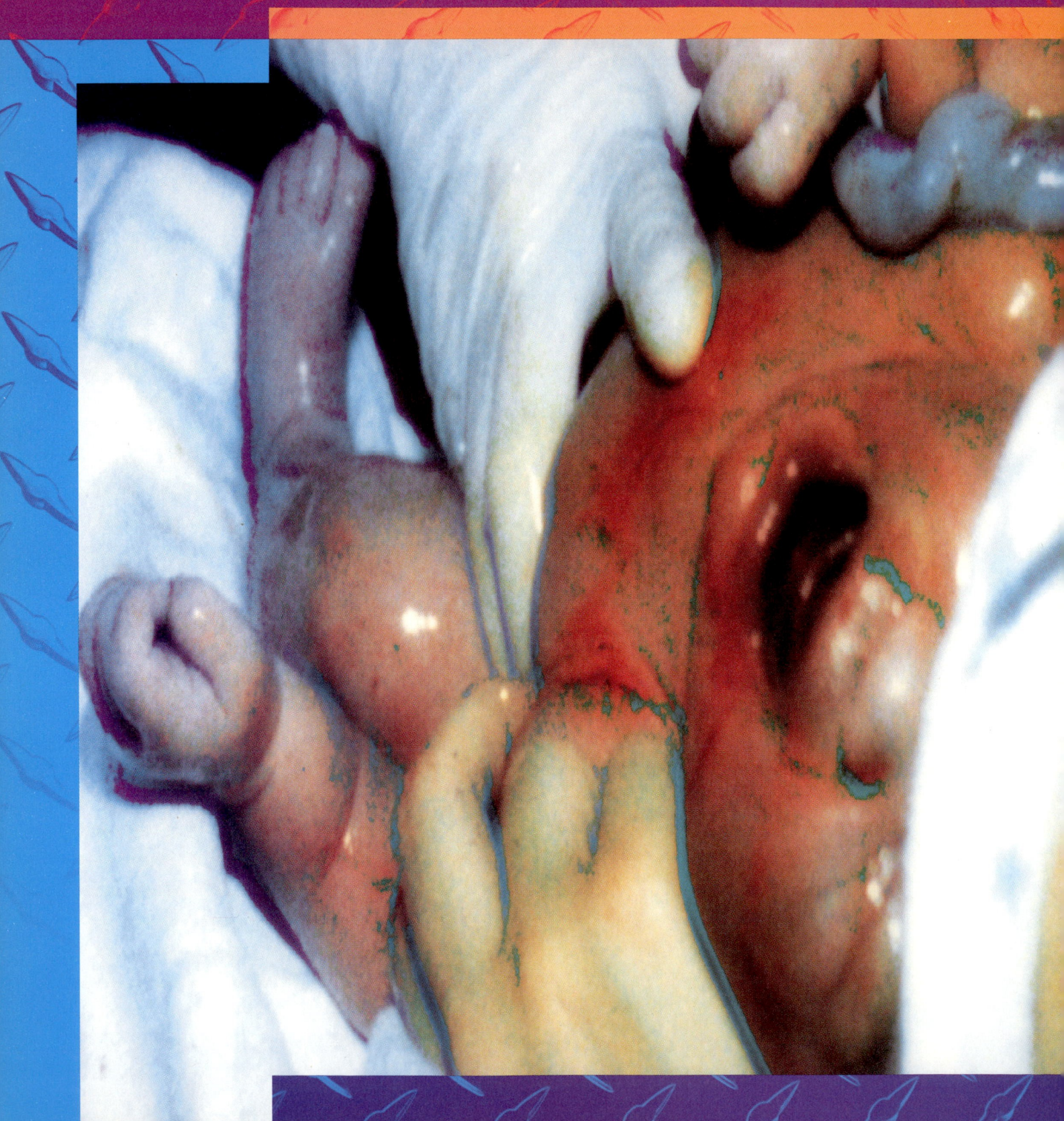

objectives

Cognitive

1. Identify the following structures: uterus, vagina, fetus, placenta, umbilical cord, amniotic sac, perineum.

2. Identify and explain the use of the contents of an obstetrics kit.

3. Identify predelivery emergencies.

4. State indications of an imminent delivery.

5. Differentiate the emergency medical care provided to a patient with predelivery emergencies from a normal delivery.

6. State the steps in the predelivery preparation of the mother.

7. Establish the relationship between body substance isolation and childbirth.

8. State the steps to assist in the delivery.

9. Describe care of the baby as the head appears.

10. Describe how and when to cut the umbilical cord.

11. Discuss the steps in the delivery of the placenta.

12. List the steps in the emergency medical care of the mother postdelivery.

13. Summarize neonatal resuscitation procedures.

14. Describe the procedures for the following abnormal deliveries: breech birth, prolapsed cord, limb presentation.

15. Differentiate the special considerations for multiple births.

16. Describe special considerations of meconium.

17. Describe special considerations of a premature baby.

18. Discuss the emergency medical care of a patient with a gynecological emergency.

Affective

19. Explain the rationale for understanding the implications of treating two patients (mother and baby).

Psychomotor

20. Demonstrate the steps to assist in the normal cephalic delivery.

21. Demonstrate necessary care procedures of the fetus as the head appears.

22. Demonstrate infant neonatal procedures.

23. Demonstrate postdelivery care of infant.

24. Demonstrate how and when to cut the umbilical cord.

25. Attend to the steps in the delivery of the placenta.

26. Demonstrate the postdelivery care of the mother.

27. Demonstrate the procedures for the following abnormal deliveries: vaginal bleeding, breech birth, prolapsed cord, limb presentation.

28. Demonstrate the steps in the emergency medical care of the mother with excessive bleeding.

29. Demonstrate completing a prehospital care report for patients with obstetrical/gynecological emergencies.

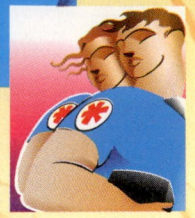

you are the emt

Rescue 6 please respond to the Jonestown Mall for a pregnant woman who is trapped in an elevator and believes she might be going into labor . . . her contractions started 20 minutes ago . . .

You may encounter any number of pregnancy-related complications in the field. Some are minor, some are serious, and some are even life-threatening for the mother, the baby, or both. This chapter will help prepare you for the miracle of birth (and its associated problems) and will help you answer the following questions:

1. When should you prepare for a field delivery rather than an immediate transport of the mother?
2. Which obstetrical/gynecological emergencies can and should be handled in the prehospital setting?

Obstetrics and Gynecological Emergencies

Most infants in the United States are delivered in a hospital, with doctors and nurses in attendance to care for not only the mother, but also the newborn infant. Occasionally, the birth process will move along faster than the mother expects, and you will find yourself with a decision to make: Should you stay on the scene and deliver the infant or transport the patient to the hospital? This chapter will tell you how to make this decision and how to proceed if on-scene delivery is necessary. It describes the normal process of childbirth and discusses common complications so that you will be prepared to handle both normal and problem deliveries. Next, it describes the evaluation and care of the newborn. Finally, the chapter discusses gynecological emergencies unrelated to childbirth.

Anatomy of the Female Reproductive System

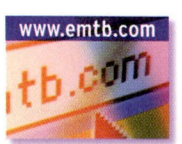

The **fetus** is the developing, unborn infant that grows inside the mother's uterus for 9 months. The **uterus**, or womb, is the muscular organ where the fetus grows (Figure 22-1). It is responsible for contractions during labor and ultimately helps to push the infant through the birth canal. The **birth canal** is made up of the vagina and the lower part or neck of the uterus, called the **cervix**. The cervix contains a mucous plug that seals the uterine opening, preventing contam-

ination from the outside world. When the cervix begins to dilate, this plug is discharged as pink-tinged mucus, or a **bloody show**. This "show" may signal the first stage of labor.

The **vagina** is the outermost cavity of a woman's reproductive system and forms the lower part of the birth canal. It is about 8 to 12 cm in length, begins at the cervix, and ends as an external opening of the body. Essentially, the vagina completes the passageway from the uterus to the outside world for the delivering infant. The **perineum** is the area of skin between the vagina and the anus. During birth, as the infant moves through the birth canal, the perineum will begin to bulge significantly.

As the fetus grows, it requires more and more nourishment, which it gets through the placenta. The **placenta**,

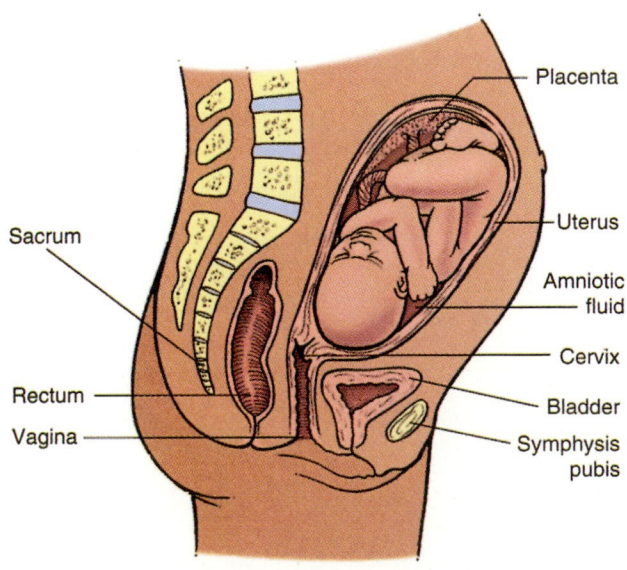

FIGURE 22-1 Anatomic structures of the pregnant woman.

originally a disk-shaped structure, is body tissue that attaches to the inner lining of the wall of the uterus. It is connected to the fetus by the umbilical cord. After delivery, the placenta, or afterbirth, separates from the uterus and is delivered. The **umbilical cord** is the infant's lifeline, connecting mother and infant through the placenta. It contains two arteries and one vein. These vessels supply blood to the fetus: the vein carries blood toward the heart (baby) and the arteries carry blood away from the heart (baby). Oxygen and other nutrients cross from the mother's circulation into the placenta and then along the umbilical cord to support the fetus as it grows. Carbon dioxide and waste products travel the same route in the opposite direction. The remarkable thing about this exchange is that the mother's blood and that of the fetus do not mix during the process.

The fetus develops inside a fluid-filled, baglike membrane called the **amniotic sac**, or bag of waters. The sac contains about 500 to 1,000 mL of amniotic fluid, which helps to insulate and protect the floating fetus as it develops. Released in a gush when the sac ruptures, usually at the onset of labor, this fluid helps to lubricate the birth canal and remove bacteria.

A full-term pregnancy is from 36 to 40 weeks, when counting from the first day of the last menstrual cycle. The pregnancy is divided into 3 trimesters of about 3 months each. Deliveries before 36 weeks are considered premature. As you will see, vaginal bleeding during the third trimester has a different significance from bleeding in the first trimester. Toward the end of the third trimester, the head of the fetus normally descends through the broad upper inlet of the mother's pelvis, positioning itself for the delivery.

Labor and Delivery

There are 3 stages of labor: dilation of the cervix, expulsion of the baby, and delivery of the placenta. The first stage begins with the onset of contractions and ends when the cervix is fully dilated. Because the cervix has to be stretched thin by uterine contractions until the opening is large enough for the infant to pass through into the vagina, the first stage is usually the longest, lasting an average of 16 hours for a first delivery. You will usually have time to transport the mother during the first stage of labor.

The onset of labor starts with contractions of the uterus. Other signs of the beginning of labor are the bloody show and the rupture of the amniotic sac, called breaking of the water. These events may occur before the first labor pain or later in the first stage of labor. The uterine contractions may not come at regular intervals at

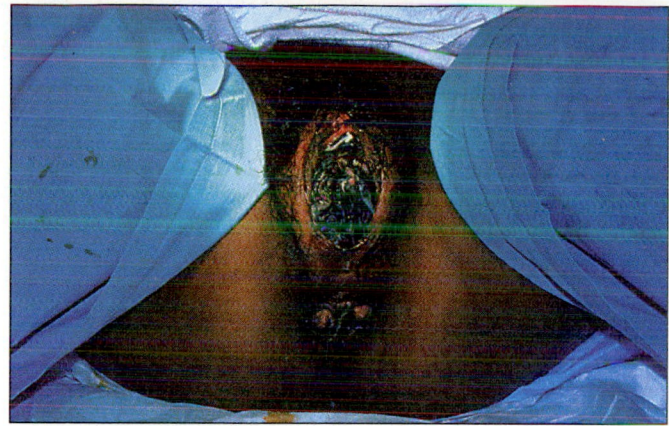

FIGURE 22-2 Crowning occurs when the infant's head appears at the vaginal opening.

first. The mother may think that she simply has a nagging backache. The frequency and intensity of true labor increase with time. The uterine contractions become more regular and last about 30 to 60 seconds each. The length of labor varies greatly. As a general rule, it is longer in a primigravida, a woman who is having her first infant, and becomes shorter in a multigravida, a woman who has previously given birth.

The second stage of labor begins when the cervix is fully dilated and ends when the infant is born. During this stage, you will have to make a decision about helping the mother to deliver at home or providing transport to the hospital. Because the infant has to move through the birth canal during this stage, the uterine contractions are usually closer together and last longer. Pressure on the rectum may make the mother feel as if she needs to have a bowel movement. She may also have the uncontrollable urge to push down. The perineum will begin to bulge significantly, and the top of the infant's head should begin to appear at the vaginal opening. This is called **crowning** (Figure 22-2).

The third stage begins with the birth of the infant and ends with the delivery of the placenta. This may take up to 30 minutes. Usually, you will not transport the mother during that time. It is important that you follow BSI techniques in all stages of labor.

Predelivery Emergencies

Most pregnant women are healthy, but some may be ill when they conceive or become ill during pregnancy. You may safely use oxygen to treat any heart or lung disease in the mother without harm to the fetus.

As the time for delivery nears, certain complications can occur. One of these is pre-eclampsia, or **pregnancy-induced hypertension**, a condition that can develop after the twentieth week of gestation, most commonly in primigravidas. This condition is characterized by the following signs and symptoms:

- Headache
- Seeing spots
- Swelling in the hands and feet
- Anxiety

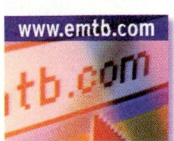 Another condition is **eclampsia**, convulsions that result from severe hypertension. To treat eclampsia, lay the mother on her side, maintain an airway, and provide supplemental oxygen; if vomiting occurs, suction the airway. Transport a pregnant patient with convulsions promptly. As usual, size up the situation and perform your initial assessment, history, and physical exam, and assess the baseline vital signs. Provide treatment based on signs and symptoms. If the patient is hypotensive, transport her on the left side. Transporting the mother in this position can prevent **supine hypotensive syndrome**, a problem in which low blood pressure develops when the mother lies supine resulting from compression by the weight of the fetus onto the inferior vena cava.

Hemorrhage from the vagina that occurs before labor begins may be very serious. In early pregnancy, it may be a sign of a spontaneous abortion, or miscarriage. Bleeding may be the sign of an **ectopic pregnancy**, a pregnancy that develops outside the uterus, most often in a fallopian tube. Ectopic pregnancy occurs about once in every 200 pregnancies. The leading cause of maternal death in the first trimester is internal hemorrhage into the abdomen following rupture of an ectopic pregnancy. For this reason, you should consider the possibility of an ectopic pregnancy in women who have missed a menstrual cycle and complain of sudden stabbing and usually unilateral pain in the lower abdomen. A history of pelvic inflammatory disease, tubal ligations, or previous ectopic pregnancies should heighten your suspicions.

In the later stages of pregnancy, hemorrhage may indicate problems with the placenta. In **placenta abruptio**, the placenta separates prematurely from the wall of the uterus (Figure 22-3). In **placenta previa**, the placenta develops over and covers the cervix (Figure 22-4).

Any bleeding from the vagina in a pregnant woman is a serious sign and should be treated in the hospital promptly. If the mother shows signs of shock, have her lie on her left side during transportation, and give her

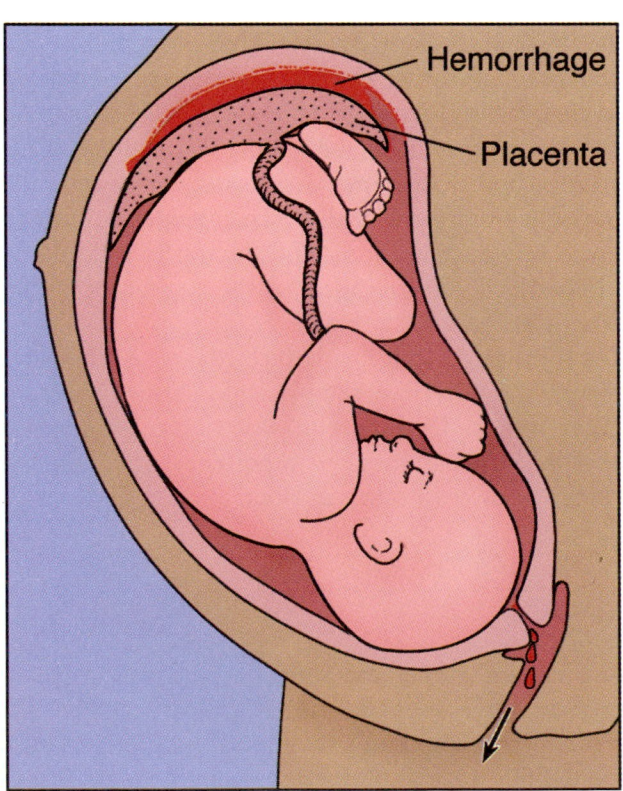

FIGURE 22-3 In placenta abruptio, the placenta separates prematurely from the wall of the uterus.

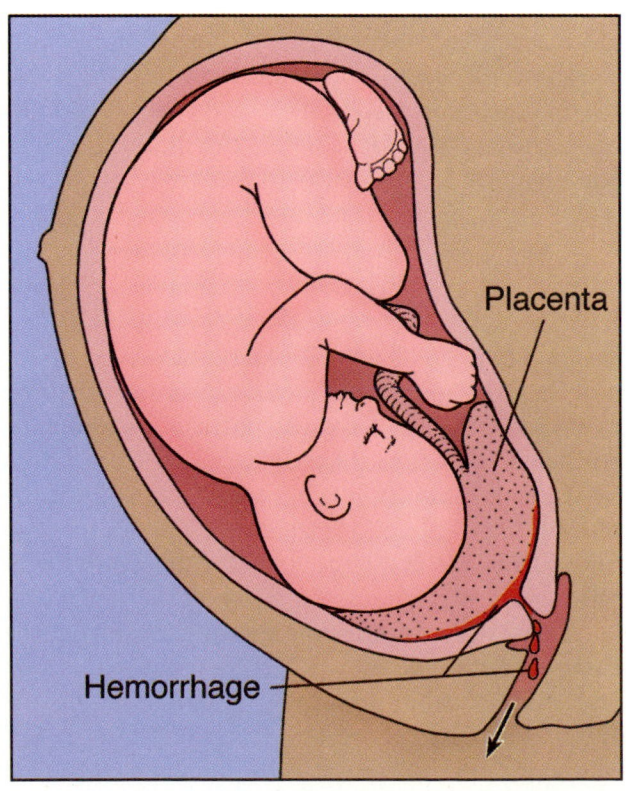

FIGURE 22-4 In placenta previa, the placenta develops over and covers the cervix.

> The leading cause of maternal death in the first trimester is internal hemorrhage into the abdomen following rupture of an ectopic pregnancy.

high-flow oxygen. Place a sterile pad or sanitary napkin over the vagina, and replace it as often as necessary. Save the pads so that hospital personnel can estimate how much blood she has lost. Also save any tissue that may be passed from the vagina. Do not put anything into the vagina.

When a pregnant woman is involved in an automobile accident, severe hemorrhage may occur from injuries to the pregnant uterus. The resulting oxygen deprivation can cause grave injury to the fetus. Promptly evaluate and transport a pregnant accident victim; support the airway, and if there is any sign of bleeding, administer high-flow oxygen. Have the mother lie on her left side rather than on her back; this will relieve the pressure of the uterus on intra-abdominal organs, especially the inferior vena cava and abdominal aorta. Pregnant women have an increased amount of blood volume. Therefore, a pregnant trauma patient may have a significant amount of blood loss before showing signs of shock. However, the infant may be in trouble well before this. Often, if the mother has sustained serious trauma, the blood supply to the fetus is reduced so that the body can supply an adequate amount of blood to the mother. In most cases, the only chance to save the infant is to adequately resuscitate the mother.

Preparing for Delivery

Consider delivering the patient at the scene in the following circumstances:

- When delivery can be expected within a few minutes
- When a natural disaster, bad weather, or some other type of catastrophe makes it impossible to reach the hospital
- When no transportation is available

How do you determine whether delivery is going to occur within a few minutes? First, look for crowning. Second, ask the mother these questions:

- How long have you been pregnant?
- When are you due?

- Is this your first baby?
- Are you having contractions? How far apart are the contractions? How long do the contractions last?
- Do you feel as though you have to strain or move your bowels?
- Have you had any showing or spotting?
- Have you had any gushing of fluid from the vagina?
- Were any of your previous children delivered by cesarean section?

Also consider asking the following questions:

- Have you had a complicated pregnancy in the past?
- What did your last ultrasound (sonogram) show?
- Do you use drugs or take any medications?
- Is there any possibility that this is a multiple birth?
- Does your doctor expect any complications?

If this is not the patient's first child, she may be able to tell you whether she is about to deliver. If she says that she is, make immediate preparations for delivery. Otherwise, does she have a rock-hard abdomen? Does she say that she has to move her bowels or feels the need to push? If so, the infant's head is probably pressing on the rectum, and delivery is about to occur. At this point, you should inspect the vagina to determine whether crowning has occurred; if so, delivery is imminent. Do not touch the vaginal area until you are sure that delivery is, in fact, imminent. In general, do not touch vaginal areas except during delivery (under certain circumstances) and when your partner is present. Spread the mother's legs apart gently, explaining that you are doing so to decide whether she should be delivered immediately or transported to the hospital.

Once labor has begun, there is no way it can be slowed down or stopped. Never attempt to hold the mother's legs together. To do so would only complicate the delivery. Do not let her go to the bathroom. Instead, reassure her that the sensation of needing to move her bowels is normal and that it means she is about to deliver.

If you decide to deliver at the scene, remember that you are only *assisting* the mother with the delivery. Your part is to help, guide, and support the infant as it is born. Remember to use BSI techniques at all times. Try to limit distractions for yourself and for the mother. You want to appear calm and reassuring while protecting the mother's modesty. Most important, recognize when the situation is beyond your level of training. If delivery is imminent with crowning, contact medical control for a decision to deliver on site. If you are on site and delivery still does not occur within 10 minutes, contact medical control again regarding permission to transport. When in doubt, contact medical control for further guidance. Always recognize your own limitations, and when unsure about what to do, transport even if delivery must occur during transport.

Delivery at the scene is usually a two-person job. If you are the only EMT-B available, you must seek assistance from a nurse, police officer, neighbor, or family member who may have had experience in childbirth. If this requires leaving the scene, you must send someone else. Never leave the mother once the decision has been made to deliver at the scene.

Your emergency vehicle should always be equipped with a sterile emergency delivery pack containing the following items (Figure 22-5):

- 1 pair of surgical scissors
- 3 hemostats or special cord clamps
- Umbilical tape
- A small rubber bulb syringe
- 5 or more towels
- 1 dozen 4" x 4" gauze sponges and/or 1 dozen 2" x 10" gauze sponges
- 2 to 4 pairs of sterile latex gloves
- 1 infant blanket
- Sanitary napkins
- An infant size breathing bag and face mask
- Goggles
- A plastic bag

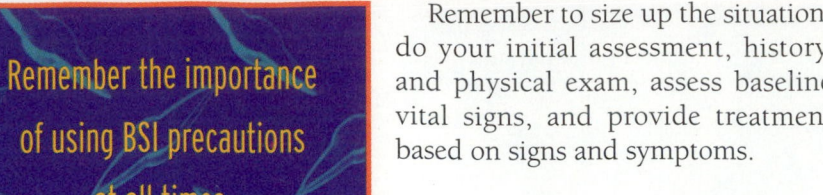

Remember the importance of using BSI precautions at all times.

Remember to size up the situation, do your initial assessment, history, and physical exam, assess baseline vital signs, and provide treatment based on signs and symptoms.

Patient position. The mother's clothing should be pushed up to her waist or, if she is wearing trousers and undergarments, removed. Remember to limit the mother's exposure and preserve her modesty as much as you can while helping her to move into a semi-Fowler's position. Place the mother on a firm surface that is padded with blankets, folded sheets, or towels. Put a pillow or blankets beneath her hips to elevate them about 2" to 4". It is sometimes better to put a pillow under one hip to allow the mother to turn to one side. This may also make it easier to suction the infant once it is born. Support the mother's head, neck, and upper back with pillows and blankets so that she does not feel as though she is being placed upside down. If delivery is occurring in an automobile, the patient should lie on the seat, with one foot on the floor and the other on the seat, with the upper knee and hip bent (Figure 22-6). A long backboard may provide the firm surface that is needed in these unusual surroundings.

If the emergency delivery is occurring at home, you should move the mother to a sturdy flat surface. You will find it easier to work on a firm surface than on a bed. Elevate the mother's hips, and support her head with one or two pillows. Have her keep her legs and hips flexed, with her feet flat on the surface beneath her and her knees spread apart. Track the progression of the delivery closely at all times; you do not want a precipitous delivery, when the crowning head pops out uncontrollably, to occur.

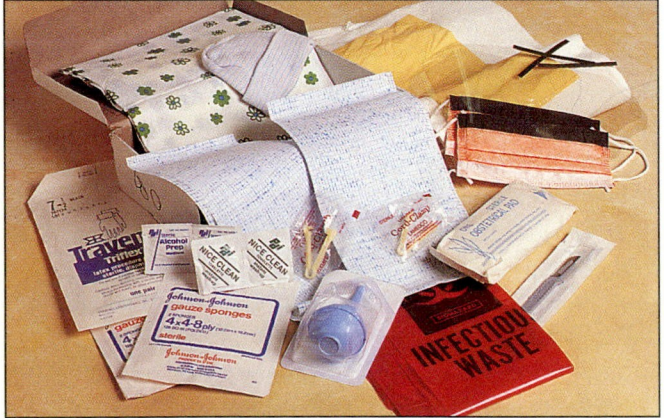

FIGURE 22-5 Your unit should contain a sterile emergency delivery pack. See the list above for the items it should include.

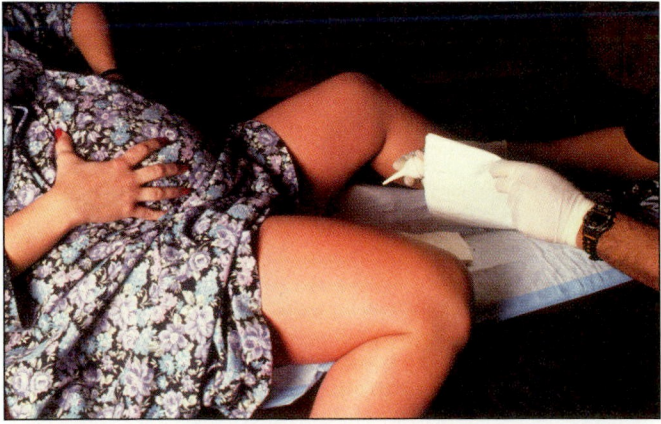

FIGURE 22-6 For delivery in a car, have the mother lie on the seat with one foot on the floor and the other on the seat. Make sure the upper knee is bent and the upper hip is flexed.

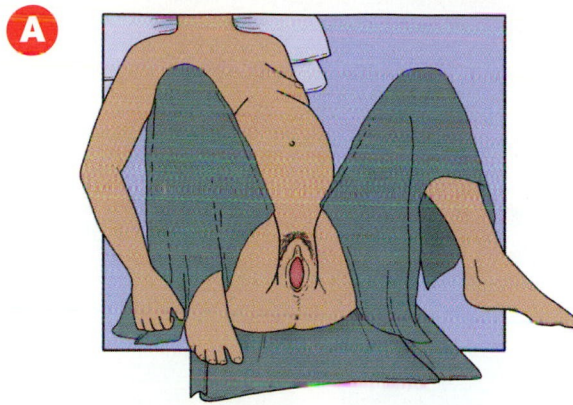

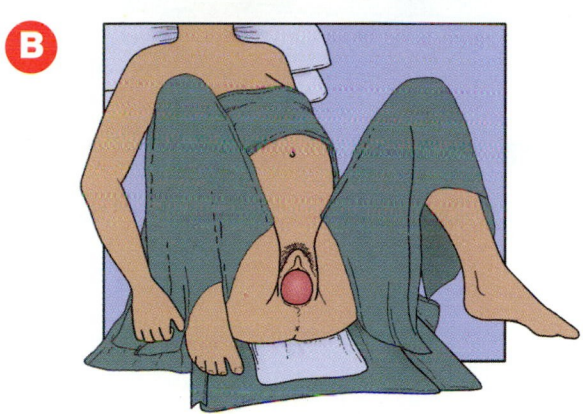

FIGURE 22-7 A: Place sheets or towels under the mother, elevate the mother's hips, and support her head with one or two pillows. **B:** Use sterile sheets and towels from the delivery pack to make a clean delivery field. Place one sheet under her buttocks, drape the other over her abdomen, and place drapes over the thighs.

Preparing the delivery field. Take the following steps to prepare the area where the infant will be born (Figure 22-7):

1. As time allows, place towels or sheets on the floor around the delivery area to help soak up the amniotic fluid that will be released when the amniotic sac ruptures. Note that the amniotic sac may have ruptured before you arrived.

2. Thoroughly wash your hands, put on goggles, mask, and gown, and open the emergency delivery pack carefully so that its contents remain sterile.

3. Put on the sterile gloves.

4. Use the sterile sheets and towels from the emergency delivery pack to make a sterile delivery field. Place 1 sheet or towel under the mother's buttocks, and unfold it toward her feet. The other sheet should be draped over her abdomen and upper legs. Alternatively, you can use 3 sheets: (1) folded under the buttocks, (2) placed between the legs, just below the vagina, and (3) placed across the abdomen.

Delivering the Baby

Be sure that your emergency delivery pack is close by for quick access, but make sure it is far enough away to avoid being contaminated by gushing amniotic fluid.

Your partner should be at the mother's head to comfort, soothe, and reassure her during the delivery. The mother may want to grip someone's hand. She may yell, cry, or say nothing at all. It is not uncommon for the mother to become nauseated and vomit. If this occurs, have your partner turn the mother's head to the side so that her mouth and airway can be cleared manually or with suction, as needed.

You must continually assess the mother for infant crowning. Do not allow a precipitous delivery to occur. Position yourself so that you can see the vagina at all times. For example, you can kneel next to the patient's right side if you are right-handed or at the left side if you are left-handed. Time the mother's contractions from the beginning of one to the beginning of the next to determine the frequency of the contractions. In addition, time the duration of each contraction. You do this by feeling the mother's abdomen from the moment the contraction begins (uterus/abdomen tightening) to the moment it ends (uterus/abdomen relaxing). Remind the patient to take quick, short breaths during each contraction but not to strain. In between contractions, encourage the mother to rest and breathe deeply through her mouth.

Delivering the Head

Watch the head as it begins to exit the vagina, as it must be supported as it emerges. See Skill Drill, "Delivering the Baby" (Figure 22-8). It may take two, three, or more contractions for the delivery of the head to occur from the time it begins to crown. Once it is obvious that the head is coming out farther with each contraction, you should place your gloved right hand (or your left hand if you are left-handed) over the emerging bony parts of the head and exert very gentle pressure on it, decreasing the pressure slightly between contractions. This will allow the head to come out smoothly and prevent it and the rest of the infant from suddenly popping out during a strong contraction, possibly causing injury. You may want to move the patient's feet so that you are between the patient's legs during the delivery. Be careful that you do not poke your fingers into the infant's eyes or into the two soft spots, called *fontanels*, on the head. One fontanel is located at the front of the head, near the brow, and one is near the back of the head. The brain is covered only by skin and membranes at these spots.

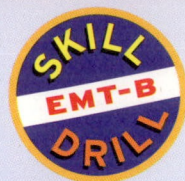

Delivering the Baby

Figure 22-8

1

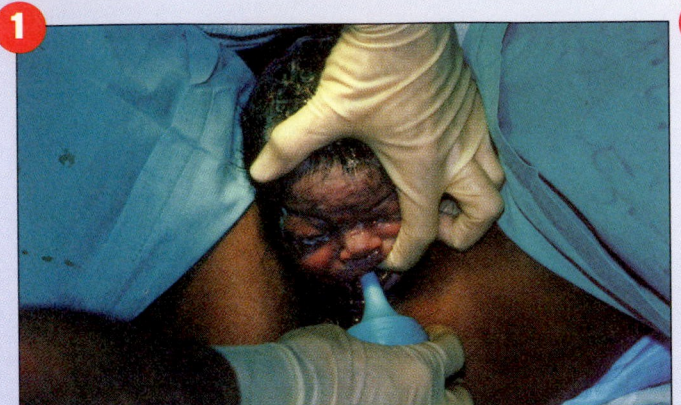

Support the head as it emerges, placing your gloved hand over the emerging bony parts of the head. Suction fluid from the mouth first, then the nostrils.

2

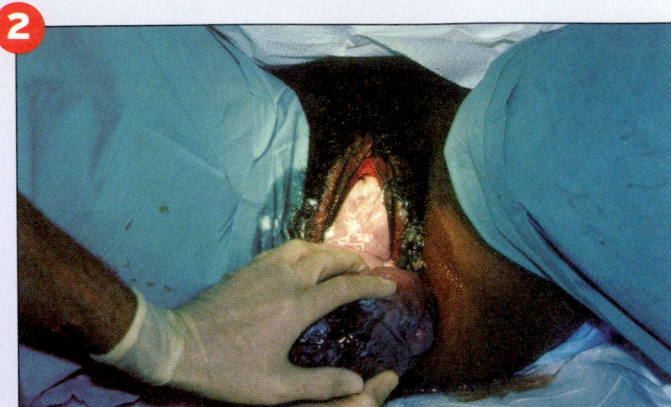

Once the head is delivered, the upper shoulder will be visible.

3

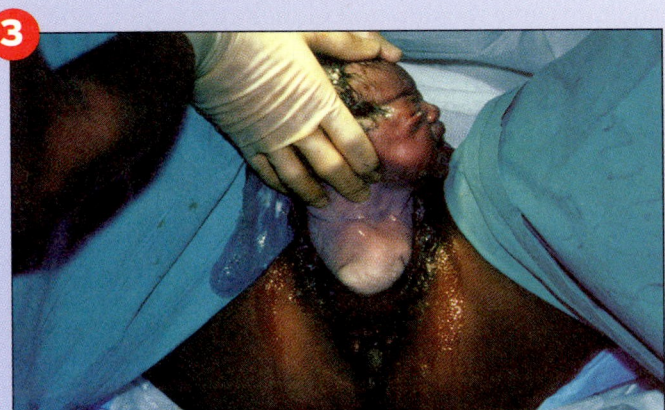

Support the head and upper body as the shoulders deliver.

4

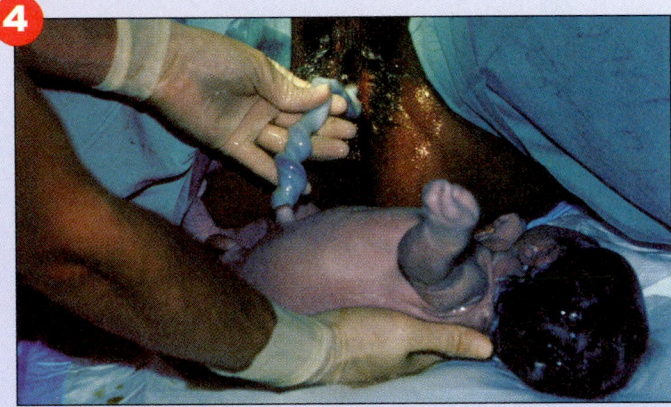

Once the body is delivered, handle the infant firmly but gently. It will be slippery. Make sure the baby's neck is in a neutral position to keep the airway open.

5

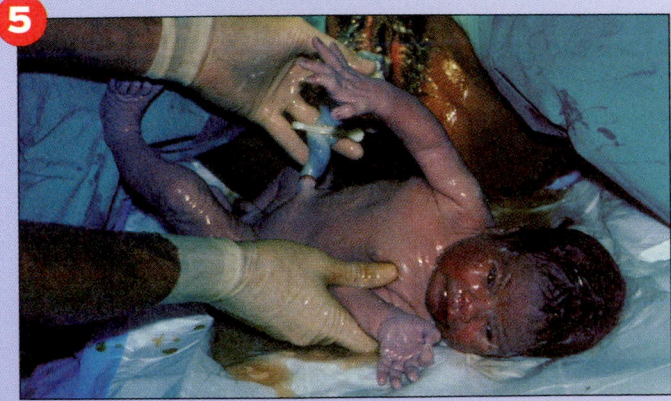

Place the clamps about 2" to 4" apart. Once they are firmly in place, cut between the clamps.

6

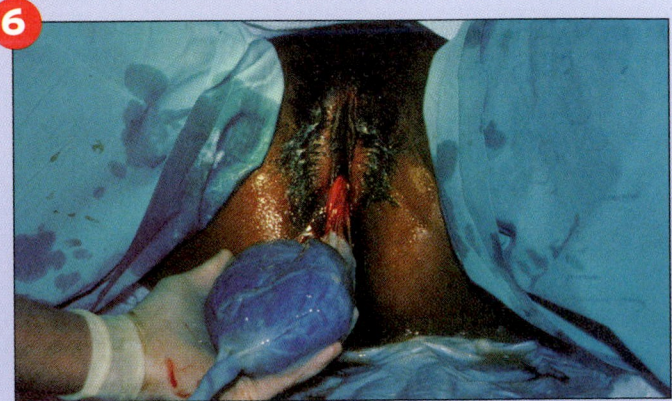

The placenta delivers itself, usually within a few minutes of birth. Never pull on the end of the umbilical cord in an attempt to speed delivery of the placenta.

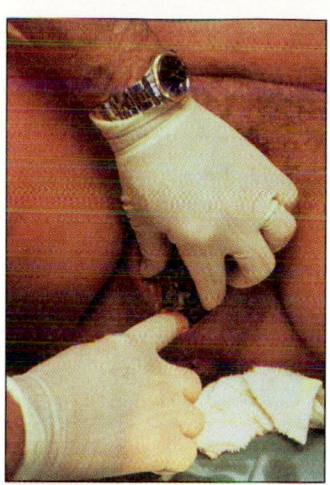

FIGURE 22-9 Applying gentle pressure on the perineum may reduce the risk of tearing as the infant emerges.

Gentle pressure, exerted horizontally across the perineum with a sterile gauze pad, may reduce the risk of tearing as the infant is emerging (Figure 22-9). Also be prepared for the possibility that feces may come out because of the pressure on the rectum.

Unruptured amniotic sac. Usually, the amniotic sac will break or rupture at the beginning of labor. The sac may also rupture during contractions. If the amniotic sac has not ruptured by this point, it will appear as a fluid-filled sac (like a water balloon) emerging from the vagina. This situation is serious, as the sac will suffocate the baby if it is not removed. If it has not spontaneously ruptured, you may puncture the sac with a clamp, away from the baby's face, only as the head is crowning, not before. As the sac is punctured, amniotic fluid will gush out. Push the ruptured sac away from the infant's face as the head is delivered. Clear the baby's mouth and nose immediately, using the bulb syringe and gauze sponge. If the amniotic fluid is greenish instead of clear or has a foul odor, make note of this in the information you will relay to medical control. Once the head has been delivered, it usually rotates to one side or the other rather than straight up and down.

Umbilical cord around the neck. As soon as the head is delivered, use the index finger of your other hand to feel whether the umbilical cord is wrapped around the neck. This commonly is called a <u>nuchal cord</u>. A nuchal cord that is wound tightly around the neck could cause the infant to strangle. It must therefore be released from the neck immediately (Figure 22-10). Usually, you can slip the cord gently over the infant's delivered head (or over the shoulder, if necessary). If not, you must cut it by placing two clamps about 2" apart on the cord and cutting the cord between the clamps. If the cord is wrapped more than once around the neck, a rare event, you have to clamp and cut only once; then you can unwrap the cord from around the neck. Handle the cord very carefully; it is fragile and easily torn. Do not let the clamps come off until the ends of the cord have been tied. Fortunately, the cord is usually not wrapped around the infant's neck and does not have to be cut until after the entire infant has been delivered. However, you must always check for a nuchal cord.

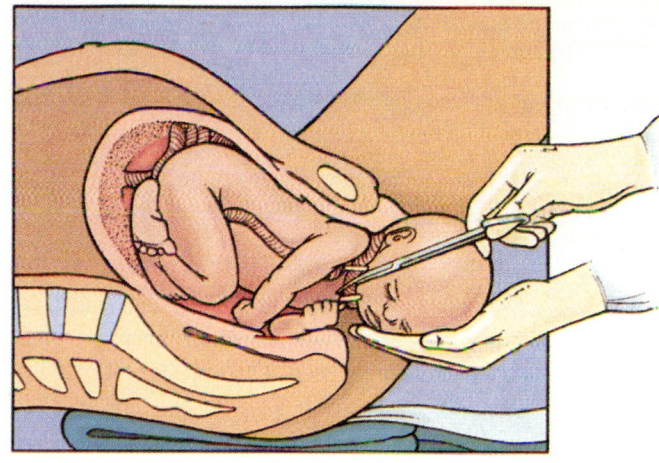

FIGURE 22-10 If the umbilical cord is wound tightly around the baby's neck, it must be released immediately by either slipping it gently over the infant's delivered head or, if necessary, by placing two clamps about 2" apart on the cord and cutting between the clamps.

Now that you have delivered the infant's head and verified that no nuchal cord is present, you will need to suction the amniotic fluids from the infant's airway before the delivery proceeds. You must ask the mother not to push while you are doing this, although her desire to do so will be very strong. While supporting the infant's head with one hand, quickly and efficiently suction the fluid from the mouth first and then the nostrils. If you suction the nostrils first, you may stimulate the infant to aspirate the fluid in the mouth or pharynx; since infants are nose breathers, any stimulation of the nose will cause a gasping response. In suctioning the airway, fully compress the bulb syringe before it is inserted 1" to $1\frac{1}{2}$" into the infant's mouth, then release the bulb to suction fluids and mucus into the syringe. Make sure the syringe does not touch the back of the mouth. Discard the fluid into a towel, and repeat the procedure, suctioning the mouth and nostrils two or three times each, or until they are clear.

Delivering the Body

By the time you are finished suctioning, the mother will most likely be pushing again, and the upper shoulder will be visible in the vagina. The infant's head is the largest part of the body. Once it is born, the rest of the infant usually delivers easily. Support the head and upper body as the shoulders deliver. Do *not* pull the infant from the birth canal. Then the abdomen and hips will appear; once these deliver, support them with your other hand. Grasp the infant's feet as they are born. Now the infant is being well supported with both hands. Handle the infant firmly but carefully. It will be slippery with a white, cheesy substance, called *vernix*

> A newborn's body temperature can drop very quickly, so dry and wrap the infant as soon as possible. Only then will you clamp and cut the umbilical cord.

caseosa. Take particular care not to squeeze the neck or chest.

Postdelivery Care

As soon as the entire infant is born, wrap it immediately in a towel, and place it on one side, with the head slightly lower than the rest of its body. Wrap the baby so that only the face is exposed, making sure that the top of the head is covered. Also make sure that the baby's neck is in a neutral position so the airway remains open. Newborn babies are very sensitive to cold, so if it is at all possible, you should keep the blanket warm before you use it. Use a sterile gauze pad to wipe the infant's mouth, and once again suction the mouth and nose. Suctioning the nose is particularly important, since babies breathe through their noses. If you prefer, you can cradle the infant in your arm while doing this, but always keep the head slightly downward to help prevent aspiration. After suctioning, keep the infant at the same level as the mother's vagina until the umbilical cord is cut. If the infant is higher than the vagina, blood will be siphoned from the infant through the umbilical cord back into the placenta.

A newborn's body temperature can drop very quickly, so dry and wrap the infant as soon as possible. Only then will you clamp and cut the umbilical cord.

Once the infant is born, the umbilical cord is of no further use to either mother or infant. Postdelivery care of the umbilical cord is important, as infection is easily transmitted through the cord to the baby. Using the two clamps in the emergency kit, clamp the cord somewhere between the mother and the infant, preferably four fingers' width from the infant. Place the clamps about 2″ to 6″ apart. Once they are firmly in place, cut the cord between them with the sterile scissors, using great care. Remember, the cord is fragile; if handled too roughly, it could be torn from the infant's abdomen, resulting in a fatal hemorrhage. Once the clamps are in place, there is no need to rush.

After you have cut the cord, tie the end coming from the infant. If it was a nuchal cord and cut during delivery, now is the time to tie it. Do not use ordinary string or twine, which will cut through the soft, fragile tissues

of the cord. Place a loop of the special "umbilical tape" around the cord about 1 inch nearer to the infant than to the clamp. Tighten the tape slowly so that it does not cut the cord, then tie it firmly with a square knot. Cut the ends of the tape, but do not remove either clamp. The part of the cord that is coming out of the mother's vagina is attached to the placenta and will be delivered when the placenta delivers.

By now, the infant should be pink and breathing on its own. Give the infant, wrapped in a warm blanket, to your partner; he or she can monitor the infant and complete its initial care. Alternatively, you can give the infant to the mother if she is alert and in stable condition, if you are allowed to do so by local protocol. The mother may want to begin breastfeeding at this time. You need to return your attention to the mother and the delivery of the placenta.

Delivery of the Placenta

The placenta is attached to the end of the umbilical cord that is coming out of the mother's vagina. Again, you need only assist. Like the infant, the placenta delivers itself, usually within a few minutes of the birth, though it may take as long as 30 minutes. You can speed up the process by gently massaging the mother's abdomen with a firm, circular motion. The abdominal skin will be wrinkled and very soft. You should be able to feel a firm, grapefruit-sized mass in the lower abdomen. This is the uterus, with the placenta inside. As you massage the uterus, it will contract and become firmer. You can also place the infant at the mother's breast to nurse, which stimulates the uterus to contract. *Never pull on the end of the umbilical cord in an attempt to speed delivery of the placenta.* You may tear the cord, the placenta, or both and cause serious, perhaps life-threatening, hemorrhage.

Once the placenta delivers, inspect it carefully. The normal placenta is round, about 7″ in diameter and about 1″ thick. One surface is smooth and covered with a shiny membrane; the other surface is rough and divided into lobes (Figure 22-11). Wrap the entire placenta and cord in a towel, place them into a plastic bag, and take them to the hospital. Hospital personnel will examine them to make certain that the entire placenta has been delivered. If a piece of the placenta has been retained inside the mother, it could cause persistent bleeding or infection.

After delivery of the placenta and before transport, place a sterile pad or sanitary napkin over the vagina and straighten the mother's legs. Before taking her, the infant, and the placenta to the hospital, take a minute to congratulate the mother and thank anyone who

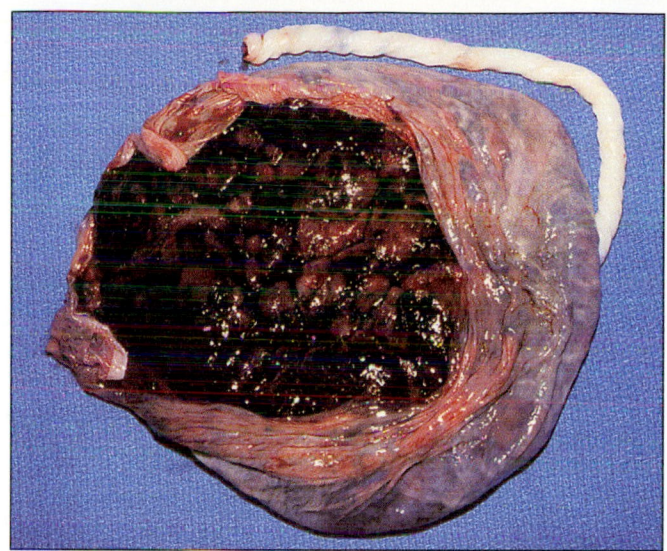

FIGURE 22-11 The normal placenta is round, about 7" in diameter and 1" thick. One surface is smooth; the other is rough and divided into lobes.

assisted. In writing your medical report, be sure to record the time of birth for the birth certificate.

Some bleeding, usually less than 250 mL (about 2 cups), occurs before the placenta delivers. The following are emergency situations:

- More than 30 minutes elapse, and the placenta has not delivered.
- There is more than 250 mL of bleeding before delivery of the placenta.
- There is significant bleeding after the delivery of the placenta.

If one or more of these events occur, transport mother and infant to the hospital promptly. Place a sterile pad or sanitary napkin over the mother's vagina, place her in Trendelenburg's (shock) position, administer oxygen, and monitor her vital signs closely. Never put anything into the vagina.

Neonatal Evaluation and Resuscitation

Remember that before you handle a newborn infant, put on gloves and follow BSI techniques. As soon as the infant is born, you must complete an initial assessment. A newborn infant will usually begin breathing spontaneously within 15 to 20 seconds after birth. If not, gently tap or flick the soles of the feet or rub the baby's back to stimulate breathing. If the baby does not breathe after 10 to 15 seconds, begin resuscitation

efforts. You should use the same scoring system that physicians in hospitals use to assess the status of the infant: the *Apgar* scoring system. This system assigns a number value (0, 1, or 2) to each of five areas of activity of the newborn infant:

- **A**ppearance. Shortly after birth, the skin of a Caucasian infant and the mucous membranes of a dark-skinned infant should turn pink. Infants often have cyanosis of the extremities for a few minutes after birth, but hands and feet should "pink up" quickly. Blue skin all over or blue mucous membranes signal a central cyanosis.

- **P**ulse. If a stethoscope is unavailable, you can measure pulsations in the umbilical cord with your fingers. Obviously, the infant with no pulse requires immediate CPR.

- **G**rimace or irritability. Grimacing, crying, or withdrawing in response to stimuli is normal in a newborn and indicates that the infant is doing well. The way to test this is to snap a finger against the sole of the infant's foot.

- **A**ctivity or muscle tone. The degree of muscle tone indicates the oxygenation of the infant's tissues. Normally, the hips and knees are flexed at birth, and, to some degree, the infant will resist attempts to straighten them out. A newborn should not be floppy or limp.

- **R**espirations. Normally, the newborn's respirations are regular and rapid, with a good strong cry. If the respirations are slow, shallow, or labored or if the cry is weak, the infant may have respiratory insufficiency and need assistance with ventilations. Complete absence of respirations or crying is obviously a very serious sign; in addition to assisted ventilations, CPR may be necessary.

APGAR scoring system

- Appearance.
- Pulse.
- Grimace or irritability.
- Activity or muscle tone.
- Respirations.

TABLE 22-1   Apgar Scoring System

Area of Activity	Score 2	Score 1	Score 0
Appearance	Entire infant is pink.	Body is pink, but hands and feet remain blue.	Entire infant is blue or pale.
Pulse	More than 100 beats/min	Fewer than 100 beats/min	Absent pulse
Grimace or Irritability	Infant cries and tries to move foot away from finger snapped against its sole.	Infant gives a weak cry in response to stimulus.	Infant does not cry or react to stimulus.
Activity or Muscle Tone	Infant resists attempts to to straighten out hips and knees.	Infant makes weak attempts to resist straightening.	Infant is completely limp, with no muscle tone.
Respiration	Rapid respirations	Slow respirations	Absent respirations

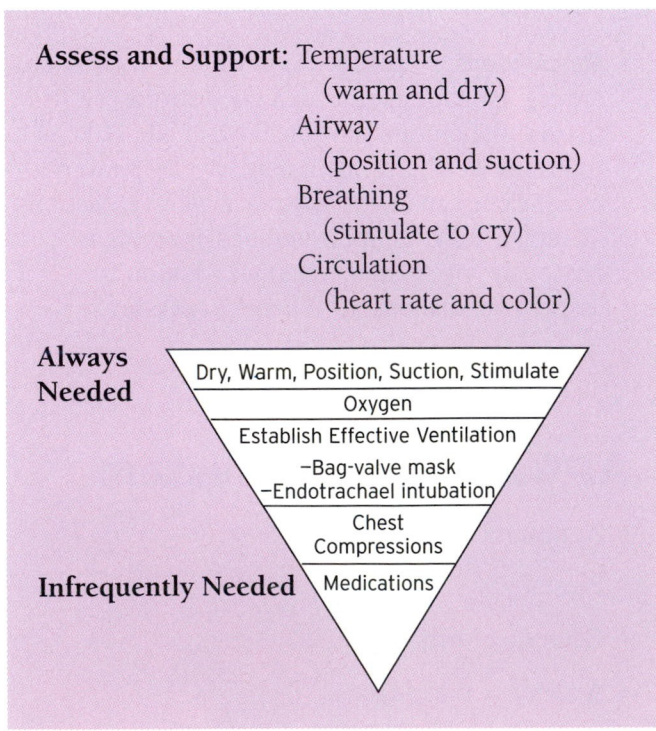

Assess and Support: Temperature
(warm and dry)
Airway
(position and suction)
Breathing
(stimulate to cry)
Circulation
(heart rate and color)

Always Needed

Dry, Warm, Position, Suction, Stimulate
Oxygen
Establish Effective Ventilation
–Bag-valve mask
–Endotrachael intubation
Chest Compressions
Medications

Infrequently Needed

FIGURE 22-12 Guidelines for neonatal resuscitation as recommended by the American Heart Association.

The total of the five numbers is the <u>**Apgar score**</u>. A perfect score is 10. The Apgar score should be calculated at 1 minute and 5 minutes after birth. Most infants will have a score of 7 or 8 at one minute and a score of 8 to 10 four minutes later. Table 22-1 shows how to calculate an Apgar score.

Consider the following delivery situation. You have assisted a delivery or arrived to find that a delivery has already taken place. You now have two patients who need assessment and care: the mother and the infant. Follow these steps in assessing the infant:

1. **Quickly calculate the Apgar score** to establish a baseline for the infant's vital functions.

2. **Suctioning and stimulation** should result in an immediate increase in respirations. If they do not, you must begin artificial ventilation. Resuscitation efforts should follow the 1994 guidelines established by the American Heart Association (Figure 22-12). Unlike adults, who may have a sudden cardiac arrest, infants who get into trouble usually have a respiratory arrest first. Therefore, it is essential to keep the infant ventilating and oxygenating well.

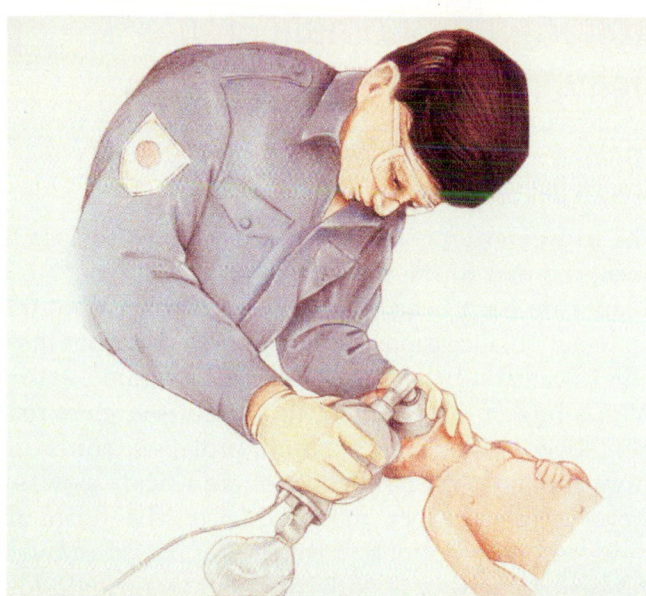

FIGURE 22-13 Use an infant mask and bag, ensuring that you cover both the infant's nose and mouth. Ventilate with high-flow oxygen at a rate of 40 to 60 breaths/min.

3. **If the infant is breathing well,** you should next check the pulse rate by feeling the brachial pulse or the pulsations in the umbilical cord. The pulse rate should be at least 100 beats/min. If it is not, begin artificial ventilation. This alone may increase the infant's heart rate. Reassess respirations and heart rate at least every 30 seconds to make sure that the pulse rate is increasing and that respirations are becoming spontaneous.

4. **Assess the infant's skin color.** You are looking for the central cyanosis. If you find it, administer high-flow oxygen (10 to 15 L/min) through oxygen tubing held close to the infant's face.

5. **Remember, you now have two patients.** You should request a second unit as soon as you determine that the infant is having problems.

In situations in which assisted ventilations are needed, you should use an infant BVM device (Figure 22-13). Cover the infant's mouth *and* nose with the mask and begin ventilations with high-flow oxygen at a rate of 40 to 60 breaths/min. Make sure you have a good mask-to-face seal. Using gentle pressure, make the chest rise with each breath. Initially, it may be necessary to bypass the pop-off valve to accomplish this. After the initial resistance, the pressures needed should not be more than 30 to 40 cm H_2O.

Assisted ventilation has been successful if you see both sides of the chest rise and hear breath sounds. If the infant starts to breathe on its own, attach an oxygen tubing mask and watch for its skin or mucous membranes to become pink. After 15 to 30 seconds of adequate respirations, assess the heart rate. If the heart rate is at least 100 beats/min and the infant is breathing spontaneously, you can stop the assisted ventilations. Do not stop suddenly. Instead, gradually decrease the rate and pressure of the assisted ventilations to determine whether the infant will continue to breathe adequately on its own. If not, continue assisted ventilations until it does. You may find that gently stimulating the infant by rubbing it will help it to maintain its respirations.

If the heart rate is less than 60 beats/min or between 60 and 80 beats/min (i.e., no increase in pulse rate), despite assisted ventilations, continue assisted ventilations and start cardiac compressions. Even though this infant has a pulse, the rate and blood output from the heart are not adequate for the needs of a newborn.

There are two ways to give chest compressions to an infant. The first way is to place both hands around the infant so that your thumbs are resting on the middle third of the sternum and the rest of your fingers encircle the thorax. This is illustrated in the Skill Drill, "Giving Chest Compressions to an Infant" (Figure 22-14). In premature or very small infants, you may have to place one thumb over the other to perform chest compressions. Your thumbs should be placed one finger width below an imaginary line drawn between the nipples on the middle third of the sternum. Press the two thumbs gently against the sternum. The newborn's chest is easy to compress. Use only enough force to compress the sternum $1/2''$ to $3/4''$. If your hands are too small to encircle the chest, you should use the middle and ring fingers of one hand to provide the compressions while your other hand supports the infant's back.

Assisted ventilation is done during a pause after every third compression. You should perform a combined total of 120 ventilations and compressions per minute, 90 compressions to 30 ventilations. Keep in mind that ventilation is absolutely crucial to the successful resuscitation of the neonate.

If the infant does not begin breathing on its own or does not have an adequate heart rate, continue CPR on the way to the hospital. Once CPR has been started, do not stop until the infant responds with adequate respirations and heart rates or is pronounced dead by a physician. Do not give up! Many infants have survived without brain damage after prolonged periods of effective CPR. If the infant presents in distress, you should not wait to measure the Apgar score at 1 minute, but begin appropriate care measures immediately.

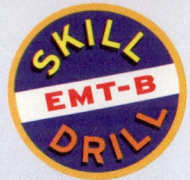

Giving Chest Compressions to an Infant
Figure 22-14

Chest compressions can be done in two ways in an infant.

1

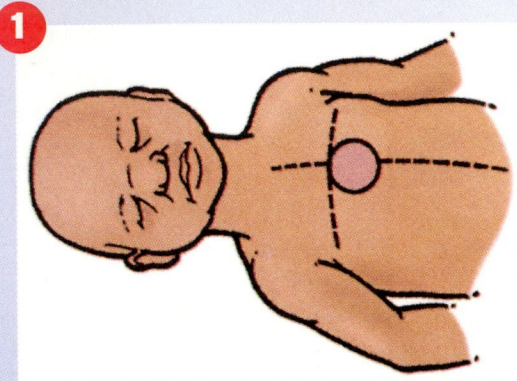

First find the proper position on the infant's chest, one finger width below an imaginary line drawn between the nipples on the middle third of the sternum.

2

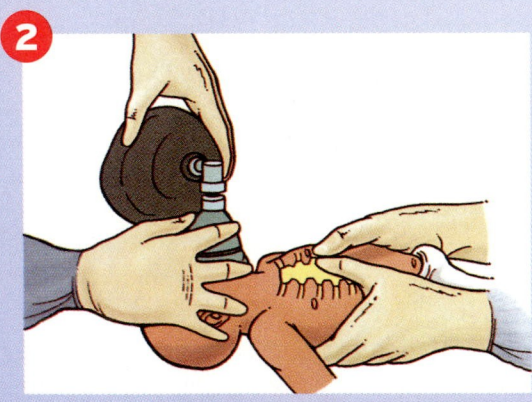

On a normal, full-term-sized infant, place both hands around the infant so that your thumbs are side by side, resting on the middle third of the sternum, and the rest of your fingers encircle the thorax.

3

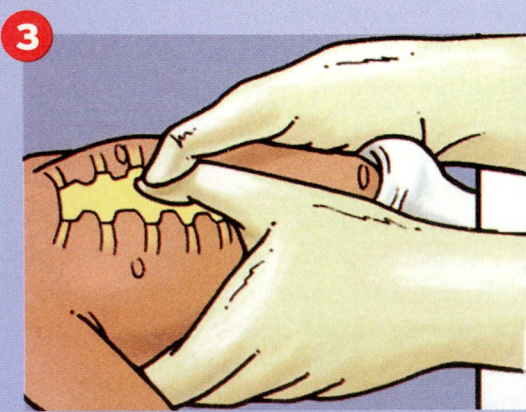

Press the two thumbs gently against the sternum.

Abnormal or Complicated Delivery Emergencies

Breech Delivery

The **presentation** is the manner in which an infant is born, the part of the body that comes out first. Most infants are born head first, in what is called a vertex presentation. Occasionally, the buttocks come out first. This is called a **breech presentation** (Figure 22-15). With a breech presentation, the infant is at great risk for delivery trauma. In addition, prolapsed cords are more common. Breech deliveries are usually slow, so there is time to get the mother to the hospital. However, if the buttocks have already passed through the vagina, delivery is underway, and you should follow emergency procedures. In general, if the mother does not deliver within 10 minutes of the buttocks presentation, provide prompt transport. Have medical control guide you in this difficult situation.

The preparations for a breech delivery are the same as those for a vertex delivery. Position the mother, unwrap the emergency delivery kit, and place yourself and your partner as you would for a normal delivery. Allow the

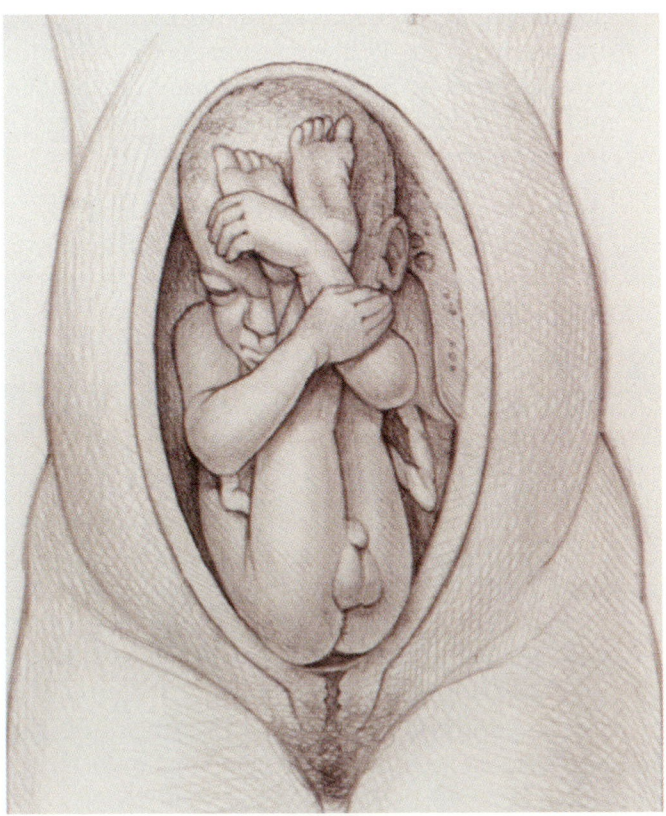

FIGURE 22-15 An infant in a breech presentation presents with the buttocks first. Breech deliveries are usually slow, so you will often have time to transport the mother to the hospital.

buttocks and legs to deliver spontaneously, supporting them with your hand to prevent rapid expulsion. The buttocks will usually come out easily. Let the legs dangle on either side of your arm while you support the trunk and chest as they are delivered. The head is almost always face down and should be allowed to deliver spontaneously. As the head is delivering, you should keep the infant's airway open: Make a "V" with your gloved fingers, and then place them into the vagina to keep the walls of the vagina from compressing the airway. *This is one of only two circumstances in which you should put your fingers into the vagina.*

Never try to pull the head out during a breech delivery. If the head is stuck in the vagina and fails to deliver, you should apply firm pressure to the uterus with the hand that is not supporting the infant. Apply the pressure to the lower abdomen, just above the pubic symphysis; you may be able to feel the head through the mother's abdominal wall. If this maneuver causes the head to be delivered spontaneously, delivery can continue as for a normal birth. If the head does not deliver spontaneously within 3 minutes, another EMT-B or an assistant will have to provide immediate transport to the hospital while you hold the infant's airway open. The mother should be given high-flow oxygen and placed in Trendelenburg's position.

Rare Presentations

On very rare occasions, the presenting part of the infant is neither the head nor buttocks, but a single arm, leg, or foot. This is called a <u>limb presentation</u> (Figure 22-16). You cannot successfully deliver such a presentation in the field. These infants usually must be delivered surgically. If you are faced with a limb presentation, you must transport the mother to the hospital immediately. If a limb is protruding, cover it with a sterile towel. Never try to push it back in, and never pull on it. Place the mother on her back, with head down and pelvis elevated. Since both mother and infant are likely to be physically stressed in this situation, remember to place the mother on high-flow oxygen.

<u>Prolapse of the umbilical cord</u>, a situation in which the umbilical cord comes out of the vagina before the infant (Figure 22-17), is another rare presentation that must be handled in the hospital. This situation is very dangerous, because the infant's head will compress the cord during birth and cut off circulation to the infant, depriving it of oxygenated blood. Do not attempt to push the cord back into the vagina. Prolapse of the umbilical cord usually occurs early in labor when the amniotic sac ruptures. As a result, there is time to get the mother to the hospital. Your job is to try to keep the infant's head from compressing the cord.

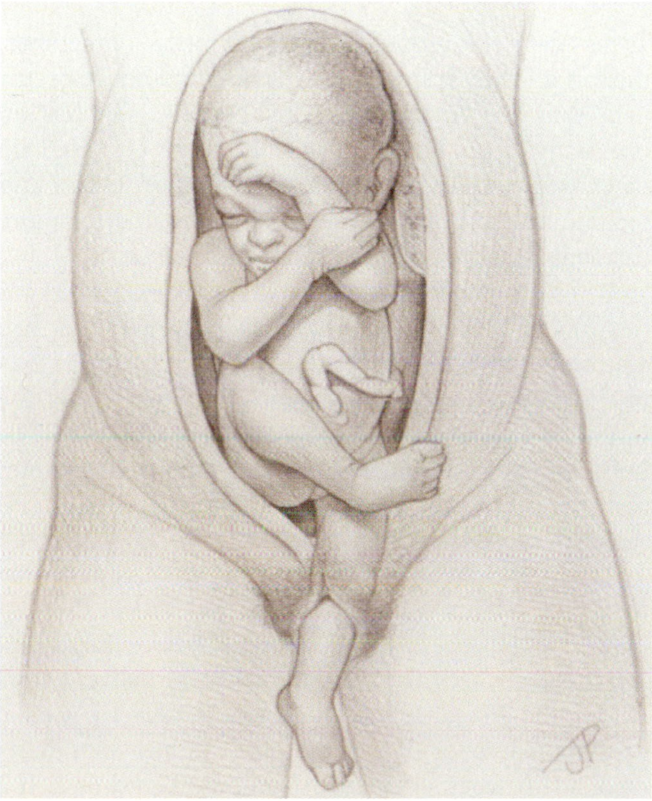

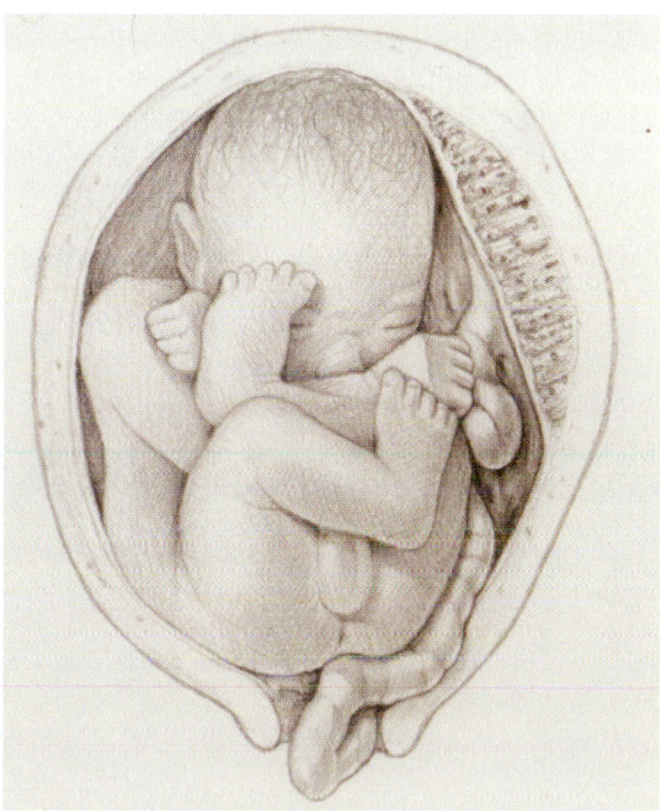

FIGURE 22-16 In very rare instances, an infant's limb, usually a single arm or leg, presents first. This is very serious situation, and you must provide prompt transport for hospital delivery.

FIGURE 22-17 A prolapsed umbilical cord, another rare situation, is very dangerous and must be cared for at the hospital.

Place the mother on a backboard in Trendelenburg's position, with her hips elevated on a pillow or folded sheet. Alternatively, the mother may be placed in a knee-chest position: kneeling and bent forward, face down. Either of these positions is meant to help keep the weight of the infant off the prolapsed cord. Carefully insert your sterile gloved hand into the vagina, and gently push the infant's head away from the umbilical cord. *Note that this is the only other occasion on which you should actually place a hand into the vagina.* Wrap a sterile towel, moistened with saline, around the exposed cord. Give the mother high-flow oxygen, and transport her rapidly.

Excessive Bleeding

Some bleeding always occurs with delivery. However, bleeding that exceeds approximately 250 mL (about 2 cups) is considered excessive. Although up to 500 mL of blood loss is tolerated, you should continue to massage the uterus. Be sure to check the massage technique if bleeding continues. If the mother appears to be in shock, treat her accordingly and transport, massaging the uterus en route. There are several other possible causes of excessive bleeding, all of which may be serious and require emergency care. Treat this condition by covering the vagina with a sterile pad, changing the pad as often as necessary. Do not discard these blood-soaked pads; hospital personnel will use them to estimate the amount of blood that the mother has lost. Also save any tissue that may have passed from the vagina.

Place the mother in Trendelenburg's position, administer oxygen, monitor vital signs frequently, and transport her immediately to the hospital. Never hold the mother's legs together in an effort to stop the bleeding, and never pack the vagina with gauze pads in an attempt to control bleeding.

Abortion (Miscarriage)

Delivery of the fetus and placenta before 20 weeks is called miscarriage or **abortion**. Abortions may be spontaneous, without any obvious known cause, or deliberate. Deliberate abortions may be self-induced, by the mother herself or by someone else, or planned and performed in a hospital or clinic. Regardless of the reasons for the abortion, it may cause complications that you may be called upon to treat.

The most serious complications of abortion are bleeding and infection. Bleeding can result from portions of the fetus or placenta being left in the uterus (incomplete abortion) or from injury to the wall of the uterus (perforation of the uterus and possibly the adjacent bowel or

bladder). Infection can result from such perforation, as well as from the use of nonsterile instruments. If the mother is in shock, treat and transport her promptly to the hospital. Collect and bring to the hospital any tissue that passes through the vagina. Never try to pull tissue out of the vagina; instead, cover it with a sterile pad.

Again, as you encounter a patient who is in shock as a result of complications of abortion, be sure to size up the situation, perform your initial assessment, history, and physical exam, and assess baseline vital signs.

In rare instances of abortion, massive bleeding may occur and cause severe hypovolemic or hemorrhagic shock. In these instances, provide immediate transport to the emergency department.

Twins

Twins occur about once in every 80 births. Sometimes, there is a family history of twins. The mother may suspect that she is having twins because she has an unusually large abdomen. Usually, however, twins are diagnosed early in pregnancy with modern ultrasound techniques. With twins, always be prepared for more than one resuscitation, and call for assistance.

Twins are smaller than single infants, and delivery is typically not difficult. Consider the possibility that you are dealing with twins any time the first infant is small or the mother's abdomen remains fairly large after the birth. If twins are present, the second one will usually be born within 45 minutes of the first. About 10 minutes after the first birth, contractions will begin again, and the birth process will repeat itself.

The procedure for delivering twins is the same as that for single infants. Clamp and cut the cord of the first infant as soon as it has been born and before the second infant is delivered. The second infant may deliver before or after the first placenta. There may be only 1 placenta, or there may be 2. When the placenta has been delivered, check whether there is 1 umbilical cord or 2. If 2 cords are coming out of 1 placenta, the twins are called identical. If only 1 cord is coming out of the placenta,

> Twins occur about once in every 80 births. With twins, always be prepared for more than one resuscitation, and call for assistance.

then the twins are called fraternal, and there will be 2 placentas. Occasionally, the 2 placentas of fraternal twins are fused, so you might think that you are dealing with identical twins. Remember, if you see only 1 umbilical cord coming out of the first placenta, there is still another placenta to be delivered. However, if both cords are attached to 1 placenta, the delivery is over. Identical twins are of the same gender; fraternal twins may be of different genders, or they may be the same.

Record the time of birth of each twin separately. Twins may be so small in weight that they look premature; handle them very carefully and keep them warm.

Delivering an Infant of an Addicted Mother

Unfortunately, more and more infants are being born to mothers who are addicted to drugs or alcohol. These mothers often have had little or no prenatal care. The effects of the addiction on the infants include prematurity, low birth weight, and severe respiratory depression. Some of these infants will die. **Fetal alcohol syndrome** is the term used to describe the condition of such infants.

If you are called to handle a delivery of a drug- or alcohol-addicted mother, pay special attention to your own safety. As with all other cases, follow BSI guidelines, and be careful not to cut or stick yourself with any needles or other sharp objects. Wear goggles and sterile gloves at all times. Clues that you are dealing with an addicted mother may include the presence of drug paraphernalia, empty wine or liquor bottles, and statements made by neighbors or by the mother herself. The newborn infant of an addicted mother will probably need immediate hospital care. Carry out the delivery as outlined earlier, but be prepared to support the infant's respirations and administer oxygen during transport. Do not judge or lecture the mother. Your job is to help deliver the infant as best you can and to get both infant and mother to the hospital.

Delivery Without Sterile Supplies

On rare occasions, you may have to deliver an infant without a sterile emergency delivery pack. Even if you do not have a sterile pack, you should always have goggles and sterile gloves with you. These are for your own protection as well as that of the mother and infant. Carry out the delivery as if sterile supplies were on hand. If you can, use clean sheets and towels that have not been used since they were laundered. As soon as the infant is born, wipe the inside of its mouth with your finger to clear away blood and mucus. Without the delivery pack, you should not cut or tie the umbilical cord. Instead, as soon as the placenta delivers, wrap it in a clean towel or put it in a plastic bag and transport it with the infant and mother to the hospital. Always keep the placenta and the infant at the same level so that blood does not drain from the infant into the placenta. Be sure to keep the infant warm. As in the case of other deliveries, note the presence of green-tinged fluid or secretions (meconium staining).

Premature Infant

The usual *gestational period,* the period of prenatal development, is 9 calendar months or 40 weeks. A normal, single infant will weigh approximately 7 lbs at birth. Any infant that delivers before 8 months (36 weeks gestation) or weighs less than 5 lbs at birth is considered *premature.* This determination is not always easy to make. Often, the exact gestation time cannot be determined. Since you probably have no scale to weigh the infant, you will have to use physical guidelines. A premature infant is smaller and thinner than a full-term infant, and its head is proportionately larger in comparison with the rest of its body (Figure 22-18). The *vernix caseosa,* a cheesy white coating on the skin that is found on the full-term infant, will be missing on the premature infant or will be very minimal. There will also be less body hair.

Premature infants need special care to survive. Often, they require resuscitation, which should be done unless physically impossible. With such care, infants as small

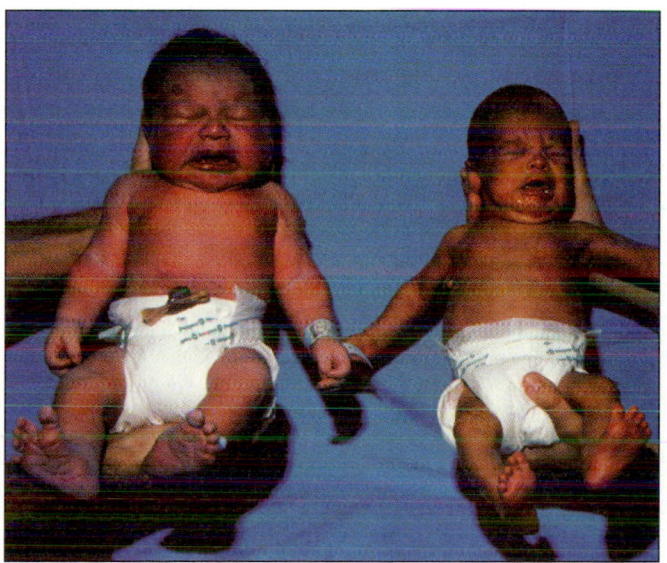

FIGURE 22-18 Premature infants are smaller and thinner than full-term infants.

as 1 lb have survived and developed normally. Follow these procedures when you are handling a premature infant:

1. **Keep the infant warm.** Dry the infant as soon as it is born, and then remove the wet towels. Wrap it in a warm blanket, exposing the face but covering the head. Keep the infant in a place where the temperature is between 90°F and 95°F (between 32.2°C and 35°C).

2. **Keep the mouth and nose clear of mucus.** Like all newborn infants, premature ones are nose breathers, and the small nasal passages can easily be obstructed. Use the bulb syringe to suction the mouth and nostrils frequently. Handle the infant and all its parts very gently.

3. **Carefully observe** the cut end of the cord attached to the infant, and be sure that it is not bleeding. The loss of even a few drops of blood can be very serious.

4. **Give oxygen.** Open the valve on your oxygen cylinder slowly to give a steady stream of oxygen (about 70 to 100 bubbles per minute through the water bottle that is attached to the oxygen tank). Direct the stream of oxygen not into the infant's mouth, but into a small tent over the infant's head; you can use a blanket or a piece of aluminum foil to make the tent. Although there is some danger to a premature infant from receiving very high concentrations of oxygen, there is no danger if it is given over a short period of time in this manner.

5. **Do not infect the infant.** Premature infants are very susceptible to infection. Protect them from contamination. Do not breathe directly into the infant's face. Your mask will help to create a barrier. Keep everyone else as far away from the infant as possible.

6. **Notify the hospital.** Does your system have a neonatal (newborn) transport team with specialized personnel and equipment for the care of premature and sick newborn infants? If so, be sure to contact the hospital before leaving the scene so that medical control can decide whether to call in the team. If not, you should still notify the hospital as soon as possible so that staff can be ready to receive the premature infant and mother. Avoid unnecessary on-scene delays.

You may have access to a specialized premature infant carrier, which can be used for immediate care as well as transport. Carrier supplies include a quilted pad, infant blanket, diaper, thermometer, suction tube and suction bulb, sterile Kelly clamp, and, most important, hot water bottles and an oxygen cylinder with the necessary attachments. Fill the hot water bottles, and pad them well so that they do not come into direct contact with the infant's skin. Place one on the bottom of the carrier and one on each side of the space for the infant. Once you have wrapped the infant in a blanket and placed it inside the carrier, secure the carrier inside the vehicle.

Keep the temperature of the vehicle at 90°F to 95°F (32.2°C to 35°C) while the infant and mother are being transported to the hospital. If a special carrier is not available, you must keep the premature infant warm with additional blankets, thermal packets, and warmed patient compartments. Any delays will lower the infant's body temperature.

Fetal Demise

Unfortunately, you may find yourself delivering an infant that has died in the mother's uterus before labor. This will be a true test of your medical, emotional, and social abilities. Grieving parents will be emotionally distraught and perhaps even hostile, requiring all your professionalism and support skills.

The onset of labor may be premature, but labor will otherwise progress normally in most cases. If an intrauterine infection has caused the demise, you may note an extremely foul odor. The delivered infant may have skin blisters, skin sloughing, and a dark discoloration, depending on the stage of decomposition. The head will be soft and perhaps grossly deformed.

Do not attempt to resuscitate an obviously dead infant. However, do not confuse such an infant with those who have had a cardiopulmonary arrest as a complication of the birthing process. You must try to resuscitate normal-appearing infants.

Gynecological Emergencies

Occasionally, women who are not pregnant will have major gynecological problems requiring urgent medical care. These include excessive bleeding and soft-tissue injuries to the external genitalia. These genital parts have a rich nerve supply, making injuries very painful.

Treat lacerations, abrasions, and tears with moist, sterile compresses, using local pressure to control bleeding and a diaper-type bandage to hold the dressings in place. Leave any foreign bodies in place after stabilizing them with bandages. Under no circumstances should you ever pack or place dressings in the vagina. Continue to assess these patients while transporting them to the emergency department. Contusions and other blunt trauma will require careful in-hospital evaluation.

Although you might not know the exact cause of a gynecological emergency, you should treat these individuals as you would any other victim of blood loss: Observe BSI, ensure maintenance of the airway, give oxygen, document vital signs, and treat for shock, while arranging for prompt transport.

Sexual Assault

Sexual assault and rape are all too common. Although most victims are women, men and children are also victims. Often, you can do little beyond providing compassion and transportation to the emergency department. On some occasions, these patients will have suffered multiple-system trauma and will also need treatment for shock.

Do not examine the genitalia of a victim of sexual assault unless obvious bleeding requires you to apply a dressing. Advise the patient not to wash, douche, urinate, or defecate until after a physician has examined him or her; this will help to preserve any evidence of a crime. If oral penetration has occurred, advise the patient not to eat, drink, brush the teeth, or use mouthwash until he or she has been examined.

Treat all other injuries according to appropriate procedures and protocols for your EMS system. Observe BSI techniques. Take the patient's history, do a limited physical exam, and provide treatment as quickly, quietly, and calmly as possible. Take care to shield the patient from curious onlookers.

The patient may refuse assistance or transport, often because he or she wants to maintain privacy and thus avoid public exposure. For adults, this is the patient's right. In such cases, you should follow your system's refusal of treatment policy or procedure for sexual assault victims without judging or being condescending to the patient. Your compassion is the best tool to gain the patient's confidence to get further help.

Offer to call the local rape crisis center for the patient. The center will have an advocate meet the patient at the hospital and provide support through the rape exam.

In addition to the usual treatment principles that apply to all victims of trauma, you should follow these special steps with patients who have been sexually assaulted:

1. Since you may have to appear in court as much as 2 or 3 years later, you must document the patient's history, assessment, treatment, and response to treatment *in detail*. Do not speculate. Record only the facts.

2. Make airway maintenance a major priority.

3. Complete the SAMPLE history in an objective and nonjudgmental fashion.

4. Follow any crime scene policy established by your system to protect the scene and any potential evidence for police, particularly that for evidence collection. If the patient will tolerate being wrapped in a sterile burn sheet, this may help investigators to find any hair, fluid, or fiber from the alleged offender.

5. Do not examine the genitalia unless there is major bleeding. If an object has been inserted into the vagina or rectum, do not attempt to remove it.

6. To reduce the patient's anxiety, make sure the EMT-B is the same gender as the patient whenever possible.

7. Discourage the patient from bathing, voiding, or cleaning any wounds until hospital staff have completed an assessment. Handle the patient's clothes as little as possible, placing articles and any other evidence in paper bags. *Do not use plastic bags.* If the female patient insists on urinating, have her do so in a sterile urine container. Also, have her deposit the toilet paper in a paper bag. Seal and mark the bag for the police. This can be critical evidence.

prep kit

ready for review

Inside the uterus, the developing fetus floats in the amniotic sac. The umbilical cord connects mother and infant through the placenta. Eventually, the uterus will propel the infant through the birth canal. The first stage of labor, dilation, begins with the onset of contractions and ends when the cervix is fully dilated. The second stage, expulsion of the baby, begins when the cervix is fully dilated and ends when the infant is born. The third stage, delivery of the placenta, begins with the birth of the infant and ends with the delivery of the placenta.

Once labor has begun, it cannot be slowed or stopped; however, there is usually time to transport the patient to the hospital during the first stage. During the second stage, you must decide whether to deliver the mother at home or transport her. During the third stage, once the infant has been born, you will probably not transport until the placenta has delivered.

Delivery at the scene is usually a two-person job. Never leave the mother once you decide to deliver her at the scene. If necessary, send someone else for help.

Use an infant BVM device to assist ventilations, starting with high-flow oxygen at a rate of 40 to 60 breaths/min. If the infant starts to breathe on its own, attach an oxygen tubing mask and watch for signs of adequate oxygenation. If the heart rate is less than 60 beats/min, start cardiac compressions, using only enough force to compress the sternum $1/2$" to $3/4$". Perform a combined total of 120 ventilations and compressions per minute, 90 compressions to 30 ventilations.

Abnormal or complicated deliveries include breech deliveries (buttocks first), limb presentations (arm, leg, or foot first), and prolapse of the umbilical cord (umbilical cord first). Quickly transport the patient with a limb presentation or prolapsed umbilical cord to the hospital. The only times you should place a finger or hand into the vagina are to keep the walls of the vagina from compressing the infant's airway during a face-down breech presentation or to push the infant's head away from the cord in a prolapse situation.

Excessive bleeding is a serious emergency. Cover the vagina with a sterile pad; change the pad as often as necessary, and take all used pads to the hospital for examination. Be prepared to support respirations during transport in an infant delivered of a drug- or alcohol-addicted mother. Also use oxygen with premature infants, and keep the temperature of the ambulance at 90°F (32.2°C) or more during transport.

Use local pressure and a diaper-type bandage to hold dressings in place when treating nonobstetric injuries to the external genitalia. Never place dressings in the vagina. Treat patients with these injuries as you would any other victim of blood loss. In the case of sexual assault or rape, treat for shock if necessary, and record all the facts in detail. Follow any crime scene policy established by your system to protect the scene and any potential evidence. Advise the patient not to wash, douche, or void until after a physician has examined him or her.

vital vocabulary

www.emtb.com

abortion Delivery of the fetus and placenta before 20 weeks; miscarriage.

amniotic sac The fluid-filled, baglike membrane in which the fetus develops.

apgar score A scoring system for assessing the status of a newborn that assigns a number value to each of five areas of activity.

birth canal The vagina and the lower part or neck of the uterus.

bloody show A plug of pink-tinged mucus that is discharged when the cervix begins to dilate.

breech presentation Delivery of an infant who comes out buttocks first.

cervix The neck of the uterus.

crowning The appearance of the infant's head at the vaginal opening during labor.

eclampsia Convulsions (seizures) resulting from severe hypertension in the pregnant woman.

ectopic pregnancy A pregnancy that develops outside the uterus, typically in a fallopian tube.

fetal alcohol syndrome A condition of infants who are born to alcoholic mothers; characterized by physical and mental retardation and a variety of congenital abnormalities.

fetus The developing, unborn infant inside the uterus.

limb presentation A delivery in which the presenting part of the infant is a single arm, leg, or foot.

multigravida A woman who has previously given birth.

nuchal cord An umbilical cord that is wrapped around the infant's neck.

perineum The area of skin between the vagina and the anus.

placenta Body tissue attached to the inner lining of the wall of the uterus, connected to the fetus by the umbilical cord.

placenta abruptio Premature separation of the placenta from the wall of the uterus.

placenta previa A condition in which the placenta develops over and covers the cervix.

presentation The manner in which an infant is born; the part of the infant that appears first.

primigravida A woman who is having her first infant.

prolapse of the umbilical cord A situation in which the umbilical cord comes out of the vagina before the infant.

supine hypotensive syndrome Low blood pressure resulting from compression by the weight of the fetus on the inferior vena cava.

umbilical cord The conduit connecting mother to infant via the placenta; contains two arteries and one vein.

uterus The muscular organ where the fetus grows, also called the womb; responsible for contractions during labor.

vagina The outermost cavity of a woman's reproductive system; the lower part of the birth canal.

assessment in action

You respond to a call to 9-1-1 requesting an ambulance for a woman having a baby "right now!" Upon arrival at a private residence, you find a 22-year-old woman lying on the bathroom floor with a small puddle of blood under her buttocks. A 2-year-old child is crying in a playpen across the hall, and you can see that history gathering will be a bit of a challenge. The patient tells you that she has been having contractions for the last hour but thought that she and her husband could get to the hospital in time. However, she states that her water "broke," and she estimates that her contractions are now only 2 to 3 minutes apart. She also says that because of financial difficulties, she has not seen a physician since she first found out that she was pregnant again.

On examination, you see what appears to be part of the baby's head showing from the vagina. Your partner obtains baseline vital signs. The patient has a blood pressure of 118/68 mm Hg, a pulse of 138 beats/min, and respirations of 32 breaths/min. The local hospital is approximately 20 minutes away.

1. Given the situation described, your most appropriate action at this time is to:
   A. perform a detailed physical examination.
   B. prepare for the imminent delivery of the baby.
   C. transport the patient to the hospital for the delivery.
   D. administer high-flow oxygen and recheck the patient's vital signs.

2. Which of the following items would **NOT** be found in the emergency delivery kit carried in the ambulance?
   A. Bulb syringe
   B. Sterile gloves
   C. Baby blanket
   D. Assorted pain medications

3. What should you do if one of the baby's legs is presenting from the vagina instead of the baby's head?
   A. Elevate the mother's head, and wait for the baby to deliver.
   B. Place the mother on her side, and wait for the baby to deliver.
   C. Give oxygen, elevate the mother's head, and recheck vital signs.
   D. Place the mother in a head-down position, give oxygen, and provide immediate transport.

4. Which of the following descriptions best characterizes a healthy newborn?
   A. No crying, pink from head to toe, and a pulse of 60 to 80 beats/min
   B. Very little crying, pink head and trunk, and a pulse of 80 to 100 beats/min
   C. Crying when stimulated, pink head and trunk, and a pulse of less than 100 beats/min
   D. Good loud cry, pink from head to toe, and a pulse of greater than 100 beats/min

5. How would you administer oxygen to a newborn with central cyanosis, adequate respirations, and a strong pulse of 20 beats/min?
   A. BVM device at 4 to 6 L/min
   B. Nonrebreathing mask at 2 to 4 L/min
   C. Nasal cannula at no more than 2 L/min
   D. Blow-by technique using oxygen tubing at more than 10 L/min

points to ponder

You respond to a woman in labor in a local supermarket. You find her seated in a chair near the checkout stands. The look on her face tells you that she is definitely in labor. She tells you that her due date was three days ago, her bag of waters broke about an hour ago, and she has had a small amount of blood appear about 1 1/2 hours ago. The man with her is encouraging her to go home. He insists that they had planned a home delivery, and that is what they should still do. The man is quite insistent, and the woman appears scared and confused. This is their first child.

- What other signs and symptoms would you check to determine whether the woman can be transported anywhere or whether delivery is imminent? If there is time to transport, would you support the mother going home? Why or why not?

online outlook

Watch how the fetus grows from conception through delivery from actual ultrasound images and review postdelivery care by completing Exercise 22 at www.emtb.com.

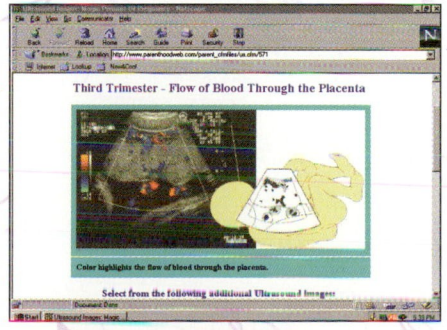

prep kit 22

Trauma

Lenworth M. Jacobs, MD, MPH, FACS

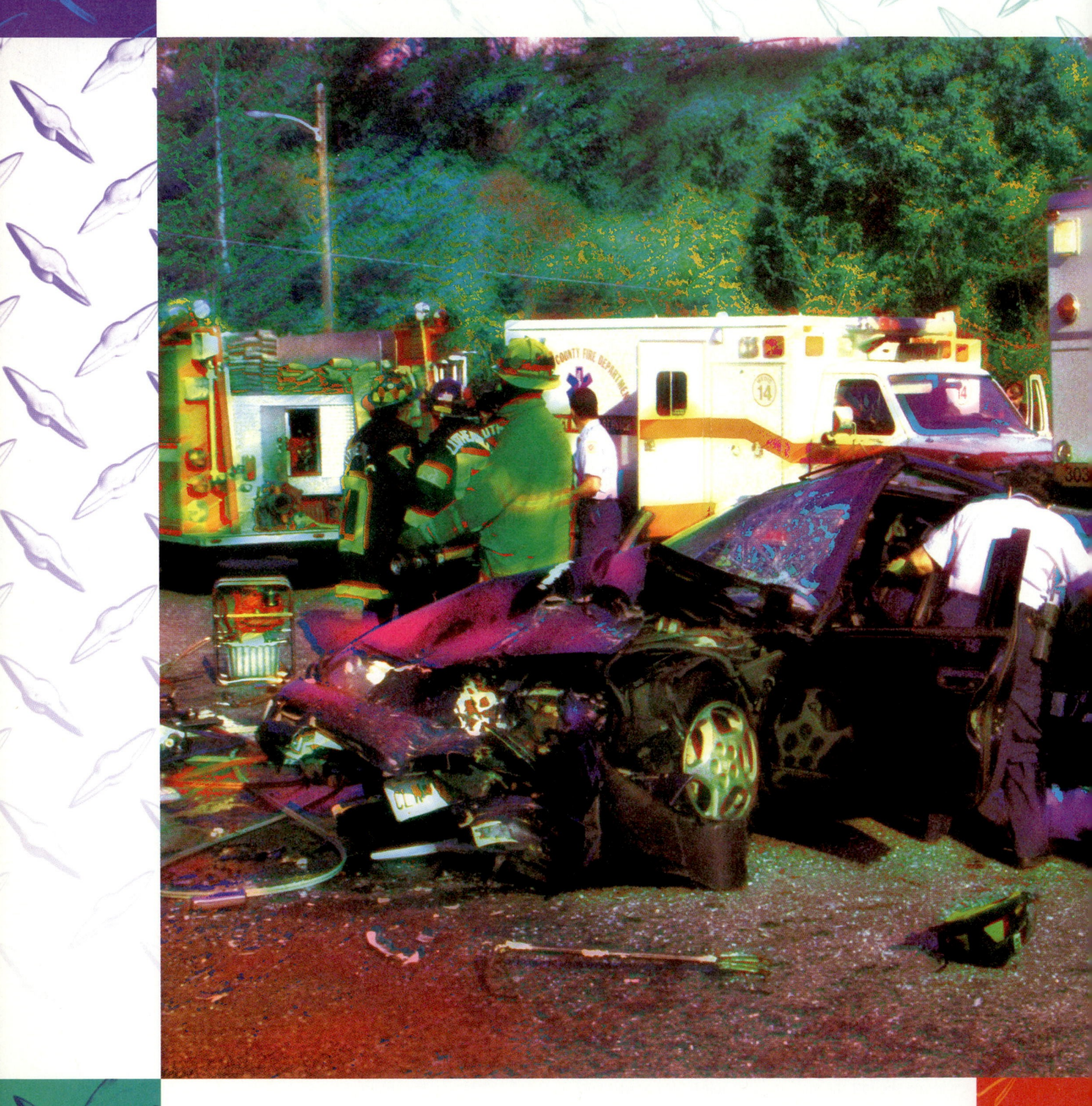

Kinematics of
Trauma

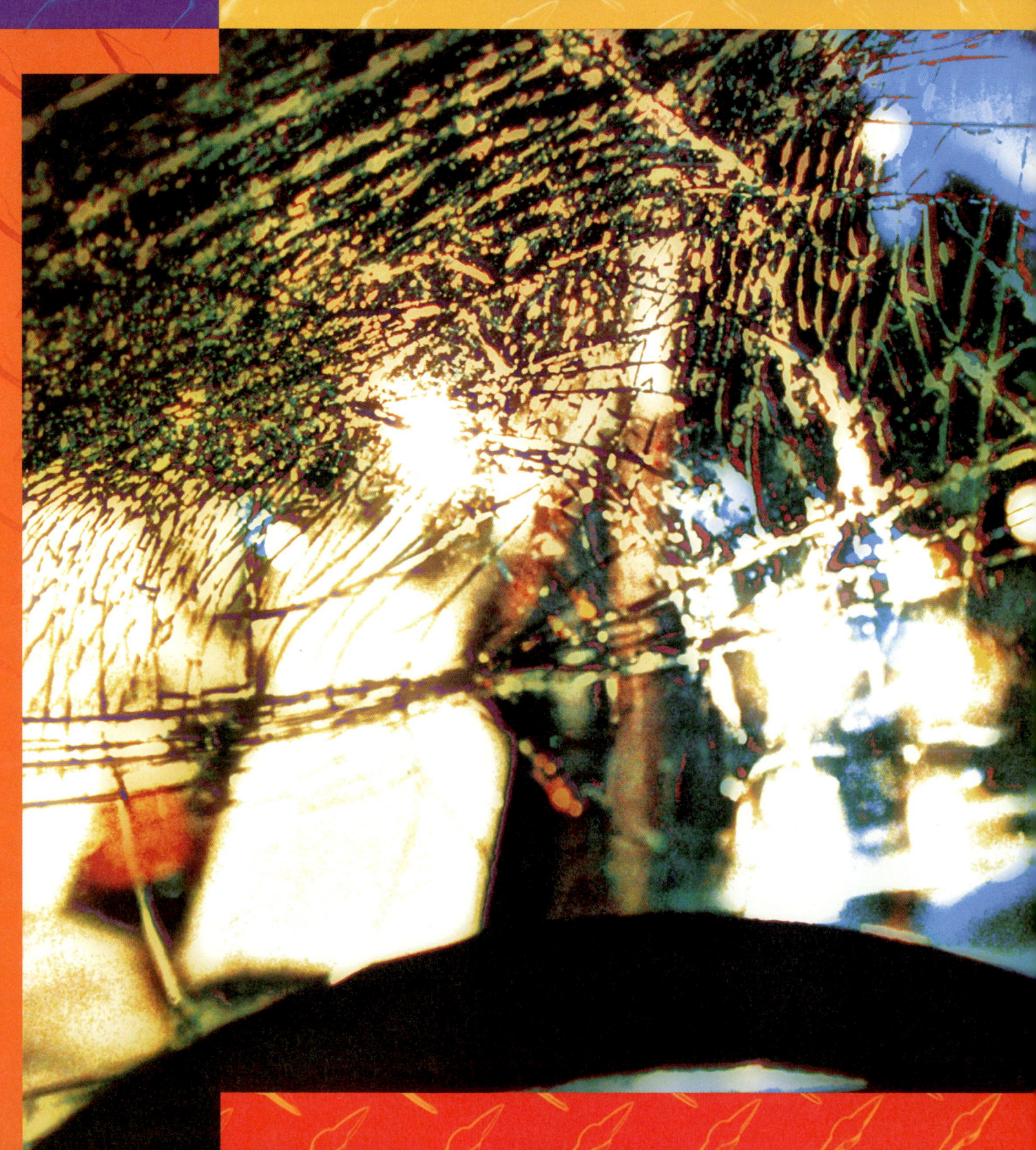

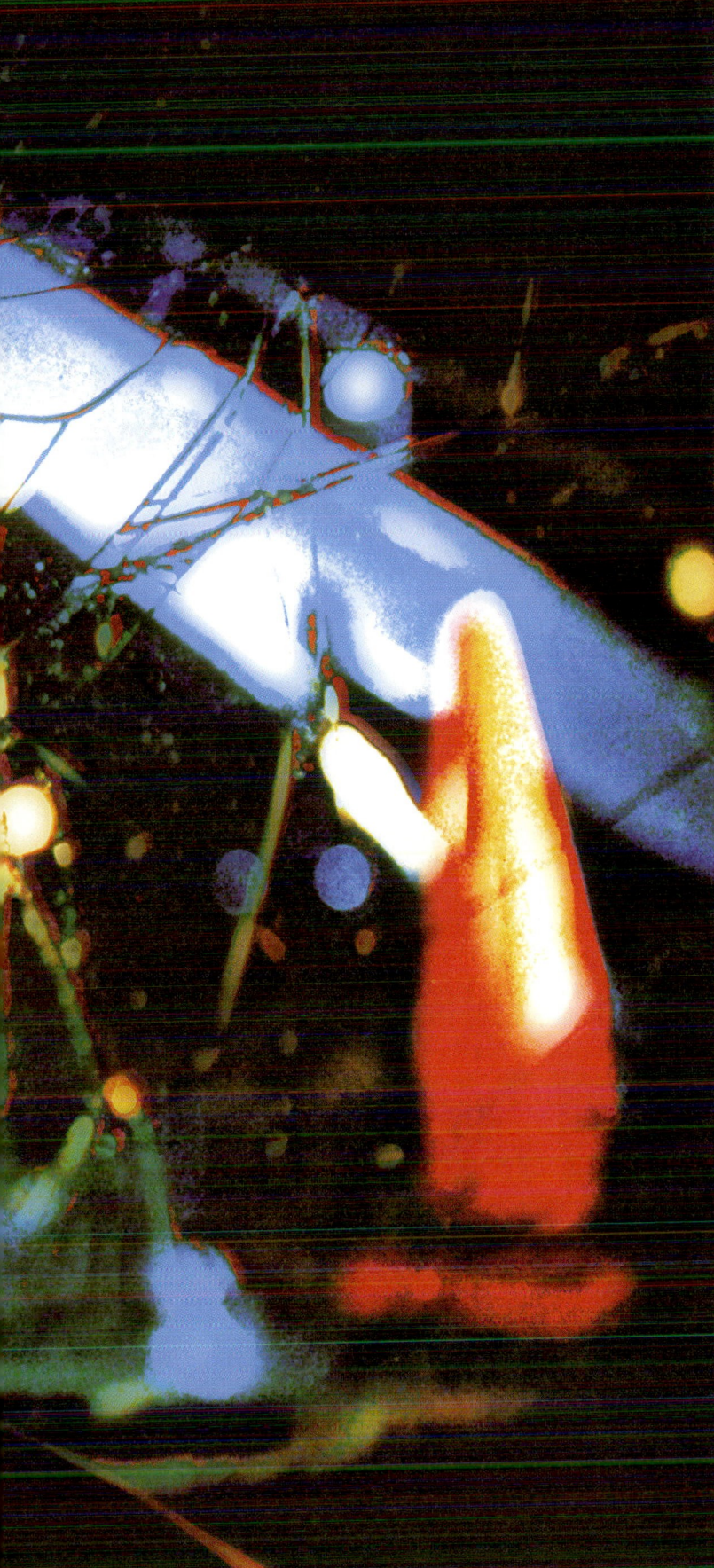

objectives*

Cognitive

1. Describe the "three collisions" associated with motor vehicle crashes.
2. Relate how the fundamental principles of physics apply to motor vehicle crashes and other types of accidents.
3. State Newton's three laws.

Affective

None

Psychomotor

4. Observe various high-energy injuries and identify potential damage to the patient.

* These are non-curriculum objectives.

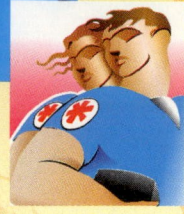

you are the emt

You hear a scream. You and your partner have just returned to quarters and are stepping out of the ambulance when you see the man who lives in the house next to the station hit the ground after falling from the top of the ladder. Even though he landed on the grass, you estimate that the ladder is close to 24' tall. He is lying on the ground and moving only a little. As you grab the jump kit, your partner notifies dispatch that you are going to check out the situation.

Traumatic incidents are one of the leading causes of death and disability in the United States. Trauma calls occur every day in EMS. This chapter will help to prepare you to assess the trauma patients. It will also help you to answer the following questions:

1. What does it mean to have a "high index of suspicion"?
2. Why is some care, such as spinal immobilization, best termed "preventive?" How is preventive care associated with evaluating the mechanism of injury?

Kinematics of Trauma

Injuries are the leading cause of death and disability in the United States among children and young adults (ages 1 to 34), claiming 140,000 lives annually—more than all other diseases combined. Each year, one person in three sustains an injury that requires medical treatment. Proper prehospital evaluation and care can do much to minimize suffering, long-term disability, and death from trauma.

This chapter introduces the basic physical concepts that dictate how injuries occur and affect the human body. When you understand these concepts, you will be better able to size up an accident scene and use that information as a vital part of patient assessment. The chapter begins with a basic discussion of energy and trauma. Next, different types of crashes and their impact on the body are explained. By assessing the body of a vehicle that has crashed, you can often determine what happened to the passengers at the time of impact, that is, what the mechanism of injury was. Certain injury patterns occur with certain types of injury events. Answers to simple questions will provide you with information on how to identify both life-threatening and other serious injuries. The chapter concludes with a brief discussion of falls and penetrating trauma. A brief section on Newton's laws is also presented.

Energy and Trauma

Traumatic injury occurs to the body when the body's tissues are exposed to energy levels beyond their tolerance. Three concepts of energy are typically associated with injury (not including thermal energy, which causes burns): *potential energy, kinetic energy,* and *work*. In considering the effects of energy on the human body, it is important to remember that energy can be neither created nor destroyed, but can only be converted or transformed. It is not the objective of this section to help you to reconstruct the scene of a motor vehicle crash. Rather, you should have a sense of the effects of work on the body and understand, in a broad sense, how that work is related to potential and kinetic energy. For example, when you are assessing a patient who fell, you need not calculate the speed at which the person hit the ground. However, it is important to estimate the height from which he or she fell and to appreciate the injury potential of the fall.

Work is defined as *force* acting over a *distance*. For example, the force needed to bend metal multiplied by the distance over which the metal is bent is the work that crushes the front end of an automobile that is involved in a frontal impact. Similarly, forces that bend, pull, or compress tissues beyond their inherent limits result in the work that causes injury.

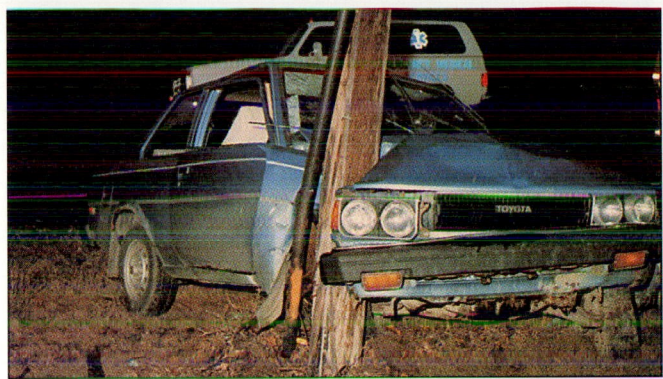

FIGURE 23-1 The kinetic energy of a speeding car is converted into the work of stopping the car, usually by crushing the car's exterior.

The energy of a moving object is called **kinetic energy** and is calculated as follows: *Kinetic energy = $\frac{1}{2}mv^2$*, where m = mass (weight) and v = velocity (speed). Remember that energy cannot be created or destroyed, only converted. In the case of a motor vehicle crash, the kinetic energy of the speeding car is converted into the work of stopping the car, usually by crushing the car's exterior (Figure 23-1). Similarly, the passengers of the car have kinetic energy because they were traveling at the same speed as the car. Their kinetic energy is converted to the work of bringing them to a stop. It is this work on the passengers that results in injury. Notice that, according to the equation for kinetic energy, the energy that is available to cause injury doubles when an object's weight doubles but quadruples when its speed doubles. Consider the debate over raising the speed limit. Increasing a car's speed from 50 mph to 70 mph doubles the energy that is available to cause injury. This point will be even clearer in considering gunshot wounds. The speed of the bullet (high-velocity compared with low-velocity) has a greater impact on producing injury than the mass (size) of the bullet. As has already been noted, this is why it is so important to report to the hospital the type of firearm that was used in a shooting. The amount of kinetic energy that is converted to do work on the body dictates the severity of the injury. High-energy injuries often produce such severe damage that patients can be saved only by immediate transport to an appropriate facility.

Potential energy is the product of mass (weight), force of gravity, and height and is mostly associated with the energy of falling objects. A worker on a scaffold has some potential energy because he or she is some height above the ground. When the worker falls, potential energy is converted into kinetic energy. As the worker hits the ground, the kinetic energy is converted into work—that is, the work of bringing the body to a stop and thereby breaking bones and damaging tissues.

Vehicular Collisions

Motor vehicle crashes are classified traditionally as frontal (head-on), lateral (T-bone), rear-end, rotational (spins), and rollovers. The principal difference among these collision types is the direction of the force of impact; also, with spins and rollovers, there is the possibility of multiple impacts. Motor vehicle crashes typically consist of a series of 3 collisions. Understanding the events that occur during each collision will help you be alert for certain types of injury patterns. The 3 collisions in a frontal impact are as follows:

1. **The collision of the car against another car, a tree, or some other object.** Damage to the car is perhaps the most dramatic part of the collision, but it does not directly affect patient care, except possibly to make extrication difficult (Figure 23-2). However, it does provide information about the severity of the collision and therefore has an indirect effect on patient care. The greater the damage to the car, the greater is the energy that was involved and therefore the greater the potential to cause injury to the patient. By assessing the body of a vehicle that has crashed, you can often determine the **mechanism of injury**, that is, what injuries may have happened to the passengers at the time of impact. When you arrive at the scene of an accident and perform your scene size-up, quickly inspect the severity of damage to the vehicle(s). If there is significant damage to a vehicle, your index of suspicion for the presence of life-threatening injuries should automatically increase. A great

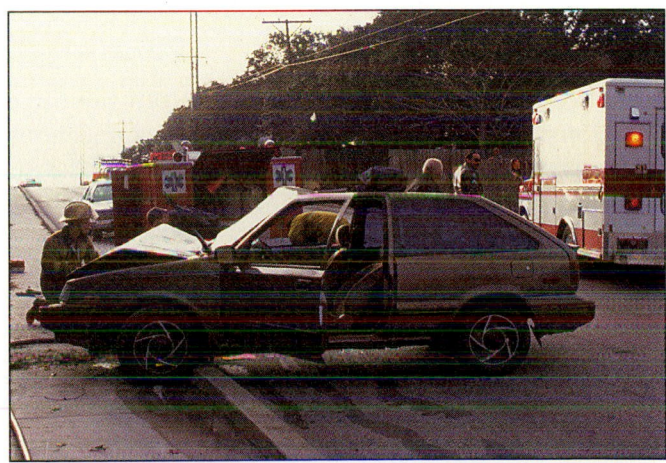

FIGURE 23-2 The first collision in a frontal impact is that of the car against another object (in this case, a utility pole). The appearance of the car can provide you with critical information about the severity of the crash. The greater the damage to the car, the greater is the energy that was involved.

amount of force is required to crush and deform the exterior of a vehicle, tear seats from their mountings, and collapse steering wheels. Such damage suggests the presence of high-energy trauma.

2. **The collision of the passenger against the interior of the car.** Just as the kinetic energy produced by the car's mass and velocity is converted into the work of bringing the car to a stop, the kinetic energy produced by the passenger's mass and velocity is converted into the work of stopping his or her body (Figure 23-3). Just like the obvious damage to the exterior of the car, the injuries that result are often dramatic and usually immediately apparent during your initial assessment. Common injuries include lower extremity fractures (knees into dashboard), flail chest (rib cage into steering wheel), and head trauma (head into windshield). Such injuries occur more frequently if the passenger is not restrained. But even when the passenger is restrained with a properly adjusted seat belt, injuries can occur, especially in lateral and rollover impacts.

3. **The collision of the passenger's internal organs against the solid structures of the body.** The injuries that occur during the third collision may not be as obvious as external injuries, but they are often the most life threatening. For example, as the passenger's head hits the windshield, the brain continues to move forward until it comes to rest by striking the inside of the skull. This results in compression injury to the anterior portion of the brain and rupture of the posterior bridging vessels (Figure 23-4). Similarly, in the thoracic cage, the heart may slam into the sternum, occasionally rupturing the aorta and causing fatal bleeding.

Understanding the relationship between the three collisions will help you to make the connections between the amount of damage to the exterior of the car and potential injury to the passenger. For example, in a high-speed collision that results in massive damage to the car, you should suspect serious injuries to the passengers, even if the injuries are not readily apparent.

> Understanding the events that occur during each collision will help you be alert for certain types of injury patterns.

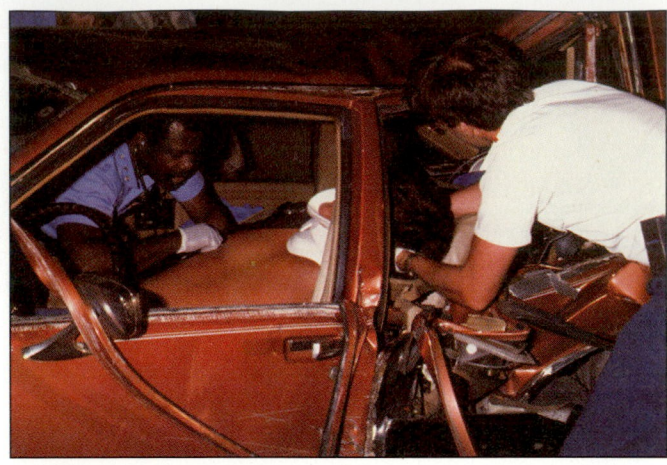

FIGURE 23-3 The second collision in a frontal impact is that of the passenger against the interior of the car. The appearance of the interior of the car can provide you with information about the severity of the patient's injuries.

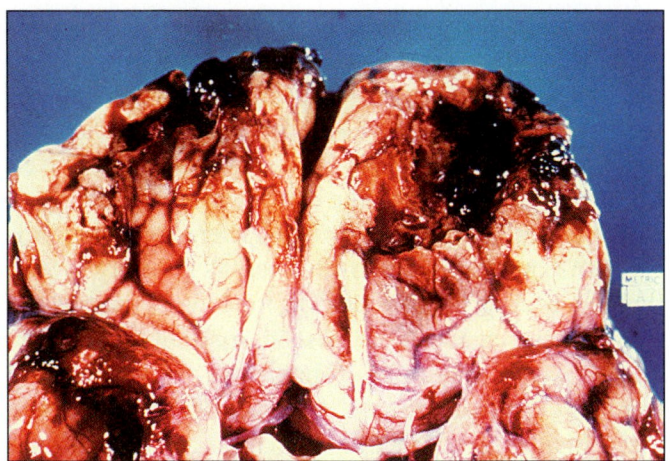

FIGURE 23-4 The third collision in a frontal impact is that of the passenger's internal organs against the solid structures of the body. In this photo of the brain, sudden deceleration of the skull resulted in fatal injury when the brain continued its forward motion and struck the inside of the skull.

A number of potential physical problems may develop as a result of traumatic injuries. Your quick initial assessment of the patient and the evaluation of the mechanism of injury can help to direct lifesaving care and provide critical information to the hospital staff (Table 23-1). Therefore, if you see a contusion on the patient's forehead and the windshield is starred and pushed out, you should strongly suspect an injury to the brain. After you inform medical control about the windshield, hospital staff can prepare the patient by ordering a CT scan of the brain. Without your input, the physician might have found the brain injury anyway, but it might have not been detected until the brain had swollen sufficiently to cause clinical signs of the injury.

TABLE 23-1   Recognizing Developing Problems in Trauma Patients

Problem	Signs and Symptoms or Mechanism of Injury
Airway Obstruction	Significant bleeding into the mouth, back of the throat, or nose
	Swelling or bleeding following blunt or penetrating trauma to the face
	Swelling about the neck (may compress the airway) following blunt or penetrating trauma to the neck
	Inability to swallow, resulting in possible choking on secretions
Breathing Problems	Significant chest pain following blunt trauma
	Any penetrating trauma to the chest, unless it is a superficial cut (Remember to check the back too.)
	Bent or crushed steering wheel, indicating blunt trauma to the chest
Hidden Blood Loss	Bruising or obvious trauma to the upper abdomen
	Significant mechanism of injury, including blunt and penetrating trauma
	Obvious bruising in the area of the pelvis
	Tenderness on gentle palpation of the pelvis
Damage to Major Vessels	Blunt or penetrating trauma to the neck, chest, or groin area (which could tear the major vessels in these areas)
	Bent or crushed steering wheel, indicating blunt trauma to the chest
Damage to the Heart	Bent or crushed steering wheel, indicating blunt trauma to the chest
Brain Injury	History of losing consciousness, inability to recall what happened, dazed appearance, confusion, disorientation, combativeness after the traumatic incident
	Slurred speech
	Difficulty moving the extremities
	Severe headache, especially if accompanied by nausea and vomiting
	Obvious blunt or penetrating trauma to the head, other than superficial cuts
	Appearance of intoxication, as signs and symptoms (especially head trauma) may be masked by the effects of alcohol
Possible Spinal Injury	Severe neck or back pain
	History of difficulty moving or feeling the extremities
	Starred windshield, indicating that the patient's head flexed forward and struck the windshield with significant force

The amount of damage that is considered significant varies, depending on the type of collision, but any substantial deformity of the vehicle should be enough cause for you to consider transporting the patient to a trauma center. Significant mechanisms of injury include the following:

- Severe deformities of the frontal part of a vehicle, with or without intrusion to the passenger compartment
- Moderate intrusions from a lateral (T-bone) type of accident
- Severe damage from the rear
- Collisions in which rotation is involved (rollover and spins)

Damage to the vehicle that was involved and information obtained from patient assessment are not the only clues to crash severity. Clearly, if one or more of the passengers are dead, you should suspect that the other passengers have sustained serious injuries, even if the injuries are not obvious. Therefore, you should focus on treating life-threatening injuries and providing transport to a trauma center, because these passengers have likely experienced the same amount of force that caused the death of the others.

Frontal Collisions

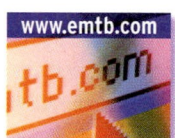

Understanding the mechanism of injury after a frontal collision first involves evaluation of the supplemental restraint system, including seat belts and air bags. You should determine whether the passenger was restrained by a full and properly applied 3-point restraint. In addition, you should determine whether the air bag was deployed. Identifying the types of restraints used and whether air bags were deployed will help you to identify injury patterns that occur related to the supplemental restraint systems.

When properly applied, seat belts are successful in restraining the passengers in a vehicle and preventing a second collision inside the motor vehicle. In addition, they may decrease the severity of the third collision, that of the passenger's organs with the chest or abdominal wall. The very presence of air bags allows seat belts to provide even more "ride down," or the gentle cushioning of the occupant as the body slows, or **decelerates**. Air bags provide the final capture point of the passengers and again decrease the severity of deceleration injuries by allowing seat belts to be more compliant and by cushioning the occupant as he or she moves forward.

Remember that air bags decrease injury to the chest, face, and head very effectively. However, you should still

suspect that other serious injuries to the extremities (resulting from the second collision) and to internal organs (resulting from the third collision) have occurred. If the accident scene indicates high energy and a significant mechanism, the patient should be treated on the basis of mechanism of injury.

You should also remember that supplemental restraint systems can cause harm when they are used improperly. For example, seat belts that buckle automatically at the shoulder but require the passengers to buckle the lap portion can result in the body "submarining" forward underneath the shoulder restraint when the lap portion is not attached. This movement of the body can cause the lower extremities and the pelvis to crash into the dashboard, as that part of the body is unrestrained. In addition, individuals of short stature can sustain significant neck and facial injuries caused by the belting systems when their lower torso is unrestrained.

When passengers are riding in vehicles equipped with air bags but are not restrained by seat belts, they are often thrown forward in the act of emergency braking. As a result, they come into contact with the air bag and/or the doors at the time of deployment. This mechanism of injury is also responsible for some severe injuries to children who are riding unrestrained in the front seats of vehicles. In addition, some passengers may pass out before impact, and you may find them lying against the air bag when it deploys. You should look for abrasions and/or traction-type injuries on the face and lower part of the neck (Figure 23-5).

Contact points are often obvious from a simple quick evaluation of the interior of the vehicle (Figure 23-6). If there is no intrusion from the second vehicle, you might see that an unrestrained front-seat passenger in a frontal collision will come into contact with the

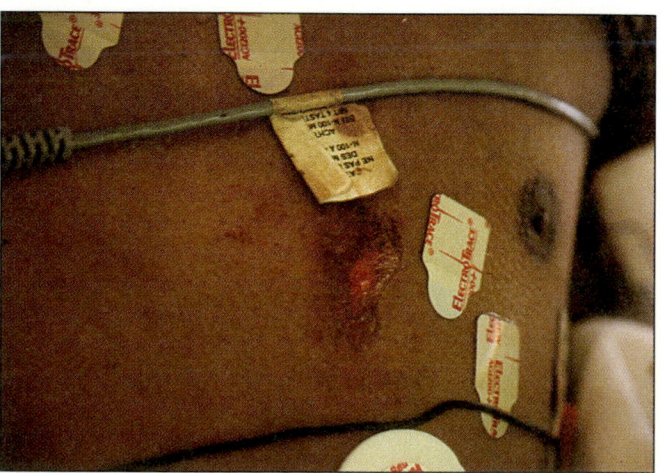

FIGURE 23-5 Air bags can cause injury in frontal collisions, specifically, abrasions and traction-type injuries to the face and neck.

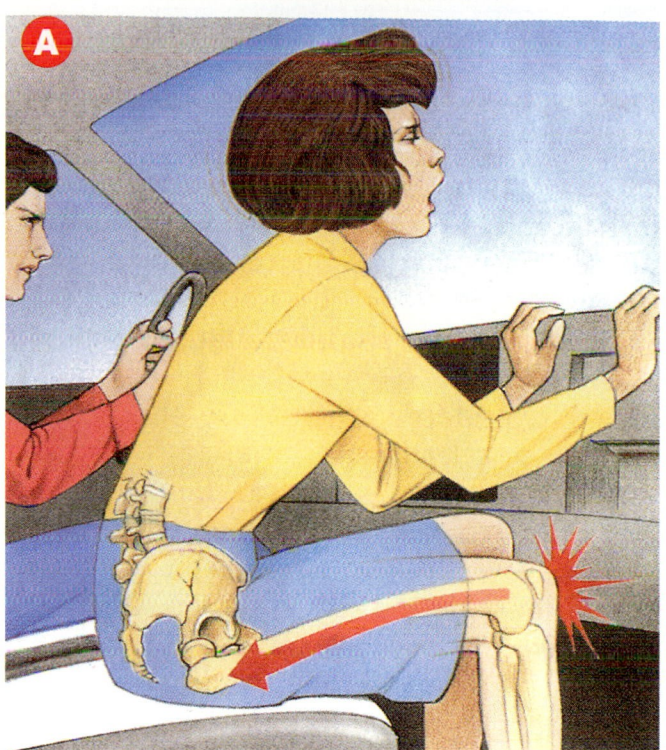

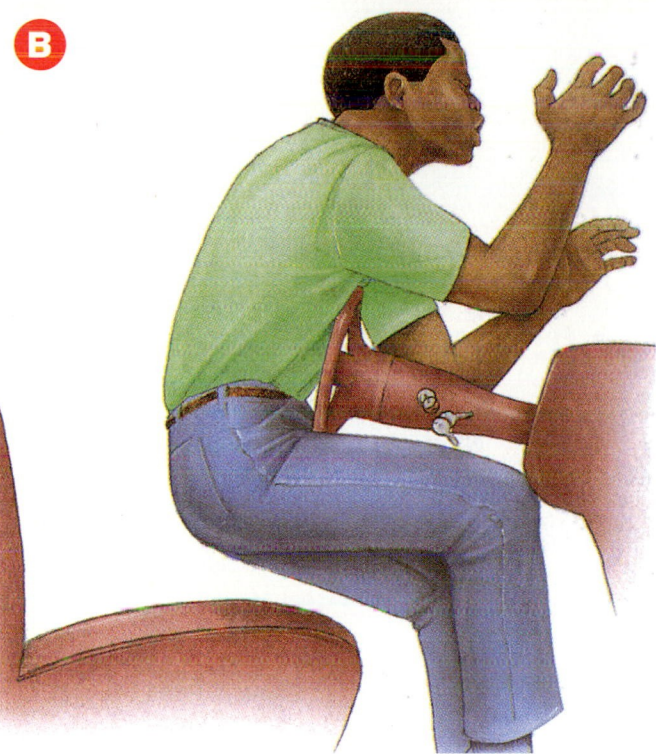

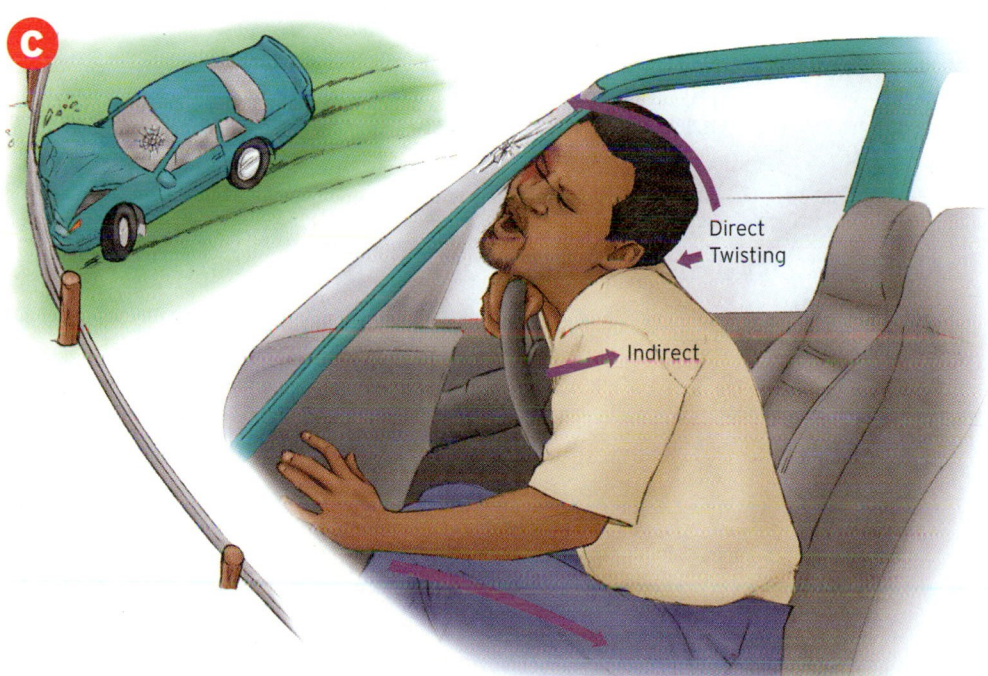

FIGURE 23-6
A: The knee can strike the dashboard resulting in a hip fracture.
B: Serious chest and abdominal injuries can result from striking the steering wheel.
C: Head and spinal injuries can result when the face and head strike the windshield.

> Contact points are often obvious from a simple quick evaluation of the interior of the vehicle.

dashboard or instrument panel at the knees and transfer loads from the knees through the femur to the pelvis and hip joint. The chest and/or abdomen may also hit the steering wheel. In addition, the passenger's face often hits the steering wheel or may launch forward and up, hitting the windshield and/or the roof header in the area of the visors. Signs of most of these injuries can be found by simply inspecting the interior of the vehicle during extrication of the patient.

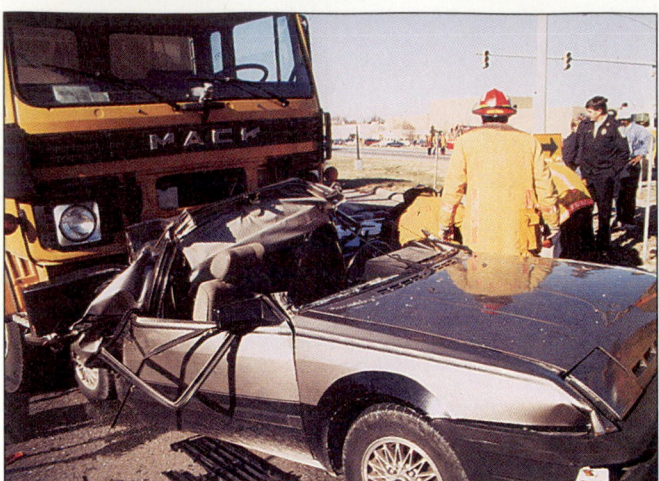

FIGURE 23-7 Rear-end impacts often cause whiplash type injuries, particularly when the head and/or neck is not restrained by a headrest.

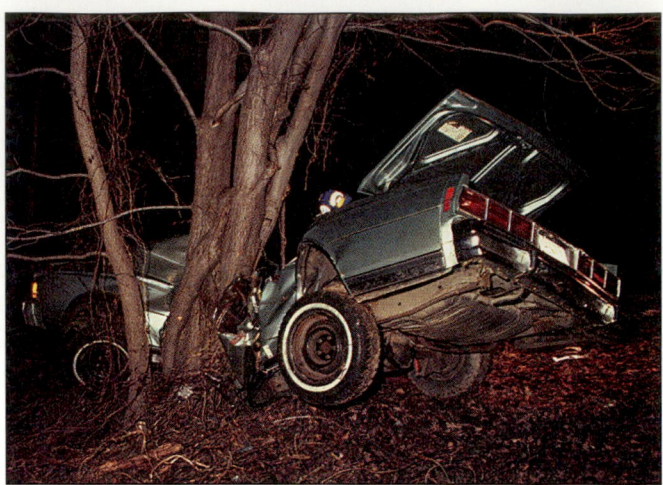

FIGURE 23-8 In a lateral collision, the car is typically struck above its center of gravity and begins to rock away from the side of impact. This causes a type of lateral whiplash in which the passenger's shoulders and head whip toward the intruding vehicle.

Rear-End Collisions

Rear-end impacts are known to cause whiplash-type injuries, particularly when the head and/or neck is not restrained by an appropriately placed headrest (Figure 23-7). Upon impact, the body and torso move forward. As the body is propelled forward, the head and neck are left behind because they are not restrained by a headrest, and they appear to be whipped back relative to the torso. As the vehicle comes to rest, the unrestrained passenger moves forward, striking the dashboard. In this type of collision, the cervical spine and surrounding area may be injured. The cervical spine is less tolerant to damage when it is bent back (in extension). Other parts of the spine and the pelvis may also be at risk for injury. In addition, the patient may sustain an acceleration-type injury to the brain, that is, the third collision of the brain within the skull. Passengers in the back seat wearing only a lap belt might have a higher incidence of injuries to the thoracic and lumbar spine.

Lateral Collisions

Lateral impacts are probably now the number one cause of death associated with motor vehicle crashes. When a vehicle is struck from the side, it is typically struck above its center of gravity and begins to rock away from the side of the impact. This results in a lateral whiplash injury (Figure 23-8). The movement is to the side, and the passenger's shoulders and head whip toward the intruding vehicle. This action may thrust the shoulder, thorax, and upper extremity and, more important, the skull against the B-pillar or the window. The cervical spine has little tolerance for lateral bending.

If there is substantial intrusion by the other vehicle into the passenger compartment, you should suspect possible fractures of the lower extremities, pelvis, and ribs. In addition, the organs within the abdomen are at risk because of a possible third collision. Approximately 25% of all severe injuries to the aorta that occur in motor vehicle crashes are a result of lateral collisions.

Rollover Crashes

Injury patterns that are commonly associated with rollover crashes differ, depending on whether the passenger was restrained. The most unpredictable are rollover crashes in which an unrestrained passenger may have sustained multiple strikes within the interior of the vehicle as it rolled 1 or more times. The most common life-threatening event in a rollover is ejection or partial ejection of the passenger from the vehicle (Figure 23-9). Passengers who have been ejected may have struck the interior of the vehicle many times before ejection. The passenger may also have struck several objects, such as trees, a guardrail, or the vehicle's exterior, before landing. Passengers who have been partially ejected may have struck both the interior and exterior of the vehicle and may have been sandwiched between the exterior and the environment as the vehicle rolled. Ejection and partial ejection are significant mechanisms of injury; in these instances, you should prepare to care for life-threatening injuries.

Even when restrained, passengers can sustain severe injuries during a rollover crash, although the patterns of injury tend to be more predictable, and when properly used, the restraint system will prevent ejection

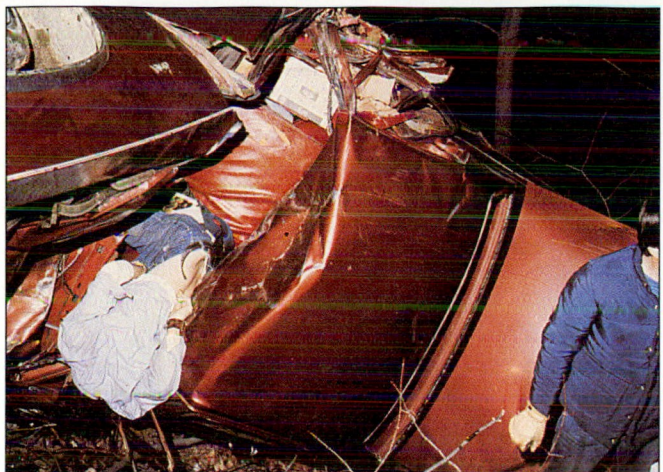

FIGURE 23-9 Passengers who have been ejected or partially ejected may have struck the interior of the car many times before ejection.

from the vehicle. A passenger on the outboard side of a vehicle that rolls over is at high risk for injury because of the centrifugal force (the patient is pinned against the door of the vehicle). When the roof hits the ground during a rollover, a passenger who is restrained can still move far enough toward the roof to make contact and sustain a spinal cord injury. Therefore, rollover crashes are particularly dangerous for both restrained and, to a greater degree, unrestrained passengers because these crashes provide multiple opportunities for second and third collisions.

Spins

Spins are conceptually similar to rollovers. The rotation of the vehicle as it spins provides opportunities for the vehicle to strike objects such as utility poles. For example, as a vehicle spins and strikes a pole, the passengers experience not only the rotational motion, but also a lateral impact.

Falls

The injury potential of a fall is related to the height from which the patient fell. The greater the height of the fall, the greater the potential for injury. A fall from more than 15′ or 3 times the patient's height is considered to be significant. Although there is no first collision in a fall, per se, there are second and third collisions. In the second collision, the patient lands on the surface just as an unrestrained passenger smashes into the interior of a vehicle. The third collision is similar. The internal organs travel at the speed of the patient's body before it

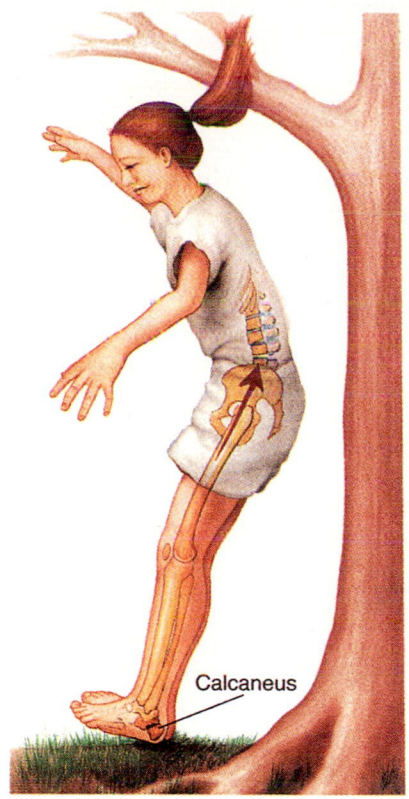

FIGURE 23-10 When a patient falls and lands on his or her feet, the energy is transmitted to the spine, sometimes producing a spine injury as well as injuries to the legs.

hits the ground and stop by smashing into the interior of the body. Again, as in a motor vehicle crash, it is these third collision internal injuries that are the least obvious on assessment but pose the gravest threat to life. Therefore, you should suspect internal injuries in a patient who has fallen from a significant height, just as you would in a patient who has been in a high-speed motor vehicle crash.

Patients who fall and land on their feet may have less severe internal injuries because their legs may have absorbed much of the energy of the fall (Figure 23-10). Of course, as a result, they may have very serious injuries to the lower extremities. Patients who fall onto their heads, as do victims of diving accidents, will likely have serious head and/or spinal injuries. In either case, a fall from a significant height is a serious event with great injury potential, and the patient should be evaluated thoroughly. Take the following factors into account:

- The height of the fall
- The surface struck
- The part of the body that hit first, followed by the path of energy displacement

Some texts consider falls to be the most common form of trauma. Many falls, especially those by the elderly, are not considered "true" trauma, even though bones may be broken. Often, these falls occur as a result of a fracture. Elderly patients often have osteoporosis, a condition in which their musculoskeletal system can fail under relatively low stress. Because of this condition, an elderly patient can sustain a fracture while in a standing position and then fall as a result. Therefore, an elderly patient may have actually sustained a fracture before the fall. These instances do not constitute true high-energy trauma unless the patient fell from a significant height.

Penetrating Trauma

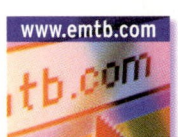

Penetrating trauma is the second largest cause of death in the United States after blunt trauma. Low-energy penetrating trauma may be caused accidentally by impalement or intentionally by a knife, ice pick, or other weapon (Figure 23-11). Once you have identified the entrance wound and the exit wound (if one exists), you know some important things about the path of the penetrating object. With low-energy penetrations, injuries are caused by the sharp edges of the object moving through the body and are therefore close to the object's path. Weapons such as knives, however, may have been deliberately moved around internally, causing more damage than the entrance and exit wounds might suggest.

In medium-velocity and high-velocity penetrating trauma, the path of the object (usually a bullet) may not be as easy to predict. This is because the bullet may flatten out, tumble, or even ricochet within the body before exiting. Also, because of its speed, pressure waves emanate from the bullet, causing damage remote from its path. This phenomenon, called **cavitation**, can result in serious injury to internal organs distant to the actual path of the bullet. Much like a boat moving through water, the bullet disrupts not only the tissues that are directly in its path but also those in its wake. Therefore, the area that is

> Penetrating trauma is the second largest cause of death in the United States after blunt trauma.

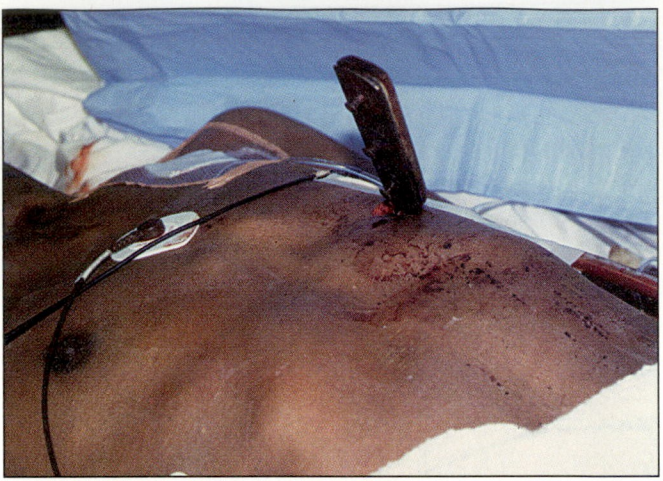

FIGURE 23-11 Injuries from low-energy penetrations, such as a stab wound, are caused by the sharp edges of the object moving through the body.

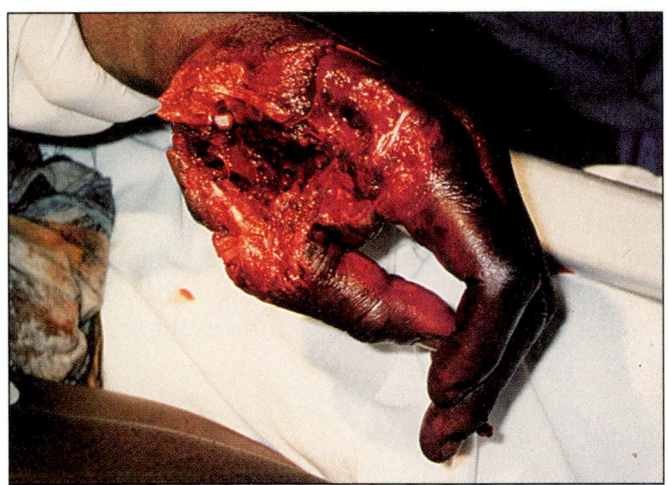

FIGURE 23-12 The area damaged by high-velocity projectiles, such as bullets, can be many times larger than the diameter of the projectile itself.

damaged by medium- and high-velocity projectiles can be many times larger than the diameter of the projectile itself (Figure 23-12). This is one reason that exit wounds are often many times larger than entrance wounds. As with motor vehicle crashes, the energy available for a bullet to cause damage is more a function of its speed than its mass (weight). If the mass of the bullet is doubled, the energy that is available to cause injury is doubled. If the speed (velocity) of the bullet is doubled, the energy that is available to cause injury is quadrupled. For this reason, it is important for you to try to determine the type of weapon that was used. Although it is not necessary (or always possible) for you to distinguish between medium- and high-velocity injuries, any information regarding the type of weapon that was used should be relayed to medical control.

Newton's laws

Newton's First Law

Newton's first law states that *objects at rest tend to stay at rest and objects in motion tend to stay in motion unless acted upon by some force.* The first part of the law is fairly clear. An object such as a empty soda can will not move spontaneously unless some force, such as a gust of wind, acts on it. An example will help to illustrate the second part. In a car going 30 mph, the passengers as well as the car are moving at 30 mph. The passengers do not feel as though they are moving because they are not moving relative to the car. However, when the car strikes a concrete barrier and comes to a sudden stop, the passengers continue to travel at 30 mph. They stay in motion until they are acted on by an external force—most likely the windshield, steering wheel, or dashboard. To appreciate the severity of the impact, think of the driver as sitting motionless while a steering wheel rams into his or her chest at 30 mph. Now consider that the same thing happens to the driver's internal organs. They also are in motion, traveling at 30 mph relative to the ground, until they are acted on by an external force, in this case the sternum, rib cage, or other body structure. This scenario illustrates the three collisions that are associated with blunt trauma.

Newton's Second Law

Newton's second law states that *force (F) equals mass (M) times acceleration (A), that is, F = MA,* in which acceleration is the change in velocity (speed) that occurs over time. Therefore, it is not so much that "speed kills" but that the change in velocity with respect to time generates the forces that cause injury. Simply put, it is not the fall, but the sudden stop at the bottom, that hurts.

In the example of the car traveling at 30 mph, it takes about 3 seconds for the car to decrease its speed from 30 mph to 0 mph when the driver applies the brakes smoothly. If he or she is properly restrained by well-adjusted seat belts, the driver slows, or decelerates, at the same rate as the car. But if the car is stopped not by braking but by hitting a large tree and the driver is not restrained, his or her body will continue to stay in motion at 30 mph until it is stopped by an external force—in this case, the steering wheel. Although the change in the body's velocity is the same as when the car was braking smoothly over 3 seconds (30 to 0 mph), that change now takes place in about 0.01 second. Because the time period of deceleration is 300 times less, the average force of impact is 300 times greater. This means that the force is approximately 150 times the force of gravity. Imagine a force 150 times your body weight slamming into your chest.

Now consider the same car striking the same tree, but this time, the driver is restrained with a shoulder and lap belt. The driver is essentially tied to the car and stops during the same period the car stops. It takes some time, although brief, to crush the front of the car and bring it to a halt. The car comes to a stop in approximately 0.05 second. The change in the driver's velocity is the same (30 to 0 mph), but the longer period of deceleration results in a g-force of only 30 times that of gravity. This is still a substantial force, but it is much less than the force that is experienced by the unrestrained driver. More to the point, it is survivable.

In a final example, the car and driver, as before, are traveling at 30 mph, and the driver is properly restrained with a 3-point belt. In this case, however, the car is also equipped with an air bag. When the car hits the tree and suddenly stops, the driver's upper body initially continues forward at 30 mph. The body is partially slowed by the lap and shoulder belts but is finally brought to rest by the air bag. The upper body compresses the air bag, which stops the body's forward motion in about 0.1 second. Thus, the air bag stretches the duration of impact by 0.05 second, buying the body even more time, and the force on the upper body drops to approximately 15 times that of gravity.

The air bag has another advantage. The force of its impact is applied over a much larger area than the area that is affected by the steering wheel or the shoulder belt, shrinking the force per unit area. This point can be illustrated by an analogy. A person standing on one toe on a sheet of ice applies a concentrated load in a very small area, thus breaking the ice and falling through. If the person lies flat on the ice, he or she greatly expands the contact area and reduces the stress on the ice, which, depending on conditions, should not break. The dual action of the air bag (distributing the force of impact over a greater area and increasing the duration of impact) results in less severe injuries.

Newton's Third Law

Newton's third law states that *for every action, there is an equal and opposite reaction.* Therefore, if you push on a door, the door pushes back (reacts) with an equal force but in the opposite direction. In the case of a dented A-pillar, the force of the driver's head was sufficient to dent the strong metal. But in terms of patient assessment, the more important point is the reaction force of the pillar on the head. Newton's third law states that the 2 forces are equal but occur in opposite directions. In other words, the head was essentially hit by an A-pillar traveling at 30 mph. Similarly, it takes a substantial force to collapse a steering wheel. When you notice a collapsed steering wheel during scene size-up, you should suspect serious chest injuries even if the driver initially has no visible signs of chest injury. Often, reading the scene and understanding the basic principles of energy transfer will give you as clear a picture of the patient's potential injuries and injury severity as the actual physical patient assessment.

prep kit

ready for review

Obtaining information about the mechanism of injury—that is, how the injuries occurred and what forces were likely involved—can be just as important as obtaining vital signs in assessing the patient. This information can help hospital staff to focus their attention on damage that may not be immediately obvious. Motor vehicle crashes are the leading cause of unintentional injury. In every crash, there are really three collisions: the collision of the car against another car or some other object, the collision of the passenger's against the interior of the car, and the collision of the passenger's internal organs against the solid structures of the body. You should suspect serious injuries in passengers who have been involved in a high-speed collision that results in massive damage to the car. The same is true of a patient who has fallen from a significant height or sustained a high-velocity penetrating injury.

points to ponder

Object. 3-2.5, 5-4.4, 5-4.5, 5-4.9

As you approach an auto-pedestrian accident you see a 4-year-old child lying on the pavement about 10' in front of the car. You also notice a person who appears to be a parent running toward the child. Before you can respond, the parent picks the child up to comfort the child. The child immediately goes limp, and you suspect that this is because of a severed spine caused by the movement.

- Would you tell the parent what he or she just did? Would you have the parent lay the child back down? If the parent asks why the child suddenly went limp, what would you say? Would you report the parent's actions? If so, to whom would you report them?

vital vocabulary *www.emtb.com*

cavitation A phenomenon in which speed causes a bullet to generate pressure waves, which cause damage distant from the bullet's path.

deceleration The slowing of an object.

kinetic energy The energy of a moving object.

mechanism of injury The way in which traumatic injuries occur; the forces that act on the body to cause damage.

potential energy The product of mass, gravity, and height, which is converted into kinetic energy and results in injury, such as from a fall.

online outlook

Injuries are the leading cause of death and disability in the United States among children and young adults (ages 1 to 34). To learn more about the specific injuries and their frequencies, complete Exercise 23 at www.emtb.com.

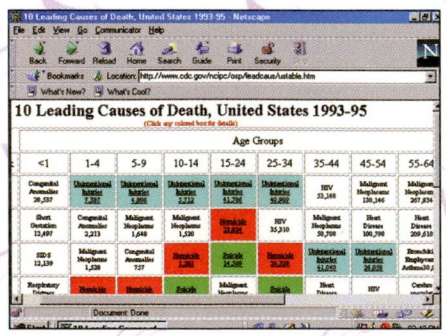

assessment in action

About 2:30 A.M. on a foggy Sunday morning, you and your partner are dispatched to a motor vehicle crash on Mountain View Road. As you pull up, you see that a pickup truck is lying on its roof partway down the embankment. The county sheriff has secured the scene and tells you that there are 2 patients. One is still inside the truck, and the other is lying approximately 50' from the truck after he was apparently ejected from the vehicle. Your partner goes to assess the second patient while you check on the driver. Your partner yells to you that the second patient is in full arrest. The driver, who was also unbelted at the time of the crash, responds minimally to voice commands and reports pain in the right shoulder and chest as well as in the right hip area. He also states that his head is throbbing.

1. Which of the following statements about injuries that result from ejection from a motor vehicle during a crash is **FALSE**?
   A. Spinal injuries are common.
   B. Head injuries are common.
   C. Injuries are not likely if the patient lands on a soft surface.
   D. Fatal injuries can occur because of rapid deceleration after an ejection.

2. Given the mechanism of injury, the unbelted driver is **LEAST** likely to have sustained which of the following injuries?
   A. Rib fracture
   B. Cervical spine injury
   C. A pelvic or hip injury
   D. Bruises to the sternum

3. Which of the following statements about the mechanisms of injury in this situation is true?
   A. The multiple mechanisms of injury increased the risk of injury.
   B. Almost all crashes involving pickup trucks result in fatalities.
   C. This crash was more severe because it occurred in the evening.
   D. Collisions on winding roads almost always occur at the highest speeds.

4. A second ambulance was requested, but you are advised by dispatch that it is delayed for 20 minutes because it had to stop for a train. On the basis of this information, the most appropriate course of action is to:
   A. ask the sheriff to assign the treatment priorities.
   B. treat the driver but not the patient who is in cardiac arrest.
   C. transport the patient who is in cardiac arrest and leave the driver at the scene.
   D. perform 2-person CPR on the patient who is in cardiac arrest and let the driver wait.

5. The fact that one of the patients has sustained fatal wounds suggests that the:
   A. mechanism of injury was quite severe.
   B. backup ambulance was not necessary.
   C. index of suspicion for trauma should be lower.
   D. other passenger probably has minor injuries.

prep kit

23

Bleeding

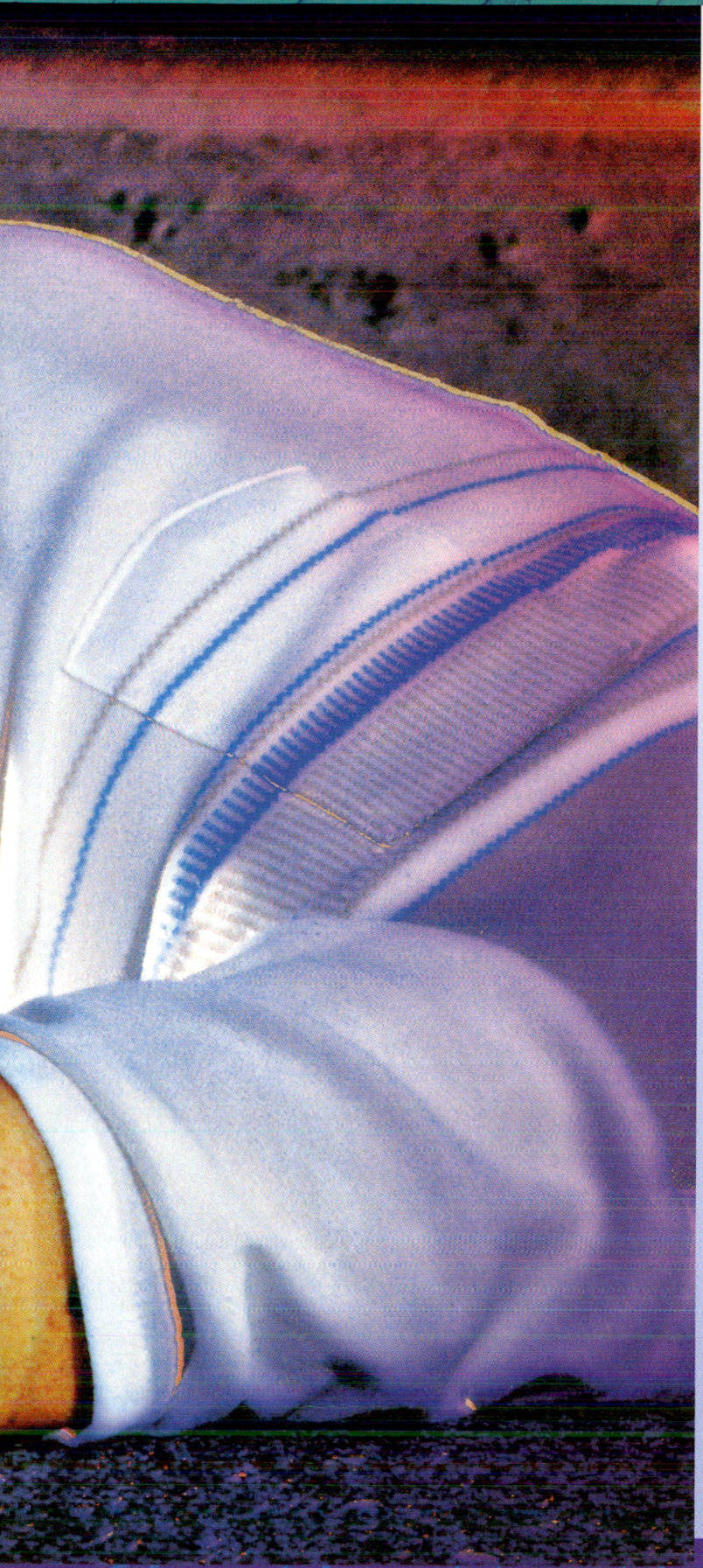

objectives

Cognitive

1. List the structure and function of the circulatory system.

2. Differentiate between arterial, venous, and capillary bleeding.

3. State methods of emergency medical care of external bleeding.

4. Establish the relationship between body substance isolation and bleeding.

5. Establish the relationship between airway management and the trauma patient.

6. Establish the relationship between mechanism of injury and internal bleeding.

7. List the signs of internal bleeding.

8. List the steps in the emergency medical care of the patient with signs and symptoms of internal bleeding.

Affective

9. Explain the sense of urgency to transport patients that are bleeding and show signs of shock (hypoperfusion).

Psychomotor

10. Demonstrate direct pressure as a method of emergency medical care of external bleeding.

11. Demonstrate the use of diffuse pressure as a method of emergency medical care of external bleeding.

12. Demonstrate the use of pressure points and tourniquets as a method of emergency medical care of external bleeding.

13. Demonstrate the care of the patient exhibiting signs and symptoms of internal bleeding.

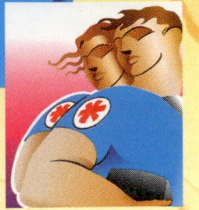

you are the emt

Squad 14, respond to the train station for a man "bleeding to death" in the first floor bathroom.

The term "bleeding to death" is an overused phrase, as the lay public often uses it to describe even minimal bleeding. However, bleeding control is a key part of good prehospital care, especially for victims of trauma. This chapter will present several different methods for controlling bleeding, and it will also help you to answer the following questions:

1. How important are BSI techniques and universal precautions when attempting to control bleeding?

2. What is the sequence of events that occurs physiologically to a patient whose serious bleeding is not controlled quickly and effectively?

Bleeding

After managing the airway, recognizing bleeding and understanding how it affects the body are perhaps the most important skills you will learn as an EMT-B. Bleeding can be external and obvious or internal and hidden. Either way, it is potentially dangerous, causing first weakness and, if left uncontrolled, eventually shock and death. The most common cause of shock after trauma is bleeding.

The purpose of this chapter is to help you understand how the cardiovascular system reacts to blood loss. The chapter begins with a brief review of the anatomy and function of the cardiovascular system. It then describes the signs, symptoms, and emergency medical care of both external and internal bleeding. The chapter concludes with a discussion on the relationship between bleeding and hypovolemic shock.

Anatomy and Physiology of the Cardiovascular System

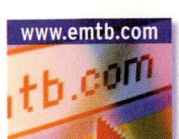

The cardiovascular system circulates blood to all of the body's cells and tissues, delivering oxygen and nutrients and carrying away metabolic waste products (Figure 24-1). Certain parts of the body, such as the brain and spinal cord, require a constant flow of blood to live. The cells in these organs cannot tolerate a lack of blood for more than a few minutes. Other organs, such as the heart, lungs, and kidneys, can sur-

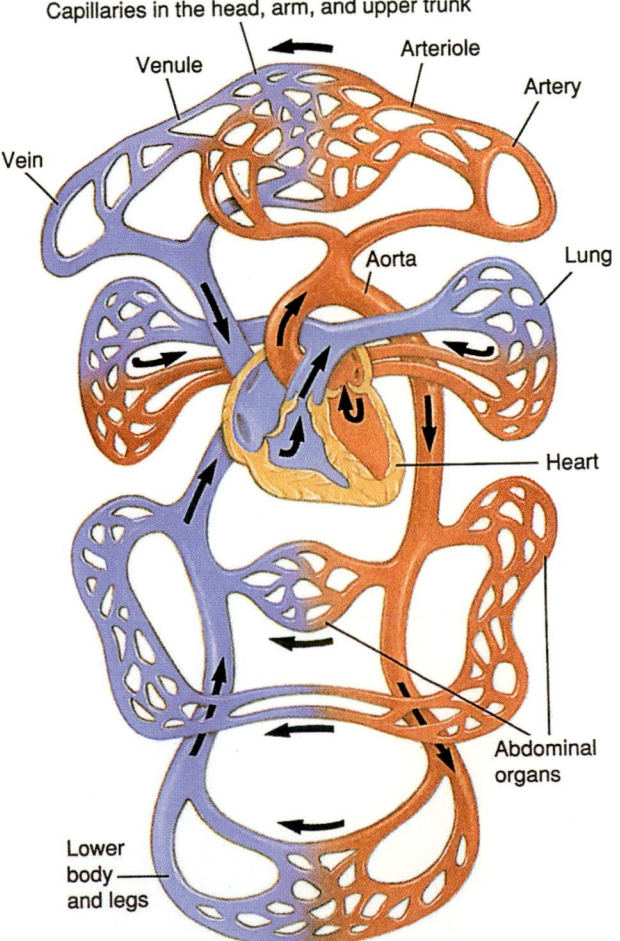

FIGURE 24-1 The cardiovascular system includes the heart, arteries, veins, and interconnecting capillaries. The exchange of nutrients and waste products occurs in the capillaries.

vive only for short periods of time without adequate blood flow. After that, their cells begin to die. This can lead to a permanent loss of function or, if enough cells die, death.

The cardiovascular system, the main system responsible for supplying and maintaining adequate blood flow, consists of 3 parts:

- The pump (the heart)
- A container (the blood vessels that reach every cell in the body)
- The fluid (blood and body fluids)

The Heart

The heart is a hollow muscular organ about the size of a clenched fist. It is an involuntary muscle that is under the control of the autonomic nervous system, but it has its own regulatory system. Thus, it can function even if the nervous system shuts down.

The heart is always working; all other organs depend on it to provide a rich blood supply. For this reason, it has a number of special features that other muscles do not. First, because the heart can tolerate a serious interruption of its blood supply for only a few seconds, its blood supply is as rich and well distributed as possible. Second, the heart works as 2 paired pumps (Figure 24-2). Each side of the heart has an upper chamber (atrium) and a lower chamber (ventricle), both of which pump blood. Blood leaves each chamber of the heart

through a one-way valve, which keeps the blood moving in the proper direction by preventing a back flow.

The right side of the heart receives oxygen-poor (deoxygenated) blood from the veins of the body. Blood enters into the right atrium from the vena cava, then fills the right ventricle. After the right ventricle contracts, blood flows into the pulmonary artery and the pulmonary circulation. The now oxygen-rich (oxygenated) blood returns to the left side of the heart from the lungs through the pulmonary veins. Blood enters the left atrium, then passes into the left ventricle. This side of the heart is more muscular than the other because it must pump blood into the aorta and on to the arteries.

Blood Vessels and Blood

There are 5 types of blood vessels:

- Arteries
- Arterioles
- Capillaries
- Venules
- Veins

As blood flows out of the heart, it passes into the aorta, the largest artery in the body. The arteries become smaller as they move away from the heart. The smaller vessels that connect the arteries and capillaries are called arterioles. Capillaries are small tubes, with the diameter of a single red blood cell, that pass among all the cells in

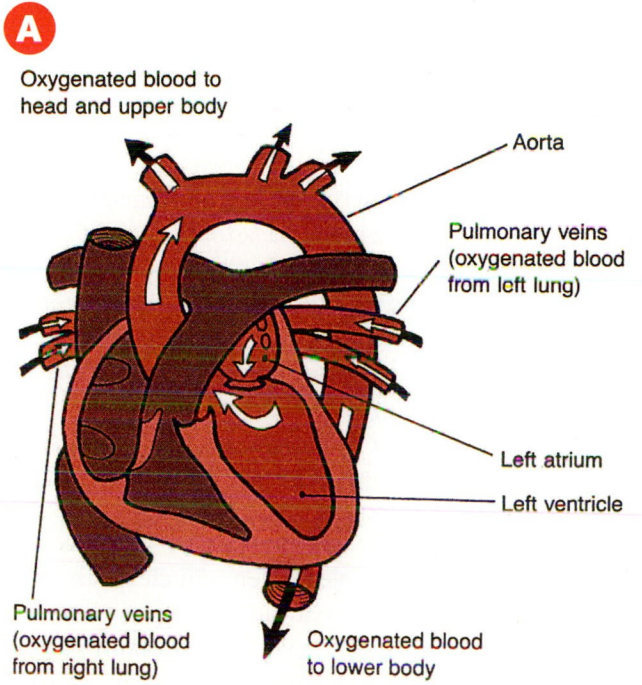

A Oxygenated blood to head and upper body

Aorta

Pulmonary veins (oxygenated blood from left lung)

Left atrium

Left ventricle

Pulmonary veins (oxygenated blood from right lung)

Oxygenated blood to lower body

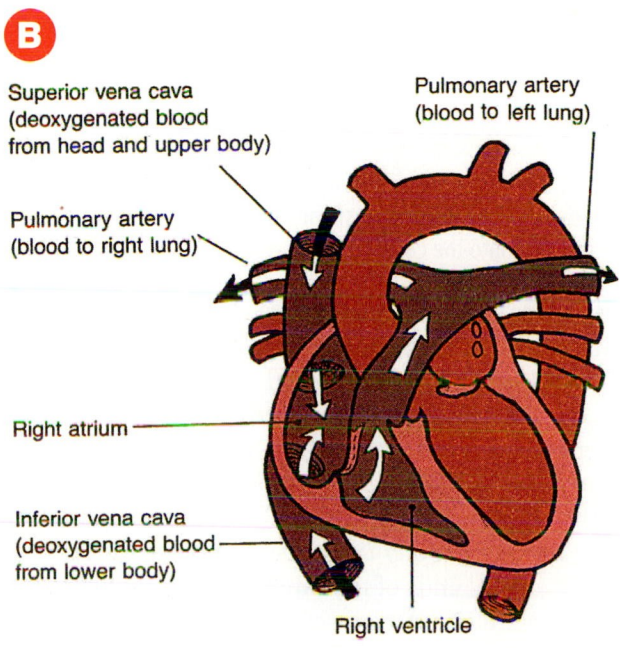

B Superior vena cava (deoxygenated blood from head and upper body)

Pulmonary artery (blood to left lung)

Pulmonary artery (blood to right lung)

Right atrium

Inferior vena cava (deoxygenated blood from lower body)

Right ventricle

FIGURE 24-2 A: The left side of the heart circulates oxygen-rich blood to all parts of the body. It is the more muscular of the two pumps, as it must pump blood into the aorta and into the arteries. **B:** The right side of the heart circulates blood from the body to the lungs.

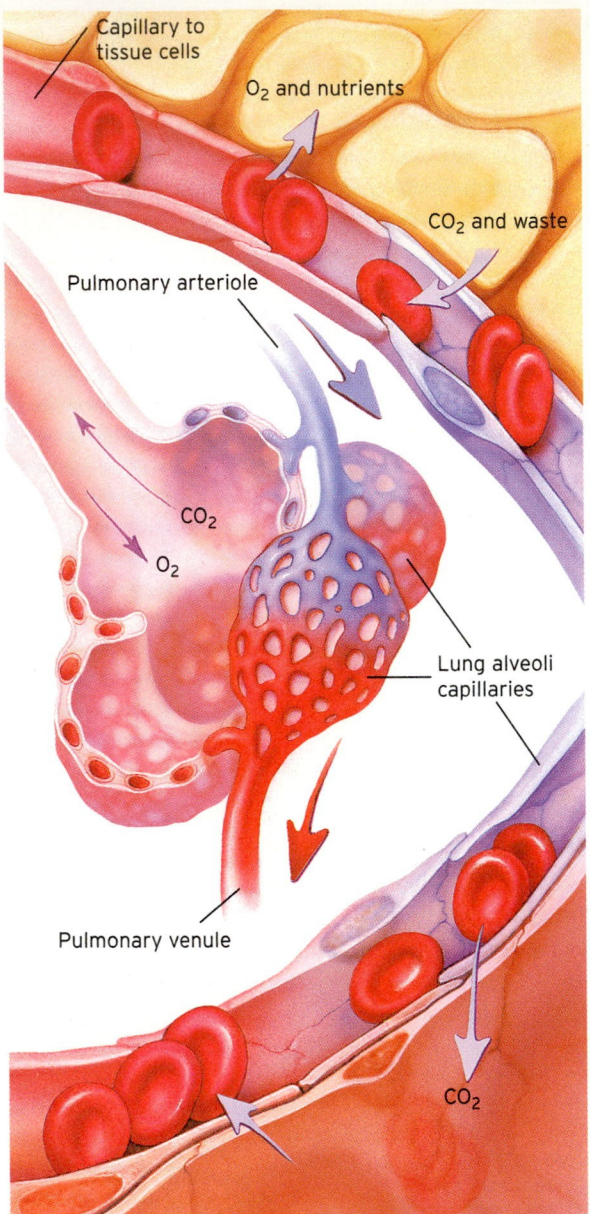

FIGURE 24-3 Oxygen and nutrients pass easily from the capillaries into the cells, and waste and carbon dioxide move out of the cells and into the capillaries.

the body, linking the arterioles and the venules. Blood leaving the distal side of the capillaries flows into the venules. These small, thin-walled vessels empty into the veins, which return the blood to the heart. Oxygen and nutrients easily pass from the capillaries into the cells, and waste and carbon dioxide move out of the cells and into the capillaries (Figure 24-3). This transportation system allows the body to rid itself of waste products.

At the arterial ends of the capillaries and in the arteries themselves are circular muscular walls, which constrict and dilate automatically under the control of the autonomic nervous system. When these muscles open (dilate), blood passes into the capillaries into close proximity to each cell of the surrounding tissue; when the

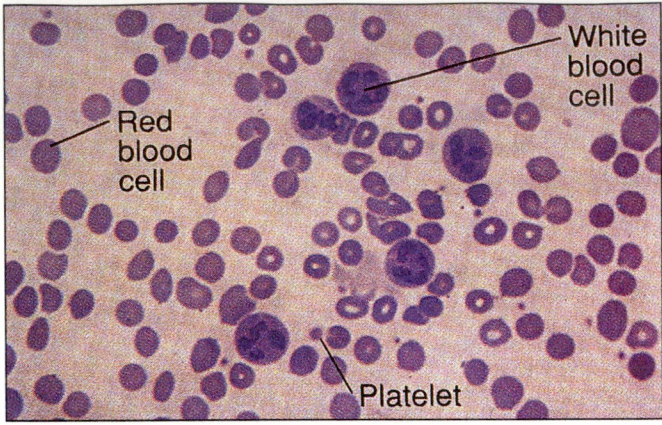

FIGURE 24-4 The microscopic appearance of the three major elements in blood: red blood cells, white blood cells, and platelets.

muscles are closed (constricted), there is no capillary blood flow. The muscles dilate and constrict in response to conditions such as fright, heat, cold, a specific need for oxygen, and the need to dispose of metabolic waste. In a healthy individual, all the vessels are never fully dilated or fully constricted at the same time.

The last part of the cardiovascular system is the contents of the container, or the blood. Blood contains red cells, white cells, and platelets and a liquid, called plasma (Figure 24-4).

Physiology and Perfusion

Perfusion is the circulation of blood within an organ or tissue in adequate amounts to meet the cells' current needs for oxygen, nutrients, and waste removal. Blood enters an organ or tissue first through the arteries, then the arterioles, and finally the capillary beds (Figure 24-5). While passing through the capillaries, the blood delivers nutrients and oxygen to the surrounding cells and picks up the wastes they have generated. Then the blood leaves the capillary beds through the venules and finally reaches the veins, which take the blood back to the heart. Oxygen and carbon dioxide exchange takes place in the lungs.

Blood must pass through the cardiovascular system at a speed that is fast enough to maintain adequate circulation throughout the body and slow enough to allow each cell time to exchange oxygen and nutrients for carbon dioxide and other waste products. While some tissues, such as the lungs and kidneys, never rest and require a constant blood supply, most require circulating blood only intermittently, especially when active. Muscles are a good example. When you sleep, they are at rest and require a minimal blood supply. However, during exercise, they need a very large blood supply. The gastrointestinal tract requires a high flow of blood after a meal. After digestion is completed, it can do quite well with a small fraction of that flow.

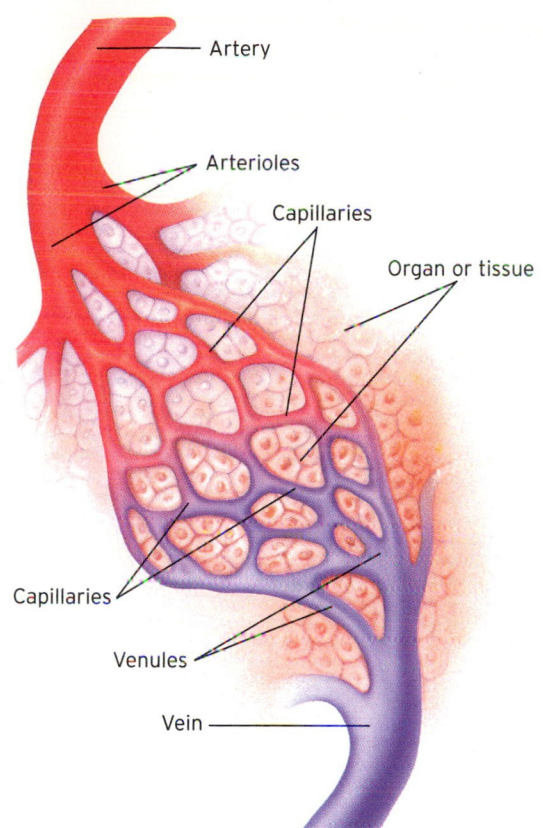

FIGURE 24-5 Perfusion occurs when blood circulates through tissues or an organ, to provide the necessary oxygen and nutrients and remove waste products.

The autonomic nervous system monitors the body's needs from moment to moment and adjusts the blood flow as required. During emergencies, the autonomic nervous system automatically redirects blood away from other organs to the heart, brain, lungs, and kidneys. Thus, the cardiovascular system is dynamic, constantly adapting to changing conditions. At times, the system fails to provide sufficient circulation for every body part to perform its function. This condition is called hypoperfusion, or __shock__.

Knowing which organs need adequate perfusion is the foundation on which your treatment of patients is based. Emergency medical care is designed to support the following systems in the following order:

- The heart (cardiovascular system)
- The brain (central nervous system)
- The lungs (respiratory system)
- The kidneys

The heart requires constant perfusion, or it will not function properly. The brain and spinal cord cannot go for more than 4 to 6 minutes without perfusion, or the nerve cells will be permanently damaged. The kidneys will be permanently damaged after 45 minutes of inadequate perfusion. Skeletal muscles cannot tolerate more than 2 hours of inadequate perfusion. The gastrointestinal tract can exist with limited (but not absent) perfusion for several hours. These times are based on a normal body temperature (98.6°F [37.0°C]). An organ or tissue that is considerably colder is much better able to resist damage from hypoperfusion.

External Bleeding

__Hemorrhage__ means "bleeding." External bleeding is a visible hemorrhage. Examples include nosebleeds and bleeding from open wounds. As an EMT-B, you must understand how to control external bleeding.

EMT-B safety

Remember that a bleeding patient may expose you to potentially infectious body fluids; therefore, you must always follow BSI techniques in treating patients with external bleeding. Wear gloves and eye protection in all situations, and wear a gown and mask if there is a risk of blood splatter (Figure 24-6). Avoid direct contact with body fluids if possible. Take special care if you have an open sore, cut, scratch, or ulcer. Also remember that frequent, thorough handwashing between patients and after every run is a simple yet important protective measure.

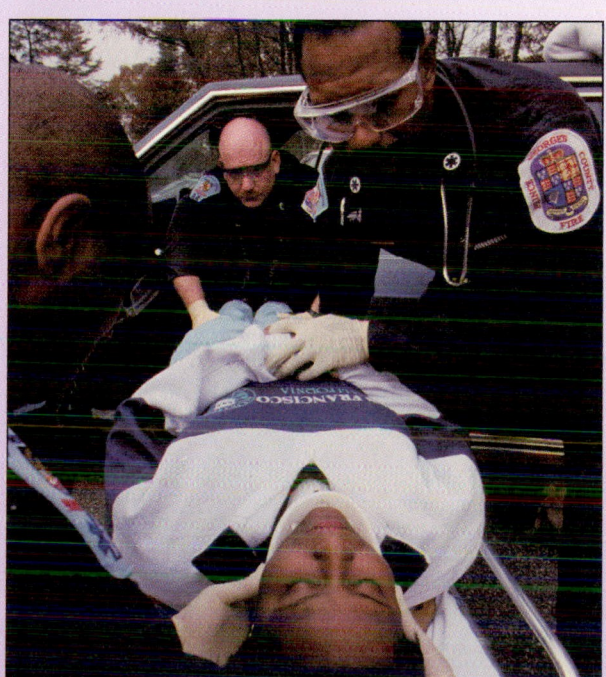

FIGURE 24-6 Your safety is paramount; therefore, you should always wear proper protective equipment when caring for a patient who is bleeding.

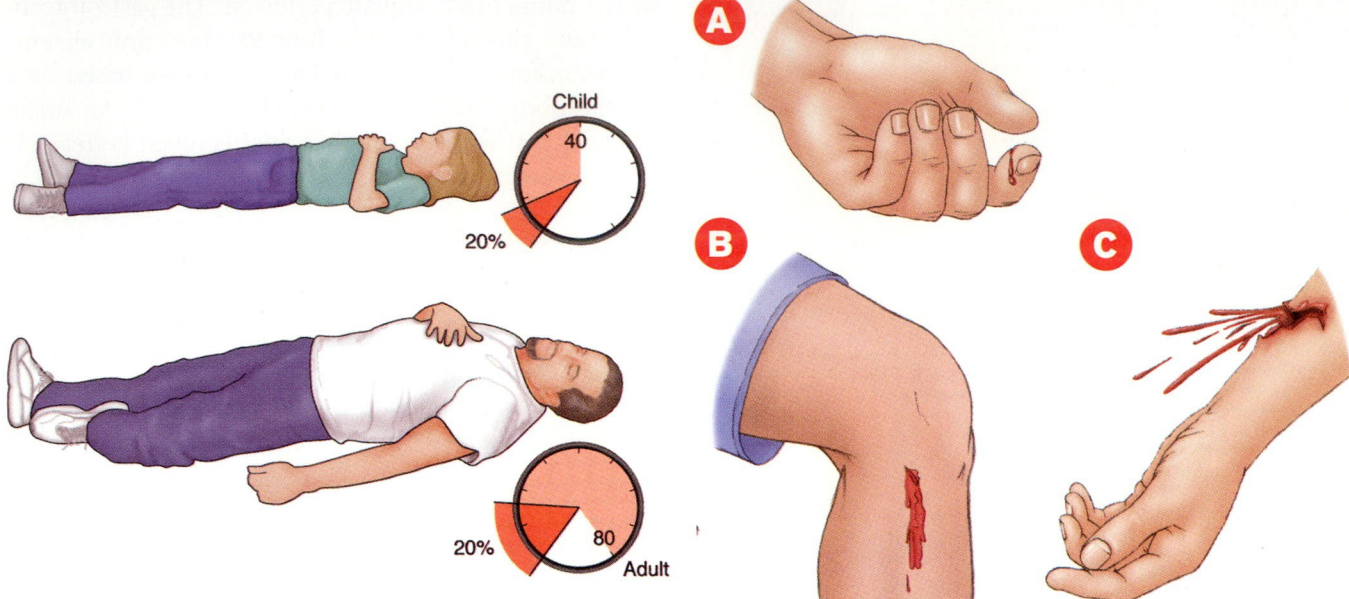

FIGURE 24-7 Loss of approximately 1 L of blood will cause significant changes in an adult; a much lesser blood loss will result in shock in a child or infant.

FIGURE 24-8 A: Bleeding from capillary vessels is dark red and oozes from the wound slowly but steadily. **B:** Venous bleeding is darker in color and flows steadily. **C:** Arterial bleeding is characteristically bright red and spurts in time with the pulse.

The Significance of Bleeding

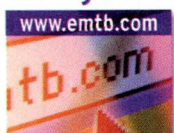

The body will not tolerate an acute blood loss of greater than 20% of blood volume (Figure 24-7). The typical adult has approximately 70 mL of blood per kilogram of body weight, or 6 L (10 to 12 pints) in a body weighing 80 kg. If the typical adult loses more than 1 L of blood (about 2 pints), significant changes in vital signs will occur, including increasing heart rate and decreasing blood pressure. Because infants and children have less blood volume to begin with, the same effect is seen with smaller amounts of blood loss. For example, a 1-year-old infant has a total blood volume of about 800 mL. Significant symptoms of blood loss will occur after only 100 to 200 mL of blood loss.

How well a person compensates for blood loss is related to how rapidly they bleed. A normal, healthy adult can comfortably donate 1 unit (500 mL) of blood over a period of 15 to 20 minutes, adapting well to this decrease in blood volume. However, if a similar blood loss occurs in a much shorter period of time, the person may rapidly develop **hypovolemic shock**, a condition in which low blood volume results in inadequate perfusion and even death. The body simply cannot compensate for such a rapid blood loss.

You should consider bleeding to be serious if the following conditions are present:

- It is associated with a significant mechanism of injury.
- The patient has a poor general appearance.

- Assessment reveals signs and symptoms of shock (hypoperfusion).
- You note a significant amount of blood loss.
- You cannot control the bleeding.

In any situation, blood loss is an extremely serious problem. It demands your immediate attention as soon as you have cleared the airway and managed the patient's breathing.

Characteristics of Bleeding

Injuries and some illnesses can disrupt blood vessels and cause bleeding. Typically, bleeding from an open artery is bright red (high in oxygen) and spurts in time with the pulse (Figure 24-8). The pressure that causes the blood to spurt also makes this type of bleeding difficult to control. As the amount of blood circulating in the body drops, so does the patient's blood pressure and, eventually, the arterial spurting.

Blood from an open vein is much darker (low in oxygen) and flows steadily. Because it is under less pressure, most venous blood does not spurt and is easier to manage. Bleeding from damaged capillary vessels is dark red and oozes from a wound steadily but slowly. It may clot spontaneously.

On its own, bleeding tends to stop rather quickly, within about 10 minutes, in response to internal mechanisms. When we are cut, blood flows rapidly from the open vessel. Soon afterward, the cut ends of the vessel begin to narrow, reducing the amount of bleeding.

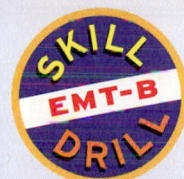

Using Direct Pressure to Control Bleeding

Figure 24-9

1

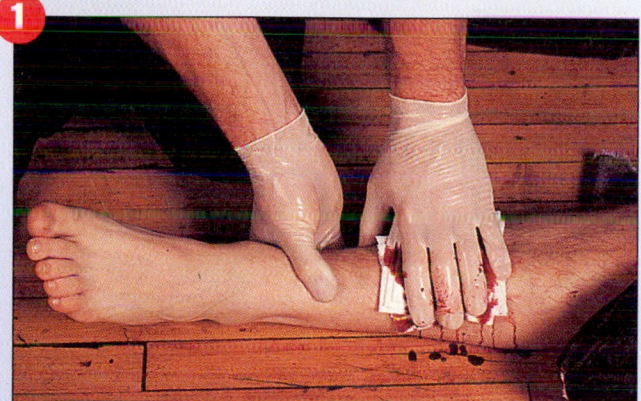

Apply direct pressure, as pressure stops the flow of blood and permits normal coagulation to occur.

2

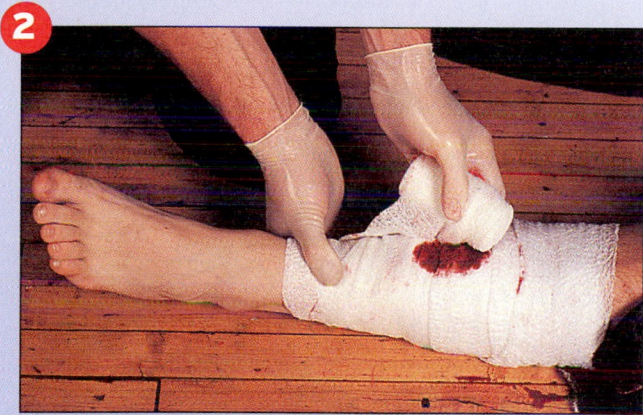

Maintain the pressure by firmly wrapping a sterile, self-adhering roller bandage around the entire wound. Cover the entire dressing, above and below the wound but not so tightly as to decrease blood flow to the extremity. You should still be able to feel a distal radial pulse.

3

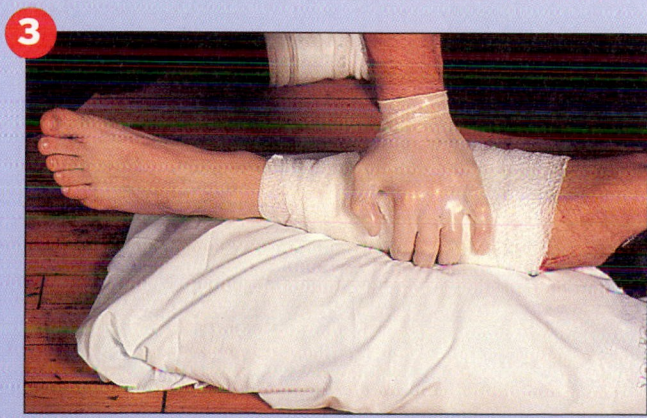

Elevate the extremity about 6″ and continue to apply pressure.

Then a clot forms, plugging the hole and sealing the injured portions of the vessel. This process is called **coagulation**. Bleeding will never stop if a clot does not form, unless the injured vessel is completely cut off from the main blood supply. Direct contact with body tissues and fluids or the external environment commonly triggers the blood's clotting factors.

Despite the efficiency of this system, it may fail in certain situations. A number of medications, including aspirin, interfere with normal clotting. With a severe injury, the damage to the vessel may be so large that a clot cannot completely block the hole. Sometimes, only part of the vessel wall is cut, preventing it from constricting. In these cases, bleeding will continue unless it is stopped by external means. Occasionally, blood loss occurs very rapidly. In these instances, the patient might die before the body's defenses, such as clotting, could help.

A very small portion of the population lacks one or more of the blood's clotting factors. This condition is called **hemophilia**. There are several forms of hemophilia, most of which are hereditary and some of which are severe. Sometimes, bleeding may occur spontaneously in hemophilia. Because the patient's blood does not clot, all injuries, no matter how trivial, are potentially serious. A patient with hemophilia should be transported immediately.

Emergency Medical Care

As you begin to care for a patient with obvious external bleeding, remember to follow BSI techniques. As with all patient care, make sure that the patient has an open airway and is breathing adequately. Provide oxygen if it is needed. You may then concentrate on controlling the bleeding.

Several methods are available to control external bleeding. Starting with the most commonly used, these include the following:

- Direct local pressure and elevation
- Pressure points (for upper and lower extremities only)
- Splints
- Air splints
- Pneumatic antishock garment
- Tourniquets (last resort)

Direct pressure and elevation. Almost all instances of external bleeding can be controlled simply by applying direct local pressure to the bleeding site (Figure 24-9). This method is by far the most effective way to control local external bleeding. Pressure stops the flow of blood and permits normal coagulation to occur. You may apply pressure with your gloved finger or hand, followed by application of a pressure dressing. Use 4″ x 4″ or 4″ x 8″

The typical adult has approximately 70 mL of blood per kilogram of body weight.

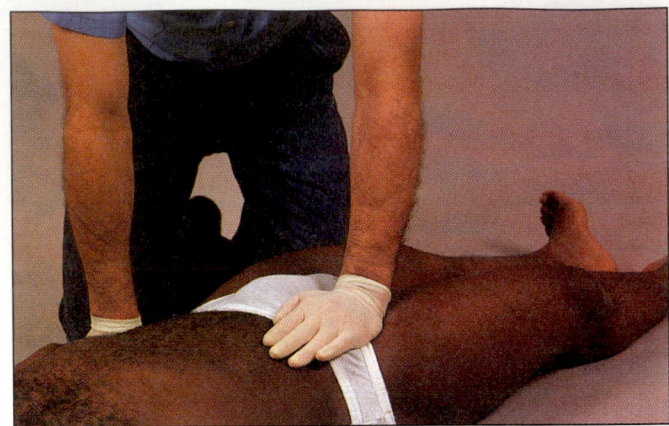

FIGURE 24-10 If a wound continues to bleed despite the use of direct local pressure, you can try placing additional pressure over a proximal pulse point.

sterile gauze pads for small wounds and sterile universal dressings for large wounds. If sterile gauze pads are not immediately available, use a clean handkerchief, sanitary napkin, or clean cloth. If no material is available, use your gloved hand to continue to provide the necessary pressure.

Once you have controlled the bleeding, you can maintain the pressure by firmly wrapping a sterile, self-adhering roller bandage around the entire wound. Cover the entire dressing, above and below the wound. Stretch the bandage tight enough to control bleeding but not so tight as to decrease blood flow to the extremity. You should be able to palpate a distal pulse on the injured extremity after applying the pressure dressing.

If bleeding continues, the dressing is probably not tight enough. Do not remove a dressing until a physician has evaluated the patient. Instead, apply additional manual pressure through the dressing. Then add additional gauze pads over the first dressing, and secure them both with a second, tighter, roller bandage. Bleeding will almost always stop when the pressure of the dressing exceeds arterial pressure. On those rare occasions when direct pressure fails to stop bleeding from a large gaping wound, you may need to pack the wound with sterile gauze pads.

Elevating a bleeding extremity by as little as 6″ often stops venous bleeding. Whenever possible, use both techniques: direct pressure and elevation. In most cases, this will stop the bleeding. However, if it does not, you still have several options.

Pressure points. If a wound continues to bleed despite use of direct local pressure, you should elevate the extremity and try placing additional pressure over a proximal pulse point. The larger the blood vessel that is involved, the more likely it is that this will occur. A pulse point, or **pressure point**, is a spot where a blood vessel lies near a bone. This technique is also useful if you have no material on hand to use for a dressing. Because a wound usually draws blood from more than one major artery, proximal compression of a major artery rarely stops bleeding completely, but it helps to slow the loss of blood (Figure 24-10). You must be thoroughly familiar with the location of the pulse points for this to work (Figure 24-11).

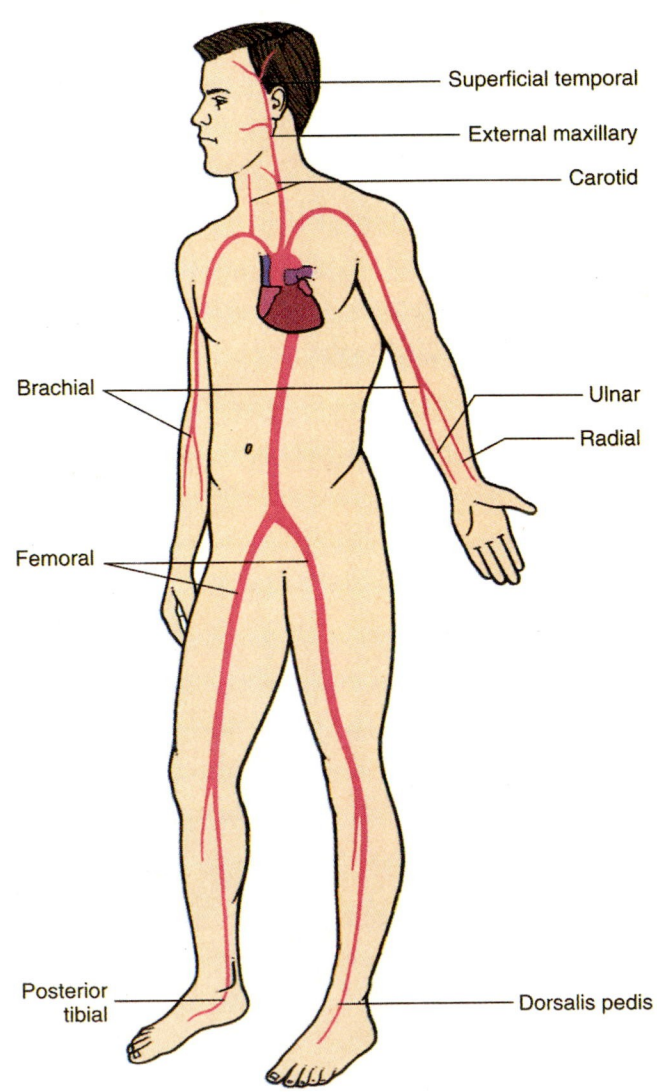

FIGURE 24-11 You should be familiar with the locations of arterial pressure points.

Splints. Much of the bleeding associated with broken bones occurs because the sharp ends of the bones cut muscles and other tissues. As long as a fracture remains unstable, the bone ends will move and continue to injure partially clotted vessels. Therefore, stabilizing a serious fracture is a high priority in the prompt control of bleeding. Often, simple splints will quickly control bleeding associated with a fracture (Figure 24-12). If not, you may need to use pressure splints, either air splints or a pneumatic antishock garment.

Air splints. Air splints can control the bleeding associated with severe soft-tissue injuries, such as massive or complex lacerations, or fractures (Figure 24-13). They also stabilize the fracture itself. An air splint acts like a pressure bandage applied to an entire extremity rather than to a small, local area. Once you have applied an air splint, be sure to monitor circulation in the distal extremity. Use only BSI-approved, clean or disposable valve stems when orally inflating air splints.

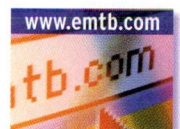 **Pneumatic antishock garments.** If a patient has injuries to the lower extremities, you may be able to use a pneumatic antishock garment (PASG) to prevent or minimize hypovolemic shock, if local protocol allows. Situations in which use of a PASG is allowed vary widely by locale. Be sure to check with medical control in every case.

Following are the few, very specific instances in which a PASG is effective:

- To stabilize fractures of the pelvis and proximal femurs

- To control significant internal bleeding associated with fractures of the pelvis and proximal femurs

- To control massive soft-tissue bleeding of the lower extremities when direct pressure is not effective

- To control shock due to significant internal bleeding

Do not use the PASG if any of the following conditions exist:

- Pregnancy (do not use the abdominal portion, but can inflate the legs)
- Chronic pulmonary edema secondary to longstanding heart disease
- Acute heart failure
- Penetrating chest injuries
- Groin injuries
- Major head injuries
- A transport time of less than 30 minutes

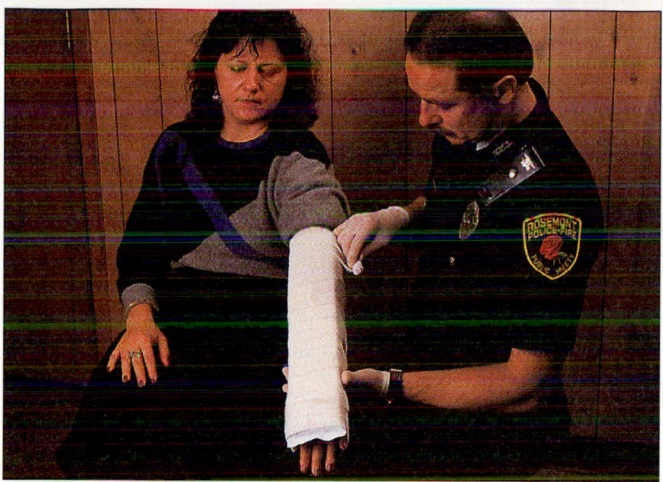

FIGURE 24-12 Use of a simple splint will often quickly control bleeding associated with a fracture. As long as a fracture is not immobilized, the bone ends are free to move and may continue to injure partially clotted vessels.

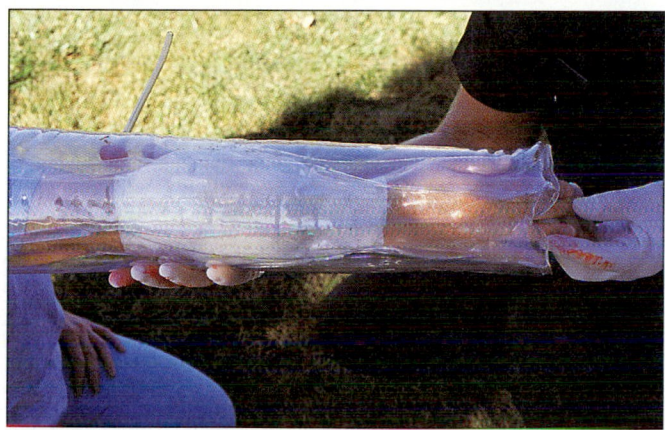

FIGURE 24-13 Air splints can also be used to control bleeding as they act as a pressure bandage for the entire extremity.

In these situations, the PASG may worsen or complicate the patient's condition. Consult with medical control if you think prolonged use or use in unusual circumstances may be necessary.

The PASG works by compressing the abdomen and lower extremities, increasing peripheral resistance in the circulatory system. This increases the amount of blood that is available to perfuse the vital organs. In applying the PASG, you should carefully inflate the device in increments (Figure 24-14). As a general rule, gradually inflate the legs of the PASG before inflating the abdominal portion. If you are using the device to stabilize a possible pelvic fracture, you must inflate all compartments.

Remember that the PASG's pressure gauges measure the air pressure in the device. They in no way reflect the

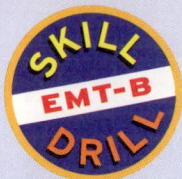

Applying a Pneumatic Antishock Garment
Figure 24-14

1

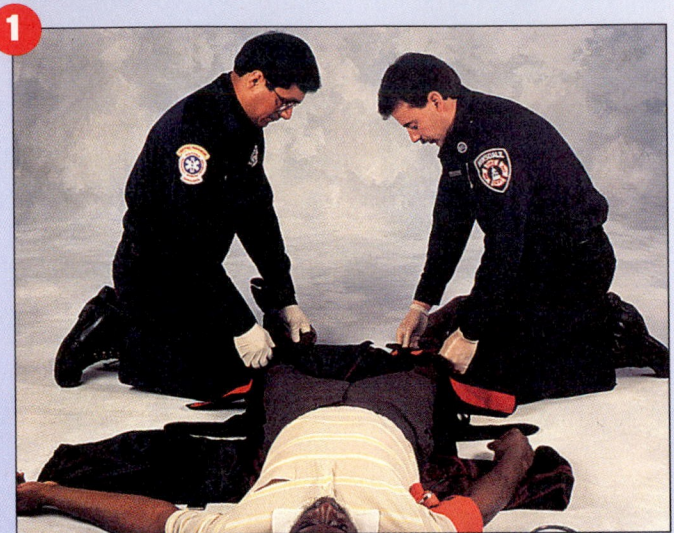

Apply the garment so that the top is below the last rib.

2

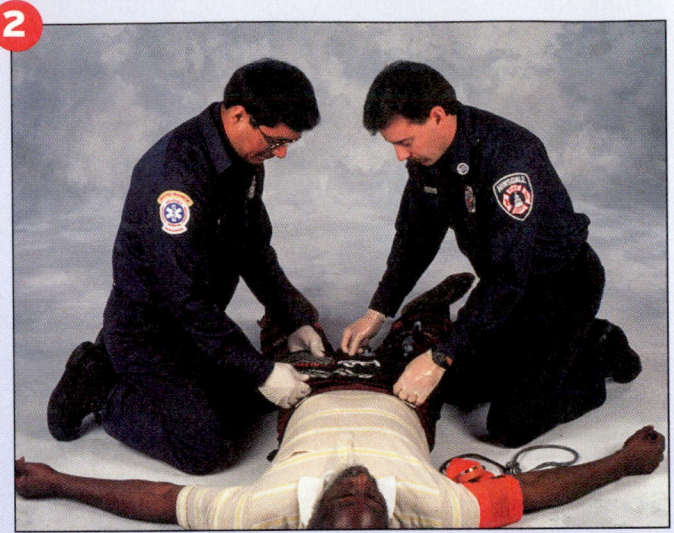

Enclose both legs and abdomen.

3

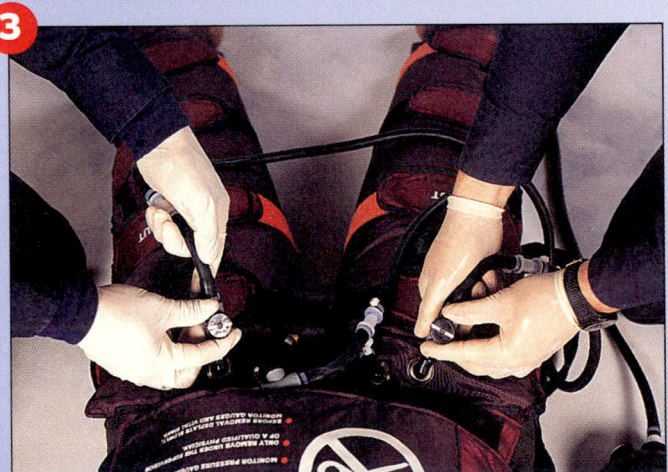

Open the stopcocks.

4

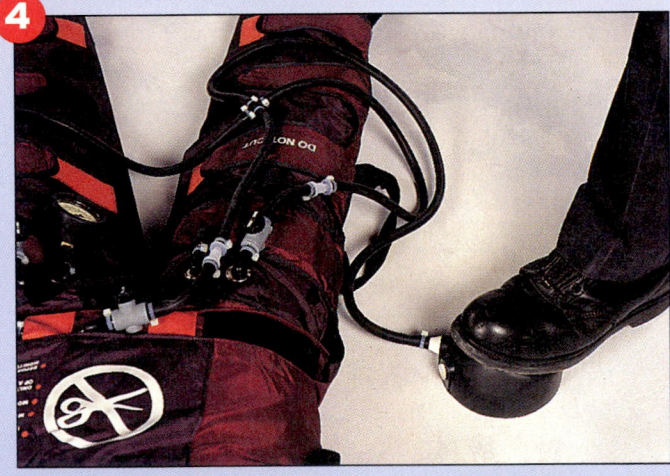

Inflate with the foot pump.

5

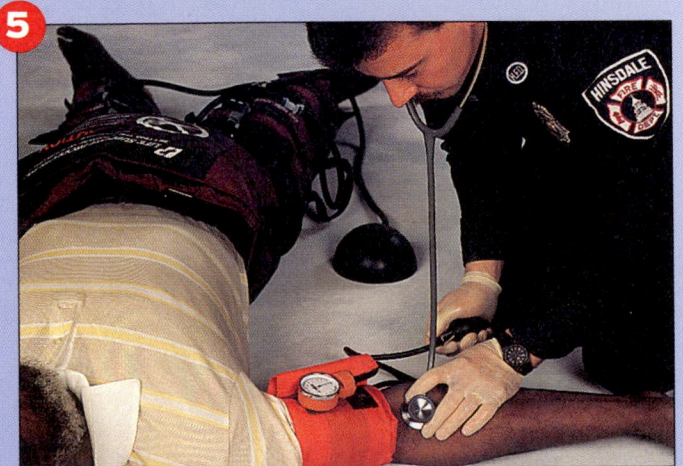

Check the patient's blood pressure, and close the stopcocks either when the patient's systolic blood pressure reaches 100 mm Hg or the Velcro snaps. Monitor the patient's vital signs en route.

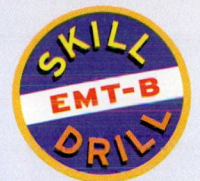

Applying a Tourniquet

Figure 24-15

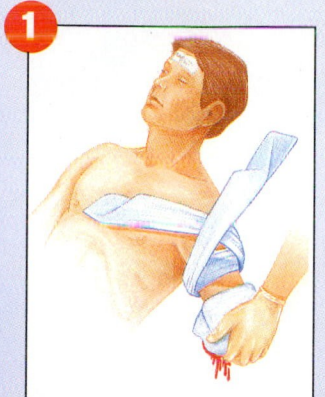

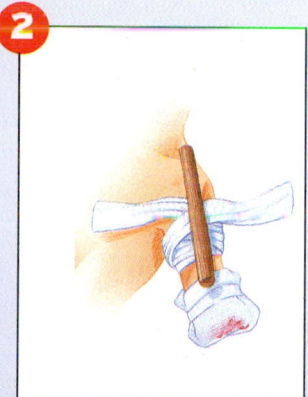

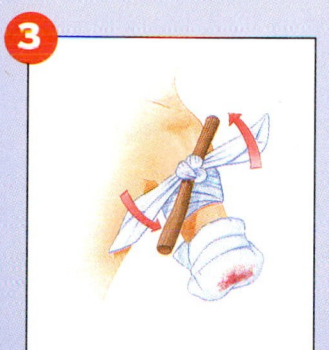

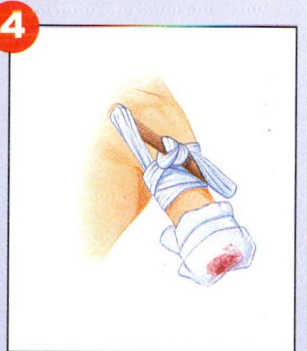

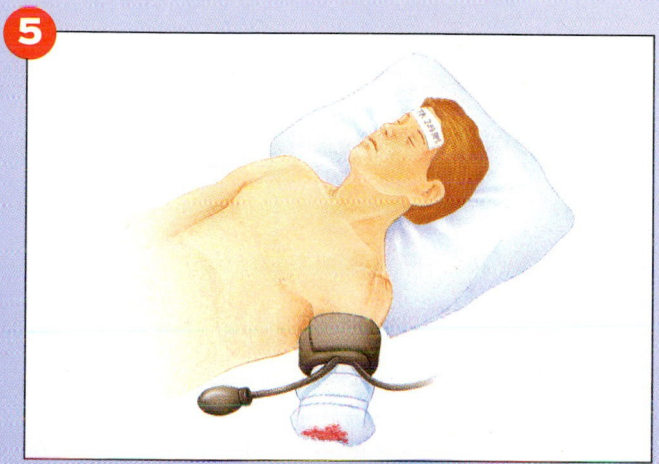

1: Wrap a 4"-wide bandage twice around the extremity, just above the bleeding site. **2:** Tie a single knot, and place a stick on the top of it. **3:** Tie a square knot over the stick, and then twist the stick until the bleeding stops. **4:** Secure the stick so that it will not unwind. Be sure to write "TK" and the exact time you applied the tourniquet on a piece of adhesive tape, and fasten the tape to the patient's forehead. **5:** You can also use a blood pressure cuff as an effective tourniquet.

patient's blood pressure. Therefore, you should monitor and record the patient's blood pressure at least every 5 minutes before, during, and after applying the device. Do not increase the garment's pressure any more than necessary. A PASG is adequately inflated when the Velcro snaps and you can dent the garment with your thumb. Higher pressures will damage tissue locally. Always stop inflating the PASG once the patient's systolic blood pressure exceeds 100 mm Hg.

If the PASG has no pressure gauges, you must monitor the distal neurovascular status of the limbs. Make sure that you can still detect pulses, sensation, and motion. You will know that the device has worked if the patient's blood pressure increases and the vital signs stabilize.

Do not remove a PASG in the field. It must be deflated gradually in the hospital under careful supervision by a physician and only after appropriate IV solutions have been given. Before turning your patient over to hospital personnel, report the patient's blood pressure, the time you applied the PASG, and the results.

Tourniquets. Tourniquets are rarely needed to control bleeding. Applying a tourniquet is considered a last resort, because it is rarely necessary and is effective for only a very limited number of injuries. Thus, a tourniquet often creates, rather than solves, problems. Application of a tourniquet can cause permanent damage to nerves, muscles, and blood vessels, resulting in the loss of an extremity. In addition, tourniquets are often improperly applied.

If you cannot control bleeding from the major vessel in an extremity in any other way, a properly applied tourniquet may save a patient's life. Specifically, the tourniquet is useful if a patient is bleeding severely from a partial or complete amputation.

Follow these steps to apply a tourniquet (Figure 24-15):

1. **Fold a triangular bandage** until it is 4" wide and 6 to 8 layers thick.

2. **Wrap the bandage** around the extremity twice. Choose an area proximal to the bleeding to reduce the amount of tissue damage to the extremity.

3. **Tie one knot** in the bandage. Then place a stick or rod on top of the knot, and tie the ends of the bandage over the stick in a square knot.

4. **Use the stick as a handle,** and twist it to tighten the tourniquet until the bleeding has stopped; then stop twisting. Secure the stick in place, and make the wrapping neat and smooth.

5. **Write "TK"** and the exact time (hour and minute) that you applied the tourniquet on a piece of adhesive tape. Use the phrase "time applied." Securely fasten the tape to the patient's forehead.

6. **Notify hospital personnel** on your arrival that your patient has a tourniquet in place. Record this same information on the ambulance run report form.

You can also use a blood pressure cuff as an effective tourniquet. Position the cuff proximal to the bleeding point, and inflate it just enough to stop the bleeding. Leave the cuff inflated. If you use a blood pressure cuff, monitor the gauge continuously to make sure that the pressure is not gradually dropping. You may have to clamp the tube with a hemostat leading from the cuff to the inflating bulb to prevent loss of pressure.

Whenever you apply a tourniquet, make sure you observe the following precautions:

- Do not apply a tourniquet directly over any joint. Keep it as close to the injury as possible.

- Use the widest bandage possible. Make sure that it is tightened securely.

- Never use wire, rope, a belt, or any other narrow material. It could cut into the skin.

- Use wide padding under the tourniquet if possible. This will protect the tissues and help with arterial compression.

- Never cover a tourniquet with a bandage. Leave it open and in full view.

- Do not loosen the tourniquet after you have applied it. Hospital personnel will loosen it once they are prepared to manage the bleeding.

Bleeding from the Nose, Ears, and Mouth

Several conditions can result in bleeding from the nose, ears, and/or mouth, including the following:

- Skull fracture

- Facial injuries, including those caused by a direct blow to the nose

- Sinusitis, infections, nose drop use and abuse, dried or cracked nasal mucosa, or other abnormalities

- High blood pressure

- Coagulation disorders

- Digital trauma (nose picking)

> Applying a tourniquet is considered a last resort, because it is rarely necessary and is effective for only a very limited number of injuries.

Epistaxis, or nosebleed, is a common emergency. Occasionally, it can cause enough of a blood loss to send a patient into shock. Keep in mind that the blood you see may be only a small part of the total blood loss. Much of the blood may pass down the throat into the stomach as the patient swallows. A person who swallows a large amount of blood may become nauseated and start vomiting the blood, which is sometimes confused with internal bleeding. Most nontraumatic nosebleeds occur from sites in the septum, the tissue dividing the nostrils. You can usually handle this type of bleeding effectively by pinching the nostrils together.

Follow these steps to treat a patient with epistaxis (Figure 24-16):

1. **Follow BSI techniques.**

2. **Help the patient to sit,** leaning forward, with the head tilted forward. This position stops the blood from trickling down the throat or being aspirated into the lungs.

3. **Apply direct pressure** for at least 15 minutes by pinching the fleshy part of the nostrils together. This is the preferred method.

4. **Placing a rolled 4" x 4" gauze bandage** between the upper lip and the gum is another option. Have the patient apply pressure by stretching the upper lip tightly against the rolled bandage and pushing it up into and against the nose. If the patient is unable to do this effectively, use your gloved fingers to press the gauze against the gum.

5. **Keep the patient calm and quiet,** especially if he or she has high blood pressure or is anxious. Anxiety tends to increase blood pressure, which could worsen the nosebleed.

6. **Apply ice over the nose.**

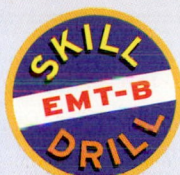

Controlling Epistaxis
Figure 24-16

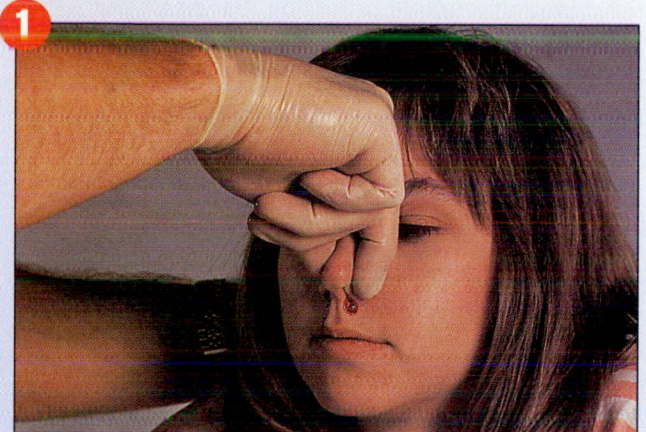

1 Help the patient to sit leaning forward with the head tilted forward. The preferred method is to apply direct pressure by pinching the fleshy part of the nostrils.

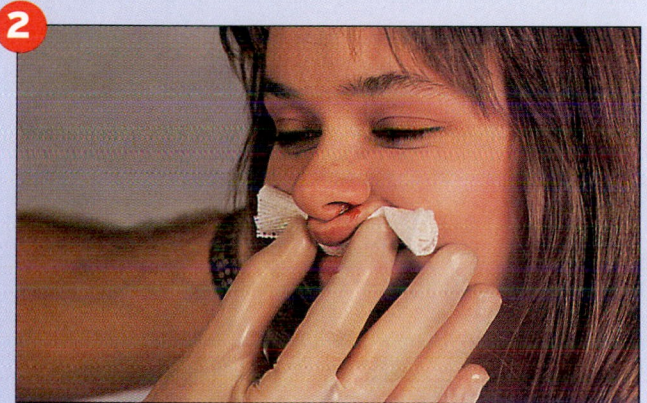

2 Another method is to place a rolled gauze bandage between the upper lip and gum and have the patient apply pressure by stretching the upper lip tightly against the bandage and pushing it up into and against the nose. (The illustration shows an EMT-B doing the same; this is also acceptable.)

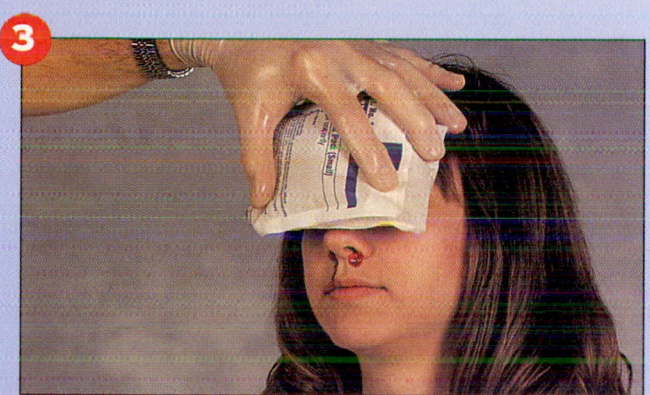

3 Apply ice over the nose.

7. **Maintain the pressure** until the bleeding is completely controlled, usually no more than 15 minutes (assuming that this is the patient's only problem). Most often, failure to stop a nosebleed is the result of releasing the pressure too soon.

8. **Provide prompt transport** once the bleeding has stopped.

9. **If you cannot control the bleeding,** if the patient has a history of frequent nosebleeds, or there is a significant amount of blood loss, transport the patient immediately. Assess the patient for signs and symptoms of shock.

Bleeding from the nose or ears following a head injury may indicate a skull fracture. In these instances, you should not attempt to stop the blood flow. First, such bleeding is difficult to control. Second, applying excessive pressure to the injury may force the blood leaking through the ear or nose to collect within the head. This could increase the pressure on the brain and possibly cause permanent damage.

If you suspect a skull fracture, loosely cover the bleeding site with a sterile gauze pad to collect the blood and help keep contaminants away from the site. There is always a risk that infection will enter the brain and lead to meningitis. Apply light compression by wrapping the dressing loosely around the head (Figure 24-17). If blood or drainage contains cerebrospinal fluid, a characteristic staining of the dressing, much like a target, will occur.

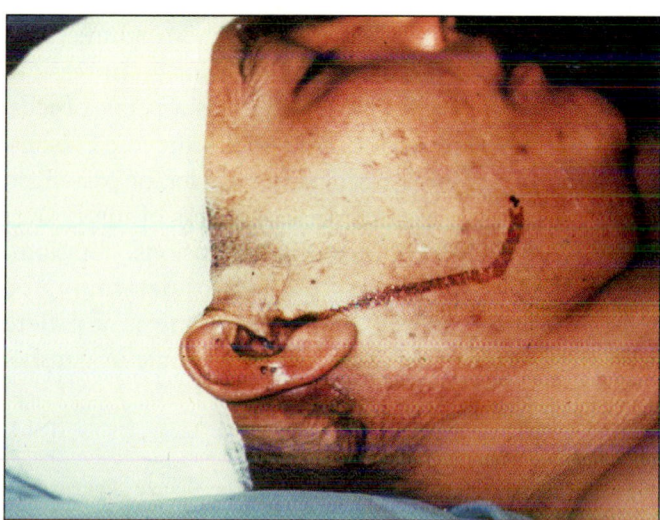

FIGURE 24-17 Bleeding from the ear after a head injury may indicate a skull fracture. Loosely cover the bleeding site with a sterile gauze pad, and apply light compression by wrapping the dressing loosely around the head.

Internal Bleeding

Internal bleeding can be very serious, especially because you might not be aware that it is happening. Injury or damage to internal organs commonly results in extensive internal bleeding, which can cause hypovolemic shock before you realize the extent of blood loss. A person with a bleeding stomach ulcer may lose a large amount of blood very quickly. Similarly, a person who has a lacerated liver or a ruptured spleen may lose a considerable amount of blood within the abdomen. Yet the patient has no outward signs of bleeding.

Broken bones, especially broken ribs, also may cause serious internal blood loss. Sometimes this bleeding extends into the chest cavity and the soft tissues of the chest wall. A broken femur can easily result in the loss of 1 L or more of blood into the soft tissues of the thigh. Often, the only signs of such bleeding are local swelling and bruising due to the accumulation of blood around the ends of the broken bone.

You must always be alert to the possibility of internal bleeding and assess the patient for related signs and symptoms, particularly if the mechanism of injury is severe. If you suspect that a patient is bleeding internally, you should promptly transport him or her to the hospital.

Mechanism of Injury

Internal bleeding is possible whenever the mechanism of injury suggests that severe forces affected the abdomen and/or the chest. These forces include rapid acceleration, deceleration, shearing, or compression. Internal bleeding commonly occurs as a result of falls, blast injuries, and automobile or motorcycle crashes, whether the patient is a pedestrian, driver, or passenger.

As you assess a patient, look for signs of injury over the chest or abdomen, including contusions, abrasions, lacerations, or other signs of injury or deformity. You should always suspect internal bleeding in a patient who has a penetrating injury, such as a knife or gunshot wound.

Nature of Illness

Nontraumatic internal bleeding can lead to shock just as easily as bleeding caused by injury. Usually, internal bleeding occurs in the abdomen as a result of irritable bowel syndrome, an aneurysm, a ruptured ectopic pregnancy, or another condition. Abdominal pain and distention are frequent in these situations but are not always present. In older patients, dizziness, faintness, or weakness may be the first sign of nontraumatic internal bleeding. Ulcers or other gastrointestinal problems may cause vomiting of blood or bloody diarrhea.

It is not as important for you to know the specific organ involved as it is to recognize that the patient is in shock and respond appropriately.

Signs and Symptoms

The most common symptom of internal abdominal bleeding is acute abdominal pain. Another common sign is bruising around the abdomen. This can occur with or without trauma. Bruising is also called contusion or **ecchymosis**. A **hematoma**, a mass of blood in the soft tissues beneath the skin, indicates bleeding into soft tissues and may be the result of either a minor or a severe injury.

Bleeding, however slight, from any body opening is serious. It usually indicates internal bleeding that is not easy to see or control. Bright red bleeding from the mouth, or rectum (hematochezia) or blood in the urine (hematuria) may suggest serious internal injury or disease. Nonmenstrual vaginal bleeding is always significant.

Other signs and symptoms of internal bleeding in both trauma and medical patients include the following:

- Hematemesis. This is vomited blood. It may be bright red or dark red, or if the blood has been partially digested, it may look like coffee ground vomitus.

- Melena. This is a black, foul-smelling, tarry stool that contain digested blood.

- Hemoptysis. This is bright red blood that is coughed up by the patient.

- Pain, tenderness, bruising, or swelling. These signs and symptoms may mean that a closed fracture is bleeding.

- Broken ribs, bruises over the lower chest, or a rigid, distended abdomen. These signs and symptoms may indicate a lacerated spleen or liver. Patients with an injury to either organ may have referred pain in the right shoulder (liver) or left shoulder (spleen). You should suspect internal abdominal bleeding in a patient with referred pain.

The first sign of hypovolemic shock (hypoperfusion) is a change in mental status, such as anxiety, restlessness, or combativeness. In nontrauma patients, weakness, faintness, or dizziness on standing is another early sign. Changes in skin color, or pallor, are seen often in both trauma and medical patients. Later signs of hypoperfusion suggesting internal bleeding include the following:

- Tachycardia
- Weakness, fainting, or dizziness at rest
- Thirst
- Nausea and vomiting
- Cold, moist (clammy) skin
- Shallow, rapid breathing
- Dull eyes
- Slightly dilated pupils that are slow to respond to light
- Capillary refill in infants and children of more than 2 seconds
- Weak, rapid (thready) pulse
- Decreasing blood pressure
- Altered level of consciousness

Patients with these signs and symptoms are at risk. Some may be in danger. Even if their bleeding stops, it could begin again at any moment. Therefore, prompt transport is necessary.

Emergency Medical Care

Controlling internal bleeding or bleeding from the major organs usually requires surgery or other procedures that must be done in the hospital. Your role as an EMT-B in these cases is to keep the patient still to promote clot formation and to provide high-flow oxygen and prompt transport. However, you can usually control internal bleeding into the extremities quite well in the field simply by splinting the extremity, usually most effectively with an air splint. You will rarely need to use a PASG, and you should never use a tourniquet to control the bleeding from closed, internal, soft-tissue injuries.

Follow these steps to care for patients with possible internal bleeding:

1. **Follow BSI techniques.**
2. **Maintain the airway** with cervical spine immobilization if the mechanism of injury suggests the possibility of spinal injury.
3. **Administer high-flow oxygen** and provide artificial ventilation as necessary.
4. **Control** all obvious external bleeding.
5. **Treat suspected internal bleeding** in an extremity by applying a splint or an air pressure splint.
6. **Monitor and record the vital signs** at least every 5 minutes.
7. **Give the patient nothing** (not even small sips of water) by mouth.
8. In nontrauma patients, **elevate the patient's legs** 6″ to 12″ to help the blood return to the vital organs.
9. **Keep the patient warm.**
10. **Provide immediate transport** for all patients with signs and symptoms of shock (hypoperfusion).

prep kit

ready for review

Perfusion is the circulation of blood in adequate amounts to meet the cells' current needs for oxygen, nutrients, and waste removal. Hypoperfusion or shock occurs when the cardiovascular system fails to provide adequate perfusion. Both internal and external bleeding can cause shock. You must know how to recognize and control both.

In the order of preference, the six methods for controlling external bleeding are direct local pressure and elevation, pressure points, splints, air splints, pneumatic antishock garment (PASG), and tourniquets. Do not remove a dressing until a physician has evaluated the patient; instead, apply additional dressings as needed. Stabilizing a serious fracture has a high priority in the control of bleeding. Use a PASG to prevent or minimize hypovolemic shock only when there is internal bleeding, massive soft-tissue bleeding of the lower extremities that cannot be otherwise controlled, or bleeding associated with fractures of the pelvis and proximal femurs. Use a tourniquet only as a last resort, typically with amputations.

Bleeding from the nose, ears, and/or mouth may result from skull fracture, facial injuries, sinusitis, high blood pressure, and coagulation disorders. To treat epistaxis, apply direct pressure for at least 15 minutes by pinching the nostrils together or using gauze between the upper lip and gum. Do not attempt to stop bleeding from the nose or ears. If you suspect a skull fracture, cover the bleeding site loosely with a sterile gauze pad.

You should assess and promptly transport any patient who may have internal bleeding, particularly if the mechanism of injury is severe and has affected the abdomen and/or the chest. The most common sign of internal abdominal bleeding is acute abdominal pain. Bleeding from any body opening is serious. Signs of internal bleeding include hematemesis, melena, hemoptysis, broken ribs, bruised chest, distended abdomen, and referred pain. Signs of shock that suggest internal bleeding include change in mental status, pallor, weakness and dizziness, tachycardia, thirst, nausea and vomiting, and shallow, rapid breathing. If you suspect that a patient is bleeding internally, maintain the airway, administer high-flow oxygen, keep the patient still, apply a splint to the affected extremity, monitor vital signs at least every 5 minutes, and, in nontrauma patients, elevate the legs.

vital vocabulary

www.emtb.com

coagulation Formation of clots to plug openings in injured blood vessels and stop blood flow.

ecchymosis Discoloration of the skin associated with a closed wound.

epistaxis Nosebleed.

hematoma Mass of blood in the soft tissues beneath the skin.

hemophilia A congenital condition in which the patient lacks one or more of the blood's normal clotting factors.

hemorrhage Bleeding.

hypovolemic shock A condition in which low blood volume, due to either massive internal or external bleeding or extensive loss of body water, results in inadequate perfusion.

perfusion Circulation of blood within an organ or tissue in adequate amounts to meet the cells' current needs.

pressure point A point where a blood vessel lies near a bone.

shock A condition in which the circulatory system fails to provide sufficient circulation so that every body part can perform its function; also called hypoperfusion.

assessment in action

It's 10 hours into a 12-hour shift when you are finally dispatched to a call. "Rescue 8, respond to Mark's Machinery for a man injured in an explosion." On arrival, a security guard leads you to the fabrication department where you find a 27-year-old man lying next to the smoking remains of his machine. The patient is conscious and answering questions, though he appears somewhat disoriented. Given what he has just been through, you consider that normal.

A co-worker is kneeling in a puddle of blood as he holds a shop towel around the injured man's arm. You look quickly under the towel and see a 5" laceration from which blood immediately spurts. The patient has multiple small cuts on his face and arms, but his safety glasses have protected his eyes, and his shop apron seems to have done the same for his chest and abdominal area.

1. Your first priority on this call is to:
   A. evaluate the patient's level of consciousness.
   B. quickly open and maintain the patient's airway.
   C. ensure that the scene is safe and secured.
   D. call for law enforcement officers to respond.

2. Blood continues to spurt from the laceration on the patient's arm primarily because:
   A. profuse bleeding is common in young men.
   B. muscle spasms in the patient's arm are forcing the blood out.
   C. there is a surge in arterial pressure with each contraction of the heart.
   D. it is a common occurrence after any injury in which the patient goes into shock.

3. Which artery in the patient's arm has most likely been injured?
   A. Jugular
   B. Carotid
   C. Brachial
   D. Femoral

4. When obtaining a blood pressure on a patient, you are measuring the pressure that the circulating blood is exerting on the walls of the:
   A. veins when the right atrium contracts.
   B. veins when the right ventricle contracts.
   C. arteries when the left ventricle contracts.
   D. arteries when the left atrium contracts.

5. What is the main reason that loss of red blood cells from bleeding has such an impact on the patient's overall condition?
   A. They are unable to fight infection as they recover.
   B. Red blood cells carry oxygen throughout the body.
   C. Chronic hypertension will usually develop in a week or two.
   D. The body is unable to replace them once they are gone.

points to ponder

Object. 1-1.3, 1-2.9, 1-2.10, 1-2.11, 5-1.3, 5-1.4

You are called to a local jewelry store in response to a patient who slipped and fell. You are led into the rear of the store, where you find that the patient not only fell, but fell through a display case and is bleeding severely. You immediately recognize the need for much more BSI protection. Your goggles, mask, and gown are out in the truck.

- Would you leave this severely bleeding patient to get more protection for yourself? If so, why? If you did leave and the patient died, would you be liable?

online outlook

Six ways to control external bleeding are presented in this chapter. Test your ability to choose the appropriate way to control bleeding for different situations by completing Exercise 24 at www.emtb.com.

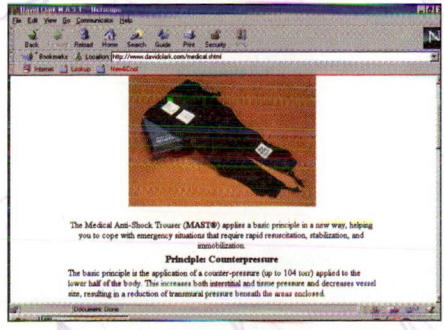

prep kit

24

Shock

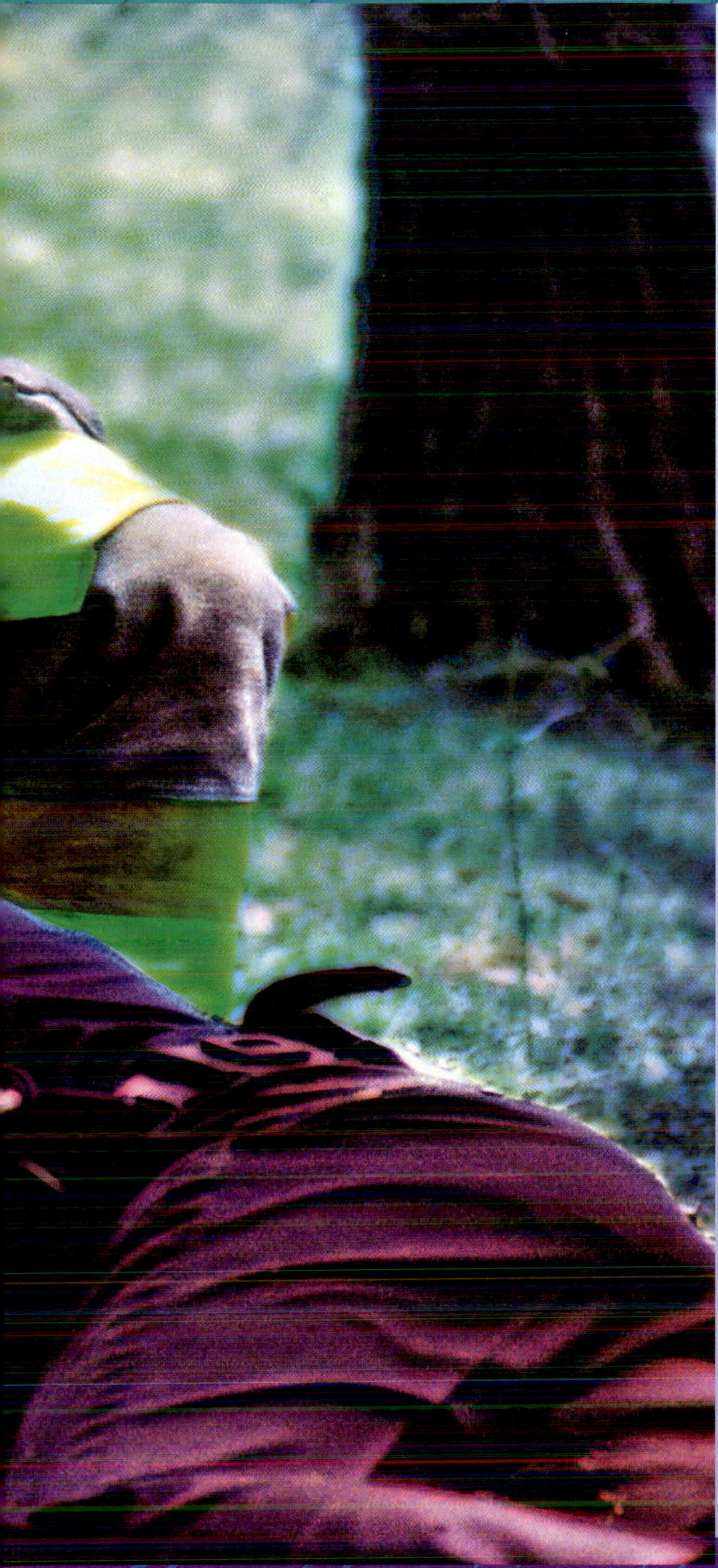

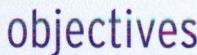

objectives

Cognitive

1. List signs and symptoms of shock (hypoperfusion).
2. State the steps in the emergency medical care of the patient with signs and symptoms of shock (hypoperfusion).

Affective

3. Explain the sense of urgency to transport patients that are bleeding and show signs of shock (hypoperfusion).

Psychomotor

4. Demonstrate the care of the patient exhibiting signs and symptoms of shock (hypoperfusion).
5. Demonstrate completing a prehospital care report for the patient with bleeding and/or shock (hypoperfusion).

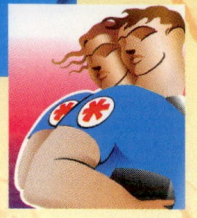

you are the emt

Medic 7, respond with Engine 2 and Rescue 1 for a man crushed by a fork lift. At the scene, you find that the situation is just as it was dispatched. However, you are surprised to find the patient alert and oriented and still pinned up against the wall.

Multiple questions cross your mind: Is he going to make it? Should we pull the forklift away now? If not, what should be done before moving the forklift? This chapter will introduce one of the most fascinating and challenging aspects of medicine: recognizing and treating shock. It will also help you to answer the following questions:

1. What are the three main types of shock? How is each unique?

2. After a patient has gone into shock, at what point is survival not a possibility?

Shock

Shock has a number of meanings. For example, we often say that a person who has received a fright or a piece of bad news is in shock. An electric current passing through the body delivers a shock. In this chapter, shock describes a state of collapse and failure of the cardiovascular system in which blood circulation slows and eventually ceases. If not treated promptly, shock can be fatal.

Shock often accompanies the events, such as heart attacks and automobile crashes, to which you will respond as an EMT-B. Therefore, you should always be able to anticipate, recognize, and treat shock in order to manage patients effectively.

This chapter begins with a close-up look at perfusion, the function that fails in shock. Next it looks at the physiologic causes of shock, describing each of its major forms. Finally, it discusses the emergency treatment of shock in general and of each kind of shock in particular.

Perfusion

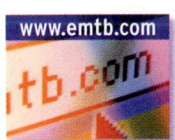

Shock, or hypoperfusion, refers to a state of collapse and failure of the cardiovascular system that leads to inadequate circulation. Like internal bleeding, shock cannot be seen. It is not a specific disease or injury. However, it is a dangerous condition that results in the inadequate flow of blood to the body's cells and failure to rid cells of metabolic wastes. As the cells begin to die, the body attempts to compensate by redirecting blood flow from nonessential organs (skin and intestines) to essential organs (heart, lungs, and brain). If the conditions causing shock are not promptly addressed, the patient will soon die.

As we have seen, the cardiovascular system consists of three parts: a pump (heart), a container (vessels), and the container's contents (blood) (Figure 25-1). The blood is the vehicle for carrying oxygen and nutrients through the vessels to the capillary beds, where these supplies are exchanged for waste products. The blood keeps moving as a result of pressure that is generated by the contractions of the heart and affected by the dilating and constricting of the vessels. This pressure, which we call blood pressure, is usually carefully controlled by the body so that there is always sufficient circulation, or **perfusion**, in the various tissues and organs. Blood pressure is, in fact, a rough measure of perfusion. It tells us how well the body's oxygen, nutrient, and waste removal needs are being met.

Remember that blood pressure is really the pressure of blood within the vessels at any one time. The systolic pressure is the arterial pressure, or pressure generated every time the heart contracts; the diastolic pressure is the pressure maintained within the system.

Blood flow through the capillary beds is regulated by the capillary **sphincters**, circular muscular walls that constrict and dilate. These sphincters are under the control of the **autonomic nervous system**, which regulates involuntary functions such as sweating and digestion. Capillary sphincters also respond to other stimuli such as heat, cold, the need for oxygen, and the need for waste removal. Keep in mind that, under normal circumstances, not all cells have the same needs at the same time. For example, the stomach and intestines have a high need for blood flow during and shortly after eating, when digestion is at a peak. Between meals, blood flow is lessened, and blood is diverted to other areas. The brain, by contrast, needs a constant and consistent supply of blood to function.

Thus, regulation of blood flow is determined by cellular need and is accomplished by vessel constriction or dilation, together with sphincter constriction or dilation. Maintenance of blood flow, or perfusion, is accomplished by the heart, blood vessels, and blood, working together.

Perfusion requires more than just having a working cardiovascular system, however. It also requires adequate oxygen exchange in the lungs, adequate nutrients in the form of glucose in the blood, and adequate waste removal, primarily through the lungs. Therefore, the respiratory system is also a major contributor to maintaining adequate perfusion.

In addition, the body also has mechanisms in place to help support the respiratory and cardiovascular systems when the need for perfusion of vital organs is increased. These mechanisms, including the autonomic nervous system and certain chemicals called hormones, are triggered when the body senses that the pressure in the system is falling. The action of the hormones stimulates an increase in heart rate and in the strength of cardiac contractions and vasoconstriction in nonessential areas, primarily in the skin and gastrointestinal tract (peripheral vasoconstriction). Together, these actions are designed to maintain pressure in the system and, as a result, perfusion of all vital organs.

Eventually, there is also a shifting of body fluids to help maintain pressure within the system. However, the response of the autonomic nervous system and hormones comes within seconds. It is this response that causes all the signs and symptoms of a patient in shock.

Causes of Shock

Shock can result from many different conditions, including respiratory failure, acute allergic reactions, and overwhelming infection. In all cases, however, the damage occurs because of insufficient perfusion of organs and tissues. As soon as perfusion stops or becomes impaired, tissues start to die, affecting all local body processes. If the conditions causing shock are not promptly arrested and reversed, death soon follows.

Understanding the basic physiologic causes of shock will better prepare you to treat it (Figure 25-2).

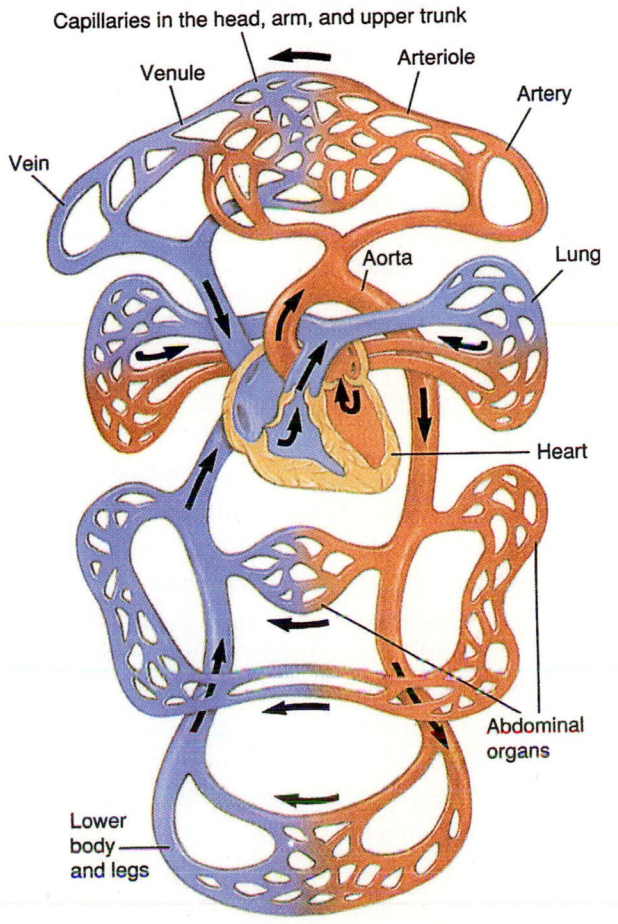

FIGURE 25-1 The cardiovascular system consists of three parts: the pump (heart), the container (vessels), and the contents (blood). The blood carries oxygen and nutrients through the vessels to the capillary beds, where they are exchanged for waste products.

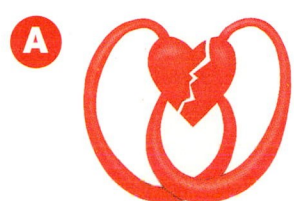

1. Poor pump function
Causes: Heart attack, trauma to heart

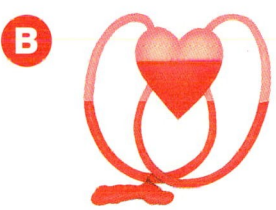

2. Blood or fluid loss from blood vessels
Causes: Trauma to vessels or tissues, fluid loss from GI tract (vomiting/diarrhea can also lower the fluid component of blood)

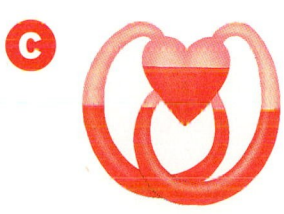

3. Blood vessels dilate
Causes: Infection, drug overdose (narcotic), spinal cord injury

FIGURE 25-2 There are three basic causes of shock and impaired tissue perfusion. **A:** Pump failure occurs when the heart is damaged by disease or injury. The heart does not generate enough energy to move the blood through the system. **B:** Decreased blood volume, usually a result of bleeding, results in inadequate perfusion. **C:** The blood vessels can dilate enough that the blood within them, even though it is of normal volume, is inadequate to fill the system and provide efficient perfusion.

> Edema is the presence of abnormally large amounts of fluid between cells in body tissues, causing swelling of the affected area. Pulmonary edema leads to impaired ventilation.

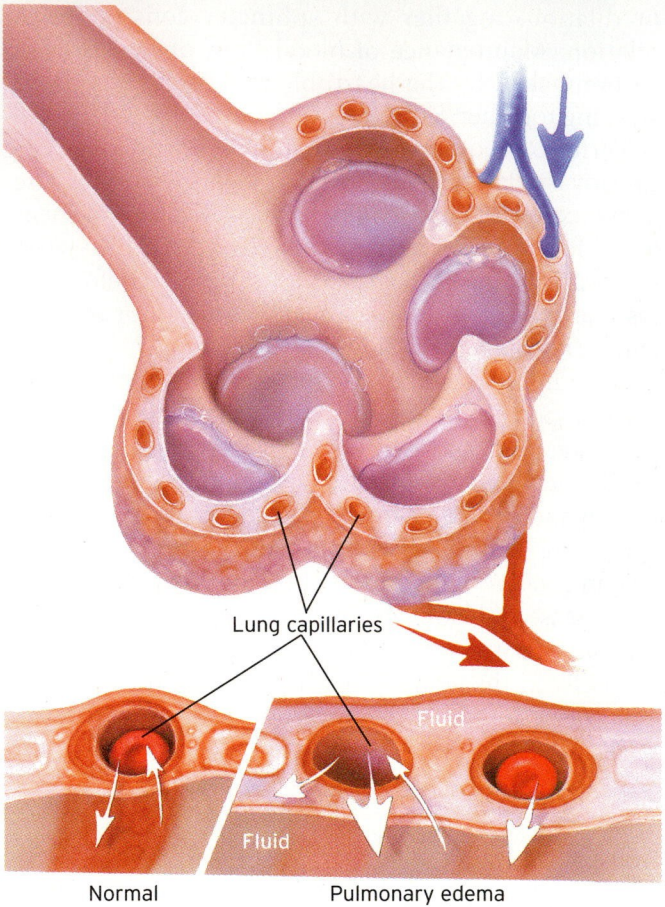

Lung capillaries

Normal   Pulmonary edema

FIGURE 25-3 Pulmonary edema develops as a result of fluid buildup within the pulmonary tissue. The edema causes swelling and leads to impaired ventilation.

There are both cardiovascular and noncardiovascular causes of shock. The three major cardiovascular causes of shock are as follows:

- **Poor pump function.** If damaged by muscular disease or injury, the heart may fail to perform properly as a pump. That is, it does not generate sufficient energy to move blood through the system.

- **Blood or fluid loss from blood vessels.** If enough blood or plasma is lost, the volume of fluid contained within the vascular system is insufficient to perfuse all tissues and organs.

- **Poor vessel function.** If all the blood vessels dilate at once, the normal volume of blood will be insufficient to fill the system and provide efficient perfusion.

The noncardiovascular causes of shock are respiratory insufficiency and **anaphylaxis**, an unusual or exaggerated allergic reaction to foreign protein or other substances.

Cardiovascular Causes of Shock

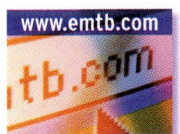

Pump failure. Cardiogenic shock is caused by inadequate function of the heart, or pump failure. Circulation of blood throughout the vascular system requires the constant pumping action of a normal and vigorous heart muscle. Many diseases can cause destruction or inflammation of this muscle. Within certain limits, the heart can adapt to these problems. If too much muscular damage occurs, however, as sometimes happens after a heart attack, the heart no longer functions well. A major effect is the backup of blood into the lungs. The resulting buildup of fluid within

the pulmonary tissue is called pulmonary edema. **Edema** is the presence of abnormally large amounts of fluid between cells in body tissues, causing swelling of the affected area (Figure 25-3). Pulmonary edema leads to impaired ventilation.

The muscular contraction of the heart moves blood through the vessels at distinct pressures. For blood to circulate efficiently throughout the entire system, there must be both the right amount of pressure and an adequate number of heartbeats. For this reason, the heart has its own electrical system that initiates and regulates its beating. Disease or injury can damage or destroy this system, causing irregular and uncoordinated beats, beats that are too slow (fewer than 50/min), or beats that are too fast (greater than 150/min).

Cardiogenic shock develops when the heart muscle can no longer generate enough pressure to circulate the blood to all organs or when the regularity of the heart-

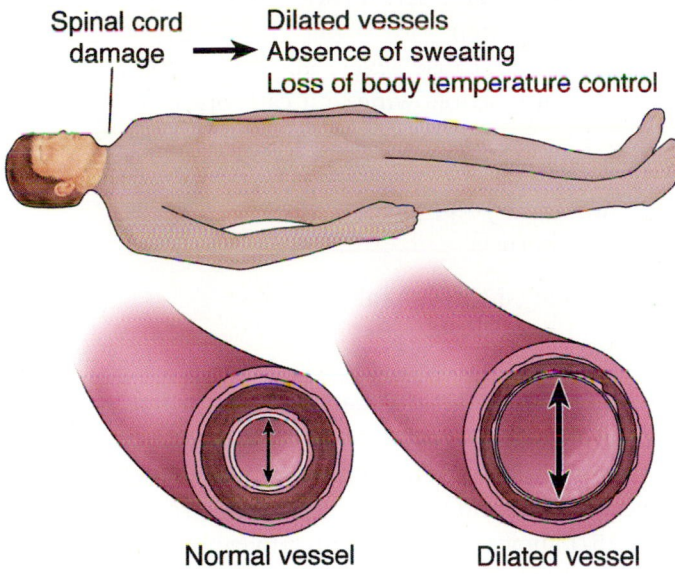

Spinal cord damage ➔ Dilated vessels
Absence of sweating
Loss of body temperature control

Normal vessel   Dilated vessel

FIGURE 25-4 Damage to the spinal cord can cause significant injury to the part of the nervous system that controls the size and muscle tone of blood vessels. If the muscles in the blood vessels are cut off from their impulses to contract, then the vessels dilate widely, increasing the size and capacity of the vascular system. The blood in the body can no longer fill the enlarged vessels, resulting in inadequate perfusion.

beat is so disrupted that the volume of blood within the system can no longer be handled efficiently. In either case, direct pump failure is the cause of shock.

Poor vessel function. Damage to the spinal cord, particularly at the upper cervical levels, may cause significant injury to the part of the nervous system that controls the size and muscular tone of the blood vessels. Neurogenic shock is usually the result. In this condition, the muscles in the walls of the blood vessels are cut off from the nerve impulses that cause them to contract. Therefore, all the vessels below the level of the spinal injury dilate widely, increasing the size and capacity of the vascular system (Figure 25-4). The available 6 L of blood in the body can no longer fill the enlarged vascular system. Even though no blood or fluid has been lost, perfusion of organs and tissues becomes inadequate, and shock occurs. In this condition, a radical change in the size of the vascular system has caused shock. A characteristic sign of this type of shock is the absence of sweating below the level of injury.

With this type of injury, many other functions that are under the control of the same part of the nervous system are also lost. The most important of them, in an acute injury setting, is the ability to control body temperature. Body temperature in the patient with neurogenic shock can rapidly fall to match that of the environment. In many situations, significant hypothermia occurs, severely complicating the situation. Hypothermia is a condition in which the internal body temperature falls below 95°F (35°C), usually after prolonged exposure to freezing temperatures.

Content failure. Following injury, shock is often a result of fluid or blood loss. This type of shock is called hypovolemic (low-volume) shock or, when caused by blood loss, hemorrhagic shock. The loss may be due to external bleeding, which is common in patients who have suffered severe lacerations or fractures. Or it may be due to internal bleeding, which follows a variety of injuries or diseases, such as rupture of the liver or the spleen, lacerations of the great vessels within the abdomen or the chest, bleeding peptic ulcers, and tumors, among others.

Hypovolemic shock also occurs with severe thermal burns. In this case, it is intravascular plasma (the colorless part of the blood) that is lost, leaking from the circulatory system into the burned tissues that lie adjacent to the injury. Likewise, crushing injuries may result in the loss of blood and plasma from damaged vessels into injured tissues. Dehydration, the loss of water from body tissues, aggravates shock.

In all these circumstances, the common factor is an insufficient volume of blood within the vascular system to provide adequate circulation to all the organs of the body.

Combined vessel and content failure. In some patients who have severe bacterial infections, toxins (poisons) generated by the bacteria or by infected body tissues produce a condition called septic shock. In this condition, the toxins damage the vessel walls, causing them to become leaky and unable to contract well. Widespread dilation of vessels, in combination with the loss of plasma through the injured vessel walls, results in shock.

Septic shock is a complex problem. First, there is an insufficient volume of fluid in the container, because much of the blood has leaked out of the vascular system (hypovolemia). Second, the fluid that has leaked out often collects in the respiratory system, interfering with ventilation. Third, there is a larger-than-normal vascular bed to contain the smaller-than-normal volume of intravascular fluid.

Septic shock is almost always a complication of some very serious illness, injury, or surgery.

Noncardiovascular Causes of Shock

There are two causes of shock that do not result from disturbances of the cardiovascular system: respiratory insufficiency and anaphylaxis.

Respiratory insufficiency. A patient with a severe chest injury or obstruction of the airway may be unable to breathe in an adequate amount of oxygen. An insufficient concentration of oxygen in the blood can produce shock as rapidly as vascular causes, even if the volume of blood, the volume of the vessels, and the action of the heart are all normal. Without oxygen, the organs in the body cannot survive, and their cells promptly start to deteriorate.

This is why the first two steps in resuscitation are always securing an airway and restoring respirations. Circulation of nonoxygenated blood will not benefit the patient.

Anaphylactic shock. Anaphylaxis, or **anaphylactic shock**, occurs when a person reacts violently to a substance to which he or she has been sensitized. **Sensitization** means becoming sensitive to a substance that did not initially cause a reaction. Do not be misled by a patient who reports no history of allergic reaction to a substance on first or second exposure. Each subsequent exposure after sensitization tends to produce a more severe reaction.

Instances that cause severe allergic reactions commonly fall into the following four categories:

- Injections (tetanus antitoxin, penicillin)
- Stings (honeybee, wasp, yellow jacket, hornet)
- Ingestion (shellfish, oral penicillin)
- Inhalation (dusts, pollens)

Anaphylactic reactions can develop in minutes or even seconds after contact with the substance to which the patient is allergic. The signs of such allergic reactions are very distinct and not seen with other forms of shock. Table 25-1 shows the signs of anaphylactic shock in the order in which they typically occur.

In anaphylactic shock, there is no loss of blood, no vascular damage, and only a slight possibility of direct cardiac muscular injury. Instead, there is widespread vascular dilation. The combination of poor oxygenation and poor perfusion in anaphylactic shock may easily prove fatal.

TABLE 25-1 Signs of Anaphylactic Shock

Skin

- Flushing, itching, or burning, especially over the face and upper chest
- Urticaria (hives), which may spread over large areas of the body
- Edema, especially of the face, tongue, and lips
- **Cyanosis** (a bluish cast to the skin resulting from poor oxygenation of circulating blood) about the lips

Circulatory System

- Dilation of peripheral blood vessels
- A drop in blood pressure
- A weak, barely palpable pulse
- Pallor
- Dizziness
- Fainting and coma

Respiratory System

- Sneezing or itching in the nasal passages
- Tightness in the chest, with a persistent dry cough
- Wheezing and **dyspnea**, or difficulty in breathing
- Secretions of fluid and mucus into the bronchial passages, alveoli, and lung tissue, causing coughing
- Constriction of the bronchi; difficulty drawing air into the lungs
- Forced expiration, requiring exertion and accompanied by wheezing
- Cessation of breathing

Psychogenic shock. A patient in **psychogenic shock** has had a sudden reaction of the nervous system that produces a temporary, generalized vascular dilation, resulting in fainting or **syncope**. Blood pools in the dilated vessels, reducing the blood supply to the brain; as a result, the brain ceases to function normally, and the patient faints. Causes of syncope range from fear, bad news, or unpleasant sights (often the sight of blood) to life-threatening cardiac arrhythmias or aneurysms.

The Progression of Shock

Although you cannot see shock, you can see its signs and symptoms (Table 25-2). The early stage of shock, while the body can still compensate for blood loss, is called **compensated shock**. The late stage, when blood pressure is falling, is called **decompensated shock**. The last stage, when shock has progressed to a terminal stage, is called **irreversible shock**. A transfusion of any type at this point will not save the patient's life.

Remember that blood pressure may be the last measurable factor to change in shock. As we have seen, the body has several automatic mechanisms to compensate for initial blood loss and to help maintain blood pressure. Thus, by the time you detect a drop in blood pressure, shock is well developed. This is particularly true of infants and children, who can maintain their blood pressure until they have lost more than half their blood volume. By the time blood pressure drops in infants and children who are in shock, they are close to death.

You should expect shock in many emergency medical situations. For example, you would expect shock to accompany massive external or internal bleeding. You should also expect shock if a patient has any one of the following conditions:

- Multiple severe fractures
- Abdominal or chest injury
- Spinal injury
- A severe infection
- A major heart attack
- Anaphylaxis

TABLE 25-2 Progression of Shock	
Compensated Shock	**Decompensated Shock**
Agitation	Falling blood pressure (systolic blood pressure of 90 mm Hg or lower in an adult)
Anxiety	Labored or irregular breathing
Restlessness	Ashen, mottled, or cyanotic skin
Feeling of impending doom	Thready or absent peripheral pulses
Altered mental status	Dull eyes, dilated pupils
Weak, rapid (thready), or absent pulse	Poor urinary output
Clammy (pale, cool, moist) skin	
Pallor, with cyanosis about the lips	
Shallow, rapid breathing	
Air hunger (shortness of breath), especially if there is a chest injury	
Nausea or vomiting	
Capillary refill in infants and children of longer than 2 seconds	
Marked thirst	

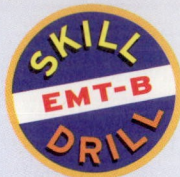

Treating Shock

Figure 25-5

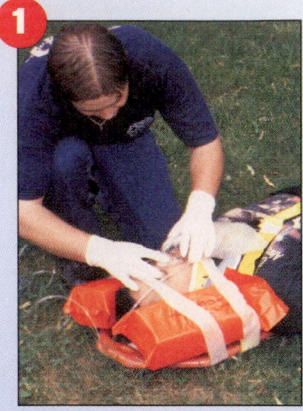

1

Keep the patient in a supine position. Provide oxygen, assist with ventilations, and monitor the patient's breathing.

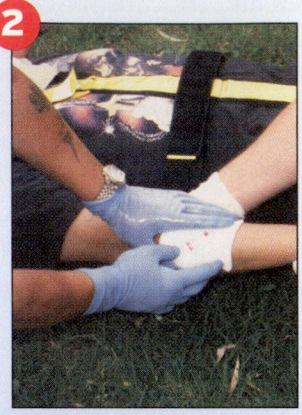

2

Control obvious external bleeding. If there are no broken bones, elevate the legs 8" to 12".

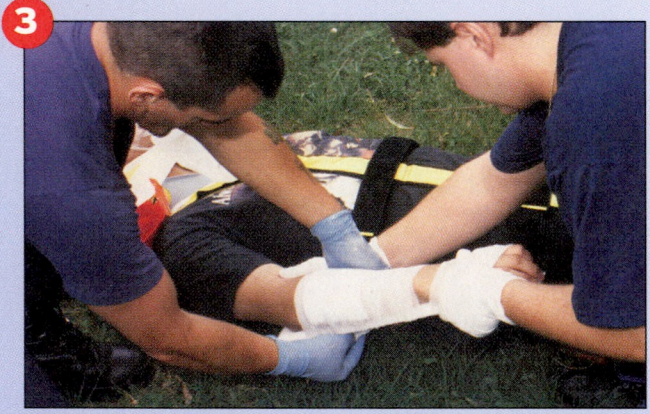

3

Splint any broken bone or joint injuries.

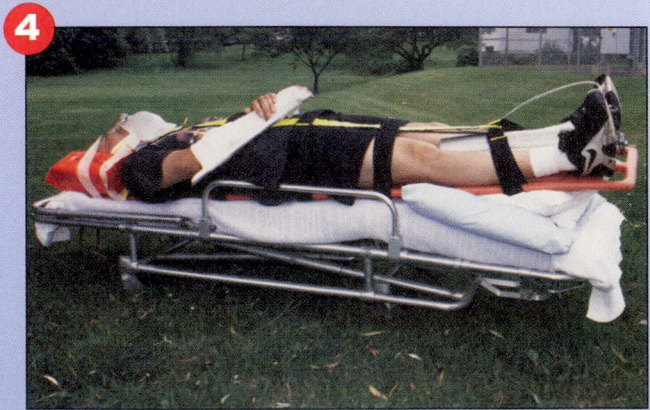

4

Place blankets under and over the patient, but do not overload the patient with covers.

Emergency Medical Care

You must begin immediate treatment for shock as soon as you realize that the condition *may* exist. As with any type of patient care, you should begin by following BSI techniques and making sure the patient has an open airway (Figure 25-5). Remember that inadequate ventilation may be the primary cause of shock or a major factor in its development. Always provide oxygen, assist with ventilations as needed, and continue to monitor the patient's breathing. In general, keep the patient in a supine position. Patients who have had a severe heart attack or who have lung disease may find it easier to breathe in a sitting or semi-sitting position.

Next, control all obvious external bleeding. Place sterile gauze compresses over the bleeding sites, and secure them with circumferential pressure dressings. If there are no broken bones, elevate the lower extremities 8" to 12". This not only stops venous bleeding in an extremity, it also allows the blood in the legs to return to the heart more rapidly.

Splint any bone or joint injuries. This minimizes pain, bleeding, and discomfort, all of which can aggravate shock. It also prevents the broken bone ends from further damaging adjacent soft tissue. In general, splinting also makes it easier to move the patient. Handle the patient gently and no more than is necessary.

There is some controversy surrounding the use of the pneumatic antishock garment (PASG). Used improperly, the device can worsen bleeding from chest injuries, interfere with adequate air exchange, and promote cardiovascular collapse. Used properly, it can effectively control bleeding from fractures and massive soft-tissue wounds. In general, the PASG should not be used without the approval of medical control or established local protocols.

The PASG is generally used for three purposes: to stabilize multiple long bone fractures of the lower extremities; to stabilize and control bleeding from pelvic fractures; and to help control massive bleeding from soft-tissue damage to the lower extremities. If the lower abdomen is tender and you suspect a pelvic injury in a patient who has no chest trauma, you should apply and inflate all three compartments of the PASG. If there are multiple fractures of the lower extremities, apply and inflate only the leg sections. If bleeding from a soft-tissue injury cannot be controlled by direct pressure or pressure points, apply and inflate the appropriate leg section(s).

To prevent the loss of body heat, place blankets under and over the patient. Be careful not to overload the patient with covers or attempt to warm the body too much. It is better for the patient to be slightly cool rather than too hot. Do not use any external heat sources, such as hot water bottles or heating pads. They may harm a patient in shock by causing vasodilation and decreasing blood pressure even more.

Do not give the patient anything by mouth, no matter how urgently you are asked. To relieve the intense thirst that often accompanies shock, give the patient a moistened piece of gauze to chew or suck. Never give a patient in shock an alcoholic drink or other depressant. A stimulant, such as coffee, also has little value in treating shock.

Accurately record the patient's vital signs approximately every 5 minutes throughout treatment and transport. It is essential to transport the trauma patient to the hospital as rapidly as possible for definitive treatment. The Golden Hour, generally thought to be the first 60 minutes after injury, is the period of time during which treatment of a patient in shock or with traumatic injuries is most critical. Remember to speak calmly and reassuringly to a conscious patient throughout assessment, care, and transport.

Table 25-3 lists the general supportive measures for the major types of shock. Not every measure is used for every type of shock.

> The Golden Hour, generally thought to be the first 60 minutes after injury, is the period of time during which treatment of a patient in shock or with traumatic injuries is most critical.

Treating Cardiogenic Shock

The patient who is in shock as a result of a heart attack does not require a transfusion of blood, IV fluids, elevation of the legs, or a PASG. There is already a greater volume of blood in circulation than the heart can handle. The damaged heart muscle simply cannot generate the necessary power to pump blood throughout the circulatory system.

Keep in mind that chronic lung disease will aggravate cardiogenic shock. If the patient has COPD, as well as heart disease, oxygenation of the blood passing through the lungs is impaired. Because fluid is collecting in the lungs, this patient is often able to breathe better in a sitting or semi-sitting position and may tell you so.

Usually, patients with cardiogenic shock do not have any injury, but they may be having chest pain. Such a patient may have taken nitroglycerin before your arrival and may want to take more. Before helping the patient self-administer nitroglycerin, be sure to consult with medical control for instructions. You will also need to perform an accurate assessment and to ensure that the patient's blood pressure meets the criteria for this medication. If the blood pressure is too low, nitroglycerin may worsen the problem. Remember that patients in cardiogenic shock usually have a low blood pressure. Other signs include a weak, irregular pulse, cyanosis about the lips and underneath the fingernails, anxiety, and nausea.

Treatment of cardiogenic shock should begin by placing the patient in the position in which breathing is easiest as you give high-flow oxygen. Be ready to assist ventilations as necessary, and have suction nearby in case the patient vomits. Provide prompt transport to the emergency department. Remember also to approach a patient who has had a suspected heart attack with calm reassurance.

Treating Neurogenic Shock

Shock that accompanies spinal cord injury is best treated by a combination of all the known supportive measures. The patient who has sustained this kind of injury usually will require hospitalization for a long time. Emergency treatment must be directed at obtaining and maintaining a proper airway, assisting impaired breathing as needed, conserving body heat, and providing the most effective circulation possible.

This patient usually is not losing blood. However, the capacity of his or her blood vessels has become significantly larger than the volume of blood they contain. Supplemental oxygen will boost the concentration of oxygen in the blood. If respirations are weak or inadequate, provide assisted ventilations. Keep the patient as warm as possible with blankets, because the injury may have disabled the body's normal temperature controls. Transport promptly.

TABLE 25-3 Types of Shock

Types of Shock	Causes	Signs/Symptoms	Treatment
Anaphylactic	Allergic reaction (most severe form)	Can develop within seconds Mild itching Burning skin Vascular dilation Generalized edema Profound coma Rapid death	Supply respiratory support Assist ventilations Determine cause Assist with administration of epinephrine Transport promptly
Cardiogenic	Inadequate heart function Disease of muscle tissue Impaired electrical system Disease or injury	Chest pains Irregular pulse Weak pulse Low blood pressure Cyanosis (lips, under nails) Anxiety	Position comfortably Administer oxygen Assist ventilations Transport promptly
Hypovolemic	Loss of blood or fluid	Rapid, weak pulse Low blood pressure Change in mental status Cyanosis (lips, under nails) Cool, clammy skin	Secure airway Assist ventilations Control external bleeding Elevate legs Prevent aspiration Apply PASG (if medical control approves) Transport promptly
Metabolic	Excessive loss of fluid and electrolytes due to vomiting, urination, or diarrhea	Rapid, weak pulse Low blood pressure Change in mental status Cyanosis (lips, under nails) Cool, clammy skin	Secure airway Assist ventilations Determine illness Transport promptly
Neurogenic	Damaged cervical spine, which causes blood vessels to dilate widely	Bradycardia (slow pulse) Low blood pressure Signs of neck injury	Secure airway Assist ventilations Conserve body heat Maximize circulation Apply PASG (if medical control approves) Transport promptly
Psychogenic (fainting)	Temporary, generalized vascular dilation Anxiety, bad news, sight of injury/blood, prospect of medical treatment, severe pain, illness, tiredness	Rapid pulse Normal or low blood pressure	Determine duration of unconsciousness Record initial vital signs and mental status Suspect head injury if patient is confused or slow to regain consciousness Transport promptly
Septic	Severe bacterial infection	Warm skin Tachycardia Low blood pressure	Transport promptly Administer oxygen en route Provide full ventilatory support Elevate legs Keep patient warm

Treating Hypovolemic Shock

The emergency treatment of hypovolemic or hemorrhagic shock includes the control of all obvious external bleeding. To prevent continued bleeding, you must apply sufficient pressure to control obvious external bleeding, splint any bone and joint injuries, and ensure that you use great care to handle the patient gently. If there are no fractured extremities, you should raise the legs from the hips 8″ to 12″, keeping the torso in a horizontal position. This will increase blood flow to the heart from the lower body and keep unwanted pressure off the diaphragm. This method combats shock by using the patient's own blood to its best advantage.

Although you cannot control internal bleeding in the field, you must recognize its existence and provide aggressive general support. Secure and maintain an airway, and provide respiratory support, including supplemental oxygen and, if needed, assisted ventilations. Start the oxygen as soon as you suspect shock, and continue it during transport; with too little circulating blood, additional oxygen may be lifesaving. Be sure the patient does not aspirate blood or vomitus into the lungs. Most important, you must transport the patient as rapidly as possible to the emergency department.

Treating Septic Shock

The proper treatment of septic shock requires complex hospital management. If you suspect that a patient has septic shock, you must transport him or her as promptly as possible while giving all the general support available. Use high-flow oxygen during transport. Full or partial ventilatory support may be necessary to maintain adequate tidal volume in this patient. Use blankets to conserve body heat.

Treating Respiratory Insufficiency

In treating the patient who is in shock as a result of inadequate respiration, you must immediately secure and maintain the airway. Clear the mouth and throat down to the larynx of anything obstructing the air passages, including mucus, vomitus, and foreign material. If necessary, provide manual ventilations using ventilatory aids, or administer mouth-to-mask resuscitation. Give supplemental oxygen, and transport the patient promptly.

Treating Anaphylactic Shock

The only really effective treatment for a severe, acute allergic reaction is to administer epinephrine via subcutaneous, intramuscular, or intravenous injection. In general, the IM injection of 0.3 to 1.0 mL of 1:1,000 epinephrine (0.3 mg) will alleviate the immediate signs

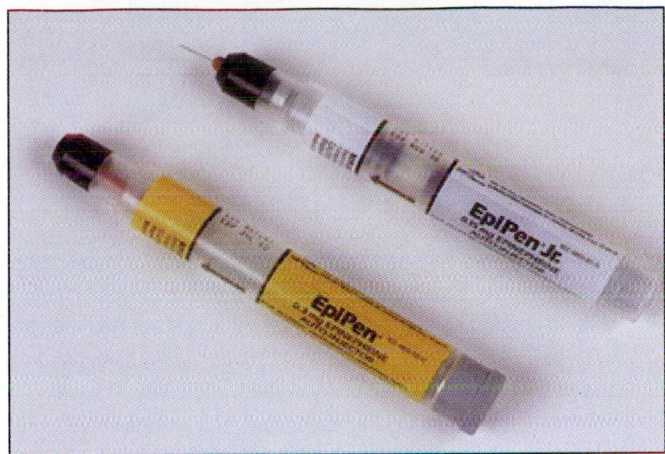

FIGURE 25-6 Patients who are allergic to bee stings often carry commercial bee sting kits, such as an IM injector or autoinjector, containing epinephrine.

and symptoms of anaphylaxis. A patient who is aware of having a specific sensitivity may carry a bee sting kit containing epinephrine (Figure 25-6). If he or she is unable to inject the medication, you may have to do so if you are allowed by local protocol. If the patient's signs and symptoms recur or worsen, you should repeat the injection after consulting with medical control.

Promptly transport the patient to the emergency department while providing all possible support, primarily supplemental oxygen and ventilatory assistance. You should also try to find out what agent caused the reaction (e.g., a drug, an insect bite or sting, a food item) and how it was received (e.g., by mouth, by inhalation, or by injection). The severity of allergic reactions can vary greatly, with symptoms ranging from mild itching to profound coma and rapid death. Keep in mind that a mild reaction may worsen suddenly or over time.

Treating Psychogenic Shock

In an uncomplicated case of fainting, once the patient collapses and becomes supine, circulation to the brain is usually restored, and with it a normal state of functioning. If the attack has caused the patient to fall, you must check for injuries, especially in older patients. However, you should also assess the patient thoroughly for any other abnormality. If, after regaining consciousness, the patient is unable to walk without weakness, dizziness, or pain, you should suspect another problem, such as head injury. You should transport this patient promptly.

Be sure to record your initial observations of vital signs and level of consciousness. In addition, try to learn from bystanders whether the patient complained of anything before fainting and how long he or she had been unconscious.

prep kit

ready for review

Shock is the collapse and failure of the cardiovascular system, in which blood circulation slows and eventually ceases. Perfusion requires a cardiovascular system with all three parts (the pump, container, and contents) working, but it also requires a functioning respiratory system. The signs and symptoms of shock are caused by the actions of the autonomic nervous system and of hormones responding to the need for additional perfusion.

The cardiovascular causes of shock include poor pump function (cardiogenic shock), blood or fluid loss from blood vessels (hypovolemic shock), and/or poor vessel function (neurogenic shock), as when all vessels dilate at once. Septic shock is a combination of vessel and content failure; it is the result of serious bacterial infection. The noncardiovascular causes of shock are respiratory insufficiency and anaphylaxis.

Signs of compensated shock include agitation or anxiety, a weak, rapid pulse, clammy skin, air hunger, nausea or vomiting, slow capillary refill in children and infants, and marked thirst. Signs of decompensated shock include labored or irregular breathing, ashen or cyanotic skin, thready or absent peripheral pulses, dilated pupils, poor urinary output, and, finally, falling blood pressure. By the time you detect a drop in blood pressure, shock is well developed. Expect shock in cases of massive internal or external bleeding, multiple severe fractures, abdominal or chest injury, spinal injury, severe infection, a major heart attack, and anaphylaxis.

Treat patients with shock by (1) opening and maintaining the airway; (2) providing oxygen and, if necessary, assisting ventilations; (3) controlling all obvious external bleeding; (4) conserving body heat with blankets; and (5) transporting promptly. Use high-flow oxygen in patients with cardiogenic or septic shock.

vital vocabulary

www.emtb.com

anaphylactic shock Severe shock caused by allergic reactions.

anaphylaxis An unusual or exaggerated allergic reaction to foreign protein or other substances.

autonomic nervous system The part of the nervous system that regulates involuntary functions, such as digestion and sweating.

cardiogenic shock Shock caused by inadequate function of the heart, or pump failure.

compensated shock The early stage of shock, while the body can still compensate for blood loss.

cyanosis Blue color of the skin resulting from poor oxygenation of the circulating blood.

decompensated shock The late stage of shock, when blood pressure is falling.

dehydration Loss of water from the tissues of the body.

dyspnea Difficulty in breathing.

edema The presence of abnormally large amounts of fluid in the extracellular spaces of body tissues, causing swelling of the affected area.

hypothermia A condition in which the internal body temperature falls below 95°F (35°C), usually as a result of prolonged exposure to freezing or near-freezing temperatures.

hypovolemic shock Shock caused by fluid or blood loss.

irreversible shock The final stage of shock, resulting in death.

neurogenic shock Circulatory failure caused by paralysis of the nerves that control the size of the blood vessels, seen in spinal cord injuries.

perfusion Circulation of blood within an organ or tissue in adequate amounts to meet the cells' current needs.

psychogenic shock Shock caused by a temporary reduction in blood supply to the brain. The common faint.

sensitization Developing a sensitivity to a substance that initially caused no allergic reaction.

septic shock Shock caused by severe bacterial infection.

shock A condition in which the circulatory system fails to provide sufficient circulation that every body part can perform its function; also called hypoperfusion.

sphincters Circular muscles that encircle and, by contracting, constrict a duct, tube, or opening.

syncope Fainting.

assessment in action

You and your partner are dispatched to a car crash out in the county. Upon arrival, you see a small sports car crushed up against a concrete bridge support. As the rescue team is working on gaining access, you look in to see the unbelted patient, who has gone down and under the steering wheel. The door is finally torn loose, and as you get your first close look at the patient, you see two obviously fractured legs and extensive soft-tissue injuries. The patient responds to voice, but just barely. He has no radial pulse but does have a weak carotid pulse at 138/min. His skin is pale, cool, and moist to the touch, and you estimate respirations of about 28 breaths/min.

1. Which of the following action plans would be most appropriate for this patient?
   A. Rapidly extricate the patient, splint the fractured legs, dress the wounds, immobilize the patient to a long backboard, and then transport.
   B. Completely immobilize the patient, extricate, initiate transport, and then dress the wounds and splint the fractured legs en route to the hospital.
   C. Rapidly extricate and then completely immobilize the patient to a long backboard, initiate transport, and then dress the wounds and splint the fractures en route to the hospital.
   D. Splint the fractures and dress the wounds while the patient is still in the car, immobilize the patient, and then extricate and initiate transport to the hospital.

2. Once the extrication is complete and the patient is accessible, scene time before initiating transport should be limited to no more than how many minutes?
   A. 10
   B. 20
   C. 30
   D. 40

3. On the basis of the patient's signs and symptoms, you should prepare to care for:
   A. hypovolemic shock.
   B. a diabetic emergency.
   C. increased intracranial pressure.
   D. hyperventilation syndrome.

4. On the basis of the patient's vital signs, you would expect capillary refill to be:
   A. almost instantaneous.
   B. about 1 to 2 seconds.
   C. about 3 to 4 seconds.
   D. virtually nonexistent.

5. The patient's respirations increase to about 40 breaths/min, and they become very shallow. To ensure adequate ventilation, you should:
   A. apply a nasal cannula with oxygen running at 8 to 10 L/min.
   B. insert a nasopharyngeal airway into either or both nostrils.
   C. administer an inhaled breathing treatment immediately.
   D. assist ventilations with a BVM device with oxygen at 15 L/min.

points to ponder

Object.4-8.1, 4-8.2, 4-8.6, 5-1.9, 5-1.10

You are treating a seriously injured motorcycle driver when the driver of the car that turned in front of the motorcycle starts asking you questions. At first, they are the kind you would expect, such as whether the motorcyclist will be okay, but they soon move to whose fault it was. Then the driver begins to get in your way, trying to help treat the patient. After you repeatedly ask the driver to step back, he threatens you and then disappears. You realize that the driver had very pale skin color and was probably suffering from hypoperfusion due to emotional stress (psychogenic shock).

- How would you deal with the driver? Would you send someone after the driver? If so, who? Is there a chance that the driver will return and carry out the threats? How does all of this affect your care of the motorcyclist?

online outlook

The signs and symptoms of shock are presented in this chapter. Test your ability to recognize shock by completing Exercise 25 at www.emtb.com.

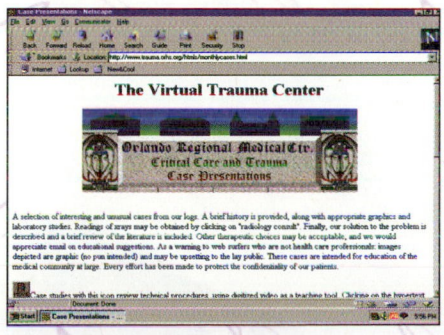

Soft-Tissue Injuries

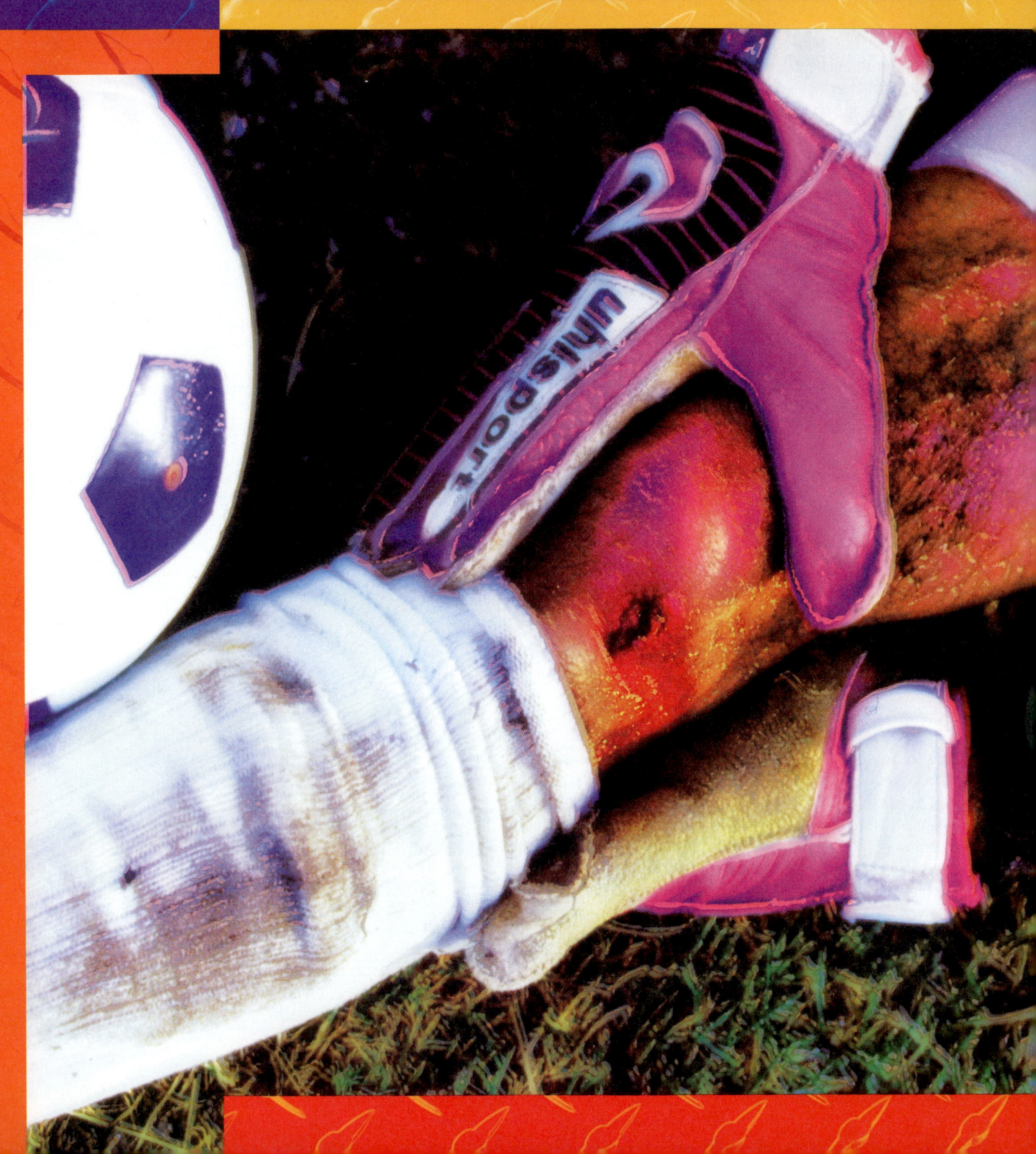

objectives

Cognitive

1. State the major functions of the skin.

2. List the layers of the skin.

3. Establish the relationship between body substance isolation (BSI) and soft-tissue injuries.

4. List the types of closed soft-tissue injuries.

5. Describe the emergency medical care of the patient with a closed soft-tissue injury.

6. State the types of open soft-tissue injuries.

7. Describe the emergency medical care of the patient with an open soft-tissue injury.

8. Discuss the emergency medical care considerations for a patient with a penetrating chest injury.

9. State the emergency medical care considerations for a patient with an open wound to the abdomen.

10. Differentiate the care of an open wound to the chest from an open wound to the abdomen.

11. List the classification of burns.

12. Define superficial burn.

13. List the characteristics of a superficial burn.

14. Define partial-thickness burn.

15. List the characteristics of a partial-thickness burn.

16. Define full-thickness burn.

17. List the characteristics of a full-thickness burn.

18. Describe the emergency medical care of the patient with a superficial burn.

19. Describe the emergency medical care of the patient with a partial-thickness burn.

20. Describe the emergency medical care of the patient with a full-thickness burn.

21. List the functions of dressing and bandaging.

22. Describe the purpose of a bandage.

23. Describe the steps in applying a pressure bandage.

24. Establish the relationship between airway management and the patient with chest injury, burns, blunt and penetrating injuries.

25. Describe the effects of improperly applied dressings, splints, and tourniquets.

26. Describe the emergency medical care of a patient with an impaled object.

27. Describe the emergency medical care of a patient with an amputation.

28. Describe the emergency care for a chemical burn.

29. Describe the emergency care for an electrical burn.

Affective

None

Psychomotor

30. Demonstrate the steps in the emergency medical care of closed soft-tissue injuries.

31. Demonstrate the steps in the emergency medical care of open soft-tissue injuries.

32. Demonstrate the steps in the emergency medical care of a patient with an open chest wound.

33. Demonstrate the steps in the emergency medical care of a patient with open abdominal wounds.

34. Demonstrate the steps in the emergency medical care of a patient with an impaled object.

35. Demonstrate the steps in the emergency medical care of a patient with an amputation.

36. Demonstrate the steps in the emergency medical care of an amputated part.

37. Demonstrate the steps in the emergency medical care of a patient with superficial burns.

38. Demonstrate the steps in the emergency medical care of a patient with partial-thickness burns.

39. Demonstrate the steps in the emergency medical care of a patient with full-thickness burns.

40. Demonstrate the steps in the emergency medical care of a patient with a chemical burn.

41. Demonstrate completing a prehospital care report for patients with soft-tissue injuries.

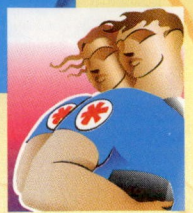

you are the emt

Your ambulance is back from maintenance after a young skater overshot a hand rail and went head-first into a clump of roses.

Athletes of all kinds sustain a myriad of soft-tissue injuries. This chapter will provide the information you will need to care for these very common injuries, as well as help you to answer the following questions:

1. Is there any practical reason that tourniquet use is still taught?
2. What is the difference between an avulsion and an amputation?

Soft-Tissue Injuries

The skin is our first line of defense against external forces. And although it is relatively tough, skin is still quite susceptible to injury. Injuries to soft tissues range from simple bruises and abrasions to serious lacerations and amputations. Soft-tissue injury may result in loss of soft tissue, exposing deep structures such as blood vessels, nerves, and bones. In all instances, you must control bleeding, prevent further contamination, and protect the wound from further damage. Therefore, you must know how to apply dressings and bandages to various parts of the body.

The Anatomy and Function of the Skin

The skin is the largest organ in the body. It varies in thickness, depending on age and its location. The skin of the very young and very old is thinner than the skin of a young adult. The skin covering your scalp, your back, and the soles of your feet is quite thick, while the skin of your eyelids, lips, and ears is very thin. Thin skin is more easily damaged than thick skin.

Anatomy of the Skin

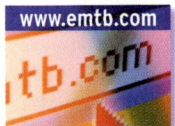

www.emtb.com

The skin has two principal layers: the epidermis and the dermis (Figure 26-1). The **epidermis** is the tough, external layer that forms a watertight covering for the body. The epidermis is itself composed of several layers. The cells on the surface layer of the epidermis are constantly worn away. They are replaced by cells that are pushed to the surface when new cells form in the germinal layer at the base of the epidermis. Deeper cells in the germinal layer contain pigment granules. Along with blood vessels in the dermis, these granules produce skin color.

The **dermis** is the inner layer of the skin. It lies below the germinal cells of the epidermis. The dermis contains the structures that give the skin its characteristic appearance: hair follicles, sweat glands, and sebaceous glands. The sweat glands act to cool the body. They discharge sweat onto the surface of the skin through small pores, or ducts, that pass through the epidermis. Sebaceous glands produce sebum, the oily material that waterproofs the skin and keeps it supple. Sebum travels to the skin's surface along the shaft of adjacent hair follicles. Hair follicles are small organs that produce hair. There is one follicle for each hair, each connected with a sebaceous gland and a tiny muscle. This muscle pulls the hair erect whenever you are cold or frightened.

Blood vessels in the dermis provide the skin with nutrients and oxygen. Small branches reach up to the germinal cells, but no blood vessels penetrate farther into the epidermis. There are also specialized nerve endings within the dermis.

The skin covers all external surfaces of the body. The various openings in our body, including the mouth, nose, anus, and vagina, are not covered by skin. Instead, these openings are lined with **mucous membranes**. These membranes are similar to skin in that they, too, provide a protective barrier against bacterial invasion. But mucous membranes differ from skin in that they secrete a watery substance that lubricates the openings. Therefore, mucous membranes are moist, while skin is dry.

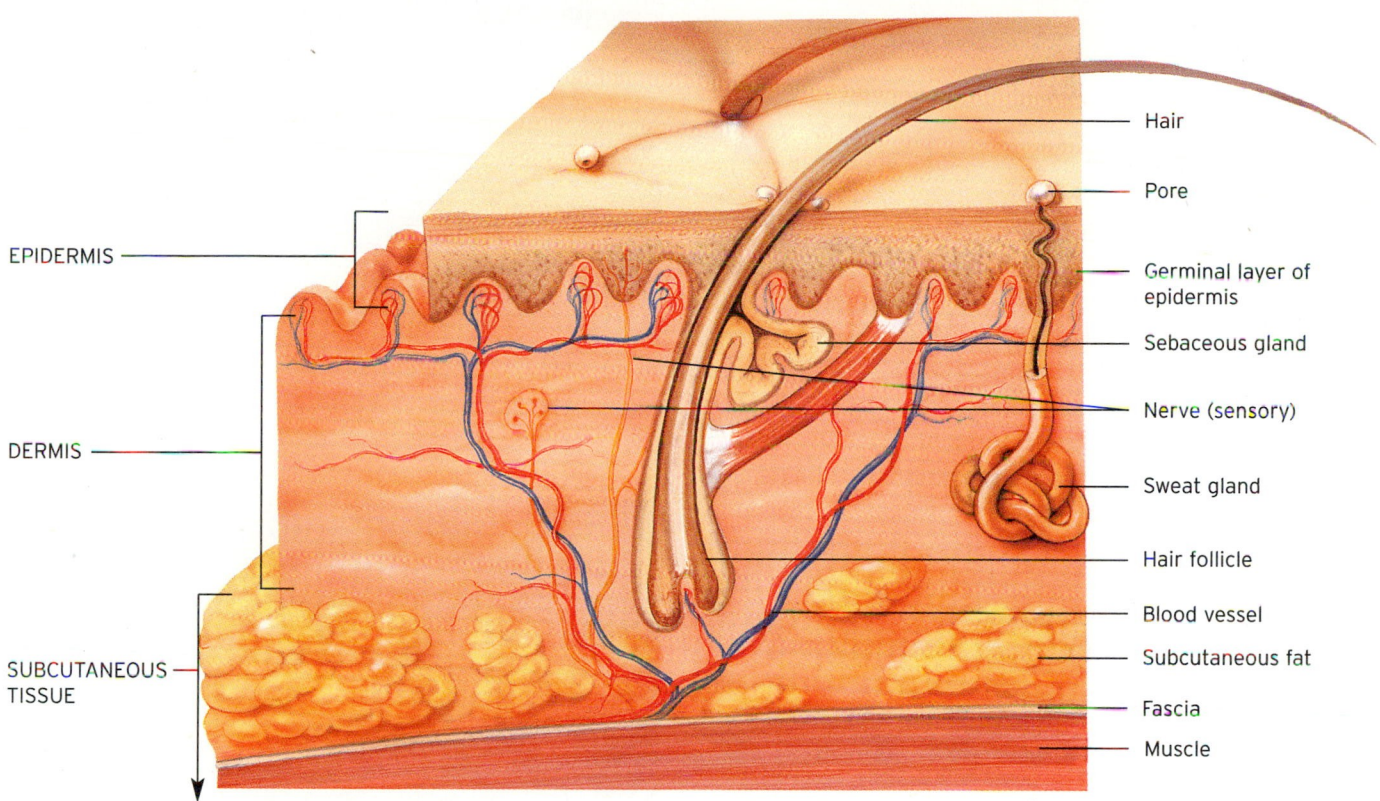

EPIDERMIS

DERMIS

SUBCUTANEOUS
TISSUE

Hair

Pore

Germinal layer of
epidermis

Sebaceous gland

Nerve (sensory)

Sweat gland

Hair follicle

Blood vessel

Subcutaneous fat

Fascia

Muscle

FIGURE 26-1 The skin is composed of a tough external layer called the epidermis and a vascular inner layer called the dermis.

Functions of the Skin

The skin serves many functions. It protects the body by keeping bacteria out and water in. The nerves in the skin report to the brain on the environment and on many sensations.

The skin is also the body's major organ for regulating temperature. In a cold environment, the blood vessels in the skin constrict, diverting blood away from the skin and decreasing the amount of heat that is radiated from the body's surface. In hot environments, the vessels in the skin dilate. The skin becomes flushed or red, and heat radiates from the body's surface. Also, sweat glands secrete sweat. As the sweat evaporates from the skin's surface, your body temperature drops, and you begin to cool down.

> The skin is our first line of defense against external forces. And although it is relatively tough, skin is still quite susceptible to injury.

Any break in the skin allows bacteria to enter and raises the possibilities of infection, fluid loss, and loss of temperature control. Any one of these problems can cause serious illness and even death.

Types of Soft-Tissue Injuries

Soft tissues are often injured because they are exposed to the environment. There are three types of soft-tissue injuries:

- **Closed injuries**, in which soft-tissue damage occurs beneath the skin or mucous membrane but the surface remains intact.

- **Open injuries**, in which there is a break in the surface of the skin or the mucous membrane, exposing deeper tissue to potential contamination.

- **Burns**, in which the soft tissue receives more energy than it can absorb without injury. The sources of this energy can be thermal heat, frictional heat, toxic chemicals, electricity, or nuclear radiation.

Closed Injuries

Closed soft-tissue injuries are characterized by a history of blunt trauma, pain at the site of injury, swelling beneath the skin, and discoloration. Such injuries can vary from mild to quite severe.

A <u>contusion</u>, or bruise, results from blunt force striking the body. The epidermis remains intact, but cells within the dermis are damaged, and small blood vessels are usually torn. The depth of the injury varies, depending on the amount of energy absorbed. As fluid and blood leak into the damaged area, the patient may have swelling and pain. The buildup of blood produces a characteristic blue or black discoloration called <u>ecchymosis</u> (Figure 26-2).

A <u>hematoma</u> is a pool of blood that has collected within damaged tissue or in a body cavity (Figure 26-3). It occurs whenever a large blood vessel is damaged and bleeds rapidly. It is usually associated with extensive tissue damage. A hematoma can result from a soft-tissue injury, a fracture, or any injury to a large blood vessel. In severe cases, the hematoma may contain more than a liter of blood.

A crushing injury occurs when a great amount of force is applied to the body for a long period of time (Figure 26-4). The extent of the damage depends on just how long that period is. In addition to causing some direct soft-tissue damage, continued compression of the soft tissues will cut off their circulation, producing further tissue destruction. For example, if a patient's legs are trapped under a collapsed pile of rocks, damage to the leg tissues will continue until the rocks are removed.

Another form of compression can result from the swelling that occurs whenever tissues are injured. The cells that are injured leak watery fluid into the spaces between the cells. If swelling is excessive or occurs in a confined space such as the skull, the tissue pressure will increase to dangerous levels. The pressure of the fluid may become great enough to compress the tissue and cause further damage. This is especially true if the blood vessels become compressed, cutting off blood flow to the tissue. This condition is called compartment syndrome. Excessive swelling often follows injury of the brain, the spinal cord, and the extremities.

Severe closed injuries can also damage internal organs. The greater the amount of energy absorbed from the blunt force, the greater is the risk of injury to deeper structures. Therefore, you must assess all patients with closed injuries for more serious hidden injuries. Remain alert for signs of shock or internal bleeding, and begin treatment of these conditions if necessary.

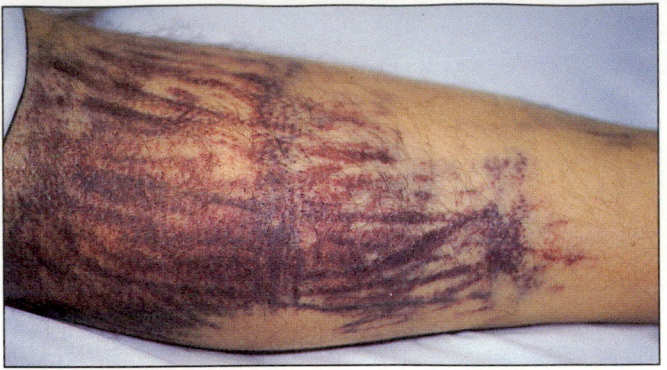

FIGURE 26-2 Contusions, more commonly known as bruises, occur as a result of a blunt force striking the body. The buildup of blood produces a characteristic blue or black discoloration.

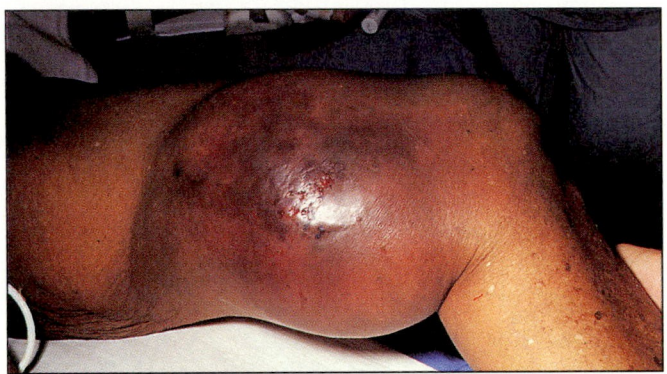

FIGURE 26-3 A hematoma develops whenever a large blood vessel is damaged and bleeds rapidly.

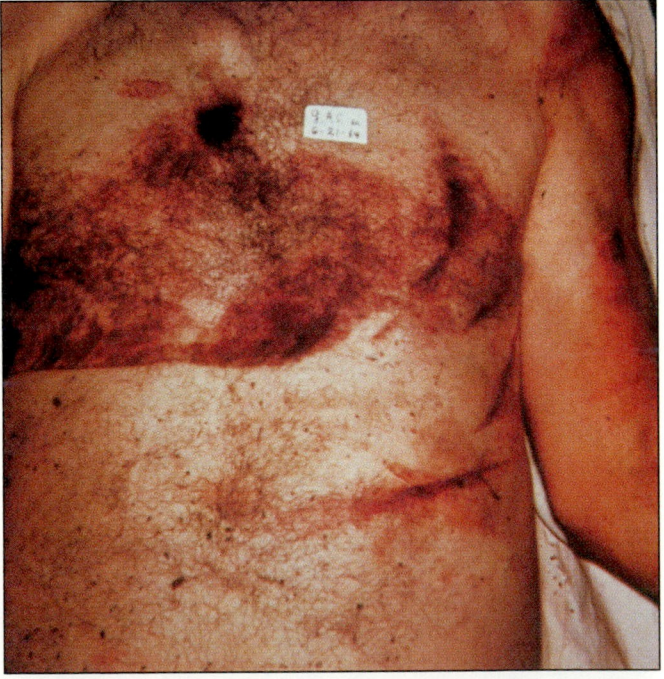

FIGURE 26-4 The damage associated with a crush or compression injury varies depending on the direct damage to the soft tissues and on how long the tissue was cut off from circulation.

Emergency Medical Care

Small contusions require no special emergency medical care. More extensive closed injuries may involve significant swelling and bleeding beneath the skin, which could lead to hypovolemic shock. Before treating a closed injury, make sure to follow BSI techniques. Wash your hands thoroughly, and wear gloves as you work with the patient.

Soft-tissue injuries may look rather dramatic. However, you must still focus on airway and breathing first. Always provide oxygen and maintain the airway in patients who need it. If the patient has difficulty breathing, you may have to assist ventilations.

Treat a closed soft-tissue injury by applying the acronym ICES:

- **Ice** (or a cold pack) slows bleeding by causing blood vessels to constrict and also reduces pain.

- **Compression** over the injury site slows bleeding by compressing the blood vessels.

- **Elevation** of the injured part just above the level of the patient's heart decreases swelling.

- **Splinting** decreases bleeding and also reduces pain by immobilizing a soft-tissue injury or an injured extremity.

In addition to using these measures to control bleeding and swelling, you should also be alert for signs of developing shock, including low blood pressure, increased heart rate, and cool or clammy skin. Any or all of these signs may indicate internal bleeding, resulting from injuries to internal organs. If the patient appears to be in shock, you should elevate his or her legs, give supplemental oxygen, and provide prompt transport to the hospital.

Open Injuries

Open injuries differ from closed injuries in that the protective layer of skin is damaged. This can produce more extensive bleeding. More important, however, a break in the protective skin layer or mucous membrane means that the wound is contaminated and may become infected. **Contamination** means that infective organisms or foreign bodies, such as dirt, gravel, or metal, are present. You must address these two problems in your treatment of open soft-tissue wounds. There are four types of open soft-tissue wounds that you must be prepared to manage: abrasions, lacerations, avulsions, and penetrating wounds.

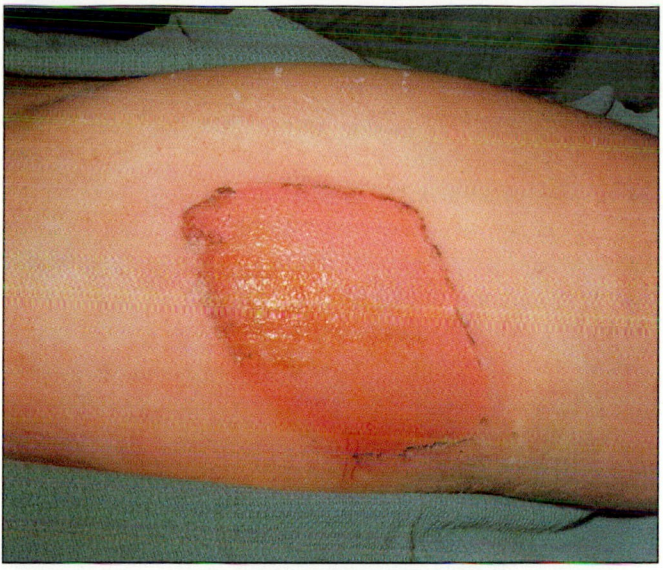

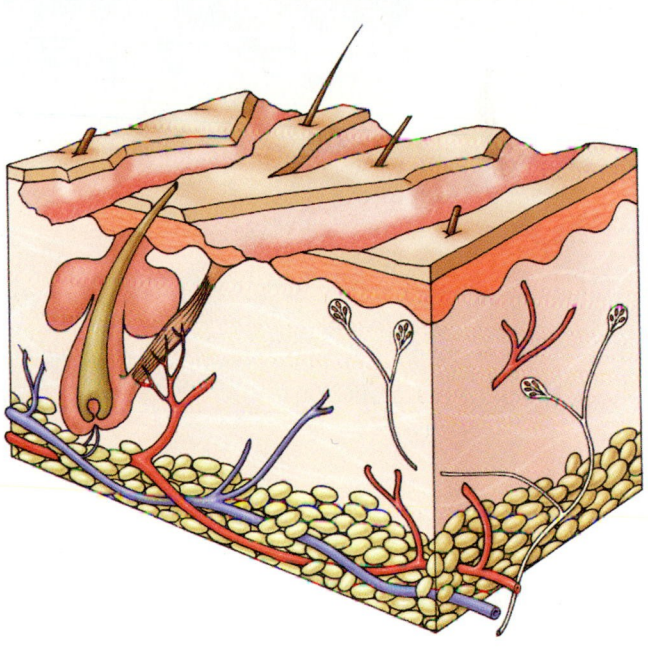

FIGURE 26-5 Abrasions usually do not penetrate completely through the dermis, but blood may ooze from the capillaries. These wounds are typically superficial and result from rubbing or scraping across a hard surface.

An **abrasion** is a wound of the superficial layer of the skin, caused by friction when a body part rubs or scrapes across a rough or hard surface. An abrasion usually does not penetrate completely through the dermis, but blood may ooze from the injured capillaries in the dermis. Known by a variety of names, including road rash, road burn, strawberry, and mat burn, abrasions can be extremely painful (Figure 26-5).

A <u>laceration</u> is a smooth or jagged cut caused by a sharp object or a blunt force that tears the tissue. The depth of the injury can vary, extending through the skin and subcutaneous tissue even into the underlying muscles and adjacent nerves and blood vessels (Figure 26-6). A laceration may appear linear (regular) or stellate (irregular) and may occur along with other types of soft-tissue injury. Lacerations that involve cut arteries may result in severe bleeding.

An <u>avulsion</u> is an injury that separates various layers of soft tissue (usually between the subcutaneous layer and fascia) so that they are either completely unattached or hanging as a flap (Figure 26-7). Usually, there is significant bleeding. If the avulsed tissue is hanging from a small piece of skin, the circulation through the flap may be at risk. If the avulsed flap can be replaced in its original position, do this. If an avulsion is complete, you should wrap the separated tissue in sterile gauze and bring it with you to the emergency department.

We usually think of amputations as involving the upper and lower extremities. But other body parts, such as the scalp, ear, nose, penis, or lips, may also be totally avulsed, or amputated. You can easily control the bleeding from some amputations, such as the fingers, with pressure dressings. But if an avulsion involves a large area of muscle mass, such as a thigh, there may be massive bleeding. In this situation, you need to treat the patient for hypovolemic shock.

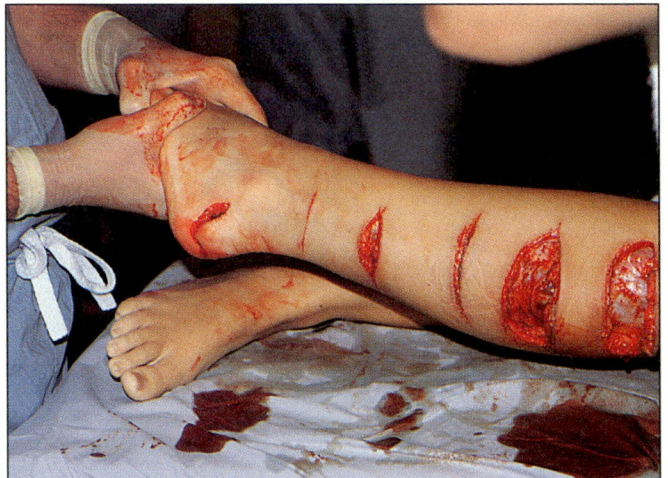

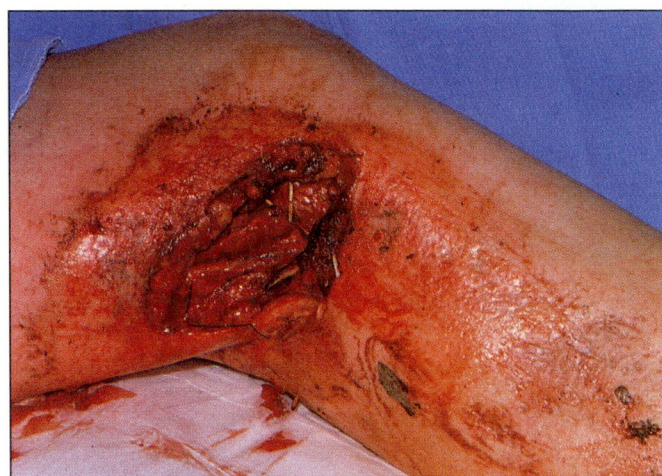

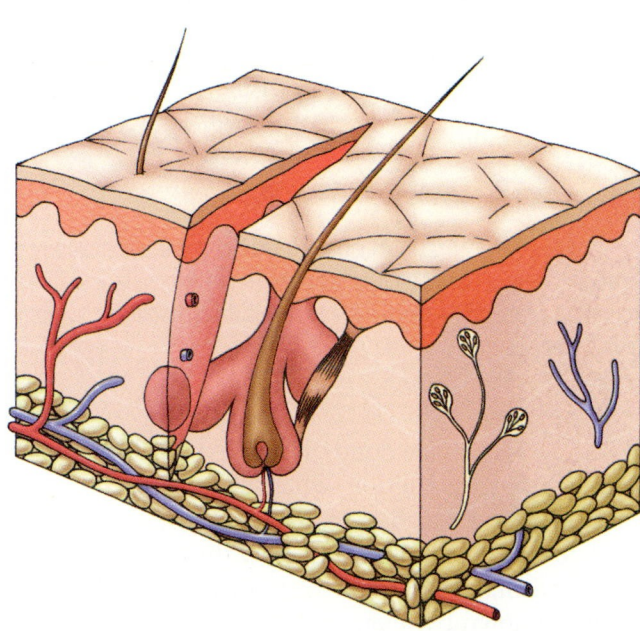

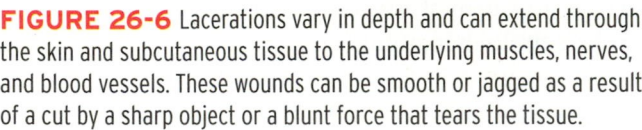

FIGURE 26-6 Lacerations vary in depth and can extend through the skin and subcutaneous tissue to the underlying muscles, nerves, and blood vessels. These wounds can be smooth or jagged as a result of a cut by a sharp object or a blunt force that tears the tissue.

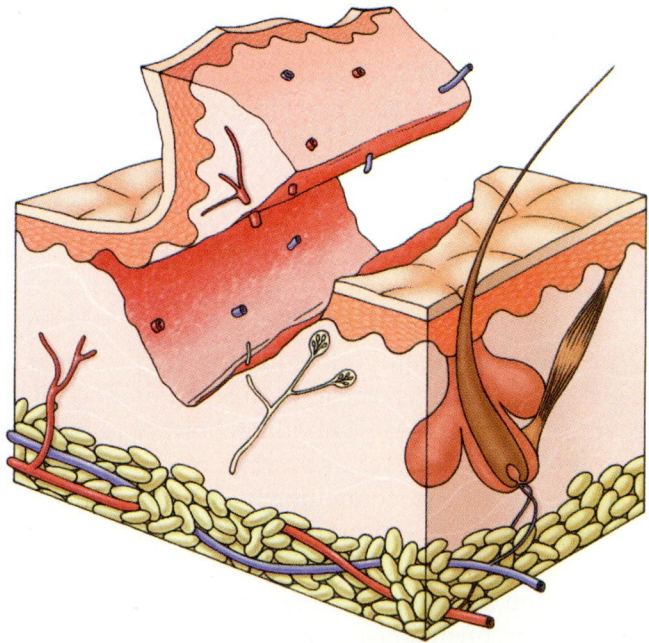

FIGURE 26-7 Avulsions are injuries characterized by either complete separation of tissue or tissue hanging as a flap. Significant bleeding is common.

A <u>penetrating wound</u> is an injury resulting from a sharp, pointed object, such as a knife, ice pick, splinter, or bullet. Such objects leave relatively small entrance wounds, so there may be little external bleeding (Figure 26-8). However, these objects can damage structures deep within the body. If the wound is in the chest or abdomen, the injury can cause rapid, fatal bleeding. Assessing the amount of damage a puncture wound has created is very difficult.

Stabbings and shootings often result in multiple penetrating injuries. You must assess these patients carefully to identify all wounds. Since a penetrating object can pass completely through the body, always look for both entrance and exit wounds, especially with gunshot wounds. An entrance wound is usually smaller than an exit wound. A gun shot at close range will leave an entrance wound with powder burns around the edges (Figure 26-9). Because of its larger size, an exit wound may bleed excessively.

Gunshot wounds have some unique characteristics that require special care. The amount of damage from a gunshot wound is directly related to the speed of the bullet. Thus, it is important to find out the type of gun that was used in the shooting. Sometimes, the patient or bystanders can tell you how many rounds were fired. This information can help hospital personnel to better care for the patient. Shotgun wounds create multiple paths of missiles (shot) and create a larger surface area and volume of tissue damage.

Most shootings end up in court at some point, and you may be called to testify. For this reason, you must carefully document the circumstances surrounding any gunshot injury, the patient's condition, and the treatment you give.

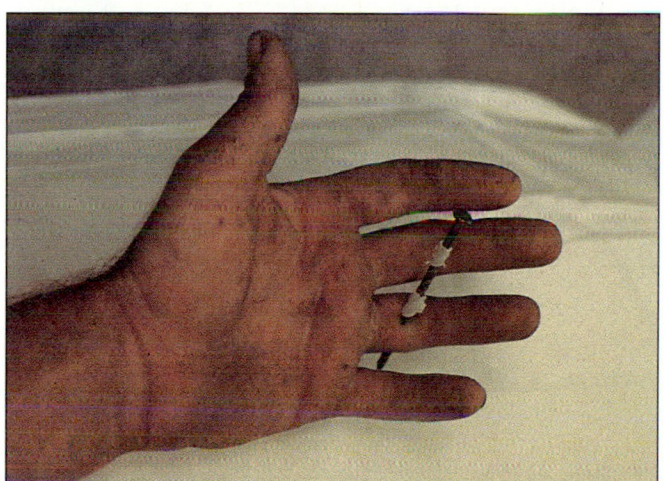

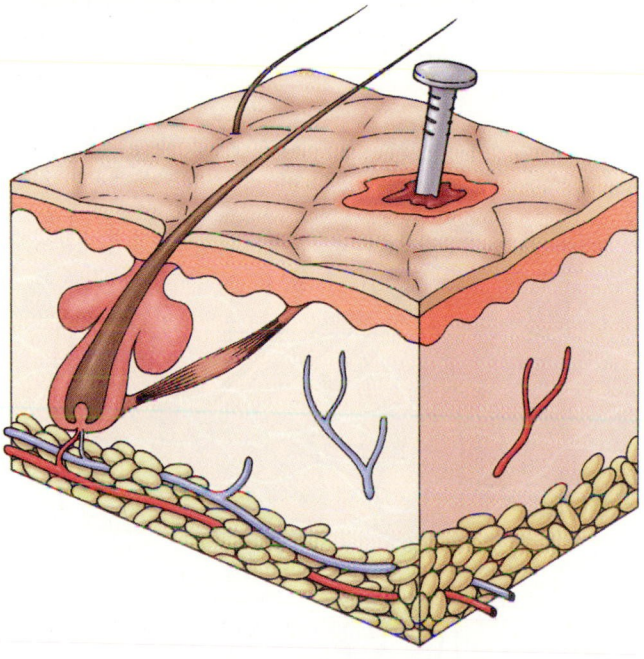

FIGURE 26-8 Puncture wounds often have very little external bleeding but can damage structures deep within the body.

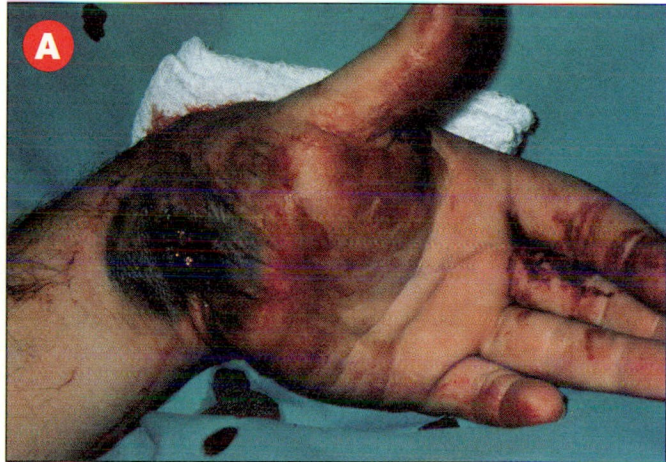

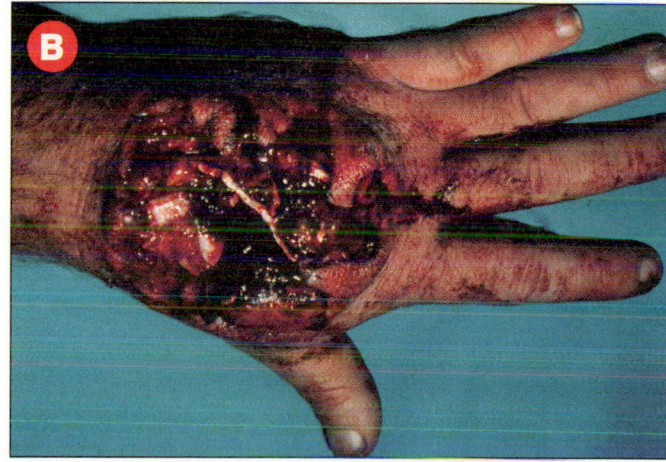

FIGURE 26-9 A: An entrance wound from a gunshot may have burns around the edges. **B:** An exit wound is larger and results in greater damage to soft tissues.

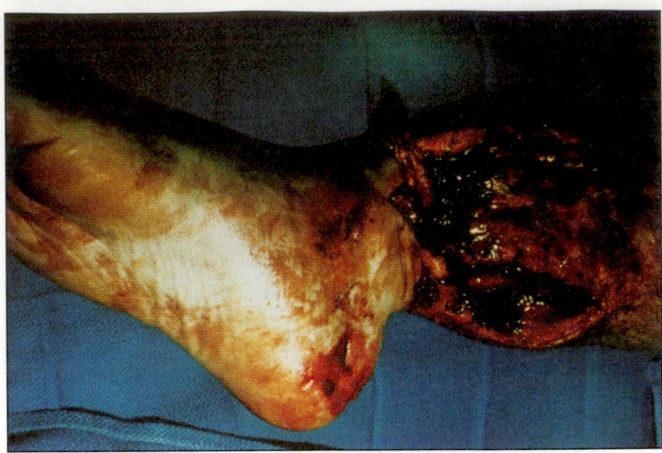

FIGURE 26-10 A crushing open wound is characterized by extensive tissue damage and deformity that is often accompanied by swelling and extreme pain.

As with closed wounds caused by crushing, open wounds caused by crushing may involve damaged internal organs or broken bones, as well as extensive soft-tissue damage (Figure 26-10). While external bleeding may be minimal, internal bleeding may be severe, even life-threatening. The crushing force damages soft tissues, as well as vessels and nerves. This frequently results in a painful, swollen, deformed area.

Emergency Medical Care

Before you begin caring for a patient with an open wound, you should be sure to protect yourself by following BSI techniques. Wear gloves, eye protection, and, if necessary, a gown. Remember that you must be sure the patient has an open airway and administer oxygen if necessary before caring for the wound. Then assess the severity of the wound, removing any clothing that may be covering it.

Your treatment priority is ABCD followed by controlling bleeding, which can be extensive and severe. To do this, apply a dry, sterile compression dressing over the entire wound. Apply pressure to the dressing with your gloved hand, and then maintain the pressure with a roller bandage (Figure 26-11). If bleeding continues or recurs, leave the original dressing in place. Apply a second dressing on top of the first, and secure it with another roller bandage. Once you have controlled the bleeding, keep the dressing in place with a splint.

All open wounds are contaminated and present a risk of infection. By applying a sterile dressing, you are preventing further contamination. This keeps foreign material, such as hair, clothing, and dirt, out of the wound and decreases the risk of secondary infection. However, do not try to remove material from an open wound, no matter how dirty the wound is. Rubbing,

brushing, or washing an open wound will only cause additional bleeding. Only hospital personnel should clean out an open wound. To prevent the wound from drying, you should apply moistened sterile sponges with sterile saline solution, if possible, then cover the wound with a dry, sterile dressing.

Often, you can better control bleeding from open soft-tissue wounds by splinting the extremity, even if there is no fracture. Splinting can also help you to keep the patient calm and quiet, as it typically reduces pain. In addition, splinting keeps sterile dressings in place, minimizes damage to an already injured extremity, and makes moving the patient easier.

Keep in mind that a patient who is bleeding significantly from an open wound can go into hypovolemic shock. You must be alert for this possibility and provide treatment, as needed.

Chest Wounds

A penetrating wound to the chest may cause air to enter the chest (pneumothorax) or blood to collect in the chest (hemothorax) (Figure 26-12). Ordinarily, the pressure inside the chest cavity is slightly lower than the pressure of the atmosphere. Inhalation further reduces

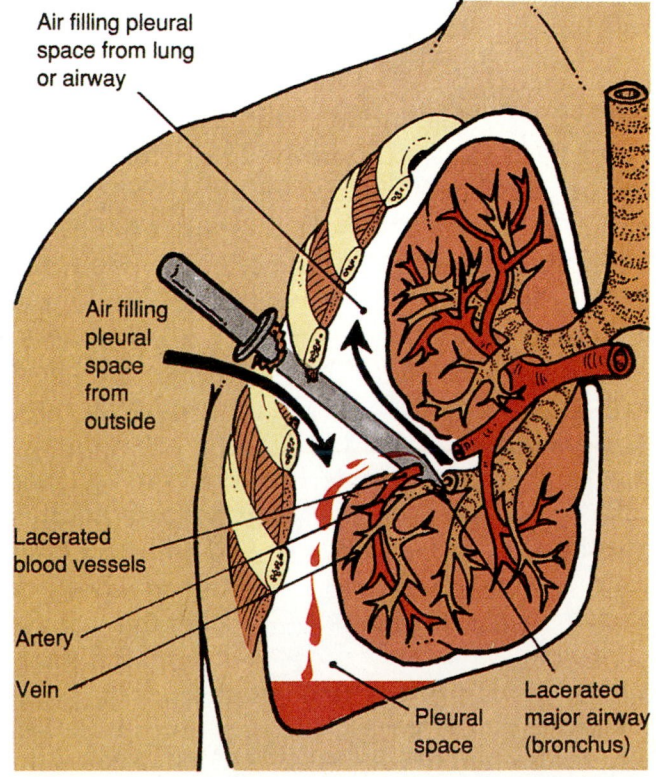

FIGURE 26-12 Penetrating wounds can cause air to enter the chest or blood to collect in the chest.

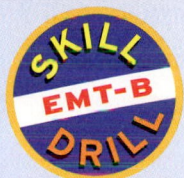

Controlling Bleeding from a Soft-Tissue Injury
Figure 26-11

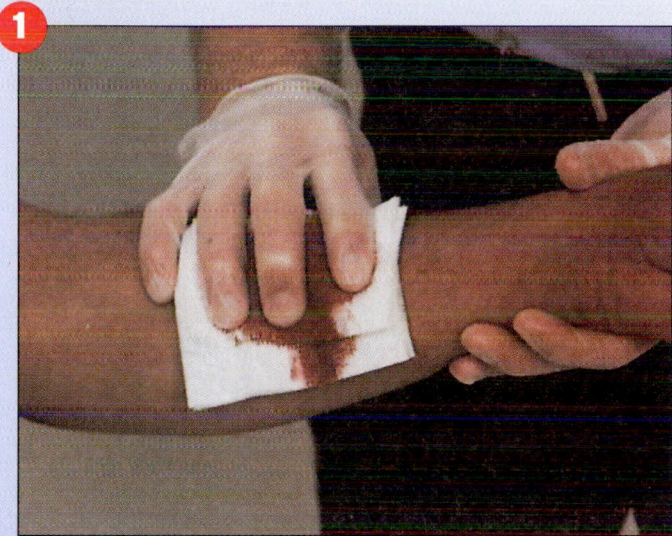

Using your gloved hand, apply direct pressure over the wound using a dry, sterile dressing.

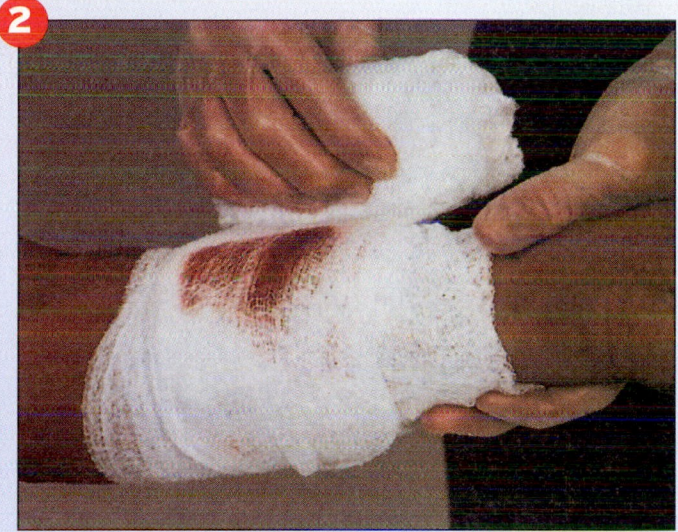

Secure the dressing in place with a roller bandage.

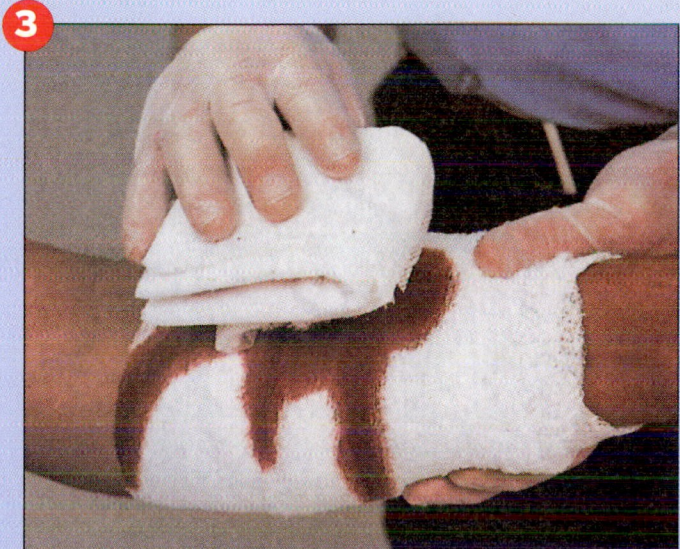

If the bleeding continues, add a second dressing on top of the first to continue to maintain direct pressure, and then secure it with another roller bandage.

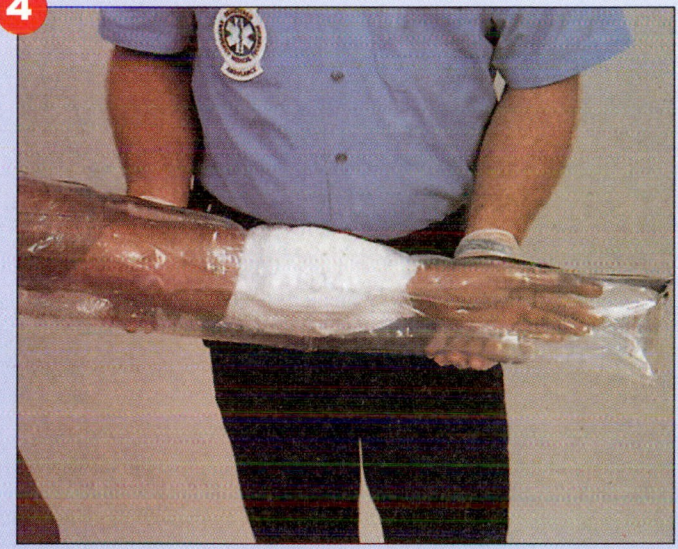

Splint the extremity to stabilize the injury even if there is no fracture, to help minimize movement, to further control the bleeding, and to keep the dressing in place.

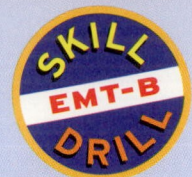

Sealing a Sucking Chest Wound
Figure 26-13

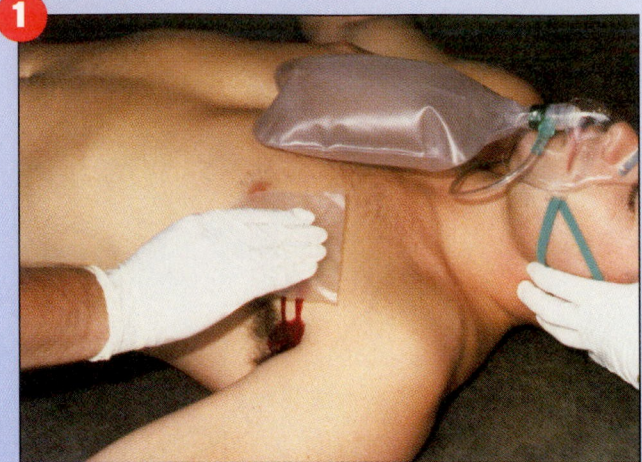

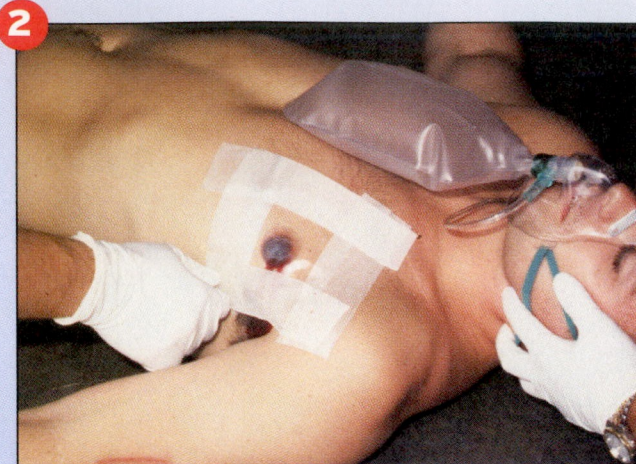

1. Place the patient in a supine position, and give supplemental oxygen.

2. Seal the wound with an airtight dressing that is large enough so that it is not pulled or sucked into the chest cavity.

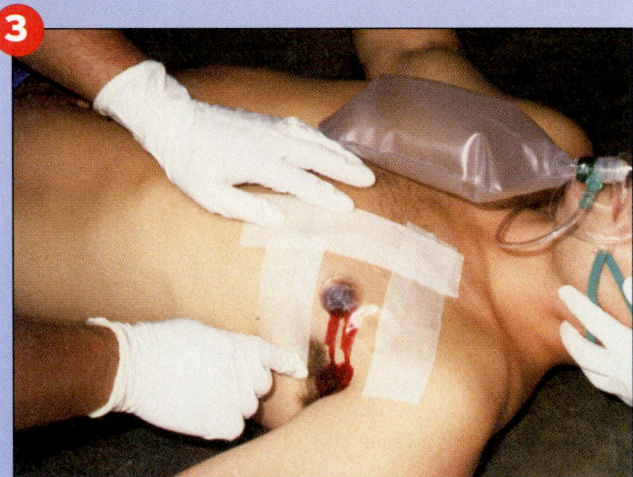

3. Depending on your local protocol, seal all four sides of the dressing, or seal three sides, creating a one-way valve that allows air to leave the chest cavity but not return.

this pressure, so air will move through a wound just as easily as it moves through the nose and mouth during normal breathing. The air that enters through the wound remains in the pleural space, and the lung does not expand; when the patient exhales, air passes back through the wound. Such "sucking chest wounds" reduce the ability of the lungs to provide fresh oxygen to the blood.

Initial emergency care should include giving supplemental oxygen and then sealing the wound with an airtight dressing (Figure 26-13). This type of dressing prevents air from being sucked into the chest through the wound. Several sterile materials, including aluminum foil, Vaseline gauze, or a folded universal dressing may be used for this purpose. Use a large enough dressing so that it is not pulled or sucked into the chest cavity. Depending on your local protocol, you may seal the dressing on all four sides, or you may seal only three sides to create a flutter valve, which is a one-way valve that allows air to leave the chest cavity but not return.

The buildup of blood in the chest can result in difficulty breathing and/or shock. Emergency medical care of this condition should include administering oxygen, elevating the patient's legs, and providing prompt transport to the nearest hospital. The patient may be placed in a position of comfort if no spinal injury is suspected.

Abdominal Wounds

An open wound in the abdominal cavity may expose internal organs. In some cases, the organs may even protrude through the wound, an injury called an eviscerration (Figure 26-14). Do not touch or move the exposed organs. Rather, cover the wound with sterile gauze compresses moistened with sterile saline solution and secured with a sterile dressing (Figure 26-15). Because the open abdomen radiates body heat very effectively, and because exposed organs lose fluid rapidly, you must keep the organs moist and warm. If you do not have gauze compresses, you may use moist sterile dressings, covered and secured in place with a bandage and tape. Do not use any material that is adher-

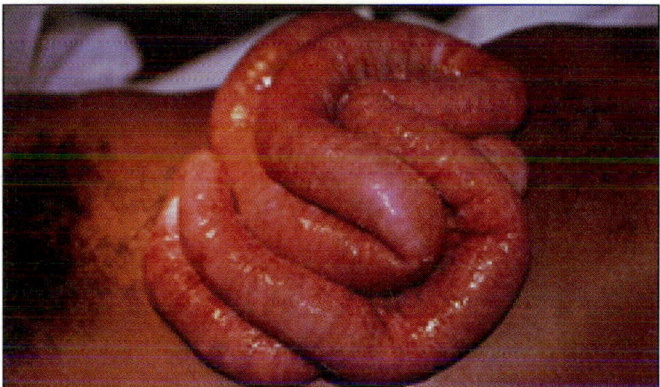

FIGURE 26-14 An abdominal evisceration is an open wound to the abdomen in which organs protrude through the wound.

ent or loses its substance when wet, such as toilet paper, facial tissue, paper towels, or absorbent cotton. If the patient's legs and knees are uninjured, flex them to relieve pressure on the abdomen. All patients with abdominal wounds require immediate transport.

Penetrating Wounds

Occasionally, a patient will have an object, such as a knife, fishhook, wood splinter, or piece of glass, impaled in his or her body. See the Skill Drill on the next page, "Stabilizing an Impaled Object" (Figure 26-16). Do not attempt to move or remove the object unless it is impaled through the cheek. Medical control should be consulted if the foreign body interferes with chest compressions or with transport. In most cases, a surgeon will have to remove the object; moving it in the field may damage nerves, blood vessels, or muscles within the wound. As with all open wounds, remove any clothing covering the injury. Control bleeding, and use a bulky dressing to stabilize the object. To prevent further injury, manually secure the object by incorporating it into the dressing.

The only exception to this rule is if the object is impaled in the cheek and obstructs breathing. In this situation, restoring the airway takes priority. If the object is very long, cut off (shorten) the exposed portion, first securing it to minimize motion and thus internal damage and pain. Once the object is secured and the bleeding is under control, provide prompt transport.

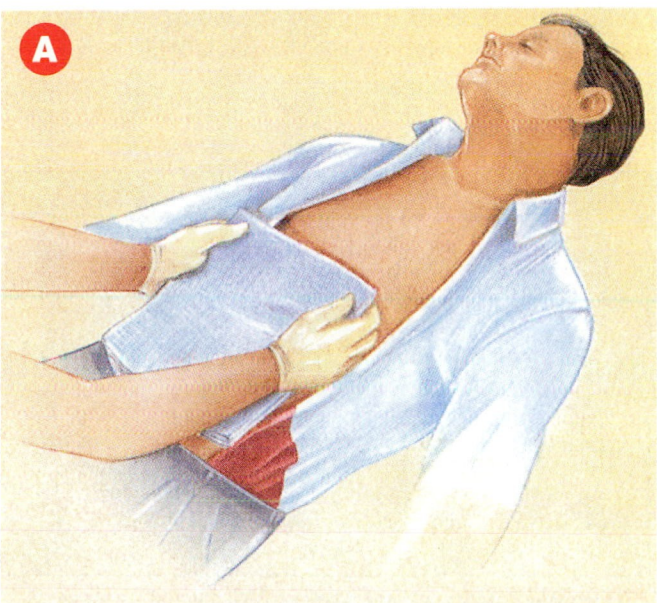

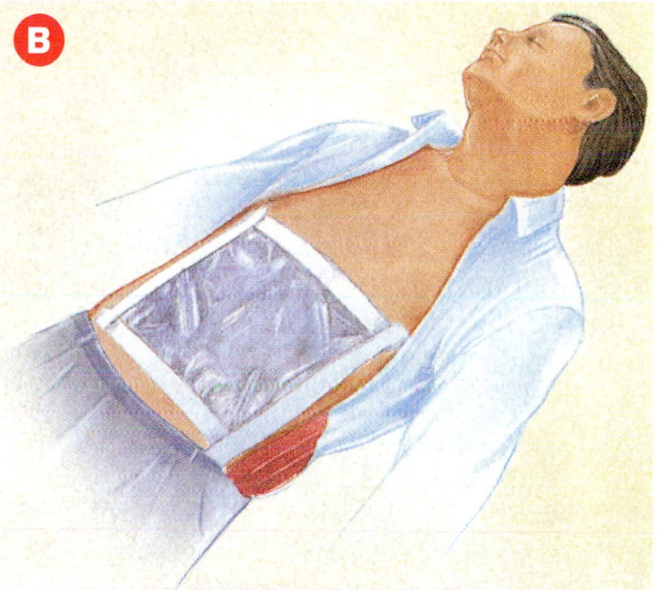

FIGURE 26-15 A: Cover exposed organs with a sterile gauze compresses moistened with sterile saline solution. **B:** Place a dressing over the compresses, and secure it in place by taping all four sides.

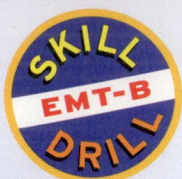

Stabilizing an Impaled Object

Figure 26-16

1

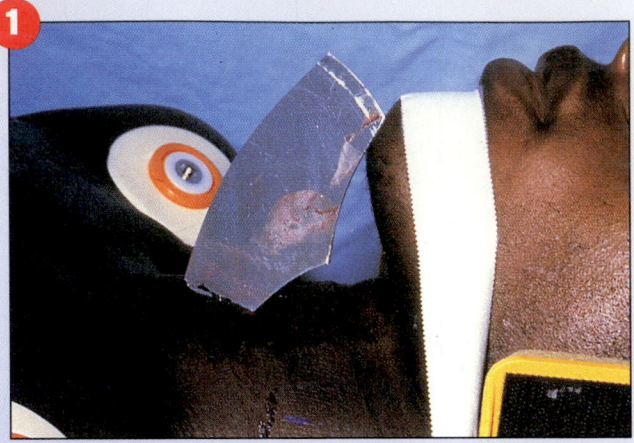

Do not attempt to remove or move an impaled object.

2

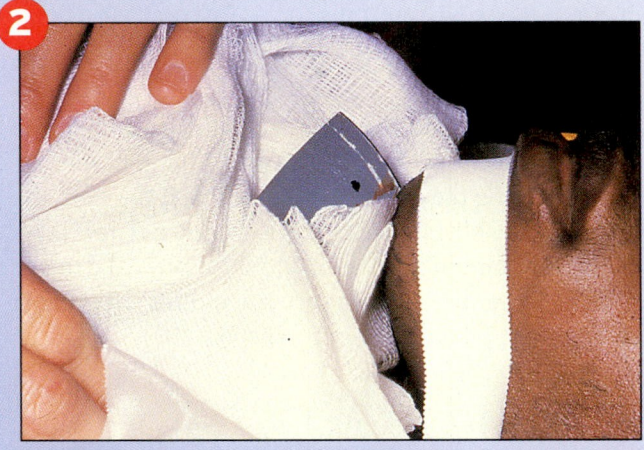

Stabilize the object in place using soft dressings, gauze, and/or tape.

3

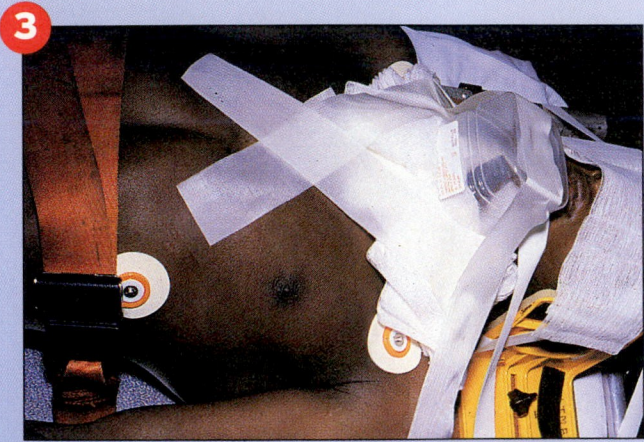

Tape a protective rigid dressing over the soft dressings to protect the object from movement during transport.

Amputations

Surgeons today can often reimplant an amputated part (Figure 26-17). However, correct prehospital care of the amputated part is vital to successful reattachment. With partial amputations, make sure to immobilize the part with bulky compression dressings and a splint to prevent further injury. Do not sever any partial amputations; this may make it impossible to reimplant the part.

With a complete amputation, make sure to wrap the part in a dry sterile dressing and place it in a plastic bag. *Follow your local protocols regarding how to preserve amputated parts. In some areas, dry sterile dressings are recommended for wrapping amputated parts; in other areas, dressings moistened with sterile saline are recommended.* Put the bag in a cool container filled with ice. The goal is to keep the part cool without allowing it to freeze or develop frostbite. The amputated part should be transported with the patient.

Neck Injuries

An open neck injury can be life threatening. If the veins of the neck are open to the environment, they may suck in air (Figure 26-18). If enough air is sucked into a blood vessel, it can actually block the flow of blood in the lungs, sending the patient into cardiac arrest. This condition is called air embolism. To control bleeding and prevent the possibility of air embolism, cover the wound with an occlusive dressing. Apply manual pressure, but do not compress both carotid vessels at the same time; if you do, this may impair circulation to the brain (Figure 26-19). Secure a pressure dressing over the wound by wrapping roller gauze loosely around the neck and then firmly through the opposite axilla.

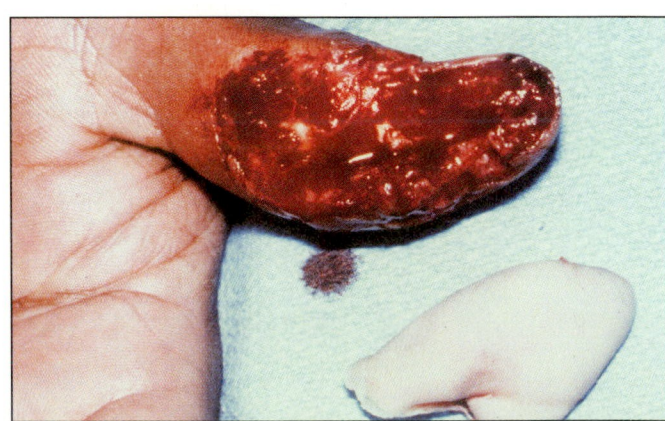

FIGURE 26-17 Amputated parts can often be reimplanted, so you should make every attempt to find the part and transport it to the emergency department along with the patient.

Burns

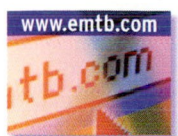
www.emtb.com
tb.com

As an EMT-B, you will often provide care to patients who have been burned. Burns account for over 10,000 deaths a year. Burns are also among the most serious and painful of all injuries. A burn occurs when the body, or a body part, receives more energy than it can absorb without injury. Potential sources of this energy include heat, toxic chemicals, and electricity. The proper emergency care of a burn may increase a patient's chances of survival and decrease the risk or duration of a long-term disability. Although a burn may be the patient's most obvious injury, you should always perform a complete assessment to determine whether there are other serious injuries.

Burn Severity

The seriousness of a burn may influence medical control's choice of a treatment facility. Five factors will help to you determine the severity of a burn:

1. What is the depth of the burn?
2. What is the extent of the burn?

These first two factors are the most important. After gauging these, ask yourself the remaining questions:

3. Are any critical areas (face, upper airway, hands, feet, genitalia) involved?
4. Are there any preexisting medical conditions or other injuries?
5. Is the patient younger than age 5 years or older than age 55 years?

If the answer to any of these last three questions is yes, you should upgrade the burn's classification (Table 26-1).

TABLE 26-1   Classification of Burns in Adults

Critical Burns

- Full-thickness burns involving the hands, feet, face, upper airway, or genitalia
- Full-thickness burns covering more than 10% of the body's total surface area
- Partial-thickness burns covering more than 30% of the body's total surface area
- Burns associated with respiratory injury (smoke inhalation)
- Burns complicated by fractures
- Burns on patients younger than age 5 years or older than age 55 years that would be classified as "moderate" on young adults

Moderate Burns

- Full-thickness burns involving 2% to 10% of the body's total surface area (excluding hands, feet, face, genitalia, or upper airway)
- Partial-thickness burns covering 15% to 30% of the body's total surface area
- Superficial burns covering more than 50% of the body's total surface area

Minor Burns

- Full-thickness burns covering less than 2% of the body's total surface area
- Partial-thickness burns covering less than 15% of the body's total surface area
- Superficial burns covering less than 50% of the body's total surface area

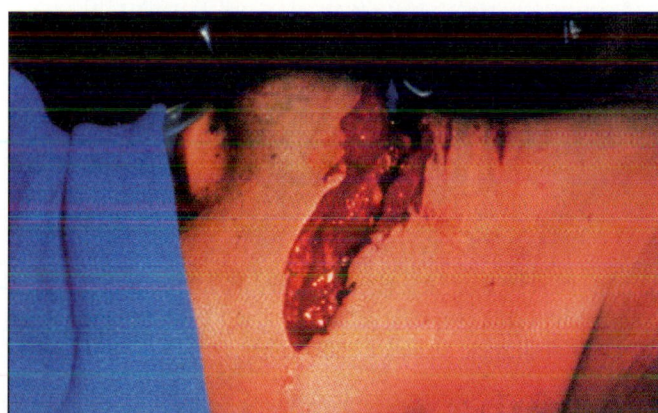

FIGURE 26-18 Open injuries to the neck can be very dangerous. If veins are open to the environment, they can suck in air, resulting in a potentially fatal condition called air embolism.

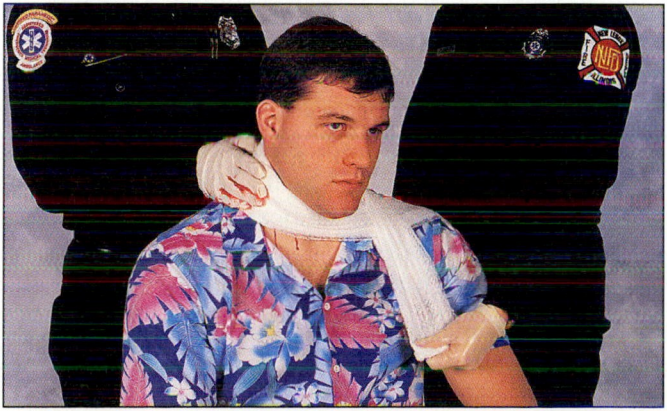

FIGURE 26-19 Cover neck wounds with an airtight dressing, and apply manual pressure. Be sure that you do not compress both carotid arteries at the same time, as this may impair circulation to the brain.

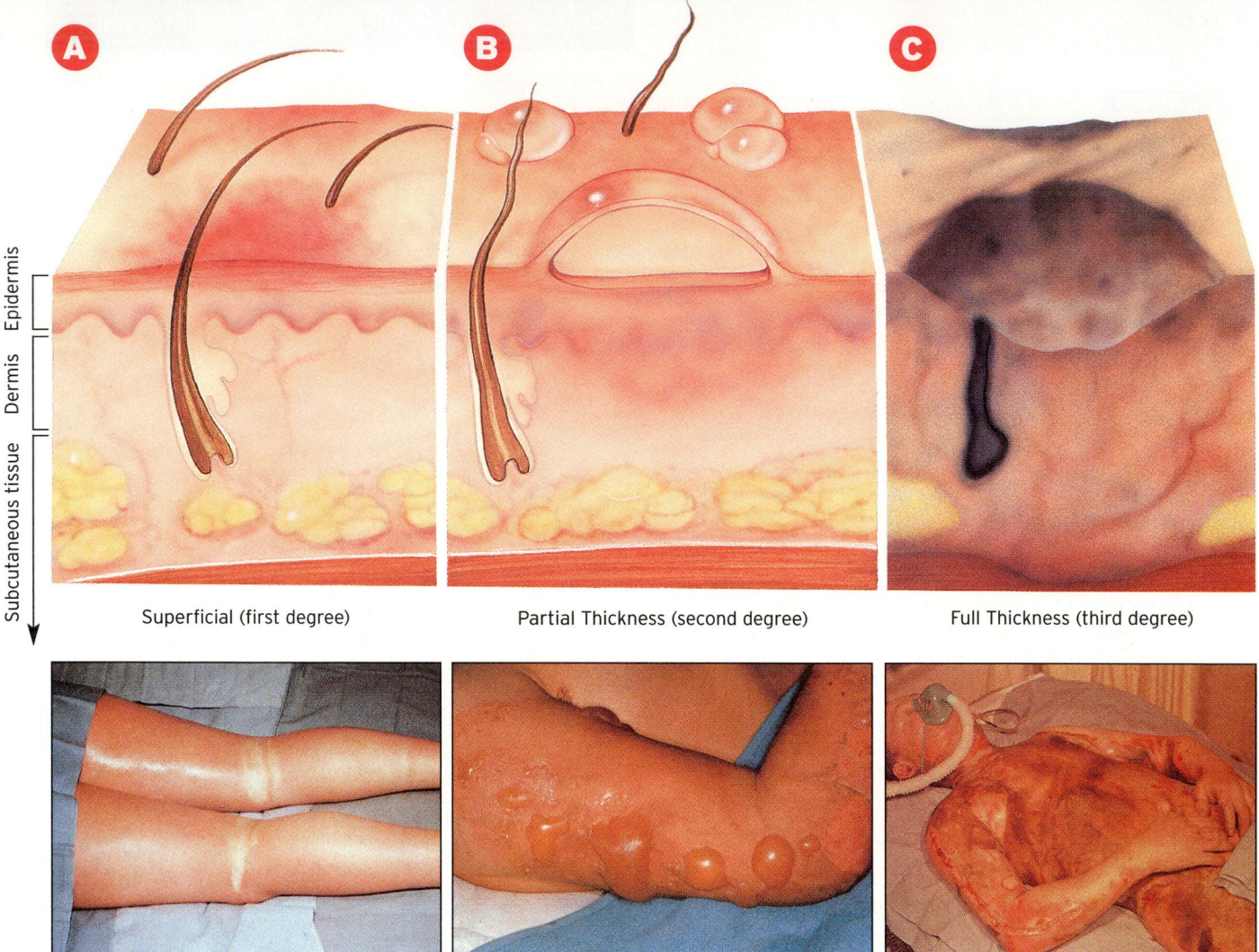

FIGURE 26-20 Classification of burns. **A:** Superficial or first-degree burns involve only the epidermis. The skin turns red but does not blister or actually burn through. **B:** Partial-thickness or second-degree burns involve some of the dermis, but they do not destroy the entire thickness of the skin. The skin is mottled, white to red, and is often blistered. **C:** Full-thickness or third-degree burns extend through all layers of the skin and may involve subcutaneous tissue and muscle. The skin is dry, leathery, and often either white or charred.

Depth. Burns are first classified according to their depth (Figure 26-20). You must be able to identify the following three types of burns:

- **Superficial (first-degree) burns** involve only the top layer of skin, the epidermis. The skin turns red but does not blister or actually burn through. The burn site is painful. A sunburn is a good example of a superficial burn.

- **Partial-thickness (second-degree) burns** involve the epidermis and some portion of the dermis. These burns do not destroy the entire thickness of the skin, nor is the subcutaneous tissue injured. Typically, the skin is moist, mottled, and white to red. Blisters are common. Partial-thickness burns cause intense pain.

- **Full-thickness (third-degree) burns** extend through all skin layers and may involve subcutaneous layers, muscle, bone, or internal organs. The burned area is dry and leathery and may appear white, dark brown, or even charred. Some full-thickness burns feel hard to the touch. Clotted blood vessels or subcutaneous tissue may be visible under the burned skin. If the nerve endings have been destroyed, a severely burned area may have no feeling. However, the surrounding, less severely burned areas may be extremely painful.

A pure full-thickness burn is unusual. Severe burns are typically a combination of superficial, partial-thickness, and full-thickness burns. Superficial burns heal well without scarring. Small partial-thickness burns also heal without scarring. However, deep partial-thickness burns and all full-thickness burns are best managed surgically.

It may be impossible to accurately estimate the depth of a particular burn. Even experienced burn surgeons sometimes underestimate or, more commonly, overestimate the extent of a particular burn.

Extent. One quick way to estimate the surface area that has been burned is to compare it to the size of the patient's palm, which is roughly equal to 1% of the patient's total body surface area. Another useful measurement system is the <u>Rule of Nines</u>, which divides the body into sections, each of which is approximately 9% of the total surface area (Figure 26-21). Remember that the head of an infant or child is relatively larger than the head of an adult, and the legs are relatively smaller.

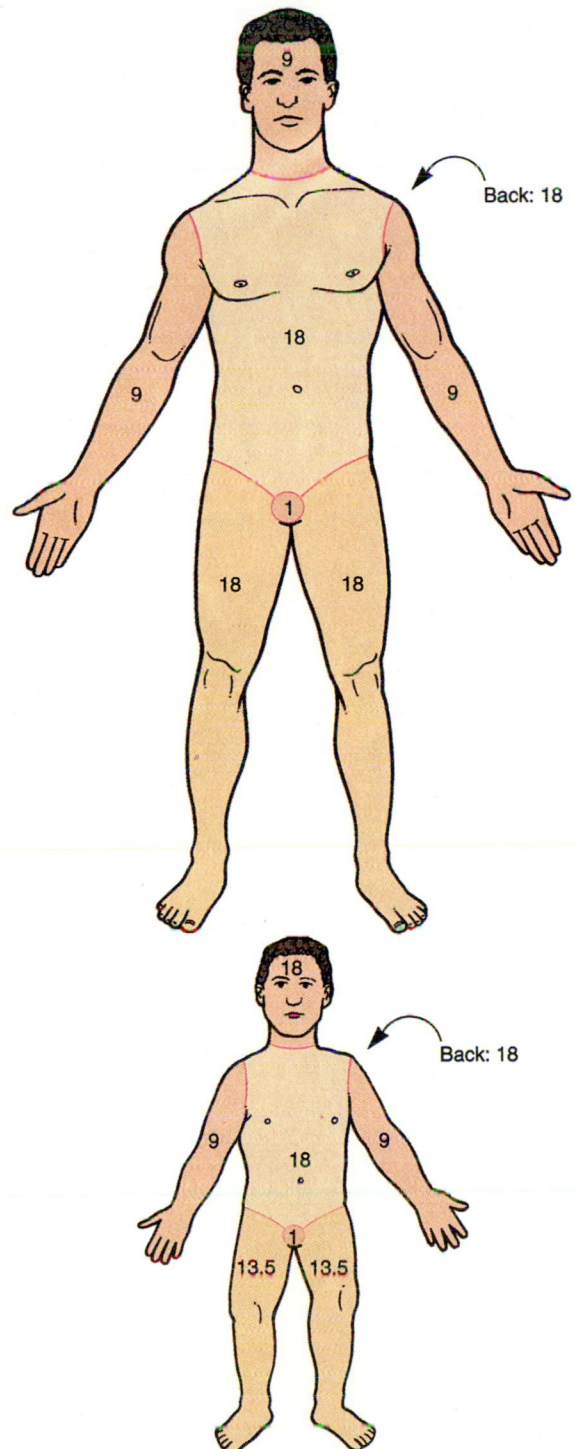

FIGURE 26-21 The Rule of Nines is a quick way to estimate the amount of surface area that has been burned. It divides the body into sections, each approximately 9% of the total body surface area.

caring for kids

Burns to children are generally considered more serious than burns to adults (Table 26-2). This is because infants and children have more surface area relative to total body mass, which means greater fluid and heat loss. In addition, children do not tolerate burns as well as adults do. Children are also more likely to go into shock, develop hypothermia, and experience airway problems.

Many burns in infants and children result from child abuse. The classic burn resulting from deliberate immersion involves the hands and wrists, as well as the feet, lower legs, and buttocks. Similarly, burns around the genitals and multiple cigarette burns should be viewed as possible abuse. You should report all suspected cases of abuse to the proper authorities.

TABLE 26-2   Classification of Burns in Infants and Children

Critical Burns

- Full-thickness or partial-thickness burns covering more than 20% of the body's total surface area
- Burns involving the hands, feet, face, airway, or genitalia

Moderate Burns

- Partial-thickness burns covering 10% to 20% of the body's total surface area

Minor Burns

- Partial-thickness burns covering less than 10% of the body's total surface area

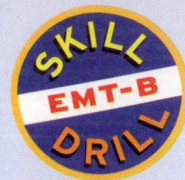

Caring for Burns
Figure 26-22

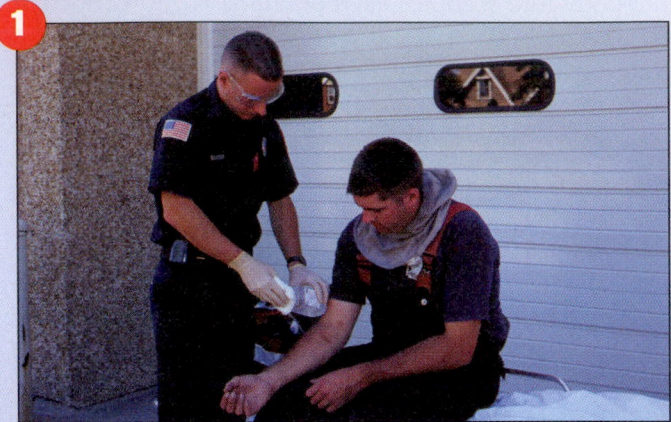

1 After the patient has been moved from the burning area, immerse hot skin or clothing in cool, sterile water, or cover the area with a wet, cool dressing to stop the burning.

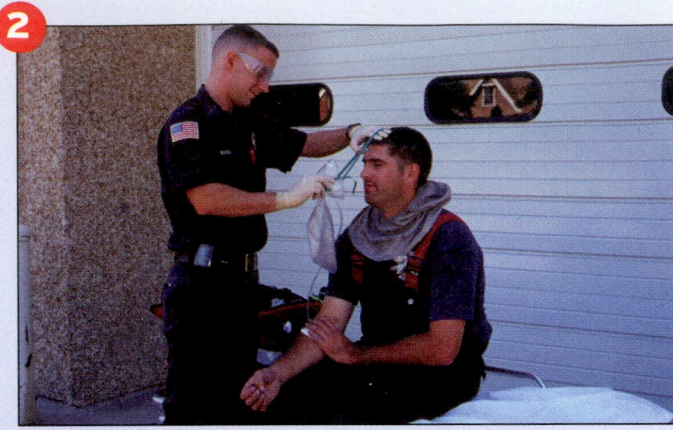

2 Assess the airway, and give the patient supplemental oxygen.

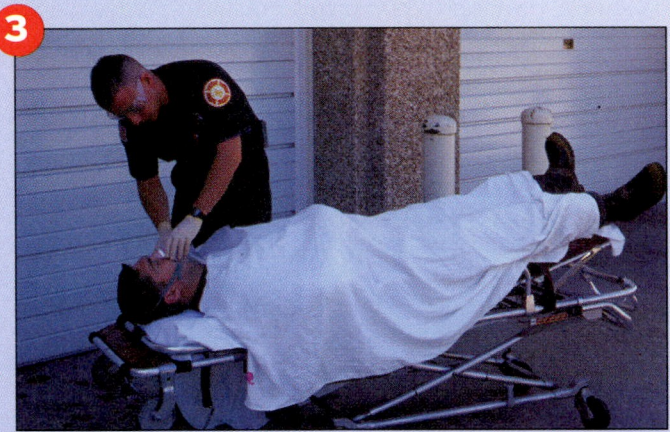

3 A patient with extensive burns may have hypothermia. Cover the patient with blankets to prevent loss of body heat.

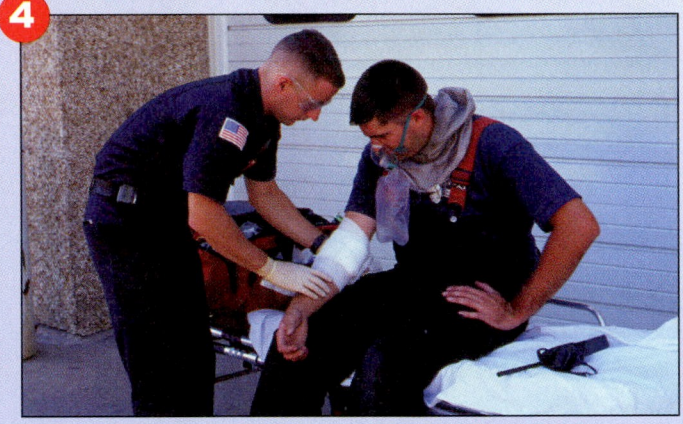

4 Estimate the severity of the burn, then cover the area with a dry dressing, such as sterile gauze, a clean sterile sheet, or a sterile burn sheet.

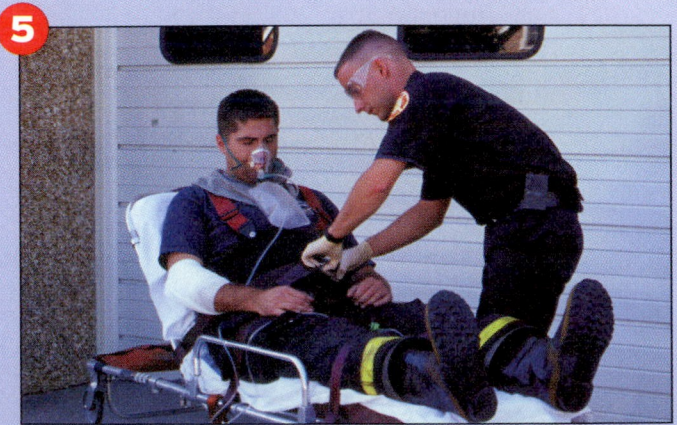

5 Assess the patient for other injuries, treating as needed. Prepare the patient for prompt transport.

Emergency Medical Care

Your first responsibility in caring for a patient with a burn is to stop the burning process and prevent additional injury, as follows (Figure 26-22):

1. **Follow BSI techniques.** Because a burn destroys the patient's protective skin layer, always wear gloves and eye protection when treating a burn patient.

2. **Move the patient away from the burning area.** If any clothing is on fire, wrap the patient in a blanket or follow specific guidelines outlined by your local fire department protocol to put out the flames, then remove any smoldering clothing and/or jewelry.

3. **Immerse the area in cool, sterile water** or saline solution, or cover with a clean, wet, cool dressing, if the skin or clothing is hot. This not only stops the burning, it also relieves pain. However, immersion increases the risk of infection. For this reason, you should not keep the affected part under water for more than 10 minutes. If the burning has stopped before you arrive, do not immerse it at all.

4. **Give oxygen if the patient has a critical burn.** Also remember that more fire victims die from smoke inhalation than from skin burns. A patient who has burns about the face or has inhaled smoke or fumes may develop respiratory distress. Therefore, you should give oxygen to these patients as well. Keep in mind that a patient who appears to be breathing well at first may suddenly develop severe respiratory distress. Therefore, you must continually assess the airway for possible problems.

5. **An extensive burn can produce hypothermia** (loss of body heat). Prevent further heat loss by covering the patient with warm blankets.

6. **Rapidly estimate the burn's severity.** Then cover the burned area with a dry, sterile dressing to prevent further contamination. Sterile gauze is best if the area is not too large. You may cover larger areas with a clean, white sheet. Most important, do not put anything else on the burned area. *Use only a dry, sterile dressing, sterile burn sheet, or clean, white sheet.* Never use ointments, lotions, or antiseptics of any kind. In addition, do not intentionally break any blisters.

7. **Check for traumatic injuries** or other medical conditions that may be more immediately life threatening. Most patients who have been burned have normal vital signs and can communicate at first, which will make your assessment easier.

8. **Treat the patient for shock** if necessary.

9. **Provide prompt transport.** If you are within 20 minutes of a hospital, do not delay transport to do a prolonged assessment or to apply coverings to burns. With pediatric burn victims, however, immediate transport is best if transport time is less than 1 hour.

general emergency medical care of burns

1. Follow BSI techniques.

2. Move the patient away from the burning area.

3. Immerse the burned skin in cool sterile water.

4. Give oxygen.

5. An extensive burn can produce hypothermia.

6. Rapidly estimate the burn's severity.

7. Check for traumatic injuries.

8. Treat the patient for shock.

9. Provide prompt transport.

Chemical Burns

A chemical burn can occur whenever a toxic substance contacts the body. Most chemical burns are caused by strong acids or strong alkalis. The eyes are particularly vulnerable to chemical burns (Figure 26-23). Sometimes, simply the fumes of strong chemicals can cause burns, especially to the respiratory tract.

To prevent exposure to hazardous materials, you must wear gloves and eye protection whenever you are caring for a patient with a chemical burn. Be particularly

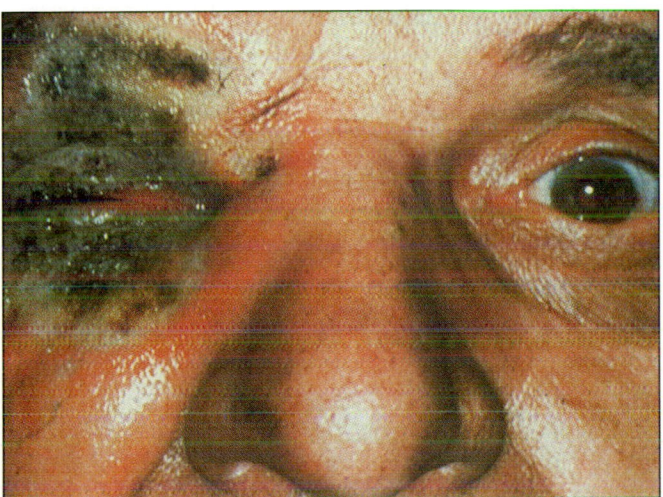

FIGURE 26-23 The eyes are particularly vulnerable to chemical burns.

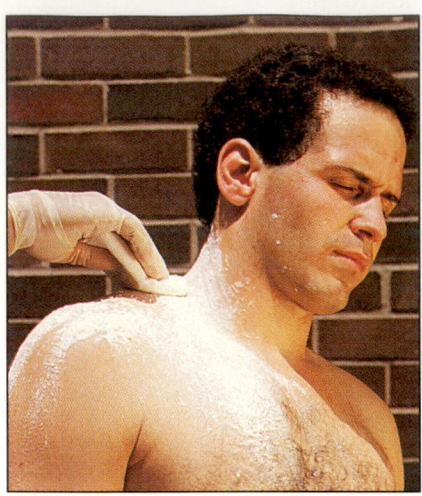

FIGURE 26-24 Brush dry chemicals off the patient before you flush the burned area with water.

careful not to get any chemical, dry or liquid, on yourself or on your uniform.

The emergency care of a chemical burn is basically the same as that for a thermal burn. To stop the burning process, remove any chemical from the patient. A dry chemical that is activated by contact with water may damage the skin more when it is wet than when it is dry. Therefore, always brush dry chemicals off the skin and clothing before flushing the patient with water (Figure 26-24). Remove the patient's clothing, including shoes, stockings, and gloves, because there may be small amounts of chemicals in the creases.

Immediately begin to flush the burned area with large amounts of water (Figure 26-25), taking care not to contaminate uninjured areas. Never direct a forceful stream of water from a hose at the patient; the extreme water pressure may mechanically injure the burned skin. Continue flooding the area with gallons of water for 15 to 20 minutes after the patient says the burning pain has stopped. If an eye has been burned, hold the eyelid open while flooding the eye with a gentle stream of water (Figure 26-26). Continue flushing the contaminated area on the way to the hospital.

> Although a burn may be the patient's most obvious injury, you should always perform a complete assessment to determine whether there are other serious injuries.

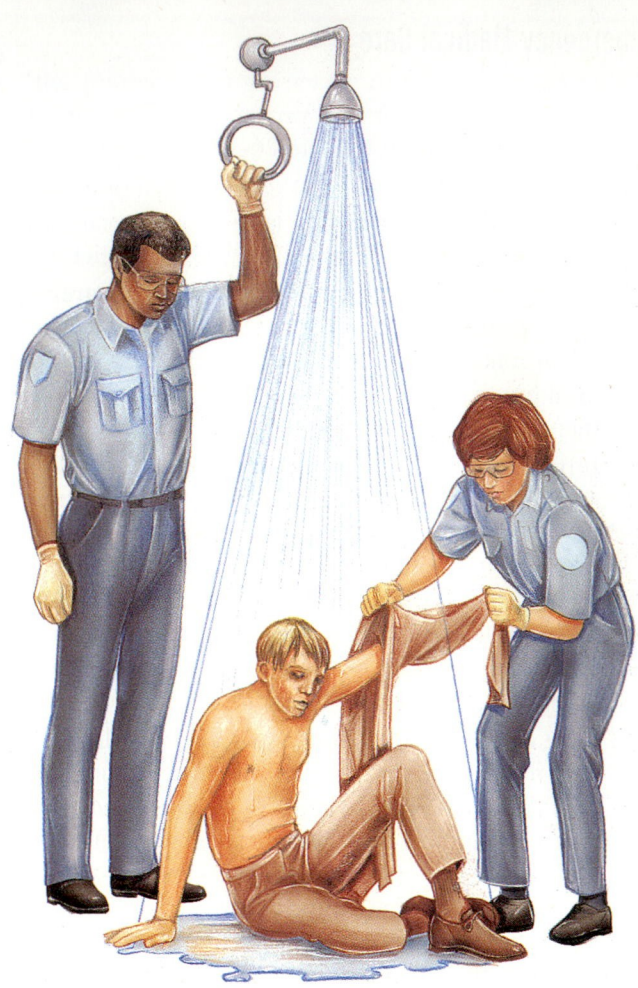

FIGURE 26-25 Flush the burned area with large amounts of water for 15 to 20 minutes after the patient says that the burning pain has stopped. Be careful to avoid contaminating uninjured areas.

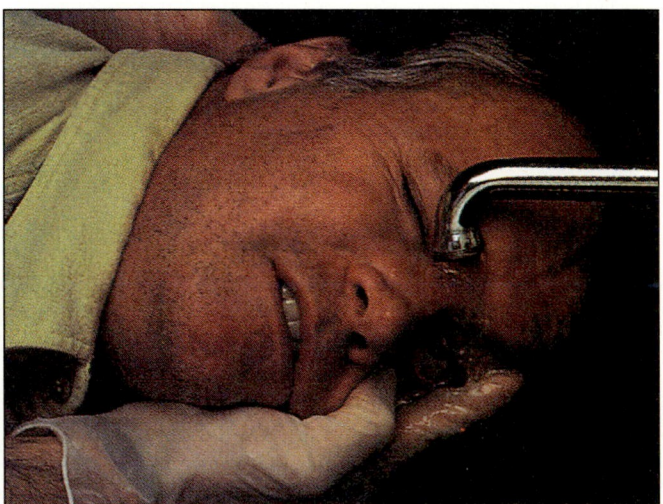

FIGURE 26-26 Flood the affected eye with a gentle stream of water. Hold the eyelids open, a challenging task because the patient's reflex is to keep the eye shut. Take care to prevent any of the chemical from getting into the other eye during flushing.

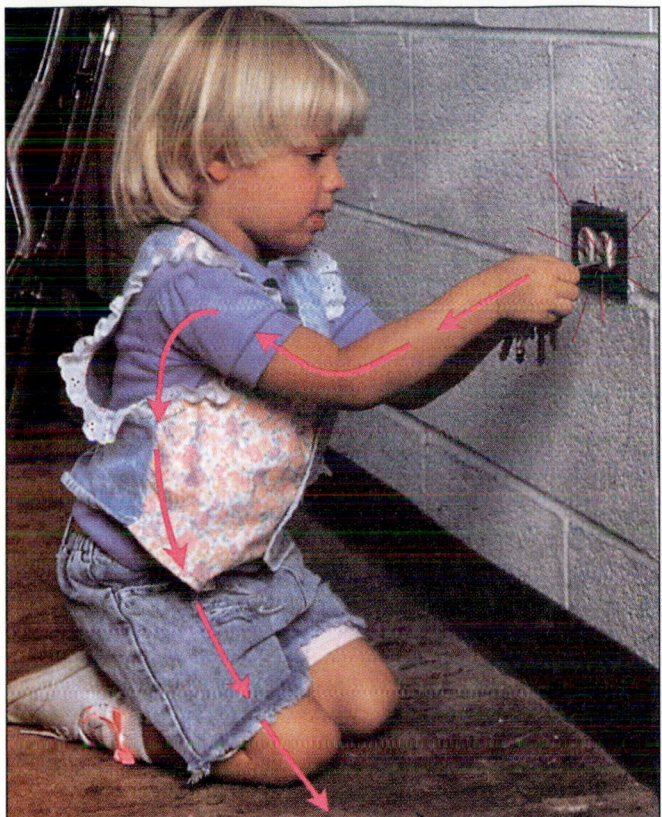

FIGURE 26-27 The human body is a good conductor of electricity. An electrical burn usually occurs when the body, acting as a conductor, completes a circuit.

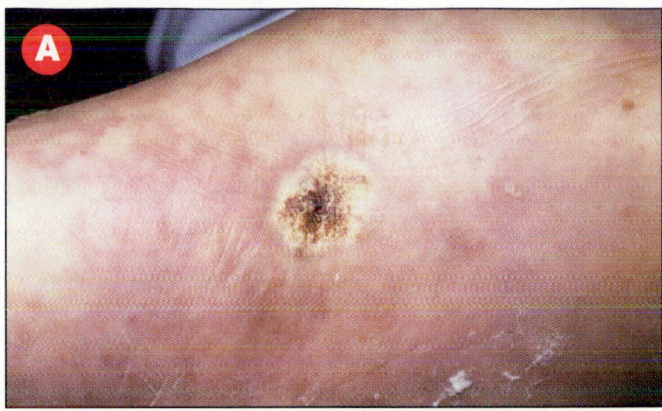

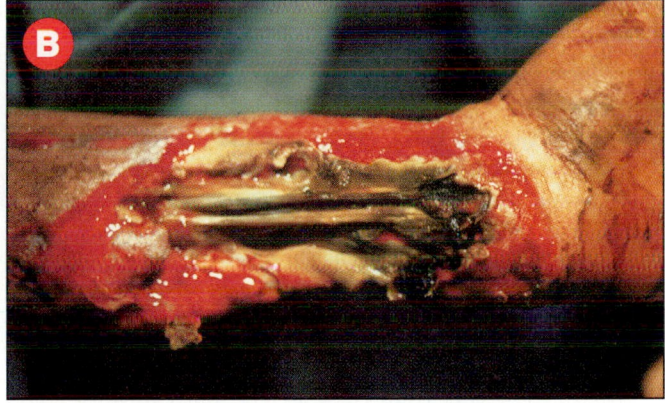

FIGURE 26-28 Electrical burns, like gunshot wounds, have entrance and exit wounds. **A:** An entrance wound is often quite small. **B:** The exit wound can be extensive and deep.

Electrical Burns

Electrical burns may be the result of contact with high- or low-voltage electricity. High-voltage burns may occur when utility workers make direct contact with power lines. However, ordinary household current is powerful enough to cause severe burns.

For electricity to flow, there must be a complete circuit between the electrical source and the ground. Any substance that prevents this circuit from being completed, such as rubber, is called an insulator. Any substance that allows a current to flow through it is called a conductor. The human body, which is primarily water, is a good conductor. Thus, electrical burns occur when the body, or a part of it, completes a circuit connecting a power source to the ground (Figure 26-27).

Your safety is of particular importance when you are called to the scene of an emergency involving electricity. Obviously, you can be fatally injured by coming into contact with power lines. But you can also be fatally injured by touching a patient who is still in contact with a live power line or any other electrical source. For this reason, you must never attempt to remove someone from an electrical source unless you are specially trained to do so. Likewise, you should never move a downed power line unless you have the special training and equipment necessary for the job or unless you are absolutely certain that the line is not live. Before even approaching someone who may still be in contact with a power line or an electrical appliance, make certain that the power is turned off.

There is always a burn injury where the electricity entered the body (an entrance wound) and another where it exited (an exit wound). The entrance wound may be quite small, but the exit wound can be extensive and deep (Figure 26-28). There are two dangers specifically associated with electrical burns. First, there may be

> Your safety is of particular importance when you are called to the scene of an emergency involving electricity.

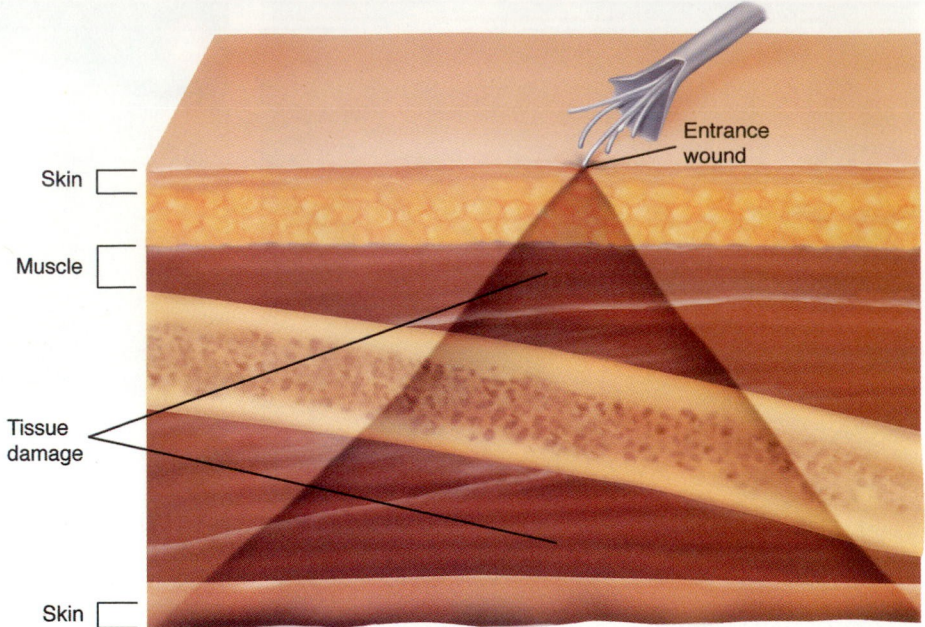

Skin

Muscle

Tissue
damage

Skin

Entrance
wound

FIGURE 26-29 External signs of an electrical burn may be deceiving. The entrance wound may be a small burn, while the damage to deeper tissue may be massive.

a large amount of deep tissue injury. Electrical burns are always more severe than the external signs indicate. The patient may have only a small burn to the skin but have massive damage to the deeper tissues (Figure 26-29). Second, the patient may go into cardiac arrest from the electric shock.

If indicated, begin CPR. Although CPR may need to be quite prolonged in electrical burn cases, it has a high success rate if started promptly. You should also be prepared to defibrillate if necessary. If neither CPR nor defibrillation is indicated, give supplemental oxygen, and monitor the patient closely for respiratory and cardiac arrest. Treat the soft-tissue injuries by placing dry, sterile dressings on all burn wounds and splinting suspected fractures. Provide prompt transport; all electrical burns are potentially severe injuries that require further treatment in the hospital.

Dressing and Bandaging

All wounds require bandaging. In most instances, splints help to control bleeding and provide firm support for the dressing. There are many different types of dressings and bandages (Figure 26-30). You should be familiar with the function and proper application of each.

In general, dressings and bandages have three primary functions:

- To control bleeding
- To protect the wound from further damage
- To prevent further contamination and infection

Sterile Dressings

Universal dressings, conventional 4 x 4″ and 4 x 8″ gauze pads, and assorted small adhesive-type dressings and soft self-adherent roller dressings will cover most wounds.

Measuring 9 x 36″ and made of thick, absorbent material, the universal dressing is ideal for covering large open wounds. It also makes an efficient pad for rigid splints. These dressings are available in compact, commercially sterilized packages. The universal dressing material is also available in 20-yard rolls, which some EMS personnel cut into 3-foot lengths, package, and sterilize themselves.

Gauze pads are appropriate for smaller wounds, and adhesive-type dressings are useful for minor wounds. Occlusive dressings, made of Vaseline gauze, aluminum foil, or plastic, prevent air and liquids from entering (or exiting) the wound. They are used to cover sucking chest wounds and abdominal eviscerations.

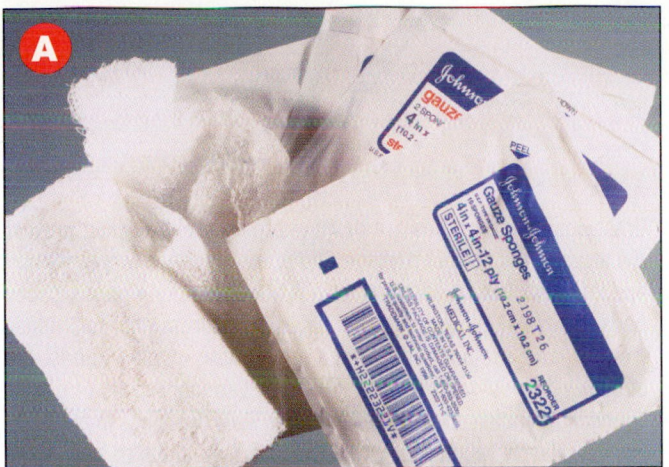

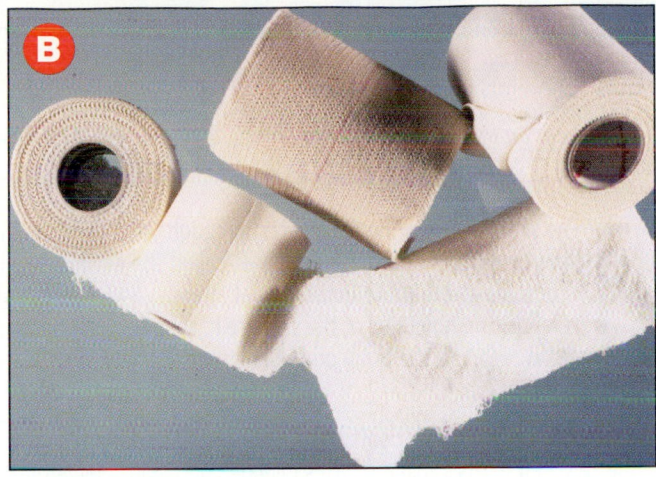

FIGURE 26-30 A: Many types of sterile dressings are used for covering open wounds, including universal dressings, gauze pads, adhesive dressings, and occlusive dressings. **B:** Bandages keep dressings in place and include soft roller bandages, triangular bandages, and adhesive tape. Splints may also be used to hold dressings in place.

Bandages

To keep dressings in place during transport, you can use soft roller bandages, rolls of gauze, triangular bandages, or adhesive tape. The self-adherent, soft roller bandages are probably easiest to use. They are slightly elastic, which makes them easy to apply, and you can tuck the end of the roll into a deeper layer to secure it in place. The layers adhere somewhat but should not be applied too tightly to one another.

Adhesive tape holds small dressings in place and helps to secure larger dressings. Some people, however, are allergic to adhesive tape. If you know that a patient has this problem, use paper or plastic tape instead.

Do not use elastic bandages to secure dressings. If the injury swells, the bandage may become a tourniquet and cause further damage. Any improperly applied bandage that impairs circulation can result in additional tissue damage or even the loss of a limb. For this reason, you should always check a limb distal to a bandage for signs of impaired circulation or loss of sensation. Air splints are useful in stabilizing broken extremities, and they can be used with dressings to help control bleeding from soft-tissue injuries.

Gas Inhalation

Poisonous gas can be just as dangerous as smoke. Fires produce two particularly dangerous gases: carbon monoxide and cyanide. There is a good chance that someone who was trapped in a burning building or room has inhaled carbon monoxide, even if he or she is unaware of it. Do not be misled by the lack of signs, such as coughing or bringing up sputum. This odorless and tasteless gas does not irritate the respiratory tract.

Cyanide gas, which is produced when plastics burn, has a characteristic odor of burnt almonds. Again, the patient may be unaware that he or she has inhaled a toxin, since many people are unfamiliar with this odor.

Both carbon monoxide and cyanide gases are poisons that interfere with the ability of red blood cells to transport oxygen. If you suspect that a patient has inhaled either gas, move him or her out of the burning area as rapidly as possible. Remember to protect yourself by wearing the proper mask system.

Once the patient is in an open area, your priority is to care for ABCD, followed by any burns. You should immediately administer 100% oxygen through a nonrebreathing mask and provide prompt transport to the hospital.

prep kit

ready for review

The skin has two principal layers: the tough outer layer, called the epidermis, and the inner layer, called the dermis, which contains the hair follicles, sweat glands, and sebaceous glands. The functions of the skin are to keep bacteria out and water in, to report to the brain on the environment, and to regulate body temperature.

There are three types of soft-tissue injuries: closed injuries, open injuries, and burns. Closed injuries include contusions, hematomas, and crushing injuries. They can be treated by applying ICES (ice, compression, elevation of the injured part, and splinting). Open injuries produce more extensive bleeding and may become infected. There are four types of open injuries: abrasions, lacerations, avulsions, and penetrating wounds. In treating these injuries, you must first control bleeding. Use a compression dressing, covered by a roller bandage, a second pressure dressing (if necessary), and a splint. Use sterile dressings moistened with sterile saline. Do not try to clean out an open wound.

Dressings and bandages are designed to control bleeding, protect the wound from further damage, and prevent further contamination and infection. Use universal dressings for large open wounds, gauze pads for smaller wounds, adhesive-type dressings for minor wounds, and occlusive dressings for sucking chest wounds and abdominal eviscerations. Use soft roller bandages, rolls of gauze, triangular bandages, or adhesive tape to keep dressings in place. Do not use elastic bandages. Always check a limb distal to a bandage for signs of impaired circulation.

vital vocabulary

www.emtb.com

abrasion Loss or damage of the superficial layer of skin as a result of a body part rubbing or scraping across a rough or hard surface.

avulsion An injury in which soft tissue either is torn completely loose or is hanging as a flap.

burns An injury in which the soft tissue receives more energy than it can absorb without injury. Types of burns include thermal heat, frictional heat, toxic chemical, electrical, and nuclear radiation burns.

closed injury Injury in which damage occurs beneath the skin or mucous membrane but the surface remains intact.

contamination The presence of infective organisms or foreign bodies such as dirt, gravel, or metal.

contusion A bruise without a break in the skin.

dermis The inner layer of the skin containing hair follicles, sweat glands, nerve endings, and blood vessels.

ecchymosis Discoloration associated with a closed wound; signifies bleeding.

epidermis The outer layer of skin that acts as a watertight protective covering.

evisceration The displacement of organs outside the body.

full-thickness burn A burn that affects all skin layers and may affect the subcutaneous layers, muscle, bone, and internal organs, leaving the area dry, leathery, and white, dark brown, or charred; traditionally called a third-degree burn.

hematoma Blood collected within the body's tissues or in a body cavity, occasionally palpable as a discrete mass.

laceration A smooth or jagged open wound.

mucous membrane The lining of body cavities and passages that are in direct contact with the outside environment.

open injury An injury in which there is a break in the surface of the skin or the mucous membrane, exposing deeper tissue to potential contamination.

partial-thickness burn A burn affecting the epidermis and some portion of the dermis but not the subcutaneous tissue, characterized by blisters and skin that is white to red, moist, and mottled; traditionally called a second-degree burn.

penetrating wound An injury resulting from a sharp, pointed object.

Rule of Nines A system that assigns percentages to sections of the body, allowing calculation of the amount of skin surface involved in the burn area.

superficial burn A burn affecting only the epidermis, characterized by skin that is red but not blistered or actually burned through; traditionally called a first-degree burn.

prep kit

26

assessment in action

It's a beautiful summer Saturday at the state park, and a group of teens has been drinking beer all day. When one teen dares another to jump the creek, another teen immediately accepts the challenge. A mighty leap later, he almost makes it to the other side, but he comes up short on the landing. His feet go out from under him, and he crashes down the bank, sideways into a boulder, and rolls off into the remains of a downed tree. The broken end of a branch leaves a 1" hole under his right scapula. The wound is still bubbling with each breath when you arrive.

1. Of the following, which is the **LEAST** important information with regard to the mechanism of injury?
   A. The approximate angle of the creek embankment
   B. A short history of any illnesses that run in his family
   C. The approximate distance the patient fell down the creek bank
   D. What the patient struck during the fall and the type surface he landed on

2. Your first step in caring for this patient is to:
   A. check pulse, sensation, and function in all four extremities.
   B. cover the open chest wound with an occlusive dressing.
   C. ask the patient to identify what he thinks is the biggest problem.
   D. ask the patient if he has a religious preference or the name of next of kin.

3. The severity of the bleeding and the patient's overall condition depends **LEAST** upon the:
   A. rate of the bleeding.
   B. total amount of blood lost.
   C. patient's blood type.
   D. patient's age and weight.

The patient is an obviously intoxicated 18-year-old man who is relatively alert and articulate. He tells you that the reason he stayed motionless by the creek edge was because it "hurt too bad" to move. He has a blood pressure of 134/70 mm Hg, a regular pulse of 126 beats/min, and shallow respirations of 40/min.

4. The patient's upper right arm and shoulder area are both quite swollen and turning dark purple, suggesting:
   A. nerve damage.
   B. systemic infection.
   C. allergic reaction.
   D. internal bleeding.

5. If this patient were to survive his first couple of days, because of the nature of his injuries, he would still be at high risk for:
   A. infection.
   B. infarction.
   C. malnutrition.
   D. hypertension.

points to ponder

Object. 1-1.6, 1-3.6, 5-2.5

You are providing medical support at a local high school football game and are called to the sideline to check out the star quarterback. He had been hurt a few plays ago and had hopped off the field. He is now able to place a little weight on the injured leg but limps badly. The game is against the rival high school and is for the league championship. The coach and player want him to return to the game. The player's parents want you to check him first. His knee has some swelling and is warm to the touch. The player is sure that he can play on it if he wears a knee brace from one of the other players. The coach has a little sports medicine training, and you are the only other medically trained person there.

• Would you allow the player to continue playing if he wants to? Would you help him put on another person's knee brace? Who else may be able to provide assistance with this decision? Do these decisions fall under EMT protocols?

online outlook

Because the soft tissues are exposed to the environment, they are often injured. Test your ability to identify different soft-tissue injuries by completing Exercise 26 at www.emtb.com.

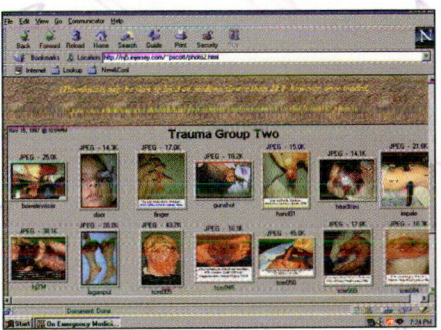

prep kit 26

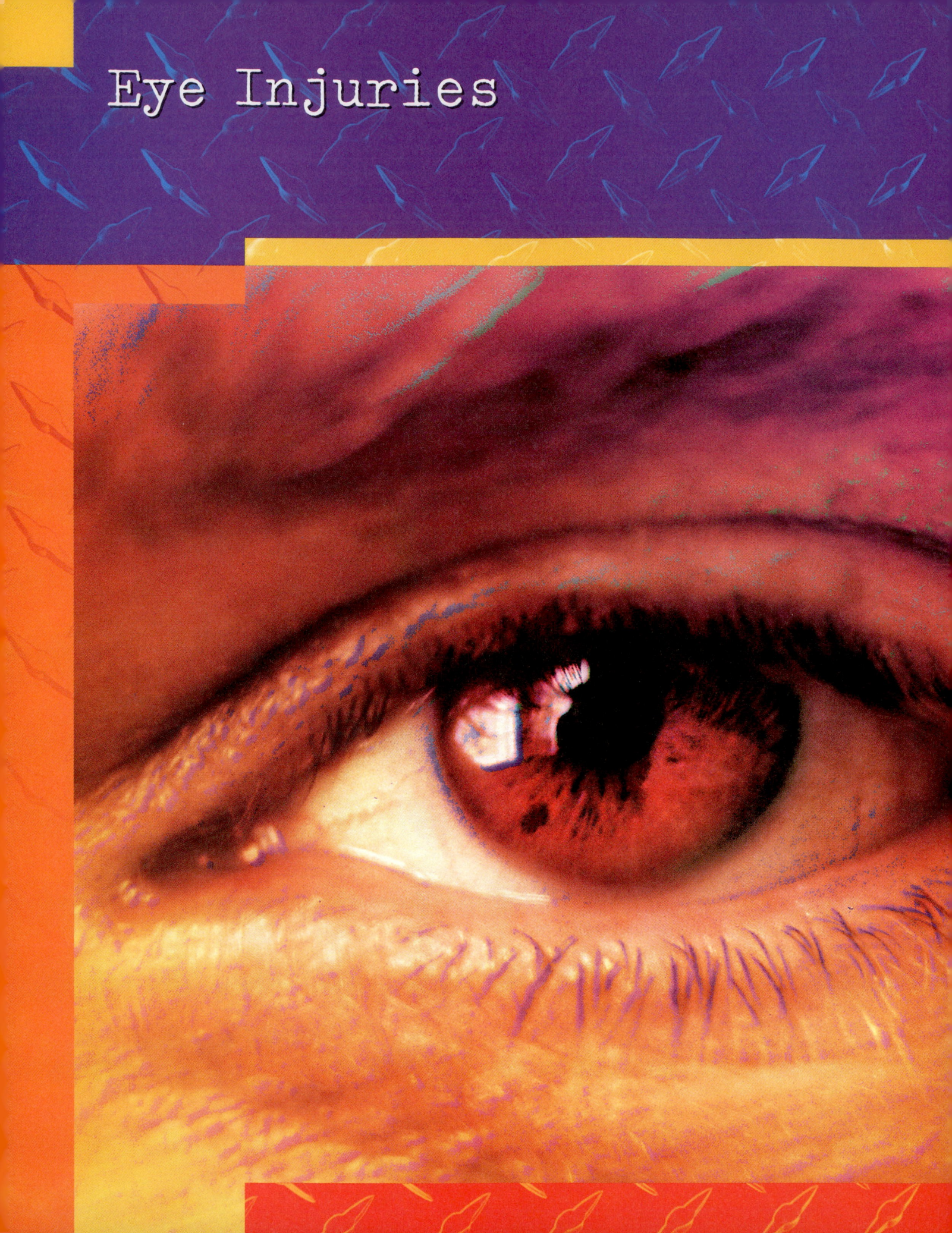

Eye Injuries

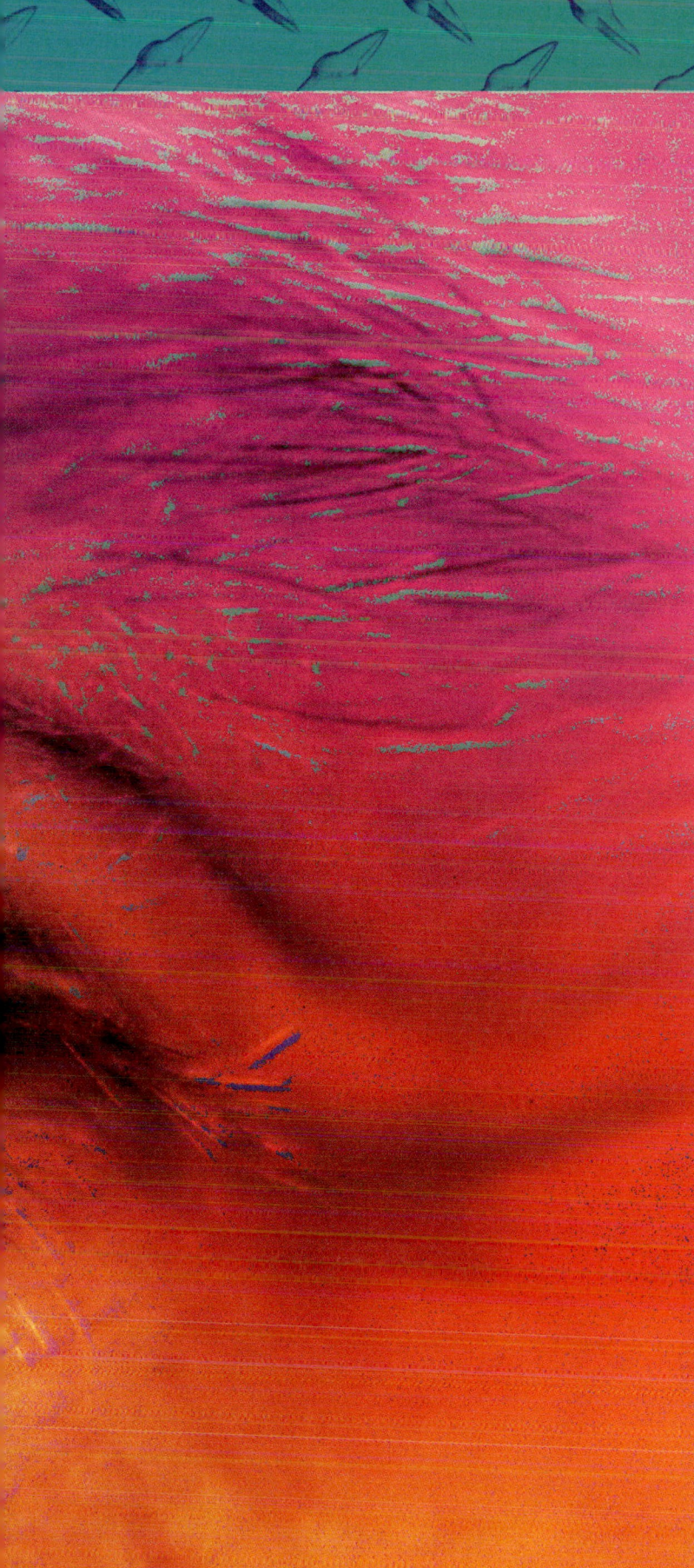

objectives*

Cognitive

1. List the main anatomical features of the eye.

2. Describe the principal functions of the eye.

3. Describe the signs and symptoms of eye injuries.

4. List the steps necessary to assess eye injuries.

5. Describe the steps for managing foreign objects in the eye.

6. Describe the steps for managing puncture wounds to the eye.

7. Describe how to manage burns to the eye.

8. Describe how to remove contact lenses from the eye.

9. Recognize abnormalities of the eyes that may indicate underlying head injury.

10. Recognize and manage a patient with an artificial eye.

Affective

None

Psychomotor

11. Demonstrate the use of irrigation to flush out foreign bodies lying on the surface of the eye.

12. Demonstrate the care of the patient with chemical burns to the eye.

13. Demonstrate the steps in the emergency care of the patient with lacerations of the eyelids.

* These are non-curriculum objectives.

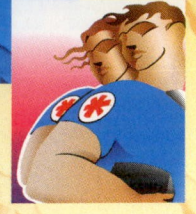

you are the emt

Squad 9, respond to the farmhouse 2 miles east of the intersection of County Road B5 and Highway 6 for an 8-year-old girl who was shot in the eye. Deer hunting season has just begun and, the first call of your shift is for an 8-year-old girl who was shot in the eye with a BB gun by her brother as a prank. You find the girl flat on her back, sobbing uncontrollably, with an obvious hole in her left eye from which fluid is leaking out.

This chapter will provide you with the tools to provide field care to one of the most fragile and least reparable organs: the eye. It will also help you to answer the following questions:

1. Does the treatment of chemical burns to the eye differ from treatment of other burns to the body?
2. Why do patients become anxious whenever someone is either touching or close to touching their eyes?

Eye Injuries

Injuries to the eye are very common, and you will encounter many in your work as an EMT-B. Proper emergency medical care for these injuries can minimize damage, which can often be severe. Fortunately, most eye injuries are relatively minor, such as foreign objects in the eye, corneal abrasions, and contusions. Some injuries are more serious, such as rupture of the globe, which requires immediate expert management. This chapter first reviews the structure and function of the eye and then looks at the different types of eye injuries, describing the emergency management of each. The handling of contact lenses and artificial eyes is also discussed.

Anatomy and Physiology of the Eye

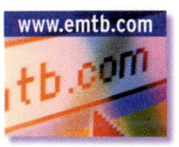

The eye is globe-shaped, approximately 1″ in diameter, and located within a bony socket in the skull called the **orbit** (Figure 27-1). The orbit is composed of the adjacent bones of the face and skull; the orbit forms the base of the floor of the cranial cavity, and directly above it are the frontal lobes of the brain. In the adult, more than 80% of the eyeball is protected within this bony orbit. Between and below the orbits are the nasal bones and the sinuses, respectively. Therefore, any severe injury to the face or head can potentially damage the eyeball or the muscles attached to the eyeball that cause the eye to move.

The eyeball, or **globe**, keeps its global shape as a result of the pressure of the fluid contained within its two chambers. The clear, jellylike fluid near the back of the eye is called the vitreous humor. If the globe is ruptured and this gel leaks out, it cannot be replaced. In front of the lens is a clear fluid called the aqueous humor, named for its watery appearance; in Latin, *aqua* means "water." In penetrating injuries of the eye, aqueous humor can also leak out, but with time and good medical treatment, the body can make more.

The inner surface of the eyelids and the surface of the eye itself, which are covered by a delicate membrane, the conjunctiva, are kept moist by fluid produced by the **lacrimal glands**, often called tear glands (Figure 27-2). Humans blink unconsciously many times per minute. This action sweeps fluid from the lacrimal glands over the surface of the eye, cleaning it. The tears drain on the inner side of the eye through two lacrimal (tear) ducts

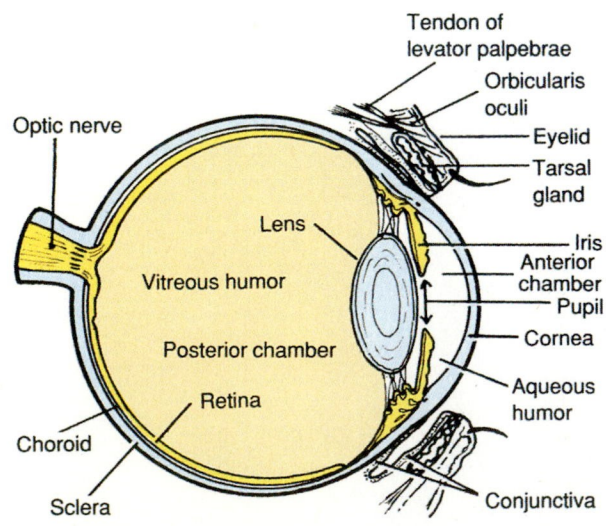

FIGURE 27-1 The major components of the eye.

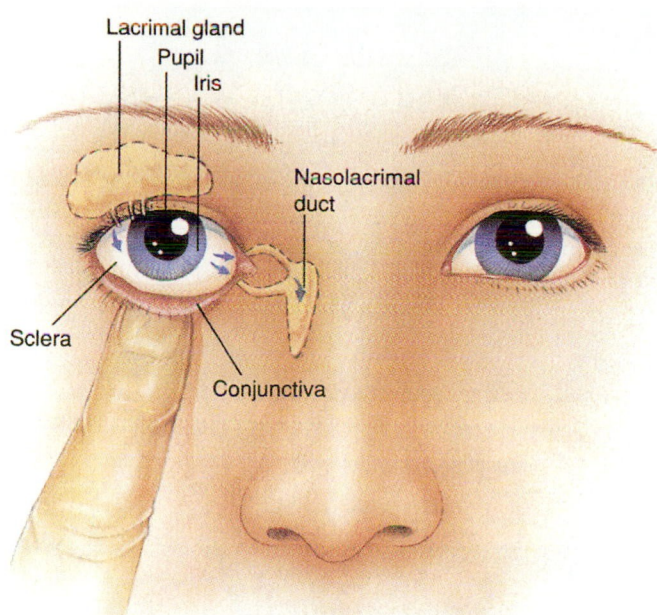

FIGURE 27-2 The lacrimal system consists of tear glands and ducts. Tears act as lubricants and keep the front of the eye from drying out.

into the nasal cavity. This is why, when people cry, they sometimes need to blow their nose.

The white of the eye, called the **sclera**, extends over the surface of the globe. This is extremely tough, fibrous tissue that helps to maintain the eye's globular shape. On the front of the eye, the sclera is replaced by a clear, transparent membrane called the **cornea**, which allows light to enter the eye. A circular muscle lies behind the cornea with an opening in its center. Like the shutter in a camera, this muscle adjusts the size of the opening to regulate the amount of light that enters the eye. This circular muscle and surrounding tissue are called the **iris**. The iris is pigmented, giving the eye its characteristic brown, green, or blue color.

The opening in the center of the iris, which allows light to move to the back of the eye, is called the **pupil**. Normally, the pupil appears black. Like the aperture in a camera, the pupil becomes smaller in bright light and larger in dim light. The pupil also becomes smaller and larger when the person is looking at objects near at hand and farther away; these adjustments occur almost instantaneously. Normally, the pupils in both eyes are equal in size. A difference between them may indicate injury to the eye or to the brain.

Behind the iris is the **lens**. Like the lens of a camera, this lens focuses an image on the light-sensitive area at the back of the globe, called the **retina**. You can think of the retina as the film in the camera. Within the retina are numerous nerve endings, which respond to light by transmitting nerve impulses through the **optic nerve** to the brain. In the brain, the impulses are interpreted as vision.

The retina is nourished by a layer of blood vessels between it and the sclera at the back of the globe. This layer is called the choroid. If, as sometimes happens, the retina detaches from the underlying choroid and sclera, the nerve endings are not nourished, and the patient then experiences blindness. This may be partial blindness, depending on how much of the retina is separated. This condition is called **retinal detachment**.

Common Eye Injuries

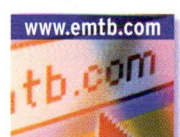

Eye injuries are common, particularly in sports. An eye injury can produce severe complications, including blindness. Proper emergency treatment will minimize pain and may very well help to prevent permanent loss of vision.

Treatment starts with a thorough examination to determine the extent and nature of any damage. Always perform your examination using BSI techniques, taking great care to avoid aggravating the problem. You are looking for specific abnormalities or conditions that may suggest the nature of the problem (Figure 27-3). For example, blunt or penetrating

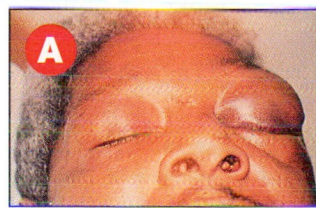
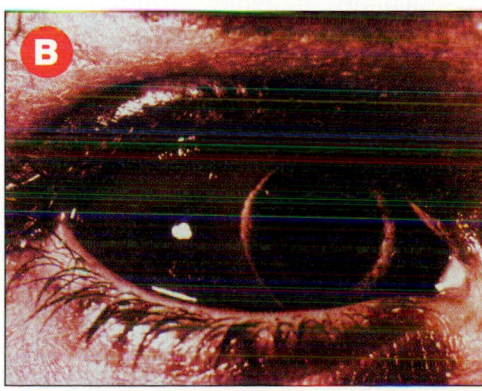
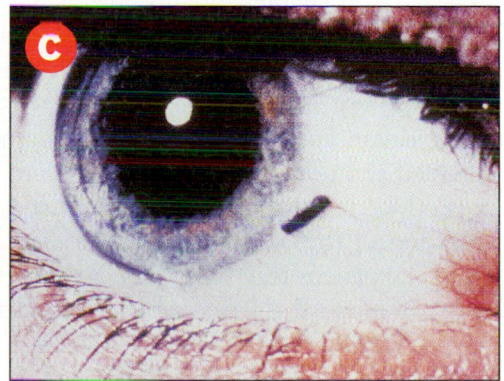

FIGURE 27-3 Injuries to the eyes are easily detected by **A:** swelling, **B:** bleeding, and **C:** the presence of foreign objects in the eye.

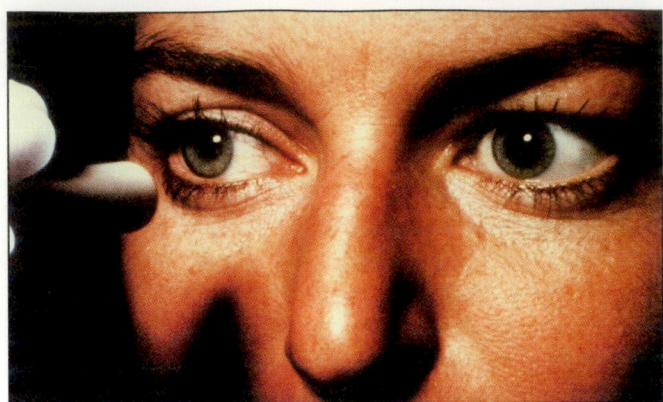

FIGURE 27-4 Normally, the pupils are round, equal in size, and react equally when exposed to light.

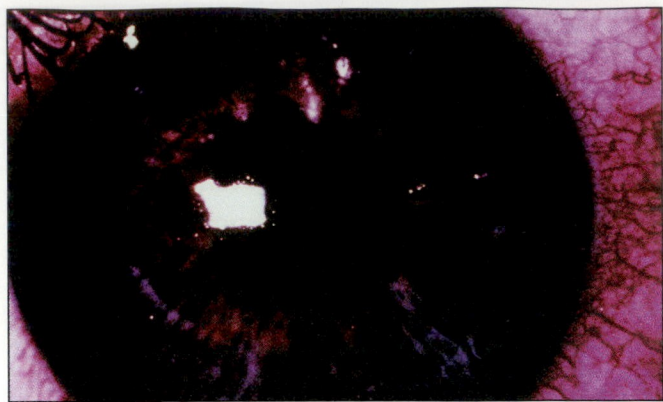

FIGURE 27-5 Conjunctivitis is often associated with the presence of a foreign object in the eye.

injuries can produce swollen or lacerated eyelids. Bleeding soon after irritation or injury can result in a bright red conjunctiva. A damaged cornea quickly loses its smooth, wet appearance.

In a normal, uninjured eye, the entire circle of the iris is visible. The pupils are round, equal in size, and react equally when exposed to light (Figure 27-4). Both eyes move together in the same direction when following your moving finger. After an injury, pupil reaction or shape and eye movement are often disturbed. Any of these conditions should cause you to suspect an injury of the globe or its associated tissues. Remember, though, that abnormal pupil reactions sometimes are a sign of brain injury rather than eye injury.

Certain elements of the patient's history are particularly important. Therefore, as you perform your assessment, always note and record the patient's signs and symptoms, including their severity and duration, the details of how the injury occurred, any reported changes in vision, the use of any eye medications, and any history of eye surgery.

Foreign Objects

Large objects are prevented from penetrating the eye by the protective orbit that surrounds it. However, moderate-sized and smaller foreign objects of many different types can enter the eye and cause significant damage. Even a very small foreign object, such as a grain of sand lying on the surface of the <u>conjunctiva</u>, may produce severe irritation (Figure 27-5). The conjunctiva becomes inflamed and red almost immediately, and the eye begins to produce tears in an attempt to flush out the object. Irritation of the cornea or conjunctiva causes intense pain. The patient may have difficulty keeping the eyelids open, because the irritation is further aggravated by bright light.

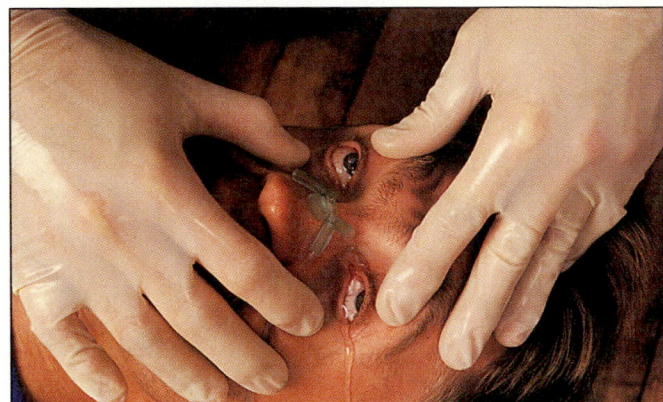

FIGURE 27-6 One method of irrigation is to direct saline into the injured eye using a round nasal airway or cannula. Always flush from the nose side of the eye toward the outside to avoid flushing material into the other eye.

If a small foreign object is lying on the surface of the patient's eye, you should use a normal saline solution to gently irrigate the eye. Irrigation with 500 to 1,000 mL of sterile saline solution will frequently flush away loose, small particles. If a small bulb syringe is at hand, you can use this, or else a round nasal airway or cannula, to direct the saline into the affected eye (Figure 27-6). Always flush from the nose side of the eye toward the outside to avoid flushing material into the other eye. After it is flushed away, a foreign body will often leave a small abrasion on the surface of the conjunctiva. For this reason, the patient will complain of irritation even when the particle itself is gone.

Gentle irrigation usually will not wash out foreign bodies that are stuck to the cornea or lying under the upper eyelid. To examine the undersurface of the upper eyelid, pull the lid upward and forward. If you spot a foreign object, you may be able to remove it with a moist, sterile, cotton-tipped applicator (Figure 27-7).

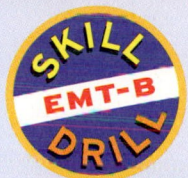

Removing a Foreign Object from Under the Upper Eyelid

Figure 27-7

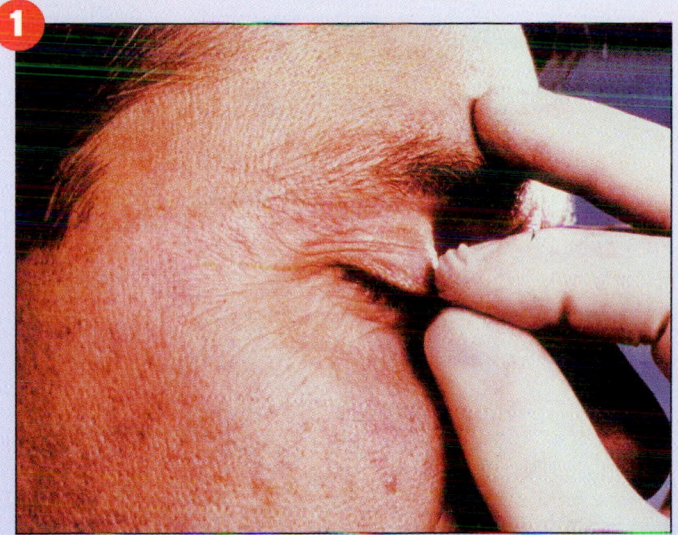

1 Tell the patient to look down while you grasp the lashes of the upper eyelid with your thumb and index finger. Gently pull the eyelid away from the eyeball.

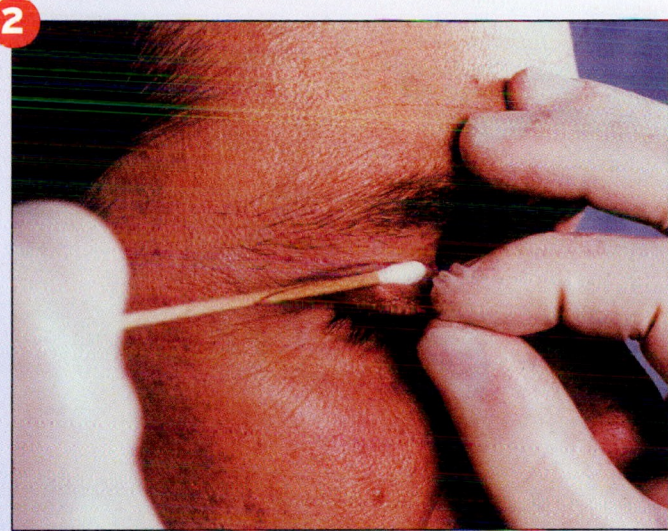

2 Gently place a cotton-tipped applicator horizontally along the center of the outer surface of the upper eyelid.

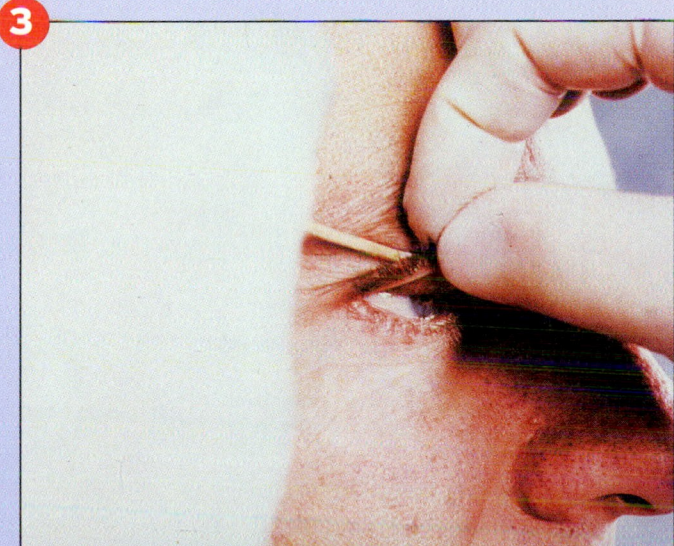

3 Pull the eyelid forward and up, which causes it to roll or fold back over the applicator, exposing the undersurface of the eyelid.

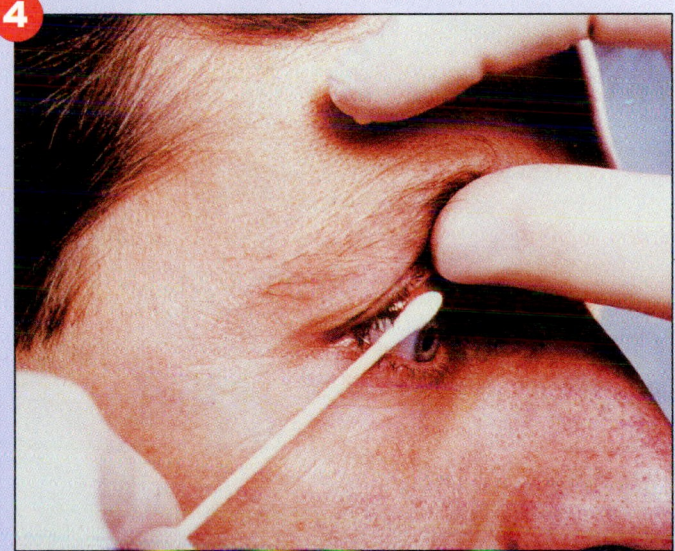

4 If you see a foreign object, gently remove it with a moistened, sterile, cotton-tipped applicator.

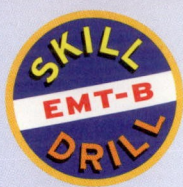

Stabilizing a Foreign Object Impaled in the Eye
Figure 27-9

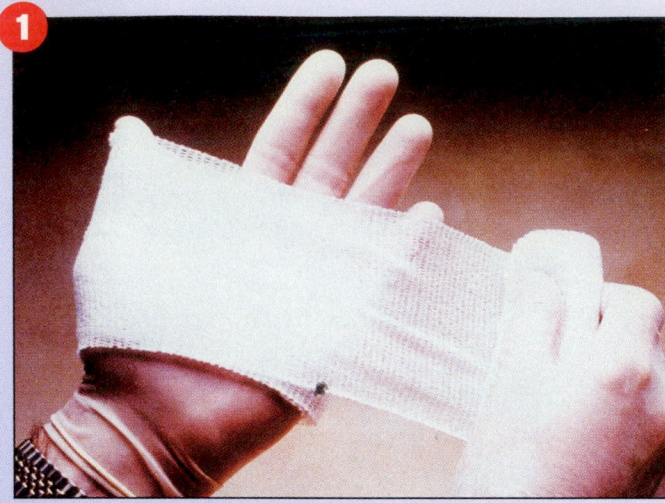

To prepare a doughnut ring, wrap a 2" roll around your fingers and thumb seven or eight times. Adjust the diameter by spreading your fingers.

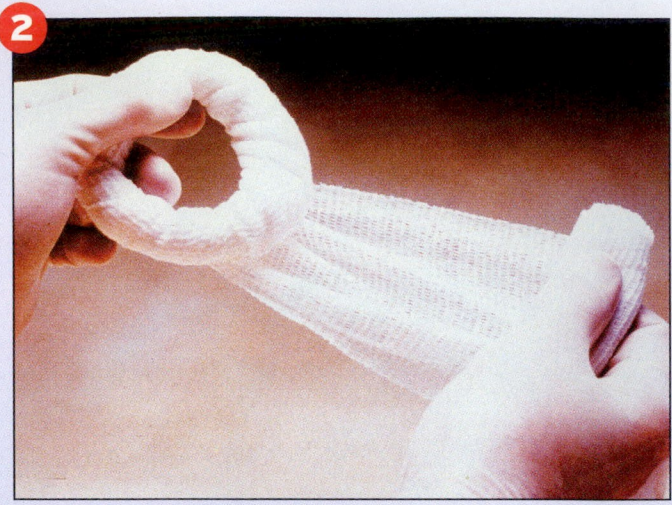

Wrap the remainder of the roll, . . .

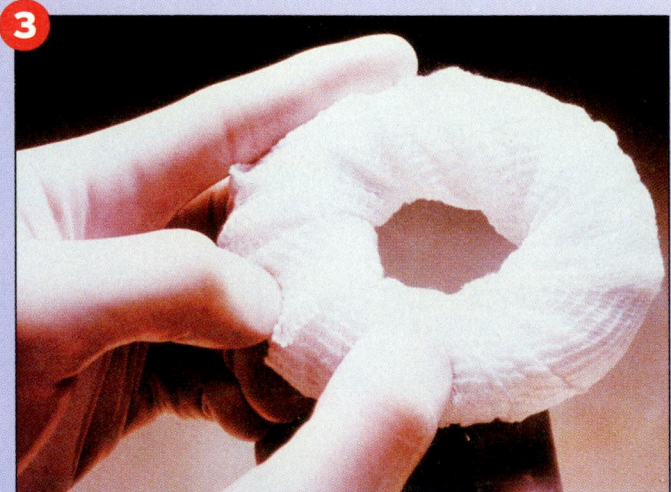

. . . working around the ring.

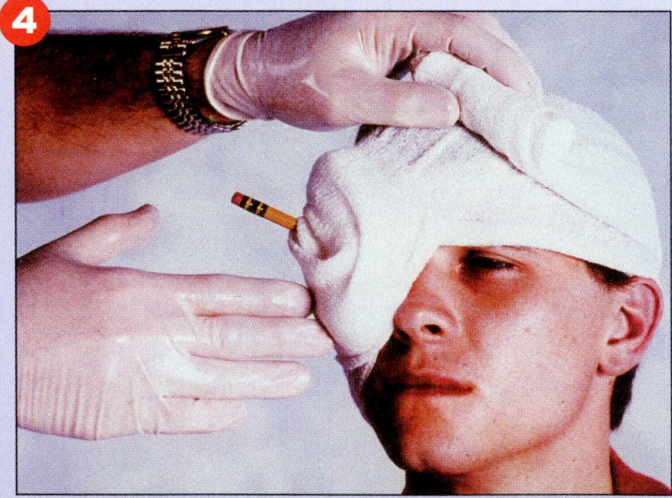

Place the dressing over the eye to hold the impaled object in place, then secure it with a gauze dressing.

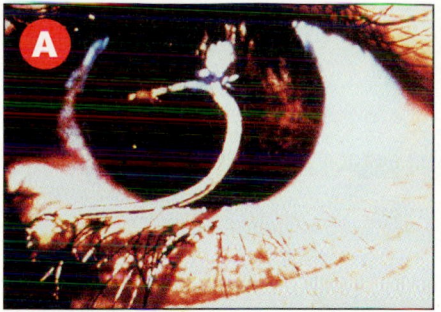 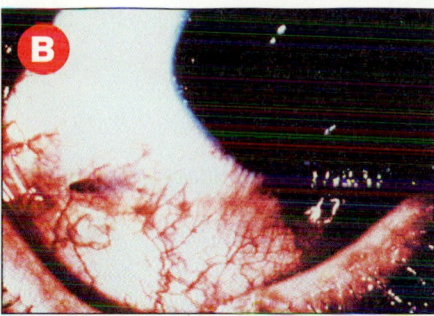 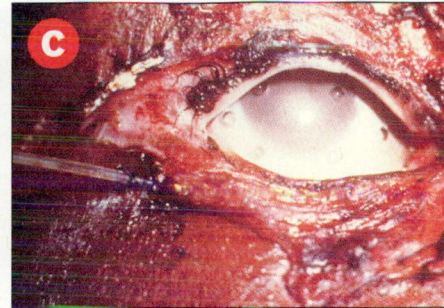

FIGURE 27-8 Any number of objects can become impaled in the eye. **A:** Fishhook. **B:** Sharp, metal sliver. **C:** Knife blade.

Never attempt to remove a foreign body that is stuck to the cornea.

Foreign bodies ranging in size from a pencil to a sliver of metal may be impaled in the eye (Figure 27-8). These objects must be removed by a physician. Your care involves stabilizing the object and preparing the patient for transport to definitive care (Figure 27-9). Bandage the object in place to support it. Cover the eye itself with a moist, sterile dressing, and then surround the object with a collar made from roller gauze or a small gauze pack. You can then stabilize the object and the gauze collar with a roller bandage surrounding the head. The greater the length of foreign object you can see sticking out of the eye, the more important stabilization becomes in avoiding further damage.

Sometimes, foreign bodies, particularly small metal fragments, become completely embedded within the eye itself. The patient may not even be aware of the cause of the problem. Suspect such an injury when the history includes metal work (e.g., hammering, exposure to splinters, vigorous filing) and when there are other signs of ocular injury. This type of injury must be handled by an ophthalmologist on an urgent basis. It may require X-rays and special equipment to find the foreign body.

Burns of the Eye

Chemicals, heat, and light rays all can burn the delicate tissues of the eye, often causing permanent damage. Your role is to stop the burn and prevent further damage.

Chemical burns. Chemical burns, usually caused by acid or alkaline solutions, require immediate emergency care (Figure 27-10). This consists of flushing the eye with water or a sterile saline irrigation solution. If sterile saline is not available, you can use any clean water.

The idea is to direct the greatest amount of solution or water into the eye as gently as possible (Figure 27-11). Because opening the eye spontaneously may cause the patient pain, you may have to force the lids open to

irrigate the eye adequately. Ideally, you will use a bulb or irrigation syringe, a nasal cannula, or some other device that will allow you to control the flow. In some circumstances, you may have to resort to pouring water into the eye by holding the patient's head under a gently running faucet. You can even have the patient immerse his or her face in a large pan or basin of water and rapidly

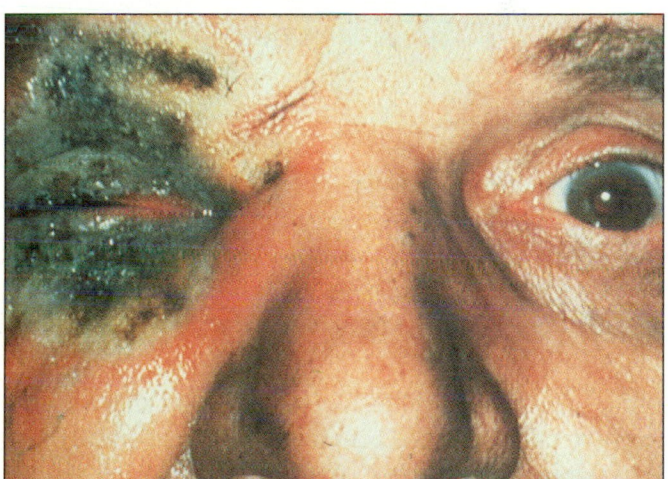

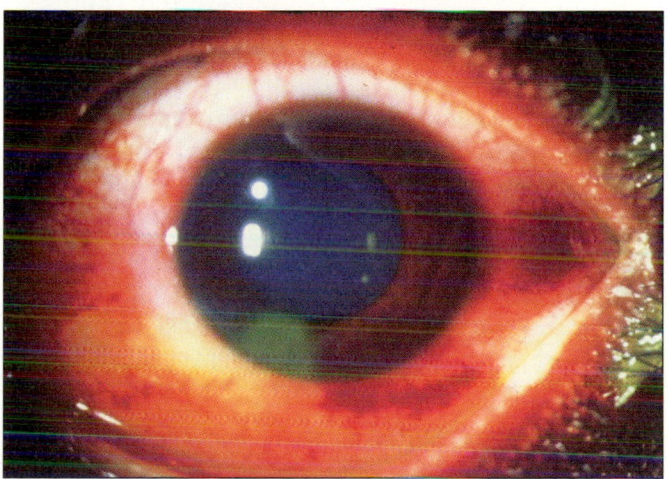

FIGURE 27-10 A: Chemical burns typically occur when an acid or alkali is splashed into the eye. **B:** This figure shows a chemical burn from lye, an alkaline solution. Because lye can continue to damage the eye even when diluted, fast action is needed.

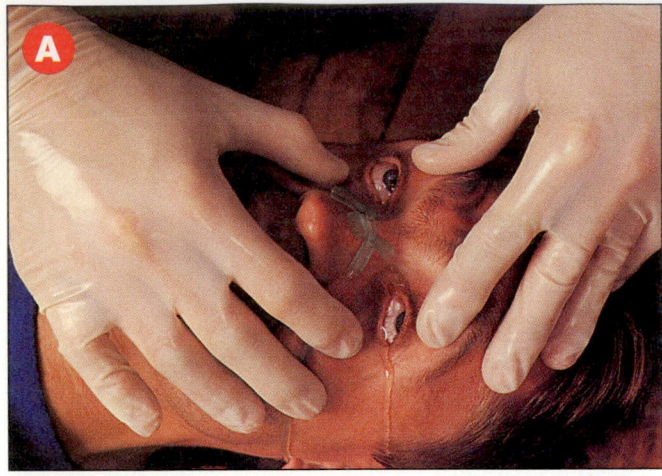
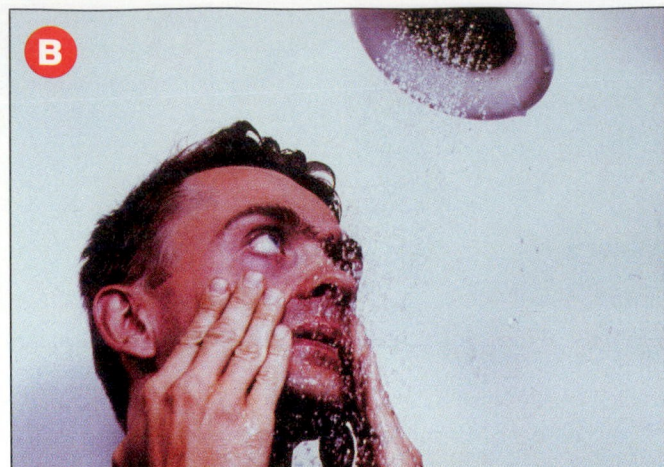
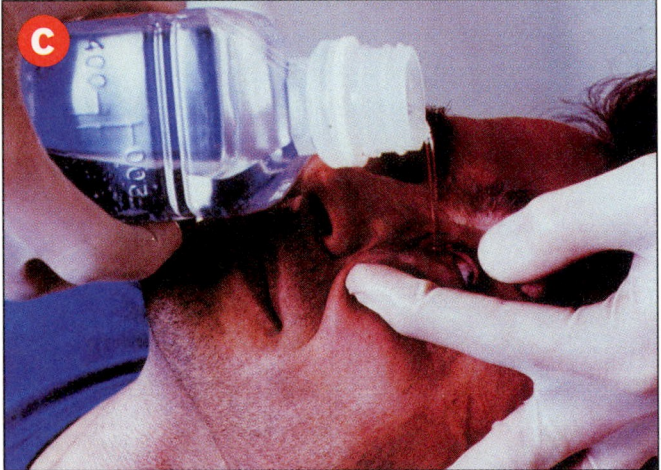
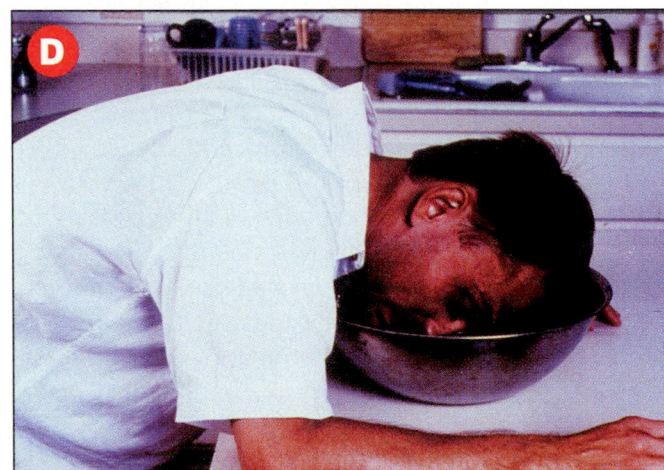

FIGURE 27-11 The following are four ways to effectively irrigate the eye. **A:** Nasal cannula. **B:** Shower. **C:** Bottle. **D:** Basin. Remember, you must protect the uninjured eye from the irrigating solution.

blink the affected eyelid. If only one eye is affected, care must be taken to avoid contaminated water from getting into the unaffected eye.

Irrigate the eye for at least 5 minutes. If the burn was caused by an alkali or a strong acid, you should irrigate the eye for 20 minutes. Strong acids and all alkaline solutions can penetrate deeply, requiring a prolonged flush. Again, always take care to protect the uninjured eye and prevent irrigation fluid from running into it.

After you have completed irrigation, apply a clean, dry dressing to cover the eye, and transport the patient promptly to the hospital for further care (Figure 27-12). If the irrigation can be carried out satisfactorily in the ambulance, it should be done during transport to save time.

Thermal burns. When a patient is burned in the face during a fire, the eyes usually close rapidly because of the heat. This reaction is a natural reflex to protect the eye from further injury. However, the eyelids remain exposed and are frequently burned (Figure 27-13). Burns of the

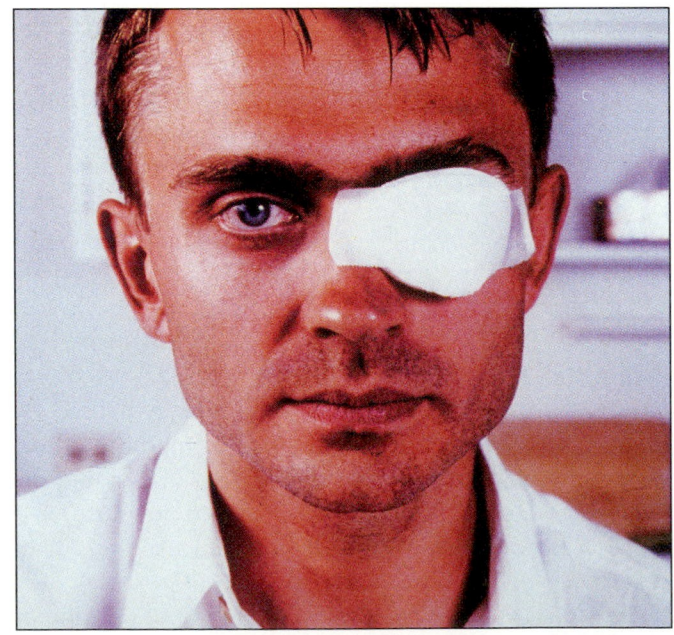

FIGURE 27-12 Apply a clean, dry dressing to cover the eye after you have finished irrigation.

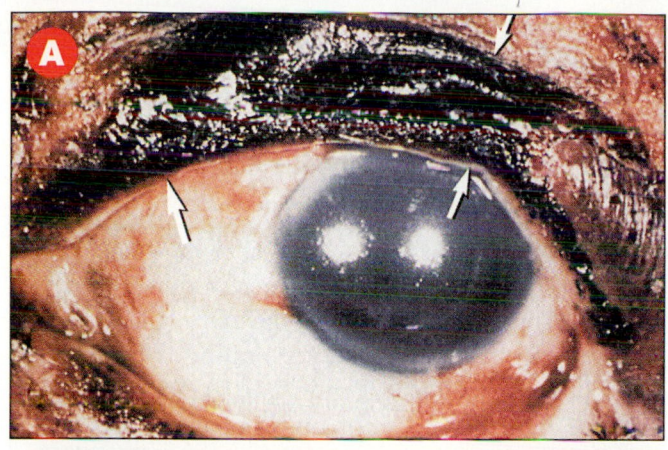

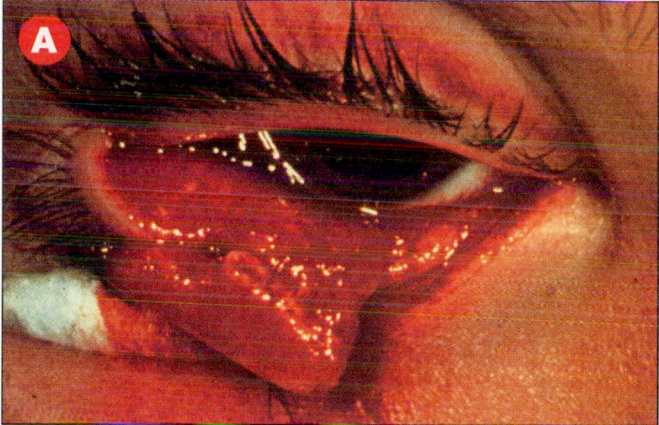

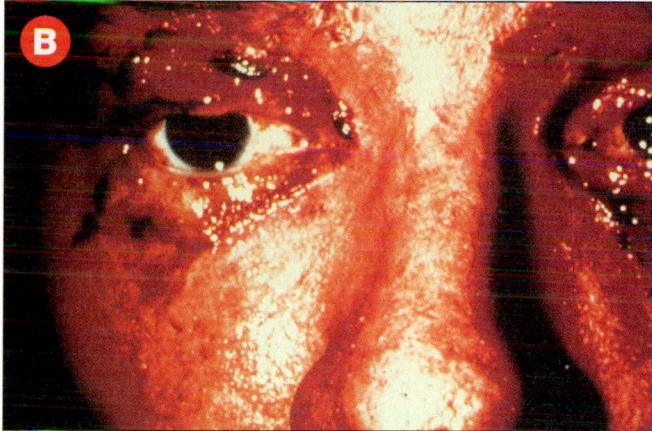

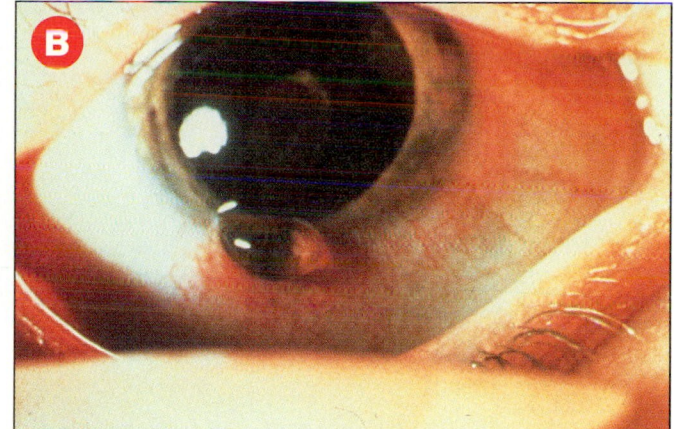

FIGURE 27-13 Thermal burns occasionally cause significant damage to the eyelids. **A:** Arrows show some full-thickness burns. **B:** Burns of the eyelids require immediate hospital care.

FIGURE 27-14 Lacerations are serious injuries that require prompt transport. **A:** While bleeding can be heavy, never exert pressure on the eye. **B:** Pressure may squeeze the vitreous humor, iris, lens, or even the retina out of the eye.

eyelids require very specialized care. It is best to provide prompt transport for these patients without further examination. First, however, you should cover both eyes with a sterile dressing moistened with sterile saline. You may apply eye shields over the dressing.

Light burns. Infrared rays, eclipse light (if the patient has looked directly at the sun), and laser burns all can cause significant damage to the sensory cells of the eye when rays of light become focused on the retina. Retinal injuries that are caused by exposure to extremes of light are generally not painful but may result in permanent damage to vision.

Superficial burns of the eye can result from ultraviolet rays from an arc welding unit, light from prolonged exposure to a sunlamp, or reflected light from a bright snow-covered area (snow blindness). This kind of burn often is not painful at first but may become so 3 to 5 hours later, as the damaged cornea responds to the injury. The patient usually develops a severe <u>conjunctivitis</u>, or inflammation of the conjunctiva, with redness, swelling, and excessive tear production. You can ease the pain from these corneal burns by covering each eye with a sterile, moist pad and an eye shield. Have the patient lie down during transport to the hospital, and protect him or her from further exposure to bright light. This patient should be examined by a physician as soon as possible.

Lacerations

Lacerations of the eyelids require very careful repair to restore both appearance and function (Figure 27-14). Bleeding may be heavy, but it usually can be controlled by gentle, manual pressure. If there is a laceration of the globe itself, apply no pressure to the eye; compression can interfere with the blood supply to the back of the eye and result in loss of vision from damage to the retina. Furthermore, pressure may squeeze the vitreous humor, iris, lens, or even the retina out of the eye and cause irreparable damage or blindness.

Follow these three important guidelines in treating penetrating injuries of the eye:

1. **Never exert pressure** on or manipulate the injured eye (globe) in any way.
2. **If part of the eyeball is exposed,** gently apply a moist, sterile dressing to prevent drying.
3. **Cover the injured eye** with a protective metal eye shield.

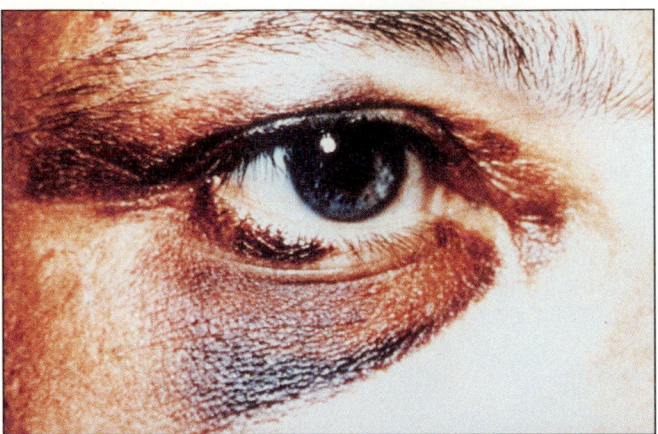

FIGURE 27-15 The typical "black eye" is caused by bleeding into the tissue around the orbit.

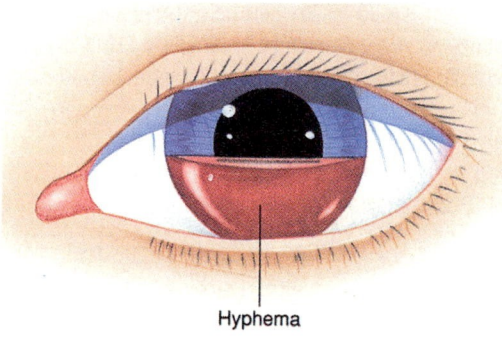

Hyphema

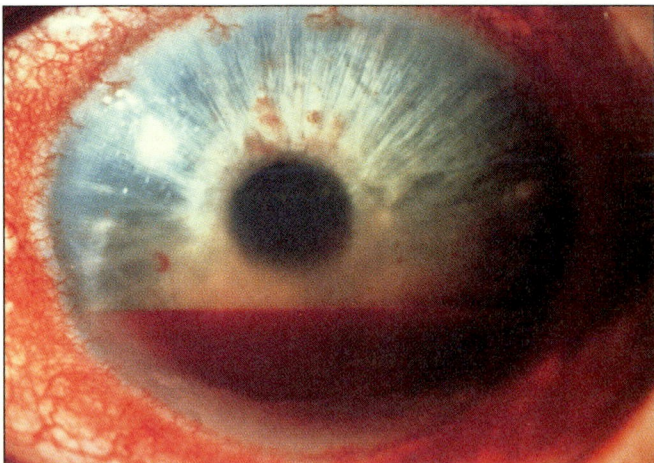

FIGURE 27-16 A hyphema, characterized by bleeding into the anterior chamber of the eye, is common following blunt trauma to the eye. This condition may seriously impair vision.

On rare occasions following a serious injury, the eyeball may be displaced out of its socket. Do *not* attempt to reposition it. Simply cover the eye, and stabilize it with a moist, sterile dressing. Have the patient lie in a supine position while en route to the hospital.

Blunt Trauma

Blunt trauma can cause a number of serious injuries of the eye. These range from the ordinary "black eye," a result of bleeding into the tissue around the orbit, to a severely damaged globe (Figure 27-15). You may see an injury called <u>hyphema</u>, or bleeding into the anterior chamber of the eye, that obscures part or all of the iris (Figure 27-16). This injury is common in blunt trauma and may seriously impair vision. It may also be a sign of a more serious injury to the globe.

Blunt trauma can also cause a fracture of the orbit, particularly of the bones that form its floor and support the globe. This injury is called a <u>blowout fracture</u> (Figure 27-17). The fragments of fractured bone can entrap some of the muscles that control eye movement, causing double vision. Any patient who reports pain, double vision, or decreased vision following a blunt injury about the eye should be placed on a stretcher and transported promptly to the emergency department. Protect the eye from further injury with a metal shield; cover the other eye to minimize movement on the injured side.

Another possible result of blunt eye injury is retinal detachment. This injury is often seen in sports, especially boxing. It is painless but produces flashing lights, specks, or "floaters" in the field of vision and a cloud or shade over the patient's vision. Because the retina is separated from the nourishing choroid, this injury requires prompt medical attention to preserve vision in that eye.

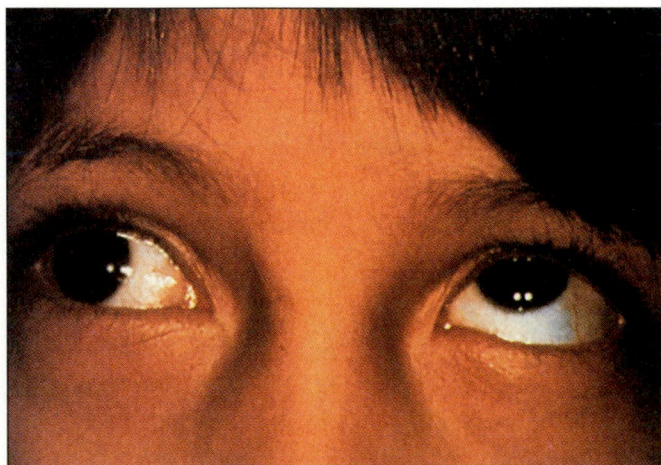

FIGURE 27-17 A patient with a blowout fracture will not move his or her eyes together because of muscle entrapment. The patient therefore sees double images of any object.

Eye Injuries Following Head Injury

Abnormalities in the appearance or function of the eyes often occur following a closed head injury. Any of the following eye findings should alert you to the possibility of a head injury:

- One pupil larger than the other (Figure 27-18)
- The eyes not moving together or pointing in different directions
- Failure of the eyes to follow the movement of your finger as instructed
- Bleeding under the conjunctiva, which obscures the sclera (white portion) of the eye
- Protrusion or bulging of one eye

Record any of these observations, along with the time that you make them. For an unconscious patient, remember to keep the eyelids closed; drying of the ocular tissue can cause permanent injury and may result in blindness. Cover the lids with moist gauze, or hold them closed with clear tape. Normal tears will then keep the tissues moist.

Contact Lenses and Artificial Eyes

Small, hard contact lenses usually are tinted, making them relatively easy to see. Large, soft ones are clear and can be very difficult to see. In general, you should not attempt to remove either kind of lens from a patient. You should *never* attempt to remove a lens from an eye that has been—or may have been—injured, since manipulating the lens can aggravate the problem. The only time that contact lenses should be removed immediately in the field is in the case of a chemical burn of the eye. In this situation, the lens can trap the chemical and make irrigation difficult.

If it is necessary to remove a hard contact lens, use a small suction cup, moistening the end with saline (Figure 27-19). To remove soft lenses, place one to two drops of saline onto the lens, gently pinch it between your thumb and index finger, and lift it off the surface of the eye.

Always advise emergency department staff if a patient is wearing contact lenses so that the patient can be properly cared for at the hospital.

Occasionally, you may find yourself caring for a patient who is wearing an eye prosthesis, an artificial eye. Many people are surprised to find that it can be difficult to distinguish a prosthesis from a natural eye. You should suspect an eye of being artificial when it does not respond to light, move in concert with the opposite eye, or appear quite the same as its mate. If you think that a patient may have an artificial eye but you are not sure, go ahead and ask about it. Although no harm will be done if you care for an artificial eye as you would a normal one, you need to be totally clear about the patient's eye function.

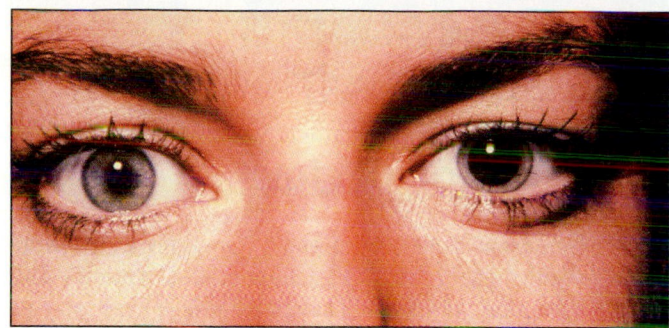

FIGURE 27-18 Variation of pupil size may indicate a head injury.

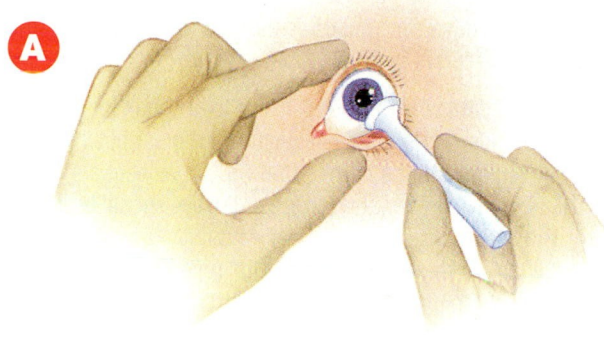

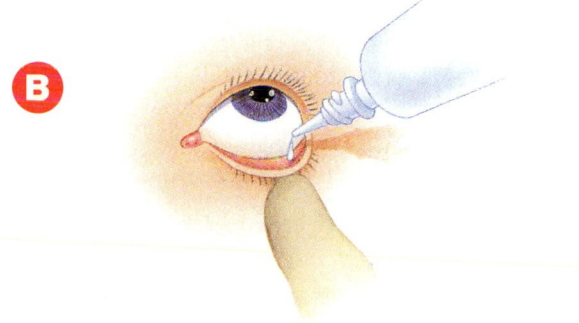

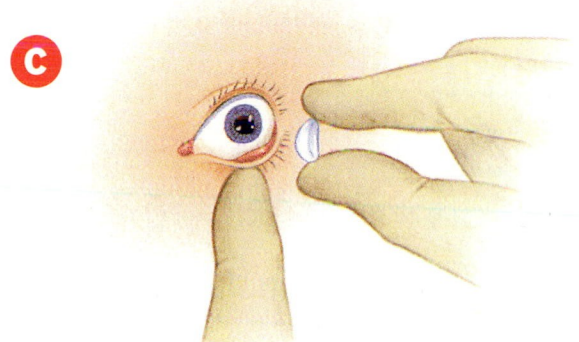

FIGURE 27-19 Removing contact lenses should be limited to patients with burn injuries. **A:** To remove hard contact lenses, use a specialized suction cup moistened with sterile saline solution. **B:** To remove soft contact lenses, instill one or two drops of saline or irrigating solution. **C:** Next, pinch off the lens with your thumb and index finger.

prep kit

ready for review

The eye is globe-shaped, about 1" in diameter, and located within a bony socket called the orbit which is actually part of the skull. Any severe injury to the face or head can potentially damage the eyeball or eye muscles. The fluid in the back of the eye is called the vitreous humor and cannot be replaced; the fluid in the front of the eye is called the aqueous humor and can be replaced. The eye works like a camera, with the iris and pupil making adjustments to light and the retina acting like film. Nerve endings in the retina send impulses through the optic nerve to the brain, which interprets them as vision.

In assessing a patient with a possible eye injury, look for swollen or lacerated eyelids, a bright red conjunctiva, irregular pupil reactions or eye movements, and a cornea that no longer appears wet and smooth. Foreign bodies on the surface of the eye should be irrigated gently with a normal saline solution; always flush from the nose side of the eye toward the outside. If a foreign body is on the undersurface of the lid, remove it with a moist, cotton-tipped applicator. Do not remove foreign bodies that are stuck to the cornea. If a foreign body is impaled in the eye, bandage the object in place, using roller gauze to create a collar around it, until it can be removed by a physician. Small metal fragments that are entirely embedded within the eye must be treated by an ophthalmologist.

Chemicals, heat, and light rays can all burn the eyes, causing permanent damage. Irrigate chemical burns with saline solution or clean water for at least 5 minutes, then apply a clean, dry dressing to the eye and transport the patient promptly. Transport the patient with heat burns of the eyelid immediately, covering both eyes with a sterile, moist dressing. Superficial burns of the eye resulting from exposure to ultraviolet rays or a sunlamp can become very painful after several hours. You can ease the pain from these corneal burns by covering the eyes with a sterile, moist pad and eye shield; the patient should lie down during transport.

Use gentle manual pressure to control bleeding from a lacerated eyelid, but do not apply pressure to a laceration of the globe itself. Instead, apply a moist, sterile dressing to prevent drying, cover the injured eye with a protective metal shield, cover the opposite eye, and transport the patient. Never attempt to reposition a displaced eyeball. Blunt trauma can cause a range of injuries, including hyphema, retinal detachment, and blowout fractures. Any patient who complains of pain, double vision, or decreased vision following a blunt injury about the eye should be placed on a stretcher and transported promptly to the emergency department.

Suspect a head injury if the patient has one pupil larger than the other, eyes not moving together, bleeding under the conjunctiva, or protrusion or bulging of one eye. Keep the eyelids closed if the patient is unconscious so that the eyes do not dry out.

Never remove contact lenses from an injured eye unless the injury is a chemical burn.

vital vocabulary

www.emtb.com

blowout fracture Fracture of the orbit or of the bones that support the floor of the orbit.

conjunctiva The delicate membrane that lines the eyelids and covers the exposed surface of the eye.

conjunctivitis Inflammation of the conjunctiva.

cornea The transparent tissue layer in front of the pupil and iris of the eye.

globe The eyeball.

hyphema Bleeding into the anterior chamber of the eye, obscuring the iris.

iris The muscle and surrounding tissue behind the cornea that dilate and constrict the pupil, regulating the amount of light that enters the eye.

lacrimal glands The glands that produce fluids to keep the eye moist; also called tear glands.

lens The transparent part of the eye through which images are focused on the retina.

optic nerve A cranial nerve that transmits visual sensations to the brain.

orbit The eye socket.

pupil The circular opening in the middle of the iris of the eye.

retina The light-sensitive area of the eye where images are projected; a layer of cells at the back of the eye that changes the light image into electrical impulses, which are carried by the optic nerve to the brain.

retinal detachment A condition in which the retina is separated from its attachments at the back of the eye.

sclera The white portion of the eye; the tough outer coat of the eye that gives protection to the delicate, light-sensitive inner layer.

prep kit 27

assessment in action

You are called to respond to a private residence for a "child who had fireworks blow up in his face." You arrive to find an alert, oriented, screaming 7-year-old boy who, according to his parents, was playing with a cherry bomb when it exploded in his face. The parents state that the child did not lose consciousness. Assessment reveals superficial and partial-thickness burns on his face, tongue, and hand. A section of his hair is singed, as are both eyebrows. He also has smoke and powder residue on the face and swelling in both eyelids.

As you progress through your assessment, you cannot convince the patient to open his eyes because "they hurt too much." However, he reports that he was able to see following the explosion. He has a blood pressure of 118/66 mm Hg, a pulse of 140 beats/min, and respirations of 28/min.

1. Intervention for the burned eyes should consist of:
   A. patching both eyes and transporting the patient in a head-down position.
   B. applying direct pressure with dry, sterile dressings for 3 to 5 minutes.
   C. irrigating both eyes for 2 to 3 minutes and leaving them uncovered.
   D. irrigating both eyes for 15 to 20 minutes, and then patching both eyes.

2. If vision testing was indicated, the most acceptable field test would consist of having the patient read:
   A. a newspaper held at arms length.
   B. road signs that are at least $1/4$ mile away.
   C. the number of fingers held up by the EMT-B.
   D. letters from a portable, office-quality eye chart.

3. Had this patient had an object impaled in his eye as a result of the explosion, the prehospital care would have changed, as the impaled object would first be:
   A. stabilized, and then the eyes patched.
   B. flushed with irrigation fluid, and then left alone.
   C. removed, and then direct pressure applied for 3 to 5 minutes.
   D. removed, irrigated, and then loose bandages applied over both eyes.

4. What is the best way to care for the patient's eyes en route?
   A. Rinse both eyes with hydrogen peroxide.
   B. Apply any over-the-counter antibiotic cream.
   C. Apply povidone-iodine cream and then bandage the eyes.
   D. No additional care is indicated at this time.

5. When irrigating a foreign substance from only one eye, you should make certain that you avoid:
   A. accidentally drowning the patient.
   B. using too much water on the patient's skin.
   C. pouring water up into the patient's nose.
   D. rinsing contaminants into the unaffected eye.

points to ponder

Object. 1-1.6

You respond to an industrial accident to find a patient with a 2" x 1" piece of metal stuck in her eye. The patient is very upset because she lost her other eye in a childhood injury and now has an artificial glass eye. It is obvious that there is a great deal of damage, and you suspect that she will lose sight in this eye. The patient asks you very directly whether she is going to lose the sight in her good eye.

- How would you answer the patient? Would it be fair to be less than honest with her? Why or why not? Would it be your role to tell her that she may end up blind?

online outlook

Injuries to the eye are very common, and you will encounter many in your work as an EMT-B. Proper emergency medical care for these injuries can minimize damage, which can often be severe. Review your knowledge of different types of eye injuries by completing Exercise 27 at www.emtb.com.

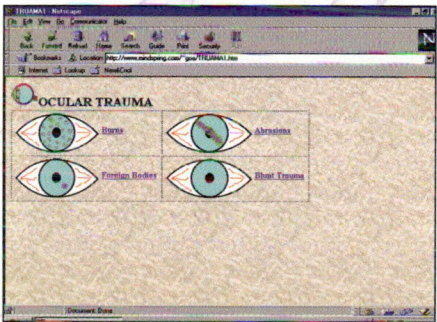

prep kit

27

Face and Throat Injuries

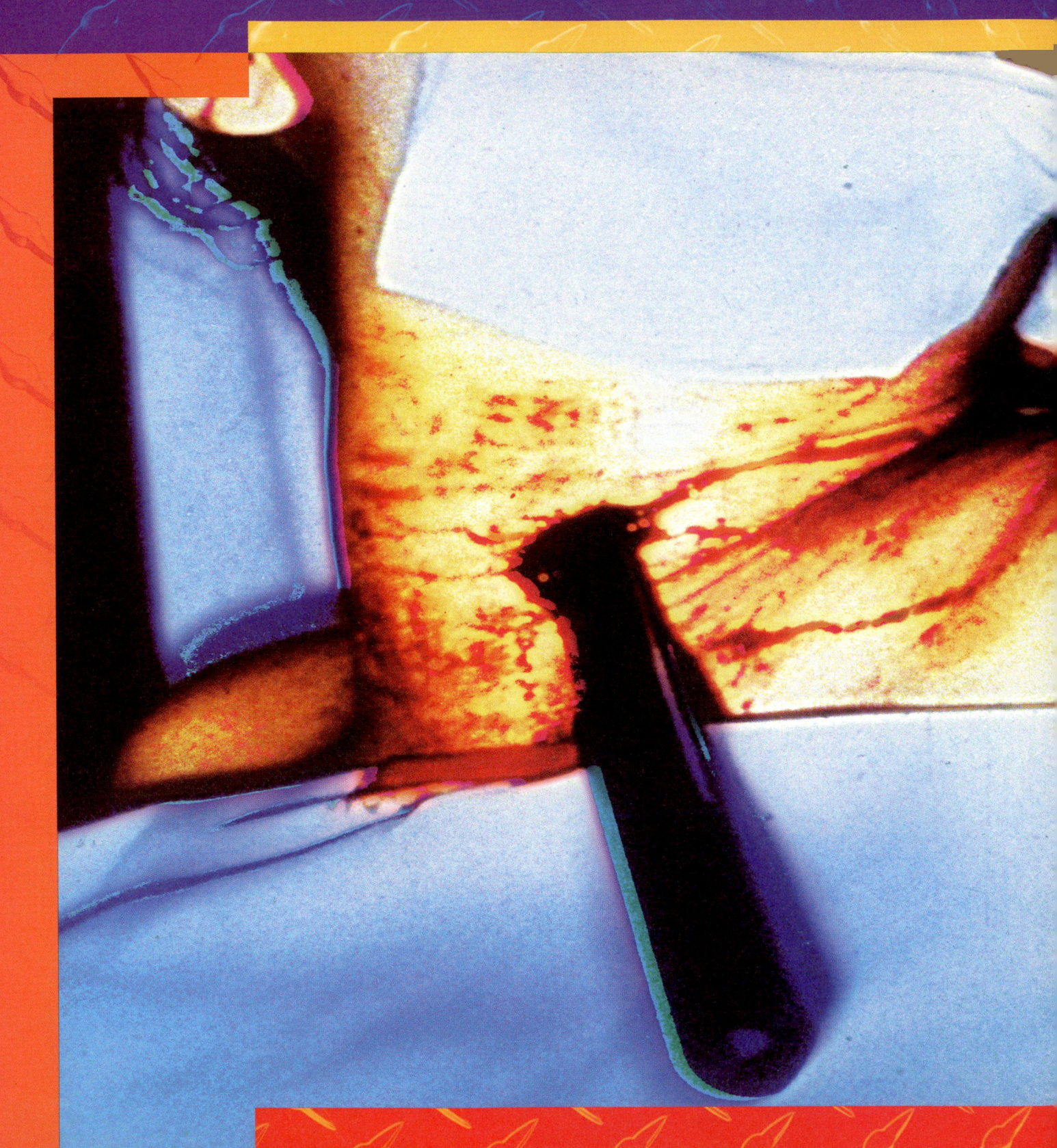

objectives*

Cognitive

1. Describe the causes of upper airway obstruction in facial injuries.

2. List the steps in the emergency medical care of the patient with soft-tissue wounds of the face and neck.

3. List the steps in the emergency medical care of the patient with injuries of the nose and ear.

4. List the physical findings of a patient with a facial fracture.

5. List the steps in the emergency medical care of the patient with a penetrating injury to the neck.

6. List the steps in the emergency medical care of the patient with an upper airway injury.

7. List the steps in the emergency medical care of the patient with dental injuries.

Affective

None

Psychomotor

8. Demonstrate the care of a patient with soft-tissue wounds of the face and neck.

9. Demonstrate the care of a patient with injuries of the nose and ear.

10. Demonstrate the care of a patient with a penetrating injury to the neck.

11. Demonstrate the care of a patient with an upper airway injury.

12. Demonstrate the care of a patient with dental injuries.

* These are non-curriculum objectives.

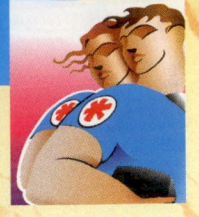

you are the emt

The doorbell rings at quarters, followed immediately by loud knocking. As you open the door, you are met by a woman who is nearly hysterical as she tells you that her husband was trying to jump start her car when the battery exploded in his face.

Any injuries to the face and/or throat have serious implications because of their potential impact on airway management. This chapter will provide the insights and techniques you will need to properly care for these injuries, and it will also help you to answer the following questions:

1. What makes the linear fractures that often accompany serious blunt trauma to the face so dangerous?

2. Describe how traumatic injuries to the face, head, and neck are related.

Face and Throat Injuries

The face and neck are particularly vulnerable to injury because of their relatively unprotected positions on the body. Soft-tissue injuries and fractures to the bones of the face are common and vary greatly in severity. Some are potentially life threatening, and many leave disfiguring scars if not treated properly. With appropriate prehospital and hospital care, what may at first seem to be a devastating injury can have a surprisingly good outcome.

As an EMT-B, your objective is to prevent further injury, particularly to the cervical spine, to manage any acute airway problems, and to control bleeding. This chapter first reviews the anatomy of the head and neck, then examines the factors that can produce upper airway obstruction. A discussion of emergency medical care of soft-tissue wounds of the face, nose, and ear; facial fractures; penetrating injuries of the neck; and dental injuries follows.

Anatomy of the Head and Neck

The head is divided into two parts: the cranium and the face. The **cranium**, or skull, contains the brain, which connects to the spinal cord through the **foramen magnum**, a large opening at the base of the skull. The most posterior portion of the cranium is called the **occiput**. On each side of the cranium, the lateral portions are called the temples or temporal regions. Between the temporal regions and the occiput lie the parietal regions. The forehead is called the frontal region. Just anterior to the ear, in the temporal region, you can feel the pulse of the superficial temporal artery. The thick skin covering the cranium, which usually bears hair, is called the scalp.

The face is composed of the eyes, ears, nose, mouth, cheeks, and jowls. Six bones—the nasal bone, the two **maxillae** (upper jawbones), the two zygomas (cheekbones), and the mandible (jawbone)—are the major bones of the face (Figure 28-1).

The orbit of the eye is composed of the lower edge of the frontal bone of the skull, the zygoma, the maxilla, and the nasal bone. The bony orbit protects the eye from injury. By viewing the face from the side, you can see the eyeball recessed in the orbit. Only the proximal one third of the nose—the bridge—is formed by bone. The remaining two thirds are composed of cartilage. Unlike the nose, the exposed portion of the ear is composed entirely of cartilage that is covered by skin. The visible part of the ear is called the **pinna**. The earlobes are the fleshy portions at the bottom of each ear. The **tragus** is a small, rounded, fleshy bulge immediately anterior to the ear canal. The superficial temporal artery can be palpated just anterior to the tragus. About 1″ posterior to the external opening of the ear is a prominent bony mass at the base of the skull called the **mastoid process** (Figure 28-2).

The **mandible** forms the jaw and chin. Motion of the mandible occurs at the **temporomandibular joint**, which lies just in front of the ear on either side of the face. Below the ear and anterior to the mastoid process, the angle of the mandible is easily palpated.

The neck also contains many important structures. It is supported by the cervical spine, or the first seven vertebrae in the spinal column (C1 through C7). The spinal

FIGURE 28-1 The face is composed of six bones: the nasal bone, two maxillae, two zygomas, and the mandible.

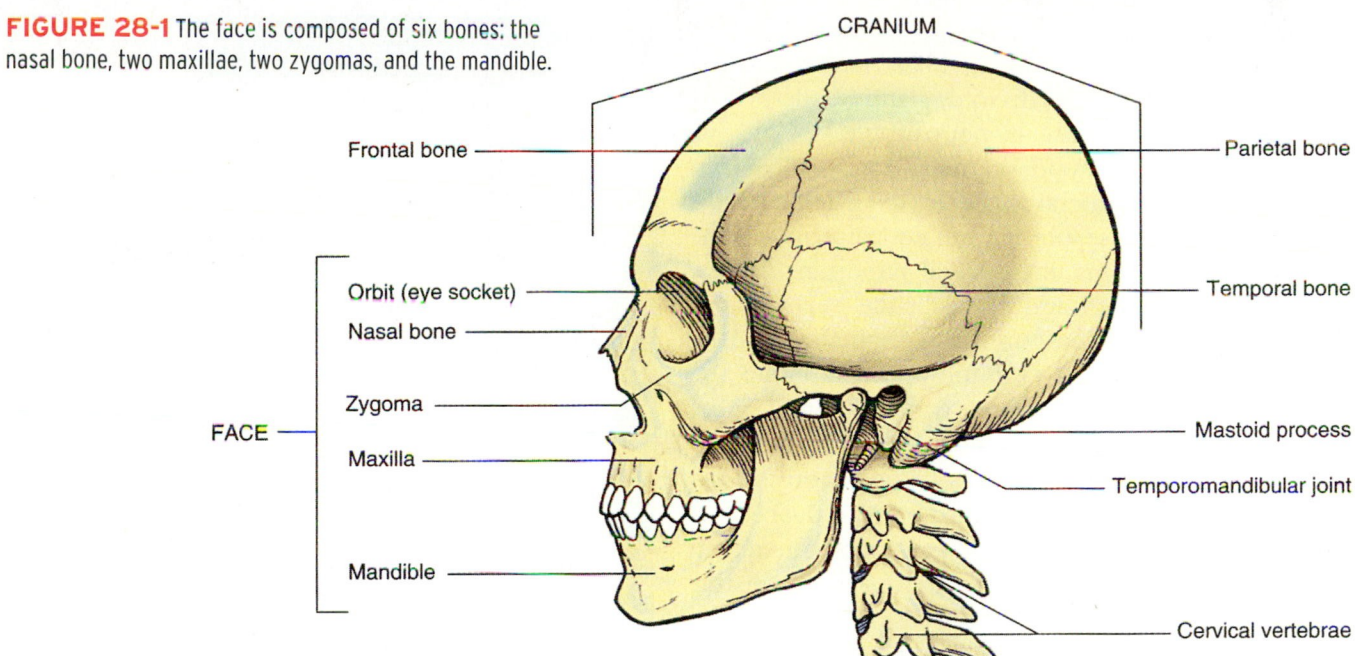

FIGURE 28-2 Principal features of the head and neck include the pinna, the tragus, the mastoid process, the occiput, the seventh cervical vertebra, and the temporomandibular joint.

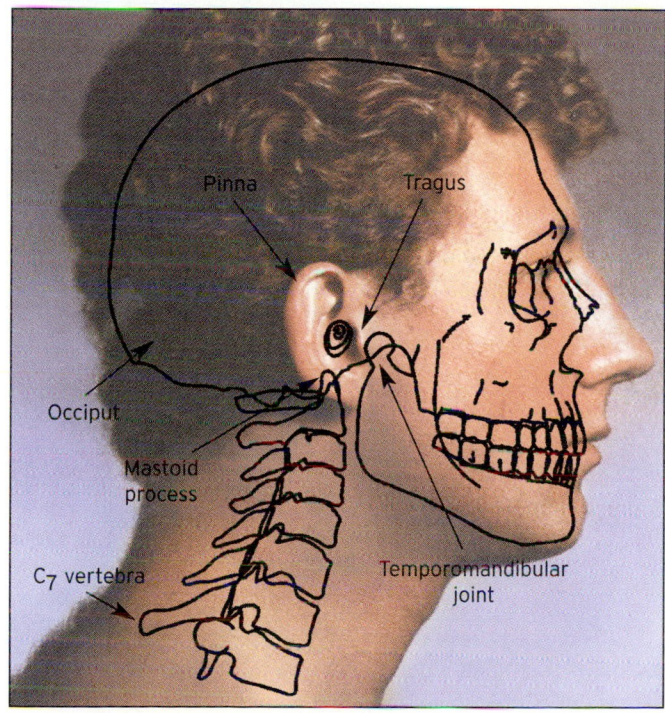

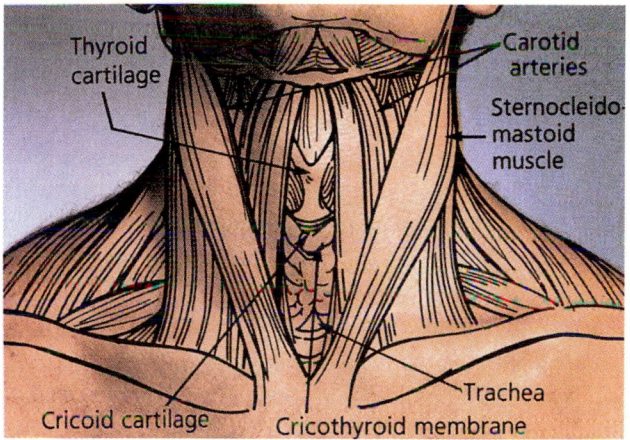

FIGURE 28-3 Important landmarks in the neck include the cricoid cartilage, the thyroid cartilage, the carotid arteries, the cricothyroid membrane, and the sternocleidomastoid muscles.

cord exits from the foramen magnum and lies within the spinal canal formed by the vertebrae. The upper part of the esophagus and the trachea lie deep in the midline of the neck. The carotid arteries may be found on either side of the trachea, along with the jugular veins and several nerves.

Several useful landmarks can be palpated and seen in the neck (Figure 28-3). The most obvious is the firm prominence in the center of the anterior surface commonly known as the **Adam's apple**. Specifically, this prominence is the upper part of the larynx, formed by the thyroid cartilage. It is more prominent in men than in women. The other portion of the larynx is the cricoid cartilage, a firm ridge of cartilage inferior to the thyroid cartilage, which is somewhat more difficult to palpate. Between the thyroid cartilage and the cricoid cartilage in the midline of the neck is a soft depression, the cricothyroid membrane. This is a thin sheet of connective tissue (fascia) that joins the two cartilages. The cricothyroid membrane is covered at this point only by skin.

Inferior to the larynx, several additional firm ridges are palpable in the anterior midline. These ridges are the cartilage rings of the trachea. The trachea connects the larynx with the main air passages of the lungs (the bronchi). On either side of the lower larynx and the upper trachea lies the thyroid gland. Unless it is enlarged, this gland is usually not palpable.

Pulsations of the carotid arteries are easily palpable in a groove 1 to 2 cm lateral to the larynx. Lying immediately adjacent to these arteries, but not palpable, are the internal jugular veins and several important nerves. Lateral to these vessels and nerves lie the <u>sternocleido-mastoid muscles</u>. These muscles originate from the mastoid process of the cranium and insert into the medial border of each collarbone and the sternum at the base of the neck. They allow movement of the head.

A series of bony prominences lie posteriorly, in the midline of the neck. They are the spines of the cervical vertebrae. The lower cervical spines are more prominent than the upper ones. They are more easily palpable when the neck is in flexion. At the base of the neck posteriorly, the most prominent spine is the seventh cervical vertebra.

Injuries to the Face

Injuries about the face often lead to partial or complete obstruction of the upper airway. Several factors may contribute to the obstruction. Bleeding from facial injuries can be very heavy, producing large blood clots in the upper airway. These clots can lead to complete obstruction, particularly in a patient who is not fully conscious. In particular, direct injuries to the nose and mouth, the larynx, or the trachea are often the source of significant bleeding. In addition, as a result of an injury, loosened teeth or dentures may become dislodged into the throat, where they may be swallowed or aspirated. The swelling that often accompanies injury to the soft tissues in these areas can also contribute to the obstruction.

The airway may also be affected when the patient's head is turned to the side, as so often is the case with a patient who has an altered level of consciousness or is unconscious. Other factors that interfere with normal respirations include possible injuries to the brain and/or cervical spine that may be associated with facial injuries. If the great vessels in the neck are injured, significant bleeding and pressure on the upper airway are common; these result in airway obstruction as well.

Soft-Tissue Injuries

Soft-tissue injuries of the face and scalp are very common. The skin and underlying tissues in these areas have a rich blood supply, so bleeding from penetrating injuries may be heavy. Indeed, even minor soft-tissue

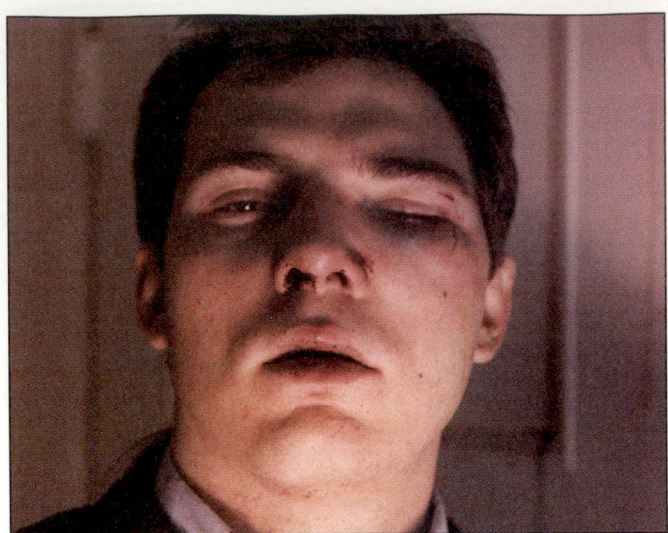

FIGURE 28-4 Facial hematoma. These injuries are often caused by interpersonal altercations.

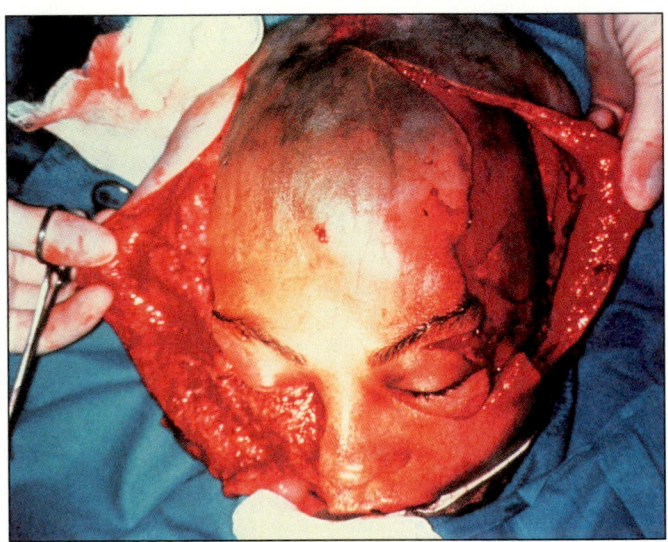

FIGURE 28-5 A major avulsion injury is characterized by a large flap of skin that is peeled back from the underlying muscle and tissue.

wounds of the face and scalp may bleed a great deal. A blunt injury that does not break the skin may cause a break in a blood vessel wall, leading blood to collect under the skin; this is called a <u>hematoma</u> (Figure 28-4). Often, a flap of skin is peeled back, or <u>avulsed</u>, from the underlying muscle and fascia (Figure 28-5).

The emergency care of soft-tissue injuries to the face and scalp is the same as treatment of soft-tissue injuries elsewhere on the body. You should assess ABCD and care for any life threats first. Remember also to follow BSI techniques in all cases.

Your first step is to open and clear the airway. Remember that blood draining into the throat can produce vomiting and airway obstruction. Take appropriate precautions if you suspect that the patient has sustained a

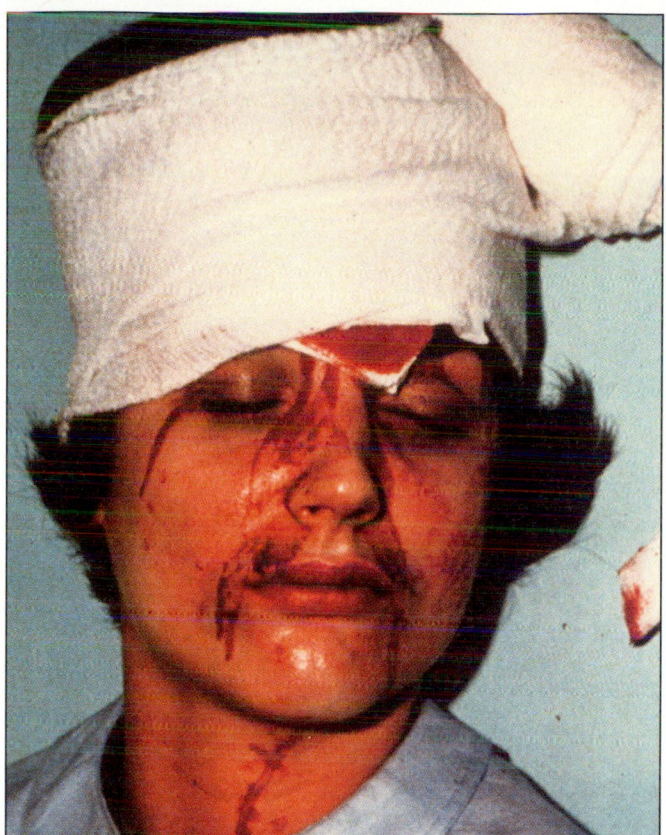

FIGURE 28-6 Use roller gauze, wrapped around the circumference of the head, to hold a pressure dressing in place.

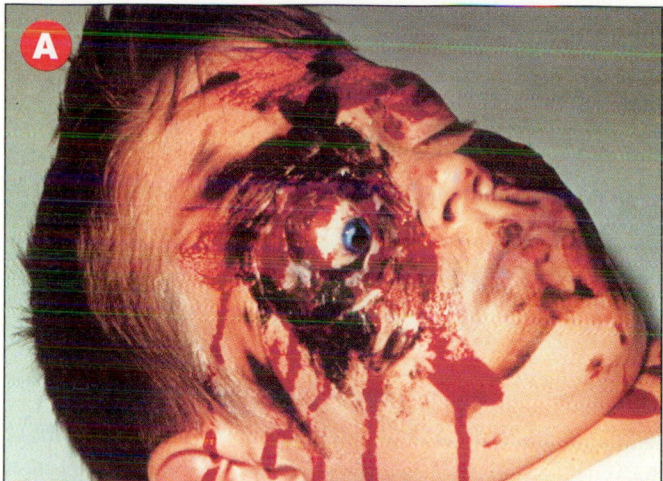

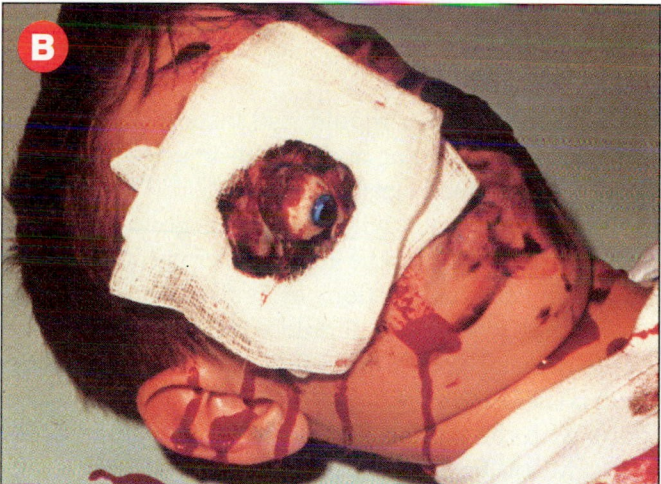

FIGURE 28-7 An injury that exposes the brain, eye, or other structures should be covered with a moist, sterile dressing to prevent further damage.

cervical spine injury; be sure to avoid moving the neck. Use the jaw-thrust or head-tilt/chin-lift maneuver, whichever is appropriate, to open the patient's airway, and then suction the mouth. Once the patient is immobilized in a cervical collar and on a backboard, you can turn him or her to one side to allow any blood or vomitus to drain out of the mouth rather than pool in the pharynx and obstruct the airway.

Control bleeding by applying direct manual pressure with a dry, sterile dressing. Use roller gauze, wrapped around the circumference of the head, to hold a pressure dressing in place (Figure 28-6). Do not apply excessive pressure if there is a possibility of underlying skull fracture. When an injury exposes the brain, eye, or other structures, cover the exposed parts with a moist, sterile dressing to protect them from further damage (Figure 28-7). For injuries in which the skin is not broken, apply ice locally to help control the swelling of bruised tissues.

For soft-tissue injuries around the mouth, you should always check for bleeding inside the mouth. Broken teeth and lacerations to the tongue may cause profuse bleeding and obstruction of the upper airway (Figure 28-8). Often, the patient will swallow the blood from lacerations inside the mouth, so the hemorrhage may

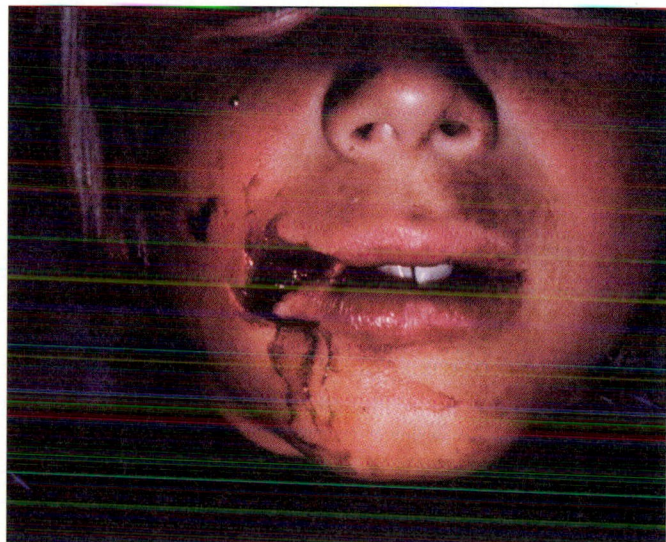

FIGURE 28-8 Soft-tissue injuries throuad the mouth can be associated with profuse bleeding inside the mouth and obstruction of the airway.

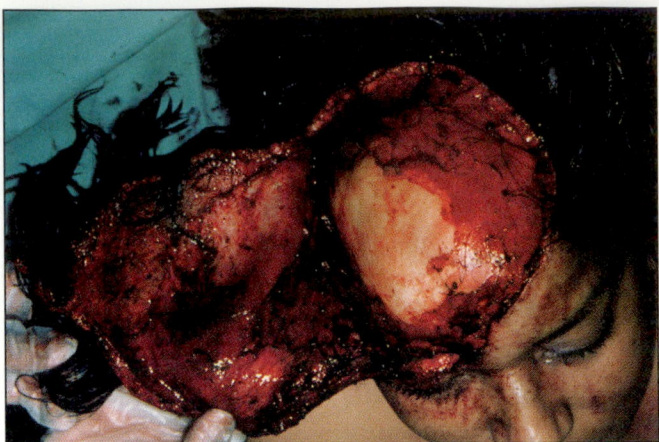

FIGURE 28-9 If avulsed skin is still attached, place the flap in a position that is as close to normal as possible, and hold it in place with a dry, sterile dressing.

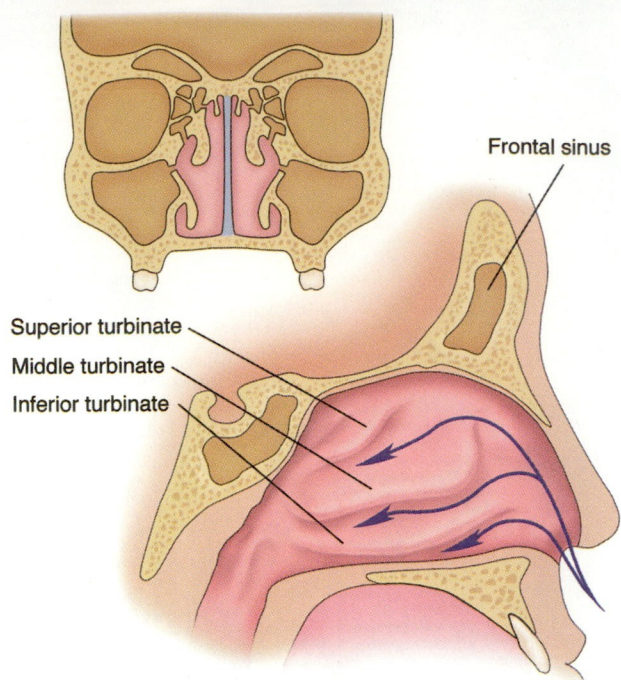

FIGURE 28-10 The nose has two chambers, divided by the septum. Each chamber is composed of layers of bone called turbinates. Above the nose are the frontal sinuses and, on either side, the orbit of the eye.

not be apparent. You should also inspect the inside of the mouth for bleeding and hidden injuries in patients who have sustained facial trauma.

Often, physicians will be able to graft a piece of avulsed skin back into the appropriate position. For this reason, if you find portions of avulsed skin that have become separated, you should wrap them in a moist, sterile dressing, place them in a plastic bag, and keep them cool. Deliver the bag to the emergency department along with the patient. In many avulsion injuries, the skin will still be attached in a loose flap (Figure 28-9). Place the flap in a position that is as close to normal as possible, and hold it in place with a dry, sterile dressing. These steps will help to increase the patient's chances of being restored to normal appearance.

Injuries of the Nose

The nose often takes the brunt of deliberate physical assaults and accidental car crashes. Blunt injuries to the nose caused by a fist or a dashboard may be associated with fractures and soft-tissue injuries of the face, head injuries, and/or injuries to the cervical spine.

In assessing injuries involving the nose, it helps to picture the inside of the nose itself (Figure 28-10). The nasal cavity is divided into two sections or chambers by the nasal septum, which is made of cartilage. Within each nasal chamber, there are layers of bone called the **turbinates**, which are covered with a moist lining. Both chambers have a superior turbinate, a middle turbinate, and an inferior turbinate. As we breathe, the air moves through the nasal chambers and is humidified as it passes over the turbinates. Directly above the nose are the frontal sinuses and, on either side, the orbit of the eye.

All these structures should be assessed for injury. In cases of severe injury, there may also be injury to the

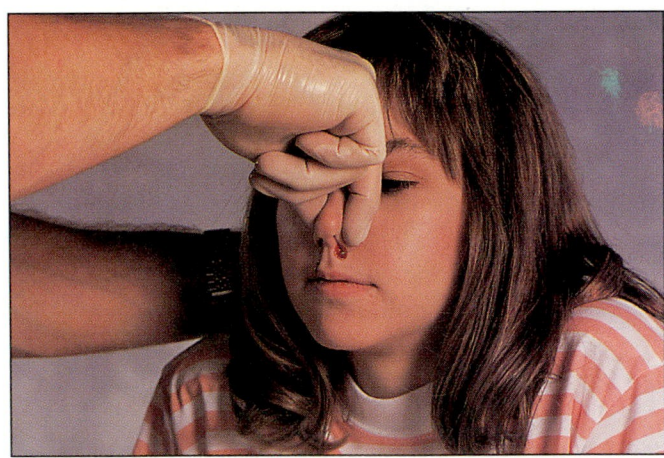

FIGURE 28-11 Control bleeding from the nose by pinching the nostrils together.

cervical spine. Keep in mind that cerebrospinal fluid (CSF) may escape down through the nose (or ears) following a fracture at the base of the skull. If blood or drainage contains CSF, a characteristic staining of the dressing will occur.

You can control bleeding from abrasions and lacerations to the nose by applying a sterile dressing. If the patient is bleeding heavily from the nose, place the patient in a sitting position leaning forward, and pinch the nostrils together (Figure 28-11). A detailed discussion of the care for epistaxis was included in Chapter 24.

Injuries of the Ear

The ear is a complex organ that is associated with both hearing and balance. The ear is divided into three parts (Figure 28-12). The external ear is composed of the pinna, or auricle, which is the part lying outside of the head, and the external auditory canal, which leads in toward the tympanic membrane, or eardrum. The middle ear contains three small bones (the hammer, anvil, and stirrup) that move in response to sound waves hitting the tympanic membrane. This is the mechanism by which we appreciate sounds. The middle ear is connected to the nasal cavity by the eustachian tube, which is the internal auditory canal. This connection permits equalization of pressure in the middle ear when external atmospheric pressure changes. The inner ear is composed of bony chambers filled with fluid. As the head moves, so does the fluid. In response, fine nerve endings within the fluid send impulses to the brain indicating both the position of the head and the rate of change of position.

Ears are often injured, but they usually do not bleed very much. If local pressure does not control the bleeding, you can apply a roller dressing (Figure 28-13). First, however, you should place a soft, padded dressing between the ear and the scalp, as bandaging the ear against the tender underlying scalp is extremely painful. In the case of an ear avulsion, you should wrap the avulsed part in a moist sterile dressing and put it in a plastic bag. Often, avulsed tissue from the ear can be reattached.

The external auditory canal is a favorite place for children to place foreign bodies such as peanuts or candy.

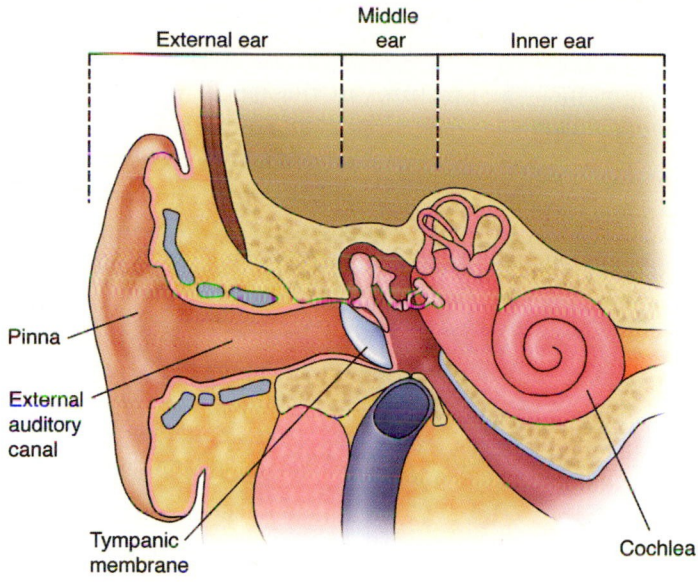

FIGURE 28-12 The ear has three principal parts: the external ear, composed of the pinna, external auditory canal, and tympanic membrane; the middle ear, including the hammer, anvil, and stirrup; and the inner ear, composed of bony chambers filled with fluid.

All such items should be removed by a physician in the emergency department. Never try to manipulate the foreign body, as you may press it further into the auditory canal and cause permanent damage to the tympanic membrane.

Again, you should note any clear fluid coming from the ear of a severely injured patient, since this may indicate a fracture at the base of the skull.

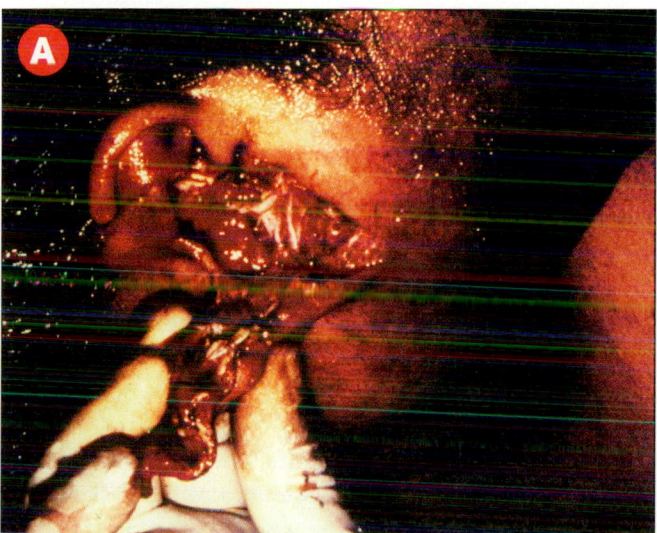
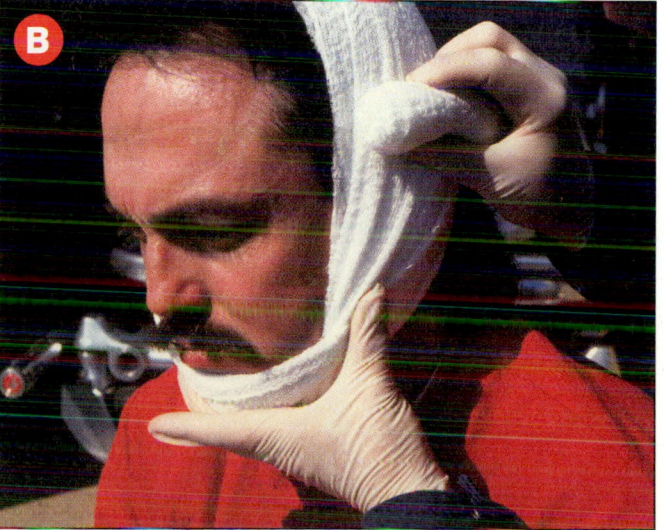

FIGURE 28-13 A: A major laceration of the ear is shown. **B:** Proper treatment includes use of a soft, sterile pad behind the ear, between it and the scalp. Then wrap a roller gauze dressing around the head to include the entire ear.

Facial Fractures

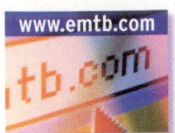

Fractures of the facial bones typically result from blunt impact. For example, the patient's head collides with a steering wheel or windshield in an automobile crash or is hit by a baseball bat or pipe in an assault (Figure 28-14). You should assume that any patient who has sustained a direct blow to the mouth or nose has a facial fracture. Other clues to the possibility of fracture include bleeding in the mouth, inability to swallow or talk, absent or loose teeth, and/or loose or movable bone fragments. Patients may also report that "it doesn't feel right" when they close their jaw, signaling an irregularity of bite.

Facial fractures alone are not acute emergencies unless there is serious bleeding. Such bleeding can be life threatening. In addition to external hemorrhage, there is the danger of blood clots in the upper airway, leading to obstruction of the upper airway. Fractures around the face and mouth can also produce deformity and loose bone fragments. However, plastic surgeons can repair the damage perfectly as long as 7 to 10 days after the injury. Be sure to remove and save loose teeth or bone fragments from the mouth; it is often possible to replant them (Figure 28-15). Remove dentures and dental bridges to protect against airway obstruction.

Another source of potential airway obstruction is swelling, which can be extreme within the first 24 hours after injury. If you notice swelling during assessment or at any time while the patient is under your care, you should check for airway obstruction.

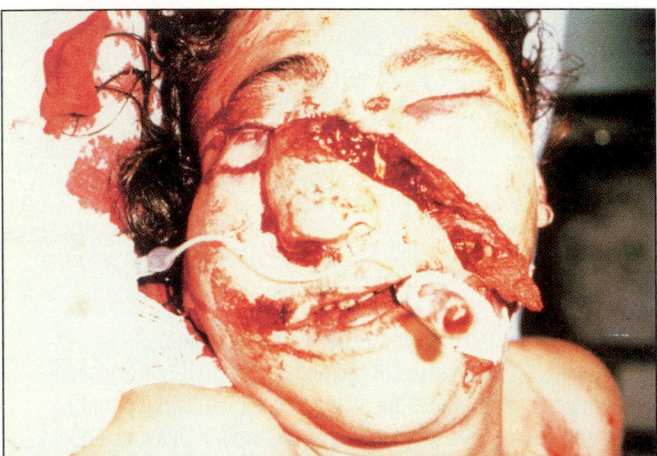

FIGURE 28-14 Bleeding following a crush injury to the face can be life threatening because, in addition to the external hemorrhage, blood clots in the airway can cause a complete obstruction.

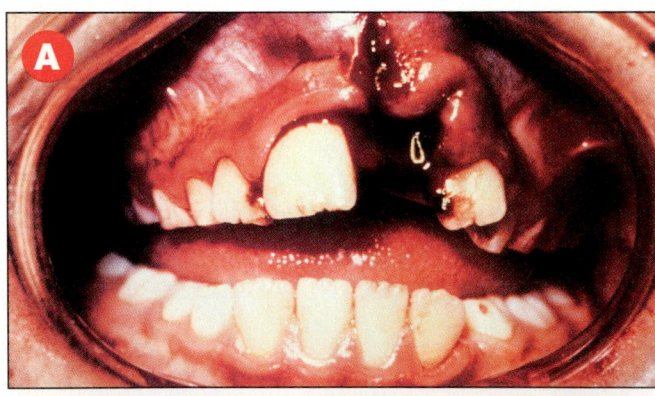

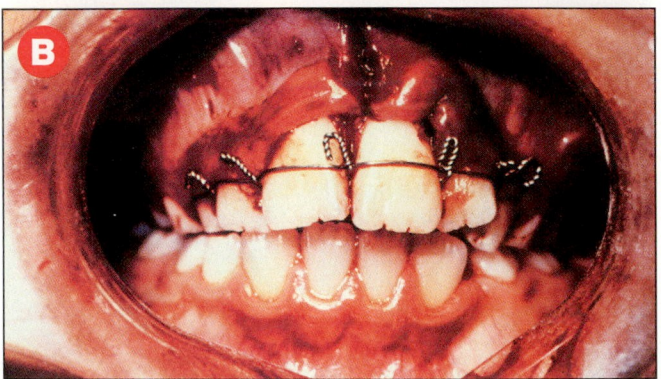

FIGURE 28-15 A: Save any lost teeth or bone fragments following an injury to the mouth, as even with traumatic loss of a tooth. **B:** The possibility of successful reimplantation is very good.

Injuries of the Neck

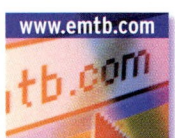

The neck contains many structures that are vulnerable to injury either by blunt trauma, such as from a steering wheel in a car crash, or by penetrating injury, such as a stab or gunshot wound. These structures include the upper airway, the esophagus, the carotid arteries and jugular veins, the thyroid cartilage or Adam's apple, the cricoid cartilage, and the upper trachea. Any injury to the neck is serious and should be considered life threatening until proven otherwise in the emergency department.

Blunt Injuries

Any crushing injury of the upper part of the neck is likely to involve the larynx or trachea. Examples include a collision with a steering wheel, an attempted suicide by hanging, and a clothesline injury sustained while riding a bicycle. Once the cartilages of the upper airway and larynx are fractured, they do not spring back to their normal position. Such a fracture can lead to loss of voice, severe and sometimes fatal airway obstruction, and leakage of air into the soft tissues of the neck (Figure 28-16). The presence of air in the soft tissues produces a characteristic crackling sensation called

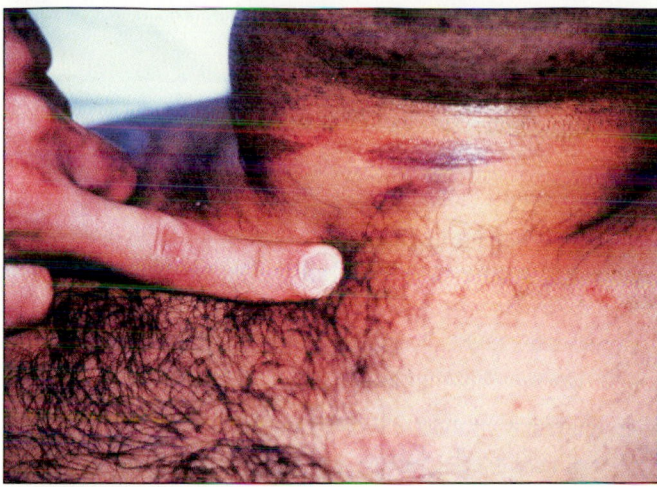

FIGURE 28-16 Fractures of the larynx or trachea can cause air to leak from the airway into the subcutaneous tissues. The presence of air in the soft tissues produces a crackling sensation called subcutaneous emphysema.

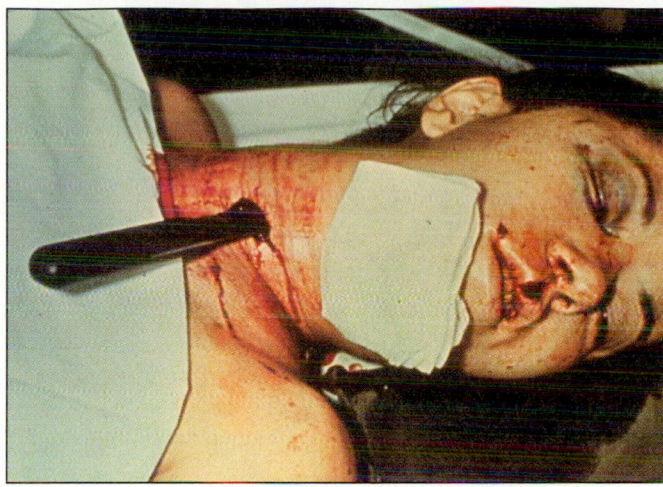

FIGURE 28-17 Penetrating injuries to the neck can result in profuse bleeding if the carotid artery or the jugular vein is damaged.

<u>subcutaneous emphysema</u>. If you feel this sensation when you palpate the neck, you should maintain the airway as best you can and provide immediate transport. Be aware that complete airway obstruction can develop very rapidly in these patients as a result of swelling or bleeding into underlying tissues. It may be very difficult to intubate such patients in the field; some will require a surgical airway at the hospital. You should also keep in mind that an incident involving a fracture in the neck may also have injured the cervical spine.

Penetrating Injuries

Penetrating injuries to the neck can cause profuse bleeding from laceration of the great vessels in the neck, either the carotid artery or the jugular veins (Figure 28-17). The airway, the esophagus, and even the spinal cord can also be damaged by a penetrating injury.

Direct pressure over the bleeding site will control most neck bleeding (Figure 28-18). However, the tissues within the neck may still bleed and compress the upper airway, so you should look for signs of airway obstruction. If a vein has been opened, air may be sucked through it to the heart, a clinical situation called <u>air embolism</u>. A large amount of air in the right atrium and right ventricle can lead to cardiac arrest.

You might find it necessary to apply pressure both above and below the penetrating wound to control life-threatening bleeding from the carotid artery (above) and the jugular vein (below). You may also need to treat the patient for shock.

Provide prompt transport for a patient with a neck injury, and ensure that the airway remains open en route.

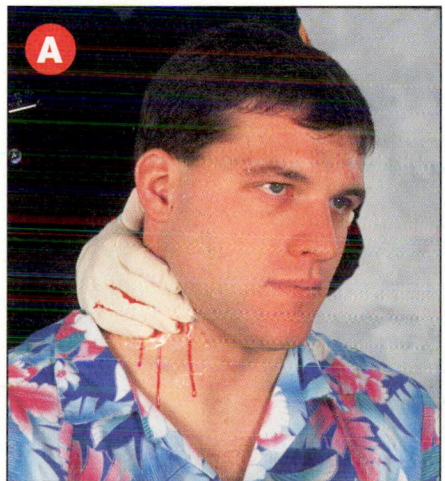

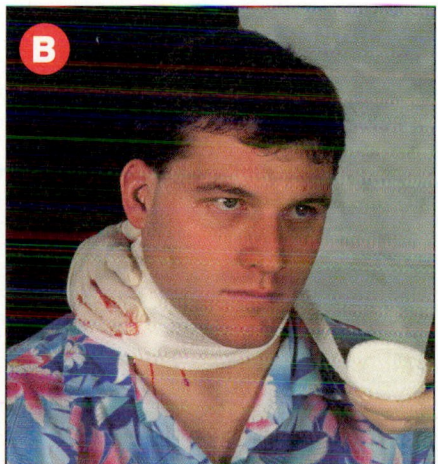

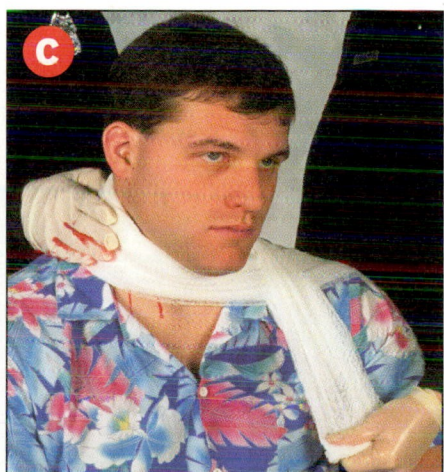

FIGURE 28-18 A: Apply direct pressure to control bleeding. **B:** Use a roller gauze to secure a dressing in place. **C:** Wrap the bandage around and under the patient's shoulder.

prep kit

ready for review

Soft-tissue injuries and fractures to the bones of the face and neck are common and vary in severity. Proper emergency care can improve the patient's chances of making a complete recovery in health and appearance. Your priorities are to prevent further injury, especially to the cervical spine, and to manage any acute airway problems. These problems can result from heavy bleeding, swelling, and injuries to the brain or cervical spine that interfere with normal respiration.

To control the often heavy bleeding from soft-tissue injuries to the face and scalp, use direct manual pressure with a dry sterile dressing, unless you suspect a skull fracture. Use a moist sterile dressing for exposed parts of the brain or eye. Always check for bleeding inside the mouth. Open and clear the airway in all patients with facial injuries. Save any pieces of avulsed skin for possible attachment later; hold any avulsed flaps in place with a dry sterile dressing. If the patient is bleeding heavily from an injury to the nose, apply a sterile dressing.

Injuries to the ear usually do not bleed very much. If local pressure does not control the bleeding, you can apply a roller dressing. Remember to place padding between the ear and the scalp, as bandaging the ear against the tender underlying scalp is extremely painful. Often, avulsed tissue from the ear can be reattached, so save any avulsed tissue. Always leave foreign bodies in the ear for a physician to remove. Watch for clear fluid coming from the ear or nose; this may indicate a basal skull fracture.

Assume that any patient who has sustained a direct blow to the nose or mouth has a facial fracture. Signs of fracture include irregularity of bite, inability to swallow or talk, and bleeding in the mouth. Check for airway obstruction if you notice swelling or if there is serious bleeding.

Both blunt and penetrating injuries to the neck can be life threatening. With blunt injuries, you should palpate the neck and feel for the characteristic crackling called subcutaneous emphysema; patients with this sign may be in danger of complete airway obstruction within minutes. Direct pressure over the bleeding site will control most neck bleeding. However, bleeding may still occur within the tissues of the neck and compress the upper airway. If a vein has been opened, be alert for the possibility of air embolism. You may have to apply pressure both above and below the penetrating wound to control life-threatening bleeding from the carotid artery and jugular vein. Patients with a neck injury require prompt transport.

vital vocabulary

www.emtb.com

Adam's apple   The firm prominence in the upper part of the larynx formed by the thyroid cartilage.

air embolism   The presence of air in the veins, which can lead to cardiac arrest if it enters the heart.

avulse   To pull or tear away.

cranium   The skull.

eustachian tube   The internal auditory canal that connects the middle ear to the nasal cavity.

external auditory canal   The ear canal.

foramen magnum   The large opening at the base of the skull through which the brain connects to the spinal cord.

hematoma   The collection of blood in a space, tissue, or organ due to a break in the wall of a blood vessel.

mandible   The bone of the lower jaw.

mastoid process   The prominent bony mass at the base of the skull about 1 inch posterior to the external opening of the ear.

maxilla   The bone that forms the upper jaw on either side of the face and contains the upper teeth, the orbit of the eye, the nasal cavity, and the palate.

occiput   The most posterior portion of the skull.

pinna   The external, visible part of the ear.

sternocleidomastoid muscles   Muscles on either side of the neck that allow movement of the head.

subcutaneous emphysema   The presence of air in soft tissues, causing a characteristic crackling sensation on palpation.

temporomandibular joint   The joint that is formed where the mandible and cranium meet, just in front of the ear.

tragus   The small, rounded, fleshy bulge that lies immediately anterior to the ear canal.

turbinates   Layers of bone within the nasal cavity.

tympanic membrane   The eardrum, which lies between the external and middle ear.

assessment in action

Thirty minutes before shift change on an unusually quiet night, you and your partner are dispatched to a duplex for a "child hemorrhaging." When you arrive you find a 3-year-old girl who, according to her parents, was running after her new puppy when she stumbled and fell onto a glass coffee table. The father stated that he saw her right after the fall and that she did not lose consciousness.

However, he admitted that he was only focusing on controlling the bleeding from the child's neck wound. Your assessment reveals that the little girl is alert and oriented, but has a 2" long laceration to the right side of her neck. The bleeding is controlled, but there is a significant amount of blood on the towel that the father used to apply pressure to the wound.

1. What is the highest priority in caring for this patient?
   A. Administering low concentrations of oxygen
   B. Treating potential or actual airway obstruction
   C. Applying sterile dressings and bandaging the wound
   D. Providing complete immobilization to a long spine board

2. Which of the following interventions is **NOT** an acceptable method for controlling bleeding in this type injury?
   A. Use of a wide band as a tourniquet
   B. Direct pressure with a sterile dressing
   C. Supplemental use of a pressure point
   D. Combination direct pressure and pressure point

3. In most cases, a patient who sustains trauma to the face or throat should be placed in what position to minimize airway obstruction?
   A. Prone
   B. Supine
   C. Sitting up
   D. Turned to the side

4. Which of the following tools is considered an essential treatment adjunct for a patient who sustained face and/or throat trauma and is spontaneously breathing but bleeding inside the mouth?
   A. A PASG
   B. A BVM device
   C. A portable suctioning unit
   D. Hemostats to clip off the artery

5. Which of the following statements about airway obstruction related to blunt trauma to the neck is true?
   A. Immediate transport is necessary because of the danger of possible obstruction.
   B. Airway obstruction is not likely to develop for at least 2 to 3 hours after the injury.
   C. Complete airway obstruction secondary to trauma is easily managed in the field by EMT-Bs.
   D. Airway obstruction rarely occurs as a complication of blunt trauma to the neck.

points to ponder

Object. 1-1.6, 1-5.3

You respond to a neighborhood park to find a patient who has been hit in the throat with a baseball. The patient's throat is quite swollen, he is cyanotic, and it does not appear that he is able to breathe. You apply a cold pack to his throat and prepare to transport. Before you are able to get him loaded into the ambulance, he loses consciousness. You are not trained to perform a cricothyrostomy (create an artificial opening in his throat), but you have seen it done in the hospital twice.

- Would you ask medical control for permission to perform a cricothyrostomy? Why or why not? If medical control authorized the procedure, who would be liable for any damages that might occur? What other treatments might you try?

online outlook

Soft-tissue injuries and fractures to the bones of the face and neck are common and vary in severity. Proper emergency care can improve the patient's chances of making a complete recovery in health and appearance. Your priorities are to prevent further injury, especially to the cervical spine, and to manage any acute airway problems. Review your knowledge of these priorities by completing Exercise 28 at www.emtb.com.

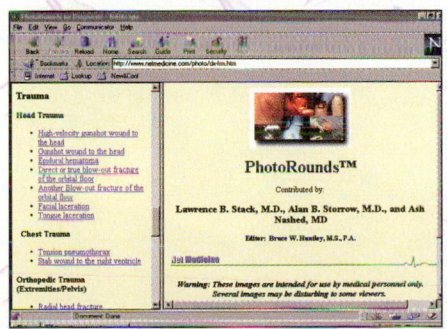

Chest Injuries

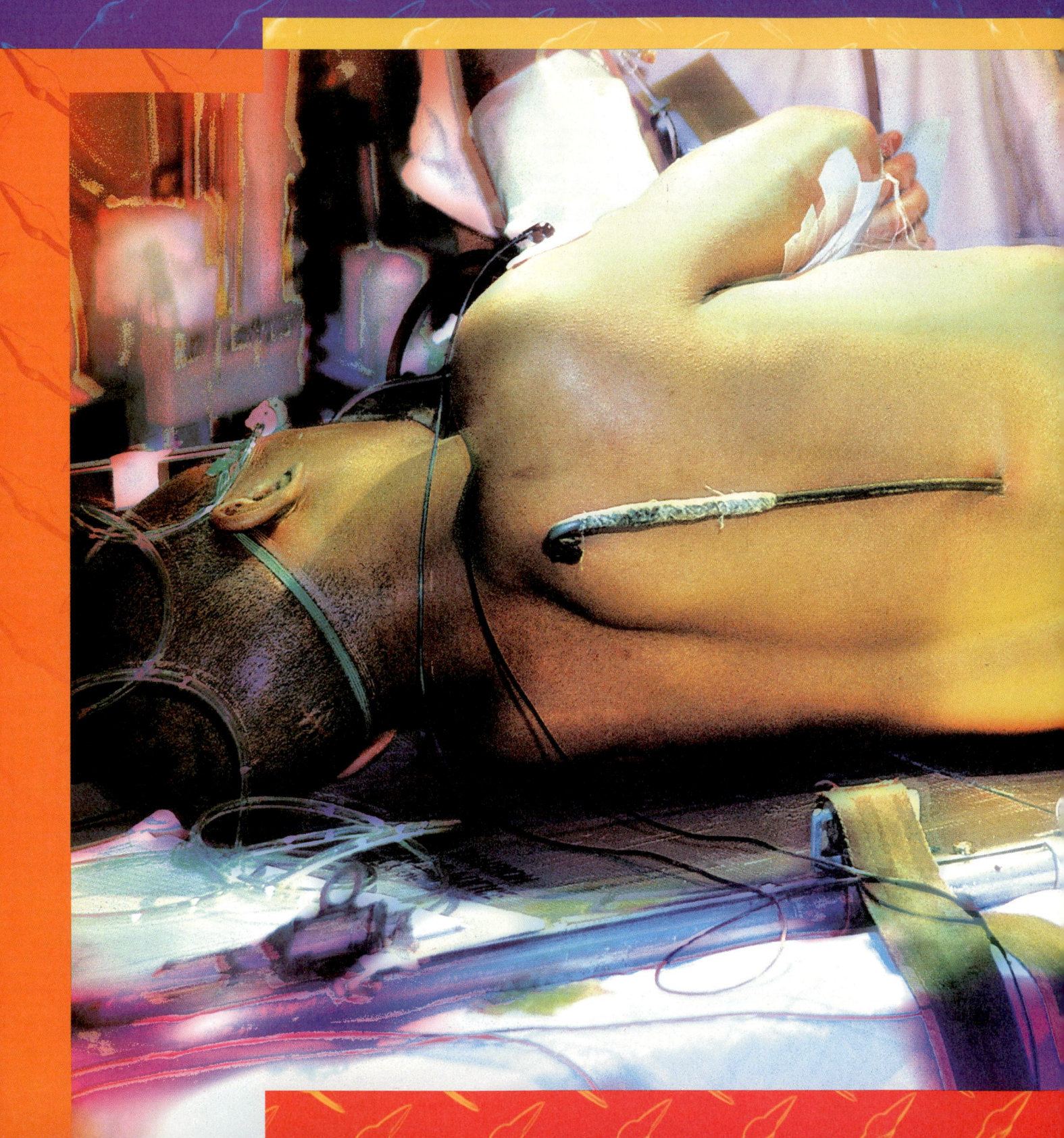

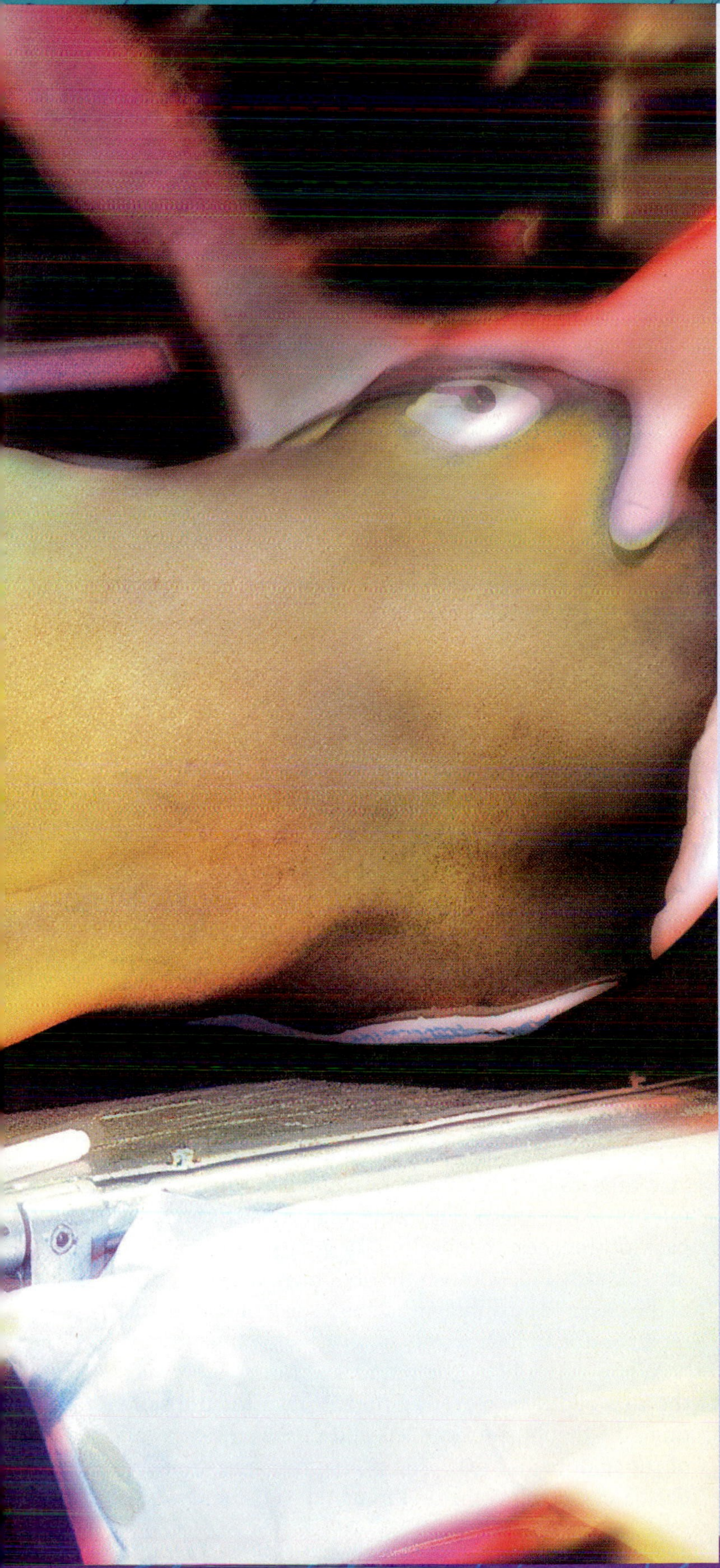

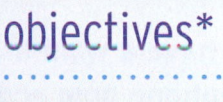
objectives*

Cognitive

1. Differentiate between an open pneumothorax, a hemothorax, a tension pneumothorax, and a closed pneumothorax.

2. Describe the emergency medical care of a patient with a flail chest.

3. Describe the emergency medical care of a patient with a sucking chest wound.

4. Describe the consequences of blunt injury to the heart.

5. List the signs of pericardial tamponade.

6. Discuss the complications that can accompany chest injuries.

Affective

None

Psychomotor

7. Demonstrate the steps in the emergency medical care of a sucking chest wound.

* These are non-curriculum objectives.

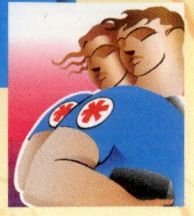

you are the emt

Dispatch, we have a walk-in patient whose car ran off the road and hit a telephone pole about a block from the station. He states that he has severe pain where his chest struck the steering wheel.

This chapter will introduce you to the complexities of chest trauma and will help you to answer the following questions:

1. How does your care of chest pain that is caused by a heart problem differ from your care of chest pain that is caused by trauma?

2. Why is trauma to the chest such a potentially serious problem?

Chest Injuries

Chest injuries are both very common and, given the likelihood of damage to the heart, lungs, or great blood vessels, very serious. Any injury that interferes with normal breathing must be treated without delay to prevent permanent damage to tissues that depend on a continuous supply of oxygen. Another major problem with chest injuries may be internal bleeding. Blood from lacerations of the thoracic organs or major blood vessels can collect in the chest cavity, compressing the lungs. Also, air can collect in the chest and prevent the lungs from expanding. Your ability to act quickly to care for patients with these injuries can make the difference between a successful outcome and death.

This chapter begins with a review of the anatomy and physiology of the chest and respiration. It then describes the common signs and symptoms of chest injuries and the proper emergency medical treatment for specific injuries.

Anatomy and Physiology of the Chest

To understand and evaluate chest injuries in the prehospital setting, you must first understand the anatomy of the chest and the mechanism by which gases are exchanged during breathing. A quick review will help you to appreciate the logic in both the emergency treatment of chest injuries and the potential complications of that treatment.

The chest (thoracic cage) extends from the lower end of the neck to the diaphragm (Figure 29-1). In an individual who is lying down or who has just completed exhalation, the diaphragm may rise as high as the nipple line. Thus, a penetrating injury to the chest, such as a gunshot or stab wound, may penetrate the lung and diaphragm and injure the liver or stomach.

The contents of the chest are partially protected by the ribs, which are connected in the back to the vertebrae and in the front, through the costal cartilages, to the sternum (Figure 29-2). The trachea, which is in the middle of the neck, divides into the left and right mainstem bronchi, which supply air to the lungs. Of course, the thoracic cage also contains the heart and the great vessels: the aorta, the right innominate and left subclavian arteries and their branches, and the superior and inferior venae cavae. The esophagus runs through the back of the chest, connecting the pharynx above with the stomach and below in the abdomen. At the bottom of the chest, the diaphragm acts as a sheet of muscle that separates the thoracic cavity from the abdominal cavity.

When you inhale, the intercostal muscles between the ribs contract, elevating the rib cage. At the same time, the diaphragm contracts and pushes the contents of the abdomen down. The pressure inside the chest decreases, and air comes in through the nose and mouth

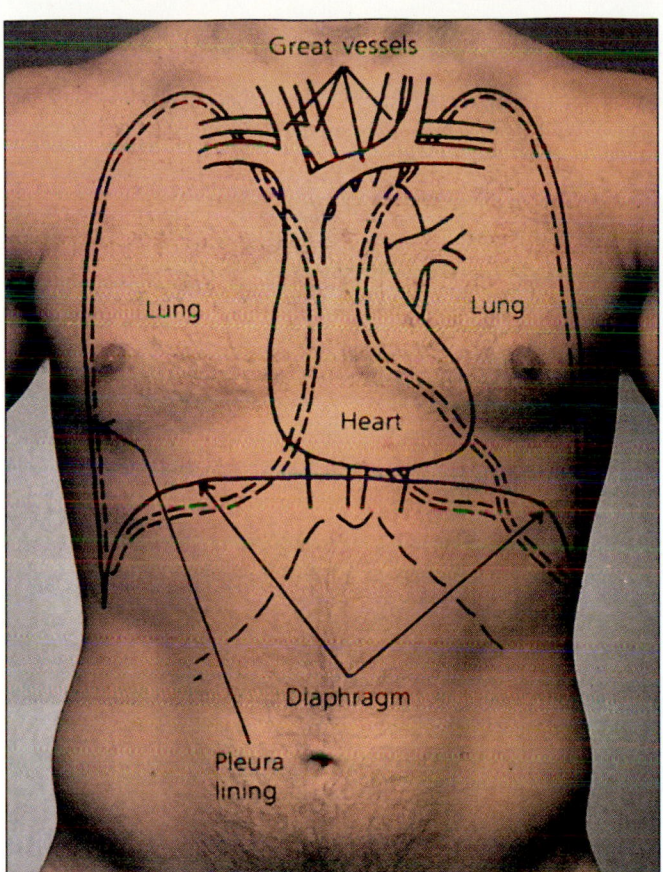

FIGURE 29-1 A view of the anterior aspect of the chest shows the major organs beneath the surface.

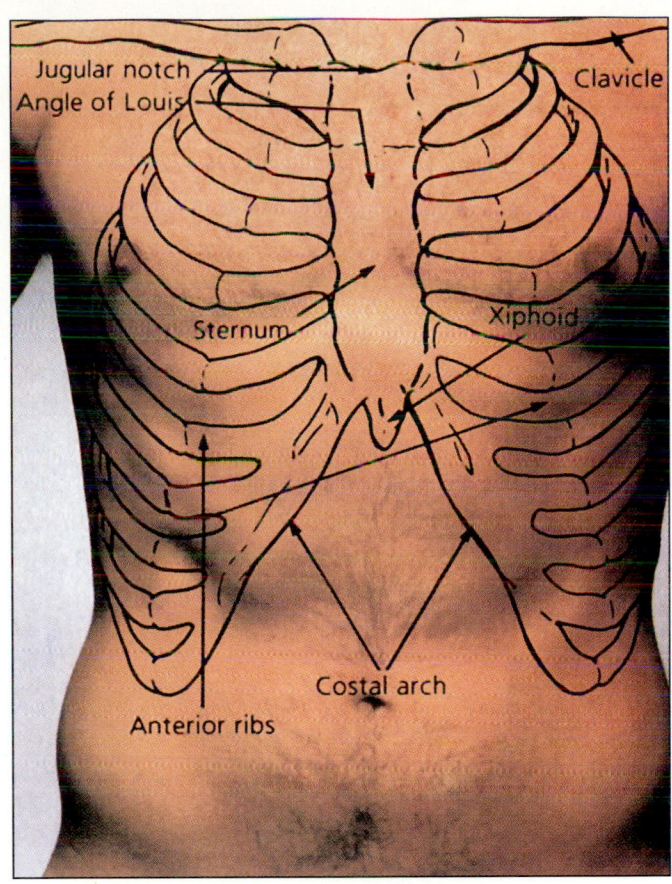

FIGURE 29-2 The organs within the chest are protected by the ribs, which are connected in back by the vertebrae and in the front, through the costal cartilages, to the sternum.

into the lungs. When you exhale, the intercostal muscles and diaphragm relax, and the tissues move back to their normal positions, allowing air to be exhaled. Note that the nerves supplying the diaphragm (the phrenic nerves) run all the way up into the neck. A patient whose neck is broken at the C5 and C6 vertebrae will lose the power to move his or her intercostal muscles, but the diaphragm will still contract, and the patient will still be able to breathe because the phrenic nerves come from the level of C4 (Figure 29-3).

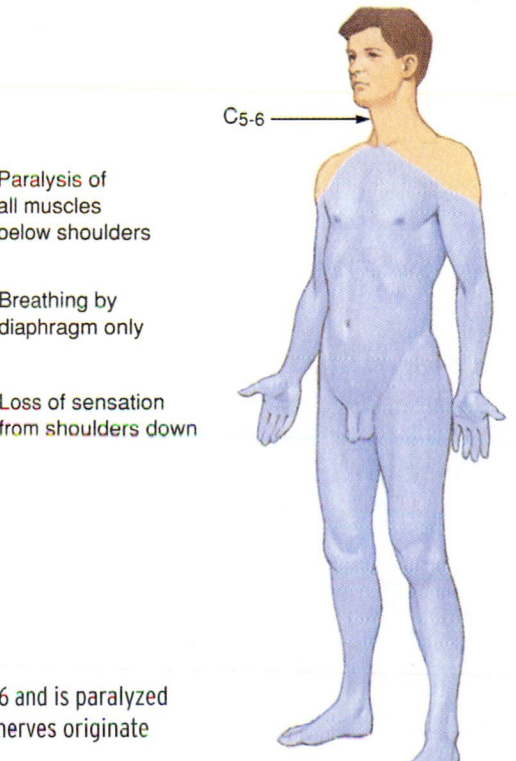

C5-6

Paralysis of
all muscles
below shoulders

Breathing by
diaphragm only

Loss of sensation
from shoulders down

FIGURE 29-3 A patient who sustains a fracture at the level of C5 to C6 and is paralyzed from the neck down can still breathe spontaneously because the phrenic nerves originate at the level of C4.

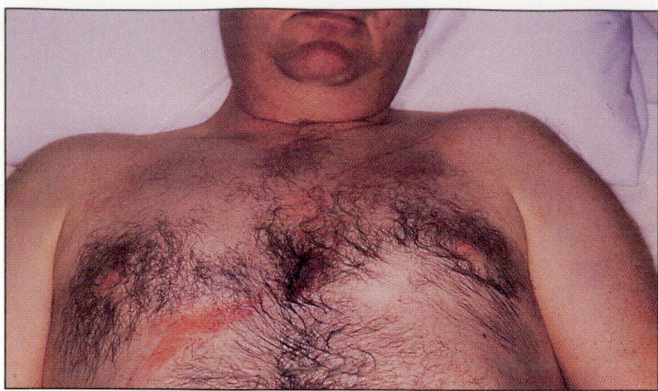

FIGURE 29-4 Closed injuries usually result from blunt trauma, such as when a patient strikes the steering wheel in a motor vehicle crash or is struck by a falling object.

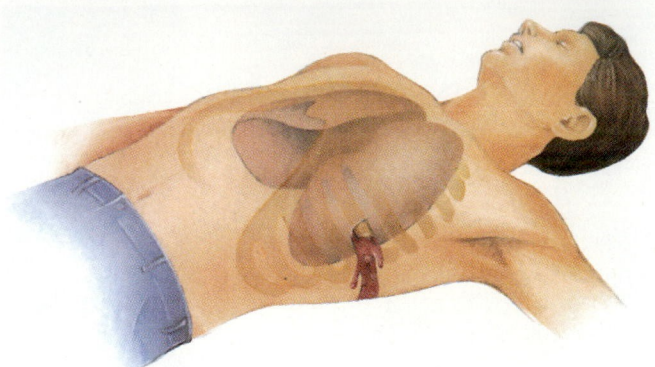

FIGURE 29-5 Open injuries occur when the chest wall is penetrated by some type of object or the broken end of a fractured rib.

Injuries of the Chest

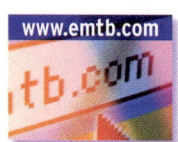
There are two types of chest injuries: penetrating, or open, injuries and blunt, or closed, injuries. As the name implies, a **closed (blunt) chest injury** is one in which the skin is not broken. This type of injury is generally caused by blunt trauma, such as when a driver strikes a steering wheel in a motor vehicle crash or is struck by a falling object (Figure 29-4). In **open chest injuries**, the chest wall itself is penetrated by some object such as a knife, a bullet, a piece of metal, or the broken end of a fractured rib (Figure 29-5).

In blunt trauma, a blow to the chest may fracture the ribs, the sternum, or whole areas of the chest wall; bruise the lungs and the heart; and even damage the aorta. Almost one third of people who are killed outright in car crashes die as a result of traumatic rupture of the aorta. Although the skin and chest wall are not penetrated in a closed injury, the contents of the chest may be lacerated by broken ribs. Indeed, vital organs can actually be torn from their attachment in the chest cavity without any break in the skin.

Signs and Symptoms

Important signs and symptoms of chest injury include the following:

- Pain at the site of injury
- Pain localized at the site of injury that is aggravated by or increased with breathing
- Dyspnea (difficulty breathing, shortness of breath)
- The coughing up of blood

- Failure of one or both sides of the chest to expand normally with inspiration
- Rapid, weak pulse and low blood pressure
- Cyanosis around the lips or fingernails

After a chest injury, any change in normal breathing is a particularly important sign. A healthy, uninjured adult usually breathes from 12 to 20 times per minute without difficulty and without pain. Respirations of fewer than 10/min or more than 24/min usually indicate respiratory distress. Patients with chest injuries often have **tachypnea** (rapid respirations) and breathe in shallow gasps because it hurts to take a deep breath.

As with any other injury, pain and tenderness are common at the point of impact as a result of a bruise or fracture. Pain is usually aggravated by the normal process of breathing. Irritation or damage of the pleural surfaces causes a characteristic sharp or sticking pain with each breath when these normally smooth surfaces must slide on one another. This sharp pain is called *pleuritic pain* or *pleurisy.*

In an injured patient, **dyspnea** (difficulty with breathing) has many causes, including airway obstruction, damage to the chest wall, improper chest expansion due to the loss of normal control of breathing, or lung compression because of accumulated blood or air. Dyspnea in an injured patient indicates significant compromise of lung function; prompt, vigorous support and transport are required.

Patient Assessment

After your initial assessment in which you quickly evaluate the patient's ABCD and treat potential life threats, carefully observe the patient's chest wall. If the chest wall does not expand on each side when the patient inhales, the chest muscles may have lost their ability to work appropriately. Loss of muscle function may be the result of a direct injury to the chest wall, or it may be related to an injury of the nerves that control those muscles.

Hemoptysis, the spitting or coughing up of blood, usually indicates that the lung itself or the air passages have been damaged. With a laceration of the lung, blood can enter the bronchial passages and is coughed up as the patient tries to clear the airway.

A rapid, weak pulse and low blood pressure are the principal signs of hypovolemic shock. Shock following a chest injury may result from insufficient oxygenation of the blood by the poorly functioning lungs. This condition can also result from extensive bleeding from lacerated structures within the chest cavity.

Cyanosis in a patient with a chest injury indicates inadequate ventilation. The classic blue appearance around the lips and fingernails indicates that blood is not being oxygenated sufficiently. Patients with cyanosis are unable to provide a sufficient supply of oxygen to the blood through the lungs and require immediate respiratory support and supplemental oxygen.

Many of these signs and symptoms occur simultaneously. When any one of them develops as a result of a chest injury, the patient requires prompt hospital care. Remember that the principal reason for concern about a patient who has a chest injury is that his or her body has no means of storing oxygen; it is supplied and used continuously, even during sleep. Any interruption in this supply can be lethal and must be treated aggressively.

Complications of Chest Injuries

Pneumothorax

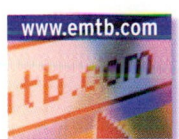

In a penetrating injury, damage to the heart, lungs, great vessels, and other organs in the chest can be complicated by the accumulation of air in the pleural space. This is a dangerous condition called a pneumothorax. In this condition, air enters through a hole in the chest wall as the patient attempts to breathe, causing the lung on that side to collapse (Figure 29-6). As a result, any blood that passes through the lung is not oxygenated, and hypoxia will develop. Depending on the size of the hole and the rate at which air fills the cavity, the lung may collapse in a few seconds or a few hours. You can actually

hear this condition in the form of a sucking sound as the patient inhales and the sound of rushing air as he or she exhales. For this reason, an open or penetrating wound to the chest wall is often called a sucking chest wound (Figure 29-7). Pneumothorax can also be caused by air leaking into the lung or bronchus into the pleural space following a laceration of either one by a fractured rib or a penetrating object.

This type of open pneumothorax is a true emergency requiring immediate emergency medical care and transport. As an initial emergency step, after clearing and

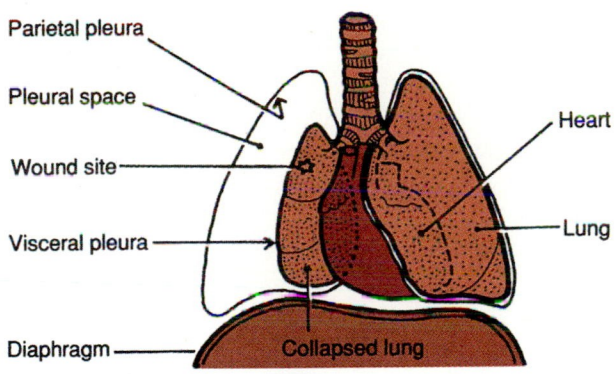

FIGURE 29-6 Pneumothorax occurs when air leaks into the pleural space from an opening in the chest wall or the surface of the lung. The lung collapses as air fills the pleural space and the two pleural surfaces are no longer in contact.

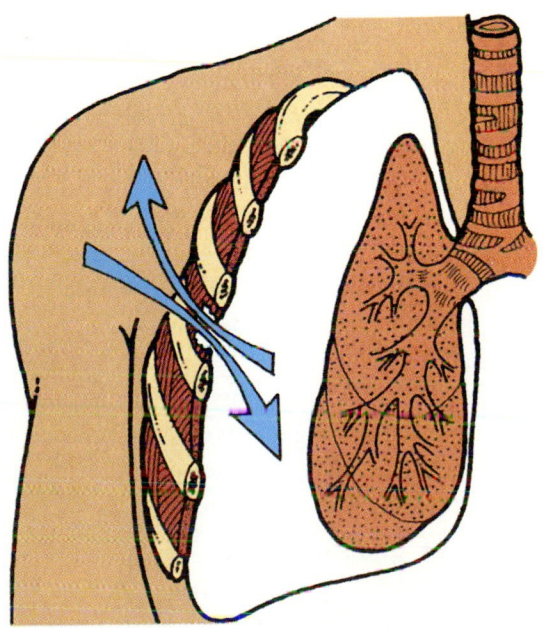

FIGURE 29-7 With a sucking chest wound, air passes from the outside into the pleural space and back out with each breath, creating the sucking sound.

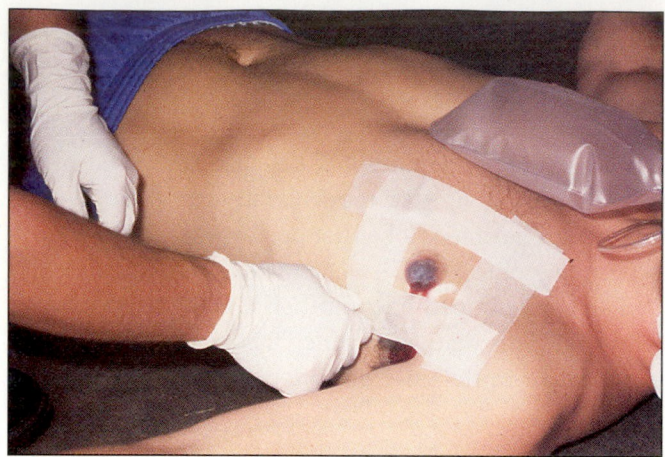

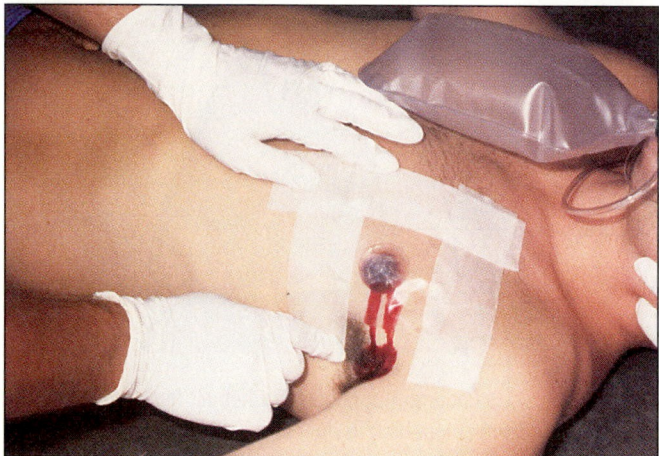

FIGURE 29-8 A sucking chest wound can be sealed with a large airtight dressing that either seals all four sides or seals three sides with the fourth side as a flutter valve. Your local protocol will dictate the way you are to care for this injury.

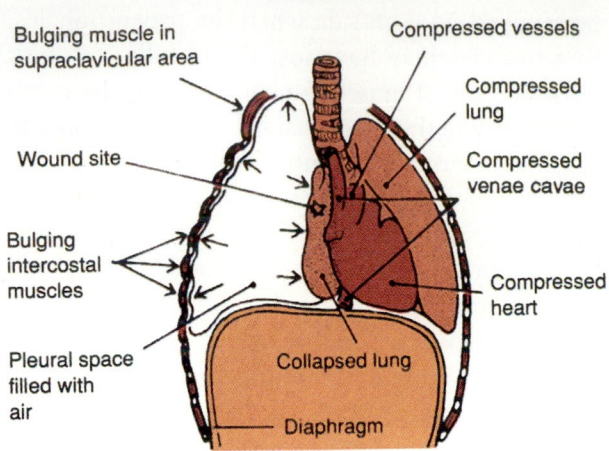

FIGURE 29-9 A tension pneumothorax can develop if a penetrating chest wound is bandaged tightly and air from a damaged lung cannot escape. The air then accumulates in the pleural space.

maintaining the airway, then providing oxygen, you must rapidly seal the open wound with a sterile airtight dressing (Figure 29-8). The purpose of the dressing is to seal the wound and prevent air from being sucked into the chest through the wound. Several sterile materials, including Vaseline gauze, aluminum foil, or a folded universal dressing may be used to seal the wound. Use a large enough dressing so that it is not pulled or sucked into the chest cavity. Depending on your local protocol, you may tape the dressing down on all four sides, or you may create a **flutter valve**, a one-way valve that allows air to leave the chest cavity but not return.

Spontaneous pneumothorax. In some individuals, congenitally weak areas exist on the surface of the lungs. Occasionally, such a weak area will rupture spontaneously, allowing air to leak into the pleural space. Usually, this event, called **spontaneous pneumothorax**, is not related to any major injury but simply happens

with normal breathing. The patient experiences sudden sharp chest pain and increasing difficulty in breathing. The affected lung collapses, losing its ability to expand normally. The amount of pneumothorax that develops varies, as does the amount of respiratory distress the patient experiences.

You should suspect a spontaneous pneumothorax in a patient who experiences sudden chest pain and shortness of breath without a specific known cause. The prehospital treatment that you can provide for this type of pneumothorax is the same as that for an open, traumatic pneumothorax.

Tension pneumothorax. A potential complication that may develop if your local protocol calls for you to seal all four sides of the dressing is called a **tension pneumothorax** (Figure 29-9). This can occur when the lung itself has been lacerated, and there is a significant ongoing air leak. In sealing the wound in the chest wall, you have effectively cut off the only escape route for air leaking into the pleural space from the lung. This air will first cause the complete collapse of the affected lung and then begin to push the mediastinum (the division between the two pleural sacs) into the opposite pleural cavity. This cuts off blood returning through the inferior vena cava to the heart and can lead to cardiac arrest.

A tension pneumothorax can also occur as a result of closed, blunt injury of the chest in which a fractured rib lacerates the lung. A tension pneumothorax may arise spontaneously. This typically happens in a young adult when a *bleb*, or blister, on the surface of the lung ruptures.

The common signs and symptoms of tension pneumothorax include increasing respiratory distress, distended neck veins, deviation of the trachea to the opposite side of the chest away from the tension pneumothorax, signs of shock, including tachycardia, low blood pressure, and cyanosis, and decreased breath sounds on the side of the pneumothorax.

If a tension pneumothorax develops as the result of sealing an open chest wound, you should partly remove the dressing to relieve the tension. As you do so, you may hear a rush of air out of the chest cavity, though this does not occur in all cases. Relieving a tension pneumothorax in a patient who does not have an open chest wound is often done by inserting a needle through the rib cage into the pleural space; however, this procedure must be performed by ALS personnel or emergency department staff.

Hemothorax

In both blunt and penetrating chest injury, blood can collect in the pleural space from a bleeding rib cage, lung, or great vessel. This condition is called a **hemothorax** (Figure 29-10). You should suspect a hemothorax if the patient has signs and symptoms of shock or decreased breath sounds on the affected side, an indication that the lung is being depressed against the mediastinum. The presence of both air and blood in the pleural space is known as a hemopneumothorax.

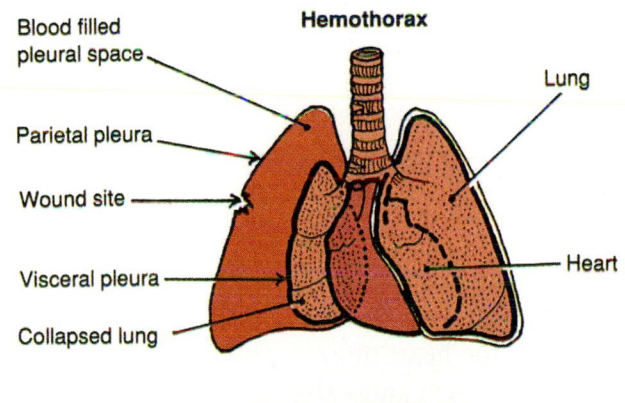

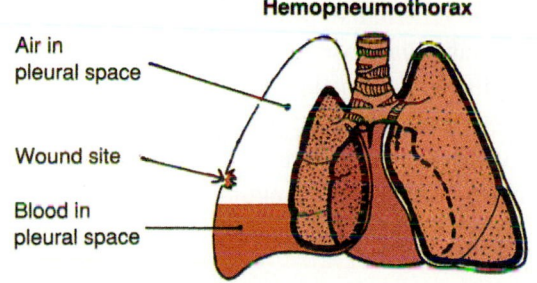

FIGURE 29-10 A hemothorax is a collection of blood in the pleural space produced by lacerated blood vessels within the chest.

Rib Fractures

Rib fractures are very common in the elderly, whose bones are brittle, but relatively uncommon in the very young, whose bones are much more supple. Because the upper four ribs are well protected by the bony girdle of the clavicle and scapula, a fracture of one of these upper ribs is considered a very severe mechanism of injury.

Be aware that a fractured rib that penetrates into the pleural space may lacerate the surface of the lung, causing a pneumothorax, a tension pneumothorax, a hemothorax, or a hemopneumothorax. One sign of this development can be a crackly feeling to the skin in the area, which indicates that air escaping from a lacerated lung is leaking into the chest wall. Be sure to relay this finding to the hospital.

Patients with one or more cracked ribs will report localized tenderness and pain on breathing. The pain is the result of broken ends of the fracture rubbing against each other with each inspiration and expiration. Patients will tend to avoid taking deep breaths, breathing rapidly and shallowly instead. They will often hold the affected portion of the rib cage in an effort to minimize the discomfort.

Flail Chest

Most often, ribs are fractured in more than one place. If three or more ribs are fractured in two or more places, or if the sternum is fractured along with several ribs, a segment of chest wall may be detached from the rest of the thoracic cage (Figure 29-11). This condition is

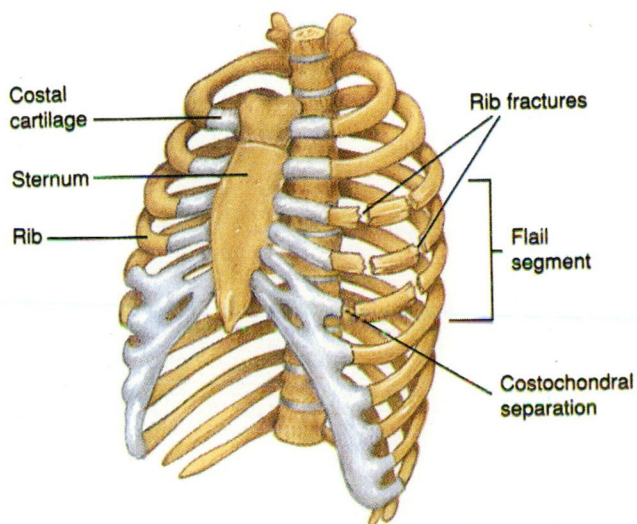

FIGURE 29-11 When three or more adjacent ribs are fractured in two or more places, a flail chest results. This segment will move paradoxically when the patient breathes.

A healthy, uninjured adult usually breathes from 12 to 20 times per minute without difficulty and without pain.

known as **flail chest**. In what is called **paradoxical motion**, the detached portion of the chest wall moves during respiration in a fashion exactly opposite of normal: in instead of out during inhalation, out instead of in during expiration. This occurs because of negative pressure that has built up in the thorax. Breathing with a flail chest can be extremely painful and rarely provides adequate oxygenation.

Your treatment of a patient with a flail chest should include maintaining the airway, providing respiratory support, giving supplemental oxygen, and performing ongoing assessments for possible pneumothorax or other respiratory compromise.

The patient may find it easier and less painful to breathe if the flail segment is immobilized. You can tape a pad against that segment of the chest for this purpose (Figure 29-12). Keep in mind that while flail chest is itself a serious condition, it suggests an injury that was forceful enough to cause other serious internal damage as well.

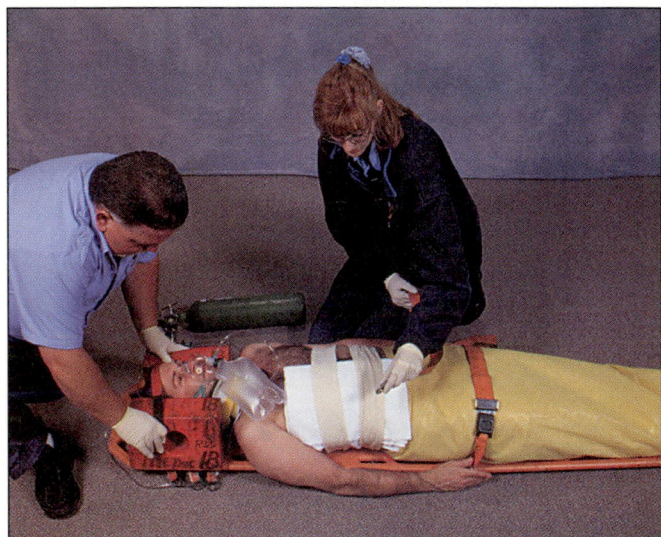

FIGURE 29-12 A flail anterior chest wall segment can be stabilized by securing (or having the patient hold) a pillow firmly against the chest wall.

Other Chest Injuries

Pulmonary Contusion

In addition to fracturing ribs, any severe blunt trauma of the chest can also injure the lung. The pulmonary alveoli become filled with blood, and edema fluid accumulates in the injured area, leaving the patient hypoxic. Severe **pulmonary contusion**, bruising of the lung, usually develops over a period of hours. If you believe that a patient may have a pulmonary contusion, you should provide respiratory support and supplemental oxygen to ensure adequate ventilation.

Traumatic Asphyxia

Sometimes, a patient will experience a sudden, severe compression of the chest, which produces a rapid increase in pressure within the chest. This may occur in an unrestrained driver who hits a steering wheel or a pedestrian who is compressed between a vehicle and a wall. The sudden increase in intrathoracic pressure results in a very characteristic appearance, including distended neck veins, cyanosis in the face and neck, and hemorrhage into the sclera of the eye, signaling the bursting of small blood vessels in the skin. These findings suggest an underlying injury to the heart and probably pulmonary contusions. You should provide ventilatory support with supplemental oxygen and monitor the patient's vital signs, as you provide immediate transport.

Blunt Myocardial Injury

As we have seen, blunt trauma to the chest may injure the heart itself, making it unable to maintain adequate blood pressure. There is much debate in the medical literature over how to assess **myocardial contusion**, or bruising of the heart muscle. Often, the pulse rate is irregular, but dangerous rhythms such as ventricular tachycardia and ventricular fibrillation are uncommon. There is no specific diagnostic test at this time, and there is no prehospital treatment for the condition. Still, you should suspect myocardial contusion in all cases of severe, blunt injury to the chest. Check the patient's pulse carefully, and note any irregularities.

Pericardial Tamponade

In pericardial tamponade, blood or other fluid collects in the pericardium, the fibrous sac surrounding the heart. This prevents the heart from filling during the diastolic phase, causing decreased cardiac output (the amount of blood the heart pumps out per minute) and decreased blood pressure. Ultimately, as blood accumulates within the pericardial cavity, it compresses the heart to the point at which cardiac output drops to zero and the patient goes into cardiac arrest. Signs and symptoms of pericardial tamponade include very soft and faint heart tones, often called muffled heart sounds, a weak pulse, low blood pressure, a narrowing of the pulse pressure, which is the difference between the systolic and diastolic pressures, and congested and distended veins in the upper part of the body, particularly the veins of the neck.

In a trauma situation, even a small amount of fluid in the pericardial sac is enough to cause pericardial tamponade and death. (Occasionally, fluid in surprisingly large amounts may collect in the pericardial sac as a chronic condition.) Pericardial tamponade is relatively uncommon, seen more often with penetrating injuries to the heart itself than with blunt injuries to the chest. If you suspect this life-threatening condition, provide vigorous respiratory support, supplemental oxygen, and prompt transport. Be sure to notify the hospital of your suspicions so that preparations can be made for immediate treatment.

Laceration of the Great Vessels

The chest contains several large blood vessels: the superior vena cava, the inferior vena cava, the main pulmonary artery, four main pulmonary veins, and the aorta, with its major arteries distributing blood throughout the body. Injury to any of these vessels may be accompanied by massive, rapidly fatal hemorrhage. Any patient with a chest wound who shows signs of shock may have an injury to one or more of these vessels. Frequently, blood loss is not obvious, because it remains within the chest cavity.

Emergency treatment for these patients includes CPR, ventilatory support, and supplemental oxygen. Here, particularly, immediate transport to the hospital may be critical. For some of these patients, a few minutes can mean the difference between life and death.

prep kit

ready for review

There are two types of chest injuries: penetrating, or open injuries and blunt, or closed, injuries. In blunt trauma, a blow to the chest may fracture the ribs, the sternum, or whole areas of the chest wall. Other problems include bruising of the lungs and the heart and possible damage to the aorta. Even if the skin and chest wall are not broken, the contents of the chest may be injured.

A sucking chest wound can result in an open pneumothorax, in which air entering through the wound accumulates in the pleural space, causing the lung to collapse. You should seal the wound with a sterile dressing, either taping it down on all four sides or creating a flutter valve. Sealing all four sides may create a tension pneumothorax, in which air leaking from a lacerated lung is unable to escape and so pressures the lung into collapsing. Eventually, this air may push the mediastinum into the opposite pleural cavity and cut off venous blood to the heart, causing cardiac arrest. A tension pneumothorax can also occur in a closed, blunt injury of the chest in which a fractured rib lacerates the surface of the lung. Look for increasing respiratory distress, distended neck veins, shock, and decreased breath sounds on one side. You may need to partly remove the dressing to relieve the underlying tension in the chest. The accumulation of blood in the chest is called a hemothorax; the collection of blood and air is called a hemopneumothorax.

A fractured rib may lacerate the surface of the lung, causing some type of pneumothorax. A sign of this is a crackly feeling to the skin in the area. Multiple rib fractures, with or without a fracture of the sternum, often result in a condition called flail chest; a portion of the chest wall is detached from the thoracic cage and moves during respiration in a fashion that is the opposite of normal. A flail chest causes very painful breathing and requires respiratory support and supplemental oxygen. It may help to immobilize the flail segment with a pad.

Other chest injuries include contusions of the lungs and heart and traumatic asphyxia, in which a sudden, severe compression of the chest produces a rapid increase in intrathoracic pressure. Signs of this condition include distended neck veins, cyanosis in the face, and hemorrhage in the sclera. Provide ventilatory support, monitor vital signs, and provide immediate transport. In pericardial tamponade, blood collects in the pericardium, preventing the heart from filling during the diastolic phase and eventually causing cardiac arrest. Signs include muffled heart sounds, a weak pulse, low blood pressure, and distended neck veins. Here as well, you should provide vigorous respiratory support and immediate transport. Laceration of the large blood vessels in the chest can cause a fatal hemorrhage. Suspect such a wound in any patient with a chest wound who shows signs of shock, even if you see little blood; it may be collecting within the chest cavity. This person needs CPR, ventilatory support, supplemental oxygen, and immediate transport.

vital vocabulary

closed (blunt) chest injury Injury to the chest in which the skin is not broken, usually due to blunt trauma.

dyspnea Difficulty with breathing.

flail chest A condition in which three or more ribs are fractured in two or more places, or in association with a fracture of the sternum so that a segment of chest wall is effectively detached from the rest of the thoracic cage.

flutter valve A one-way valve that allows air to leave the chest cavity but not return.

hemoptysis The spitting or coughing up of blood.

hemothorax A collection of blood in the pleural cavity.

myocardial contusion A bruise of the heart muscle.

open chest injury Injury to the chest in which the chest wall itself is penetrated by some object.

paradoxical motion The motion of the portion of the chest wall that is detached in a flail chest; the motion is exactly the opposite of normal motion during breathing: in during inhalation, out during exhalation.

www.emtb.com

pericardial tamponade Acute compression of the heart due to a buildup of blood or other fluid in the pericardial sac.

pericardium The fibrous sac that surrounds the heart.

pneumothorax An accumulation of air or gas in the pleural cavity.

pulmonary contusion A bruise of the lung.

spontaneous pneumothorax Pneumothorax that occurs when a weak area on the lung ruptures spontaneously, allowing air to leak into the pleural space.

sucking chest wound An open or penetrating chest wall wound through which air passes during inspiration and expiration.

tachypnea Rapid respirations.

tension pneumothorax An accumulation of air or gas in the pleural cavity that progressively increases and causes a rise in intrathoracic pressure.

assessment in action

You and your partner are dispatched to a local liquor store for a shooting. En route, you recall reading in the newspaper that the same store was robbed 3 weeks ago. You learn upon arrival that the store owner had purchased a handgun and shot the robber twice in the chest.

You find the 22-year-old patient lying on the floor in a large puddle of blood. He has one entrance wound in the left shoulder and a second wound just under the left clavicle, which is bleeding profusely. During your initial assessment, you are unable to palpate a radial pulse, but you manage to find a fast, weak carotid pulse. Between the patient's moaning and crying, you determine that he has respirations of more than 40 breaths/min.

1. Because the patient is moaning, crying, and talking, you know that his airway is open. However, he reports that he is having difficulty breathing and has shoulder pain. Your first step in caring for the patient is to:
   A. apply and quickly inflate all three compartments of the PASG.
   B. cover the wounds, give oxygen, and prepare to transport.
   C. obtain a complete set of vital signs and then check breath sounds.
   D. complete a detailed physical examination and prepare to transport.

2. What additional intervention has a high priority at this time?
   A. Obtaining the patient's name and Social Security number
   B. Checking for equal grip strength in the patient's hands
   C. Determining whether the patient has insurance coverage
   D. Contacting the receiving hospital to report on the patient

3. The patient has very minimal breath sounds on the left side and appears to be very anxious and seems to be struggling to breathe. His neck veins are distended, and his pulse is so fast and weak that it is almost imperceptible. These signs and symptoms suggest:
   A. fractured ribs.
   B. a serious infection.
   C. a tension pneumothorax.
   D. an upper airway obstruction.

4. The principal reason for placing occlusive dressings over gunshot wounds is to help prevent:
   A. scarring.
   B. air from entering the chest.
   C. the patient from seeing them.
   D. serious heat loss from the chest.

5. Which of the following findings would be considered the **LEAST** significant aspect of this call?
   A. The patient was found in a supine position.
   B. The patient has two open chest wounds.
   C. The patient is having difficulty breathing.
   D. You could not obtain a radial pulse initially.

points to ponder

Object. 1-3.6, 1-5.28, 3-3.2, 3-3.4, 3-3.7

You are assessing a middle-aged woman with chest injury and difficulty breathing. She has cyanosis around her lips, her respirations are 44/min, and they are shallow and labored. She was thrown against the dashboard during an automobile accident. During the trauma assessment, you ask to bare her chest to look for discoloration, deformity, or paradoxical breathing because you suspect a flail chest. The patient refuses to allow you to open her blouse or even lift it up to look. You ask whether a woman at the scene could look for you, and the patient refuses to allow that also.

- How would you adequately assess this woman's injuries? How else might you convince her to allow you to look at the injuries? How would you treat this injury if you could not look for paradoxical breathing? What are some possible reasons why the patient would refuse to be examined?

online outlook

Chest injuries are both very common and, given the likelihood of damage to the heart, lungs, or great blood vessels, very serious. Test your ability to anticipate and identify different chest injuries by completing Exercise 29 at www.emtb.com.

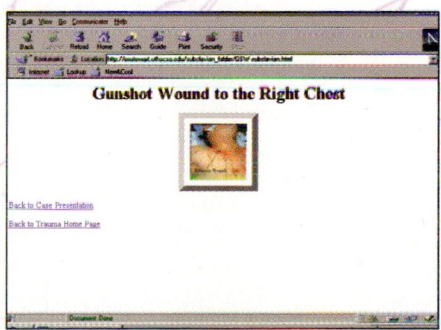

prep kit 29

Abdomen and Genitalia Injuries

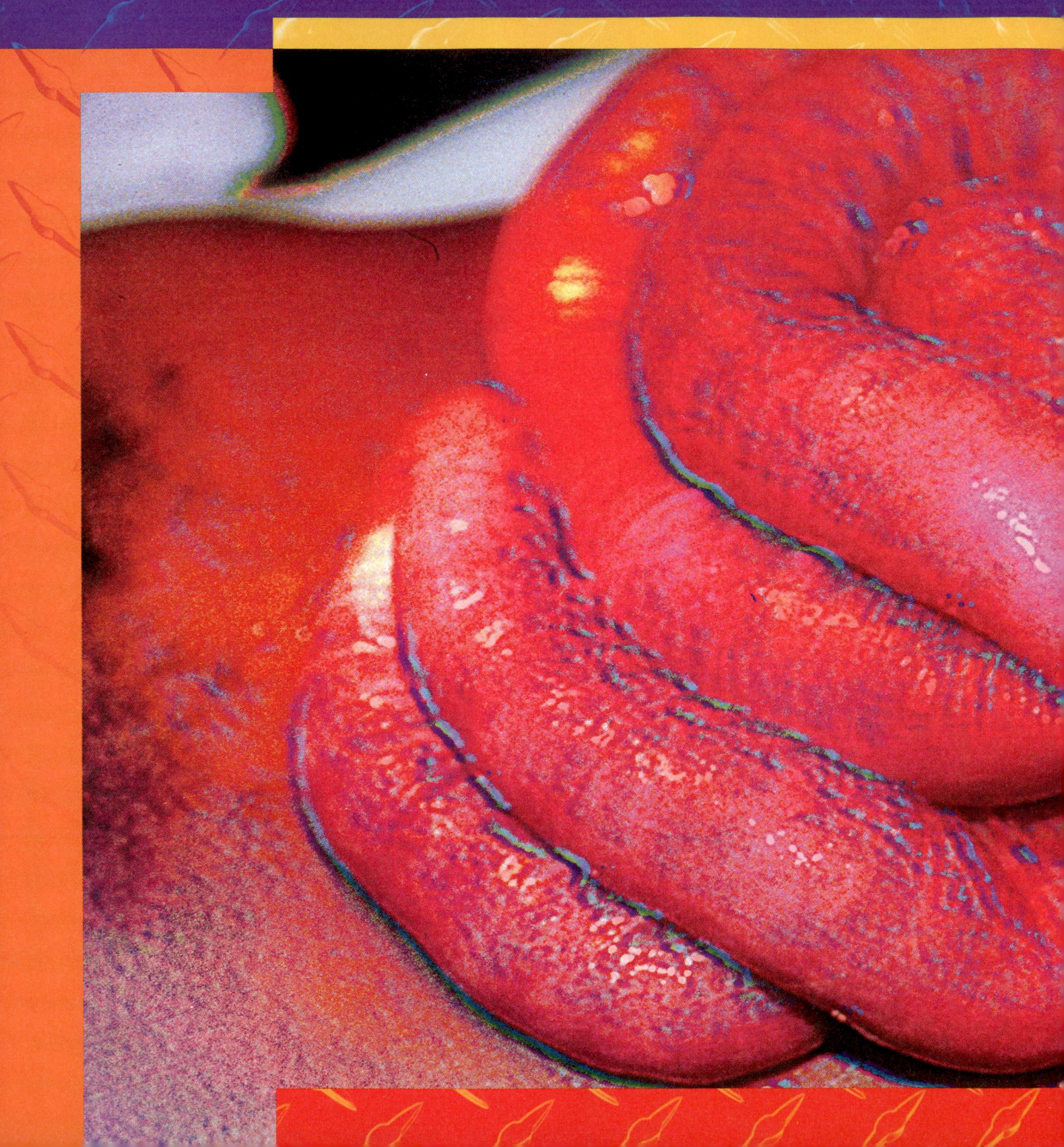

objectives*

Cognitive

1. State the steps in the emergency medical care of a patient with a blunt or penetrating abdominal injury.

2. Describe how solid and hollow organs can be injured.

3. State the steps in the emergency medical care of a patient with an object impaled in the abdomen.

4. State the steps in the emergency medical care of a patient with an abdominal evisceration wound.

5. State the steps in the emergency medical care of the patient with a genitourinary injury.

Affective

None

Psychomotor

6. Demonstrate proper treatment of a patient who has an object impaled in the abdomen.

7. Demonstrate how to apply a dressing to an abdominal evisceration wound.

* These are non-curriculum objectives.

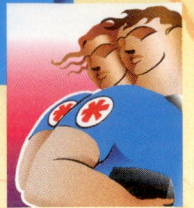

you are the emt

Squad 6, respond to the George Washington High School cafeteria for a girl with abdominal pain. Your partner laughs and comments that the girl probably has nothing more than an upset stomach from lunch.

A number of very serious conditions may first appear as abdominal pain. Therefore, you should not make any assumptions on calls of this nature because abdominal complaints are often complex problems. This chapter will help to prepare you to assess and manage abdominal problems. It will also help you to answer the following questions:

1. Why is assessing abdominal pain so difficult?
2. Do abdominal conditions more commonly affect women? If so, why?

Abdomen and Genitalia Injuries

The abdomen is the lower of the two major body cavities, extending from the diaphragm to the pelvis. It contains several organs that make up the digestive, urinary, and genitourinary systems. Although any of these organs may be injured, some are better protected than others. You must know where these organs are located within the abdominal or pelvic cavities. You must also understand their functions so that when an illness or injury occurs, you can assess its seriousness.

This chapter begins with a brief review of the anatomy of the abdomen, followed by a discussion of common types of abdominal injuries. Next, patient assessment strategies are discussed, followed by a description of specific abdominal injuries that you are likely to encounter and how to treat each. The genitourinary system is then described, and common injuries and treatment are discussed.

The Anatomy of the Abdomen

The abdomen contains both hollow and solid organs, any of which may be damaged. **Hollow organs**, including the stomach, intestines, ureters, and bladder, are actually tubes through which materials pass (Figure 30-1). They usually contain food that is in the process of being digested, urine that is being passed to the bladder for release, or bile. When ruptured or lacerated, these organs

spill their contents into the **peritoneal cavity** (the abdominal cavity), causing an intense inflammatory reaction called **peritonitis**. The first signs of peritonitis are severe abdominal pain, tenderness, and muscular spasm. Later, normal bowel sounds diminish or disappear as the bowel stops functioning. A patient may feel nauseous and may vomit; the abdomen becomes distended and firm to touch.

The **solid organs**, as their name suggests, are solid masses of tissue. They include the liver, spleen, pan-

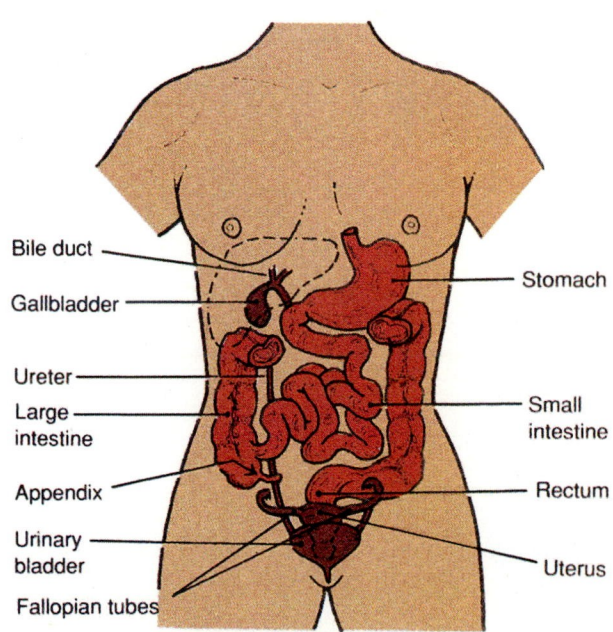

FIGURE 30-1 The hollow organs in the abdominal cavity are actually tubes through which materials pass.

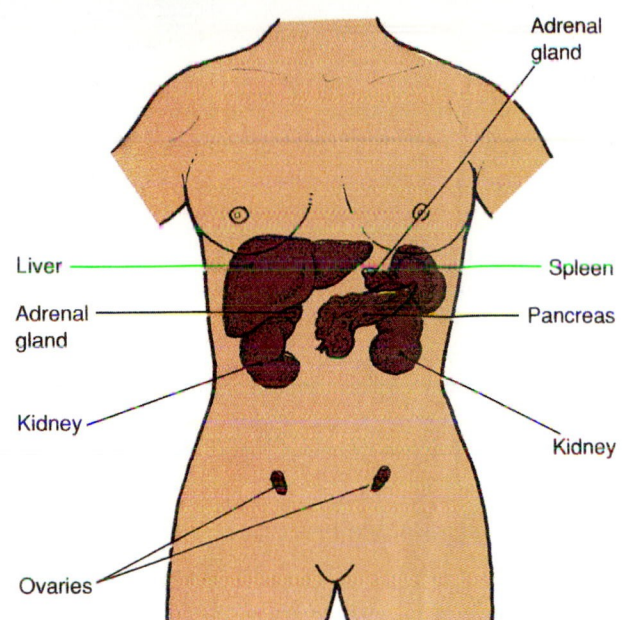

FIGURE 30-2 The solid organs are solid masses of tissue that do much of the chemical work in the body.

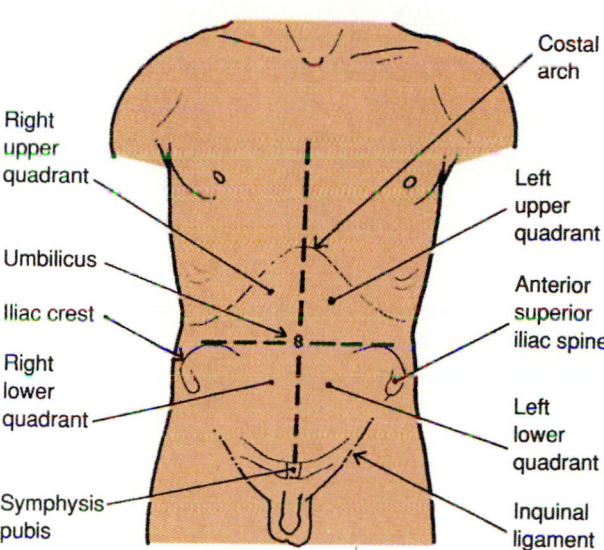

FIGURE 30-3 The abdominal cavity is divided into four quadrants, which serve as your means of identifying and reporting problems in the abdomen.

creas, and kidneys (Figure 30-2). It is here that much of the chemical work of the body—digestion, excretion, and energy production—takes place. Solid organs have a rich blood supply, so injury can cause severe hemorrhage. The same is true of the aorta or inferior vena cava, whether the injury is open or closed. Unlike gastric juices and bacteria, blood within the peritoneal cavity does not provoke an inflammatory response. Therefore, the absence of pain and tenderness does not necessarily mean the absence of major bleeding in the abdomen.

The bony landmarks in the abdomen include the symphysis pubis, the costal arch, the iliac crests, and the anterior superior iliac spines. The major soft-tissue landmark is the umbilicus, which overlies the fourth lumbar vertebra. The abdomen is divided arbitrarily into quadrants by two perpendicular lines that intersect at the umbilicus (Figure 30-3).

Injuries of the Abdomen

Abdominal injuries may be as obvious as loops of intestines protruding from a stab wound or as subtle as a laceration to the liver or spleen. Remember to follow BSI techniques as you begin your initial assessment; these injuries often bleed profusely, and even if they do not, some blood or other body fluid is likely to be present. Injuries of the abdomen are considered open or closed and can involve hollow and/or solid organs.

Closed abdominal injuries are those in which a severe blow damages the abdomen without breaking the skin; these are also known as blunt injuries. Such a blow might come from the patient's striking the handlebar of a bicycle or the steering wheel of a car (Figure 30-4). **Open abdominal injuries** are those in which a foreign object enters the abdomen and opens the peritoneal

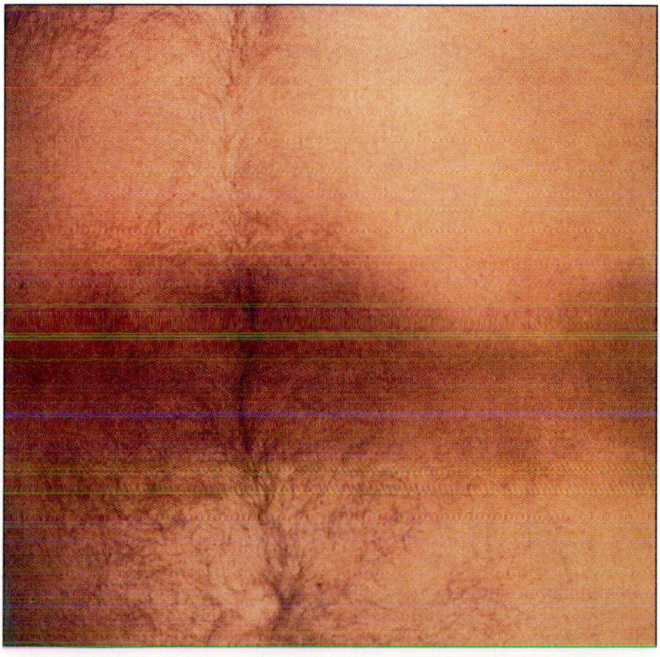

FIGURE 30-4 Blunt trauma to the abdomen can occur when a patient strikes the steering wheel of an automobile as a result of a crash.

cavity to the outside; these are also known as penetrating injuries (Figure 30-5). Stab wounds and gunshot wounds are examples of open injuries.

Signs and Symptoms

Patients with abdominal injuries generally have one principal complaint: pain. But other significant injuries may mask the pain at first, and some patients may not be able to tell you about pain because they are unconscious or unresponsive, such as after a head injury or drug or alcohol overdose. The most common sign of significant abdominal injury is an elevated heart rate. Later signs are those of shock: decreased blood pressure and pale, cool, moist skin. In some cases, the abdomen may become distended from the accumulation of blood and fluid. As an EMT-B, you must look for other clues. Blunt injuries

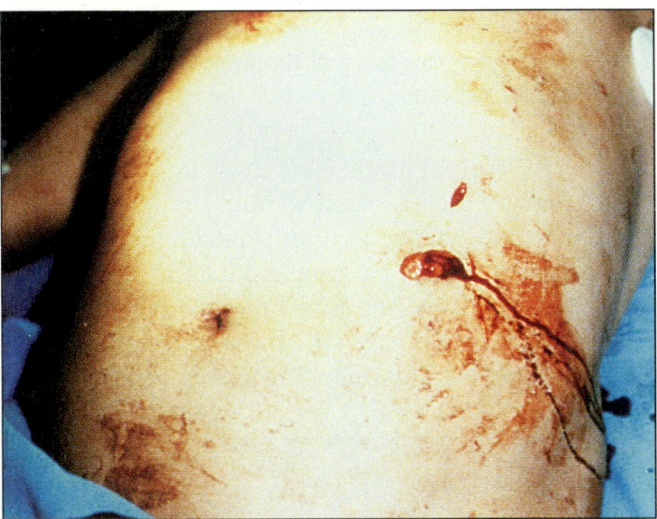

FIGURE 30-5 Penetrating injuries might not go deeper than the wall of the abdomen, but this is difficult to determine. Therefore, you must assume the worst—that organs have been damaged—and provide prompt transport.

include bruises or other visible marks, whose location should guide your attention to adjacent structures (Figure 30-6). For example, bruises in the right upper quadrant, left upper quadrant, or flank might suggest an injury to the liver, spleen, or kidney, respectively.

The signs of abdominal injury are usually more definite than the symptoms, including firmness on palpation of the abdomen, obvious entry and exit wounds, bruises, and altered vital signs such as low blood pressure, a rapid pulse, and rapid, shallow respirations (although this might not appear until later). Common symptoms include abdominal tenderness, particularly localized tenderness, and difficulty with movement because of pain.

Evaluating Abdominal Injuries

Your goal in initial assessment is to evaluate the patient's ABCD and then immediately care for any life threats. You should then begin the focused history and physical exam to determine the type of abdominal injury (open or closed), the extent of the damage, and the presence of shock. Note that patients may or may not be able to tell you about the severity and location of their pain. However, they may report that they feel nauseous, and they may vomit. Remember to keep the airway clear of vomitus so that it is not aspirated into the lungs, especially in a patient who is unconscious or has an altered level of consciousness. Turn the patient to one side, using spinal precautions if necessary, and try to clear any material from the throat and mouth. Note the nature of the vomitus: undigested food, blood, mucus, or bile.

Normally, you will evaluate all patients with abdominal injuries in the same manner. First, you should place the patient in a supine position with the knees slightly flexed and supported (Figure 30-7). Remove or loosen clothes. Then, before you do anything else, assess and record baseline vital signs. Many abdominal emergen-

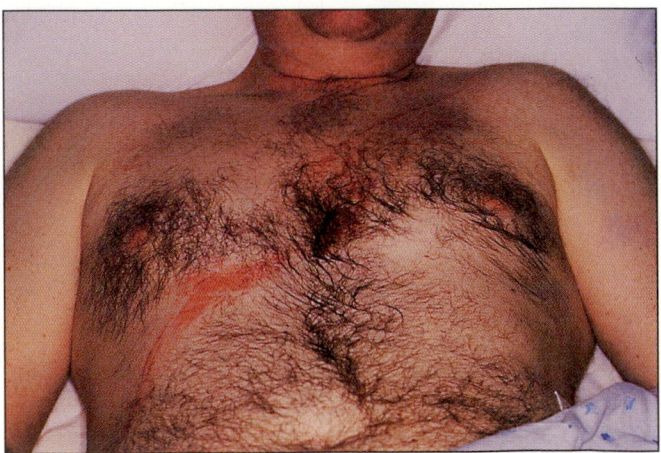

FIGURE 30-6 Bruising on the abdomen can provide clues to the possibility of injury to the underlying organs.

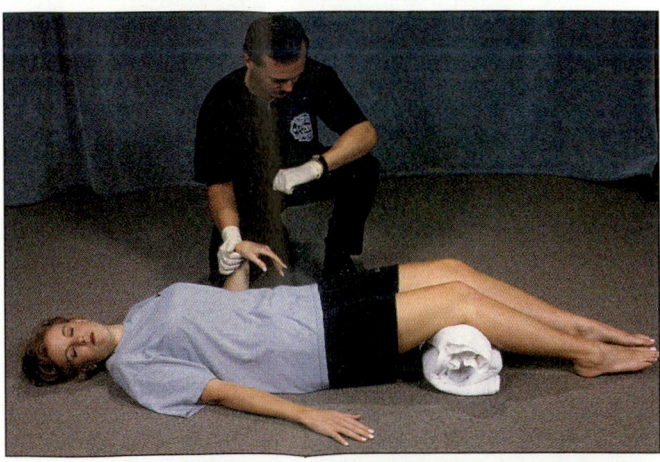

FIGURE 30-7 Patients with abdominal injuries should be placed in a supine position with the knees slightly flexed and supported.

cies, aside from those that cause severe bleeding, can cause a rapid pulse and low blood pressure. Your record of vital signs, made as early as possible and periodically thereafter, will be of tremendous help to physicians in evaluating the problem when the patient arrives in the emergency department.

Quickly assess the patient's condition with a simple inspection, noting the manner in which he or she is lying. Movement of the body or the abdominal organs irritates the inflamed peritoneum, causing additional pain. To minimize this pain, patients will lie still, usually with the knees drawn up, and breathe rapidly and shallowly. For the same reason, they will contract their abdominal muscles, a sign called **guarding**.

Next, inspect the skin of the abdomen for holes through which bullets, knives, or other missile-type foreign bodies may have passed. Keep in mind that the size of the wound does not necessarily indicate the extent of underlying injuries. If you find an entry wound, you must always check for a corresponding exit hole in the patient's back or sides. If the injury was caused by a very high-velocity missile from a rifle, you may see a small, harmless-looking entrance wound with a large, gaping exit wound. Do not attempt to remove a knife or other object that is impaled in the patient. Instead, stabilize the object with supportive bandaging. Bruises or other visible marks are important clues to the cause and severity of any blunt injury. Steering wheels and seat belts produce characteristic patterns of bruising on the abdomen or chest.

Types of Abdominal Injuries

Blunt Abdominal Wounds

A patient with a blunt abdominal wound may have one or some combination of the following:

- Severe bruises of the abdominal wall
- Laceration of the liver and spleen
- Rupture of the intestine
- Tears in the *mesentery*, membranous folds that attach the intestines to the walls of the body, and injury to blood vessels within them
- Rupture of the kidneys, or tearing of the kidneys from their arteries and veins
- Rupture of the bladder, especially in a patient who had been drinking and therefore had a full and distended bladder at the time of the crash
- Severe intra-abdominal hemorrhage
- Peritoneal irritation and inflammation in response to the rupture of hollow organs

A patient who has sustained a blunt abdominal injury should be log rolled to a supine position on a backboard. Ensure that you protect the spine as you do so. If the patient vomits, turn him or her to one side and clear the mouth and throat of vomitus. Monitor the vital signs for any indication of shock such as pallor; cold sweat; rapid, thready pulse; or low blood pressure. If you see any of these signs, administer supplemental oxygen via nonrebreathing mask, and take all the appropriate measures to combat shock. Keep the patient warm with blankets, and provide prompt transport to the emergency department.

Injuries from Seat Belts and Airbags

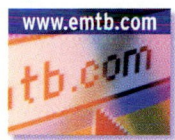

Seat belts have prevented many thousands of injuries and saved many lives, including those of people who otherwise would have been thrown out of a smashed car. However, seat belts occasionally cause blunt injuries of the abdominal organs. When worn properly, a seat belt lies below the anterior superior iliac spines of the pelvis and against the hip joints. If the belt lies too high, it can squeeze abdominal organs or great vessels against the spine when the car suddenly decelerates or stops (Figure 30-8). Occasionally, fractures of the lumbar spine have been reported. If you are called to the scene of such an accident, keep in mind that the use of seat belts in many cases turns what could have been a fatal injury into a manageable one.

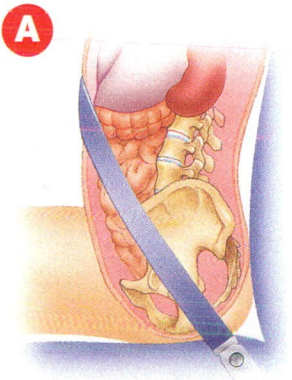
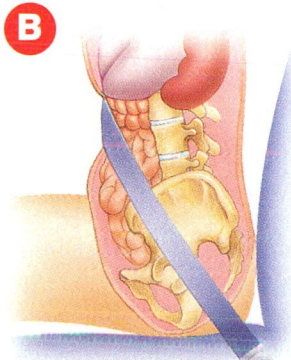
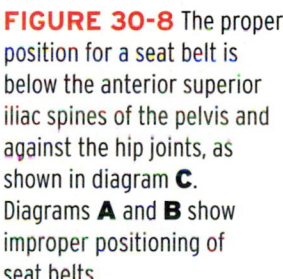
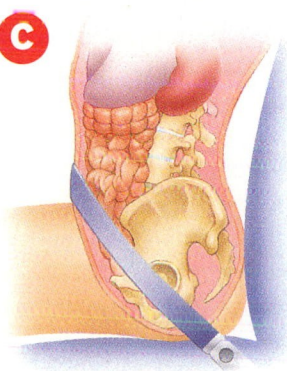

FIGURE 30-8 The proper position for a seat belt is below the anterior superior iliac spines of the pelvis and against the hip joints, as shown in diagram **C**. Diagrams **A** and **B** show improper positioning of seat belts.

In all current-model automobiles, the lap and diagonal (shoulder) safety belts are combined into one so that they may not be used independently. Of course, people can still place the diagonal portion of the belt behind the back, significantly reducing the effectiveness of this design. In some older cars, only lap belts or two separate belts are provided. Used alone, diagonal shoulder safety belts can cause injuries of the upper part of the trunk, such as a bruised chest, fractured ribs, lacerated liver, or even decapitation. Far fewer head and neck injuries are seen when this belt is used in combination with a lap belt and a head rest.

The airbag, which is standard in today's vehicles, is a great advance in automotive safety. In head-on collisions, it can be a genuine lifesaver. However, because frontal airbags provide no protection in a side impact or rollover accident, they must be used in combination with safety belts. Small children and short individuals who are in the front seat of the automobile may be at risk of injury when the airbag is deployed. Special attention should be used in evaluating these patients when a deployed airbag is noted.

Penetrating Abdominal Injuries

Patients with penetrating injuries generally have obvious wounds and external bleeding. A large wound may have bowel, fat, or a fold of peritoneum protruding from it. In addition to pain, these patients often report nausea and vomiting. Patients with peritonitis generally prefer to lie very still with their legs drawn up because it hurts to move or straighten their legs. They may complain about every bump in the road during transport.

Some penetrating injuries go no deeper than the abdominal wall, but the severity of the injury can be hard to determine. Only a surgeon can accurately assess the damage. Therefore, as you care for a patient with this type of wound, you should assume that the object has penetrated the peritoneum, entered the abdominal cavity, and possibly injured one or more organs even if there are no immediate obvious signs.

If major blood vessels are cut or major solid organs are lacerated, bleeding may be rapid and severe. Other signs of intra-abdominal injuries may develop slowly, particularly in penetrating wounds to hollow organs. Once such an organ is punctured and its contents are discharged into the abdominal cavity, peritonitis will follow. But this may take several hours.

In caring for a patient with a penetrating wound of the abdomen, you should follow the same steps that are prescribed for care of a blunt abdominal wound (Figure 30-9):

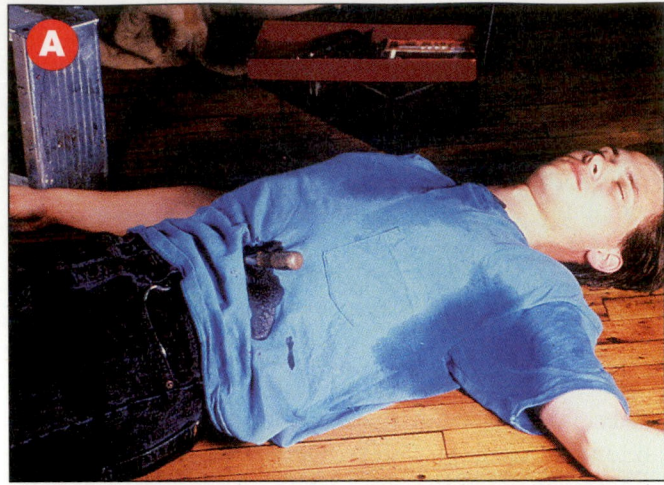

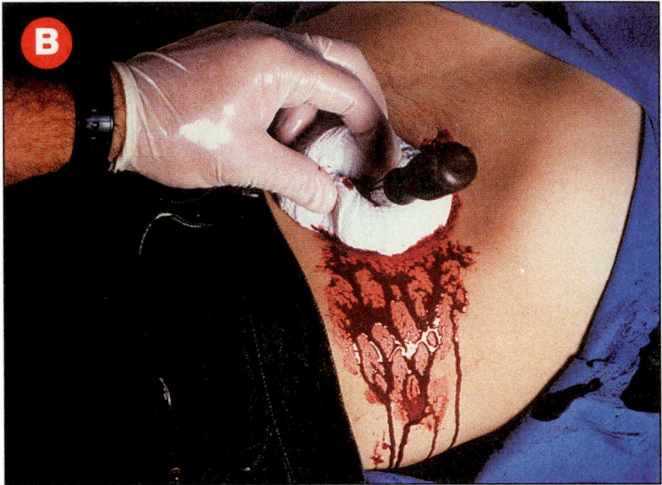

FIGURE 30-9 A: Penetrating injuries have obvious wounds and may also have external bleeding. **B:** If the penetrating object is still in place, use a roller bandage to stabilize the object and to control bleeding.

1. Inspect the patient's back and sides for exit wounds.
2. Apply a dry, sterile dressing to all open wounds.
3. If the penetrating object is still in place, apply a stabilizing bandage around it to control external bleeding and to minimize movement of the object.

Abdominal Evisceration

Severe lacerations of the abdominal wall may result in an **evisceration**, in which internal organs or fat protrude through the wound (Figure 30-10). Never try to replace an organ that is protruding from an abdominal laceration, whether it is a small fold of peritoneum or nearly all of the intestines. Instead, cover it with sterile gauze compresses moistened with sterile saline solution, and secure them with a sterile dressing. Because the open abdomen radiates body heat very effectively, and because exposed organs lose fluid rapidly, you must keep the organs moist and warm. If you do not have gauze compresses, you may use moist, sterile dressings, covered and secured in place with a bandage and tape (Figure 30-11). Do not use any material that is adherent or loses its substance when wet, such as toilet paper, facial tissue, paper towels, or absorbent cotton.

Once you have covered the extruding organ, you should provide other emergency care as necessary and provide prompt transport to the emergency department.

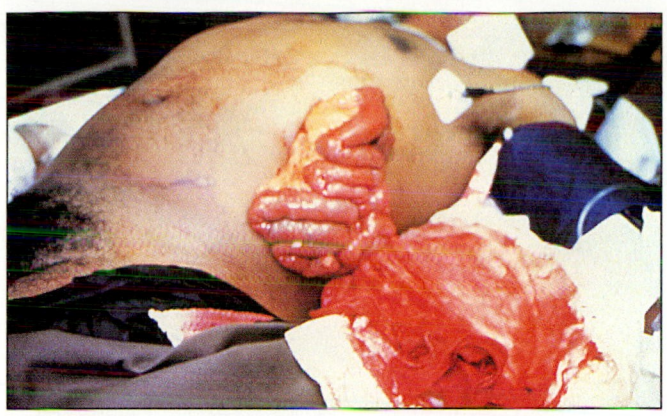

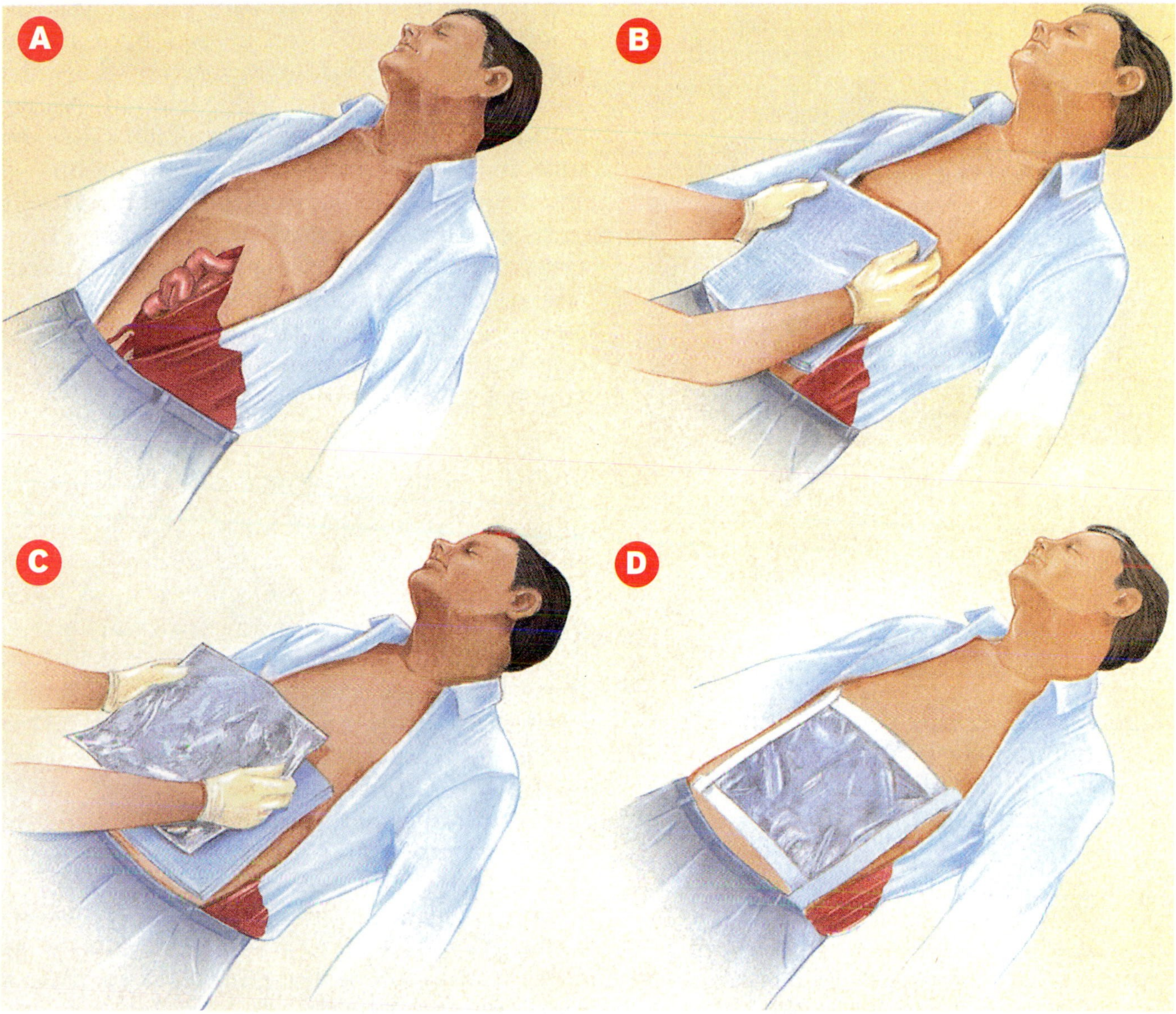

FIGURE 30-10 An abdominal evisceration is an open wound in the abdominal cavity in which internal organs or fat protrude from the wound.

FIGURE 30-11 A: The open abdomen radiates body heat rapidly and must be covered. **B:** Cover the wound with moistened sterile gauze. **C:** Secure the dressing with a bandage. **D:** Secure the bandage with tape.

Anatomy of the Genitourinary System

The genitourinary system controls both the reproductive functions and the waste discharge system, which are generally considered together.

The urinary system controls the discharge of certain waste materials filtered from the blood by the kidneys. In the urinary system, the kidneys are solid organs; the ureters, bladder, and urethra are hollow organs (Figure 30-12).

The genital system controls the reproductive processes from which life is created. The male genitalia, except for the prostate gland and the seminal vesicles, lie outside the pelvic cavity (Figure 30-13). The female genitalia, except for the vulva, clitoris, and labia, are contained entirely within the pelvis (Figure 30-14). The male and female reproductive organs have certain similarities and, of course, basic differences. They allow for the production of sperm and egg cells and appropriate hormones, the act of intercourse, and, ultimately, reproduction.

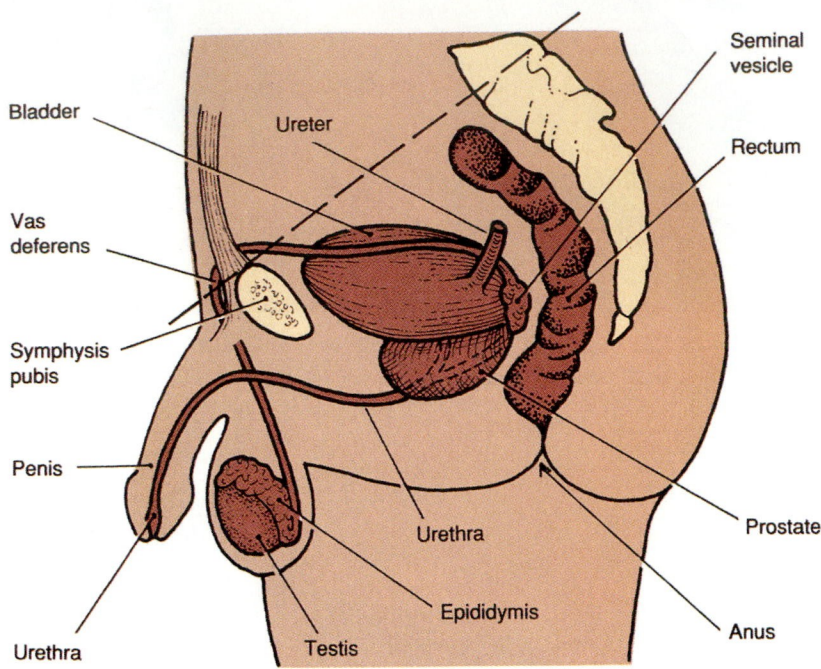

FIGURE 30-13 The male reproductive system includes the testicles, vasa deferentia, seminal vesicles, prostate gland, urethra, and penis.

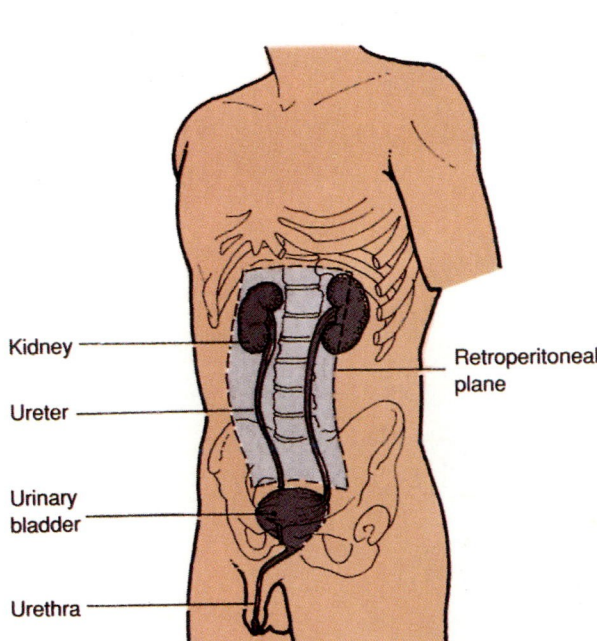

FIGURE 30-12 The urinary system lies in the retroperitoneal space behind the digestive tract. The kidneys are solid organs; the ureter, bladder, and urethra are hollow organs.

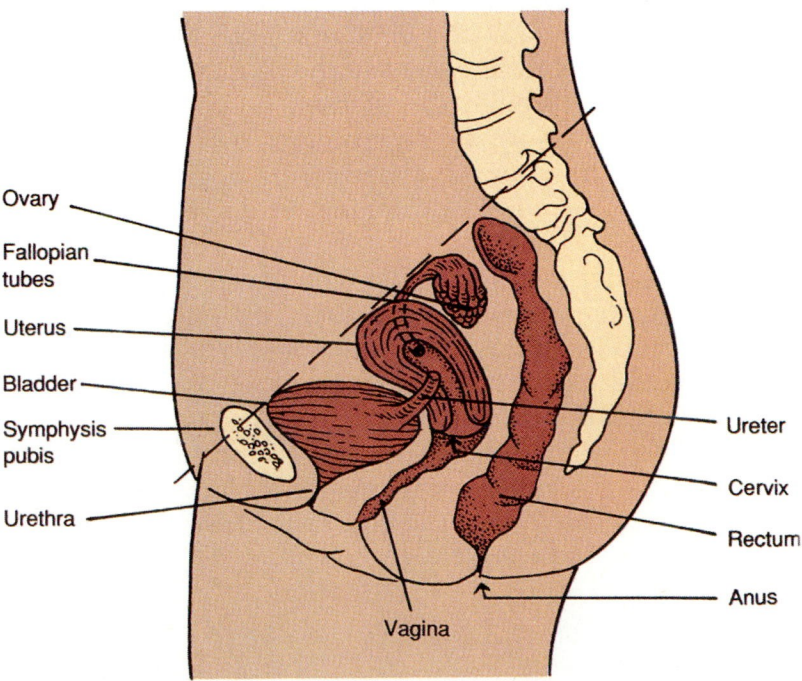

FIGURE 30-14 The female reproductive system includes the ovaries, fallopian tubes, uterus, cervix, and vagina.

Injuries of the Genitourinary System

Injuries of the Kidney

Injuries of the kidney are not unusual and rarely occur in isolation. This is because the kidneys lie in such a well-protected area of the body. A penetrating wound that reaches the kidneys almost always involves other organs. The same is true with blunt injuries. A blow that is forceful enough to cause significant kidney damage almost always damages other intra-abdominal organs, often fracturing a rib as well. Less significant injuries to the kidneys may result from a direct blow or even from a tackle in football (Figure 30-15). Suspect kidney damage if the patient has a history or physical evidence of any of the following findings:

- An abrasion, laceration, or contusion in the flank
- A penetrating wound in the region of the lower rib cage (the flank) or the upper abdomen
- Fractures on either side of the lower rib cage or of the lower thoracic or upper lumbar vertebrae

Damage to the kidneys may not be obvious on inspection of the patient. You may or may not see bruises or lacerations on the overlying skin. However, you will see signs of shock if the injury is associated with significant blood loss. Because one of the functions of the kidney is the formation of urine, another sign of kidney damage is blood in the urine, called **hematuria**. Treat shock and associated injuries in the appropriate manner. Provide prompt transport to the hospital, monitoring the patient's vital signs carefully en route.

Injury of the Urinary Bladder

Injury of the urinary bladder, either blunt or penetrating, may result in its rupture. When this happens, urine spills into the surrounding tissues, and any urine that passes through the urethra is likely to be bloody. Blunt injuries of the lower abdomen or pelvis often cause rupture of the urinary bladder, particularly when the bladder is full and distended. Sharp, bony fragments from a fracture of the pelvis often perforate the urinary bladder (Figure 30-16). Penetrating wounds of the lower midabdomen or the *perineum* (the pelvic floor and associated structures that occupy the pelvic outlet) can directly involve the bladder. In the male, sudden deceleration from a motor vehicle or motorcycle crash can literally shear the bladder from the urethra.

Suspect a possible injury of the urinary bladder if you see blood at the urethral opening or physical signs of trauma on the lower abdomen, pelvis, or perineum. There may be blood at the tip of the penis or a stain on the patient's underwear. If possible, save any urine passed by a patient with suspected bladder injury for detailed analysis in the emergency department, even if the urine does not look bloody. Under a microscope, even a tiny number of red blood cells will show up.

The presence of associated injuries or of shock will dictate the urgency of transport. In most instances, provide prompt transport, and monitor the patient's vital signs en route.

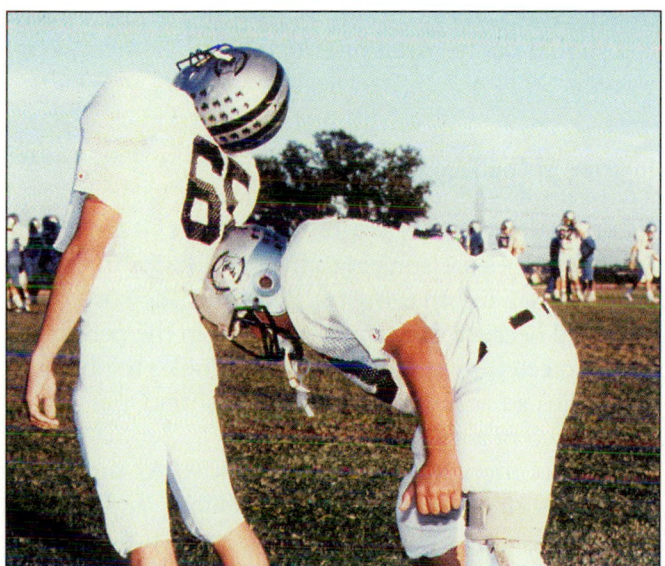

FIGURE 30-15 A tackle in football can result in blunt trauma to the lower rib cage or the flank, resulting in kidney injury.

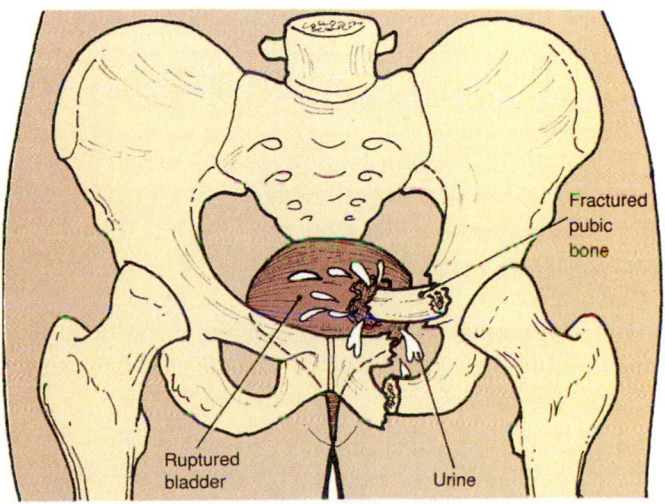

FIGURE 30-16 Fracture of the pelvis can result in a laceration of the bladder by the bony fragments. Urine then leaks into the pelvis.

Injuries of the External Male Genitalia

Injuries of the external male genitalia include all types of soft-tissue wounds. Although these injuries are uniformly painful and generally a source of great concern to the patient, they are rarely life threatening. Especially in industrial accidents, avulsion (tearing away) of the skin of the penis can occur, particularly in the uncircumcised male. If you encounter a patient with such an injury, wrap the penis in a soft, sterile dressing moistened with sterile saline solution, and transport the patient promptly. Use direct pressure to control any bleeding. You should try to save and preserve the avulsed skin, but do not delay treatment or transport for more than a few minutes to do so.

Managing blood loss is your top priority in amputation of the penile shaft, whether partial or complete. You should use local pressure with a sterile dressing on the remaining stump. Never apply a constricting device to the penis to control bleeding. Surgical reconstruction of even a completely amputated penis is possible if you can locate the amputated part. Wrap it in a moist, sterile dressing; place it in a plastic bag; and transport it in a cooled container without allowing it to come in direct contact with ice.

If the connective tissue surrounding the erectile tissue in the penis is severely damaged, the shaft of the penis can be fractured or severely angled, sometimes requiring surgical repair. The injury may occur during particularly active sexual intercourse. It is associated with intense pain, bleeding into the tissues, and fear. Provide prompt transport to the emergency department.

Accidental laceration of the skin about the head of the penis usually occurs when the penis is erect and is associated with heavy bleeding. The injury usually appears worse than it actually is; once the penis becomes flaccid, the size of the laceration decreases. Local pressure with a sterile dressing is usually sufficient to stop the hemorrhage.

It is not uncommon for the skin of the shaft of the penis or the foreskin to get caught in the zipper of pants. If a small segment of the zipper is involved (one or two teeth), you can try to unzip the pants. If a longer segment is involved or the patient is agitated, use heavy scissors to cut the zipper out of the pants to make the patient more comfortable during transport. Be sure to explain what the scissors are for before you begin cutting.

Urethral injuries in the male are uncommon. Lacerations of the urethra can result from straddle injuries, pelvic fractures, or penetrating wounds of the perineum. These injuries may bleed quite a lot, although this may not be evident externally. Direct pressure with a dry, sterile dressing usually controls any external hemorrhage. Because the urethra is the channel for urine, it is very important to know whether the patient can urinate and whether hematuria is present. For this reason, you should save any voided urine for later examination at the hospital. Any foreign bodies that may be protruding from the urethra will have to be removed in a surgical setting.

Avulsion of the skin of the scrotum may damage the scrotal contents. If possible, preserve the avulsed skin in a moist, sterile dressing for possible use in reconstruction. Wrap the scrotal contents or the perineal area with a sterile, moist compress, and use a local pressure dressing to control bleeding. Transport this patient promptly to the emergency department.

Direct blows to the scrotum can result in the rupture of a testicle or significant accumulation of blood around the testes. In either case, you should apply an ice pack to the scrotal area while transporting the patient.

A few general rules apply to the treatment of injuries involving the external male genitalia:

- These injuries are very painful. Make the patient as comfortable as possible.

- Use sterile, moist compresses to cover areas that have been stripped of skin.

- Apply direct pressure with dry, sterile gauze dressings to control bleeding.

- Never move or manipulate impaled instruments or foreign bodies in the urethra.

- If possible, always identify and bring avulsed parts to the hospital with the patient.

Remember, these are rarely life-threatening injuries and should not be given priority over other, more severe wounds.

Injuries of the Female Genitalia

Internal female genitalia. The uterus, ovaries, and fallopian tubes are subject to the same kinds of injuries as any other internal organ. However, they are rarely damaged because they are small, deep in the pelvis, and well protected by the pelvic bones. Unlike the bladder, which lies adjacent to the bony pelvis, they are usually not injured in a pelvic fracture.

An exception is the pregnant uterus. As pregnancy progresses, the uterus enlarges substantially and rises out of the pelvis, becoming vulnerable to both penetrating and blunt injuries. These injuries can be particularly severe because the uterus has a rich blood supply during pregnancy. You must also keep in mind that another life—that of the unborn child—is at risk. You can expect to see the signs and symptoms of shock with these patients; be prepared to provide all necessary support and prompt transport. Note that contractions may begin as well. If possible, ask the patient when she is due, and report this information to the hospital.

In the last trimester of pregnancy, the uterus is large and may obstruct the vena cava, decreasing the amount of blood returning to the heart if the patient is placed in a supine position. As a result, blood pressure may decrease. The patient should be carefully placed on her left side so that the uterus will not lie on the vena cava.

External female genitalia. The external female genitalia include the vulva, the clitoris, and the major and minor labia (lips) at the entrance of the vagina. The female urethra enters the anterior vagina. Injuries of the external female genitalia can include all types of soft-tissue injuries. Because these genital parts have a rich nerve supply, injuries are very painful. Lacerations, abrasions, and avulsions should be treated with moist, sterile compresses. Use local pressure to control bleeding and a diaper-type bandage to hold dressings in place. Under no circumstances should you pack or place dressings into the vagina. Leave any foreign bodies in place after you stabilize them with bandages.

In general, although these injuries are painful, they are not life threatening. Bleeding may be heavy, but it can usually be controlled by local compression. Contusions and other blunt injuries all require careful in-hospital evaluation. However, the urgency of the need for transport will be determined by associated injuries, the amount of hemorrhage, and the presence of shock.

Remember that victims of sexual assault, whether they are male or female, need medical assistance. In these cases, you must treat the medical injuries but also provide privacy, support, and reassurance.

prep kit

ready for review

Abdominal injuries are classified as either open (penetrating) or closed (blunt) in origin. Either type can damage both hollow organs, such as the stomach and ureters; and solid organs, such as the liver, spleen, and kidneys. Penetrating injuries are most frequently caused by knives or handguns; blunt injuries are often the result of a collision with a steering wheel. Both types of injury cause pain, although this may be masked at first.

These injuries are evaluated in a similar fashion. Place the patient in a supine position, assess and record vital signs, and perform a visual inspection. Always assume that major damage has occurred to abdominal organs, even if there are no obvious signs. Look for bruises or other marks that may point you toward underlying damage: a firm abdomen, difficulty in moving, abdominal tenderness and guarding, obvious entry and exit wounds, and altered vital signs. If hollow organs have spilled their contents into the peritoneal cavity, peritonitis will develop. In an effort to minimize the pain of this condition, patients will want to lie still with their knees drawn up. Treat for shock as necessary, keep the throat clear of vomitus, keep the patient warm, and promptly transport him or her to the emergency department.

Never try to replace an eviscerated organ; keep it warm and moist with sterile gauze compresses. Injuries to the kidneys or bladder will not have obvious external signs, but there are usually more subtle clues such as lower rib pain or a possible pelvic fracture. Always save urine passed by a patient with a suspected kidney or bladder injury so that it can be inspected later for hematuria. The external genitalia in both males and females can sustain injuries that can be extremely painful, but these are rarely life threatening.

vital vocabulary

www.emtb.com

closed abdominal injury   Any injury of the abdomen caused by a nonpenetrating instrument or force in which the skin remains intact. Also called blunt abdominal injury.

evisceration   The displacement of organs outside of the body.

guarding   Contracting the stomach muscles to minimize the pain of abdominal movement; a sign of peritonitis.

hematuria   The presence of blood in the urine.

hollow organs   Tubes through which materials pass, such as the stomach, small intestines, large intestines, ureters, and bladder.

open abdominal injury   Any injury of the abdomen caused by a penetrating or piercing instrument or force in which the skin is lacerated or perforated and the cavity itself is opened to the atmosphere. Also called penetrating injury.

peritoneal cavity   The abdominal cavity.

peritonitis   Inflammation of the peritoneum.

solid organs   Solid masses of tissue where much of the chemical work of the body takes place (e.g., the liver, spleen, pancreas, and kidneys).

prep kit
30

assessment in action

It's a hot, humid July evening, and you and your partner are covering the local rodeo. The bull-riding competition begins as the bull twists and turns out of the chute, launching the rider into the air and tossing him onto a fence. The 27-year-old cowboy falls on the other side of the fence, well away from the bull. Assessment reveals a large bruise developing across his abdomen. He states that, while he is having difficulty breathing, his chief complaint is abdominal pain. He has a blood pressure of 148/92 mm Hg, a pulse of 140/min, and respirations of 32/min. His skin is flushed and moist, and his pupils are equal and reactive to light.

1. Given the patient's mechanism of injury, manual immobilization of the cervical spine should be applied:
   A. immediately after the airway is secured.
   B. only after the detailed physical examination is completed.
   C. only after determining whether a physician is present at the scene.
   D. after the patient is in the ambulance and ready to transport.

2. Which of the following steps is the most important part of your examination of the patient's abdomen?
   A. Flexion
   B. Inspection
   C. Massage
   D. Auscultation

3. You should evaluate breath sounds:
   A. whenever you have time.
   B. as soon as the airway is open.
   C. only if the patient's respiratory status begins to deteriorate.
   D. once you have immobilized the patient to a long backboard.

4. The bruising over the patient's abdomen is becoming more prominent, and the abdomen is beginning to feel tight, suggesting:
   A. a punctured lung.
   B. a rapidly spreading infection.
   C. decreasing oxygen levels.
   D. continued internal bleeding.

5. The patient becomes very anxious en route to the hospital. His skin is cool and slightly moist. He has a blood pressure of 110/66 mm Hg, a pulse of 140/min, and respirations of 32/min. You suspect that the patient may:
   A. have heat exhaustion and require observation only.
   B. have a head injury and increasing intracranial pressure.
   C. be going into shock as a result of his injuries.
   D. be experiencing a normal response to his fear of the ambulance.

points to ponder

Object. 1-1.1, 1-1.2, 1-1.6, 1-3.7, 1-3.8,

You respond to a person in an alley near the homeless shelter who has been stabbed multiple times in the abdomen. You recognize the patient as a street person who has been around for a couple of years. You have talked with the patient many times before and have enjoyed those encounters. You contact the nearest hospital and establish medical control. It has been a relatively slow night, but when medical control finds out where the patient is located, they assume that the patient is homeless and unable to pay for services. The hospital immediately reports being overloaded and refers you to another hospital that is farther away.

• Would you immediately question their decision? If so, how? Would you report this action? If so, to whom? Is there a legal responsibility to accept all patients in the emergency department? Are these wounds possibly life threatening? If so, does that affect the hospital's ability to deny treatment? Does a prehospital response agency fall under these same requirements?

online outlook

The abdomen is the lower of the two major body cavities, extending from the diaphragm to the pelvis. You must know where the organs are located within the abdominal or pelvic cavities. Review your knowledge by completing Exercise 30 at www.emtb.com.

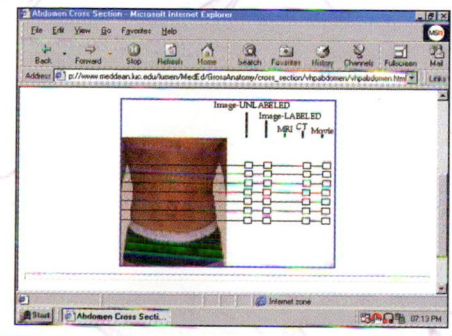

Musculoskeletal Care

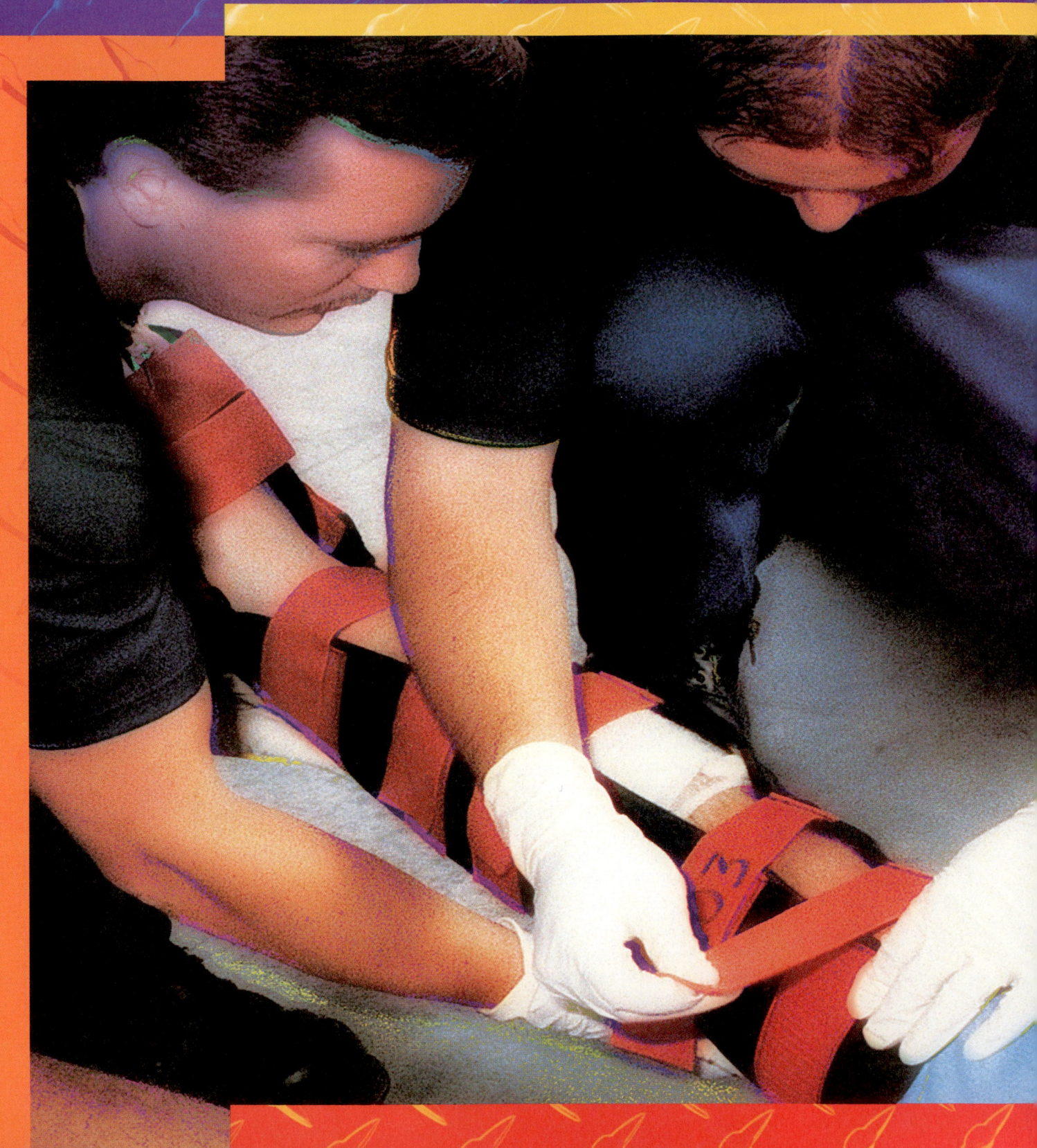

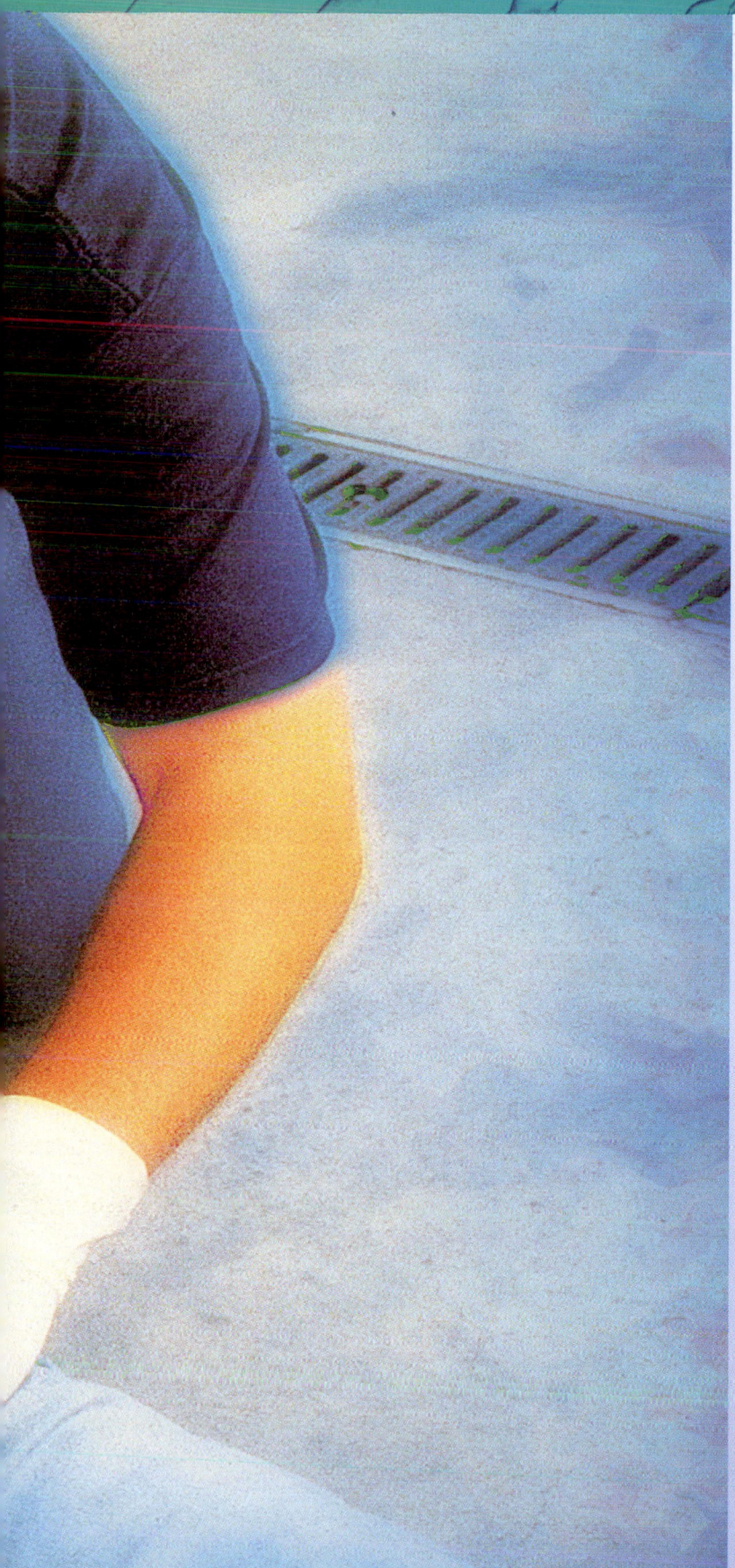

objectives

Cognitive

1. Describe the function of the muscular system.

2. Describe the function of the skeletal system.

3. List the major bones or bone groupings of the spinal column, the thorax, the upper extremities, the lower extremities.

4. Differentiate between an open and closed painful, swollen, deformed extremity (fracture).

5. State the reasons for splinting.

6. List the general rules of splinting.

7. List the complications of splinting.

8. List the emergency medical care for a patient with a swollen, painful, deformed extremity (fracture).

Affective

9. Explain the rationale for splinting at the scene versus load and go.

10. Explain the rationale for immobilization of the painful, swollen, deformed extremity (fracture).

Psychomotor

11. Demonstrate the emergency medical care of a patient with a painful, swollen, deformed extremity (fracture).

12. Demonstrate completing a prehospital care report for patients with musculoskeletal injuries.

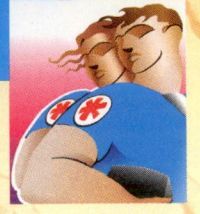

you are the emt

Squad 4, this is dispatch. Do you copy? We copy loud and clear dispatch. Go ahead. What's your status, 4? We are available. Please respond to Branson Park for a mountain bike crash. Meet the officer at the gate and he'll lead you in. Squad 4 en route to Branson Park.

The mountain bike has gained in popularity over the past 20 years. With its increase in popularity has been an increase in a variety of musculoskeletal injuries. Given the off-road locations in which individuals use these bikes, the potential for severe injuries increases accordingly.

This chapter will introduce you to the principles and practices of caring for musculoskeletal injuries and will also help you to answer the following questions:

1. What types of fractures are most stable? Most unstable?
2. Why are there so many choices when it comes to splinting?

Musculoskeletal Care

The human body is a well-designed system whose form, upright posture, and movement are provided by the musculoskeletal system, which also protects the vital internal organs of the body. As its combination form suggests, the term "musculoskeletal" refers to the bones and voluntary muscles of the body. However, the bones and muscles themselves are susceptible to external forces that can cause injury. Also at risk are the tendons that attach muscles to bones, the joints that form wherever two bones come into contact, and the ligaments that hold the bone ends of a joint together.

As an EMT-B, you must be familiar with the basic anatomy of the body's musculoskeletal system. Although muscles are technically soft tissue, they are discussed in this chapter because of their close relationship to the skeleton. Therefore, the chapter begins with a review of the musculoskeletal anatomy. Various types and causes of musculoskeletal injuries in general are identified, and the assessment and treatment process for each are explained, followed by a detailed discussion of splinting. The chapter then focuses on specific musculoskeletal injuries, beginning at the clavicle and ending at the feet.

Anatomy and Physiology of the Musculoskeletal System

Muscles

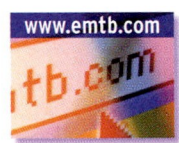

The musculoskeletal system is composed of three types of muscles: skeletal, smooth, and cardiac (Figure 31-1). **Skeletal muscle**, also called striated muscle because of its characteristic stripes, attaches to the bones and usually crosses at least one joint, forming the major muscle mass of the body. This type of muscle is also called voluntary muscle, because it is under direct voluntary control of the brain, responding to commands to move specific body parts. Usually, movement is the result of several muscles contracting and relaxing simultaneously.

All skeletal muscles are supplied with arteries, veins, and nerves. Blood from the arteries bring oxygen and nutrients to the muscles (Figure 31-2). Waste products, including carbon dioxide and lactic acid, are carried away in the veins. Either disease or trauma can result in the loss of a muscle's nervous energy; this, in turn, can lead to *atrophy,* or a wasting of the muscle. Muscle tissue is directly attached to the bone by tough, ropelike fibrous structures known as **tendons**, which are extensions of the fascia that covers all skeletal muscle.

Smooth muscle, also called involuntary muscle, performs much of the automatic work of the body. This type of muscle is found in the walls of most tubular structures of the body, such as the gastrointestinal tract and the blood vessels. Smooth muscle contracts and

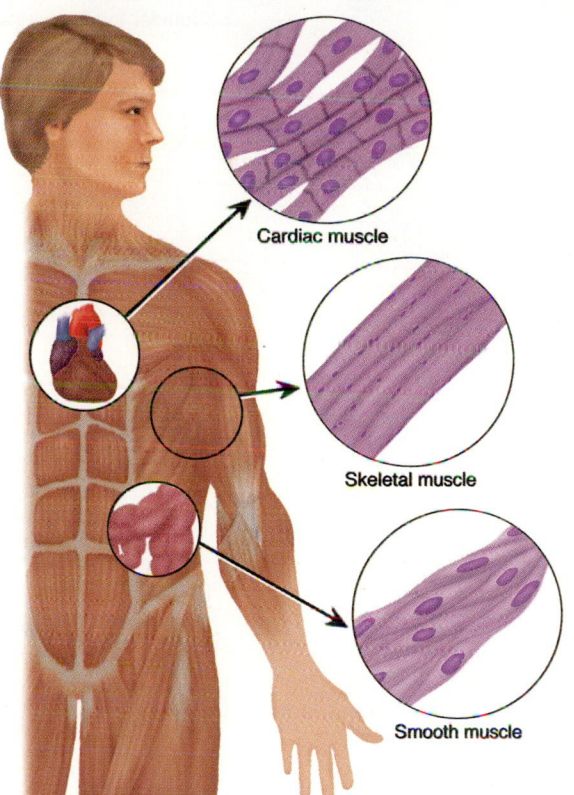

FIGURE 31-1 The musculoskeletal system includes three types of muscle: skeletal or voluntary muscles, smooth or involuntary muscles, and cardiac muscle.

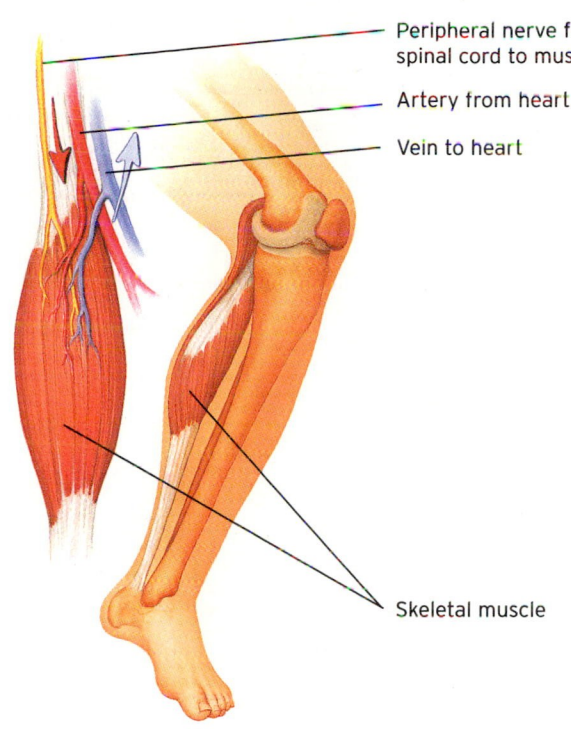

FIGURE 31-2 Skeletal muscles are supplied with arteries, veins, and nerves that bring oxygen and nutrients, carry away waste products, and supply nervous stimuli.

relaxes to control the movement of the contents of these structures (Figure 31-3).

The heart neither looks nor acts like skeletal or smooth muscle. It is a specially adapted involuntary muscle with its own regulatory system.

The remainder of this chapter is concerned exclusively with skeletal muscle.

The Skeleton

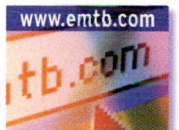

The skeleton, which gives us our recognizable human form, protects our vital internal organs, and allows us to move, is made up of approximately 206 bones (Figure 31-4). The bones in the skeleton also produce blood cells (in the bone marrow) and serve as a reservoir for important minerals and electrolytes.

The skull surrounds and protects the brain. The thoracic cage protects the heart, lungs, and great vessels, and the lower ribs protect much of the liver and spleen. The bony spinal canal formed by vertebrae encases and protects the spinal cord. The upper extremity extends from the shoulder girdle to the fingertips and is composed of the arm, elbow, forearm, wrist, hand, and

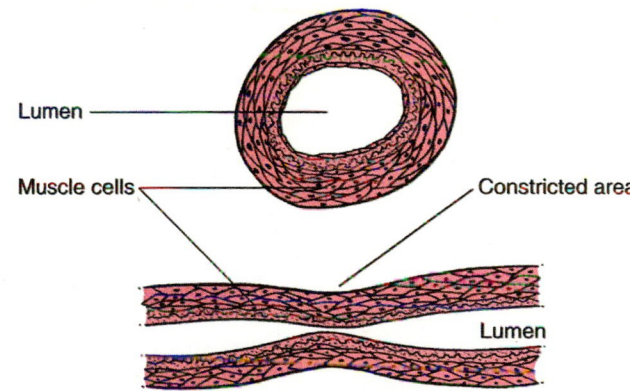

FIGURE 31-3 Smooth muscle is found in the walls of most tubular structures in the body. These muscles contract and relax to control the movement of the contents of these structures.

fingers. The arm extends from the shoulder to the elbow. The pelvic ring supports the body weight and protects the structures within the pelvic structure, bladder, rectum, and female reproductive organs. The lower extremity consists of the thigh, leg, and foot. The joint between the pelvis and the thigh is the hip; the joint

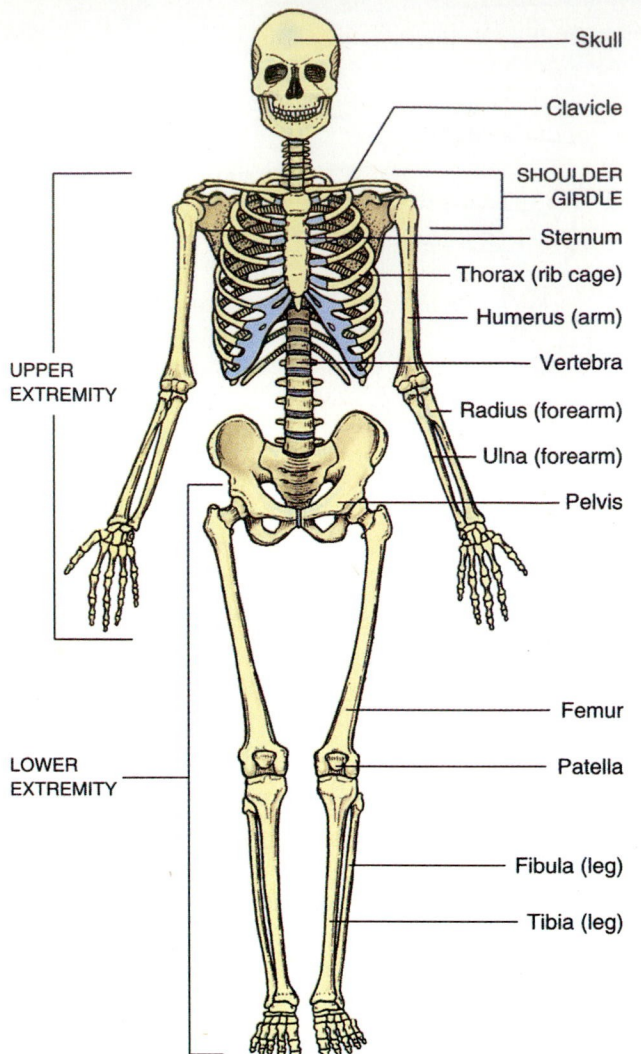

FIGURE 31-4 The human skeleton, consisting of 206 bones, gives us our form and protects our vital organs.

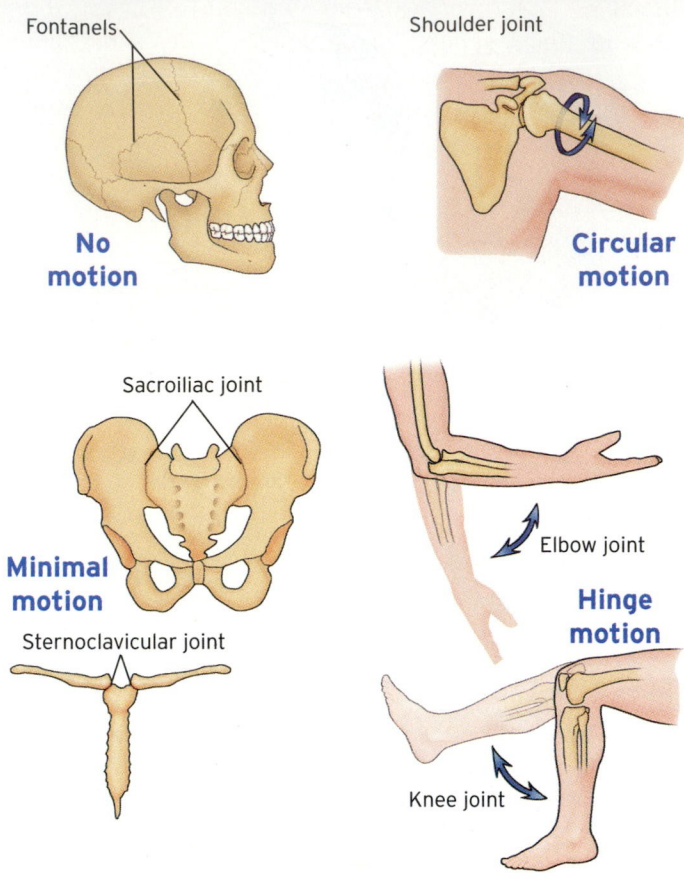

FIGURE 31-5 Joints have many functions. Some joints allow for motion to occur in a circular fashion; others act as hinges. Still others allow only a minimum amount of motion.

between the thigh and lower leg is the knee, and the joint between the lower leg and foot is the ankle.

The bones of the skeleton provide a framework to which the muscles and tendons are attached. Bone is a living tissue that contains nerves and receives oxygen and nutrients from the arterial system. Therefore, when a bone breaks, a patient typically experiences severe pain and bleeding. Bone marrow, located in the center of each bone, is constantly producing red blood cells to provide oxygen and nourishment to the body and remove waste.

A **joint** is formed wherever two bones come into contact. The sternoclavicular joint, for example, is where the sternum and the clavicle come together. Joints are held together in a tough fibrous structure known as a capsule, which is supported and strengthened in certain key areas by bands of fibrous tissue called **ligaments**. In moving joints, the ends of the bones are covered with

a thin layer of cartilage known as **articular cartilage**. This cartilage is a pearly substance that allows the ends of the bones to glide easily. Joints are bathed and lubricated by synovial fluid.

Most joints, such as the shoulder, allow motion to occur in a circling fashion. Other joints, such as the knee and elbow, act as hinges. Still other joints, including the sacroiliac joint in the lower back and sternoclavicular joints, allow only a minimum amount of motion. Certain joints, such as the fontanels in the skull, fuse two bones together to create a solid, immobile, bony structure (Figure 31-5).

Musculoskeletal Injuries

A **fracture** is a broken bone. More precisely, it is a break in the continuity of the bone often occurring as a result of an external force (Figure 31-6). The break can occur anywhere on the surface of the bone.

A **dislocation** is a disruption of a joint, so that the bone ends are no longer in contact. The supporting ligaments are torn, usually completely, allowing the bone ends to separate completely from each other (Figure 31-7). A fracture-dislocation is a combination injury at the joint in which the joint is dislocated and there is a fracture of the end of the bone.

A <u>sprain</u> is a joint injury in which there is both some partial or temporary dislocation of the bone ends and partial stretching or tearing of the supporting ligaments. After the injury, the joint surfaces generally fall back into alignment, so the joint is not significantly displaced. Sprains can range from mild to severe, depending on the amount of damage done to the supporting ligaments. The most severe sprains involve complete dislocation of the joint; mild sprains typically heal rather quickly.

A <u>strain</u>, or muscle pull, is a stretching or tearing of the muscle, causing pain, swelling, and bruising of the soft tissues in the area. Unlike a sprain, no ligament or joint damage occurs.

Injury to bones and joints is often associated with injury to the surrounding soft tissues, especially to the adjacent nerves and blood vessels. The entire area is known as the zone of injury (Figure 31-8). Depending on the amount of kinetic energy the tissues absorb from forces acting on the body, the zone may extend to a distant point. For this reason, you should not focus on a patient's obvious injury without first completing an initial assessment to check for associated injuries, which may be even more serious. This is especially true in assessing damage from gunshots and falls from a height.

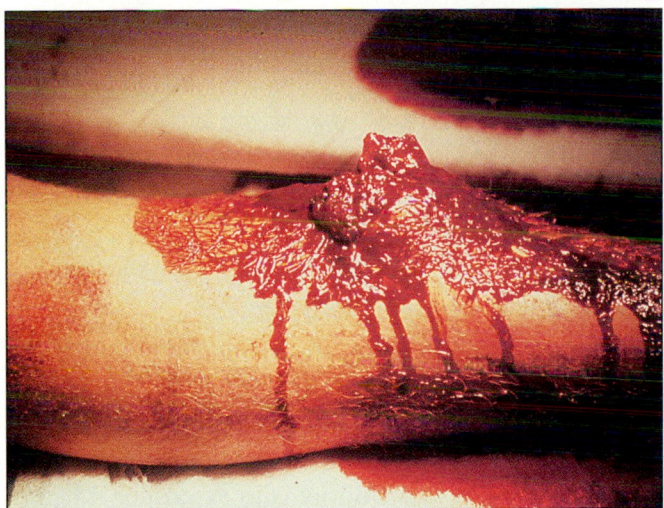

FIGURE 31-6 A fracture can occur anywhere on the surface of a bone and may or may not break the skin.

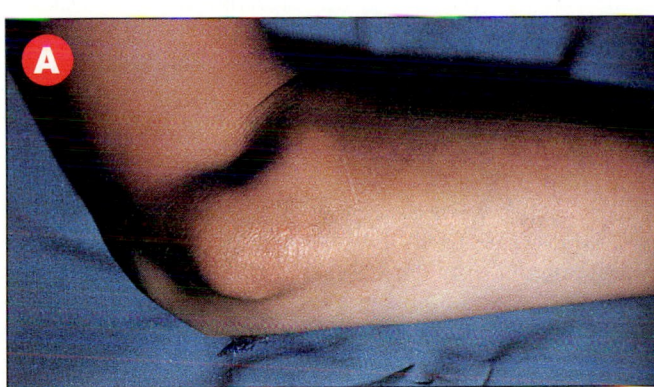

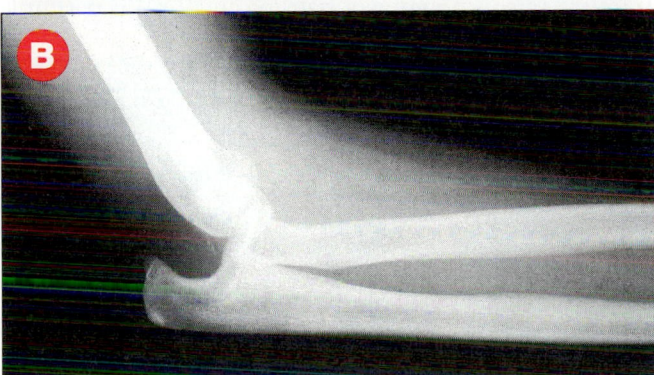

FIGURE 31-7 A dislocation is a disruption of a joint in which the bone ends are no longer in contact. **A:** The clinical appearance of an elbow dislocation. **B:** X-ray appearance of the same elbow.

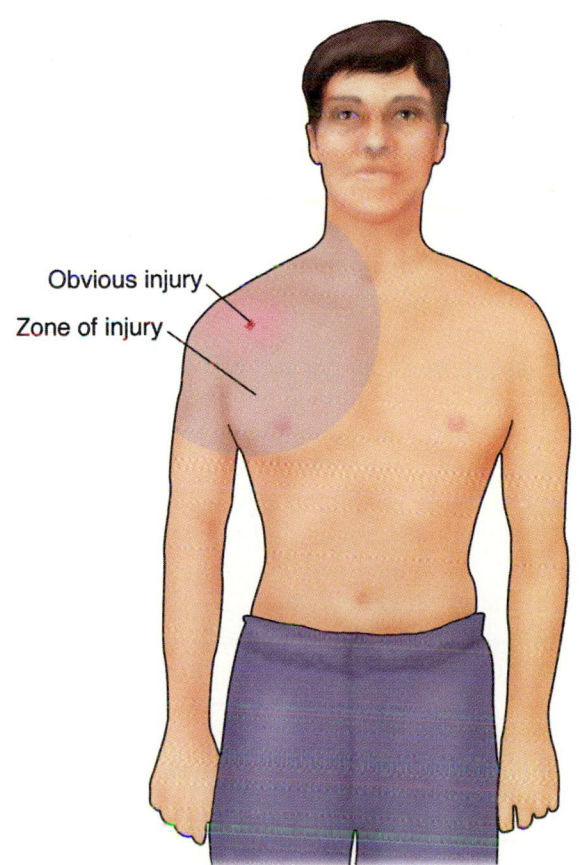

FIGURE 31-8 The zone of injury includes the area of soft tissue, including the adjacent nerves and blood vessels, that surrounds the bone or joint that has been injured.

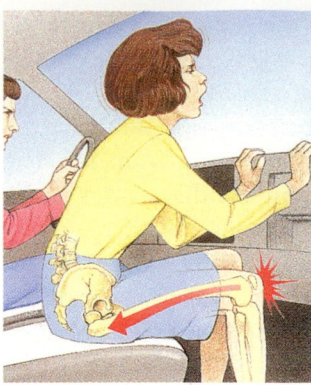
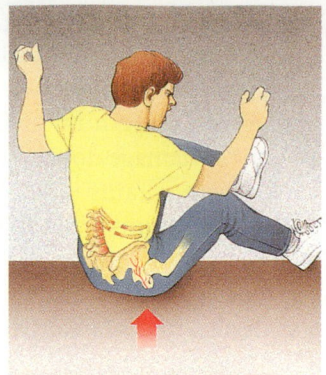
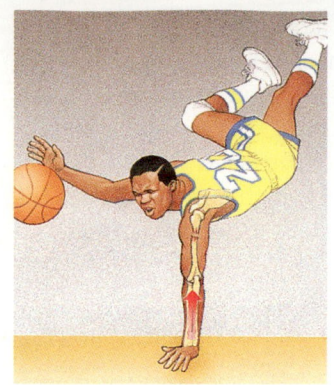
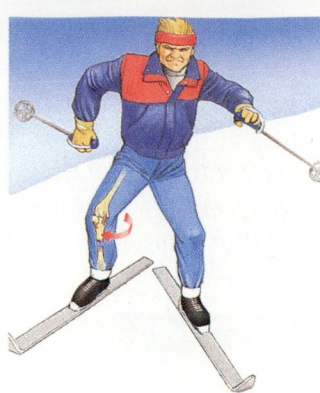

FIGURE 31-9 Significant force is required to cause fractures or dislocations. Among these are direct blows, indirect forces, high-energy injuries, and twisting forces.

Mechanism of Injury

Significant force is generally required to cause fractures or dislocations. This force may be applied to the limb in any of the following ways (Figure 31-9):

- Direct blows
- Indirect forces
- Twisting forces
- High-energy injury

A direct blow fractures the bone at the point of impact. An example is the **patella** (kneecap) that fractures when it strikes the dashboard in an automobile crash.

Indirect force may cause a fracture or dislocation at a distant point, as when a person falls and lands on an outstretched hand. The direct impact may cause a wrist fracture, but the indirect force can cause dislocation of the elbow or a fracture of the forearm, humerus, or even clavicle. Therefore, when caring for patients who have fallen, you must identify the point of contact and the mechanism of injury so that you will not overlook associated injuries.

Twisting forces are a common cause of musculoskeletal injury, especially to the anterior cruciate ligament at the knee. Skiing injuries often happen this way. A ski becomes caught, and the skier falls, applying a twisting force to the lower extremity.

High-energy injuries, such as those that occur in automobile crashes, falls from heights, gunshot wounds, and other extreme forces, produce severe damage to the skeleton, surrounding soft tissues, and vital internal organs. A patient may have multiple injuries to many body parts, including more than one fracture or dislocation in a single limb.

Violence is not necessary to fracture a bone. A slight force can easily fracture a bone that is weakened by a tumor or *osteoporosis,* a generalized bone disease that is common tramong postmenopausal women. In elderly patients with osteoporosis, minor falls, simple twisting injuries, or even a muscle contraction can cause a frac-ture, most often of the wrist, spine, or hip. You should suspect the presence of a fracture in any older patient who has sustained even a mild injury.

Fractures

Fractures are classified as either closed or open. In assessing and treating patients with possible fractures or dislocations, your first priority is to determine whether the overlying skin has been damaged. If it is not, the patient has a **closed fracture**. However, making this determination is not always as easy as it sounds. With an **open fracture**, there is an external wound, caused either by the same blow that fractured the bone or by the broken bone ends lacerating the skin. The wound may vary in size from a very small puncture to a gaping tear that exposes bone and soft tissue. Regardless of the extent and severity of the damage to the skin, you should treat any injury that breaks the skin as a possible open fracture. Greater blood loss and a higher likelihood of infection, possibilities that you must try to prevent, tend to occur with open fractures.

Fractures are also described by whether the bone is moved from its normal position. A **nondisplaced fracture** (also known as a hairline fracture) is a simple

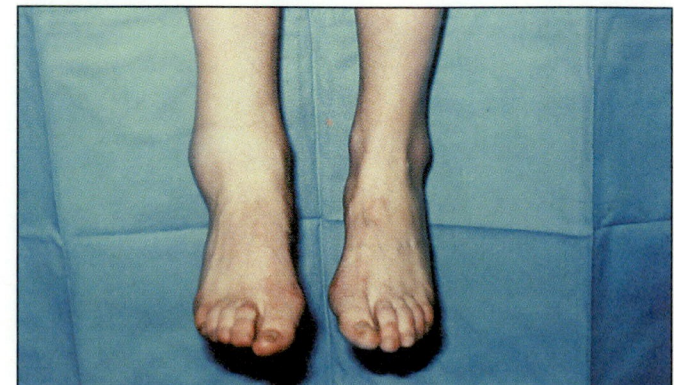

FIGURE 31-10 You should always compare the injured limb with the uninjured limb when checking for deformity.

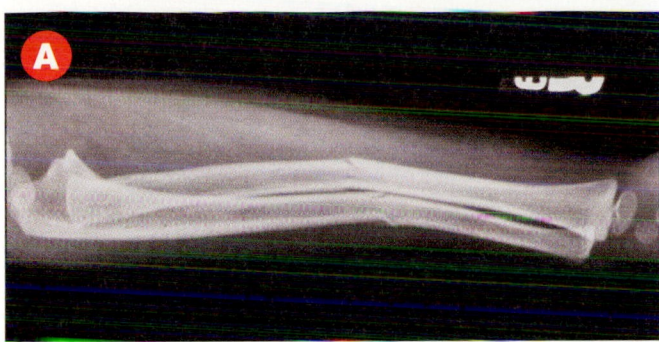

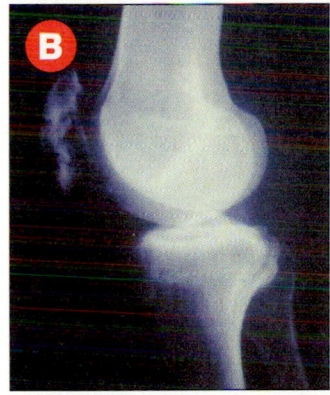

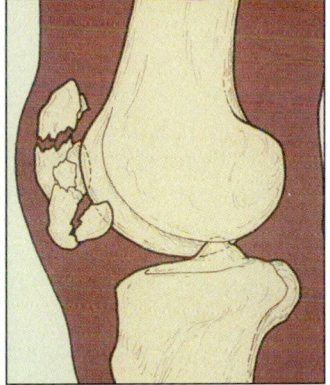

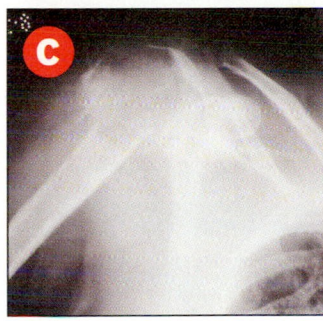

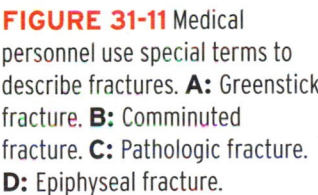

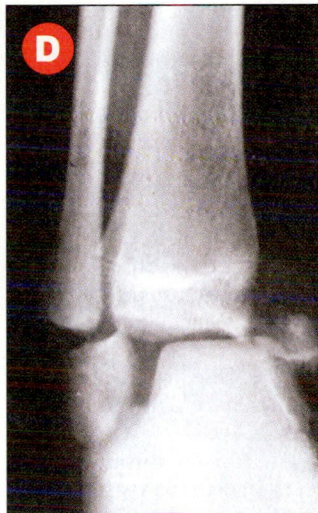

FIGURE 31-11 Medical personnel use special terms to describe fractures. **A:** Greenstick fracture. **B:** Comminuted fracture. **C:** Pathologic fracture. **D:** Epiphyseal fracture.

crack of the bone that may be difficult to distinguish from a sprain or simple contusion. In fact, X-rays may be required for hospital personnel to diagnose a nondisplaced fracture. A <u>**displaced fracture**</u> produces actual deformity, or distortion, of the limb by shortening, rotating, or angulating it. Often, the deformity is very obvious and can be associated with crepitus; however, in some cases, the deformity is minimal. Be sure to look for differences between the injured limb and the opposite uninjured limb in any patient with a fracture of an extremity (Figure 31-10).

Medical personnel often use the following special terms to describe particular types of fractures (Figure 31-11):

- **Greenstick fracture.** An incomplete fracture that passes only partway through the shaft of a bone but may still cause severe angulation; occurs in children.

- **Comminuted fracture.** A fracture in which the bone is broken into more than two fragments.

- **Pathologic fracture.** A fracture of weakened or diseased bone, seen in patients with osteoporosis or cancer; generally produced by minimal force.

- **Epiphyseal fracture.** A fracture that occurs in a growth section of a child's bone, which may prematurely stop growth if not properly treated.

You should suspect a fracture if one or more of the following signs is present in any patient who has a history of injury and reports pain.

Deformity. The limb may appear to be shortened, rotated, or angulated at a point where there is no joint. Always use the opposite limb as a mirror image for comparison (Figure 31-12).

Tenderness. <u>**Point tenderness**</u> on palpation in the zone of injury is the most reliable indicator of an underlying fracture, although it does not tell you the type of fracture (Figure 31-13). Be sure to wear gloves if there are any open wounds.

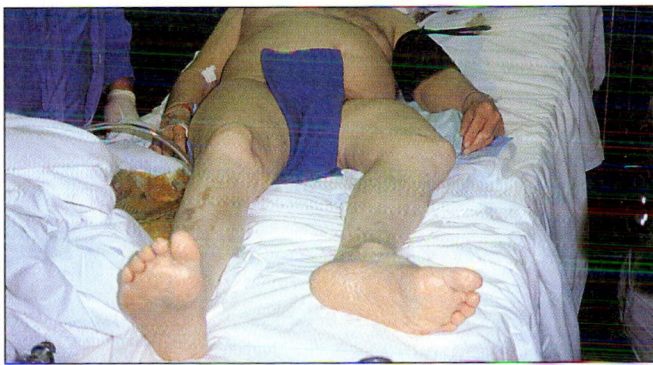

FIGURE 31-12 Obvious deformity, shortening, rotation, or angulation suggests a fracture. Remember to compare the injured limb with the opposite, uninjured limb.

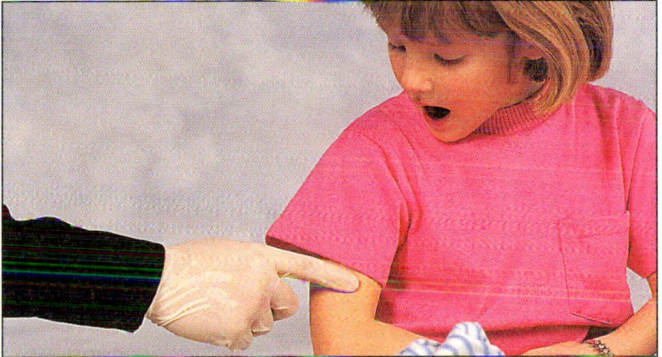

FIGURE 31-13 Point tenderness is the sensitive spot at the site of injury that can be located by gentle palpation along the bone with the tip of your finger.

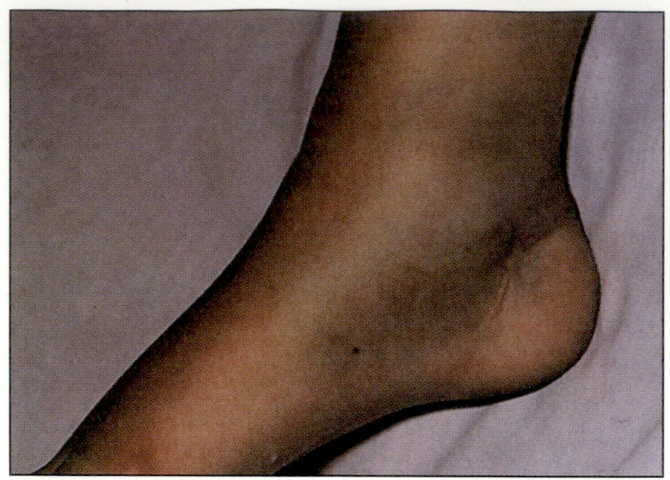

FIGURE 31-14 Swelling that occurs in association with a fracture can often mask deformity of the limb.

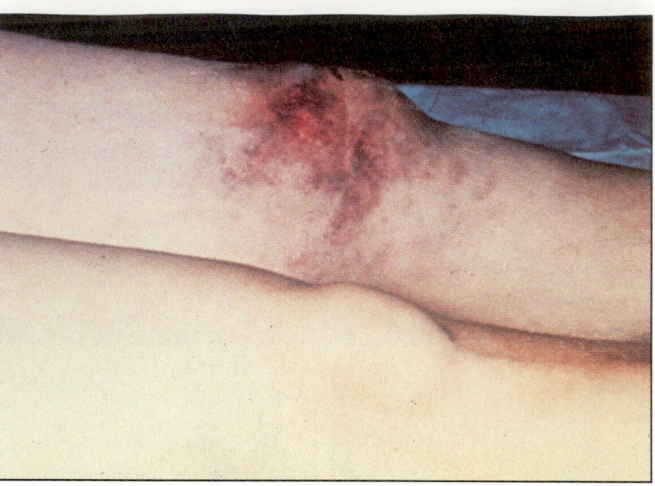

FIGURE 31-15 Fractures almost always have associated bruising into the surrounding soft tissue.

Guarding. An inability to use the extremity is the patient's way of immobilizing it to minimize pain. The muscles around the fracture contract in an attempt to prevent any movement of the broken bone. Guarding does not occur with all fractures; some patients may continue to use the injured part for a period of time. Occasionally, nondisplaced fractures are not very painful, and there is minimal soft-tissue damage.

Swelling. Rapid swelling usually indicates bleeding from a fracture site and is typically followed by severe pain (Figure 31-14). Often, if the swelling is severe enough, it may mask deformity of the limb. Generalized swelling from fluid buildup may occur several hours after an injury.

Bruising. Fractures are almost always associated with ecchymosis (discoloration) of the surrounding soft tissues (Figure 31-15). Bruising may be present after almost any injury; it is not specific for bone or joint injuries.

Crepitus. A grating or grinding sensation known as crepitus can be felt and sometimes even heard when fractured bone ends rub together.

False motion. Motion at a point in the limb where there is no joint is a positive indication of a fracture.

Exposed fragments. In open fractures, bone ends may protrude through the skin or be visible within the wound (Figure 31-16).

Pain. Pain, along with tenderness and bruising, commonly occurs in association with fractures.

Locked joint. A joint that is locked into position makes any attempt to move the joint both difficult and painful.

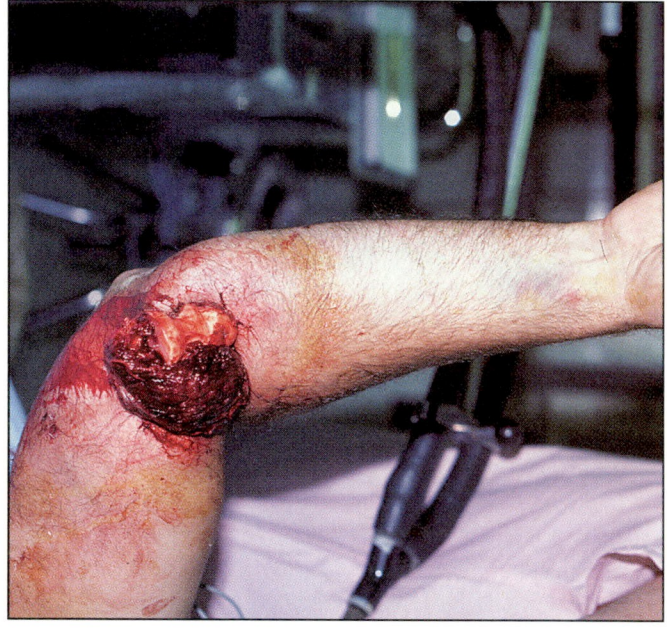

FIGURE 31-16 Bone ends may protrude through the skin or be visible within the wound of an open fracture.

Keep in mind that crepitus and false motion appear only when a limb is moved or manipulated and are associated with injuries that are extremely painful. Do not manipulate the limb excessively in an effort to elicit these signs.

Dislocations

A dislocated joint sometimes will spontaneously reduce, or return to its normal position, before your assessment. In this situation, you will be able to confirm the dislocation only by taking a patient history. Often, however, injury to the supporting ligaments and capsule is so severe that the joint surfaces remain completely separated from one another. A dislocation that does not spontaneously reduce is a serious problem. The ends of the bone can be locked in a displaced position, making any attempt at motion of the joint very difficult and very painful. The most commonly dislocated joints are the fingers, shoulder, elbow, hip, and ankle.

The signs and symptoms of a dislocated joint are similar to those of a fracture (Figure 31-17):

- Marked deformity

- Swelling

- Pain that is aggravated by any attempt at movement

- Tenderness on palpation

- Virtually complete loss of normal joint motion (locked joint)

- Numbness or impaired circulation to the limb or digit

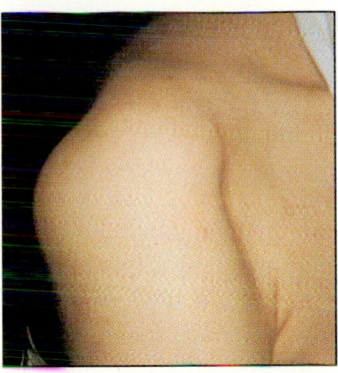

FIGURE 31-17 Joint dislocations, such as this shoulder, are characterized by deformity, swelling, pain with any movement, tenderness, locking, and impaired circulation.

Sprains

A sprain occurs when a joint is twisted or stretched beyond its normal range of motion. As a result, the supporting capsule and ligaments are stretched or torn. A sprain should be considered a partial dislocation or subluxation. The alignment generally returns to a fairly normal position, although there may be some displacement. Note that severe deformity does not typically occur with a sprain. Sprains most often occur in the knee and the ankle, but a sprain can occur in any joint. The following signs and symptoms often indicate that the patient may have a sprain (Figure 31-18):

- Point tenderness can be elicited over the injured ligaments.

- Swelling and ecchymosis appear at the point of injury to the ligament as a result of torn blood vessels.

- Pain prevents the patient from moving or using the limb normally.

- Instability of the joint is indicated by increased motion, especially at the knee; however, this may be masked by severe swelling and guarding.

A fracture can look like a sprain, and vice versa. You will not be able to distinguish a nondisplaced fracture from a sprain, especially at the ankle. *Therefore, remember to document the mechanism of injury, as certain sprains and fractures occur more consistently with certain mechanisms. This is especially true at the ankle.* In general, your approach should always be to try to rule out the possibility of fracture first. The basic principles of field management for sprains, dislocations, and fractures are essentially the same.

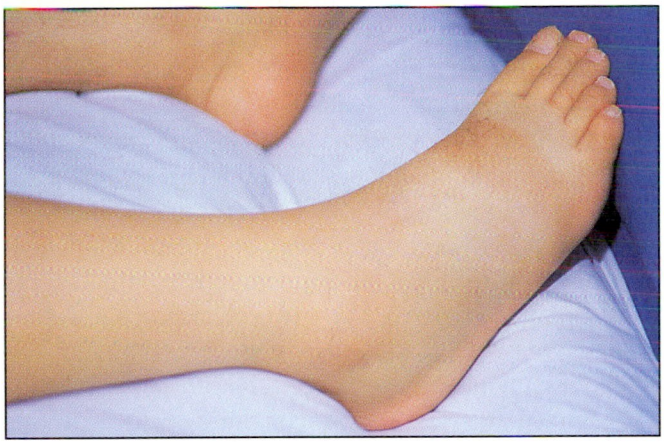

FIGURE 31-18 Sprains most often occur in the knee or ankle and are characterized by swelling, bruising, point tenderness, pain and joint instability.

Assessing Musculoskeletal Injuries

As an EMT-B, you are the point person in the team approach to the trauma patient. Therefore, your assessments, attempts at simple reduction and splinting, and work to stabilize the patient are very important. Look at the big picture, evaluating the overall complexity of the situation. Always carefully assess the mechanism of injury to try to determine the amount of kinetic energy that an injured limb has absorbed.

Assessment of patients with musculoskeletal injuries must include a rapid initial assessment of the patient, followed by a focused physical exam of the affected limb, including evaluation of neurovascular function. Be sure to follow BSI techniques. If oxygen is indicated and you have not already applied it, be sure to do so.

Because patients often have multiple injuries, you must assess their overall condition, stabilize their vital functions, and control any serious bleeding before further treating the injured extremity. If you cannot stabilize the vital functions of a critically injured patient, you should secure the patient to a long spine board to rapidly immobilize the spine, pelvis, and extremities and provide prompt transport to a trauma center. In this situation, extensive evaluation and splinting of limb injuries in the field are a waste of valuable time.

If the patient has no life-threatening injuries, you may take extra time at the scene to stabilize the patient's overall condition and more completely evaluate the injured extremity. During the detailed physical exam, you can inspect and gently palpate the other extremities and the spine to identify areas of point tenderness that may indicate underlying fractures, dislocations, or sprains. Remember to compare the injured limb with the opposite, uninjured limb. If possible, gently and carefully remove the patient's clothing to look for open fractures or dislocations, severe deformity, swelling, and/or ecchymosis.

Again, it is not important to distinguish among fractures, dislocations, sprains, and contusions. In most instances, your assessment will be reported as an "injury to the limb." However, you must be able to distinguish mild injuries from severe injuries, since some severe injuries may compromise neurovascular functioning.

If your assessment turns up no external signs of injury, ask the patient to move each limb carefully, stopping immediately if a movement causes pain. Skip this step in your evaluation if the patient reports neck or back pain; even the slightest motion could cause permanent damage to the spinal cord.

Be on the alert for compartment syndrome, which most commonly occurs in the fractured tibia or forearm of children and is often overlooked, especially in patients with an altered level of consciousness. The name "compartment syndrome" refers to elevated pressure in the fascial compartment, which is the fibrous tissue that surrounds and supports the muscles and neurovascular structures. <u>Compartment syndrome</u> occurs within 6 to 12 hours after injury, usually as a result of excessive bleeding, a severely crushed extremity, or the rapid return of blood to an ischemic limb. This syndrome is characterized by pain that is out of proportion to the injury, pallor, decreased sensation, and decreased power (ranging from decreased strength and movement of the limb to complete palsy).

If you suspect that a patient has compartment syndrome, splint the affected limb, keeping it at the level of the heart, and provide immediate transport, checking neurovascular status frequently during transport. Compartment syndrome must be managed surgically.

Evaluating Neurovascular Function

Many important blood vessels and nerves lie close to the bone, especially around the major joints. Therefore, any injury or deformity of the bone may have associated vessel or nerve injury. For this reason, you must assess neurovascular function during the detailed physical exam, repeating it every 5 to 10 minutes, depending on the patient's condition, until the patient is at the hospital. Always recheck the neurovascular function before and after you splint or otherwise manipulate the limb. Manipulation can cause a bone fragment to press against or impale a nerve or vessel. Failure to restore circulation in this situation can lead to death of the limb. Always give priority to patients with impaired circulation resulting from bone fragments.

Examination of the injured limb should include assessments of the following (Figure 31-19):

1. **Pulse.** Palpate the pulse distal to the point of injury. Palpate the radial pulse in the upper extremity and the posterior tibial pulse and dorsalis pedis pulse in the lower extremity.

2. **Capillary refill.** Note and record the skin color, identifying any pallor or cyanosis. Then apply firm pressure to the tip of the fingernail or toenail, which will cause the skin to blanch (turn white). If normal color does not return within 2 seconds after you release the nail, you can assume that circulation is impaired. This test is typically recommended for use in children, although it can be used in adults as well.

3. **Sensation.** In the hand, check the feeling on the pulp of the index finger and thumb, as well as the little finger. In the foot, check the feeling on the pulp of the big toe and on the dorsum of the foot laterally. The patient's ability to sense light touch in the fingers or toes distal to the site of a fracture is a good indication that the nerve supply is intact.

4. **Motor function.** Evaluate muscular activity when the injury is proximal to the patient's hand or foot. Ask the patient to open and close a fist for an upper extremity injury and to wiggle the toes and move the foot up and down for a lower extremity injury. Sometimes, an attempt at motion will produce pain at the injury site. If this happens, do not continue this part of the examination. To avoid causing pain, do not perform this test at all if the injury involves the hand or foot itself.

Because many of the steps require patient cooperation, you will not be able to assess sensory and motor function in an unconscious patient, but you can still evaluate the limb for deformity, swelling, ecchymosis, false motion, and crepitus. If a patient is unconscious, first perform an initial assessment and stabilize the vital functions, then examine the extremities. Assume that an unconscious patient has a spinal fracture, and immobilize the spine.

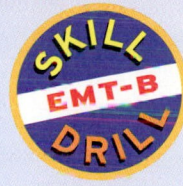

Evaluating Neurovascular Function
Figure 31-19

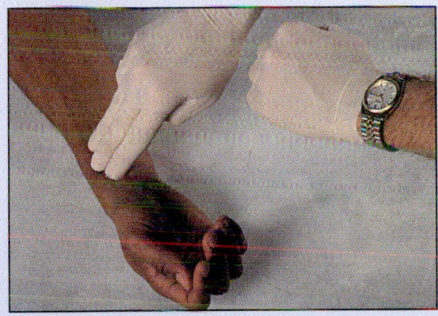

Evaluate the pulse distal to the site of injury. Palpate the radial pulse in the upper extremity.

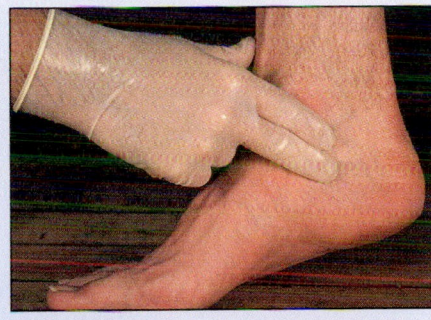

Palpate the posterior tibial pulse in the lower extremity.

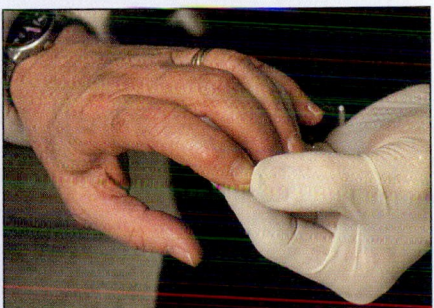

Although assessing capillary refill is usually limited to children, it is also a valid second step in the evaluation of neurovascular function in adults.

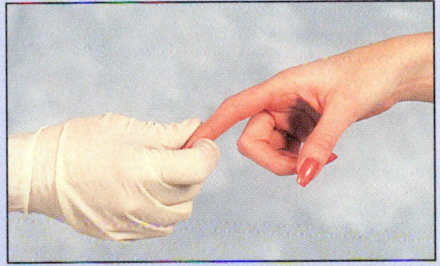

Assess sensation on the pulp of the index finger in the hand.

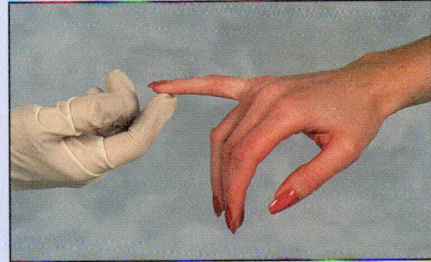

Check sensation on the pulp of the little finger.

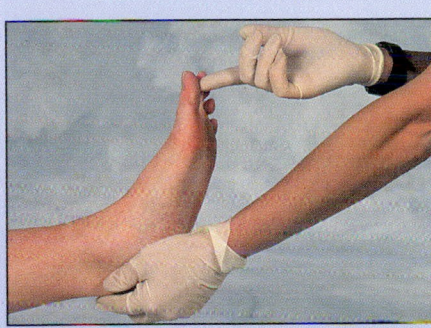

Check sensation on the pulp of the great toe in the foot.

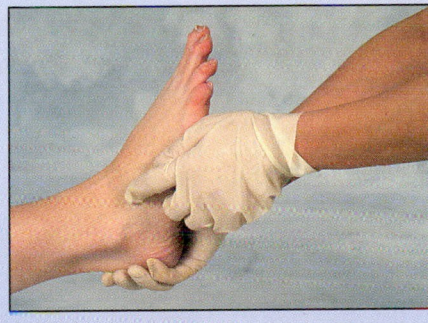

Check sensation on the dorsum of the foot laterally.

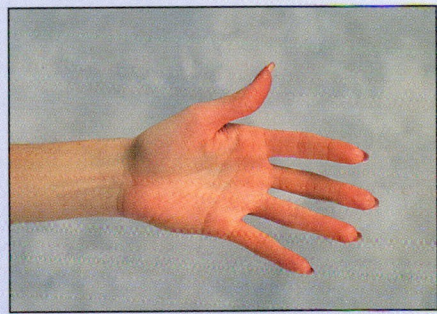

Evaluate motor function by asking the patient to open his or her hand.

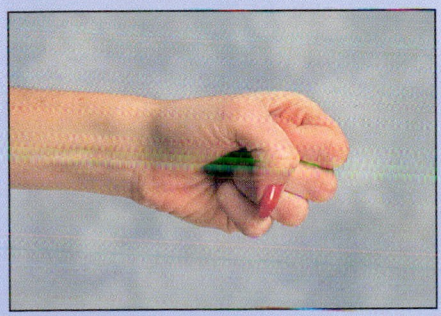

Ask the patient to make a fist and open and close the fist.

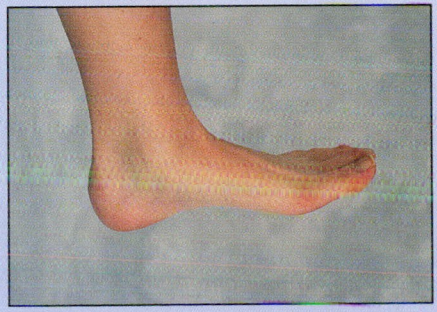

Ask the patient to extend the foot to evaluate motor function in the foot.

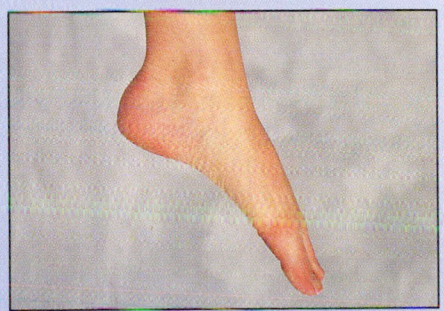

Ask the patient to flex the foot and wiggle the toes.

Assessing the Severity of Injury

You must become skilled at quickly and accurately assessing the severity of injury. The Golden Hour is critical not just for life, but for limb as well. In an extremity with anything less than complete circulation, prolonged hypotension can cause significant damage. For this reason, any suspected open fracture or vascular injury is considered a medical emergency, especially in a patient with multiple trauma.

Remember that most injuries are not critical; you can identify critical injuries by using the musculoskeletal injury grading system shown in Table 31-1.

Emergency Medical Care

Your first steps in providing care for any patient are the initial assessment and stabilizing the patient's ABCD. After you have done so, you can focus on specific injuries. Remember to always follow BSI techniques.

You should take the following steps when caring for patients with musculoskeletal injuries (Figure 31-20):

1. **Completely cover open wounds** with a dry, sterile dressing, and apply local pressure to control bleeding. Once you have applied a sterile compression dressing, you should treat an open fracture in the same way as a closed fracture.

2. **Apply the appropriate splint,** and elevate the extremity. Patients with lower extremity injuries should lie supine with the limb elevated about 6″ to minimize swelling. For any patient, be sure to position the injured limb slightly above the level of the heart. Never allow the injured limb to flop about or dangle from the edge of the backboard.

3. **If swelling is present,** apply cold packs to the area; however, avoid placing cold packs directly on the skin or other exposed tissues. Placing a cold pack on top of an air splint or other thick, insulating material will not help to reduce swelling.

4. **Prepare the patient for transport.** A patient with an isolated upper extremity will most likely be more comfortable in a semiseated position rather than lying flat; however, either position is acceptable.

5. **Always inform hospital personnel** about all wounds that have been dressed and splinted.

Splinting

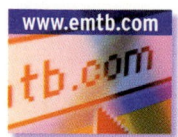

A **splint** is a flexible or rigid device that is used to protect and maintain the position of an injured extremity (Figure 31-21). Unless the patient's life is in

TABLE 31-1	Musculoskeletal Injury Grading System

Minor Injuries
- Minor sprains
- Fractures or dislocations of digits

Moderate Injuries
- Open fractures of digits
- Nondisplaced long bone fractures
- Nondisplaced pelvic fractures
- Major sprains of a major joint

Serious Injuries
- Displaced long bone fractures
- Multiple hand and foot fractures
- Single open long bone fractures
- Displaced pelvic fractures
- Dislocations of major joints
- Multiple digit amputations
- Laceration of major nerve or blood vessels

Severe, Life-Threatening Injuries (survival is probable)
- Multiple closed fractures
- Limb amputations

Critical Injuries (survival is uncertain)
- Multiple open fractures of the limbs
- Pelvic fractures with hemodynamic instability

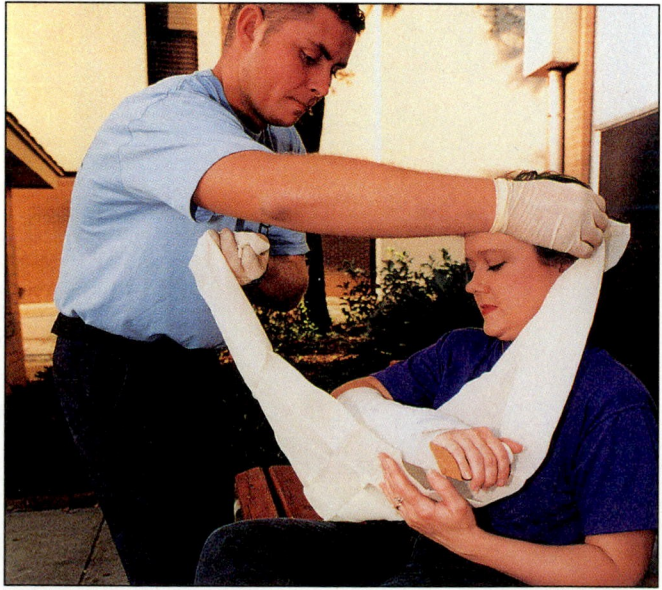

FIGURE 31-21 Splinting reduces pain and prevents additional damage to the injured extremity.

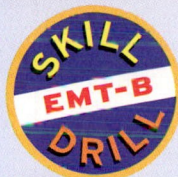

Caring for Musculoskeletal Injuries
Figure 31-20

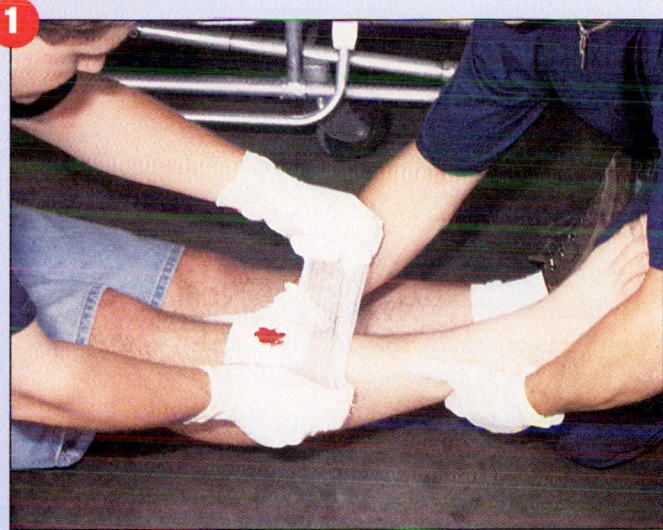

Cover open wounds with a dry, sterile dressing, and apply local pressure to bleeding.

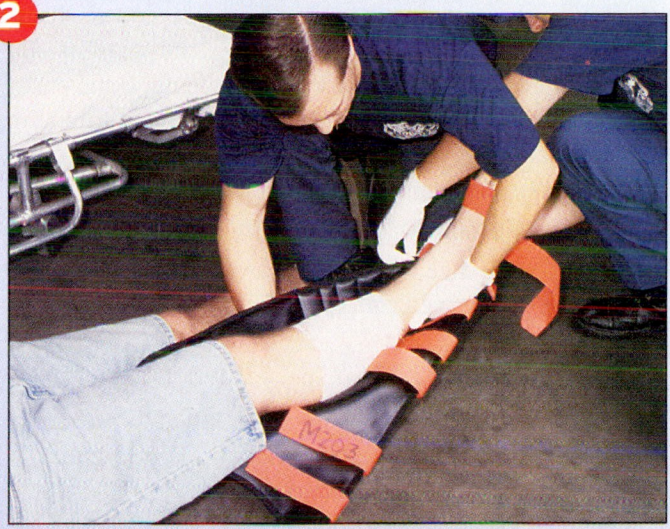

Apply a splint, and elevate the extremity about 6" (so that it is slightly above the level of the heart) to minimize swelling.

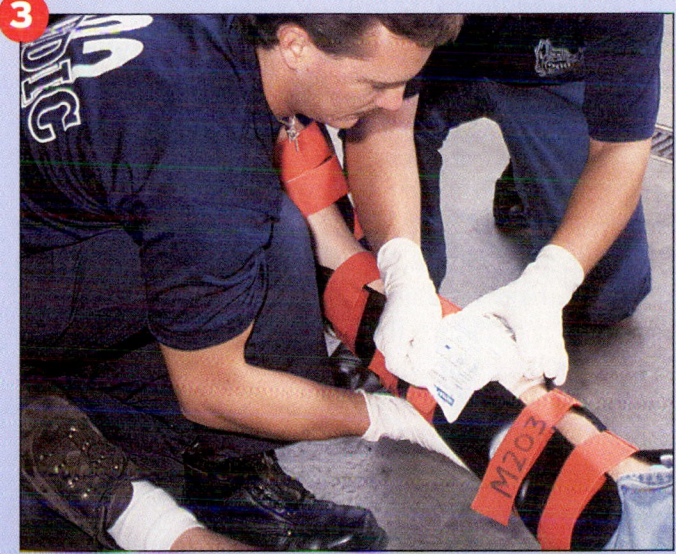

Apply cold packs to the area if there is swelling present, but do not place them directly on the skin.

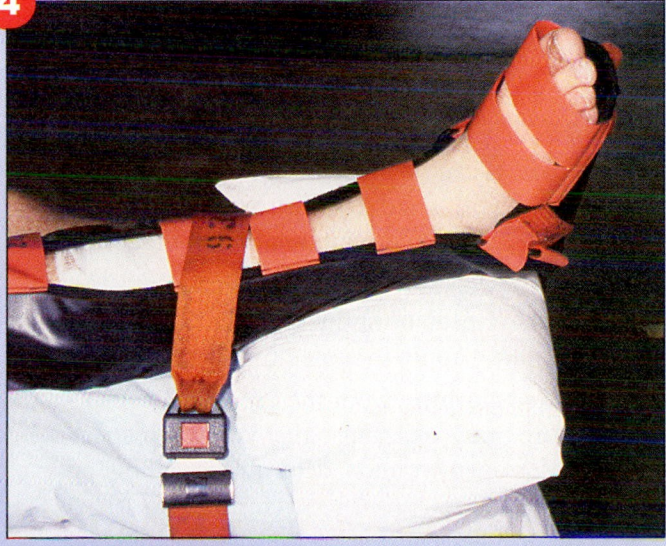

Prepare the patient for transport. Ensure that the extremity is elevated above the level of the heart and secured so that it does not dangle from the edge of the backboard.

> **The three basic types of splints are rigid, formable, and traction splints.**

immediate danger, you should splint all fractures, dislocations, and sprains before moving the patient. By preventing movement of fracture fragments, bone ends, a dislocated joint, or damaged soft tissues, splinting reduces pain and makes it easier to transfer and transport the patient. In addition, splinting will help to prevent the following:

- Further damage to muscles, the spinal cord, peripheral nerves, and blood vessels from broken bone ends

- Laceration of the skin by broken bone ends. One of the primary indications for splinting is to prevent a closed fracture from becoming an open fracture (conversion)

- Restriction of distal blood flow resulting from pressure of the bone ends on blood vessels

- Excessive bleeding of the tissues at the injury site caused by broken bone ends

- Increased pain from movement of bone ends

- Paralysis of extremities resulting from a damaged spine

A splint is simply a device to prevent motion of the injured part. It can be made from any material on occasions when you need to improvise. However, you should have an adequate supply of standard commercial splints on hand.

General principles of splinting. The following principles of splinting apply to most situations:

1. **Remove clothing from the area** of any suspected fracture or dislocation so that you can inspect the limb for open wounds, deformity, swelling, and ecchymosis.

2. **Note and record the patient's neurovascular status** distal to the site of the injury, including pulse, capillary refill, sensation, and movement. Continue to monitor the neurovascular status until the patient reaches the hospital.

3. **Cover all wounds with a dry, sterile dressing** before splinting. Be sure to follow BSI techniques. Do not intentionally replace protruding bones. Notify the receiving hospital of all open wounds.

4. **Do not move the patient before splinting** an extremity unless there is an immediate hazard to the patient or yourself.

5. In a suspected fracture of the shaft of any bone, be sure to **immobilize the joints** above and below the fracture.

6. With injuries in and around the joint, be sure to **immobilize the bones** above and below the injured joint.

7. **Pad all rigid splints** to prevent local pressure and discomfort to the patient.

8. While applying the splint, **use your hands** to minimize movement of the limb and to support the injury site.

9. If fracture of a long bone shaft has resulted in severe deformity, **use constant, gentle manual traction** to align the limb so that it can be splinted. This is especially important if the distal part of the extremity is cyanotic or pulseless.

10. **If you encounter resistance** to limb alignment, splint the limb in its deformed position.

11. **Immobilize all suspected spinal injuries** in a neutral in-line position.

12. **If the patient has signs of shock** (hypoperfusion), align the limb in the normal anatomic position and provide transport (total body immobilization).

13. **When in doubt, splint.**

General principles of in-line traction splinting.
In-line traction is the act of exerting a pulling force on an object. It is the most effective way to realign a fracture of the shaft of a long bone so that the limb can be splinted more effectively. Excessive traction can be very harmful to an injured limb. When applied correctly, however, traction stabilizes the bone fragments and improves the overall alignment of the limb. You should not attempt to reduce the fracture or force all the bone fragments back into alignment. This is the physician's responsibility. In the field, the goals of in-line traction are as follows:

1. To **stabilize the fracture** fragments to prevent excessive movement

2. To **align the limb** sufficiently to allow it to be placed in a splint

3. To **avoid** potential neurovascular compromise

The amount of pull that is required to accomplish these objectives varies but rarely exceeds 15 lb. You should use the least amount of force necessary. Grasp the foot or hand at the end of the injured limb firmly; once you start pulling, you should not stop until the limb is fully splinted. The direction of traction pull is always along the long axis of the limb. Imagine where the normal, uninjured limb would lie, and pull gently along the line of that imaginary limb until the injured limb is in approximately that position (Figure 31-22). Grasping the foot or hand and the initial pull of traction usually cause some discomfort as the bone fragments move. It helps if a second person can support the injured limb directly under the site of the fracture. This initial discomfort quickly subsides, and you can then apply further gentle traction. However, if the patient strongly resists the traction or if it causes more pain that persists, you must stop and splint the limb in the deformed position.

Remember that many different materials can be used as splints if necessary. When no splinting materials are available, the arm can be bound to the chest wall, and an injured leg can be bound to the uninjured leg to provide at least temporary stability. The three basic types of splints are rigid, formable, and traction splints.

Rigid splints. Rigid (nonformable) splints are made from firm material and are applied to the sides, front, and/or back of an injured extremity to prevent motion at the injury site. Common examples of rigid splints include padded board splints, molded plastic and metal splints, padded wire ladder splints, and folded card-board splints. As always, be sure to follow BSI techniques. It takes two EMT-Bs to apply a rigid splint, as follows (Figure 31-23 on the next page):

1. First EMT-B: **Gently support the limb** at the site of injury. Apply steady, in-line traction if necessary. Maintain this support until the splint is completely applied.

2. Second EMT-B: **Place the rigid splint** under or alongside the limb.

3. Second EMT-B: **Place padding between the limb** and the splint to make sure there is even pressure and even contact. Look for bony prominences, and pad them.

4. Second EMT-B: **Apply bindings** to hold the splint securely to the limb.

5. Second EMT-B: **Check and record** the distal neurovascular function.

There are two situations in which you must splint the limb in the position of deformity: when the deformity is severe, as is the case with many dislocations, or when you encounter resistance or extreme pain when applying gentle traction to the fracture of a shaft of a long bone. In either situation, you should apply padded board splints to each side of the limb and secure them with soft roller bandages (Figure 31-24).

Formable splints. The most commonly used formable or soft splint is the precontoured, inflatable, clear plastic *air splint*. These are available in a variety of sizes and shapes, with or without a zipper that runs the length of

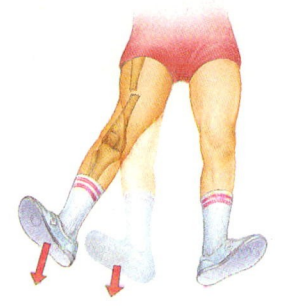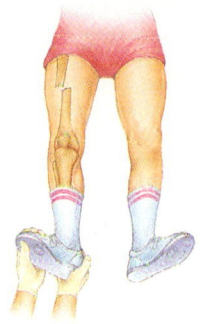

FIGURE 31-22 To apply traction, imagine the position where the normal uninjured limb would lie, and then gently pull along that line until the injured limb is in that position.

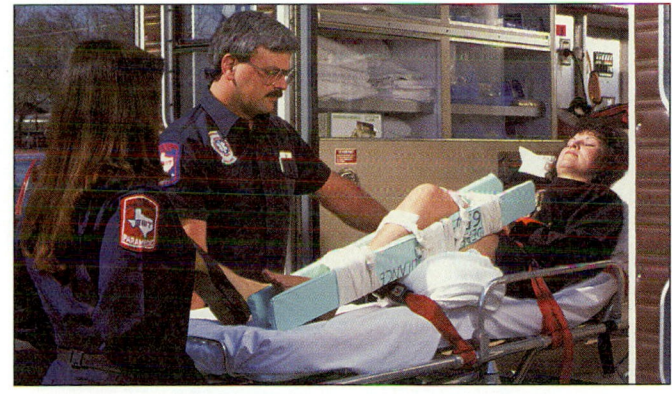

FIGURE 31-24 If you encounter resistance or extreme pain when applying traction to a long bone, apply padded board splints to each side of the limb, and secure them with soft roller bandages, securing the limb in its deformed position.

the splint. After applying the splint, you inflate it with your mouth, never with a pump. The air splint is comfortable, provides uniform contact, and has the added advantage of applying firm pressure to a bleeding wound. Air splints are used to immobilize injuries below the elbow or below the knee.

Air splints have some drawbacks, particularly in cold weather areas. The zipper can stick, clog with dirt, or freeze. Significant changes in the weather affect the pressure of the air in the splint, decreasing as the environment grows colder and increasing as the environment grows warmer. The same thing happens when there are changes in altitude, which can be a problem with helicopter transport of patients. Therefore, you should carefully monitor the splint and let air out if the splint becomes overinflated.

The method of applying an air splint depends on whether it has a zipper. With either type, you must first cover all wounds with a dry, sterile dressing, making sure that you use BSI techniques. Then, if the splint has a zipper, hold the injured limb slightly off the ground, applying gentle traction and supporting the site of

SKILL DRILL EMT-B

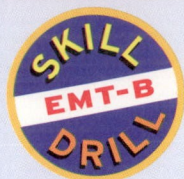

Applying a Rigid Splint

Figure 31-23

1

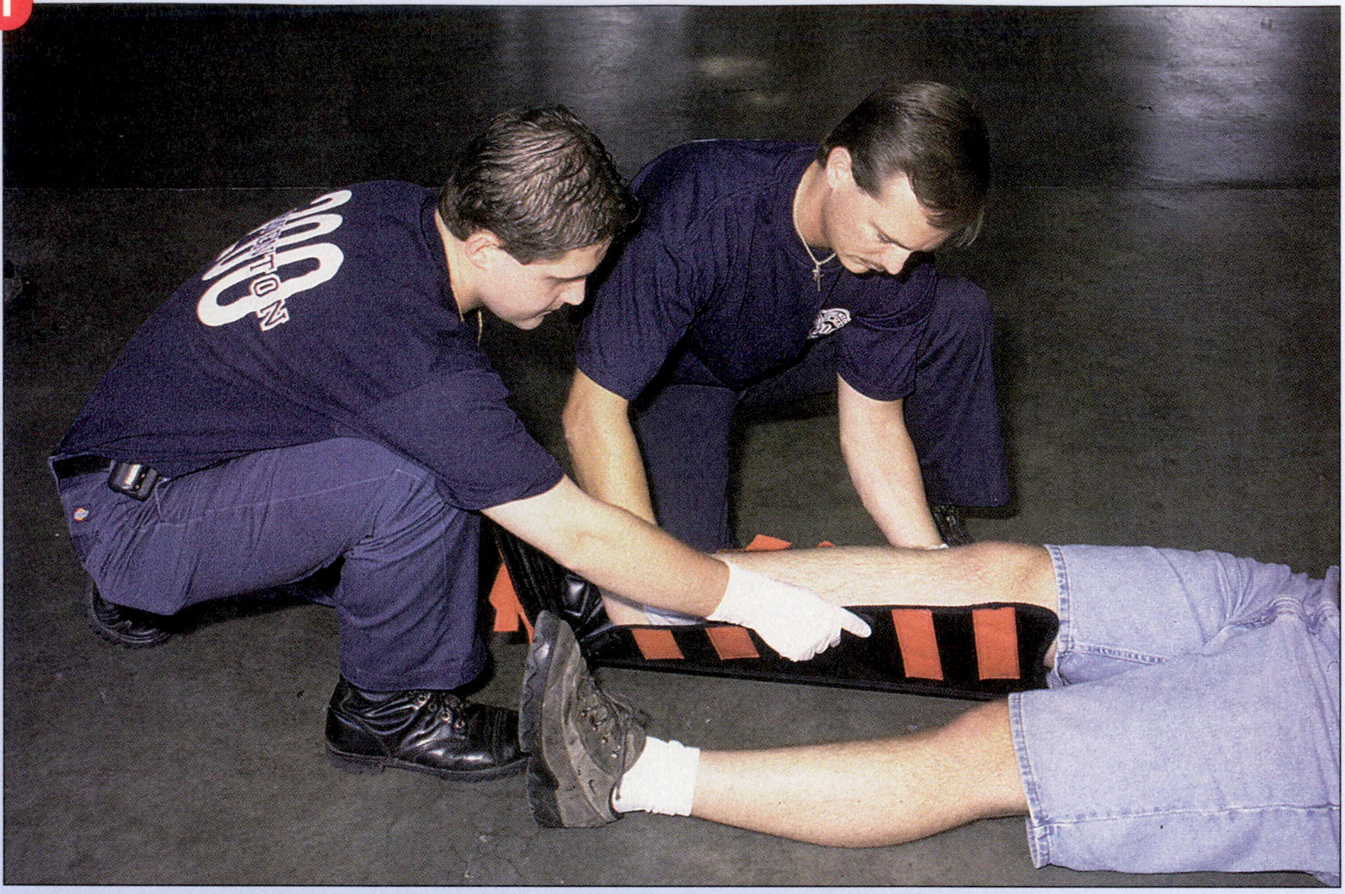

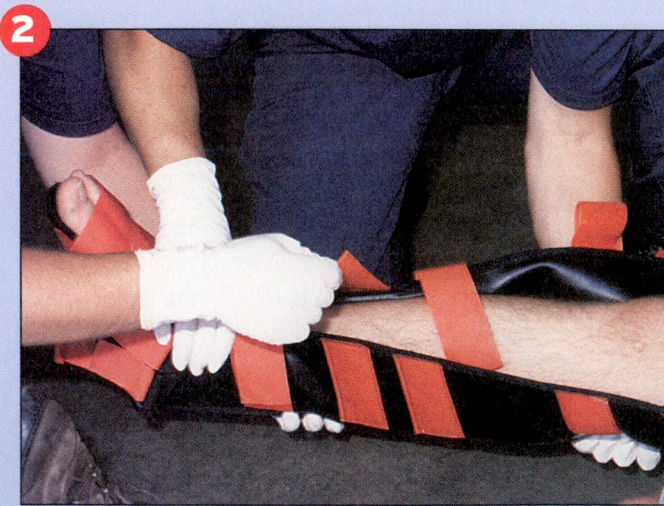

Provide gentle support and in-line traction to the limb as your partner prepares the splint alongside or under the limb. With some splints you may need to place a pad between the limb and the splint to ensure there is even pressure and even contact.

2

Apply bindings to secure the splint to the limb.

3

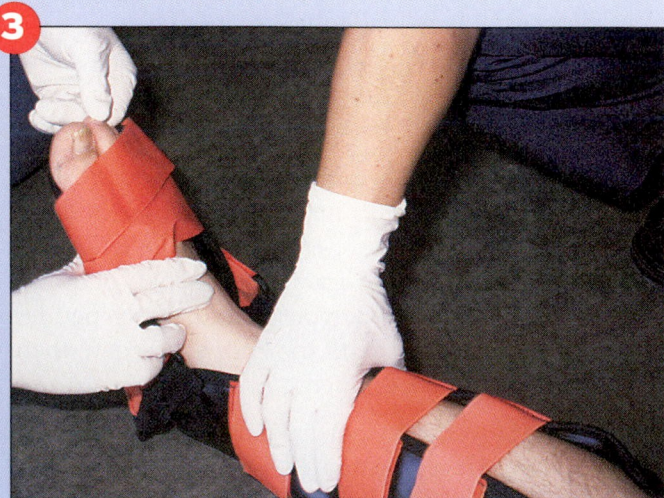

Assess neurovascular function distal to the splint.

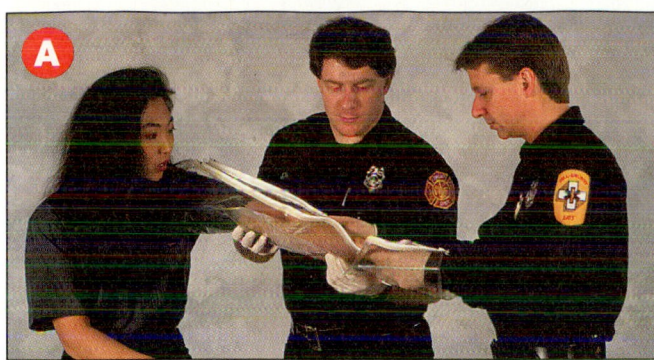

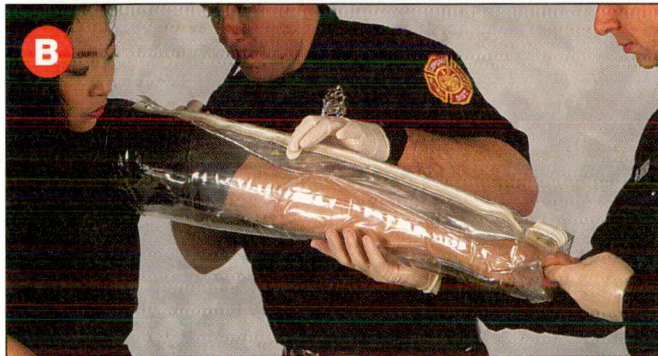

FIGURE 31-25 A: Support the injured limb, applying gentle traction as your partner places the open deflated splint around the limb. **B:** Zip up the splint, and then inflate it by mouth.

injury. Place the open, deflated splint around the limb, zip it up, and inflate it by mouth (Figure 31-25). When this is done, test the pressure in the splint.

If you use a nonzippered or partially zippered type of air splint, have another person help you follow these steps (Figure 31-26):

1. First EMT-B: **Place your arm** through the splint. Extend your hand beyond the splint, and grasp the hand or foot of the injured limb.

2. Second EMT-B: **Support the patient's injured limb** until splinting is accomplished.

3. First EMT-B: **Apply gentle traction** to the hand or foot while sliding the splint onto the injured limb. The hand or foot of the injured limb should always be included in the splint.

4. Second EMT-B: **Inflate the splint** by mouth.

5. First EMT-B: **Test the pressure** in the splint. This is something that you must do with either type of air splint. With proper inflation, you should just be able to compress the walls of the splint together with a firm pinch between the thumb and index finger near the edge of the splint.

6. First EMT-B: As with any other splint, **check and record** the distal neurovascular function and monitor it periodically until the patient reaches the hospital.

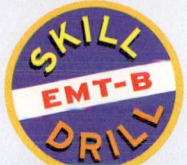

Applying an Air Splint
Figure 31-26

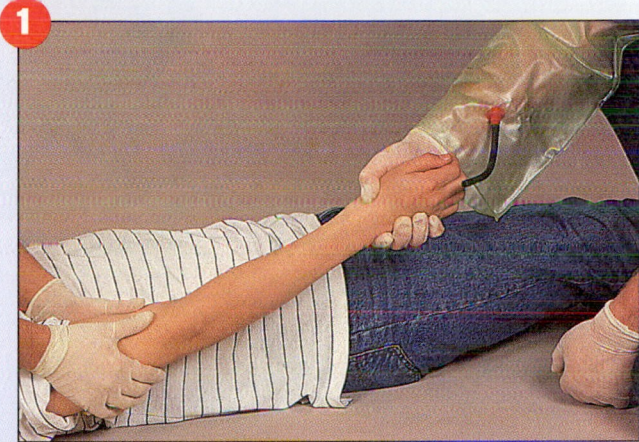

Support the injured limb as your partner places his or her arm through the splint to grasp the patient's hand.

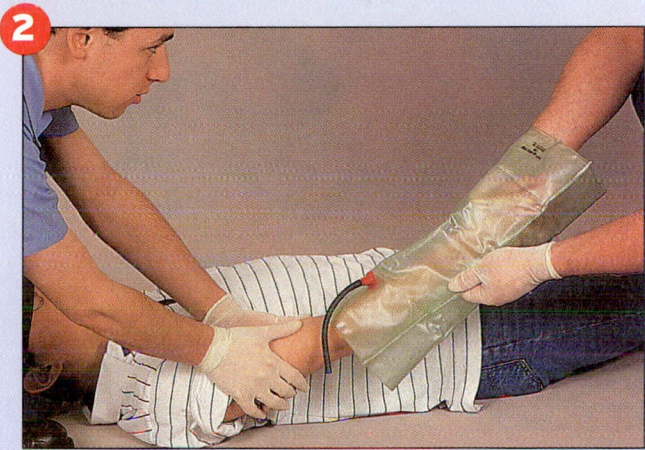

Continue to support the limb as your partner applies gentle traction while sliding the splint onto the injured limb.

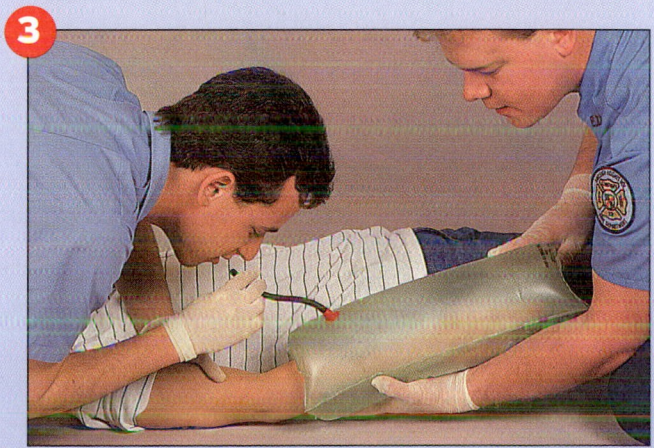

Inflate the splint by mouth.

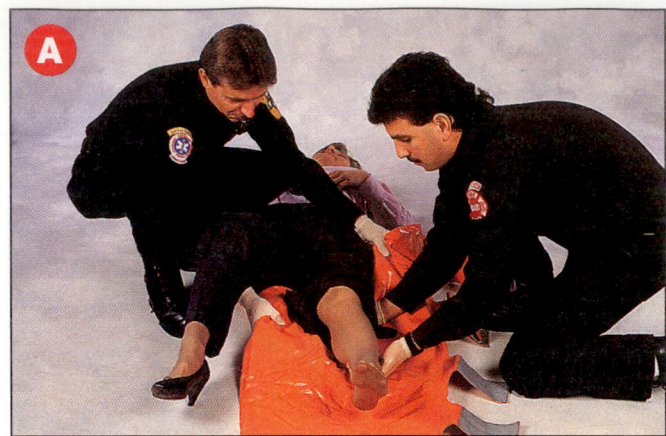

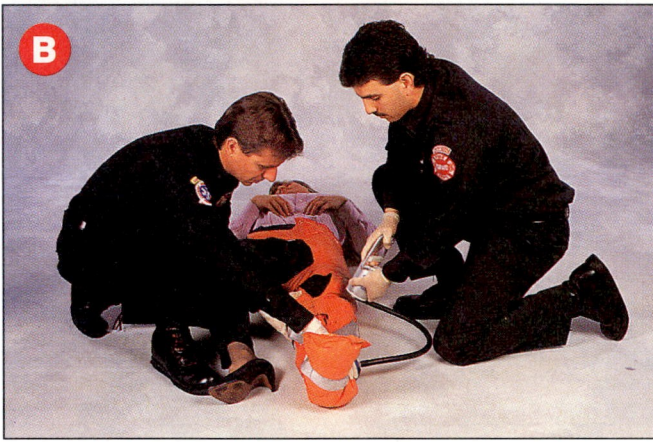

FIGURE 31-27 A: Gently place the injured limb onto the vacuum splint. **B:** Wrap the splint around the limb, draw the air out of the splint through the suction valve with your mouth, and then seal the valve.

Other formable splints include pillow splints, SAM splints, a sling and swathe, and the pneumatic antishock garment (PASG) for pelvic fractures. Just like an air splint, a vacuum splint can be easily shaped to fit around a deformed limb. Instead of pumping air in, however, you suck it out through a valve. Once the valve is sealed, the vacuum splint becomes rigid, conforming to the shape of the deformed limb and immobilizing it (Figure 31-27).

Traction splints. Traction splints are used primarily to secure fractures of the shaft of the femur, which are characterized by pain, swelling, and deformity of the midthigh. A traction splint should not be used if the patient has a joint or lower leg injury. Several different types of lower extremity traction splints are commercially available, such as the Hare traction splint, the Sager splint, and the Kendrick splint, each with its own unique method of application with which you must be familiar. The use of the Hare and Sager splints is described in this chapter.

The Hare traction splint uses a force called countertraction, which is applied by the upper end of the splint

against the ischial tuberosity of the patient's pelvis. This splint is not suitable for use on the upper extremity because the major nerves and blood vessels in the patient's axilla cannot tolerate countertraction forces.

Do not use traction splints for any of the following conditions:

- Injuries of the upper extremity
- Injuries close to or involving the knee
- Injuries of the hip
- Injuries of the pelvis
- Partial amputations or avulsions with bone separation
- Lower leg or ankle injury

Proper application of a traction splint requires two well-trained EMT-Bs working together. Practice the following steps with your partner until the sequence and necessary teamwork have become routine (Figure 31-28):

1. **Cut open the patient's pant leg,** or otherwise expose the injured lower extremity. Follow BSI techniques as needed. Be sure to assess and record the pulse, motor function, and sensation distal to the injury.

2. **Place the splint beside the patient's uninjured leg,** and adjust it to the proper length, with the ring at the ischial tuberosity and the splint extending 12″ beyond the foot. Open and adjust the four Velcro support straps, which should be positioned at the midthigh, above the knee, below the knee, and above the ankle.

3. First EMT-B: **Manually support and stabilize** the injured limb so that no motion will occur at the fracture site while the second EMT-B fastens the appropriate-sized ankle hitch about the patient's ankle and foot. Normally, the patient's shoe is removed for this procedure.

4. First EMT-B: **Support the leg at the site of the suspected injury** while the second EMT-B manually applies gentle longitudinal traction to the ankle hitch and foot. Use only enough to force to align (reposition) the limb so that it will fit into the splint; do not attempt to align the fracture fragments anatomically.

5. First EMT-B: **Slide the splint into position** under the patient's injured limb, making certain that the ring is seated well on the ischial tuberosity. Pad the groin, and gently apply the ischial strap.

6. First EMT-B: While the second EMT-B continues to maintain traction, **connect the loops of the ankle hitch** to the end of the splint. Then apply

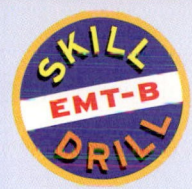

Applying a Hare Traction Splint
Figure 31-28

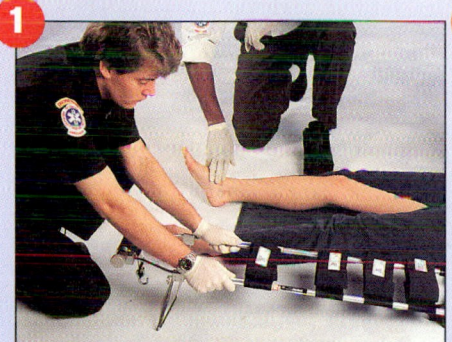

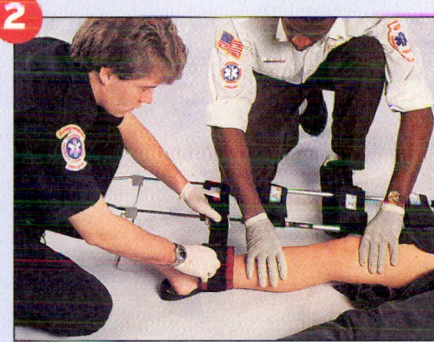

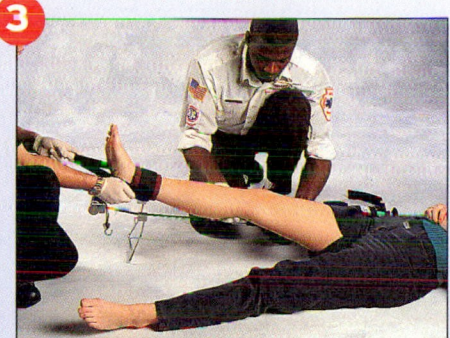

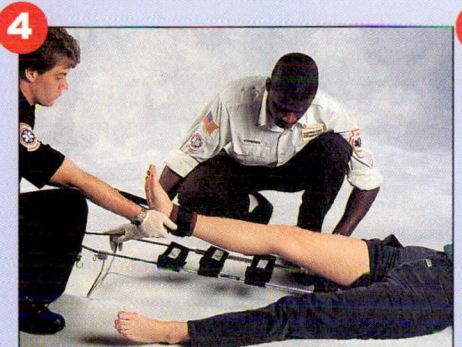

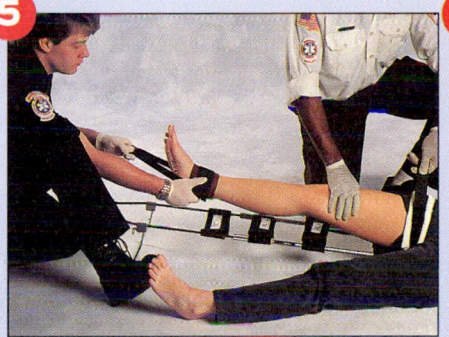

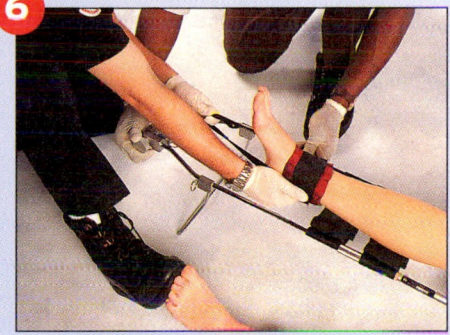

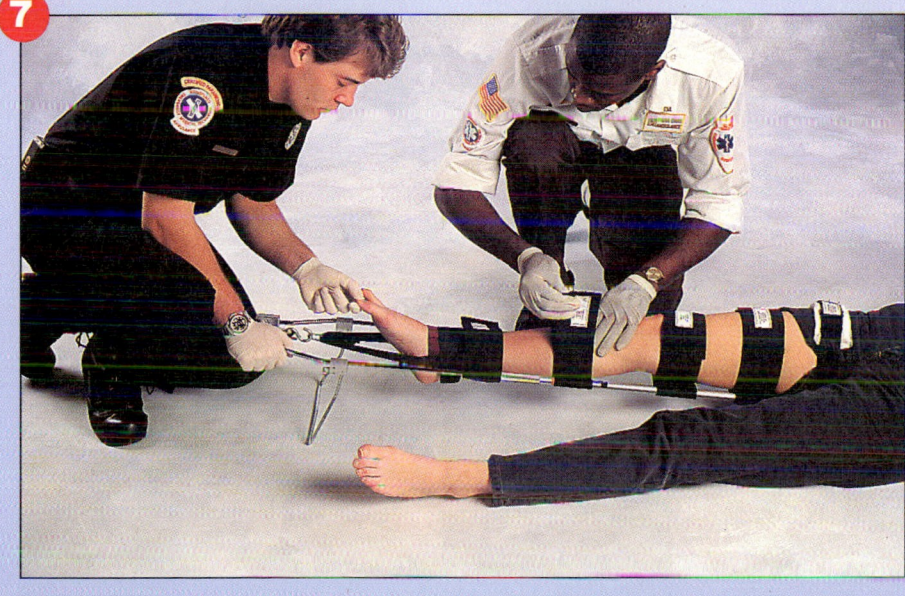

1 Cut open the patient's pant leg, or otherwise expose the injured limb. Then place the splint beside the patient's uninjured limb, and adjust it to the proper length.

2 Support the injured limb as your partner fastens the ankle hitch about the patient's foot and ankle.

3 Continue to support the limb as your partner applies gentle in-line traction to the ankle hitch and foot.

4 Slide the splint into position under the injured limb.

5 Pad the groin area, and fasten the ischial strap.

6 Connect the loops of the ankle hitch to the end of the splint as your partner continues to maintain traction.

7 Fasten the support straps so that the limb is secured in the splint, and assess distal pulses. Secure the patient to a long spine board for transport.

gentle traction to the connecting strap between the ankle hitch and the splint, just strongly enough to maintain limb alignment. Use caution: This splint comes with a ratchet mechanism to tighten the strap, which can overstretch the limb and further injure the patient.

7. Once proper traction has been applied, **fasten the support straps** so that the limb is securely held in the splint. Check *all* proximal and distal support straps to make sure they are secure.

8. At this point, **reassess distal pulses,** motor function, and sensation.

9. **Place the patient securely on a long spine board** for transport to the emergency department. You may need to load the patient feet first into the ambulance so that you do not shut the door against the splint.

Because this traction splint immobilizes the limb by producing countertraction on the ischium and in the groin, use care to pad these areas well. You must avoid excessive pressure on the external genitalia. Always use commercially available padded ankle hitches rather than pieces of rope, cord, or tape. Such improvised hitches can sometimes be painful and can potentially obstruct circulation in the foot.

Hazards of improper splinting. You must be aware of the hazards associated with the improper application of splints, including the following:

- Compression of nerves, tissues, and blood vessels
- Delay in transport of a patient with a life-threatening injury
- Reduction of distal circulation if the splint is too tight
- Aggravation of the injury
- Injury to tissue, nerves, blood vessels, or muscles as a result of excessive movement of the bone or joint

Transportation

Once an injured limb is adequately splinted, the patient is ready to be transferred to a backboard or stretcher and transported.

Very few, if any, musculoskeletal injuries justify the use of excessive speed during transport. The limb will be stable once a dressing and splint have been applied. However, the patient with a pulseless limb must be given a higher priority. Still, if the hospital is only a few minutes away, speeding to the emergency department will make little or no difference to the patient's eventual outcome. If the treatment facility is an hour or more away, the patient with a pulseless limb should be transported by helicopter or immediate ground transportation. If circulation in the distal limb is impaired, always notify medical control so that proper steps can be taken quickly once the patient arrives in the emergency department.

Specific Musculoskeletal Injuries

Injuries to the Clavicle and Scapula

The <u>clavicle</u>, or collarbone, is one of the most commonly fractured bones in the body. Fractures of the clavicle occur most often in children when they fall on an outstretched hand. They can also occur with crushing injuries of the chest. A patient with a fracture of the clavicle will report pain in the shoulder and will usually hold the arm across the front of his or her body. A young child often reports pain throughout the entire arm and is unwilling to use any part of that limb. These complaints may make it difficult to localize the point of injury, but, generally, swelling and point tenderness occur over the clavicle (Figure 31-29). Because the clavicle is subcutaneous (just beneath the skin), the skin will occasionally "tent" over the fracture fragment. The clavicle lies directly over major arteries, veins, and nerves; therefore, fracture of the clavicle may lead to neurovascular compromise.

Fractures of the <u>scapula</u>, or shoulder blade, occur much less frequently because this bone is well protected by many large muscles. Fractures of the scapula are almost always the result of a forceful, direct blow to the back, directly over the scapula, which may also injure the thoracic cage, lungs, and heart. For this reason, you must carefully assess the patient for signs of breathing problems. Provide supplemental oxygen and prompt transport for patients who are having difficulty

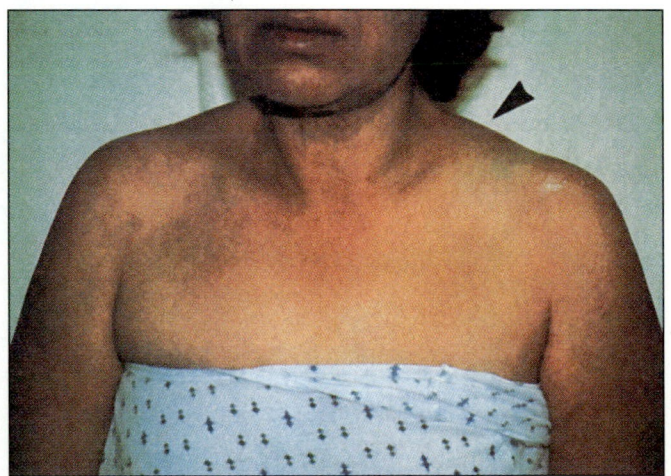

FIGURE 31-29 A clavicle injury is characterized by swelling, point tenderness, and "tenting" over the fracture fragment.

breathing. Remember, it is the associated chest injuries, not the fractured scapula, that pose the greatest threat of long-term disability.

Abrasions, contusions, and significant swelling may also occur, and the patient will often limit use of the arm because of pain at the fracture site (Figure 31-30). The scapula also has bony projections that may be fractured with a lesser degree of force.

The joint between the outer end of the clavicle and the acromion process of the scapula is called the acromio-clavicular (A/C) joint. This joint is frequently separated during football and hockey play when a player falls and lands on the point of the shoulder, driving the scapula away from the outer end of the clavicle. This dislocation is often called an A/C separation. The distal end of the clavicle will usually stick out, and the patient will complain of pain, including point tenderness over the A/C joint (Figure 31-31).

Fractures of the clavicle and scapula and A/C separations can all be splinted effectively with a sling and swathe (Figure 31-32). A sling is any bandage or material that helps support the weight of an injured upper extremity, relieving the downward pull of gravity on the injured site. To be effective, a sling must apply gentle upward support to the olecranon process of the ulna. The knot of the sling should be tied to one side of the neck so that it does not press uncomfortably on the cervical spine.

To fully immobilize the shoulder region, a swathe, a bandage that passes completely around the chest, must be used to bind the arm to the chest wall. The swathe should be tight enough to prevent the arm from swinging freely but not so tight as to compress the chest and compromise breathing. Leave the patient's hand exposed so that you can assess neurovascular function at regular intervals.

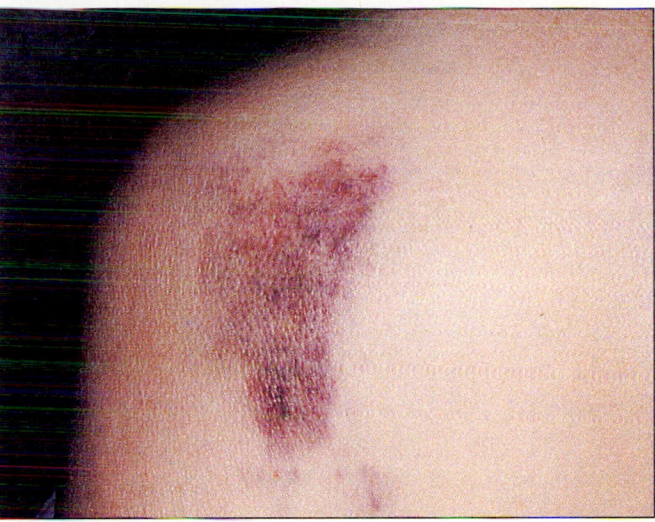

FIGURE 31-30 Contusions or abrasions over the scapular area may indicate a fracture.

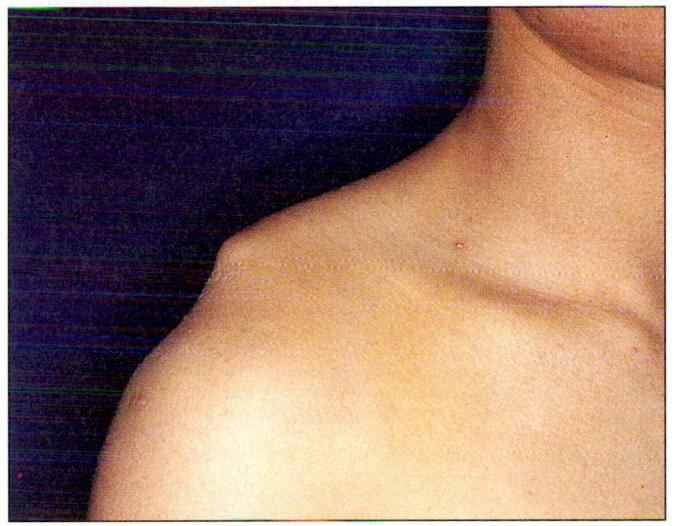

FIGURE 31-31 With A/C separations, the distal end of the clavicle usually sticks out.

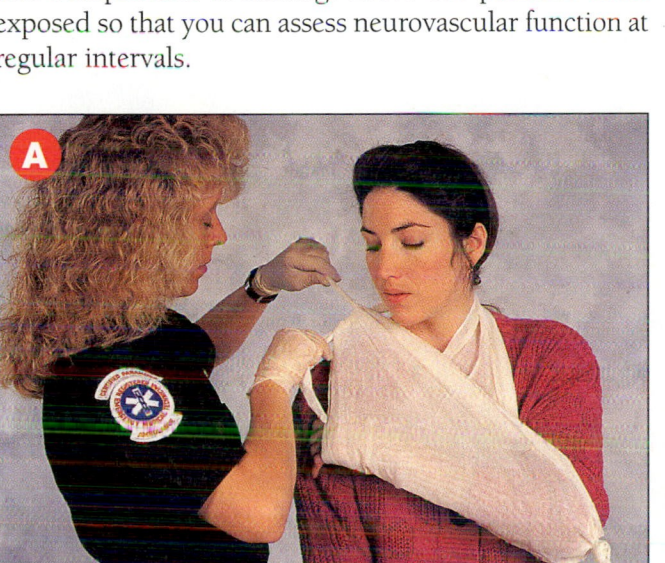
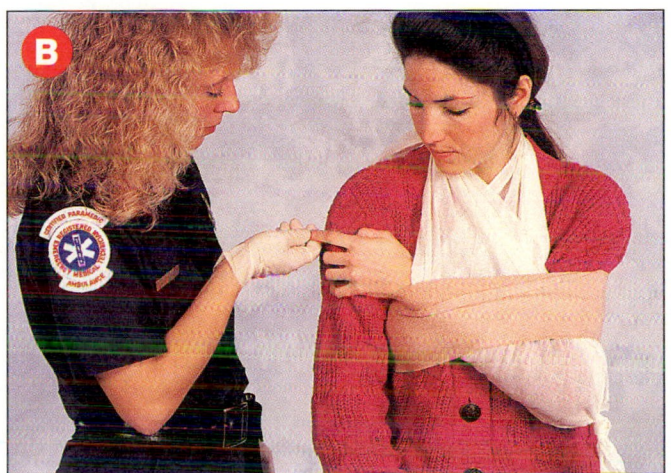

FIGURE 31-32 A: Apply the sling so that the knot is tied to one side of the neck. **B:** Bind the arm to the chest wall with a swathe so that the arm cannot swing freely. Leave the patient's hand exposed so that you can assess distal circulation.

Commercially available shoulder immobilizers or slings will provide adequate splinting for injuries of the shoulder region, as will triangular bandage slings. When all else fails, place a T-shirt over the arm.

Dislocation of the Shoulder

The glenohumeral joint (shoulder joint) is where the head of the <u>humerus</u>, the supporting bone of the upper arm, meets the glenoid fossa of the scapula. The <u>glenoid fossa</u> joins with the humeral head to form the glenohumeral joint. It is the most commonly dislocated large joint in the body. Almost always, the humeral head will dislocate anteriorly, coming to lie in front of the scapula as a result of forced abduction (away from the midline) and external rotation of the arm (Figure 31-33).

Shoulder dislocations are extremely painful. The patient will guard the shoulder and try to protect it by holding the dislocated arm in a fixed position away from the chest wall (Figure 31-34). The shoulder joint will usually be locked, and the shoulder will appear squared off or flattened. The humeral head will protrude anteriorly underneath the pectoris major on the anterior chest wall. As a result, the axillary nerve may be compressed, causing a numb patch on the outer aspect of the shoulder. Be sure to document this finding. Some patients may also report some numbness in the hand because either the nerves or the circulation is compromised.

Immobilizing an anterior shoulder dislocation is difficult, because any attempt to bring the arm in toward the chest will produce pain. You must splint the joint in whatever position is most comfortable for the patient. If necessary, place a pillow or rolled blankets or towels between the arm and chest to fill up the space between them (Figure 31-35). Once the arm is stabilized in this way, the elbow can usually be flexed to 90° without causing further pain. At this point, you can apply a sling to the forearm and wrist to support the weight of the arm. Finally, secure the arm in the sling to the pillow and chest with a swathe. Transport the patient in a sitting or semiseated position.

Dislocation of the shoulder disrupts the supporting ligaments of the anterior aspect of the shoulder. Often, these ligaments fail to heal properly, so dislocation recurs, each time causing further neurovascular compromise and joint injury. In certain cases, surgical repair may be required. Some patients are able to reduce (set) their own dislocated shoulders. Generally, however, this maneuver must be done in a hospital setting and only after X-rays have been obtained.

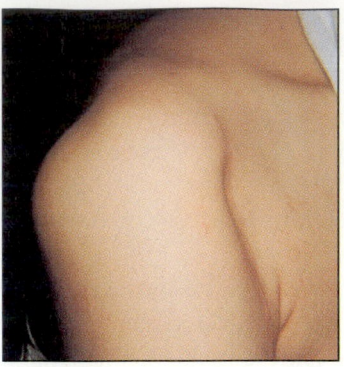

FIGURE 31-33 The shoulder almost always dislocates anteriorly. Note the absence of the normal rounded appearance of the shoulder.

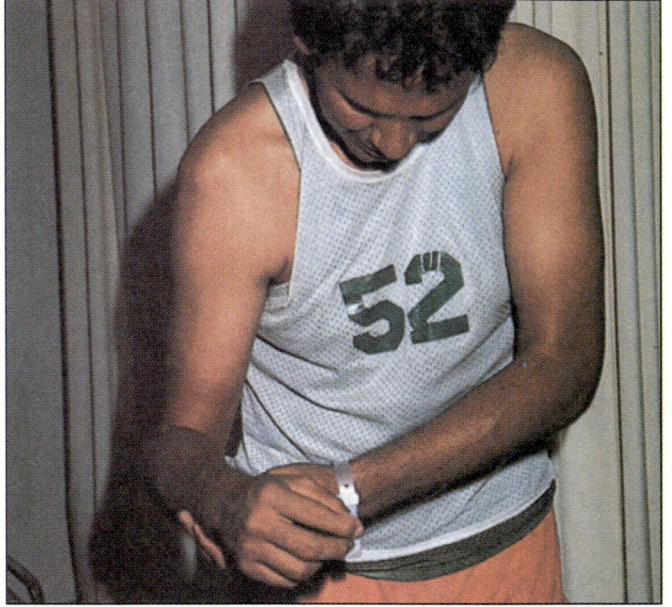

FIGURE 31-34 A patient with a dislocated shoulder will guard the shoulder, trying to protect it by holding the arm in a fixed position away from the chest wall.

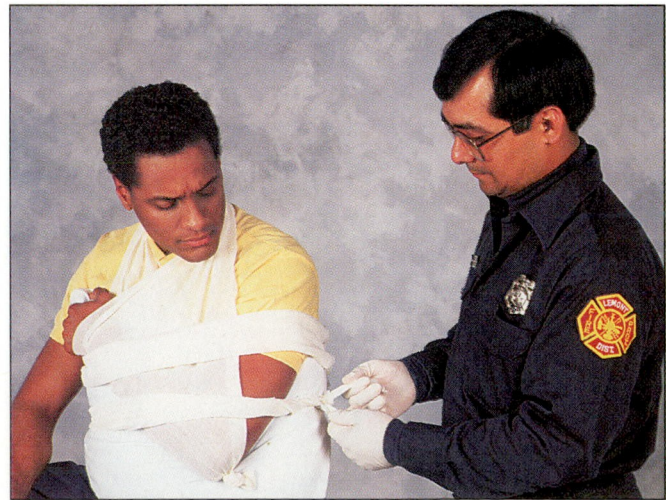

FIGURE 31-35 Splint the joint in a position of comfort, and place a pillow or towel between the arm and the chest wall to stabilize the arm, after which the elbow can be flexed to 90°. Apply a sling, and secure the arm to the chest with a swathe.

A shoulder will dislocate posteriorly instead of anteriorly about once in every 20 occurrences. Football players, especially linemen, are susceptible to this injury. The arm will often be locked in an adduction (toward the midline), so it cannot be rotated. Reducing the dislocation usually requires medical supervision. Afterward, the patient will need a modified airplane or gunslinger splint, because a sling may cause dislocation to recur.

Fracture of the Humerus

Fractures of the humerus occur either proximally, in the midshaft, or distally at the elbow (Table 31-2). Fractures of the proximal humerus resulting from falls are common among the elderly. Fractures of the midshaft occur more often in young patients, usually as the result of a violent injury.

With any severely angulated fracture, you should apply traction to realign the fracture fragments before

TABLE 31-2	Characteristics and Treatment of Fractures of the Humerus	
Type	**Characteristics**	**Treatment**
Proximal Humeral Fractures	• Significant swelling, but no deformity, of the upper arm • Neurovascular compromise • Any or all of the brachial plexus affected, depending on the degree of displacement • Concurrent soft-tissue injuries • Possible rotator cuff injury (if X-rays show no fracture, a tear of the rotator cuff is possible, especially if the patient cannot move the arm toward the medial plane)	• Immobilize in a sling and swathe or a shoulder immobilizer. • Use the chest wall as a splint and secure the injured arm to the chest wall. • Place a short, padded board splint on the lateral side of the arm under the sling and swathe for additional support.
Midshaft Fractures	• Gross angulation of the arm • Marked instability and crepitus of fracture fragments • Possible neurovascular compromise • Possible entrapment of the radial nerve (The patient cannot extend or dorsiflex the wrist or fingers and may report numbness on the dorsum of the hand; classic "wrist drop.")	• Immobilize with a sling and swathe or a shoulder immobilizer. • Use the chest wall as a splint, and secure the injured arm to the chest wall. • Place a short, padded board splint on the lateral side of the arm under the sling and swathe for additional support.
Distal Humeral Fractures	• Significant swelling at the elbow • Possible neurovascular compromise • Possible injury to the ulnar or median nerves (document nerve status before and after any attempt to reduce the fracture)	• Immobilize in a splint, in addition to a sling and swathe or a shoulder immobilizer.

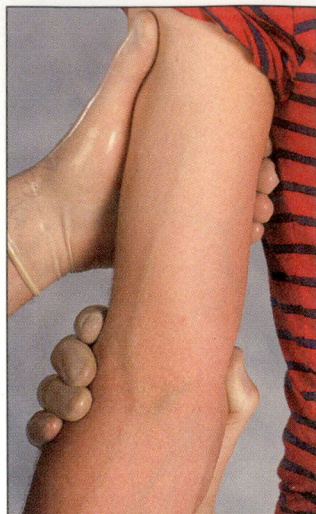

FIGURE 31-36 To align a severe deformity associated with a humeral shaft fracture, apply gentle pressure to the humeral condoyles, as shown in this uninjured arm.

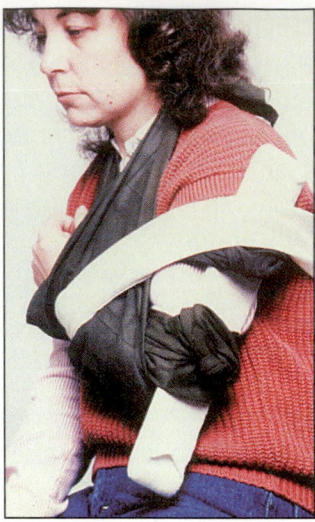

FIGURE 31-37 Splint a humeral shaft fracture with a sling and swathe supplemented by a padded board splint on the lateral aspect of the arm.

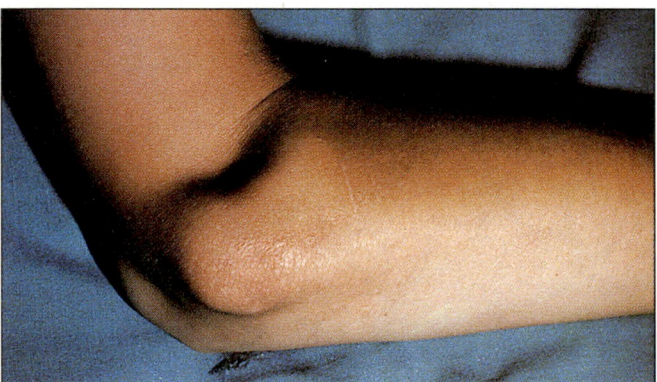

FIGURE 31-38 Posterior dislocation of the elbow makes the olecranon process of the ulna much more prominent.

splinting them. Support the site of the fracture with one hand, and with the other hand, grasp the two humeral condyles just above the elbow. Pull gently in line with the normal axis of the limb (Figure 31-36). Once you achieve gross alignment of the limb, splint the arm with a sling and swathe, supplemented by a padded board splint on the lateral aspect of the arm (Figure 31-37). If the patient reports significant pain or resists gentle traction, splint the fracture in the deformed position with a padded wire ladder or a padded board splint, using pillows to support the injured limb. Note that compartment syndrome can develop in the forearm in children with these fractures.

Elbow Injuries

Fractures and dislocations often occur around the elbow, and the different types of injuries are difficult to distinguish without X-rays. However, they all produce similar limb deformities and require the same emergency care. Injuries to nerves and blood vessels are quite common in this region. Such injuries can be caused or worsened by inappropriate emergency care, particularly by excessive manipulation of the injured joint.

Fracture of the distal humerus. This type of fracture, also known as a supracondylar or intercondylar fracture, is common in children. Frequently, the fracture fragments rotate significantly, producing deformity and causing injuries to nearby vessels and nerves. Swelling occurs rapidly and is often severe.

Dislocation of the elbow. This type of injury typically occurs in athletes and does not appear in young children. The ulna and radius are most often displaced posteriorly. The <u>ulna</u>, the bone on the small finger side of the forearm, and the <u>radius</u>, the bone on the thumb side of the forearm, both join the distal humerus. The posterior displacement makes the olecranon process of the ulna much more prominent (Figure 31-38). The joint is usually locked, with the forearm moderately flexed on the arm; this position makes any attempt at motion extremely painful. As with a fracture of the distal humerus, there is swelling and significant potential for vessel or nerve injury.

Elbow joint sprain. This injury is rare and is usually diagnosed by X-ray. Often, the real problem is a hard-to-detect fracture.

Fracture of the olecranon process of the ulna. This fracture is usually the result of a direct blow and is often characterized by lacerations and abrasions. Often, the patient will be unable to extend the elbow.

Fracture of the radial head. Often missed during diagnosis, this fracture generally occurs as a result of a fall on an outstretched arm or a direct blow to the lateral aspect of the elbow. Attempts to rotate the elbow or wrist are very uncomfortable.

Care of elbow injuries. All elbow injuries are serious and require careful management (Figure 31-39). Always assess distal neurovascular functions periodically in patients with elbow injuries. If you find strong pulses and good capillary refill, then splint the elbow injury in the position in which you found it, adding a wrist sling if this seems helpful. Two padded board splints, applied to each side of the limb and secured with soft roller bandages, usually are enough to stabilize the arm. Make sure the board extends from the shoulder joint to the wrist joint, immobilizing the entire bone above and below the injured joint. Alternatively, you can mold a padded wire ladder splint or a SAM splint® to the shape of the limb. If necessary, you may add further support to the limb with a pillow.

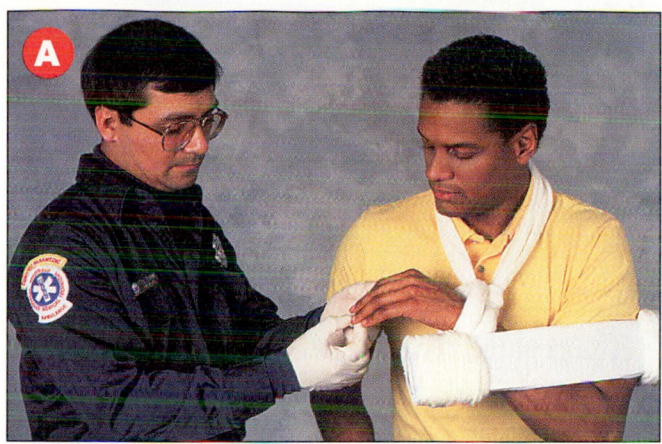
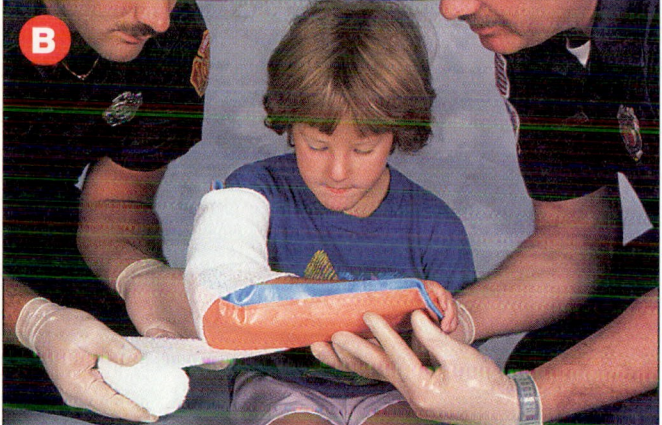

FIGURE 31-39 A: Two padded board splints provide adequate stabilization for an injured elbow. The addition of a wrist sling provides additional support. **B:** A SAM splint® can be molded to the shape of the limb so that you can splint it in the position in which it was found.

A cold, pale hand or a weak or absent pulse and poor capillary refill indicate that the blood vessels have likely been injured. Further care of this patient must be dictated by a physician. Notify medical control immediately. If you are within 10 to 15 minutes of the hospital, splint the limb in the position in which you found it and provide prompt transport. Otherwise, medical control may direct you to try to realign the limb to improve circulation in the hand.

If the limb is pulseless and significantly deformed at the elbow, apply gentle manual traction in line with the long axis of the limb to decrease the deformity. This maneuver may restore the pulse. Be careful, as excessive manipulation will only worsen the vascular problem. If no pulse returns after one attempt, splint the limb in the most comfortable position for the patient. If the pulse is restored by gentle longitudinal traction, splint the limb in whatever position allows the strongest pulse. Provide prompt transport for all patients with impaired distal circulation.

Fractures of the Forearm

Fractures of the shaft of the radius and ulna are common in people of all age groups but are seen most often in children. Usually, both bones break at the same time when the injury is the result of a fall on an outstretched hand. An isolated fracture of the shaft of the ulna may occur as the result of a direct blow to it; this is known as a nightstick fracture (Figure 31-40).

Fractures of the distal radius, which are especially common in elderly patients with osteoporosis, are often known as Colles fractures. The term "silver fork deformity" is used to describe the distinctive appearance of the patient's arm (Figure 31-41). In children, this fracture may occur through the growth plate and can have long-term consequences.

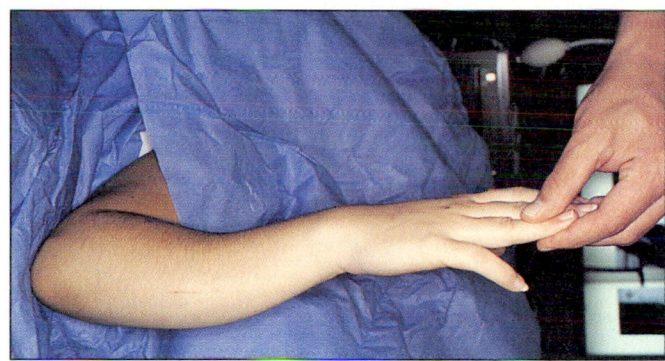

FIGURE 31-40 Fractures of the forearm often occur in children as a result of a fall on an outstretched hand.

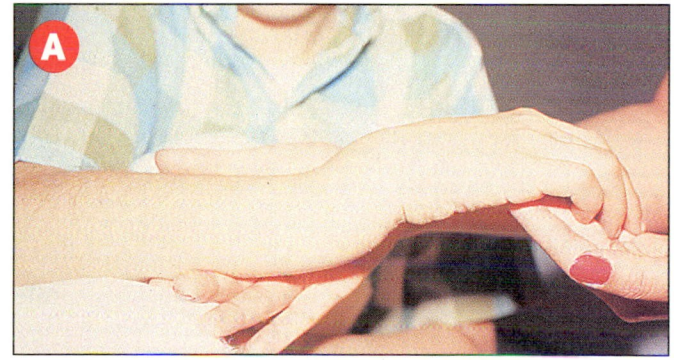

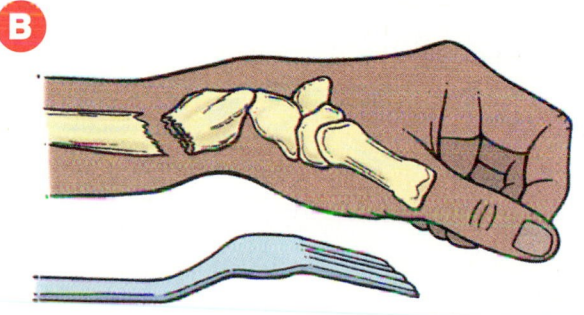

FIGURE 31-41 A: Fractures of the distal radius produce a characteristic silver fork deformity. **B:** An artist's illustration of same.

To immobilize fractures of the forearm or wrist, you can use a padded board, air, vacuum, or pillow splint. If the shaft of the bone has been fractured, be sure to include the elbow joint in the splint. Splinting of the elbow joint is not essential with fractures near the wrist; however, the patient will be more comfortable if you add a sling or pillow for more support.

Injuries to the Wrist and Hand

Injuries of the wrist, ranging from dislocations to sprains, must be confirmed by X-ray. Dislocations are usually associated with a fracture, resulting in a fracture-dislocation. Another common wrist injury is the isolated, nondisplaced fracture of a carpal bone, especially the scaphoid. Any questionable wrist sprain must be splinted and evaluated in the emergency department.

There is a great variety of hand injuries, some with potentially serious consequences. Industrial, recreational, and home accidents often result in dislocations, fractures, lacerations, burns, and amputations. Because the fingers and hands are required to function in such intricate ways, any injury that is not treated properly may result in permanent disability, as well as deformity. For this reason, all injuries to the hand, including simple lacerations, must be evaluated promptly by a physician. For example, you should not attempt to "pop" a dislocated finger joint back in place (Figure 31-42). Always bring any amputated parts to the hospital with the patient. Be sure to wrap the amputated part in a dry, sterile dressing and place it in a dry plastic bag. Put the bag in a cool container; *do not soak the part in water or allow it to freeze.*

A bulky forearm dressing makes an effective splint for any hand or wrist injury, as follows (Figure 31-43):

1. **Follow BSI techniques.**
2. **Cover all wounds** with a dry, sterile dressing.
3. **Form the injured hand** into the **position of function**, that is, with the wrist slightly dorsiflexed and all finger joints moderately flexed. This is the position that is used to hold a can most comfortably.

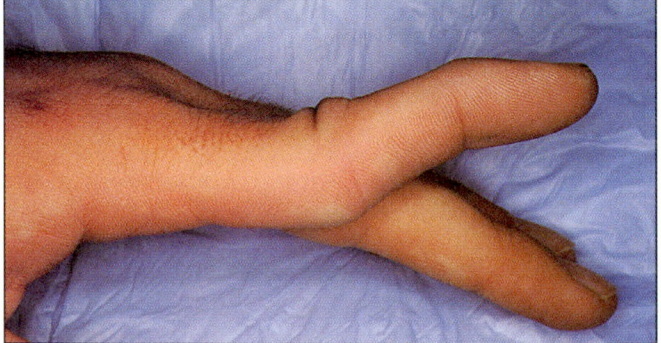

FIGURE 31-42 Dislocation of the finger joint. Do not be tempted to try to "pop" the joint back into place.

4. **Place a soft roller bandage** into the palm of the hand.
5. **Apply a padded board splint** to the palmar side of the wrist, and secure the entire length of the splint with a soft roller bandage.
6. **Prop the splinted hand** and wrist on a pillow or on the patient's chest during transport to the hospital.

Fractures of the Pelvis

Fracture of the pelvis is most often a result of direct compression in the form of a heavy blow that literally crushes the pelvis. The blow may be from a motor vehicle accident or a weapon used deliberately, a falling object, or a fall from a height. Injuries to the pelvis can also be caused by indirect forces. For example, when the knee strikes the dashboard in an automobile accident, the impact of the force is transmitted along the line of the **femur**, the thigh bone, which is the longest and largest bone in the body. The head of the femur is driven into the pelvis, causing it to fracture. However, not all pelvic fractures result from violent trauma. Even a simple fall can produce a fracture of the pelvis, especially in elderly individuals with osteoporosis.

Fractures of the pelvis may be accompanied by life-threatening loss of blood from the laceration of blood vessels affixed to the pelvis at certain key points. Up to several liters of blood may drain into the pelvic space and the **retroperitoneal space**, which lies between the abdominal cavity and the posterior abdominal wall. The kidneys, stomach, spleen, and intestines are contained in the retroperitoneal space. The result is significant hypotension, shock, and sometimes death. For this reason, you must take immediate steps to combat shock, even if there is only minimal swelling. Often, there are no visible signs of bleeding until severe blood loss has occurred. You should be prepared to resuscitate the patient rapidly if this becomes necessary.

Because the pelvis is surrounded by heavy muscle, open fractures of the pelvis are quite uncommon. However, pelvis fracture fragments can lacerate the rectum and vagina, creating an open fracture that is often overlooked. Once the protective pelvic ring is broken, the structures it is designed to protect, including the urinary bladder, are open to injury. The bladder may be lacerated by pelvic bone fragments, but more often, it tears or ruptures as a result of tension on either the bladder or the urethra.

You should suspect a fracture of the pelvis in any patient who has sustained a high-velocity injury and complains of discomfort in the lower back or abdomen. Because the area is covered by heavy muscle and other soft tissue, deformity or swelling may be very difficult to see. The most reliable sign of fracture of the pelvis is

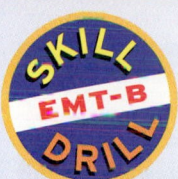

Splinting the Hand and Wrist

Figure 31-43

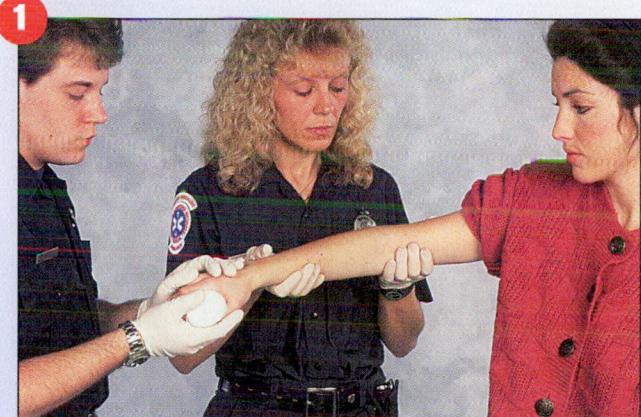

Support the injured limb as your partner forms the hand into the position of function, with the wrist slightly dorsiflexed and all finger joints moderately flexed. Place a soft roller bandage into the palm of the hand.

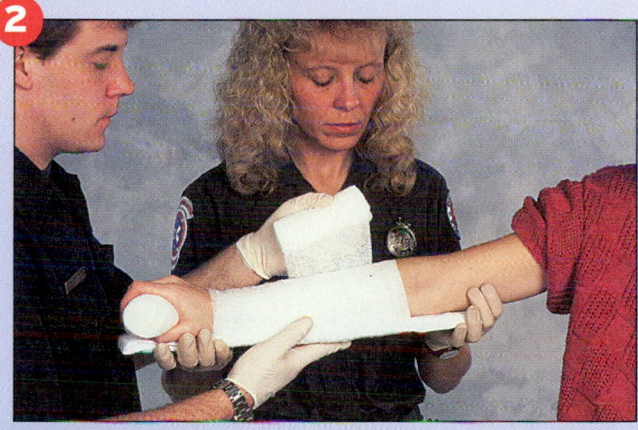

Apply a padded board splint to the palmar side of the wrist.

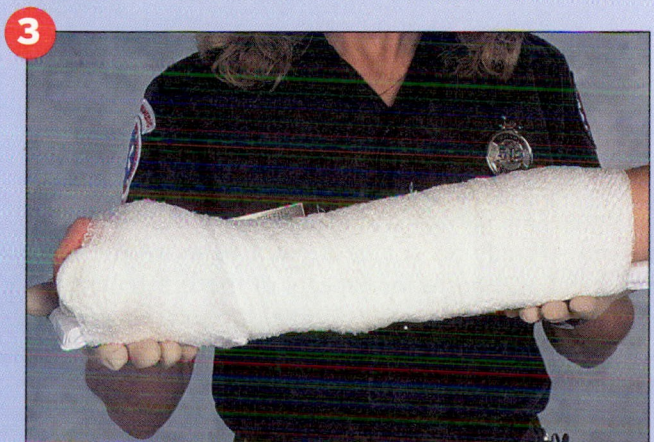

Secure the entire length of the splint with a soft roller bandage.

simple tenderness on firm compression and palpation. Firm compression on the two iliac crests will produce pain at a fracture site in the pelvic ring. Assess for tenderness by taking the following steps (Figure 31-44):

1. **Place the palms of your hands** over the lateral aspect of each iliac crest, and apply firm but gentle inward pressure on the pelvic ring.

2. **With the patient lying supine**, place a palm over the anterior aspect of each iliac crest, and apply firm downward pressure.

3. **Use the palm of your hand** to firmly but gently palpate the symphysis pubis, the firm cartilaginous joint between the two pubic bones. This area will be tender if there is injury to the anterior portion of the pelvic ring.

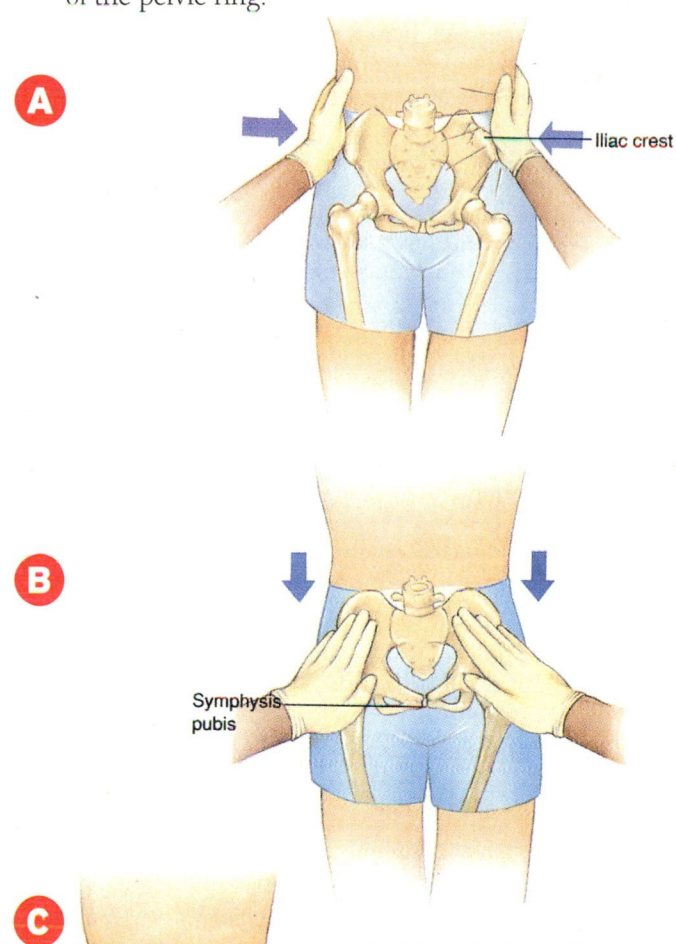

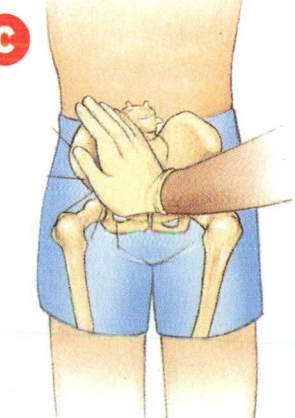

FIGURE 31-44 A: To assess for tenderness in the pelvic region, place your hands over the lateral aspect of each iliac crest, and gently compress the pelvis. **B:** With the patient in a supine position, place your palms over the anterior aspect of each iliac crest, and apply firm but gentle downward pressure. **C:** Palpate the symphysis pubis with the palms of your hand.

If there has been injury to the bladder or the urethra, the patient will have lower abdominal tenderness and may have evidence of <u>hematuria</u> (blood in the urine) or blood at the urethral opening.

Perform an initial assessment, and carefully monitor the general condition of any patient who you suspect has a pelvic fracture, because he or she is at high risk for hypovolemic shock. Stable patients can be secured to a long spine board or a scoop stretcher to immobilize isolated fractures of the pelvis. Place a PASG on the spine board or stretcher before transferring the patient to the backboard (Figure 31-45). The PASG will be ready to apply and inflate if the patient develops signs of shock. Remember, the PASG is only a temporary stabilization device and must be removed within 24 hours. Such a critically injured patient must be transferred to the hospital immediately.

Dislocation of the Hip

The hip joint is a very stable ball-and-socket joint that dislocates only after significant injury. Almost all dislocations of the hip are posterior. The femoral head is displaced posteriorly to lie in the muscles of the buttock. Posterior dislocation of the hip most commonly occurs during automobile accidents in which the knee meets with a direct force, such as the dashboard, and the entire femur is driven posteriorly, dislocating the joint (Figure 31-46). Thus, you should suspect a hip dislocation in any patient who has been in an automobile accident and has a contusion, laceration, or obvious fracture in the knee region. Very rarely does the femoral head dislocate anteriorly; in this circumstance, the legs are suddenly and forcibly spread wide apart and locked in this position.

Posterior dislocation of the hip is frequently complicated by injury to the sciatic nerve, which is located directly behind the hip joint. The <u>sciatic nerve</u> is the most important nerve in the lower extremity; it controls the activity of muscles in the thigh and below the knee, as well as sensation in the entire leg and foot. When the head of the femur is forced out of the hip socket, it may compress or stretch the sciatic nerve, leading to partial or complete paralysis of the nerve. The result is decreased sensation in the leg and foot and frequently weakness in the foot muscles. Generally, only the dorsiflexors, the muscles that raise the toes or foot, are involved, causing the "foot drop" that is characteristic of damage to the peroneal portion of the sciatic nerve.

Patients with a posterior dislocation of the hip typically lie with the hip joint flexed (the knee joint drawn up toward the chest) and the thigh rotated inward toward the midline of the body over the top of the opposite thigh (Figure 31-47). With the rare anterior dislocation, the limb is in the opposite position, extended straight out, rotated, and pointing away from the midline of the body.

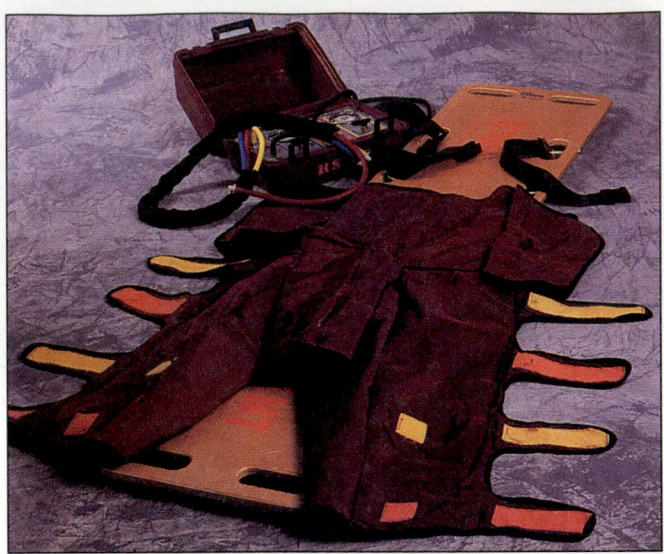

FIGURE 31-45 Place a PASG on the spine board before log-rolling a patient with a suspected pelvic fracture.

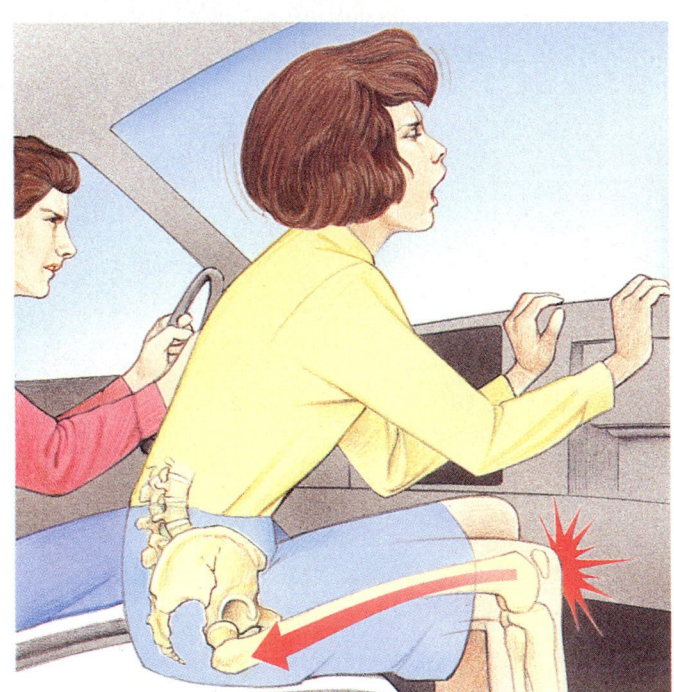

FIGURE 31-46 Posterior dislocation of the hip can occur as a result of the knee hitting the dashboard in an automobile crash. The impact drives the femur posteriorly (see arrow), dislocating the joint.

Dislocation of the hip is associated with very distinctive signs. The patient will have severe pain in the hip and will strongly resist any attempt to move the joint. The lateral and posterior aspects of the hip region will be tender on palpation. With some thin individuals, you can palpate the femoral head deep within the muscles of the buttock. Check for a sciatic nerve injury by carefully assessing sensation and motor function in the lower extremity. Occasionally, sciatic nerve function will be normal at first and then slowly diminish.

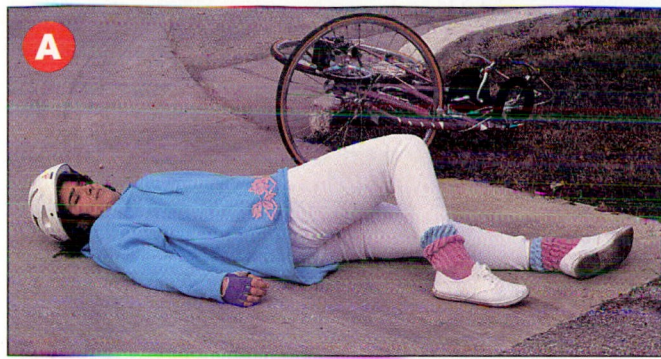

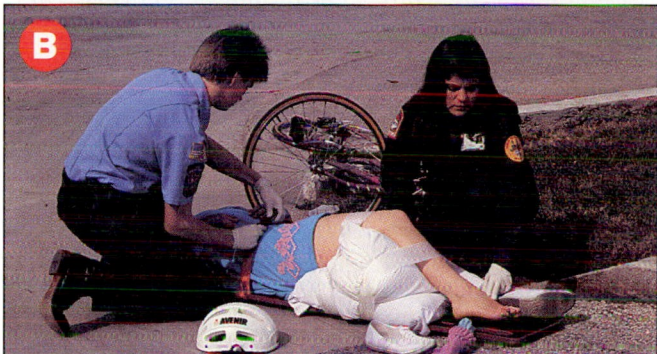

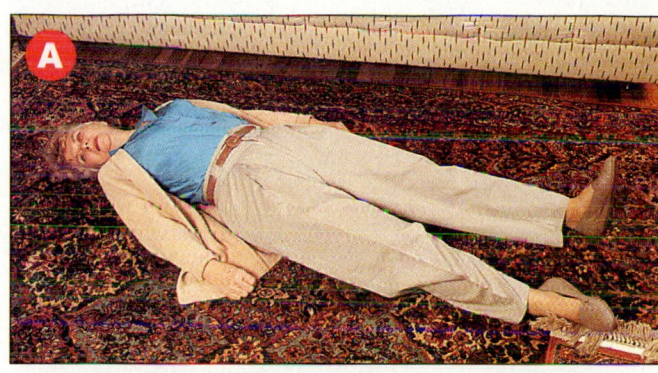

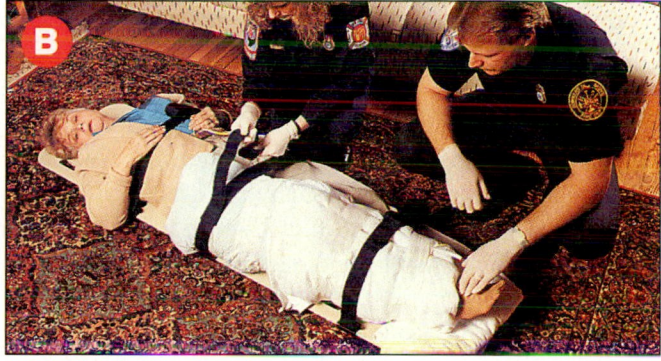

FIGURE 31-47 A: The usual position of a patient with a posterior dislocation of the hip. The hip joint is flexed, and the thigh is rotated inward and adducted across the midline of the body. **B:** Support the affected limb with pillows and blankets, particularly under the flexed knee. Secure the entire limb to a long board with long straps to prevent movement during transport.

FIGURE 31-48 A: A patient with a fracture of the proximal femur will typically lie with the leg externally rotated, and the injured leg usually appears shorter than the opposite uninjured leg. **B:** Immobilize the patient on a long backboard, using pillows or rolled blankets to support the injured limb in the deformed position.

As with any other dislocated joint, you should make no attempt to reduce the dislocated hip in the field. Splint the dislocation in the position of the deformity and place the patient supine on a long spine board. Support the affected limb with pillows and rolled blankets, particularly under the flexed knee. Then secure the entire limb to the spine board with long straps so that the hip region will not move. Be sure to provide prompt transport.

Fractures of the Proximal Femur

Fractures of the proximal (upper end) of the femur are among the most common fractures, especially in elderly people. Although they are usually called hip fractures, they rarely involve the hip joint. Instead, the break goes through the neck of the femur, the intertrochanteric (middle) region, or across the proximal shaft of the femur (subtrochanteric fractures). Although these three fracture types occur most often in older patients, particularly patients with osteoporosis, they may also be seen as a result of high-energy injuries in young adults.

All patients with displaced fractures of the proximal femur display a very characteristic deformity. They lie with the leg externally rotated, and the injured leg is usually shorter than the opposite, uninjured limb. When the fracture is not displaced, this deformity is not

present. With any kind of hip fracture, patients typically are unable to walk or move the leg because of pain in the hip region or in the groin or inner aspect of the thigh. The hip region is usually tender on palpation, and gentle rolling of the leg will cause pain but will not do further damage. On occasion, the pain is referred to the knee, and it is not uncommon for an elderly patient with a hip fracture to complain of knee pain after a fall. You should splint the lower extremity of an elderly patient who has fallen and complains of pain in either the hip or the knee, even if there is no deformity, and then transport the patient to the emergency department.

The age of the patient and the severity of the injury will dictate how you splint the fracture. With young people, fractures of the hip resulting from violent injury are best immobilized with a traction splint or the combination of a PASG and a spine board. The PASG offers an added advantage: It will help to control bleeding in the region. Apply the traction splint as you would for a femoral shaft fracture, taking special care to protect the injured region from excessive pressure from the ring of a Hare traction splint.

An elderly patient with an isolated hip fracture does not require a traction splint (Figure 31-48). You can effectively immobilize such a fracture by placing the patient on a long spine board or scoop stretcher, using pillows or rolled blankets to support the injured limb in the deformed position. Then secure the injured limb carefully to the stretcher with long straps.

All patients with hip fractures may lose significant amounts of blood. Therefore, you should watch for shock and monitor the patient's vital signs frequently.

Femoral Shaft Fractures

Fractures of the femur can occur in any part of the shaft, from the hip region to the femoral condyles just above the knee joint. Following a fracture, the large muscles of the thigh spasm in an attempt to "splint" the unstable limb. The muscle spasm often produces significant deformity of the limb, with severe angulation or external rotation at the fracture site. Usually, the limb shortens significantly as well. Fractures of the femoral shaft are often open, and fragments of bone may protrude through the skin.

There is always a significant amount of blood loss, as much as 500 to 1,000 mL, after a fracture of the shaft of the femur. With open fractures, the amount of blood loss may be even greater. Thus, it is not unusual for hypovolemic shock to develop. Handle these patients with extreme care, because any extra movement or fracture manipulation will increase the amount of blood loss.

Because of the severe deformity that occurs with these fractures, bone fragments may penetrate or press on important nerves and vessels and produce significant damage. For this reason, you must carefully and periodically assess the distal neurovascular function in patients who have sustained a fracture of the femoral shaft. Remove the clothing from the affected limb so that you can adequately inspect the injury site for any open wounds. Remember to follow BSI techniques when any blood or body fluids are present. Monitor the patient's vital signs closely, and continue to watch for the onset of hypovolemic shock. You must provide immediate transport in this situation.

Cover any wound with a dry sterile compression dressing. If the foot or leg below the level of the fracture shows signs of impaired circulation (is pale, cold, or pulseless), apply gentle longitudinal traction to the deformed limb in line with the long axis of the limb. Gradually turn the leg from the deformed position to restore the limb's overall alignment. Often, this restores or improves circulation to the foot. If it does not, the patient may have sustained a serious vascular injury and is in need of prompt medical attention.

A fracture of the femoral shaft is best immobilized with a traction splint, such as a Hare traction splint or a Sager splint. The Sager splint is lightweight, is easy to store, applies a measurable amount of traction, and can be used with a PASG. Best of all, you can apply it by yourself when necessary. As with any splint, in addition to knowing the precise sequence of steps to apply the splint properly, you must practice the splinting technique frequently to maintain the necessary skills. Take the following steps to apply a Sager splint (Figure 31-49):

1. Before applying the splint, **adjust the thigh strap** so that it will lie anteriorly when secured in place.

2. **Estimate the proper splint length** by placing it alongside the injured limb, so that the wheel is at the level of the heel.

3. **Arrange the ankle pads** to fit the size of the patient's ankle.

4. **Place the splint** along the inner aspect of the limb, and slide the thigh strap around the upper thigh so that the perineal cushion is snug against the groin and the ischial tuberosity. Tighten the thigh strap snugly.

5. **Secure the ankle harness** tightly around the patient's ankle just above the malleoli.

6. **Pull the cable ring** snugly up against the bottom of the foot.

7. **Pull out the inner shaft** of the splint to apply traction of approximately 10% of body weight, using a maximum of 15 lb.

8. **Secure the limb** to the splint using elasticized cravats.

9. **Secure the patient** to a long spine board.

Injuries of Knee Ligaments

The knee is very vulnerable to injury; therefore, many different types of injuries occur in this region. Ligament injuries, for example, range from mild sprains to complete dislocation of the joint. The patella can also dislocate. In addition, all the bony elements of the knee (distal femur, upper tibia, and patella) can fracture.

The knee is especially susceptible to ligament injuries, which occur when abnormal bending or twisting forces are applied to the joint. Such injuries are often seen in both recreational and competitive athletes. The ligaments on the medial side of the knee are the ones that are most frequently injured, typically when the foot is fixed to the ground and the lateral aspect of the knee is struck by a heavy object, such as when a football player is clipped or tackled from the side.

Usually, the patient with a knee ligament injury will report pain in the joint and be unable to use the extremity normally. When you examine the patient, you will

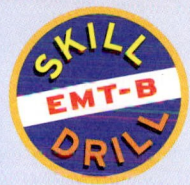

Applying a Sager Traction Splint

Figure 31-49

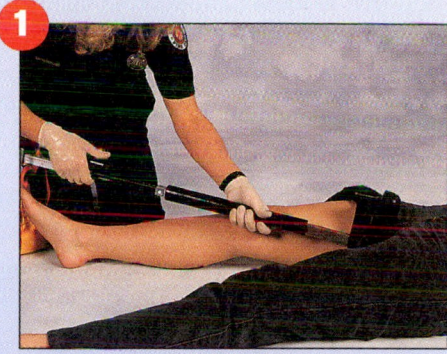

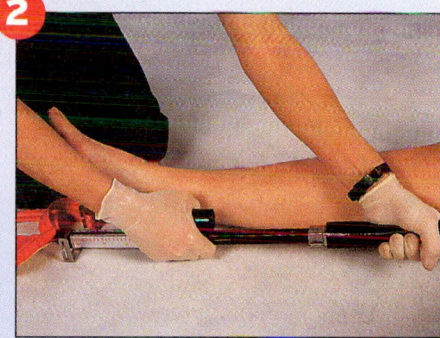

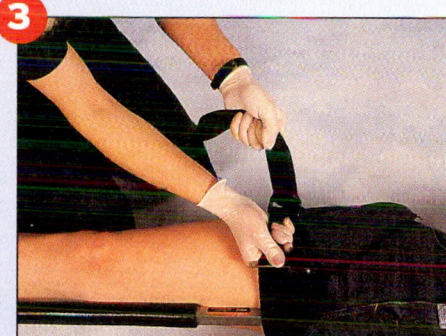

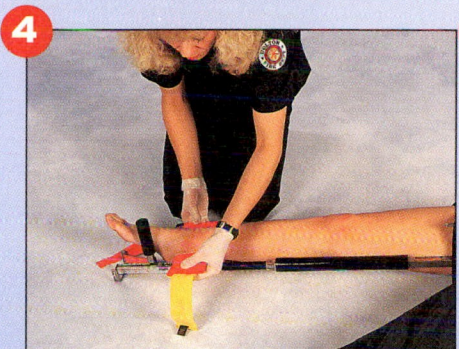

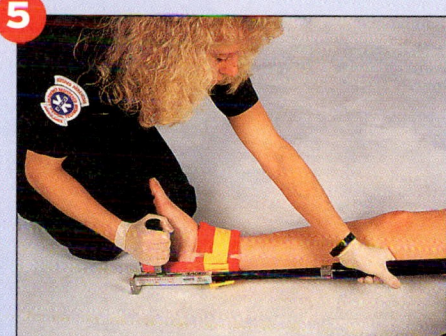

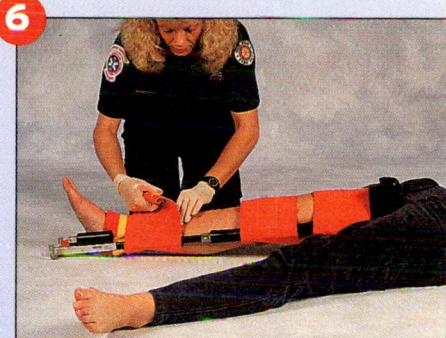

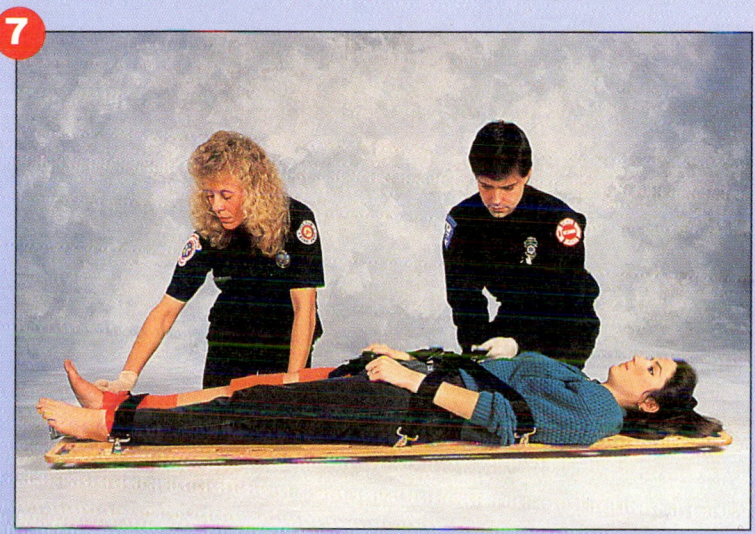

1 Adjust the thigh strap so that it lies anteriorly when secured in place.

2 Estimate the proper length of the splint by placing it next to the injured limb.

3 Place the splint along the inner aspect of the thigh, slide the thigh strap around the upper part of the thigh, and secure snugly.

4 Secure the ankle harness tightly around the ankle just above the malleoli.

5 Pull out the inner shaft of the splint to apply traction of approximately 10% of body weight.

6 Secure the limb to the splint using elasticized cravats.

7 Secure the patient to a long spine board.

generally find swelling, occasional ecchymosis, point tenderness at the injury site, and joint effusion (excess fluid in the joint).

You must splint all suspected knee ligament injuries. The splint should extend from the hip joint to the foot, immobilizing the bone above the injured joint (the femur) and the bone below it (the tibia). A variety of splints can be used, including a padded, rigid, long leg splint or two padded board splints securely applied to the medial and lateral aspects of the limb. A long spine board, a pillow splint, or simply binding the injured limb to its uninjured mate are acceptable but less effective splinting techniques. The patient will usually be able to straighten the knee to allow you to apply the splint. However, if you encounter resistance or pain when trying to straighten the knee, splint it in the flexed position. Then continue to monitor the distal neurovascular function until the patient reaches the hospital.

Dislocation of the Knee

Complete disruption of the ligaments supporting the knee may result in dislocation of the joint. When this happens, the proximal end of the tibia completely displaces from its juncture with the lower end of the femur, usually producing a significant deformity. Although substantial ligament damage always occurs with a knee dislocation, the more urgent injury is to the popliteal artery, which is often lacerated or compressed by the displaced tibia. When gross deformity, severe pain, and an inability to move the joint cause you to suspect a dislocation of the knee, always check the distal circulation carefully before taking any other step. If the distal pulses are absent, contact medical control immediately for further stabilization instructions.

If adequate distal pulses are present, splint the knee in the position in which you found it, and transport the patient promptly (Figure 31-50). Do not attempt to manipulate or straighten any severe knee injury if there are good distal pulses. If the limb is straight, apply standard rigid long leg splints to at least two sides of the limb to immobilize it. If the knee is bent and the foot has a good pulse, splint the joint in the bent position, using parallel padded board splints secured at the hip and ankle joint to provide a stable A-frame. Secure the limb to a spine board or stretcher with pillows and straps to eliminate any motion during transport.

On rare occasions, medical control may instruct you to realign a deformed, pulseless limb to reduce compression of the popliteal artery and thus restore distal circulation. You should make only one attempt to do this. First, straighten the limb by applying gentle longitudinal traction in the axis of the limb. Once you apply manual traction, maintain it until the limb is fully

splinted; otherwise, the limb will return to its deformed position. If traction significantly increases the patient's pain, do not continue. As you apply traction, monitor the posterior tibial pulse to see whether it returns. Splint the limb in the position in which you feel the strongest pulse. If you are unable to restore the distal pulse, splint the limb in the position that is most comfortable for the patient, and then provide prompt transport to the hospital. Notify medical control of the status of the distal pulse so that arrangements to treat the patient can be made in advance.

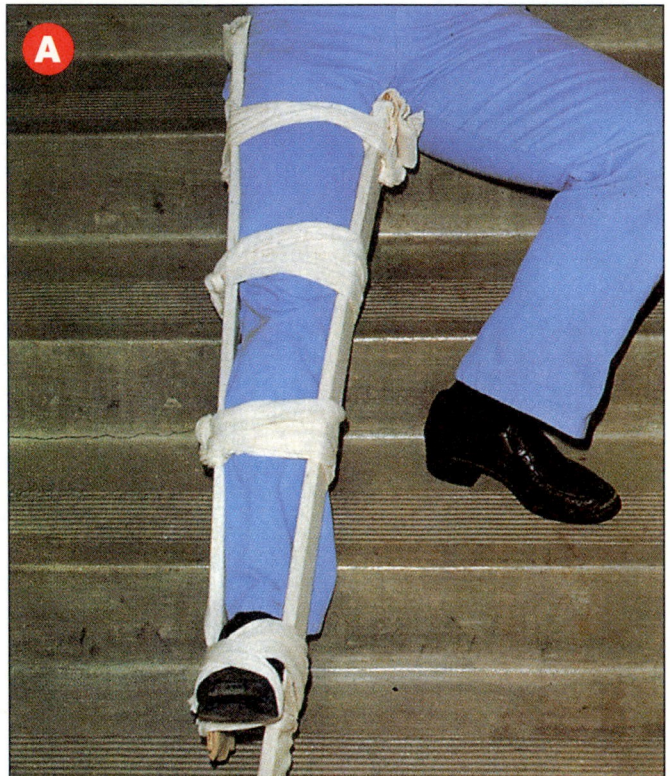

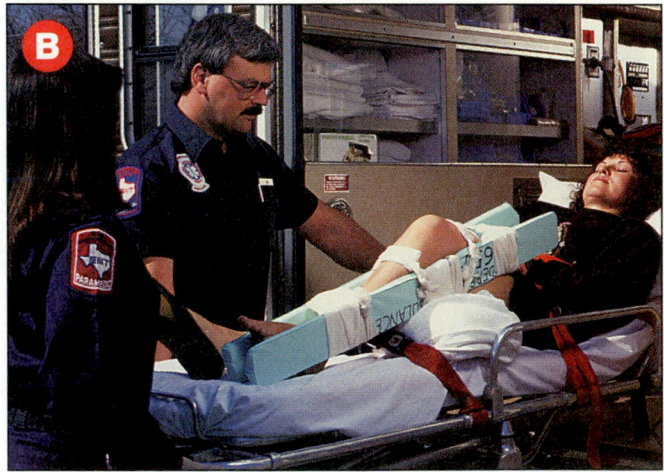

FIGURE 31-50 A: When the injured knee is straight, apply padded board splints extending from the hip to the ankle. **B:** If the knee is flexed and the foot has good pulses, apply padded board splints with the knee in the flexed position.

Fractures About the Knee

Fractures about the knee may occur at the distal end of the femur, at the proximal end of the tibia, or in the patella. Because of local tenderness and swelling, it is easy to confuse a nondisplaced or minimally displaced fracture about the knee with a ligament injury. Likewise, a displaced fracture about the knee may produce significant deformity that makes it look like a dislocation. Management of the two types of injuries is as follows:

- If there is an adequate distal pulse and no significant deformity, splint the limb with the knee straight.

- If there is an adequate pulse and significant deformity, splint the joint in the position of deformity.

- If the pulse is absent below the level of the injury, contact medical control immediately for further instructions.

Dislocation of the Patella

A dislocated patella most commonly occurs in teenagers and young adults who are engaged in athletic activities. Some patients have recurrent dislocations of the patella. As with recurrent dislocation of the shoulder, a minor twisting may be enough to produce the problem. Usually, the dislocated patella displaces to the lateral side, and the knee is held in a partially flexed position. The displacement of the patella produces a significant deformity in which the knee is held in a moderately flexed position and the patella is displaced to the lateral side of the knee (Figure 31-51).

Splint the knee in the position in which you found it; most often, this is with the knee flexed to a moderate degree. To immobilize the knee, apply padded board splints to the medial and lateral aspects of the joint, extending from the hip to the ankle. Use pillows to support the limb on the stretcher.

Occasionally, as you apply the splint, the patella will return to its normal position spontaneously. When this occurs, immobilize the limb as for a knee ligament injury, in a padded long leg splint. The patient still needs to be transported to the emergency department. Report the spontaneous reduction as soon as you arrive at the hospital so that the medical staff is aware of the severity of the injury.

Injuries to the Tibia and Fibula

The <u>tibia</u> is the larger of the two leg bones that are responsible for supporting the major weight-bearing surface of the knee and ankle; the <u>fibula</u> is the smaller of them. Fracture of the shaft of the tibia or the fibula may occur at any place between the knee joint and the ankle joint. Usually, both bones fracture at the same time. Even a single fracture may result in severe deformity, with significant angulation or rotation. Because the tibia is located just beneath the skin, open fractures of this bone are quite common (Figure 31-52).

Fractures of the tibia and fibula should be immobilized with a padded, rigid long leg splint or an air splint that extends from the foot to the upper thigh. You can also use a traction splint; however, constant traction is not usually necessary to maintain limb alignment with isolated tibial fractures. When both the tibia and the femur in the same limb have been fractured, a properly applied traction splint will provide sufficient immobilization for both bones. As with most other fractures of the shaft of long bones, you should correct severe deformity before splinting by applying gentle longitudinal

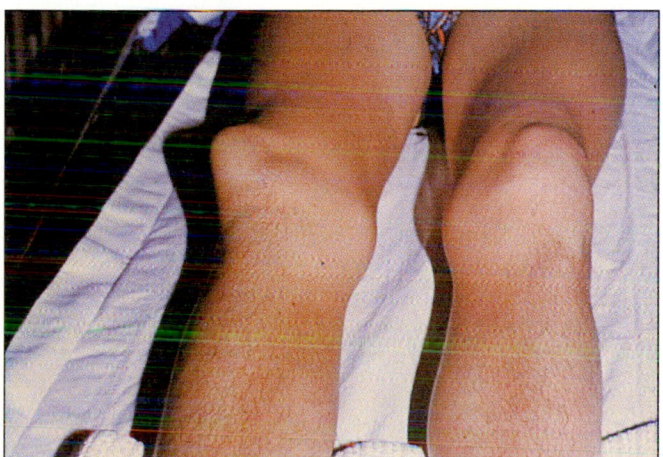

FIGURE 31-51 A dislocated patella will typically appear with the patella displaced lateral to the knee and with the knee moderately flexed.

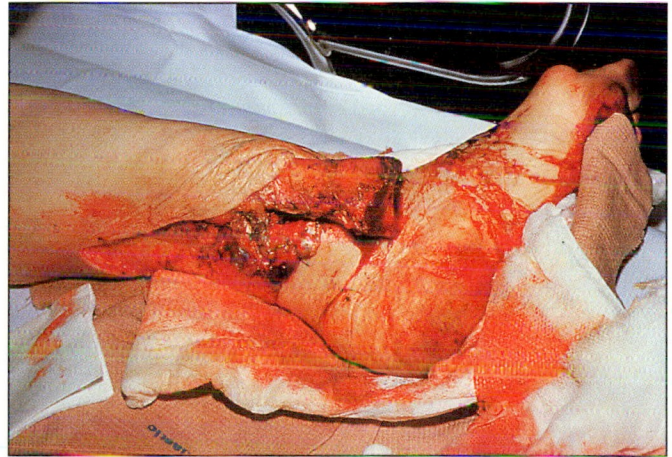

FIGURE 31-52 Because the tibia is so close to the skin, open fractures are quite common.

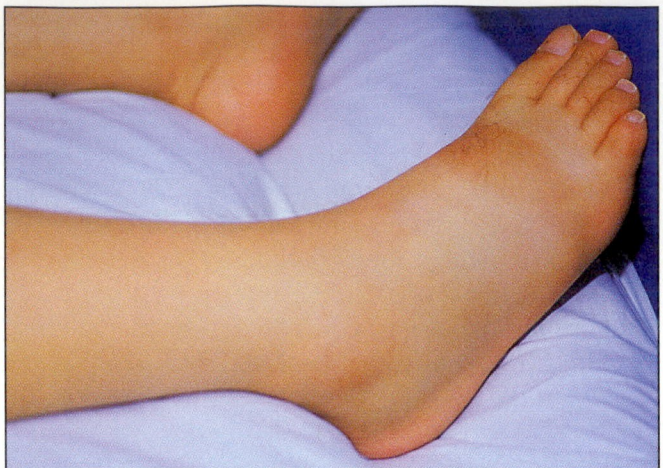

FIGURE 31-53 Swelling about the ankle is characteristic of both sprains and fractures.

traction. The goal here is to restore a position that will take a standard splint; it is not necessary to replace the fracture fragments in their anatomic position.

Fractures of the tibia and fibula are often associated with vascular injury as a result of the distorted position of the limb following injury. Realigning the limb frequently restores an adequate blood supply to the foot. If it does not, transport the patient promptly and notify medical control while you are en route.

Ankle Injuries

The ankle is the most commonly injured joint. Ankle injuries occur in individuals of all ages and range in severity from a simple sprain, which heals after a few days' rest, to severe fracture-dislocations. As with other joints, it is sometimes difficult to tell a nondisplaced ankle fracture from a simple sprain without X-rays (Figure 31-53). Therefore, any ankle injury that produces pain, swelling, localized tenderness, or the inability to bear weight must be evaluated by a physician. The most frequent mechanism of ankle injury is twisting, which stretches or tears the supporting ligaments. A more extensive twisting force may result in fracture of one or both malleoli. Dislocation of the ankle is usually associated with fractures of both malleoli.

You can manage the wide spectrum of injuries to the ankle in the same way, as follows:

1. Dress all open wounds.

2. Assess distal neurovascular function.

3. Correct any gross deformity by applying gentle longitudinal traction to the heel.

4. Before releasing traction, apply a splint.

You can use a padded rigid splint, an air splint, or a pillow splint. Just make sure it includes the entire foot and extends up the leg to the level of the knee joint.

Foot Injuries

Injuries to the foot can result in the fracture of one or more of the tarsals, metatarsals, or phalanges of the toes. Toe fractures are especially common.

Of the tarsal bones, the <u>calcaneus</u>, the heel bone, is the most frequently fractured. Injury usually occurs when the patient falls or jumps from a height and lands directly on the heel. The force of injury compresses the calcaneus, producing immediate swelling and ecchymosis. If the force of impact is great enough, as from a fall from a roof or tree, there may be other fractures as well.

Frequently, the force of injury is transmitted up the legs to the spine, producing a fracture of the lumbar spine (Figure 31-54). When a patient who has jumped or fallen from a height complains of heel pain, be sure to question him or her about back pain and carefully check the spine for tenderness or deformity.

Injuries of the foot are associated with significant swelling but rarely with gross deformity. Vascular injuries are not common. As in the hand, lacerations about the ankle and foot may damage important underlying nerves and tendons. Puncture wounds of the foot

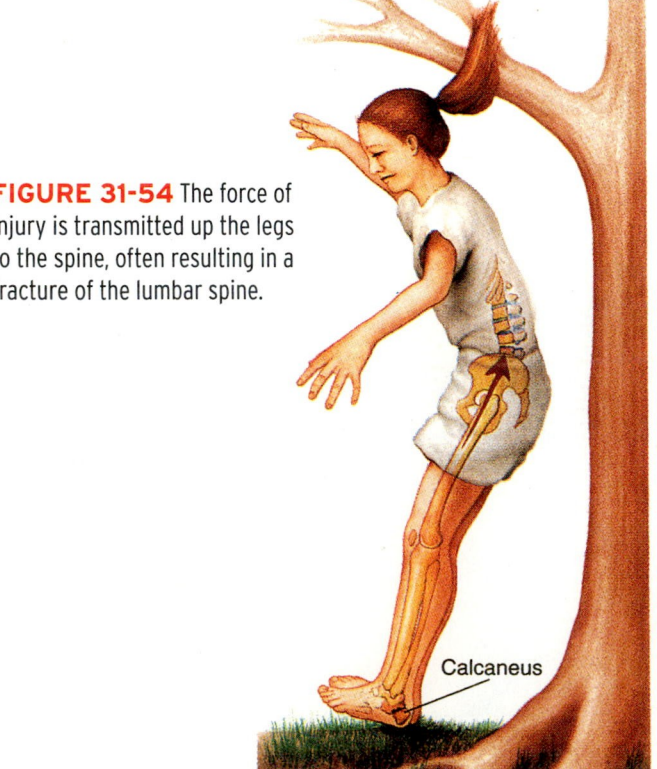

FIGURE 31-54 The force of injury is transmitted up the legs to the spine, often resulting in a fracture of the lumbar spine.

Calcaneus

are common and may cause serious infection if not treated early. All of these injuries must be evaluated and treated by a physician.

To splint the foot, apply a rigid padded board splint, an air splint, or a pillow splint, immobilizing the ankle joint as well as the foot (Figure 31-55). Leave the toes exposed so that you can periodically assess neurovascular function.

When the patient is lying on the stretcher, elevate the foot approximately 6" to minimize swelling. All patients with lower extremity injuries should be transported in the supine position to allow for elevation of the limb. Never allow the foot and leg to dangle off the stretcher onto the floor or ground.

If a patient has fallen from a height and complains of heel pain, use a long spine board to immobilize any possible spinal injury in addition to splinting the foot.

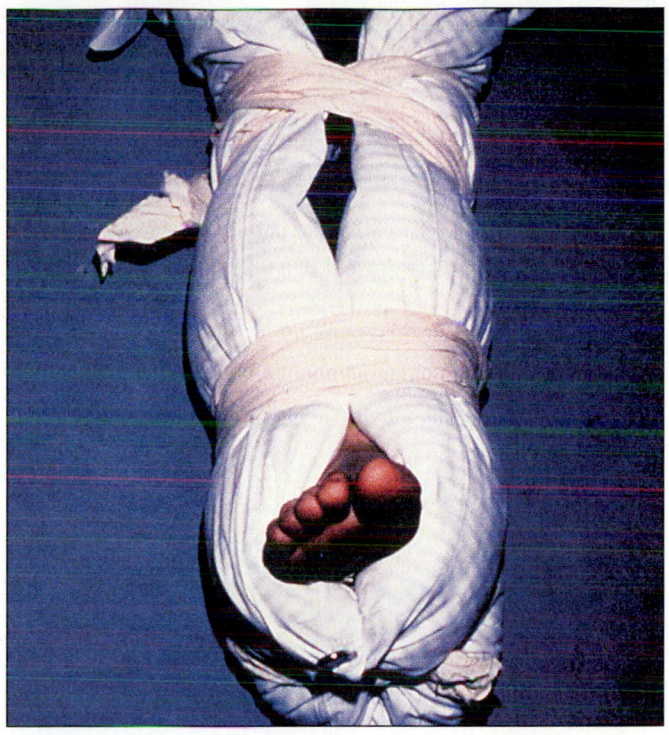

FIGURE 31-55 A pillow splint provides excellent immobilization of the foot.

prep kit

ready for review

Skeletal or voluntary muscle, which attaches to bone and forms the major muscle mass of the body, is supplied with arteries, veins, and nerves. The 206 bones of the skeleton are living tissue that, when fractured, can bleed and cause severe pain. Wherever two bones come into contact, a joint is formed, strengthened in key areas by ligaments. A fracture is a broken bone; a dislocation is a disruption of a joint; a sprain is a joint injury that involves partial or temporary dislocation of bone ends and partial stretching or tearing of ligaments; and a strain is a muscle pull. Depending on the amount of kinetic energy absorbed by the tissues, the zone of injury may extend to a distant point, so you must always check for associated injuries beyond the obvious ones. Fractures are either open or closed, displaced or nondisplaced. Signs of fracture and dislocation include pain, deformity, point tenderness, guarding, swelling, crepitus, and false motion. Signs of sprain include ecchymosis and instability of the joint.

Your approach to patients with musculoskeletal injuries should include a rapid initial assessment, stabilization of vital functions and control of serious bleeding, focused physical exam of the injured body part, assessment of neurovascular function in the affected limb, an attempt to reduce fractures and dislocations, splinting to immobi-lize the affected part, and prompt transport to the hospital. For each limb, your neurovascular examination should include pulse, capillary refill, sensation, and motor function. Repeat this exam every 5 to 10 minutes.

The principles of splinting include the following: If you suspect a fracture of the shaft of any bone, make sure the splint immobilizes the joints above and below the fracture; with injuries in and around a joint, make sure the splint immobilizes the bones above and below the injured joint; where fracture of a long bone shaft has resulted in severe deformity, use constant, gentle, manual traction (pull) to align the limb so that it can be splinted, unless this is too painful. There are three types of splints: rigid splints and traction splints, which require two people to apply, and formable splints, including air splints. In addition, slings and swathes are used to help support the weight of an injured upper extremity and immobilize the shoulder region, respectively.

Provide immediate transport to any patient if you are unable to restore a pulse to a pulseless limb by applying traction. The only life-threatening musculoskeletal injuries are multiple fractures, fractures with arterial injuries, severe open fractures, limb amputations, and pelvic fractures with hemodynamic instability.

prep kit

vital vocabulary

acromioclavicular (A/C) joint   A simple joint where the bony projections of the scapula and the clavicle meet at the top of the shoulder.

articular cartilage   A pearly layer of specialized cartilage covering the articular surface of bones in synovial joints.

calcaneus   The heel bone.

clavicle   The collarbone.

closed fracture   Any fracture in which the skin is not broken.

compartment syndrome   An elevation of pressure within the fibrous tissue that surrounds and supports muscles and neurovascular structures, characterized by extreme pain, hypesthesia (decreased pain sensation), pain on stretching of affected muscles, and decreased power; most frequently seen in fractures below the elbow or knee in children.

crepitus   A grating or grinding sensation caused by fractured bone ends or joints rubbing together.

dislocation   Disruption of a joint in which ligaments are damaged and the bone ends are completely displaced.

displaced fracture   A fracture in which fracture fragments are separated from one another and not in anatomic alignment.

ecchymosis   Bruising or discoloration associated with bleeding within or under the skin.

femur   The thigh bone, which extends from the pelvis to the knee and is responsible for formation of the hip; the longest and largest bone in the body.

fibula   The outer and smaller bone of the two bones of the leg.

fracture   Any break in the continuity of a bone.

glenoid fossa   The part of the scapula that joins with the humeral head to form the glenohumeral joint.

hematuria   Discharge of blood in the urine.

humerus   The supporting bone of the upper arm that joins with the scapula (glenoid) to form the shoulder joint and with the ulna and radius to form the elbow joint.

joint   The place where two bones come into contact.

ligament   A band of fibrous tissue that connects bones to bones. It supports and strengthens a joint.

nondisplaced fracture   A simple crack in the bone that has not caused the bone to move from its normal anatomic position; also called a hairline fracture.

open fracture   Any break in the bone in which the overlying skin has been damaged.

patella   The kneecap.

point tenderness   Tenderness that is sharply localized at the site of the injury and is found by gently palpating along the bone with the tip of one finger.

position of function   A hand position in which the wrist is slightly dorsiflexed and all finger joints are moderately flexed.

www.emtb.com

radius   The bone on the thumb side of the forearm; most important in wrist function.

reduce   Return a dislocated joint or fractured bone to its normal position; set.

retroperitoneal space   The space between the abdominal cavity and the posterior abdominal wall containing the kidneys, certain large vessels, and parts of the gastrointestinal tract.

scapula   Shoulder blade.

sciatic nerve   The major nerve to the lower extremity.

skeletal muscle   Striated muscles that are attached to bones and usually cross at least one joint.

sling   Any bandage or material that helps to support the weight of an injured upper extremity.

splint   A flexible or rigid appliance used to protect and maintain the position of an injured extremity.

sprain   Any joint injury involving damage to supporting ligaments.

strain   Stretching or tearing of a muscle; also called a muscle pull.

swathe   A bandage that passes around the chest to secure an injured arm to the chest.

symphysis pubis   The firm cartilaginous joint between the two pubic bones.

tendon   A tough ropelike cord of fibrous tissue that attaches a skeletal muscle to a bone.

tibia   The larger of the two leg bones responsible for supporting the major weight-bearing surface of the knee and the ankle; the shinbone.

traction   The act of exerting a pulling force on a structure.

ulna   The bone on the small finger side of the forearm; most important for elbow function.

assessment in action

A young kitten has climbed a tree and, for now, refuses to come down. Seeing no other option, a man brings an extension ladder in preparation for climbing the tree. About 12' into the climb, his foot slips off the rung and his leg slides through. He turns and falls toward the ground, pulling the ladder after him. His wife calls 9-1-1.

You arrive to find a 35-year-old man, still tangled in the ladder, lying on the ground, complaining of severe pain. Injured areas include his right lower leg, hip, and shoulder. His skin is warm and moist; respirations and pulse are present but fast. He is alert to person, place, and time. An obvious bone end protrudes through the leg of his sweatpants.

1. What is the most accurate description of the mechanism of injury?
   - A. Direct force only
   - B. Twisting and direct force
   - C. Twisting force only
   - D. None of the above

2. Which of the following is **NOT** considered one of the rules of splinting?
   - A. Gently push protruding bone ends back into place.
   - B. When in doubt, splint the injury.
   - C. Cover open wounds with sterile dressings.
   - D. Remove or cut away clothing from around open injuries.

3. What type of splint is the best choice for the patient's upper leg fracture?
   - A. Ladder
   - B. Pillow
   - C. Traction
   - D. Cardboard

4. After splinting the patient's leg, you determine that the pulse by the ankle still feels weak. You should document this finding by recording that the patient has a:
   - A. dermal pulse.
   - B. despondent pulse.
   - C. delineated, dominant pulse.
   - D. diminished distal pulse.

5. You are riding a crowded elevator back down to the emergency department when your partner exclaims how stupid the man was to fall off the ladder, and he even mentions the patient's name. This type of behavior can lead to charges of:
   - A. proximate cause.
   - B. assault and battery.
   - C. medical malnutrition.
   - D. breach of confidentiality.

points to ponder

Object. 1-3.1, 1-3.6, 5-3.4, 5-3.5, 5-3.8, 5-3.10

You respond to a roller rink to find a patient with a dislocated shoulder. The patient is complaining of pain and asks you to "pop it back in." The patient explains that the shoulder has dislocated a couple times before, but she has always been able to get it back into joint. The patient has good circulation and neurologic function in the arm. She explains how to pull gently and rotate the arm to get it to pop back in. The patient refuses to go to the hospital.

- Would you assist the patient in reducing the dislocated shoulder? If so, how? Should the patient be seen by a care provider? Why or why not?

online outlook

Because musculoskeletal injuries occur so often, you must be able to evaluate them properly. Injury to the bones and joints is often associated with injury to the surrounding soft tissue. To improve your knowledge of injuries to the skeletal system, complete Exercise 31 at www.emtb.com.

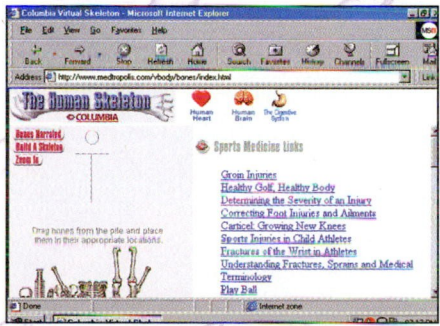

Head and Spine Injuries

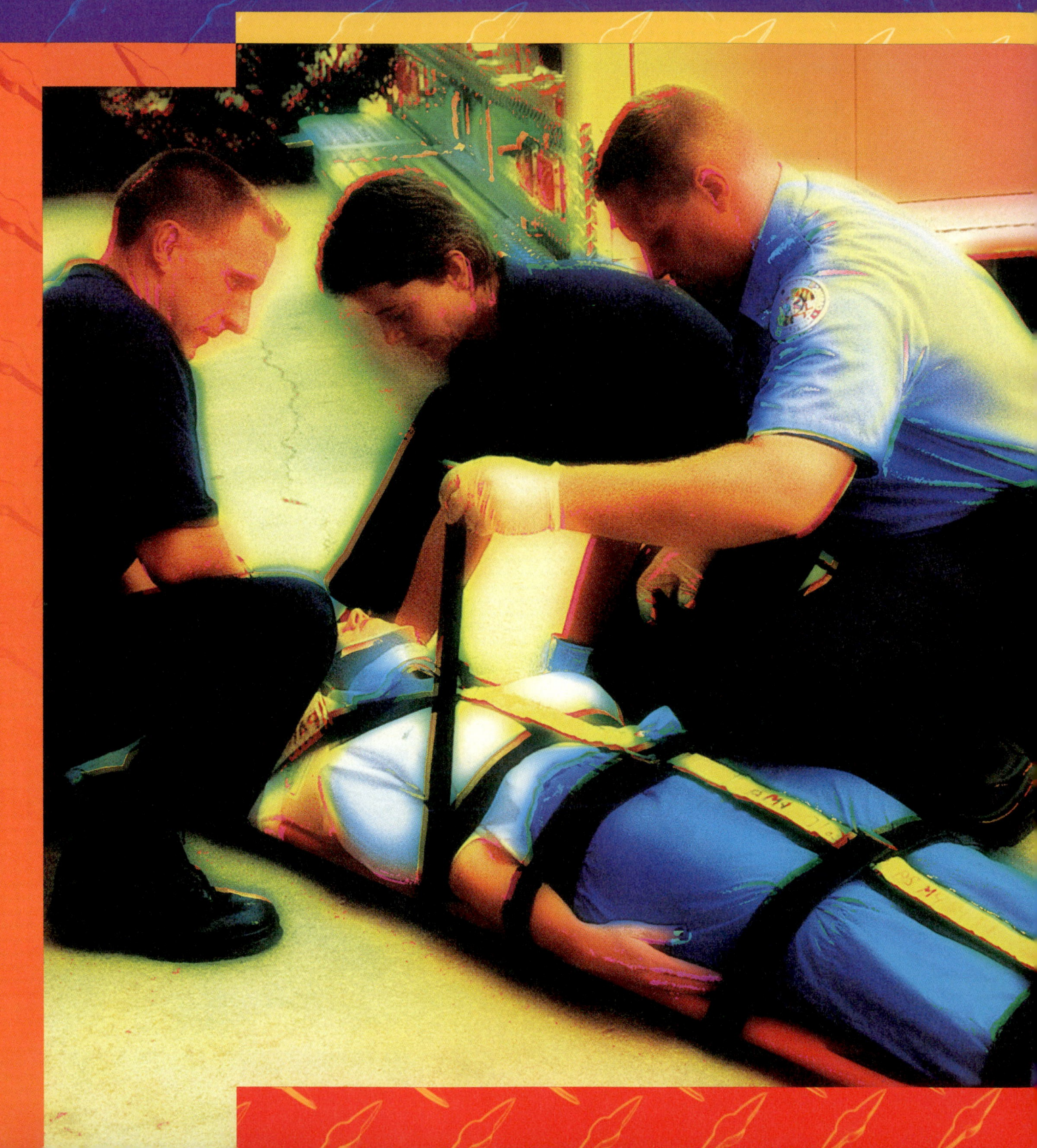

objectives

Cognitive

1. State the components of the nervous system.

2. List the functions of the central nervous system.

3. Define the structure of the skeletal system as it relates to the nervous system.

4. Relate mechanism of injury to potential injuries of the head and spine.

5. Describe the implications of not properly caring for potential spinal injuries.

6. State the signs and symptoms of a potential spinal injury.

7. Describe the method of determining if a responsive patient may have a spinal injury.

8. Relate the airway emergency medical care techniques to the patient with a suspected spinal injury.

9. Describe how to stabilize the cervical spine.

10. Discuss indications for sizing and using a cervical spine immobilization device.

11. Establish the relationship between airway management and the patient with head and spinal injuries.

12. Describe a method for sizing a cervical spine immobilization device.

13. Describe how to log roll a patient with a suspected spinal injury.

14. Describe how to secure a patient to a long spine board.

15. List instances when a short spine board should be used.

16. Describe how to immobilize a patient using a short spine board.

17. Describe the indications for the use of rapid extrication.

18. List the steps in performing rapid extrication.

19. State the circumstance when a helmet should be left on the patient.

20. Discuss the circumstances when a helmet should be removed.

21. Identify different types of helmets.

22. Describe the unique characteristics of sports helmets.

23. Explain the preferred methods to remove a helmet.

24. Discuss alternative methods for removal of a helmet.

25. Describe how the patient's head is stabilized to remove the helmet.

26. Differentiate how the head is stabilized with a helmet compared to without a helmet.

Affective

27. Explain the rationale for immobilization of the entire spine when a cervical spine injury is suspected.

28. Explain the rationale for utilizing immobilization methods apart from the straps on the cots.

29. Explain the rationale for utilizing a short spine immobilization device when moving a patient from the sitting to the supine position.

30. Explain the rationale for utilizing rapid extrication approaches only when they indeed will make the difference between life and death.

31. Defend the reasons for leaving a helmet in place for transport of a patient.

32. Defend the reasons for removal of a helmet prior to transport of a patient.

Psychomotor

33. Demonstrate opening the airway in a patient with a suspected spinal cord injury.

34. Demonstrate evaluating a responsive patient with a suspected spinal cord injury.

35. Demonstrate stabilization of the cervical spine.

36. Demonstrate the four-person log roll for a patient with a suspected spinal cord injury.

37. Demonstrate how to log roll a patient with a suspected spinal cord injury using two people.

38. Demonstrate securing a patient to a long spine board.

39. Demonstrate using the short board immobilization technique.

40. Demonstrate the procedure for rapid extrication.

41. Demonstrate preferred methods for stabilization of a helmet.

42. Demonstrate helmet removal techniques.

43. Demonstrate alternative methods for stabilization of a helmet.

44. Demonstrate completing a prehospital care report for patients with head and spinal injuries.

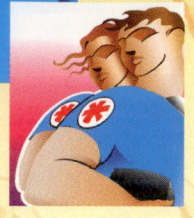

you are the emt

You and your partner are leaving a restaurant when you see a motorcycle race by, run a red light, and crash into the passenger-side door of a pickup truck. You see the biker crash to the ground about 20' past the truck. The biker is not moving when your partner calls dispatch.

Injuries to the head and spine produce some of the most tragic outcomes of all trauma patients, often producing profound effects for both them and for those who may have suddenly inherited a lifetime of care giving. This chapter will prepare you to meet the challenges of caring for the patient with brain or spinal trauma and will also help you to answer the following questions:

1. Does the size of a patient's cervical collar really make a difference?
2. Is a fixed and dilated pupil a serious sign worth noting?

Head and Spine Injuries

The nervous system is a complex network of nerve cells that enables all parts of the body to function. It includes the brain, the spinal cord, and several billion nerve fibers that carry information to and from all parts of the body. Because the nervous system is so vital, it is well protected. The brain lies within the skull, and the spinal cord is inside the bony spinal canal. Despite this protection, serious blows can damage the nervous system.

This chapter first briefly reviews the anatomy and function of the central and peripheral nervous systems and of the skeletal system, knowledge that you will need to make an accurate assessment of injuries to these systems. It then discusses specific head and spinal injuries, including signs, symptoms, and treatment. Extrication of patients with possible spinal injuries and removal of helmets are also described.

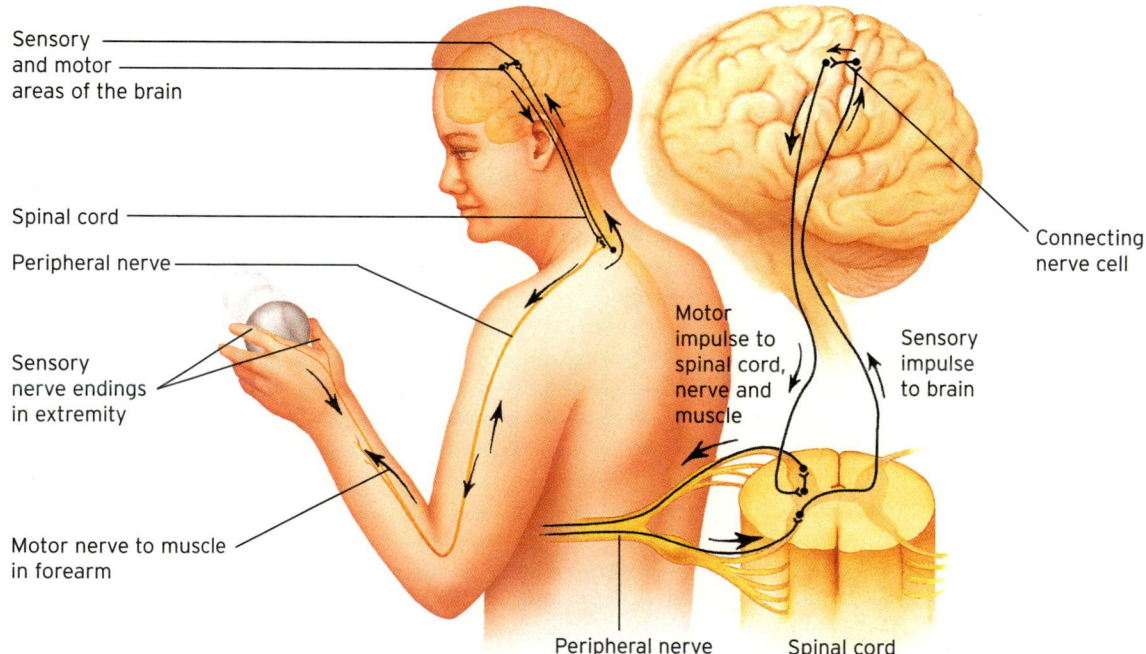

FIGURE 32-1 The body has two nervous systems: the central nervous system and the peripheral nervous system. The central nervous system is composed of the brain and the spinal cord. The peripheral nervous system conducts sensory and motor impulses from the skin and other organs to the spinal cord.

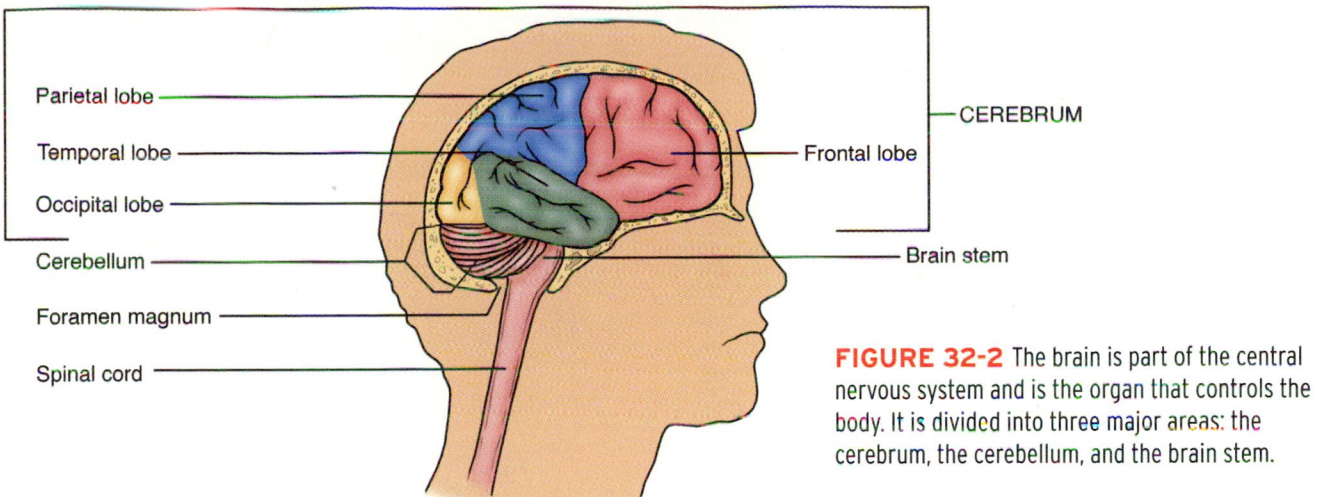

FIGURE 32-2 The brain is part of the central nervous system and is the organ that controls the body. It is divided into three major areas: the cerebrum, the cerebellum, and the brain stem.

Anatomy and Physiology of the Nervous System

The nervous system is divided into two anatomic parts: the central nervous system and the peripheral nervous system (Figure 32-1). The **central nervous system (CNS)** consists of the parts of the nervous system that are covered and protected by bones: the brain and the spinal cord, including the nuclei and cell bodies of most nerve cells. Long fibers link these cells to the body's various organs through openings in the bony coverings. These cables of nerve fibers make up the **peripheral nervous system**.

Central Nervous System

The central nervous system (CNS) is composed of the brain and spinal cord. The brain is the organ that controls the body, the center of consciousness. It is divided into three major areas: the cerebrum, the cerebellum, and the brain stem (Figure 32-2).

The **cerebrum**, which contains about 75% of the brain's total volume, controls a wide variety of activities. Underneath the cerebrum lies the **cerebellum**, which coordinates body movements. The most primitive part of the central nervous system, the **brain stem**, controls virtually all the functions that are necessary for life, including the cardiac and respiratory systems. Deep within the cranium, the brain stem is the best-protected part of the central nervous system.

The spinal cord, the other major portion of the central nervous system, is mostly made of fibers that extend from the brain's nerve cells. The spinal cord carries messages between the brain and the body.

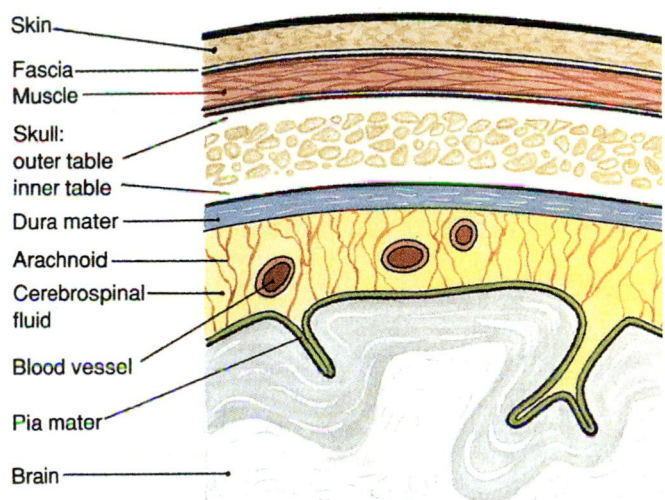

FIGURE 32-3 The central nervous system has several layers of protective coverings: the skin, muscles and their fascia, bone, and the meninges. The three layers of the meninges include the dura mater, the arachnoid, and the pia mater.

Protective Coverings

The cells of the brain and spinal cord are soft and easily injured. Once damaged, they cannot be regenerated or reproduced. Therefore, the entire central nervous system is contained within a protective framework.

The thick, bony structures of the skull and spinal canal withstand injury very well. The skull is covered by a layer of muscle fascia and, above that, the scalp, a thick vascular layer of skin. The spinal canal, too, is surrounded by a thick layer of skin and muscles.

The central nervous system is further protected by the **meninges**, three distinct layers of tissue that suspend the brain and the spinal cord within the skull and the spinal canal (Figure 32-3). The outer layer, the dura mater, is a tough, fibrous layer that closely resembles leather. This layer forms a sac to contain the central nervous system, with small openings through which the peripheral nerves exit.

The inner two layers of the meninges, called the arachnoid and the pia mater, are much thinner than the dura mater. They contain the blood vessels that nourish the brain and spinal cord. Both the arachnoid and the pia mater produce cerebrospinal fluid (CSF), which fills the spaces between them and acts as an excellent shock absorber. The brain and spinal cord essentially float in this fluid, buffered from injury.

When an injury does penetrate all these protective layers, clear, watery CSF may leak from the nose, the ears, or an open skull fracture. Therefore, if a patient with a head injury has what looks like a runny nose or has a salty taste at the back of the throat, you should assume that the fluid is CSF.

Ironically, the very layers of tissue that isolate and protect the central nervous system can lead to serious problems in closed head injuries. Severe injury may cause bleeding of the vessels under the dura mater. This, in turn, causes blood to collect in this space (a subdural hematoma), increasing the pressure inside the skull and compressing softer brain tissue. Only prompt surgery can prevent permanent brain damage.

Peripheral Nervous System

The peripheral nervous system has two anatomic parts: 31 pairs of spinal nerves and 12 pairs of cranial nerves.

The 31 pairs of spinal nerves conduct sensory impulses from the skin and other organs to the spinal cord. They also conduct motor impulses from the spinal cord to the muscles. Because the arms and legs have so many muscles, the spinal nerves serving the extremities are arranged in complex networks. The brachial plexus controls the arms, and the lumbosacral plexus controls the legs (Figure 32-4).

Cranial nerves are the 12 pairs of nerves that pass through holes in the skull and transmit sensations directly to or from the brain. For the most part, they perform special functions in the head and face, including sight, smell, taste, hearing, and facial expressions.

There are three major types of peripheral nerves. The **sensory nerves**, with endings that can perceive only one type of information each, carry that information from the body to the brain via the spinal cord. The **motor nerves**, one for each muscle, carry information from the central nervous system to the muscles. The **connecting nerves**, found only in the brain and spinal cord, connect the sensory and motor nerves with short fibers, which allow the cells on either end to exchange messages.

How the Nervous System Works

The nervous system sentrols virtually all of our body's activities, including reflex, voluntary, and involuntary activities.

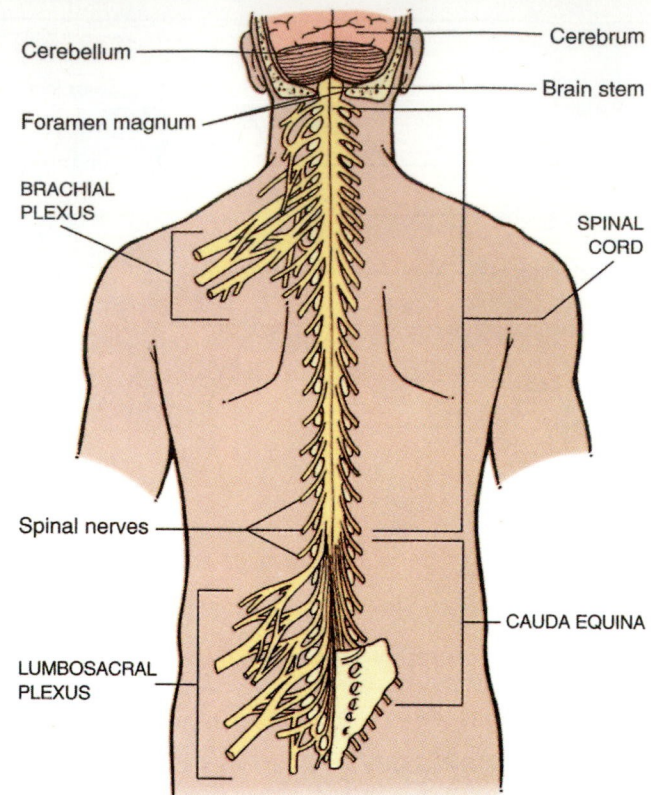

FIGURE 32-4 The peripheral nervous system is a complex network because it conducts motor and sensory nerves to organs and muscles all over the body. The brachial plexus controls the arms, and the lumbosacral plexus controls the legs.

In connecting the sensory and motor nerves of the limbs, the connecting nerves in the spinal cord form a reflex arc. If a sensory nerve in this arc detects an irritating stimulus, such as heat, it will bypass the brain and send a message directly to the motor nerve (Figure 32-5).

Voluntary activities are the actions that we consciously perform, in which sensory input determines the specific muscular activity—for example, reaching across the table for a salt shaker or to pass a dish. **Involuntary activities** are the actions that are not under the control of our will, such as breathing; in most instances, we inhale and exhale without consciously thinking about it. Many of our body's functions occur independently of thought, or involuntarily.

The part of the nervous system that regulates or controls our voluntary activities, including almost all coordinated muscular activities, is called the **somatic (voluntary) nervous system**. The mechanism of the somatic nervous system is simple. The brain interprets the sensory information that it receives from the peripheral nerves and responds by sending signals to the voluntary muscles.

The body functions that occur without conscious effort are regulated by the much more primitive **autonomic (involuntary) nervous system**. The autonomic

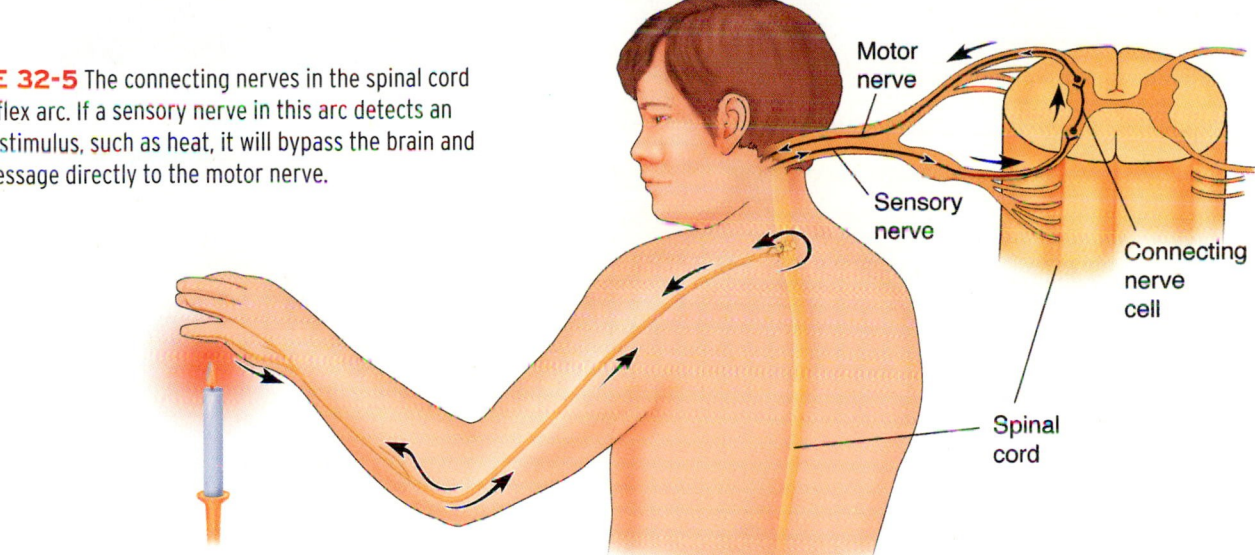

FIGURE 32-5 The connecting nerves in the spinal cord form a reflex arc. If a sensory nerve in this arc detects an irritating stimulus, such as heat, it will bypass the brain and send a message directly to the motor nerve.

nervous system controls the functions of many of the body's vital organs, over which the brain has no voluntary control.

The autonomic nervous system, like so much in our nervous system, is composed of two parts: the sympathetic nervous system and the parasympathetic nervous system. Confronted with a threatening situation, the sympathetic nervous system reacts to the stress with the fight-or-flight response. The parasympathetic nervous system has the opposite effect on the body, causing blood vessels to dilate, slowing the heart rate, and relaxing the muscle sphincters. These two divisions of the autonomic nervous system tend to balance each other so that basic body functions remain stable and effective.

Anatomy and Physiology of the Skeletal System

The skull has two layers of bone, the outer and inner tables, that protect the brain. It is divided into two large structures: the cranium and the face. The mandible (lower jaw), the only movable facial bone, is connected to the cranium by the temporomandibular joint just in front of each ear (Figure 32-6).

FIGURE 32-6 The skull has two large structures: the cranium and the face.

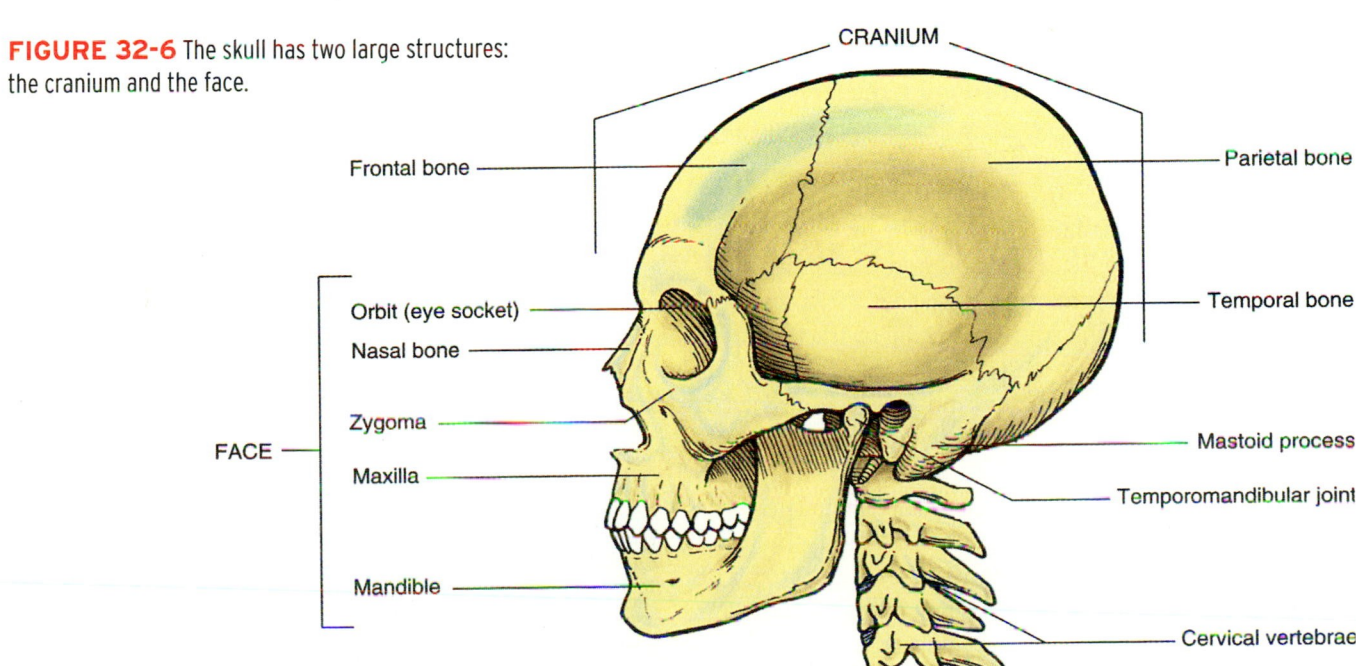

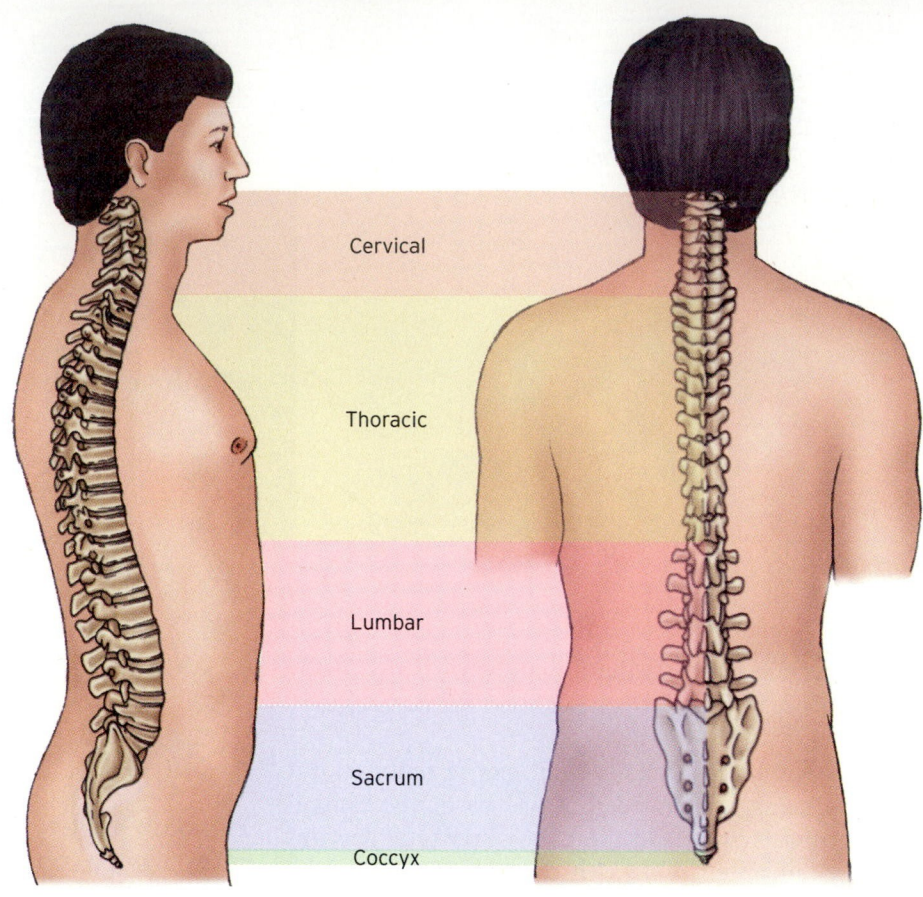

FIGURE 32-7 The spinal column is the body's central supporting system and consists of 33 bones divided into five sections: cervical , thoracic, lumbar, sacral, and coccygeal. Injury to the vertebrae, depending on the level at which the injury occurs, can result in paralysis.

Cervical

Thoracic

Lumbar

Sacrum

Coccyx

The spinal column is the body's central supporting structure. It has 33 bones, called vertebrae, and is divided into five sections (Figure 32-7).

The front part of each vertebra consists of a round, solid block of bone called the "body"; the back part forms a bony arch. From one vertebra to the next, the series of arches form a tunnel running the length of the spine. This is the spinal canal, which encases and protects the spinal cord (Figure 32-8).

The vertebrae are connected by ligaments and separated by cushions, called <u>**intervertebral disks**</u>. While allowing the trunk to bend forward and back, these ligaments and disks also limit motion so that the spinal cord is not injured. When the spine is injured or fractured, the spinal cord and its nerves are left unprotected. Therefore, until the spine is stabilized, you must keep it aligned as best you can to prevent further injury to the spinal cord.

The spinal column itself is almost entirely surrounded by muscles. However, you can palpate the posterior spinous process of each vertebra, which lies just under the skin in the midline of the back. The most prominent and most easily palpable spinous process is at the seventh cervical vertebra at the base of the neck.

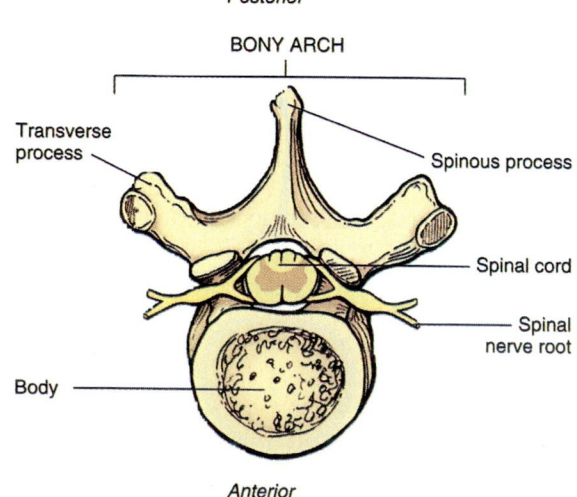

Posterior

BONY ARCH

Transverse process

Spinous process

Spinal cord

Spinal nerve root

Body

Anterior

FIGURE 32-8 The spinal canal is protected by a solid block of bone called the body of the vertebra.

If a trauma patient is unconscious and you do not know the mechanism of injury, you should always assume that he or she has a spinal injury.

Injuries of the Spine

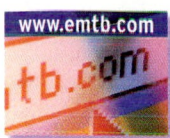

The cervical, thoracic, and lumbar portions of the spine can be injured in a variety of ways. Compression injuries can occur as a result of a fall, regardless of whether the patient landed on his or her feet, coccyx, or, as in diving accidents, top of the head. Motor vehicle crashes or other types of trauma can overextend, flex, or rotate the spine. Any one of these unnatural motions, as well as excessive lateral bending, can result in fractures or neurologic deficit.

Any time the spine is **distracted**, or pulled along its length, you can expect to find serious injuries to the spine. For example, hangings typically fracture the vertebrae high up in the cervical spine.

Assessment of Spinal Injuries

You should always suspect a possible spinal injury any time you encounter one of the following mechanisms of injury:

- Motor vehicle crashes
- Pedestrian-motor vehicle collisions
- Falls
- Blunt trauma
- Penetrating trauma to the head, neck, or torso
- Motorcycle crashes
- Hangings
- Diving accidents
- Recreational accidents

If a trauma patient is unconscious and you do not know the mechanism of injury, you should always assume that he or she has a spinal injury. Take great care to avoid any movement that could cause further injury.

In fact, this is the safest approach to *any* injured patient, conscious or unconscious. The reason is that complications of spinal cord injuries are serious, often leading to death or lifelong disability. Examples include respiratory failure resulting from direct injury to the brain stem or upper spinal cord and partial or complete paralysis below the point of injury.

When assessing a patient for possible spinal injury, you should begin with an initial assessment, focusing on ABCD. If the patient is responsive, make sure you ask about the mechanism of injury and about his or her symptoms, starting with these five questions:

1. Does your neck or back hurt?
2. What happened?
3. Where does it hurt?
4. Can you move your hands and feet?
5. Can you feel me touching your fingers? Your toes?

As part of your focused physical exam, inspect the spinal area for deformities, contusions, abrasions, punctures/penetrations, burns, tenderness, lacerations, and swelling. Make sure that you do not move any body parts excessively. Determine whether the strength in each extremity is equal by asking the patient to squeeze your hands and to gently push each foot against your hands (Figure 32-9). Finally, assess the equality of strength of the extremities by comparing the right limb to the left limb.

With unresponsive patients, you should try to identify the mechanism of injury. As part of your assessment, inspect the patient for deformities, contusions, abrasions, punctures/penetrations, burns, tenderness, lacerations, and swelling (DCAP-BTLS). First responders, family members, or bystanders may have helpful information, including when the patient lost consciousness or what his or her previous level of consciousness was.

Remember that the ability to walk, move the extremities, or feel sensation does not necessarily rule out a spinal cord injury. Nor does an absence of pain. Do not ask patients with possible spinal injuries to move as a test for pain. On the contrary, you should instruct them to be still.

However, pain or tenderness when you palpate the spinal area is certainly a warning sign that a spinal injury may exist. Patients with spinal injuries may complain of constant or intermittent pain along the spinal column or

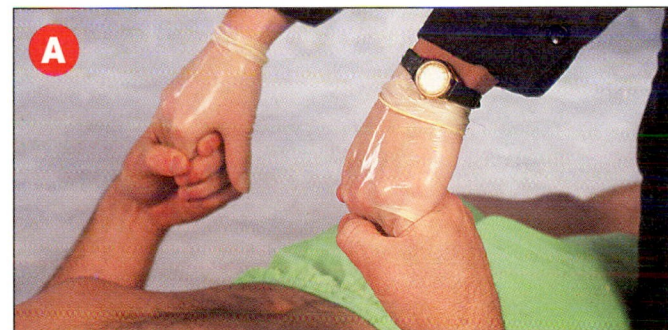

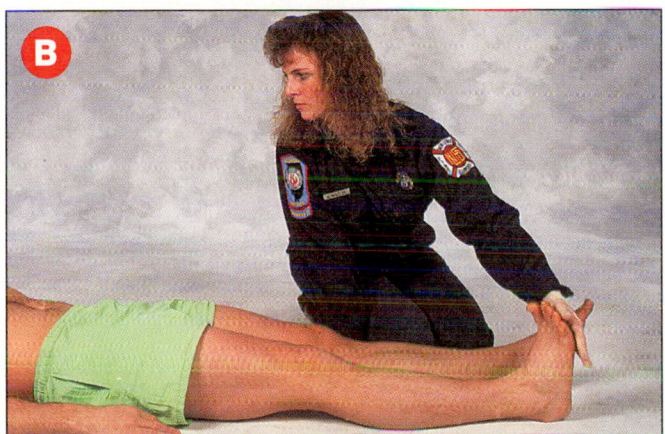

FIGURE 32-9 A: Assess the equality of strength of each extremity by asking the patient to squeeze your hands. **B:** Next, ask the patient to gently push each foot against your hands.

in their extremities. A spinal cord injury may also produce pain independent of movement or palpation.

Other signs and symptoms of spinal injury include an obvious deformity as you palpate the spine; numbness, weakness, or tingling in the extremities; and soft-tissue injuries in the spinal region. Patients with severe spinal injury may lose sensation or experience paralysis below the suspected level of injury or be incontinent (Figure 32-10). Obvious injury to the head and neck may indicate injury to the cervical spine. Injury to the shoulders, back, or abdomen may indicate injury to the thoracic or lumbar spine. Injuries of the lower extremities may indicate a problem with the lumbar spine or sacrum.

Emergency Medical Care

Emergency medical care of a patient with a possible spinal injury begins, as does all patient care, with your protection; therefore, you must remember to follow BSI techniques. Next, you must maintain the airway in the proper position, assess respirations, and give supplemental oxygen.

Restoring the airway. Knowing that improper handling of a spinal injury can leave a patient permanently paralyzed should not paralyze *you* in the presence of an airway obstruction. Remember, all patients without an airway will die. If a patient with a spinal injury has an airway obstruction, you should perform the jaw-thrust maneuver to open the airway (Figure 32-11). Do not use the head-tilt/chin-lift maneuver, as it extends the neck and may further damage the cervical spine. If the patient is unconscious, you can lift or pull the tongue forward so that you do not have to move the neck. Once the airway is open, hold the head still, in a neutral, in-line position, until it can be fully immobilized.

After you open the airway, consider inserting an oropharyngeal airway. If you do so, be sure to monitor the airway closely and have a suctioning unit available, as you will often need to clear away blood, saliva, or vomitus. Give oxygen to any patient who is having trouble breathing.

If you cannot open the airway because of the position of the head, realign the neck. Firmly grasp the patient's head with both hands, pull the head gently and firmly away from the trunk, and turn it to the front. Maintain the head in this position while you or your partner repeats the jaw-thrust maneuver.

Immobilization of the cervical spine. Stabilizing the airway is your first priority. You must then stabilize the head and trunk so that bone fragments do not do further damage (Figure 32-12). Even small movements can significantly injure the spinal cord. Begin manual in-line immobilization by holding the head firmly with both

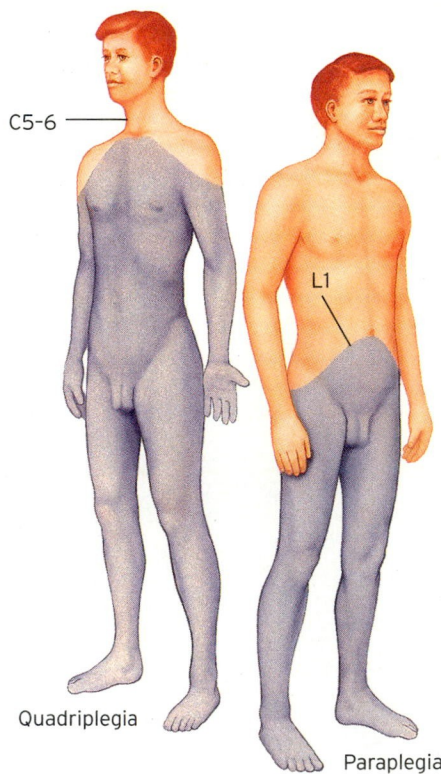

FIGURE 32-10 With severe spinal injuries, patients may lose sensation or experience paralysis below the suspected level of injury.

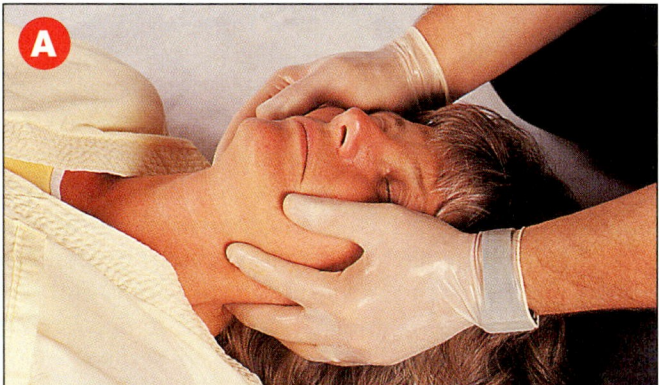

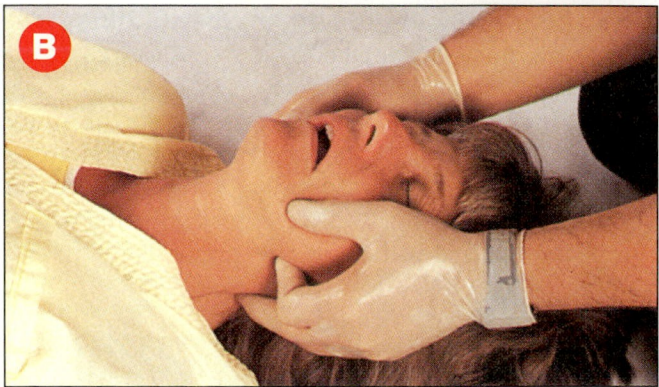

FIGURE 32-11 Jaw-thrust maneuver. **A:** Stabilize the neck in a neutral, in-line position. **B:** Push the angle of the lower jaw forward.

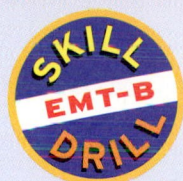

Performing Manual In-Line Immobilization

Figure 32-12

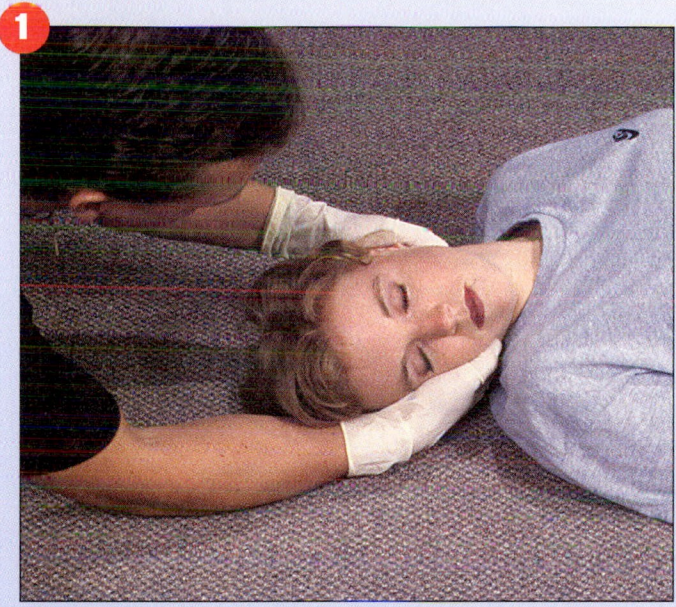

Kneel behind the patient, and place your hands firmly around the base of the skull on either side.

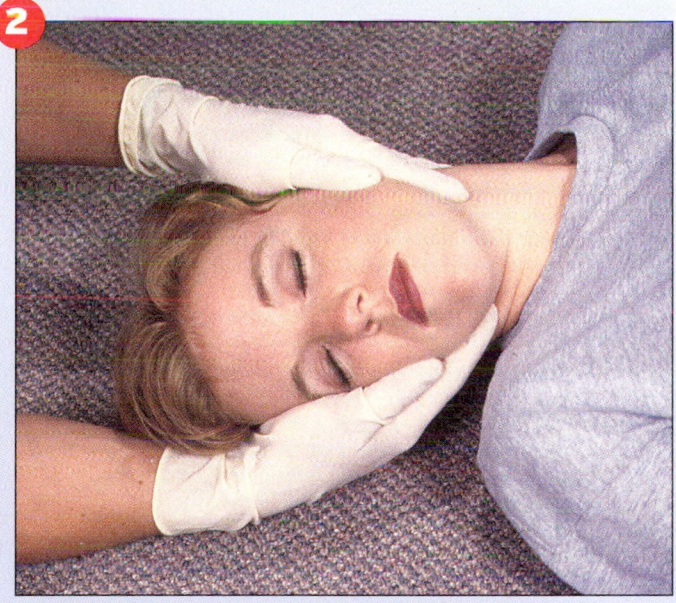

Support the lower jaw with your index and long fingers as you support the head with your palms.

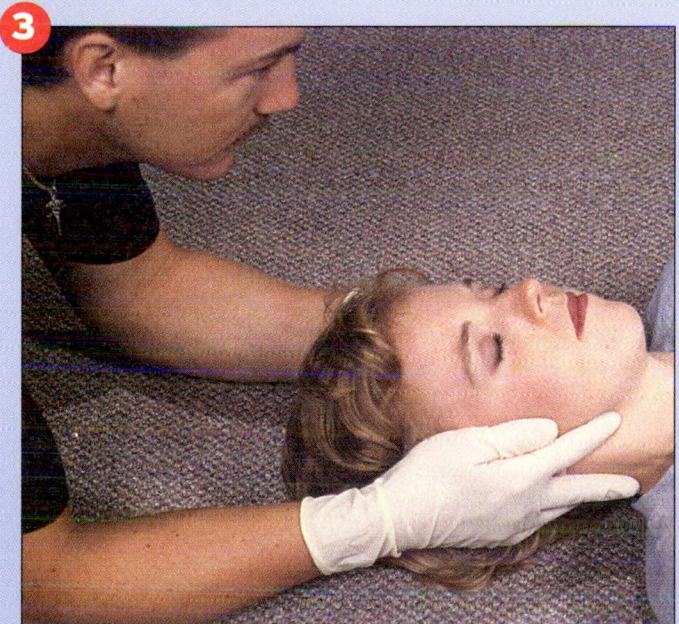

Gently lift the head until the patient's eyes are looking straight ahead and the head and torso are in line. Align the nose with the navel. Make sure that you do not twist, flex, or extend the head or neck excessively.

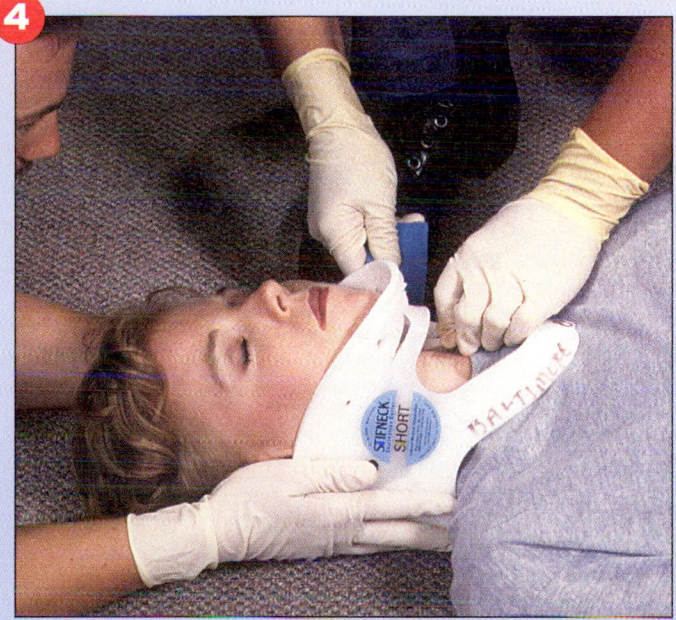

As you continue to support the head manually, have your partner place a rigid cervical collar around the neck to provide more stability.

> Even small movements can significantly injure the spinal cord.

hands. Whenever possible, kneel behind the patient, and place your hands around the base of the skull on either side. Support the lower jaw with your index and long fingers, while you are supporting the head with your palms.

Then gently lift the head until the patient's eyes are looking straight ahead and the head and torso are in line. This neutral **eyes forward position** makes immobilization easier. Align the nose with the navel. Never twist, flex, or extend the head or neck excessively. Manually maintain this position as you continue to maintain the airway and ventilate the patient. Do not remove your hands from the patient's head until the patient is properly secured to a backboard and the head is immobilized. The patient must remain immobilized until he or she is examined at the hospital.

Once the patient's head and neck are manually immobilized, assess the pulse, motor functions, and sensation in all extremities. Then assess the cervical spine area and neck. As you continue to support the head manually, your partner should place a rigid spinal immobilization collar (cervical collar) around the neck to provide some stability. This is in addition to, not instead of, manual support. Remember that an improperly fitting collar will do more harm than good. If you do not have the proper size, place a rolled towel around the head, and tape it to the backboard as you immobilize the patient on the board. In any case, maintain manual support until the patient is fully secured to a backboard.

There are some situations in which you should not force the head into a neutral, in-line position. Do not move the head if any of the following causes the patient to complain of pain:

- Muscle spasms in the neck
- Increased pain
- Numbness, tingling, or weakness
- Compromised airway or ventilations

In these situations, immobilize the patient in the position in which you found him or her.

Preparation for Transport

Supine Patients

A patient who is supine can be effectively immobilized by securing him or her to a long backboard. The ideal procedure for moving a patient from the ground to a backboard is the **four-person log roll**. This procedure is recommended any time you suspect a cervical spine injury. In other cases, you may choose instead to slide the patient onto a backboard or use a scoop stretcher. The patient's condition, the scene, and the available resources will dictate the method you choose.

You should direct the team from a kneeling position by the patient's head so that you can maintain manual in-line immobilization. Your job is to ensure that the head, torso, and pelvis move as a unit, with your teammates controlling the movement of the body. If necessary, you may recruit bystanders to the team, but be sure to instruct them fully before moving the patient. Proceed as follows (Figure 32-13):

1. **Quickly assess the posterior body** if this has not already been done in the focused history and physical examination.

2. **Make sure that the backboard is close at hand,** so that you can slide it under the patient's back and that a cervical collar is on the patient.

3. **The other team members** should place their hands on the far side of the patient to increase their leverage. Instruct them to use their body weight and their shoulder and back muscles to ensure a smooth, coordinated pull, concentrating their pull on the heavier portions of the patient's body.

4. **At your command,** the team should roll the patient onto the backboard, avoiding rotating the head, shoulders, or pelvis.

5. **Place foam padding or a blanket roll** under the head of an adult to support it in the in-line position. Pads may also be placed in the space between the adult patient's torso and the backboard, but be careful to avoid excessive patient movement.

6. Once the patient is centered on the backboard, **secure the upper torso** to the board with long straps. Secure the pelvis with a strap over the iliac crests or with groin loops.

7. Once the patient is adequately padded, **secure his or her head to the board** with two straps: one over the forehead and the second over the pads and cervical collar. Straps should never be placed around the chin, in case an airway problem develops.

8. **Secure the legs to the board** with straps that pass above and below the knees.

9. **Place the arms securely under a second strap** passing across the lower torso so they do not move during transport. Alternatively, you can loosely tie the patient's wrists together with a scarf or soft, rolled bandage.

10. **Reassess the patient's pulse,** motor function, and sensation periodically to make sure that the straps are not too tight.

Sitting Patients

Some patients with a possible spinal injury will be in a sitting position, such as after an automobile crash. With these patients, you should use a short backboard or other short spinal extrication device to immobilize the cervical and thoracic spines. The short board is then secured to the long board.

The exceptions to this rule are situations in which you do not have time to first secure the patient to the short board, including the following situations:

- You or the patient is in danger.
- You need to gain immediate access to other patients.
- The patient's injuries justify urgent removal.

In these situations, your team should lower the patient directly onto a long backboard, using the Rapid Extrication technique as described in chapter 6. Be sure that you provide manual immobilization of the cervical spine as you move the patient. Rapid extrication is based on time and the patient, not your preference.

In all other cases, you should handle the sitting patient as follows (Figure 32-14 on page 696):

1. As with the supine patient, you must **first stabilize the head** and then maintain manual in-line immobilization until the patient is secured to the long backboard.

2. **Secure the airway,** and apply the cervical collar.

3. **Wedge the short board** between the patient's upper back and the seat back.

4. **Open the board's side flaps (if present),** and position them around the patient's torso and snug to the armpits. Make any adjustments necessary without excessive movement of the patient.

5. Once the board is properly positioned, **secure first the upper torso straps** and then the midtorso straps. Position and fasten both groin loops. Then check all torso straps to make sure they are secure.

6. **Pad any space** between the patient's head and the board as necessary. Secure the forehead strap, and then fasten the lower head strap around the cervical collar.

7. **Place the long backboard** next to the patient's buttocks, perpendicular to the trunk. Then turn the patient parallel to the long board, and slowly lower him or her onto it.

8. **Lift the patient** (without rotating him or her), and slip the long board under the short board.

9. **Secure the short and long boards** together.

10. **Reassess the pulse,** motor function, and sensation in all four extremities. Note your findings, and prepare for immediate transport.

Standing Patients

You may arrive at a scene in which you find a patient standing or wandering around after an accident or injury. If you suspect that there may be underlying head, neck, or spinal injuries, you should immobilize the patient to a long backboard before proceeding to assess him or her. This will require three EMT-Bs, as follows (Figure 32-15 on page 698):

1. **FIRST EMT-B:** Maintain in-line immobilization and instruct the patient to remain still.

2. **SECOND EMT-B:** Apply a cervical collar and position the board upright directly behind the patient.

3. **SECOND AND THIRD EMT-Bs:** Stand on either side of the patient. Reach under the patient's arm and grasp the handhold at shoulder level.

4. **SECOND AND THIRD EMT-Bs:** Carefully lower the patient and the backboard to the ground.

5. **FIRST EMT-B:** Continue to maintain in-line immobilization as the patient is lowered to the ground.

6. **SECOND AND THIRD EMT-Bs:** With the board on the ground, assess the patient and secure the patient to the backboard.

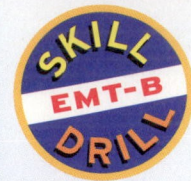

Immobilizing a Patient to a Long Backboard
Figure 32-13

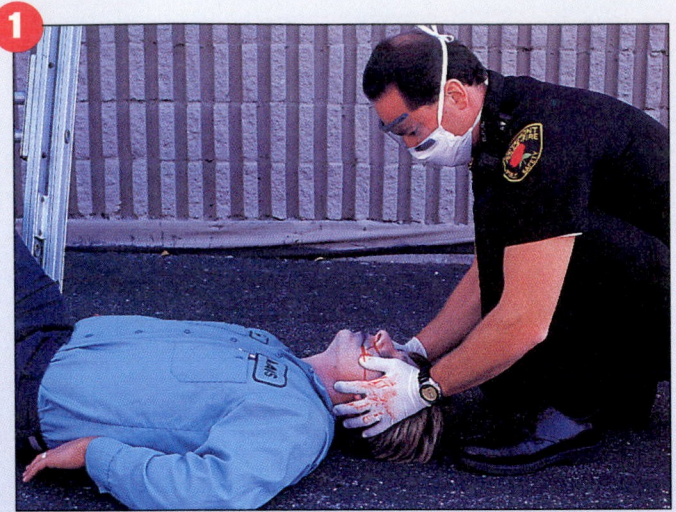

Maintain in-line immobilization from a kneeling position at the patient's head. This EMT-B directs the log roll.

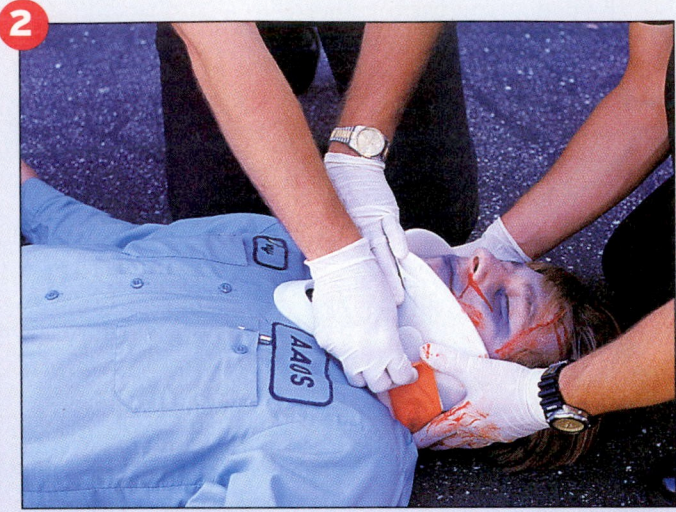

Apply a cervical collar.

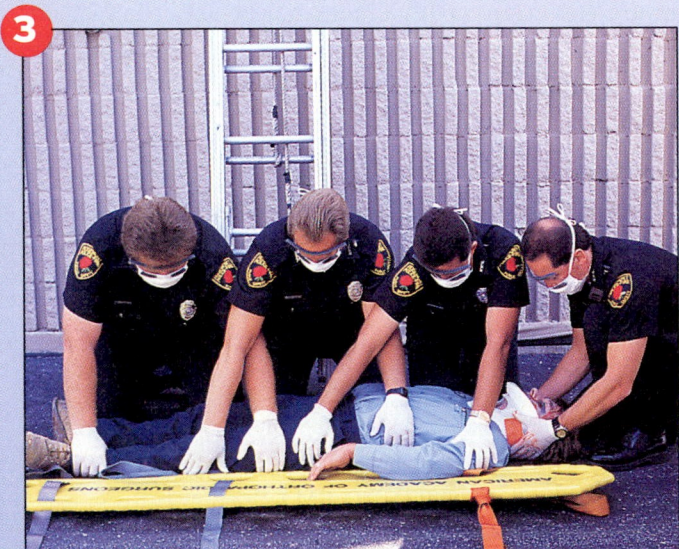

Place your hands on the far side of the patient to increase leverage as you log roll. Ensure that proper lifting techniques are used.

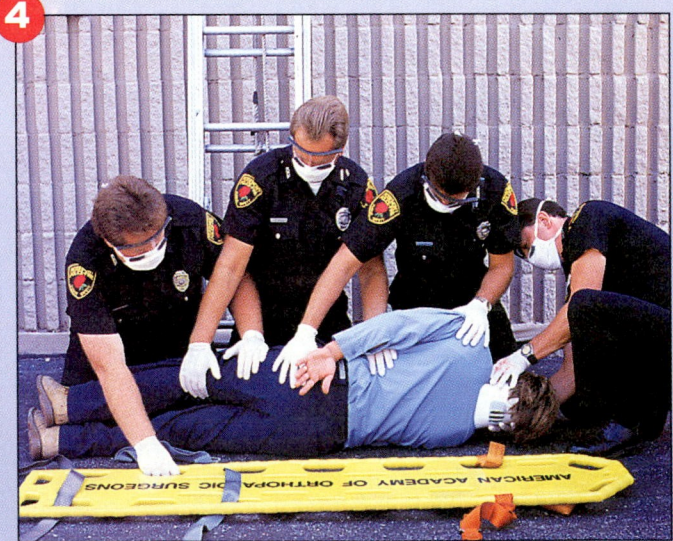

At the command of the EMT-B at the head, log roll the patient onto the backboard without rotating the head, shoulders, or pelvis.

5

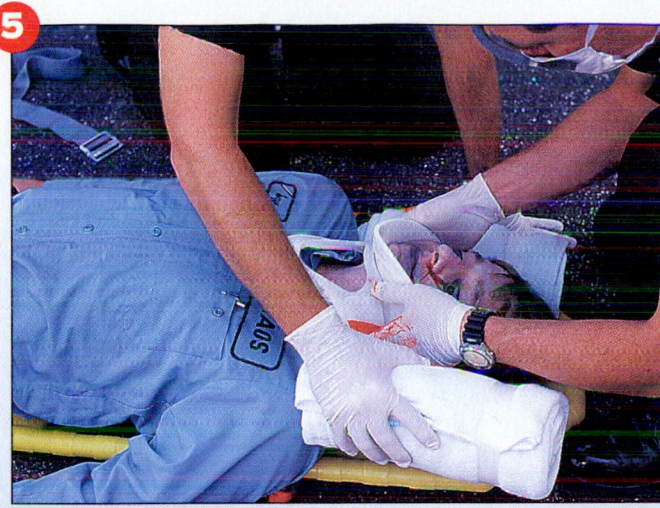

Place rolled towels or foam padding around the patient's head to maintain the in-line position.

6

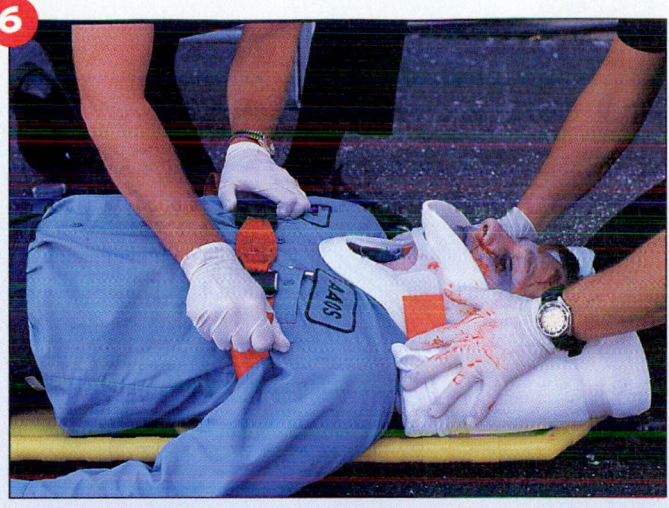

Secure the upper torso to the backboard with straps.

7

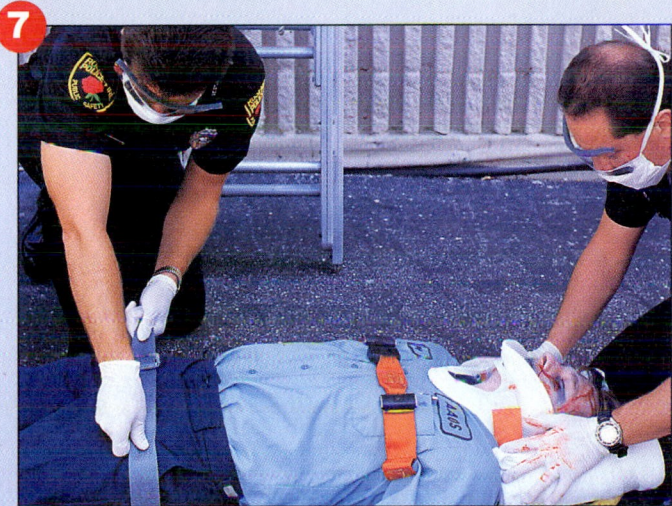

Secure the pelvis with straps over the iliac crests.

8

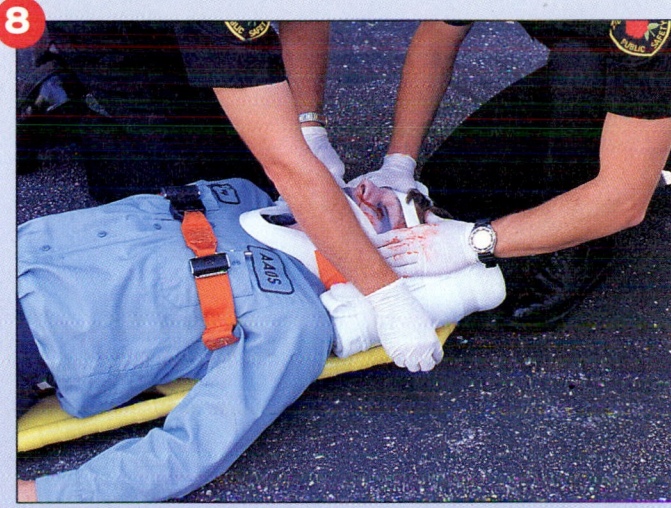

Once the patient is padded, secure the head to the backboard with two straps: one over the forehead and one over the pads and cervical collar.

9

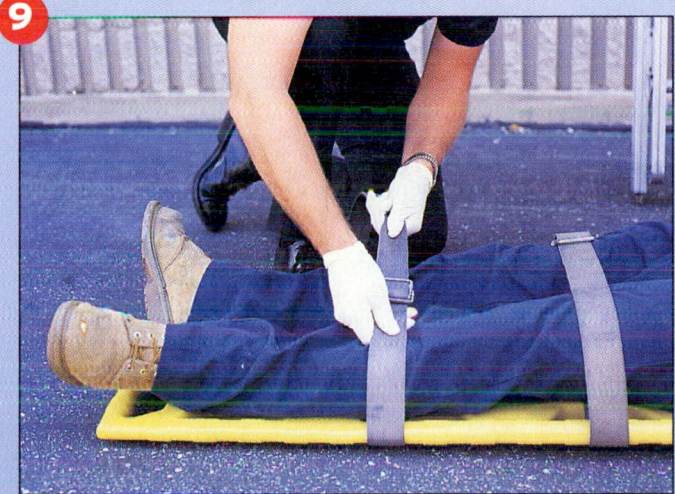

Secure the legs to the backboard.

10

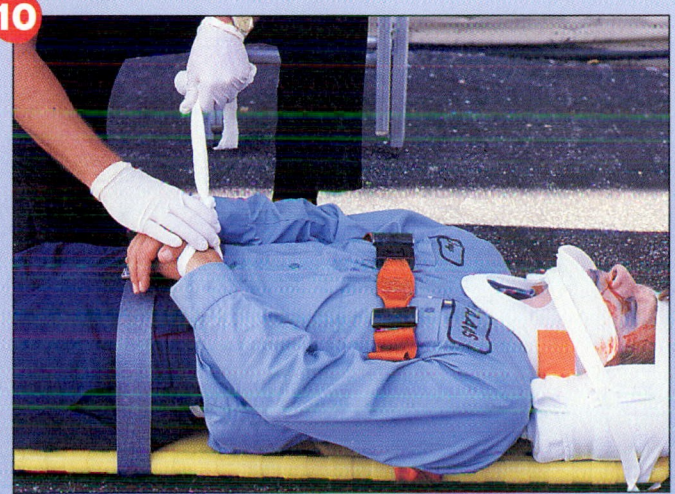

Secure the hands with a cravat or alternatively, by securing them under a second strap across the lower torso.

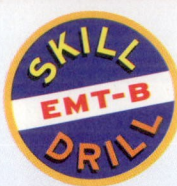

Immobilizing a Patient Found in a Sitting Position

Figure 32-14

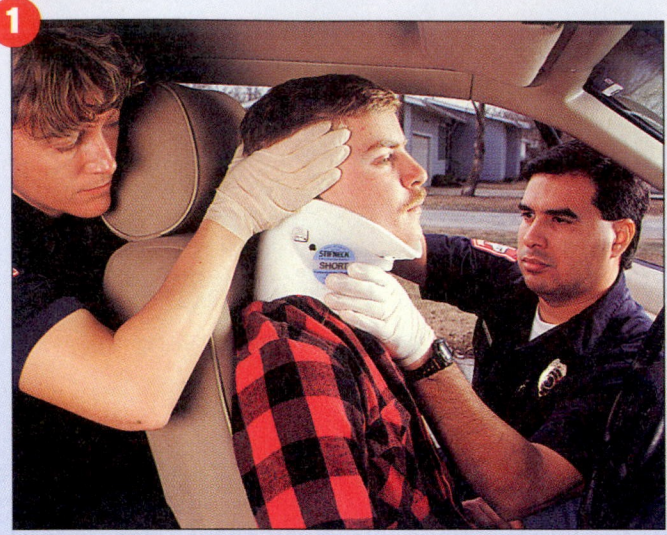

1 Stabilize the head and neck in a neutral, in-line position. Secure the airway, and apply a cervical collar.

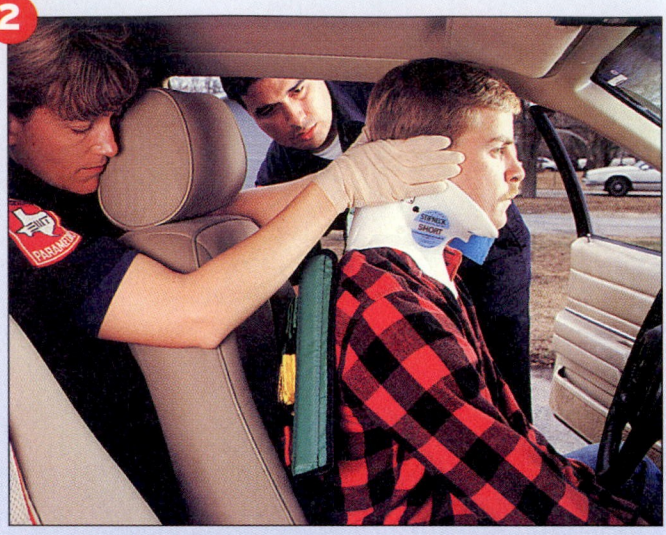

2 Insert a short spine immobilization device between the patient's upper back and the seat.

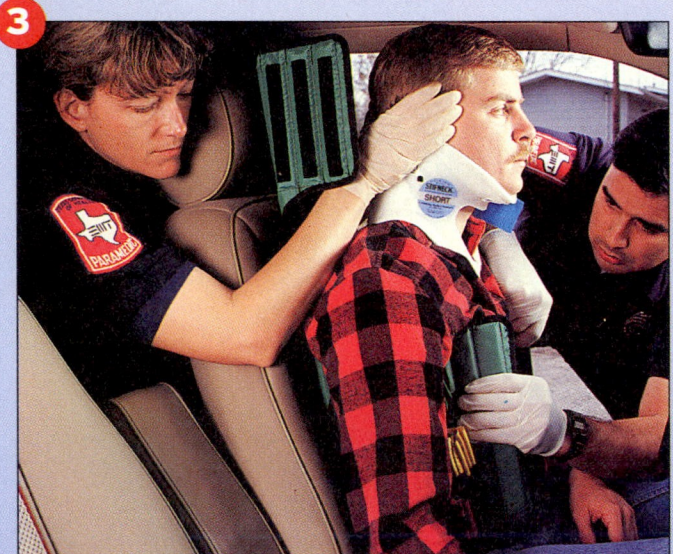

3 Open the side flaps, and position them around the patient's torso, snug around the armpits.

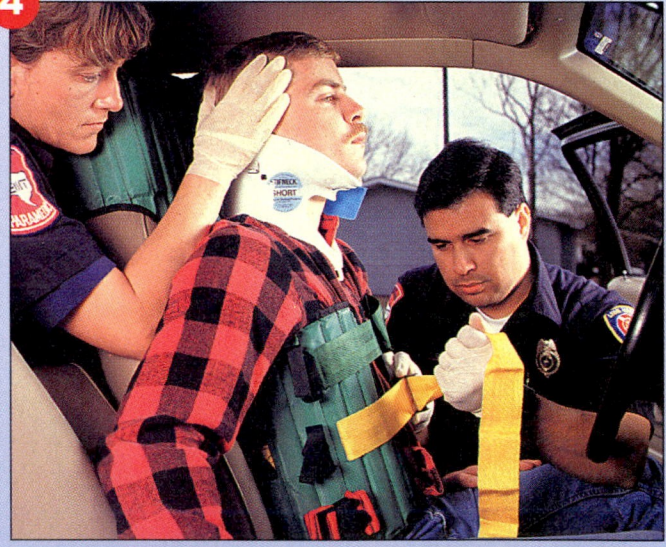

4 Once the device is positioned properly, secure the upper torso flaps and then the midtorso flaps.

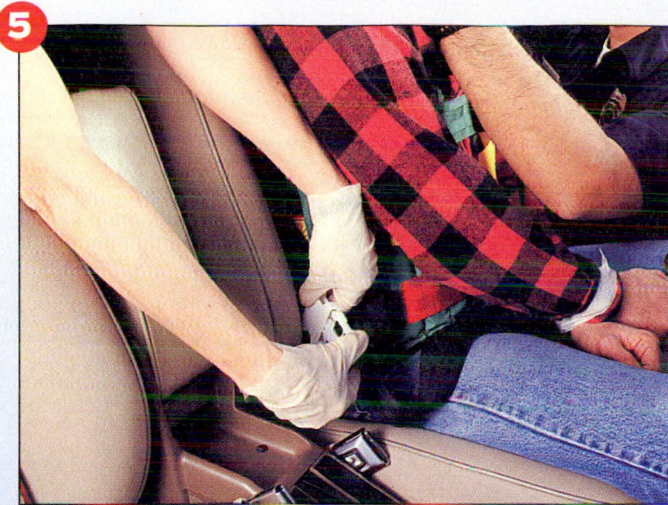

Secure the groin loops (leg straps).

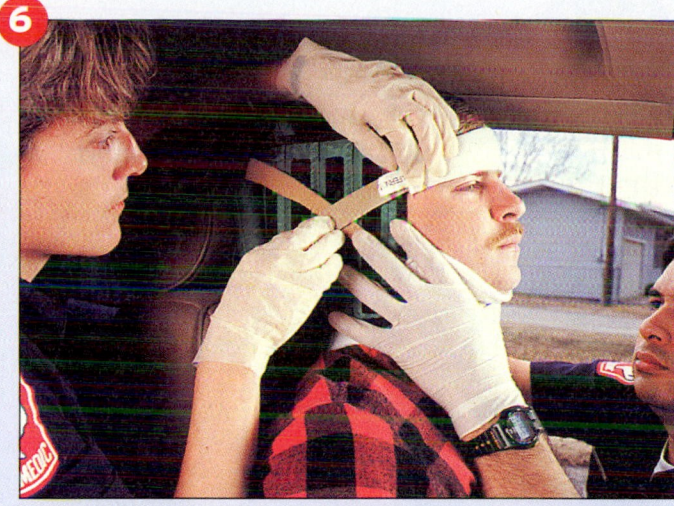

Pad any space between the patient's head and the device. Secure the forehead strap, and then fasten the lower head strap around the cervical collar.

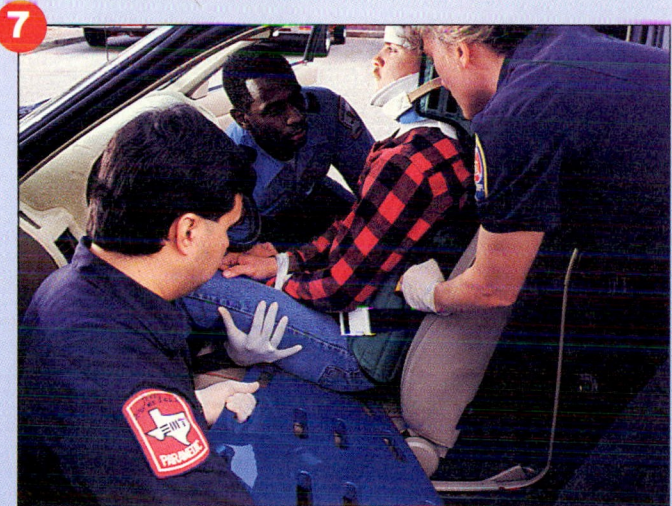

Wedge a long backboard next to the patient's buttocks, perpendicular to the trunk.

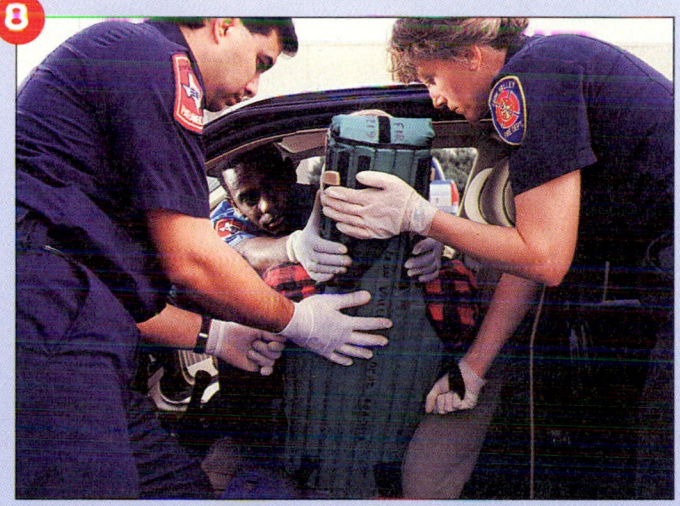

Turn the patient parallel to the long board, and slowly lower him or her onto it. Lift the patient, and slip the long board under the spine device.

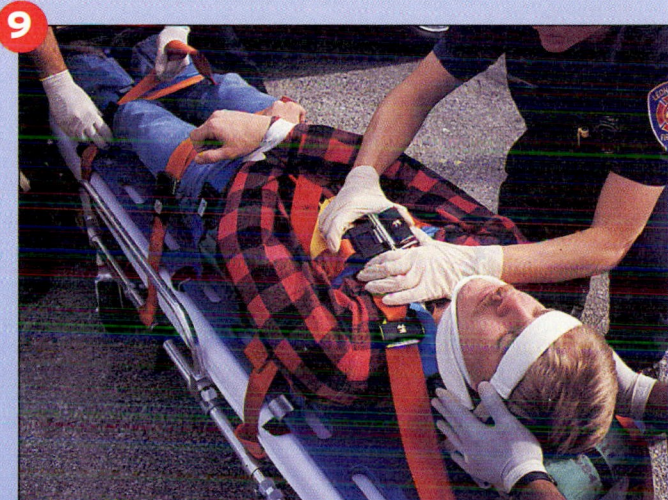

Secure the spine device to the long board.

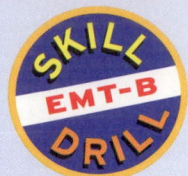

Immobilizing a Patient Found in a Standing Position
Figure 32-15

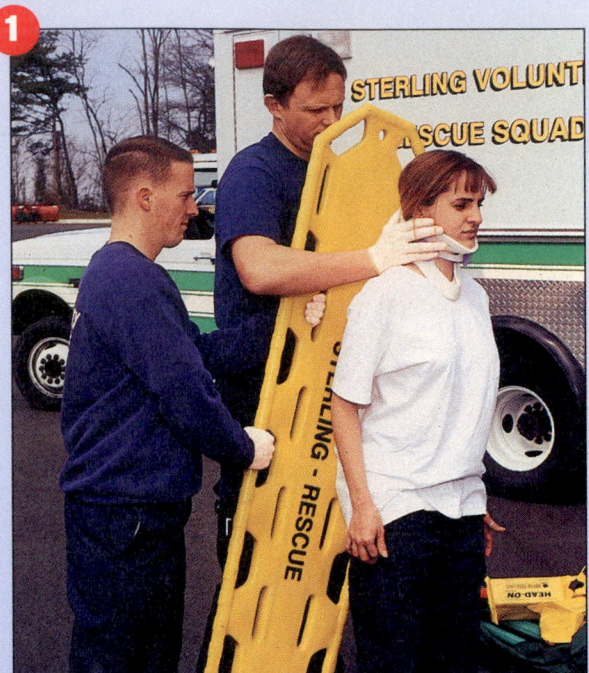

After applying a cervical collar, postion a backboard directly behind the patient.

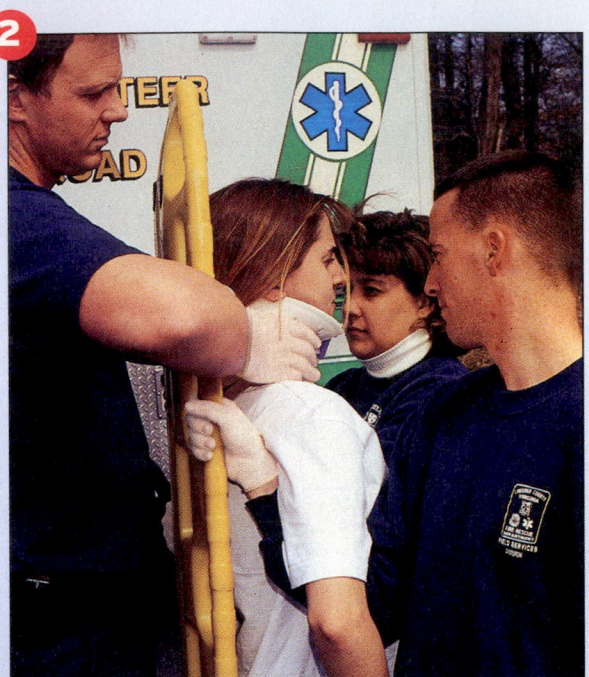

The two EMT-Bs standing on either side of the backboard should reach under the patient's arms and grasp the handholds at shoulder level.

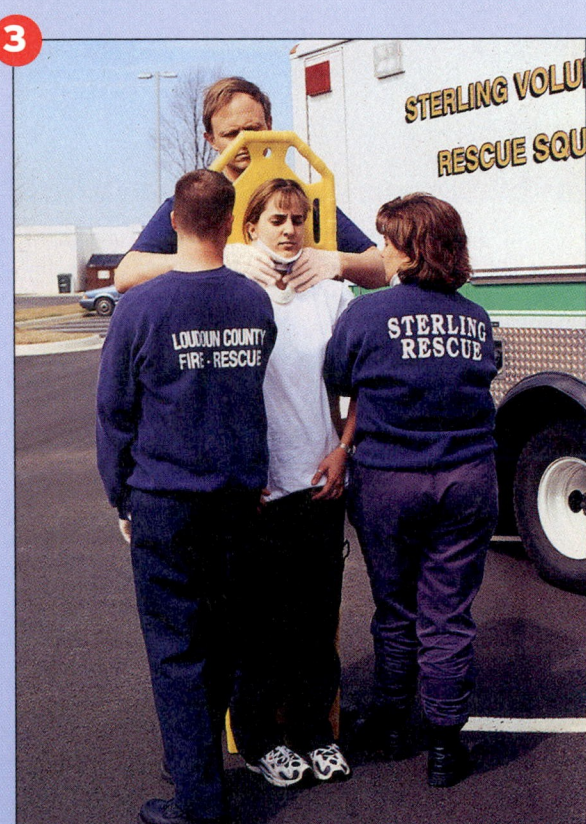

Under the direction of the EMT-B at the patient's head, prepare to lower the patient to the ground.

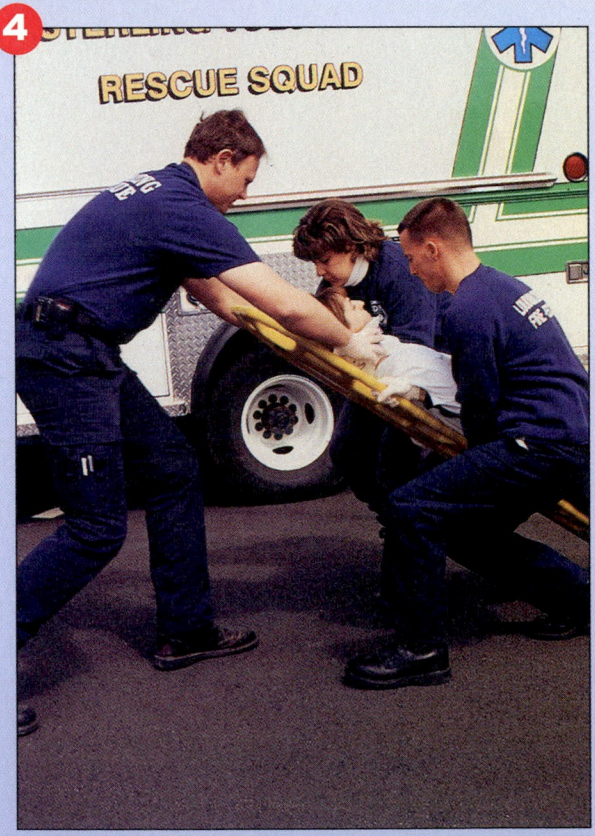

Working as a team, carefully lower the patient to the ground.

Head Injuries

All head injuries are potentially serious. If not properly treated, those that at first seem minor may end up being life threatening. On the other hand, severe lacerations of the scalp or fractures of the skull may occur with little or no brain injury and may produce minimal or no long-term problems.

Scalp Lacerations

Scalp lacerations can be minor or very serious (Figure 32-16). Because both the face and the scalp have unusually rich blood supplies, even small lacerations can quickly lead to significant blood loss. Occasionally, this blood loss may be severe enough to cause hypovolemic shock, particularly in children. In any patient with multiple injuries, bleeding from scalp or facial lacerations contributes to hypovolemia. In addition, since scalp lacerations are usually the result of direct blows to the head, they often indicate deeper, more serious injuries.

You can almost always control bleeding from a scalp laceration by applying direct pressure over the wound (Figure 32-17). Remember to follow BSI techniques. Use a dry sterile dressing, folding any torn skin flaps back down onto the skin bed before applying pressure. In some instances, you will have to apply firm compression for several minutes to control the bleeding. If you suspect a skull fracture, do not apply excessive pressure to the open wound. Otherwise, you may increase intracranial pressure or push bone fragments into the brain.

If the dressing becomes soaked, do not remove it. Instead, place a second dressing over the first. Continue applying manual pressure until the bleeding is controlled, then secure the compression dressing in place with a soft, self-adhering roller bandage.

Skull Fracture

Fracture of the skull is an indication that a significant force has been applied to the head. As with any fracture, a skull fracture may be open or closed, depending on whether there is an overlying laceration of the scalp.

You can almost always control bleeding from a scalp laceration by applying direct pressure over the wound.

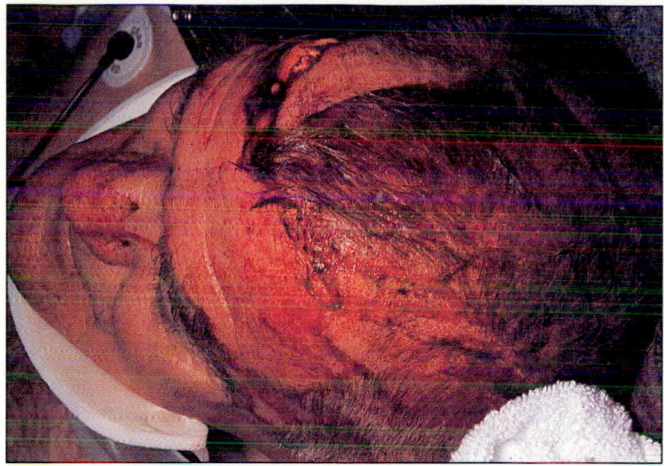

FIGURE 32-16 The scalp has an unusually rich blood supply; therefore, even small lacerations can result in significant blood loss.

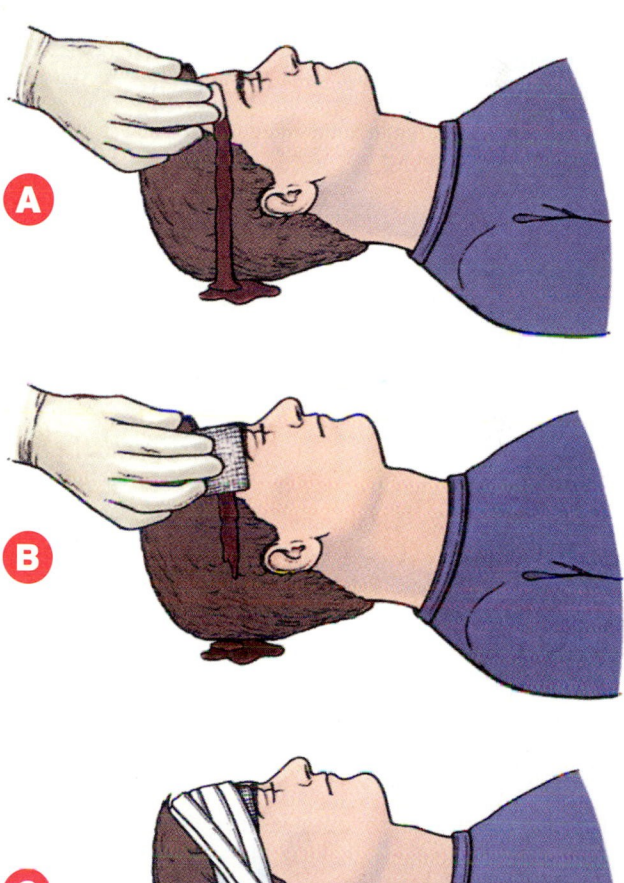

FIGURE 32-17 A: Apply pressure with a sterile dressing to fold any torn skin flaps back down onto the skin bed. **B:** Apply firm compression for several minutes to control the bleeding. **C:** Secure the compression dressing in place with a soft, self-adhering roller bandage.

Injuries from bullets or other penetrating weapons frequently result in fracture of the skull. The diagnosis of a skull fracture is usually made in the hospital by X-ray examination, but you can conclude that a fracture is present if the patient's head appears deformed or if there is a visible crack in the skull within a scalp laceration. Another sign of skull fracture that you may see is ecchymosis that develops under the eyes (raccoon eyes) or behind one ear over the mastoid process (Battle's sign) (Figure 32-18).

Brain Injuries

Concussion. A blow to the head or face may cause concussion of the brain. There is no universal agreement on the exact definition of a *concussion*, but in general, it means a temporary loss or alteration of part or all of the brain's abilities to function without actual physical damage to the brain. For example, a person who "sees stars" after being struck in the head has had a concussion that affects the occipital portion of the brain. A concussion may result in unconsciousness and even the inability to breathe for short periods of time.

A patient with a concussion may be confused or have amnesia (loss of memory). Occasionally, the patient can remember everything but the events leading up to the injury; this is called <u>retrograde amnesia</u>. Inability to remember events after the injury is called <u>anterograde (posttraumatic) amnesia</u>.

Usually, a concussion lasts only a short time. In fact, it is often over by the time you arrive. Nevertheless, you should ask about symptoms of concussion in any patient who has sustained an injury to the head; these symptoms include dizziness, weakness, or visual changes.

Contusion. Like any other soft tissue in the body, the brain can sustain a *contusion,* or bruise, when the skull is struck. A contusion is far more serious than a concussion, because it involves physical injury to the brain tissue, which may suffer long-lasting and even permanent damage. As with contusions elsewhere, there is associated bleeding and swelling from injured blood vessels. Injury of brain tissue or bleeding inside the skull will cause an increase of pressure within the skull. A patient who has had a brain contusion may exhibit any or all of the signs of brain injury described later in this chapter.

Intracranial bleeding. Laceration or rupture of a blood vessel inside the brain or in the meninges that cover the brain will produce intracranial bleeding (hematoma) in one of three areas (Figure 32-19):

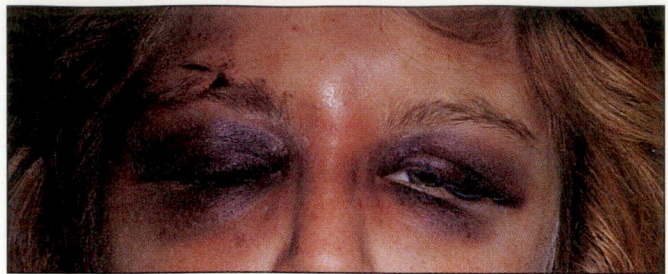
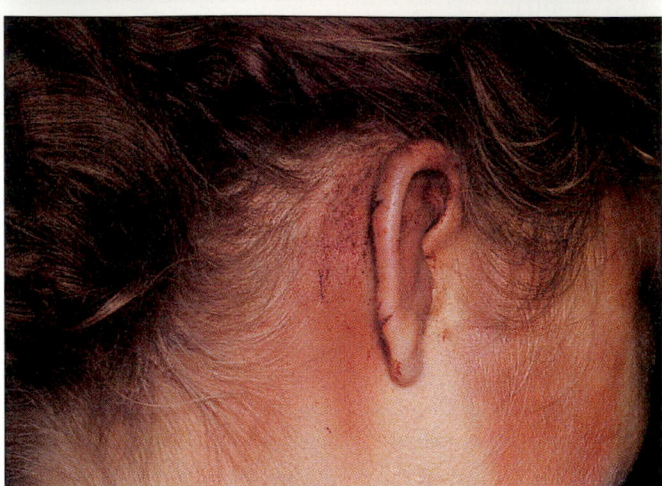

FIGURE 32-18 Skull fracture is a possibility if a patient has ecchymosis under the eyes (raccoon eyes) or behind one ear over the mastoid process (Battle's sign).

Types of intracranial hematomas

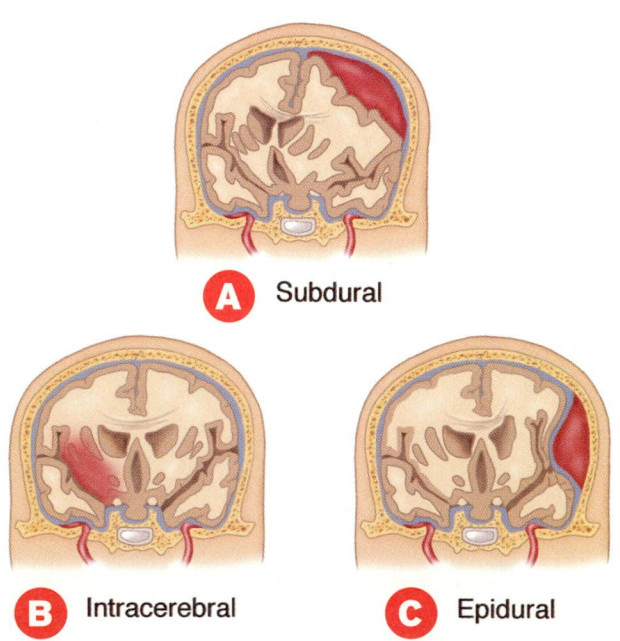

FIGURE 32-19 Intracranial bleeding can occur in one of three areas. **A:** Beneath the dura but outside the brain (subdural hematoma). **B:** Within the substance of the brain tissue (intracerebral hematoma). **C:** Outside the dura and under the skull (epidural hematoma).

- Beneath the dura but outside the brain: a subdural hematoma

- Within the substance of the brain tissue itself: an intracerebral hematoma

- Outside the dura and under the skull: an epidural hematoma

A hematoma may develop rapidly, usually because of arterial injury, as in an epidural hematoma; or it may develop very slowly, as with a subdural hematoma. In any case, because the brain occupies nearly the entire space inside the skull, the result is increased pressure inside the skull, leading to compression of the brain tissue. The expanding hematoma will cause progressive loss of brain function and, if not treated properly, death.

Rapid deterioration of neurologic signs following a head injury is a sign of intracranial hematoma. You must act quickly to evaluate and treat such patients. Provide oxygen, monitor the airway, elevate the head of the stretcher, and provide immediate transport.

Other Brain Injuries

Brain injuries are not always a result of trauma. Certain medical conditions, such as blood clots or hemorrhaging, can also cause brain injuries that produce significant bleeding or swelling. Problems with the blood vessels, high blood pressure, or any number of other causes may cause spontaneous bleeding in the brain, affecting the patient's level of consciousness. This is known as altered mental status. The signs and symptoms of nontraumatic injuries are the same as those of traumatic brain injuries, except that there is no obvious mechanism of injury or any evidence of trauma.

Complications of Head Injury

Cerebral edema, or swelling of the brain, is one of the most common complications of any head injury. It is also one of the most serious, because, as we have seen, swelling in the skull compresses the brain tissue, resulting in a loss of brain function.

Cerebral edema is aggravated by low oxygen levels in the blood and improved by high ones. For this reason, you must make sure that the airway is open and that adequate ventilations and high-flow oxygen are given to any patient with a head injury. This is especially true if the patient is unconscious. Do not wait for cyanosis or other obvious signs of hypoxia to develop.

It is not uncommon for the patient with a head injury to have a convulsion, or seizure. This is the result of excessive excitability of the brain, caused by direct injury or the accumulation of fluid within the brain (edema). You should be prepared to manage convulsions in all patients who have had a head injury.

Another common response to head injuries, even among children with very slight head injuries, is vomiting. This is usually the result of increased intracranial pressure. In managing such vomiting, you should pay particular attention to protecting the airway.

As was discussed earlier, the appearance of clear or pink watery cerebrospinal fluid from the nose, the ear, or an open scalp wound indicates that the dura and the skull have both been penetrated. You should make no attempt to pack the wound, ear, or nose in this situation. Cover the scalp wound, if there is one, with sterile gauze to prevent further contamination, but do not bandage it tightly.

Assessing Head Injuries

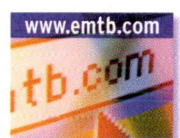

Motor vehicle crashes, direct blows, falls from heights, assault, and sports injuries are common causes of head injury. A patient who has experienced any of these events should immediately arouse your suspicion and cause you to start looking for specific signs and symptoms of head injury. A deformed windshield or dented helmet may indicate a major blow to the head, which is likely to have caused injury (Figure 32-20). It is especially important to evaluate and monitor the level of consciousness in patients with suspected head injuries, paying particular attention to any changes that may occur.

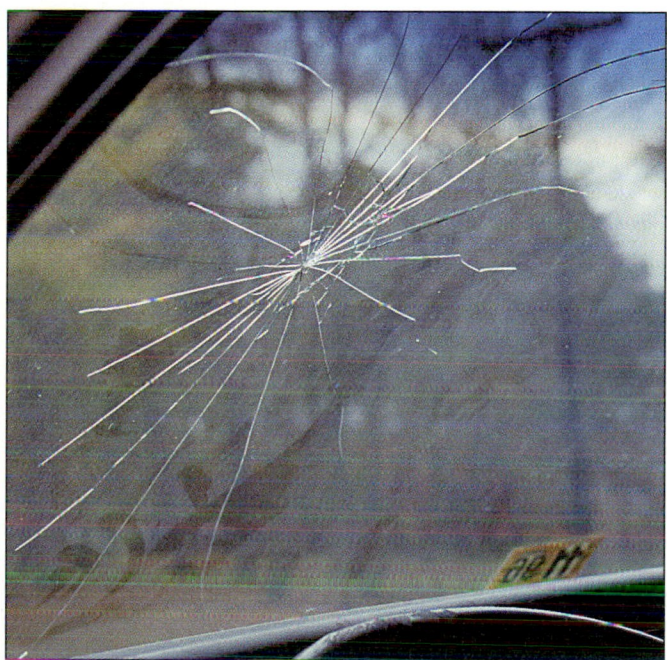

FIGURE 32-20 The classic "star" on the windshield after an automobile crash is a significant indicator of injury. Be alert for the signs and symptoms of head injury.

Types of Head Injuries

Closed head injuries, usually associated with trauma, are those in which the brain has been injured but the skin has not been broken and there is no obvious bleeding. In assessing a patient with a possible closed head injury, consider the mechanism of injury. Did the patient fall? Was he or she in an automobile crash or the victim of an assault? Was there deformity of the windshield or deformity of the helmet? Look for scalp lacerations, contusions, hematomas, or skull deformities. Sometimes, the skull will appear to have been pushed into the brain.

Decreased level of consciousness is the most reliable sign of this type of injury. Monitor the patient for changes in level of consciousness, including signs of confusion, disorientation, or deteriorating mental status. Is the patient unresponsive or repeating questions? Experiencing seizures? Nauseous or vomiting? Next, assess the patient for decreased movement and/or numbness and tingling in the extremities. Assess the vital signs carefully. People with head injuries may have irregular respirations, depending on which region of the brain is affected. Look for blood or cerebrospinal fluid leaking from the ears, nose, or mouth and for bruising around the eyes and behind the ears.

You should also evaluate the patient's pupils, especially if he or she has a decreased level of consciousness. Often, unequal pupil size after a head injury signals a serious problem. Developing blood clots may be pressing on the third cranial nerve, causing one pupil to dilate (Figure 32-21).

Scalp contusions, lacerations, hematomas, and obvious skull deformities are all signs of open head injuries, which are often caused by a penetrating object. There may be bleeding and exposed brain tissue. Do not probe open scalp lacerations with your gloved finger, as this may push bone fragments into the brain. Do not remove an impaled object.

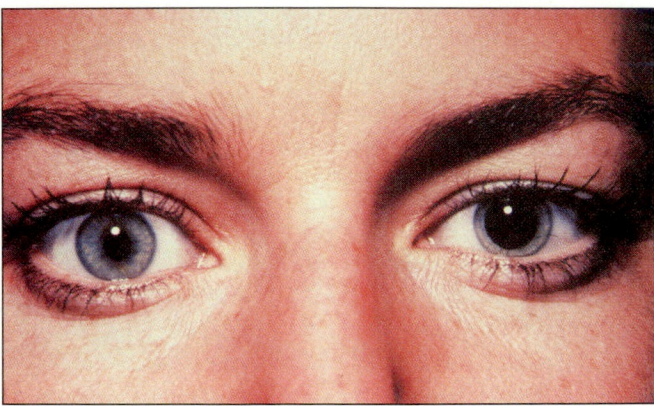

FIGURE 32-21 Assess pupil size if you suspect a head injury. Unequal pupil size may signal a serious problem.

Signs and Symptoms of Head Injury

Open and closed head injuries have essentially the same signs and symptoms.

Following an injury, any patient who exhibits one or more of these signs or symptoms should be evaluated promptly in the emergency department:

- Lacerations, contusions, or hematomas to the scalp
- Soft area or depression upon palpation
- Visible fractures or deformities of the skull
- Ecchymosis about the eyes or behind the ear over the mastoid process
- Clear or pink cerebrospinal fluid leakage from a scalp wound, the nose, or the ear
- Failure of the pupils to respond to light
- Unequal pupil size
- Loss of sensation and/or motor function
- A period of unconsciousness
- Anterograde or retrograde amnesia
- Seizures
- Numbness or tingling in the extremities
- Irregular respirations
- Dizziness
- Visual complaints
- Combative or other abnormal behavior
- Nausea or vomiting

Level of consciousness. Change in the level of consciousness is the single most important observation that you can make in assessing the severity of brain injury. Level of consciousness usually corresponds to the extent of loss of brain function. As soon as you determine that a head injury is present, you should perform a baseline assessment using the AVPU scale and record the time. Reevaluate the patient and record your observations every 15 minutes if the patient's condition is stable and at least every 5 minutes if the patient's condition is not stable, until you reach the hospital.

Frequently, the levels will fluctuate, improving, deteriorating, then improving again over time. On other occasions, there is a gradual, progressive deterioration in the patient's response to stimuli; this usually indicates serious brain damage that may need aggressive medical and/or surgical treatment. The physicians who treat the patient will need to know when loss of consciousness occurred. They will want to compare their neurologic evaluation with the one you performed in the field.

GLASGOW COMA SCALE

Eye Opening

Spontaneous	4
To Voice	3
To Pain	2
None	1

Verbal Response

Oriented	5
Confused	4
Inappropriate Words	3
Incomprehensible Words	2
None	1

Motor Response

Obeys Command	6
Localizes Pain	5
Withdraws (pain)	4
Flexion (pain)	3
Extension (pain)	2
None	1

Glasgow Coma Score Total	**15**

FIGURE 32-22 The Glasgow Coma Scale is one method of evaluating level of consciousness. Note that the lower the score, the more severe the extent of brain injury.

Your EMS system may choose to use the more detailed *Glasgow Coma Scale* instead of the AVPU scale to assess patients' level of consciousness (Figure 32-22). In either case, you should always use simple, easily understood terms when reporting the level of consciousness, such as "does not remember events immediately preceding injury" or "confused about date and time." Terms such as "obtunded" or "dazed" have different meanings to different people and should not be used in either written or verbal reports.

Changes in pupil size. The nerves that control dilation and constriction of the pupils are very sensitive to pressure within the skull. When you beam a bright light into the eye, the pupil should constrict. Failure to do so is an early and important sign of increased intracranial pressure. Unequal pupil size may indicate increased pressure on one side of the brain.

As soon as you have assessed the patient's level of consciousness, determine the reaction of each pupil to light. Sketch the size of both pupils on the ambulance report to indicate any difference between the two eyes. Continue to monitor the pupils. Any change in their reactions over time may indicate progressive brain damage.

Emergency Medical Care

Patients with head injuries often have injuries to the cervical spine as well. Therefore, when treating a patient with a head injury, you must keep in mind the need to protect and stabilize the cervical spine at all times. Avoid moving the neck unnecessarily until the spine can be appropriately splinted. An initial assessment with spinal immobilization should be done on scene with a complete, detailed physical examination en route.

Beyond this, you should treat the patient with a head injury according to three general principles, which are designed to protect and maintain the critical functions of the central nervous system:

1. **Establish an adequate airway.** If necessary, begin and maintain ventilation and always provide high-flow supplemental oxygen.

2. **Control bleeding**, and provide adequate circulation to maintain cerebral perfusion. Begin CPR, if necessary. Be sure to follow BSI techniques.

3. **Assess the patient's baseline** level of consciousness, and continuously monitor it.

As you continue to treat the patient, do not apply pressure to an open or depressed skull injury. In addition, you must assess and treat other injuries, dress and bandage open wounds as indicated in the treatment of soft-tissue injuries, splint fractures, anticipate and deal with vomiting to prevent aspiration, be prepared for convulsions and changes in the patient's condition, and transport the patient promptly and with extreme care.

Restoring the airway. The most important step in the treatment of patients with head injury, regardless of the severity, is to establish an adequate airway. If the patient has an airway obstruction, you should perform the

> Change in the level of consciousness is the single most important observation that you can make in assessing the severity of brain injury.

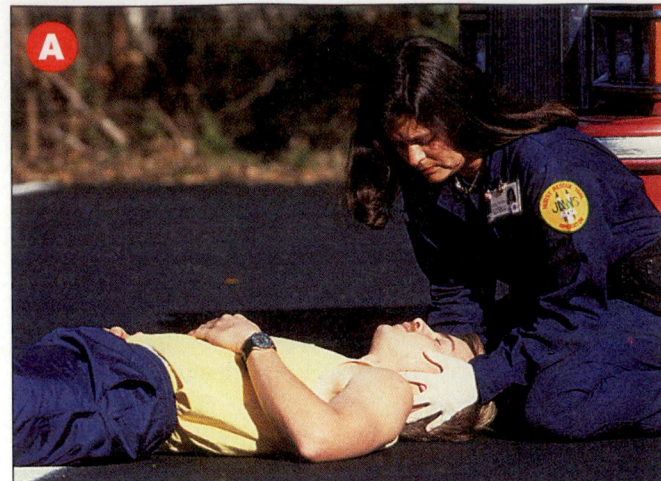

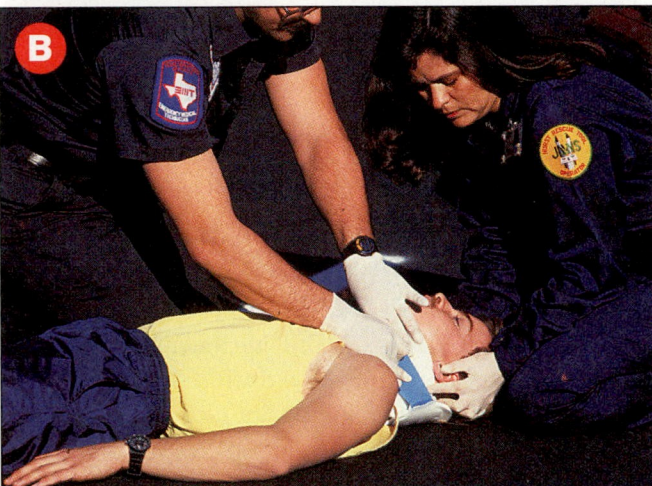

FIGURE 32-23 A. Maintain the head and cervical spine in a neutral in-line position. **B:** Apply a cervical collar as you finish the initial assessment.

jaw-thrust maneuver to open the airway. Once the airway is open, maintain the head and cervical spine in a neutral, in-line position until it can be fully immobilized with a cervical collar (Figure 32-23). Remove any foreign bodies, secretions, or vomitus from the airway. Make sure a suctioning unit is available, because you will often need to clear blood, saliva, or vomitus from the airway.

Once you have cleared the airway, check ventilation. If the respiratory control center of the brain has been injured, the rate and/or depth of breathing may be ineffective. Ventilation may also be limited by chest injuries or, if the spinal cord is injured, by paralysis of some or all of the muscles of respiration. Give high-flow oxygen to any patient who is having trouble breathing. This reduces hypoxia and possible cerebral edema. An injured brain is even less tolerant of hypoxia than a healthy brain, and studies have shown that supplemental oxygen can reduce brain damage. However, to be effective, it must be started as soon as possible. Do not wait until the patient becomes cyanotic. Continue to assist ventilations and administer supplemental oxygen until the patient reaches the hospital.

Circulation. If the heart is not beating, providing airway maintenance, ventilation, and oxygen accomplishes nothing. You must also begin CPR if the patient is in cardiac arrest.

Active blood loss aggravates hypoxia by reducing the available number of oxygen-carrying red blood cells. Although they rarely cause shock except in infants and children, scalp lacerations often cause the loss of large volumes of blood, which must be controlled. Bleeding inside the skull may cause intracranial pressure to rise to life-threatening levels, even though the actual volume of blood lost inside the skull is relatively small.

Shock that develops in a patient with a head injury is usually due to hypovolemia caused by bleeding for other injuries. As with other trauma patients, shock in these cases indicates that the situation is critical. Such patients must be transported immediately to a trauma center. Maintain the airway while you protect the patient's cervical spine, ensure adequate ventilation, administer 100% oxygen, control obvious sites of bleeding with direct pressure, place the patient supine on a spine board, keep the patient warm, and provide immediate transport.

If the patient has a medical condition or nontraumatic injury along with the head injury, place him or her on the left side to prevent aspiration if the patient happens to vomit. **Be sure to maintain the head in the in-line neutral position, with the cervical collar in place.** You should also have a suctioning unit available.

Immobilization Devices

An injured spine is often very difficult to evaluate in a patient with a head injury. Sometimes, there is no neurologic loss. Pain in the spine may be missed because of shock or because the patient's attention is directed to more painful injuries. Evaluation is even more difficult if the patient is unconscious. Because any manipulation of the unstable cervical spine may cause permanent damage to the spinal cord, you must assume the presence of spinal injury in all patients who have sustained head injuries. Use manual in-line immobilization or a cervical collar and long backboard.

Cervical collars. Rigid cervical immobilization devices, or cervical collars, provide preliminary, partial support. A cervical collar should be applied to every patient who has a possible spinal injury, based on

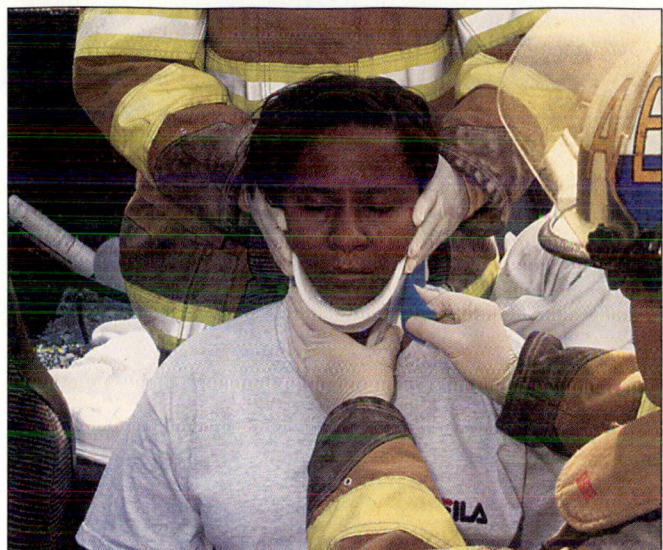

FIGURE 32-24 Proper fit is essential in applying a cervical collar. The collar should rest on the shoulder girdle and provide firm support under both sides of the mandible without obstructing the airway or any ventilation efforts.

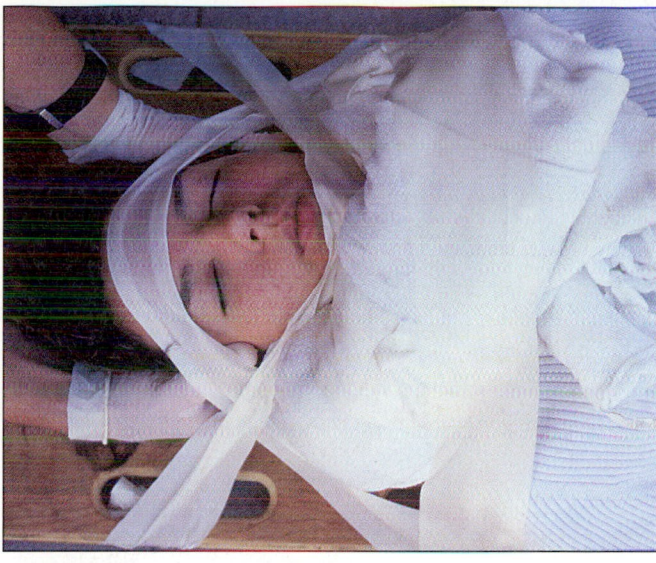

FIGURE 32-25 If you do not have an appropriately sized cervical collar, you may use a rolled towel. Tape it to the backboard around the patient's head, and provide continuous manual support.

mechanism of injury, history, or signs and symptoms. Keep in mind, however, that cervical collars do not fully immobilize the cervical spine. Therefore, you must maintain manual support until the patient is completely secured to a spinal immobilization device, such as a long or a short backboard.

To be effective, a rigid cervical collar must be the correct size for the patient. It should rest on the shoulder girdle and provide firm support under both sides of the mandible, without obstructing the airway or ventilation efforts in any way (Figure 32-24). Either you or your partner should apply the collar while the other provides continuous manual in-line support of the head. It is essential that the cervical collar fits properly. An improperly sized immobilization device has a potential for further injury. If you do not have the correct size, use a rolled towel; tape it to the backboard around the patient's head, and provide continuous manual support (Figure 32-25).

Short backboards. There are several types of short board immobilization devices. The most common are the vest-type device and the rigid short board (Figure 32-26). These devices are designed to stabilize and immobilize the head, neck, and torso. They are used to immobilize noncritical patients who are found in a sitting position and have possible spinal injuries.

As was described earlier in this chapter, the first step in securing a patient to a short board or device is to provide manual, in-line support of the cervical spine. Assess the pulse, motor function, and sensation in all

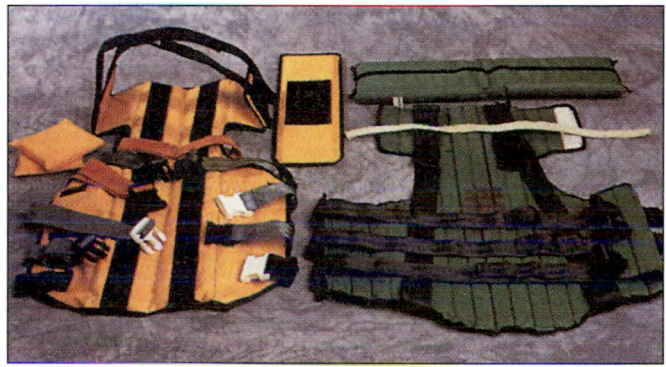

FIGURE 32-26 The most common types of short board immobilization devices are vest type devices.

extremities, and then assess the cervical area. Then apply an appropriately sized cervical collar.

Position the device behind the patient, and secure it to the torso. Evaluate how well the torso and groin are secured, and make adjustments as necessary. Avoid excessive movement of the patient. Next, evaluate the position of the patient's head. Pad behind the head as needed to maintain neutral, in-line immobilization.

Now secure the patient's head to the device. Once you have done that, you may release manual support of the head. Rotate or lift the patient to the long backboard. At this point, you must reassess the pulses, motor function, and sensation in all four extremities to determine whether the change in position has affected the patient's vital signs or neurologic status. Finally, you should immobilize the patient to the long backboard.

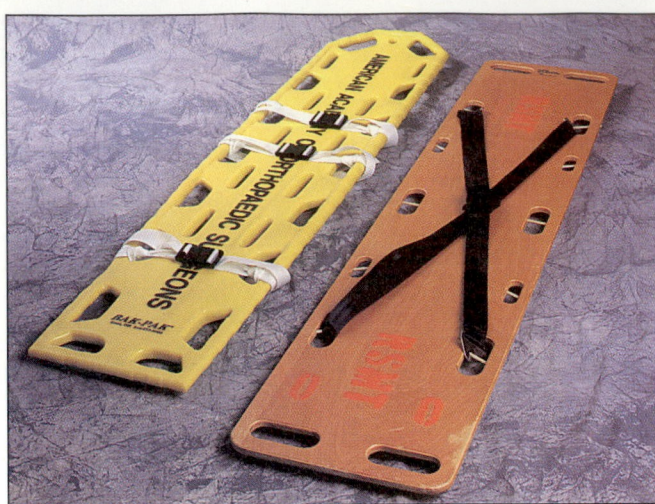

FIGURE 32-27 Long board immobilization devices provide full body spinal immobilization, including stabilization of the head, neck and torso, pelvis, and extremities.

Long backboards. There are several types of long board immobilization devices that provide full body spinal immobilization (Figure 32-27). They also provide stabilization and immobilization to the head, neck and torso, pelvis, and extremities. Long backboards are used to immobilize patients who are found in any position (standing, sitting, supine), sometimes in conjunction with short backboards.

Securing a patient to a long board was described in detail earlier in this chapter. Briefly, you should begin by providing manual, in-line support of the head. Assess pulse, motor function, and sensation in all extremities, and assess the cervical area. Then apply an appropriately sized cervical collar, and proceed as follows:

1. **Position the device.**

2. **Log roll the patient onto the device.** You may also move the patient onto the device by suitable lift or slide or by scoop stretcher. As you maintain in-line support, your partner should kneel by the patient's head and direct the other two EMT-Bs as you roll the patient. Your partner's job is to make sure that the head, torso, and pelvis move as a unit. As the patient's back comes into view, quickly assess its condition if you did not do so during initial assessment. One EMT-B should position the device under the patient. Then, at your partner's command, roll the patient onto the board.

3. **If there are spaces** between the patient's head and torso and the board, fill them with pads. In an adult, these spaces are usually under the head and torso. In a child, place padding from the shoulders to the toes to establish a neutral position.

4. **Secure the torso to the device** by applying straps across the chest and pelvis. Adjust these straps as needed. Then secure the patient's head to the board and, lastly, the legs, above and below the knees.

5. **Reassess pulse,** motor function, and sensation in all extremities.

6. **When the patient is properly secured,** you can safely lift the board or turn it on its side, if necessary.

Helmet Removal

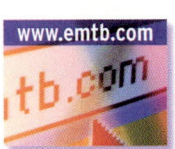

As you plan your care of a patient wearing a helmet, ask yourself the following questions:

- Is the patient's airway clear?
- Is the patient breathing adequately?
- Can you maintain the airway and assist ventilations if the helmet remains in place?
- How well does the helmet fit?
- Can the patient move within the helmet?
- Can the spine be immobilized in a neutral position with the helmet on?

A helmet that fits well prevents the patient's head from moving and should be left on, as long as (1) there are no impending airway or breathing problems, (2) it does not interfere with assessment and treatment of airway or ventilation problems, and (3) you can properly immobilize the spine. You should also leave the helmet on if there is any chance that removing it will further injure the patient.

Remove a helmet if (1) it makes assessing or managing airway problems difficult, (2) it prevents you from properly immobilizing the spine, or (3) it allows excessive head movement. Finally, always remove a helmet from a patient who is in cardiac arrest.

Sports helmets are typically open in the front and may or may not include an attached face mask. The mask can be removed without affecting helmet position or function by simply removing or cutting the straps that hold it to the helmet. In this way, sports helmets allow easy access to the airway (Figure 32-28). Motorcycle helmets often have a shield covering the face. This, too, can be unbuckled to allow access to the airway (Figure 32-29). If a shield cannot be removed, then the helmet must be removed.

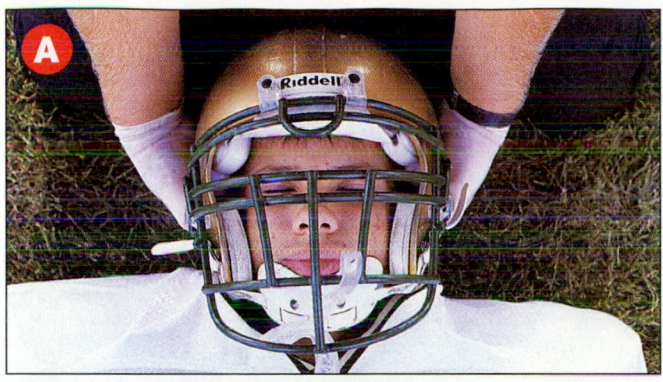

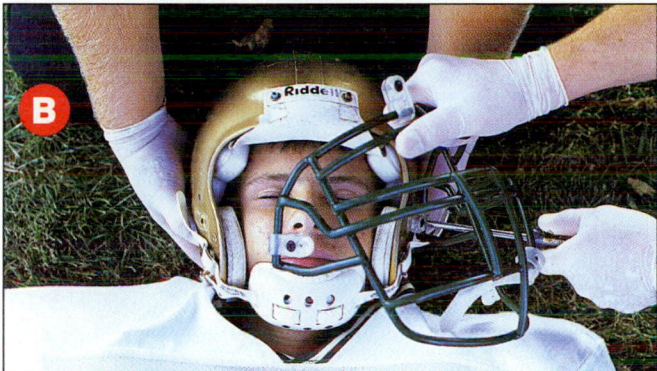

FIGURE 32-28 Removing the mask on a sports helmet can be done without affecting helmet position or function. **A:** Stabilize the neck in a neutral, in-line position. **B:** Remove or cut the straps that hold the mask to the helmet to access the airway.

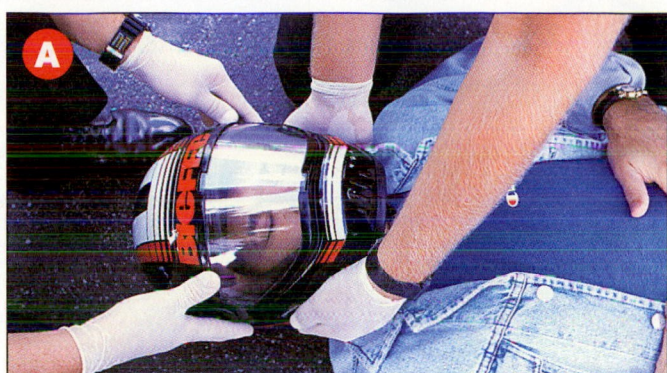

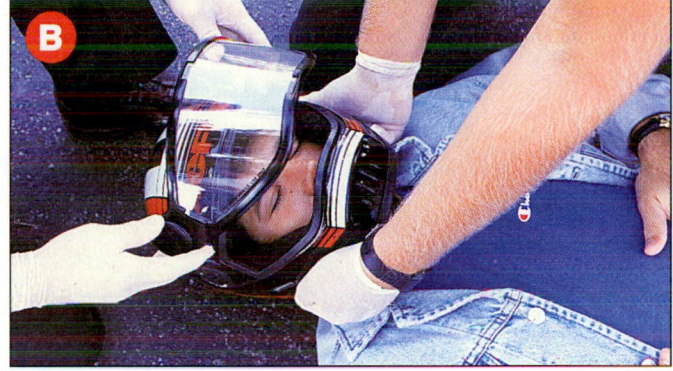

FIGURE 32-29 Motorcycle helmets often have a shield covering the face that can be removed. **A:** Stabilize the neck in a neutral, in-line position. **B:** Unbuckle or snap off the face shield to access the airway.

Preferred Method

Removing a helmet is at least a two-person job; however, the technique for helmet removal depends on the actual type of helmet worn by the patient. One EMT-B provides constant in-line support as the other moves; you and your partner should not move at the same time. You should first consult with medical control, if possible, about your decision to remove a helmet. Then proceed as follows (Figure 32-30 on the next page):

1. **Begin by kneeling down** at the patient's head. Your partner should kneel on one side of the patient, at the shoulder area.

2. **Open the face shield,** if there is one, and assess the patient's airway and breathing. Remove eyeglasses if the patient is wearing them.

3. **Stabilize the helmet** by placing your hands on either side of it, with your fingers on the patient's lower jaw to prevent movement of the head. Once your hands are in position, your partner can loosen the face strap.

4. **Once the strap is loosened,** your partner should place one hand on the patient's lower jaw at the angle of the jaw and the other behind the head at the occipital region. Once your partner's hands are

in position, you may pull the sides of the helmet away from the patient's head.

5. **Gently slip the helmet** halfway off the patient's head, stopping when the helmet reaches the halfway point.

6. **Your partner then slides** his or her hand from the occiput to the back of the head. This will prevent the head from snapping back once the helmet is completely removed.

7. With your partner's hand in place, **remove the helmet,** and immobilize the cervical spine.

8. **Apply the cervical collar,** and then secure the patient to the backboard.

9. **With large helmets** or small patients, you may need to pad under the shoulders. This will prevent flexion of the neck. If shoulder pads or a heavy jacket is in place, you may need to pad behind the patient's head to prevent extension of the neck.

Remember, you do not need to remove a helmet if you can access the patient's airway, if the head is snug inside the helmet, and if the helmet can be secured to an immobilization device.

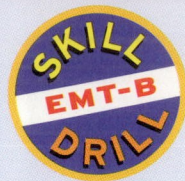

Removing a Helmet
Figure 32-30

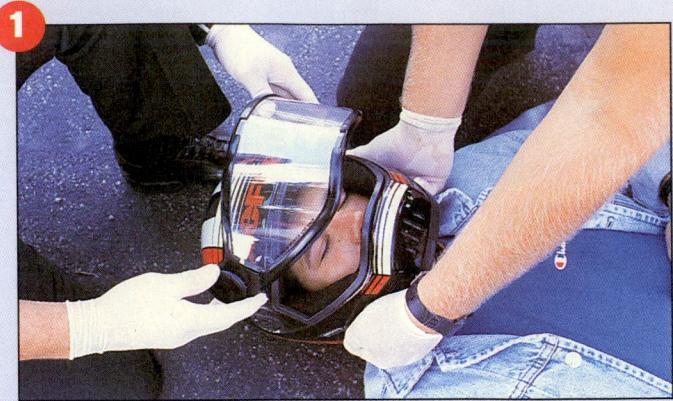

Kneel down at the patient's head, and open the face shield so that you can assess the airway and breathing. Remove eyeglasses if the patient is wearing them.

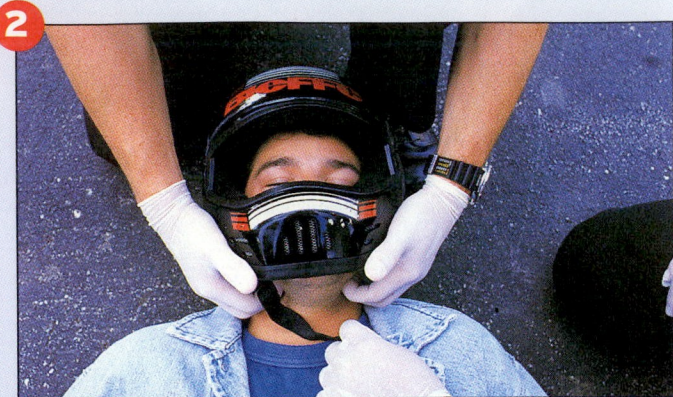

Stabilize the helmet by placing your hands on either side of it, ensuring that your fingers are on the patient's lower jaw to prevent movement of the head. Your partner can then loosen the strap.

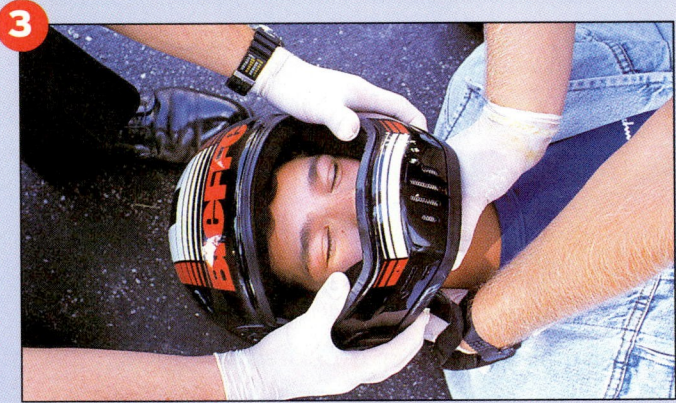

After the strap is loosened, your partner should place one hand on the patient's lower jaw and the other behind the head at the occiput.

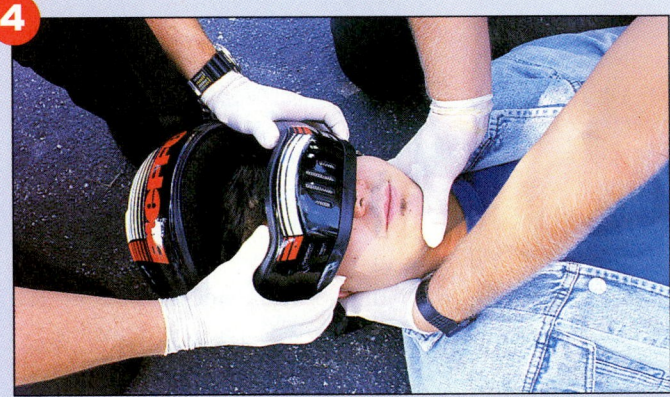

Once your partner's hands are in position, gently slip the helmet off about halfway, and then stop.

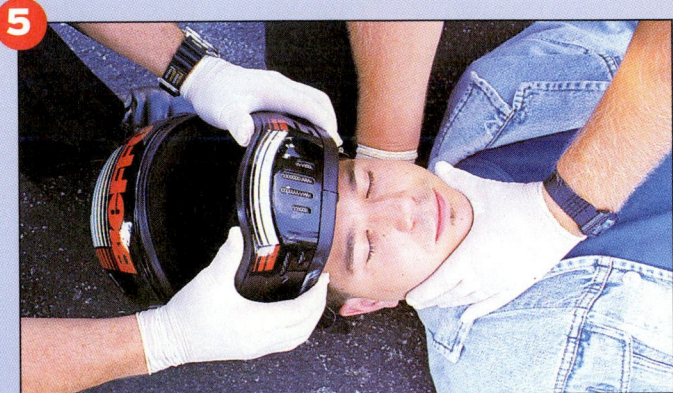

Have your partner slide his or her hand from the occiput to the back of the head to prevent the head from snapping back once the helmet is removed.

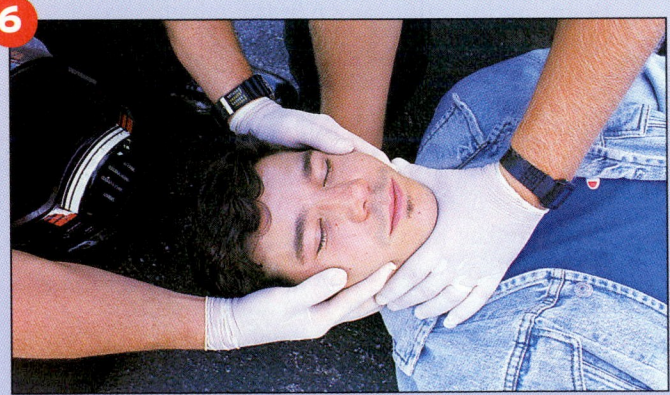

With your partner's hand in place, remove the helmet, and stabilize the cervical spine. Apply a cervical collar, and then secure the patient to a long backboard. NOTE: With large helmets or small patients, you may need to pad under the shoulders.

Alternate Method

An alternate method for removal of football helmets is possible. The advantage of this method is that it allows the helmet to be removed with less force applied, therefore causing less possibility of motion at the neck. The disadvantage of this method is that it is slightly more time consuming (Figure 32-31). The first step involves removal of the chinstrap. This can be cut or unsnapped carefully. Be careful during removal of the chinstrap to avoid jarring the neck or head and causing excessive motion. Next, remove the face mask. The face mask is anchored to the helmet by plastic clips secured with screws. These can removed with a screwdriver or, alternately, cut with a knife. After the face mask has been removed, the jaw pads can be popped out of place. This can be accomplished with the use of a tongue depressor. The fingers can be placed inside the helmet allowing greater control of the helmet during removal. If the shoulder pads are in place, appropriate padding must be applied behind the head to prevent hyperextension. Just as with the previously described method, the person over the patient's chest is responsible for making sure that the head and neck do not move during removal of the helmet.

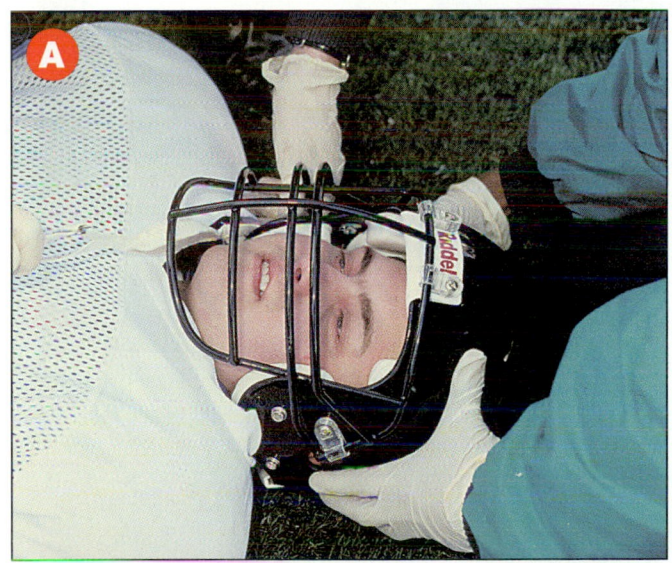
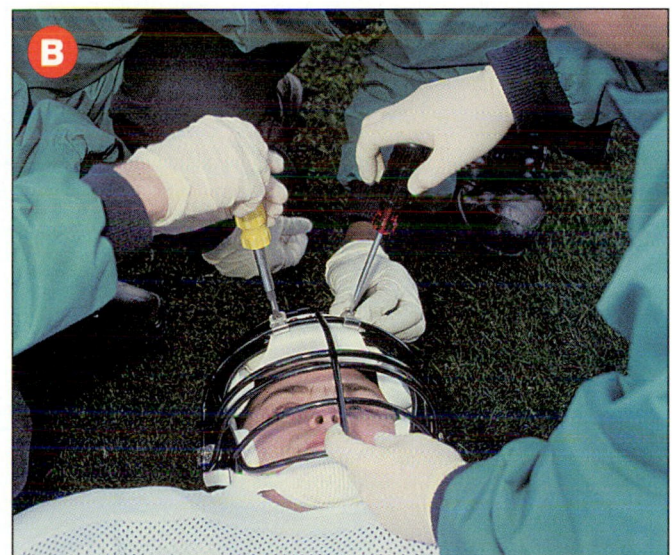
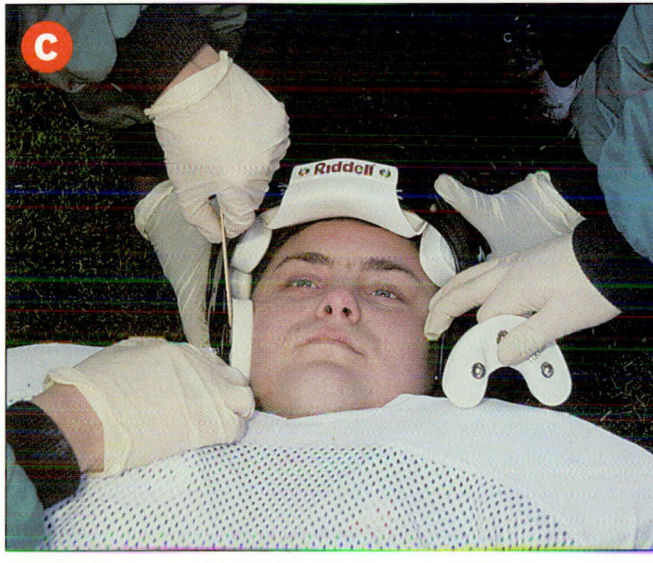
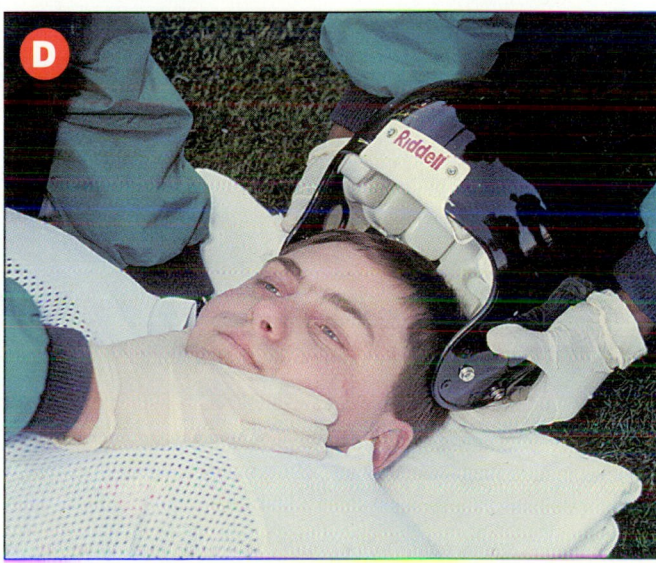

FIGURE 32-31 A: The chinstrap is removed first. Be careful when unsnapping the strap to avoid a jarring motion of the head and neck. **B:** The face mask can be removed from the helmet by releasing the clips that hold it in place. This is done with screwdrivers. **C:** The jaw pads can be removed from the inside of the helmet with the aid of a tongue depressor. **D:** The fingers can be placed inside the helmet allowing the helmet to be gently rocked out of place. The person at the foot of the patient controls the head by controlling the jaw with one hand and the occiput with the other. Padding is inserted behind the occiput to prevent neck extension.

caring for kids

You are likely to find infants and children who have been in automobile crashes still in their car seats. Your best course of action is to immobilize the child in the car seat if possible. Whenever you apply a cervical collar, make sure it is properly sized. If a properly fitting collar is not available, use a rolled towel and tape it to the car seat. Pad the sides of the car seat, if necessary, to prevent lateral movement (Figure 32-32), and place additional padding in any spaces between the patient and the car seat. If the child is not in a car seat or was removed before your arrival, use an appropriately sized immobilization device. If the cervical immobilization device does not fit, use a rolled towel, and tape it to the board and manually support the head.

Remember that small children may require additional padding to maintain the in-line neutral position. Children are not small adults. They have smaller airways, so padding is important to maintain the airway. Pad under the shoulders to the toes, as needed, to avoid excessive neck flexion (Figure 32-33). In addition, place blanket rolls between the child and the sides of an adult-sized board to prevent the child from slipping to one side or the other (Figure 32-34). Appropriately sized backboards are available for children.

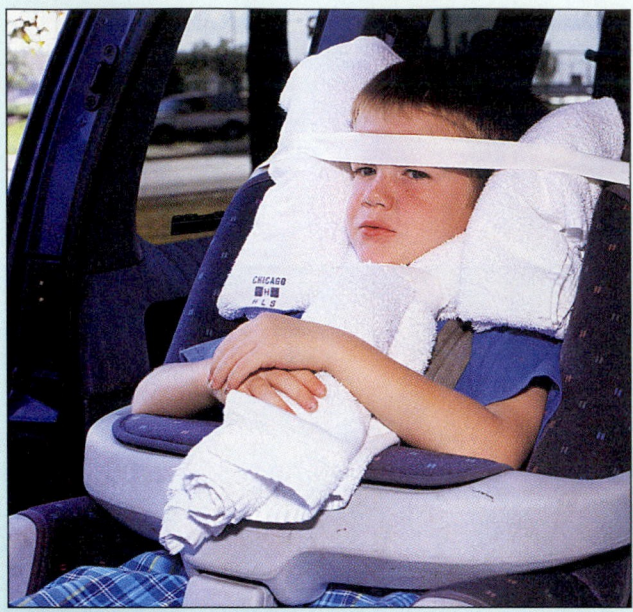

FIGURE 32-32 If you do not have an appropriately sized cervical collar for a child, you may use a rolled towel and tape it to the car seat. Pad the sides of the car seat, if needed, to prevent lateral movement.

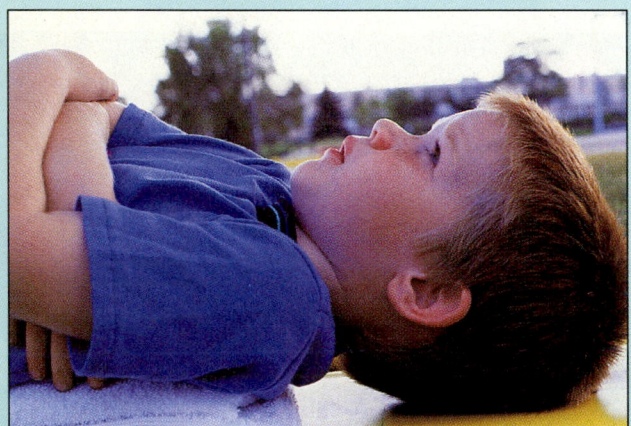

FIGURE 32-33 Children have proportionately larger heads than adults, so you may need to place padding under the shoulders to avoid excessive flexion of the head.

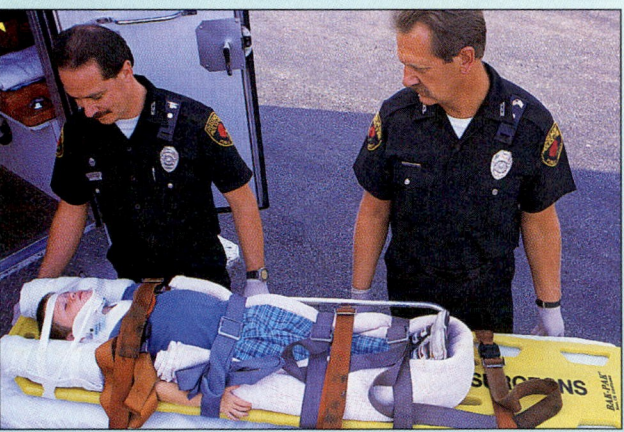

FIGURE 32-34 Place blanket rolls between the child and the sides of an adult-sized board to prevent the child from slipping to one side or the other.

prep kit

ready for review

The nervous system is divided into two parts: the central nervous system and the peripheral nervous system. The central nervous system consists of the brain and the spinal cord. The cables of nerve fibers linking nerve cells in the brain and spinal cord to the body's organs make up the peripheral nervous system. In addition to the skull and spinal canal, the central nervous system is protected by the meninges, three layers of tissue called the dura mater, arachnoid, and pia mater. The peripheral nervous system consists of 31 pairs of spinal nerves, which conduct sensory impulses from the skin and other organs to the spinal cord and conduct motor impulses from the spinal cord to the muscles, and 12 pairs of cranial nerves, which transmit sensations relating to sight, smell, taste, and hearing directly to the brain. The three major types of peripheral nerves are sensory nerves, motor nerves, and connecting nerves.

The part of the nervous system that regulates our voluntary activities is called the somatic or voluntary nervous system. The much more primitive autonomic or involuntary nervous system regulates involuntary body functions. The autonomic nervous system is composed of the sympathetic and parasympathetic nervous systems, which balance each other.

The skull is divided into two large bony structures that protect the brain: the cranium and the face. The spinal column has 33 bones, called vertebrae, in five sections: cervical, thoracic or dorsal, lumbar, sacral, and coccygeal.

The cervical, thoracic, and lumbar portions of the spine can be injured through compression resulting from a fall; through unnatural motions such as overextension caused by motor vehicle crashes and other types of trauma; and through distraction (pulling) along the length of the spine, as in hanging. Start your assessment of a patient with a possible spinal injury by focusing on ABCD and, if he or she is responsive, by asking five questions: Does your neck or back hurt? What happened? Where does it hurt? Can you move your hands and feet? Can you feel me touching your fingers and toes? Look for contusions, punctures, or skull deformities; test for strength in the extremities; ask about pain; and check for numbness, weakness, or tingling in the extremities. Patients with severe spinal injury may lose sensation or be paralyzed below the suspected injury.

Keep the head in a neutral, in-line position while you open and maintain the airway, assess respirations, and give supplemental oxygen. Provide manual immobilization until the patient is properly secured to a backboard. A patient who is supine can be immobilized with a long backboard, using the four-person log roll. With sitting patients, you should use a short backboard, then secure the short board to a long board. If the patient is standing, immobilize him or her to a long backboard before starting your assessment; this requires three EMT-Bs.

Common head injuries include skull wounds (scalp lacerations and skull fracture) and brain injuries (concussion, contusion, intracranial bleeding), typically caused by direct blows, car crashes, falls from heights, assault, and sports injuries. Cerebral edema, seizures, vomiting, and leakage of cerebrospinal fluid are common complications of both open and closed head injuries. Common signs and symptoms of head injuries include lacerations, visible deformities of the skull, ecchymosis about the eyes or behind the ear, unequal pupil size and failure of the pupils to respond to light, loss of sensation and/or motor function, visual complaints, and irregular respirations.

The single most important observation that you can make in assessing a brain injury is of change in the level of consciousness. Use the AVPU scale or the Glasgow Coma Scale to assess consciousness immediately and every 15 minutes for a stable patient and 5 minutes for an unstable patient, recording scores and times as you do so. Also monitor pupil size and reactions.

Patients with head injuries often have injuries to the cervical spine as well. Therefore, when treating a patient with a head injury, you must protect and stabilize the cervical spine at all times. Three principles govern treatment of head injuries: airway, ventilation, and high-flow supplemental oxygen; bleeding and circulation; and assessing/monitoring level of consciousness.

Immobilization devices include cervical collars, which must be the correct size; short backboards, including vest-type devices and rigid short boards; and long backboards.

A helmet that fits well prevents the patient's head from moving and should be left on, as long as it does not interfere with assessment/treatment of airway or ventilation problems and you can properly immobilize the spine. Remove a helmet if it makes assessing or managing airway problems difficult, prevents you from immobilizing the spine, or allows excessive head movement. Never remove a helmet if doing so will further injure the patient. Always remove a helmet if the patient is in cardiac arrest.

prep kit

vital vocabulary

www.emtb.com

anterograde (posttraumatic) amnesia   Inability to remember events after an injury.

autonomic (involuntary) nervous system   The part of the nervous system that regulates functions, such as digestion and sweating, that are not controlled by conscious will.

brain stem   The part of the central nervous system that controls virtually all functions that are necessary for life, including the cardiac and respiratory systems.

central nervous system (CNS)   The brain and spinal cord.

cerebellum   The part of the brain that coordinates body movements.

cerebral edema   Swelling of the brain.

cerebrum   The largest part of the brain, containing about 75% of the brain's total volume.

closed head injury   Injury usually associated with trauma in which the brain has been injured but the skin has not been broken and there is no obvious bleeding.

connecting nerves   Nerves that connect the motor and sensory nerves.

distracted   The action of pulling the spine along its length.

eyes forward position   A position in which the head is gently lifted until the patient's eyes are looking straight ahead and the head and torso are in line.

four-person log roll   The recommended procedure for moving a patient with a suspected spinal injury from the ground to a long spine board.

intervertebral disk   A cushion that lies between the vertebrae.

involuntary activity   The actions that we do not consciously control.

meninges   Three distinct layers of tissue that surround and protect the brain and the spinal cord within the skull and the spinal canal.

motor nerves   Nerves that carry information from the central nervous system to the muscles.

open head injury   Injury to the head often caused by a penetrating object in which there may be bleeding and exposed brain tissue.

peripheral nervous system   Thirty-one pairs of spinal nerves and 12 pairs of cranial nerves.

retrograde amnesia   The inability to remember events leading up to a head injury.

sensory nerves   Nerves that transmit sensory input, such as touch, taste, heat, cold, and pain, from the body to the central nervous system.

somatic (voluntary) nervous system   The part of the nervous system that regulates our voluntary activities, such as walking, talking, and writing.

voluntary activity   Actions that we consciously perform, in which sensory input determines the specific muscular activity.

assessment in action

On the first nice weekend of April, two young men take their mountain bikes to the Elk Ridge trails. With taunts as to who is "King of the Mountain," they race off down the trail. One of the cyclists loses control of his bike and crashes into the underbrush. He is launched over the handlebars and lands on the ground, shaken and confused. His friend quickly rides back to the ranger station to call 9-1-1.

You and your partner arrive to find a 17-year-old man still down the trail. He is wearing shorts, sandals, and sunglasses but no helmet. The patient responds to pain when you move his arms or legs. He has a blood pressure of 166/98 mm Hg, a regular pulse of 60 beats/min, and irregular respirations of 28 breaths/min. Additional examination shows a slightly angulated fracture of the left tibia and multiple abrasions over his entire body.

1. Based on the patient's presenting signs and symptoms, what is the most life-threatening condition?
   A. Fractured tibia
   B. Multiple abrasions
   C. Possible spinal cord injury
   D. Increasing intracranial pressure

2. In preparation for transport, you must secure the patient to a long spine board. What is the proper strapping sequence?
   A. Head first, then torso, and the legs last
   B. Torso first, then the legs, and the head last
   C. Legs first, then the head, and the torso last
   D. The sequence for strapping is unimportant.

3. Whenever possible, in what position should you immobilize a patient's head and cervical spine?
   A. Slight flexion
   B. Moderate extension
   C. Moderate flexion
   D. Neutral

4. Just as you finish securing the patient to the long spine board, he starts to retch in preparation for vomiting. You should immediately:
   A. leave him supine but prepare to suction the airway.
   B. remove all the straps and roll him over onto his stomach.
   C. keep the patient strapped to the board and turn him on his side.
   D. remove the head strap and turn the patient's head to the side.

5. En route, you notice a watery, blood-tinged fluid leaking from the patient's nose. You should respond by:
   A. placing loose sterile dressings over the area.
   B. applying direct pressure with sterile dressings.
   C. packing the nostrils and applying direct pressure.
   D. packing the nostrils with tight, sterile dressings.

points to ponder

Object. 1-6.2, 3-2.5, 5-4.4, 5-4.5, 5-4.9

You find a patient at an automobile accident on the floor in front of the front seat, curled under the dashboard. The patient is conscious and complaining of pain in his abdomen, neck, and left ankle. He also explains that every time he moves his head, a burning pain shoots down his back. The patient is able to move his fingers and toes, except right after the shooting pain. The patient now begins to complain of nausea. Within a couple minutes of complaining of nausea, the patient begins vomiting.

• Would you move this patient? Why or why not? When would you move the patient? How would you move him?

online outlook

Bleeding from a lacerated or torn brain vessel compresses the brain tissue, resulting in a loss of brain function. Review your knowledge of intracranial hematomas by completing Exercise 32 at www.emtb.com.

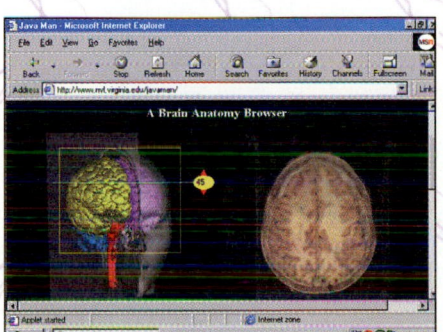

Infants
and Children

J.J. Tepas, III, MD, and James S. Seidel, MD, PhD

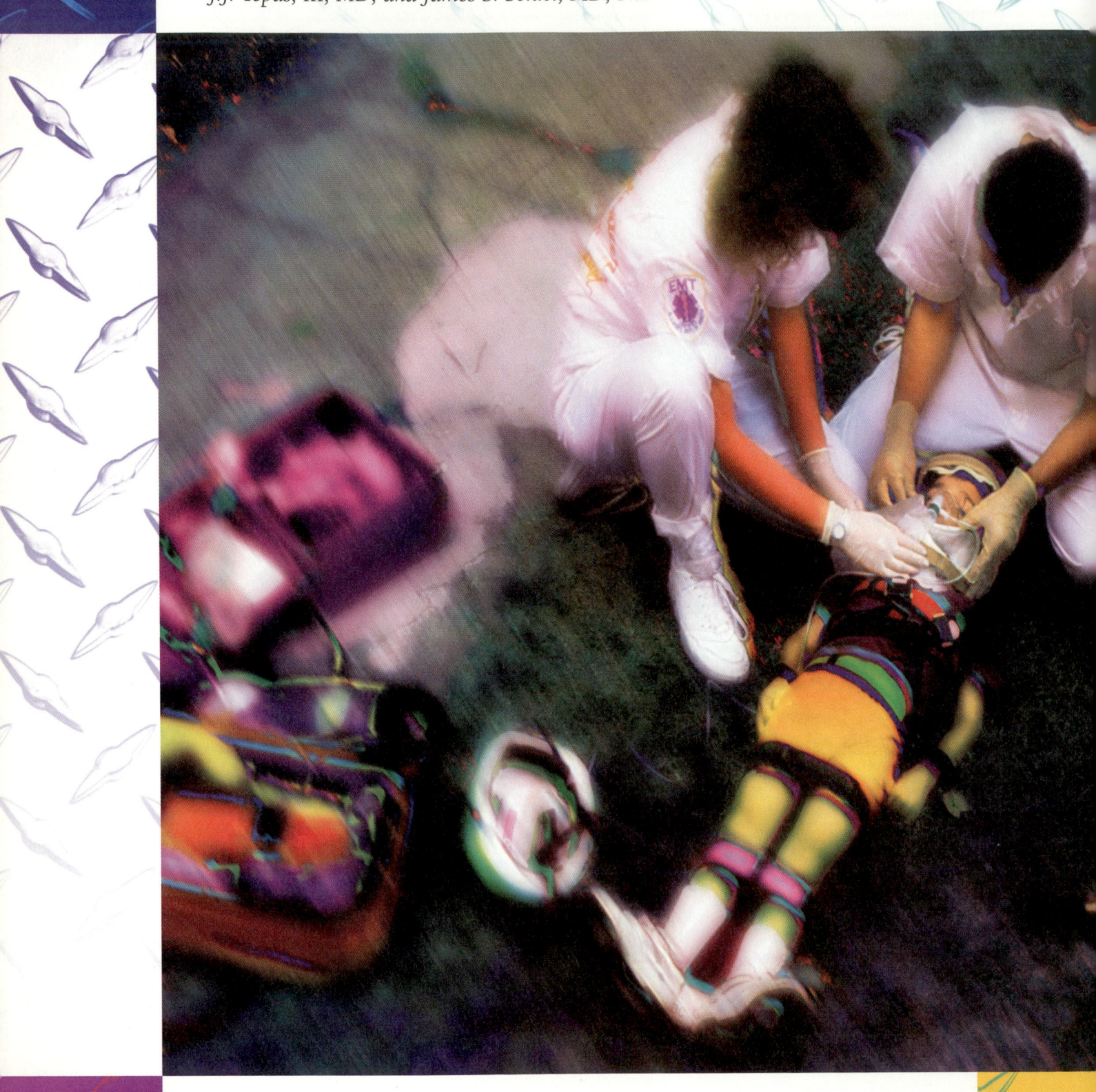

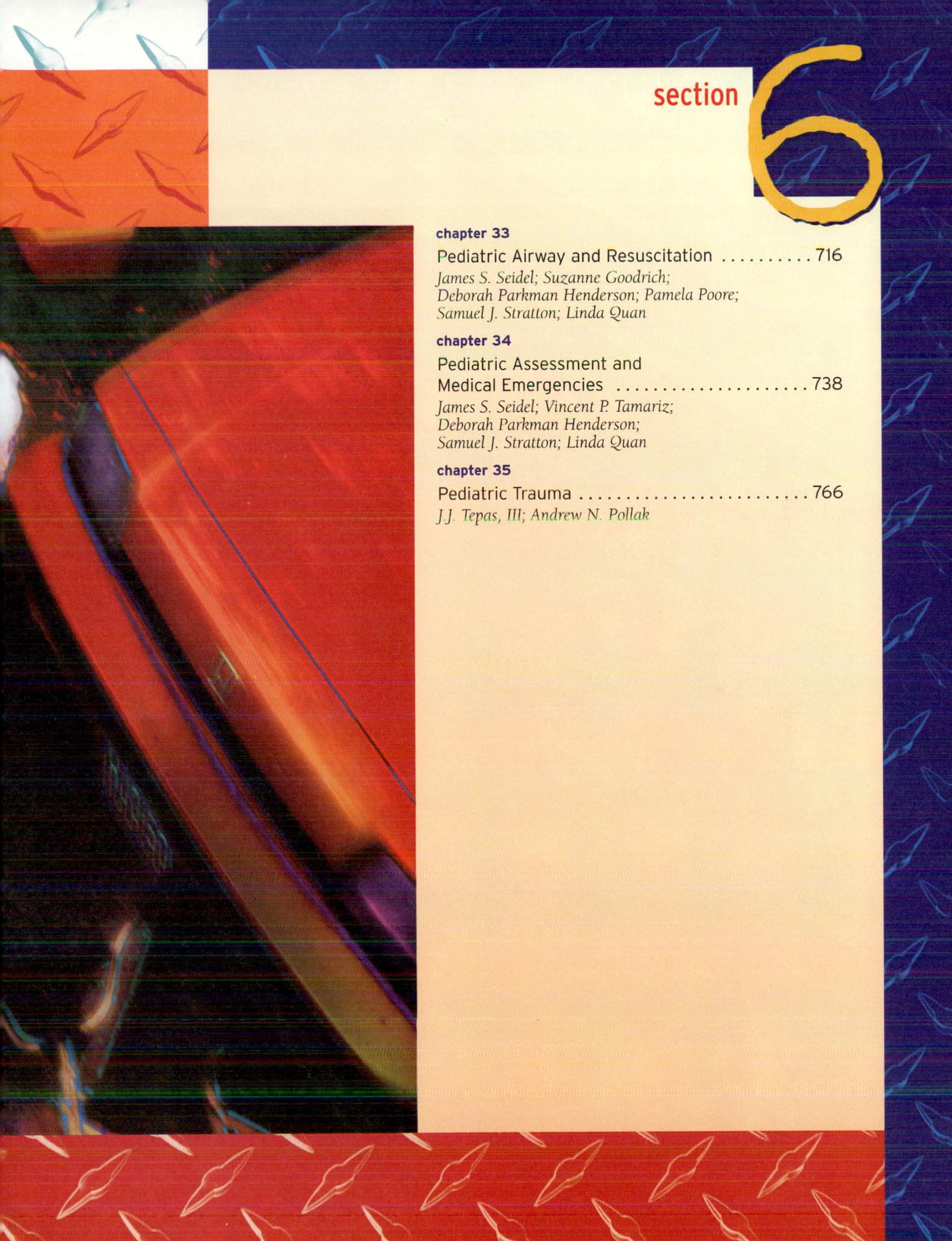

Pediatric Airway and Resuscitation

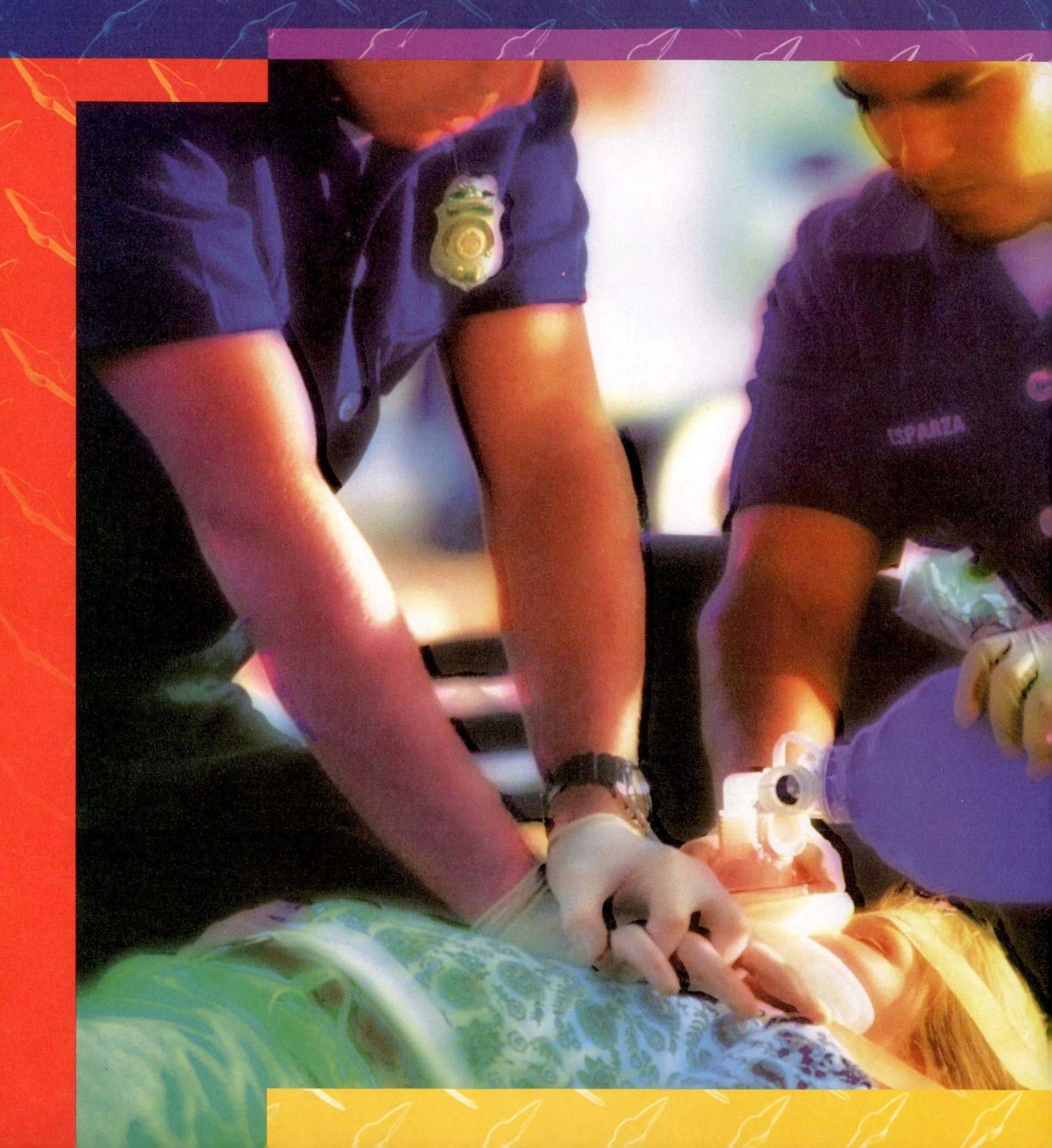

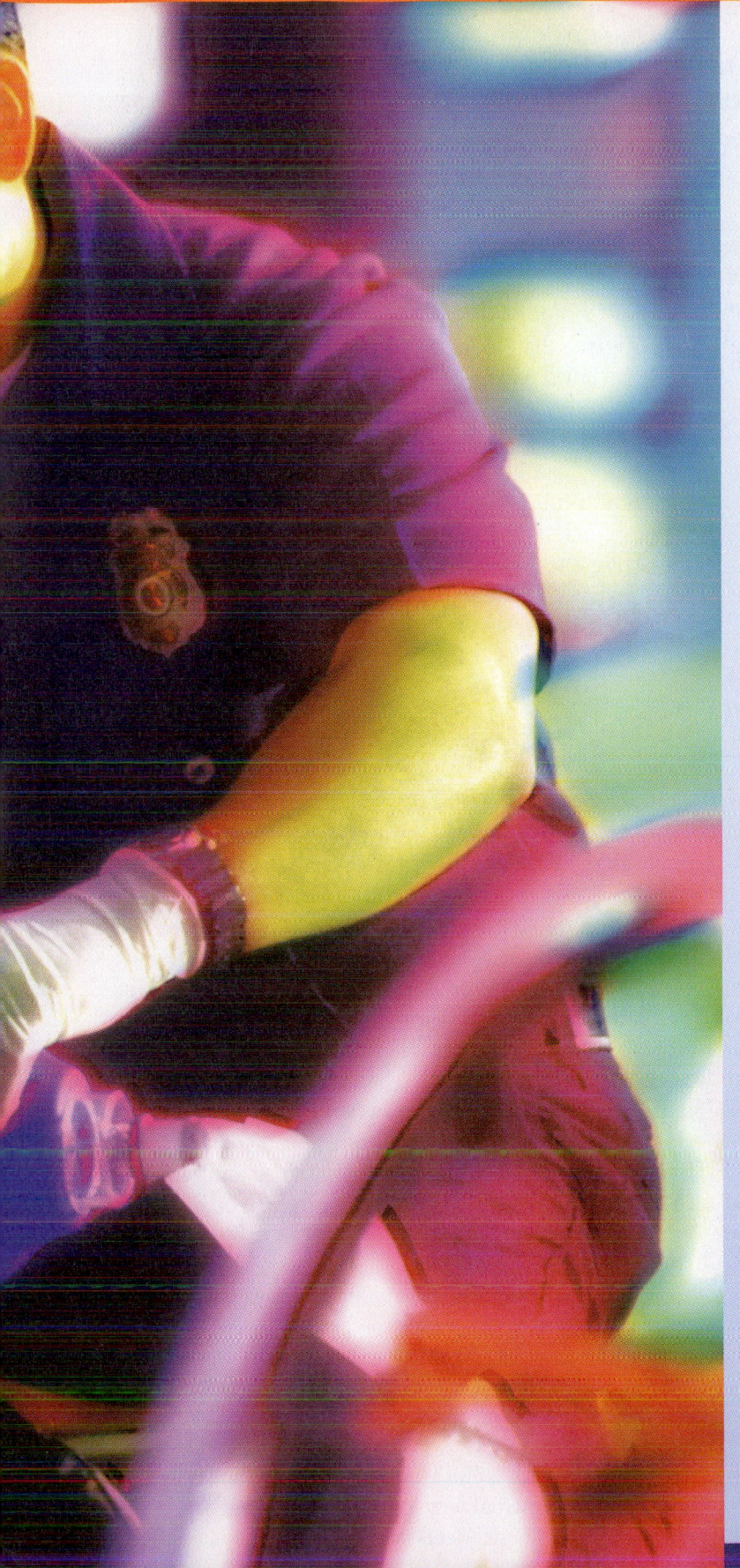

objectives

Cognitive

1. Describe differences in anatomy and physiology of the infant, child and adult patient.

2. Identify the usual cause of cardiac arrest in infants and children versus adults.

3. Describe the steps in positioning an infant and/or child to maintain an open airway.

4. Summarize neonatal resuscitation procedures.

Affective

5. Explain the rationale for having knowledge and skills appropriate for dealing with the infant and child patient.

6. Attend to the feelings of the family when dealing with an ill or injured infant or child.

Psychomotor

7. Demonstrate neonatal resuscitation techniques.

8. Demonstrate bag-valve-mask artificial ventilations for the infant.

9. Demonstrate bag-valve-mask artificial ventilations for the child.

10. Demonstrate oxygen delivery for the infant and child.

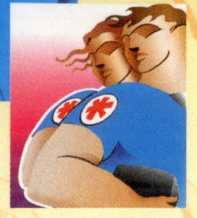

you are the emt

Squad 8, respond to the fair on County Road K57 for a child in the livestock barn having difficulty breathing. Your partner looks at you and says, "You handle this call. I don't do well with kids!" You reply, "Well, neither do I!" Now what should you do?

Of all the calls that EMS professionals handle, the most difficult are often those involving pediatric patients. This chapter will introduce you to the first component of pediatric care: airway management and resuscitation. It will also help you to answer the following questions:

1. Why is it beneficial to carry written reference material on the unit that lists normal values for vital signs and other aspects of pediatric patient care?

2. Is it true that pediatric patients are nothing more than small adults?

Pediatric Airway and Resuscitation

EMTs who are cool and calm when caring for adults often find themselves anxious when dealing with critically ill or injured infants or children. However, treatment of children is often the same as that of adults in most emergency situations. Once you understand the differences in anatomy between children and adults and learn to recognize signs of respiratory distress in children, you will find it easier to approach even the smallest patients in a professional manner.

Because a young child might not be able to speak, your assessment of his or her condition must be based in large part on what you can see and hear. In addition, families may be helpful in providing vital information about an accident or illness. You should think of families as part of the caregiving team and, whenever possible, include them in all decisions about care and transportation.

There are many causes of respiratory distress and failure in children. Although you might not be able to identify the exact cause in every patient, you must be able to intervene appropriately to restore breathing in all of them. Ensuring adequate oxygenation and ventilation will help to achieve the best possible outcome for the patient, regardless of the underlying problem.

This chapter begins by identifying the major anatomic differences, particularly at the airway, between adults and children that have a bearing on your work. It then offers some general guidelines for assessing children, including how to obtain and interpret vital signs. A discussion of how to open and maintain the airway in

infants and children follows, including placement of airway adjuncts and the use of oxygen delivery devices, including the bag-valve-mask (BVM) device. After a brief review of neonatal resuscitation, the chapter concludes with a review of BLS techniques for infants and children.

Caring for Pediatric Patients

Children have many unique health problems. Similarly, many problems that are common in adults do not occur in children. Therefore, there is a separate medical practice devoted to the care of the young, called **pediatrics**.

Handling a sick or injured child can be extremely challenging, and it is almost always a trying experience to care for a child who is seriously ill or injured. Not everyone is comfortable caring for children. In most situations, handling an infant or child means that you must manage the parents as well. Therefore, it is vital that you remain calm and professional when you care for a child (Figure 33-1). Hard as it is, you must keep your personal feelings in check as you work with infants, children, and their families. Despite these challenges, you have an opportunity to make a real difference in the lives of these children and their families.

To effectively manage the pediatric airway, you must first understand the anatomic differences between adults and children. To start with, the heart is higher in a child's chest and the lungs smaller. The opening to the trachea is higher in the neck, and the neck itself is shorter (Figure 33-2).

The anatomy of a child's airway differs from that of an adult in five principal ways. These differences will influence the treatment decisions that you make about pediatric patients, including whether or not intervention is needed and, if so, what procedure to use. The anatomy of a child's airway and other important structures differs from that of an adult's in the following ways:

- A larger, rounder **occiput**, or back of the head, which requires more careful positioning

- A proportionately larger tongue relative to the size of the mouth and a more anterior location in the mouth. The child's tongue is also large relative to the small mandible and can easily block the airway.

- A floppy, U-shaped epiglottis that is larger than an adult's, relative to the size of the airway

- Less well-developed rings of cartilage in the trachea that may easily collapse if the neck is flexed or hyperextended

- A narrower, lower airway

Because of the smaller diameter of the trachea in infants, which has about the same diameter as a drinking straw, their airway is easily obstructed by secretions, blood, or swelling. Also, since intercostal muscles are not well developed in children, movement of the diaphragm, their major muscle of respiration, dictates the amount of air they inspire. Gastric distention can interfere with movement of the diaphragm and lead to hypoventilation.

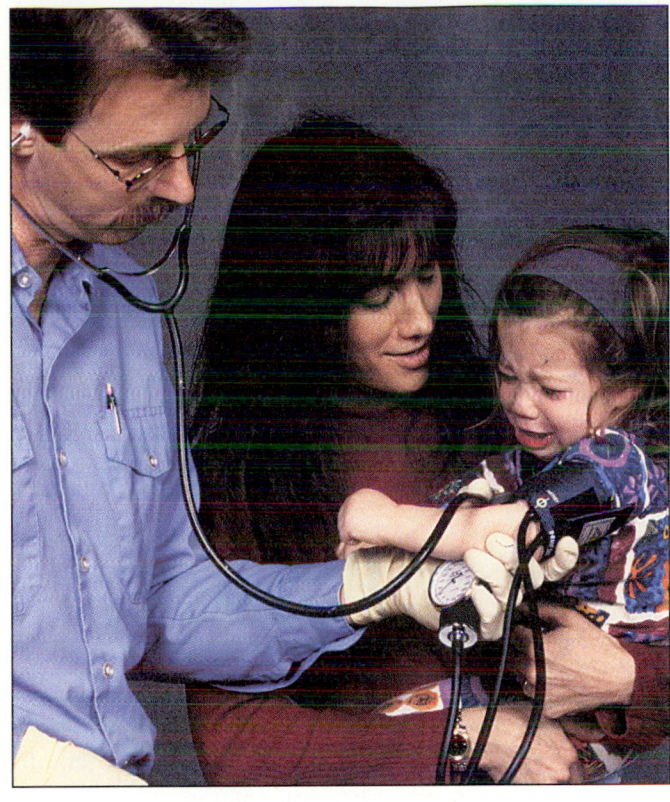

FIGURE 33-1 Handling a sick or injured child can be extremely challenging. A calm, professional demeanor is of utmost importance as you care for both the child and the parents.

FIGURE 33-2 The anatomy of a child's airway differs from that of an adult's in five principal ways: The back of the head is larger in a child, so head positioning requires more care. The tongue is proportionally larger and more anterior in the mouth. The epiglottis is larger. The trachea is smaller in diameter and more flexible. The airway itself is lower and narrower.

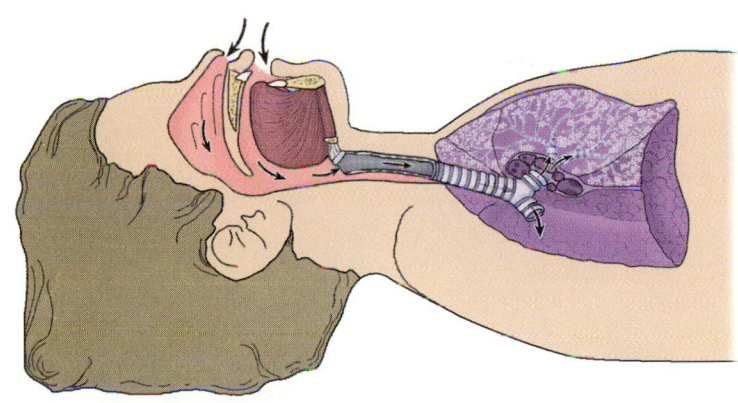

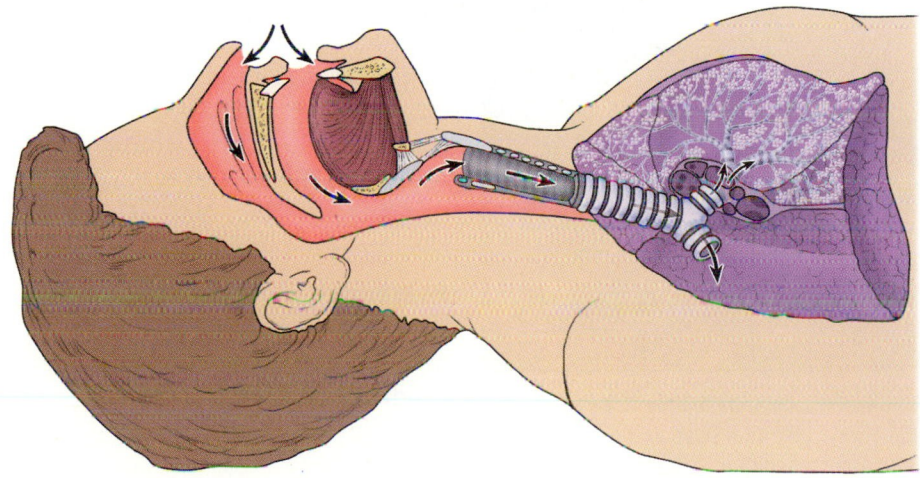

Assessing Pediatric Patients

As an EMT-B, you must be prepared to assess pediatric patients, support their vital functions, and provide transport to a facility that is capable of caring for their special needs. In doing so, you must act rapidly and pay close attention to the three fundamental elements of pediatric emergency care, as follows:

1. **Provide BLS** as needed.
2. **Prevent disability** by stabilizing the spine with a backboard and cervical collar or other restraining devices.
3. **Consult with ALS** when appropriate.

Approach to Assessment

Although each child and situation is unique, you should follow a few basic guidelines when assessing and caring for infants and children. *You should take a child's vital signs in the field because you are the eyes, ears, and hands of medical control.* During your assessment, you should obtain a complete set of baseline vital signs, including respirations, pulse, blood pressure (when possible), skin signs, level of activity, muscle tone, and movement.

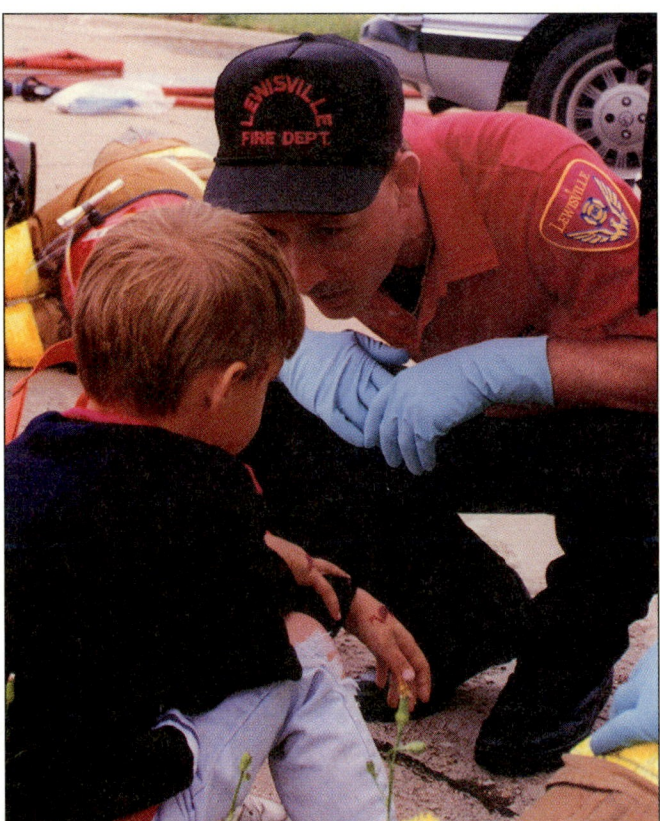

FIGURE 33-3 You are the eyes, ears, and hands of medical control. Therefore, you should always take vital signs in the field. Begin by talking to the child, then assess respirations and pulse.

> You should take a child's vital signs in the field because you are the eyes, ears, and hands of medical control.

You must also decide whether to call for ALS backup or provide immediate transport. This decision is often made with the assistance of either off-line medical direction protocols or on-line medical direction. It is always a good idea to inform the base or receiving hospital about the status of a pediatric patient so that the facility can prepare to meet the child's particular needs. The condition of infants and children may deteriorate rapidly during transport, so you should have pediatric resuscitation equipment ready to use at all times (Table 33-1). Finally, whenever possible, transport infants and children to facilities that are capable of providing the appropriate level of care. Not all community hospitals offer all higher levels of care for children. You may have to bypass closer emergency care facilities to reach a pediatric center. When this is not possible, as in many rural areas, a hospital may arrange for secondary transportation after stabilizing the child's condition.

Vital Signs

Note that normal vital signs in pediatric patients vary with the age of the child (Table 33-2). Remember that your approach to taking vital signs also varies with the age of the child. Be gentle, talk to the child, assess respirations and pulse next, and assess blood pressure last (Figure 33-3). Warm your stethoscope on your hands or a cloth before placing it on the skin. You may also want to let the child hold the equipment or stethoscope before placing it on him or her.

Respirations. Abnormal respirations are a common sign of illness or injury in children. Respirations should be counted for at least 30 seconds. However, do not base your evaluation by counting the number of times the chest rises and falls in infants and children under 3 years of age. Rather, count the rise and fall of the abdomen. This is usually easier to do with the child in the caretaker's lap. Note the effort the child makes in breathing, and listen for noises during respiration.

Pulse. Pulses may be difficult to feel if they are very weak, very fast, or slow (Figure 33-4). In infants, feel over the brachial area or in the femoral area. In older children, use the carotid artery. Count the pulse for at least 1 minute. Note the strength of the pulse: Is it weak or strong?

TABLE 33-1 Pediatric Equipment: Getting the Size Right

The best way to identify the appropriately sized equipment for a pediatric patient is to use a length-based <u>pediatric resuscitation tape measure</u>, which can determine weight as well as height in patients of up to 34 kg (see Figure 33-9). The proper sequence in which to use the tape is as follows:

1. Place the patient supine on a flat surface.
2. Lay the tape next to the patient with the multicolored side up.
3. Place the red end of the tape at the top of the patient's head.
4. Place one hand, side down, on top of the patient's head, covering the red box at the end of the tape.
5. Starting from the patient's head, run the side of your free hand down the tape.
6. Stretch the tape out the full length of the child, stopping at the heel. If the child is longer than the tape, stop here and use the appropriate adult technique.
7. Place your free hand, side down, at the bottom of the child's heel.
8. Note the color or letter block and weight range on the edge of tape where your hand is. Say the color or letter out loud.
9. Select the appropriately sized equipment by matching the color or letter on the tape to the color or letter on the equipment.

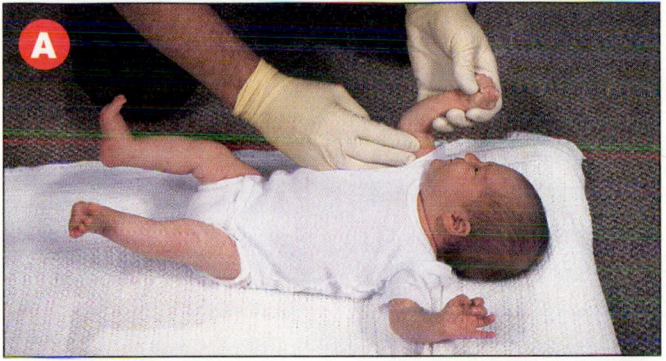

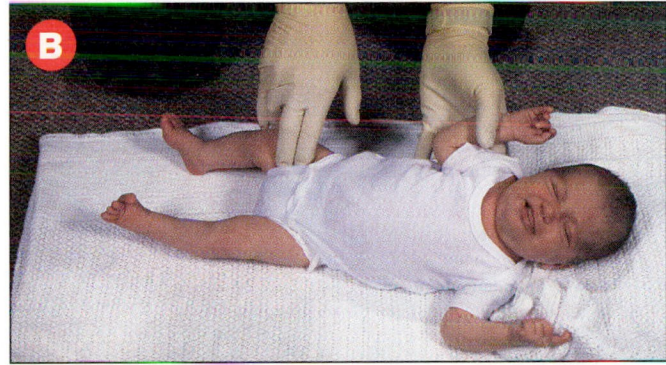

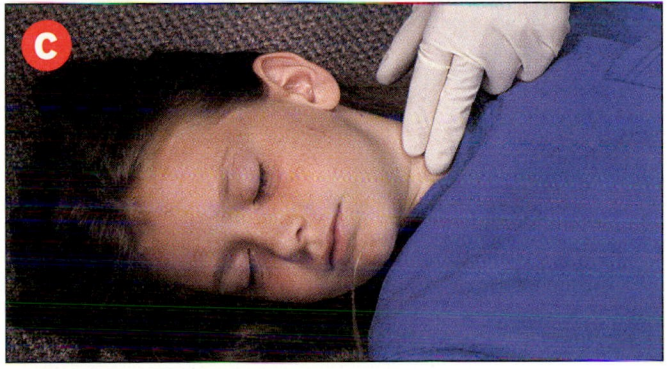

FIGURE 33-4 A: Palpate over the brachial area to assess the pulse of an infant. **B:** Palpate over the femoral area as a second choice. **C:** In older children, use the carotid artery.

TABLE 33-2 Vital Signs by Age

Age	Respirations (breaths/min)	Pulse (beats/min)	Systolic Blood Pressure (mm Hg)
Newborn	30 to 60	100 to 160	50 to 70
1 to 6 weeks	30 to 60	100 to 160	70 to 95
6 months	25 to 40	90 to 120	80 to 100
1 year	20 to 30	90 to 120	80 to 100
3 years	20 to 30	80 to 120	80 to 110
6 years	18 to 25	70 to 110	80 to 110
10 years	15 to 20	60 to 90	90 to 120

Blood pressure. Taking a child's blood pressure in the field can be tricky. To get an accurate reading, you must have a cuff that covers two thirds of the patient's upper arm (Figure 33-5). If conditions at the scene make it impossible to measure blood pressure accurately, do not waste a lot of time trying.

Skin signs. Feel the skin for temperature and moisture at the same time that you measure the other vital signs. Is the skin warm and dry, or cold and clammy? Estimate capillary refill by squeezing the end of a finger or toe for several seconds and then observing the return of blood to the area (Figure 33-6). Color should return in less than 2 seconds.

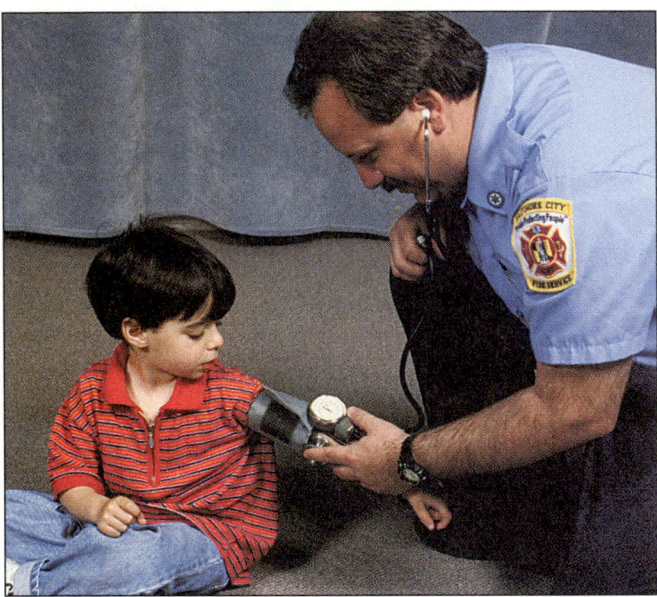

FIGURE 33-5 When taking a child's blood pressure, ensure that the cuff covers two thirds of the patient's upper arm.

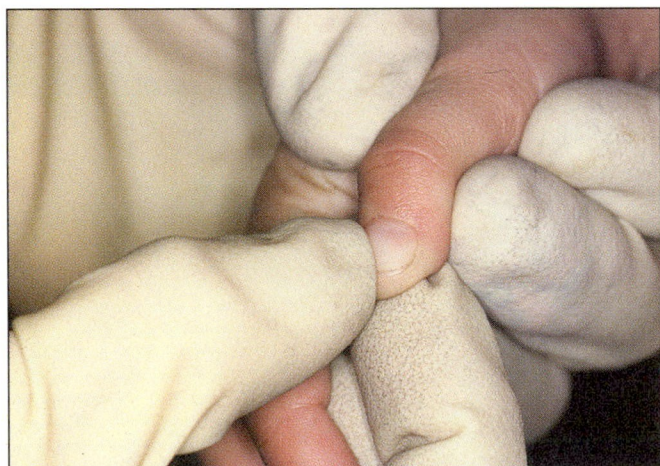

FIGURE 33-6 Estimate capillary refill by squeezing the end of a finger or toe for several seconds until the fingertip blanches. Normal color should return within 2 seconds.

Care of the Pediatric Airway

Positioning the Airway

Positioning the airway correctly is critical in pediatric emergency care. Always position the airway in a neutral sniffing position (Figure 33-7). This accomplishes two goals at once: It keeps the trachea from kinking when the neck is bent back (hyperextended) or forward (flexed), and it maintains the proper alignment if you have to immobilize the spine. If the child has been involved in trauma or trauma is suspected, use the jaw-thrust maneuver to open the airway.

Follow these steps to position the airway in a child or infant (Figure 33-8):

1. **Place the patient** on a firm surface such as a short backboard or pediatric immobilization device.
2. **Fold a small towel** to a thickness of approximately 1", and place it under the patient's shoulders and back.
3. **Place tape across the child's forehead** to limit rolling of the head during transport.

Airway Adjuncts

In children with inadequate ventilation, whatever the reason, you should use an airway adjunct to maintain an open airway. Airway adjuncts are devices that help to maintain the airway or assist in providing artificial ventilation, including oral and nasal airways, bite blocks, and BVM devices. Placing the adjuncts correctly starts with choosing the appropriately sized equipment (Figure 33-9).

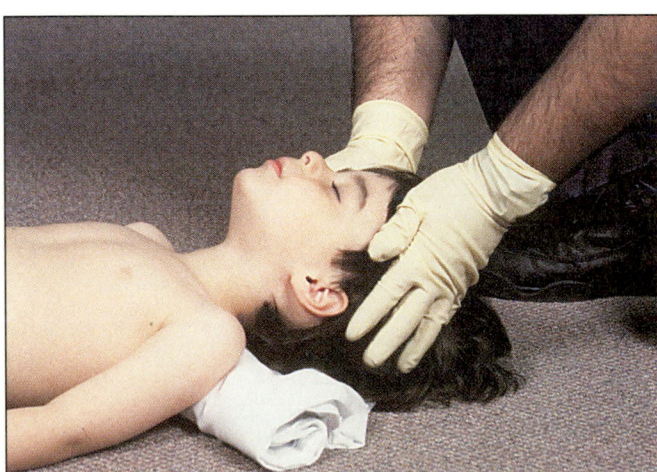

FIGURE 33-7 The airway should be placed in a neutral sniffing position to keep the trachea from kinking when the neck is flexed or hyperextended.

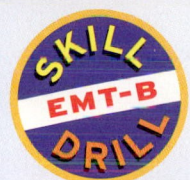

Positioning the Airway in a Child

Figure 33-8

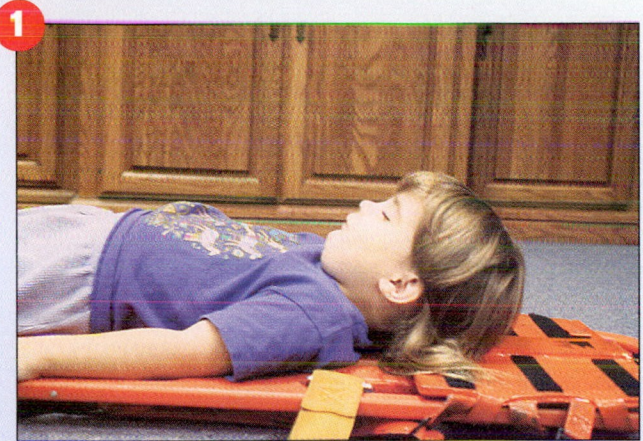

Place the patient on a firm surface such as a short backboard or pediatric immobilization device.

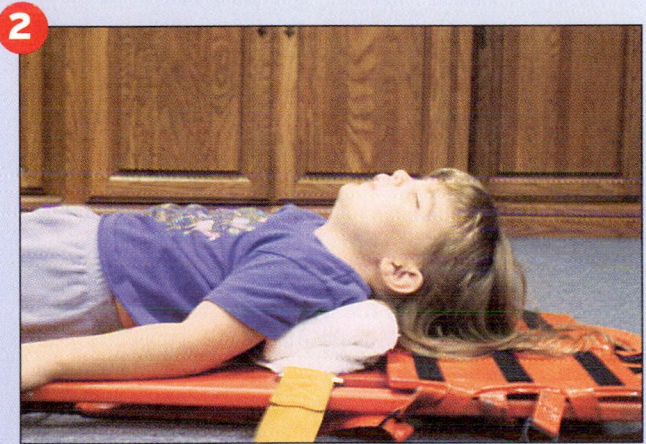

Fold a small towel to a thickness of about 1", and place it under the patient's shoulders and back.

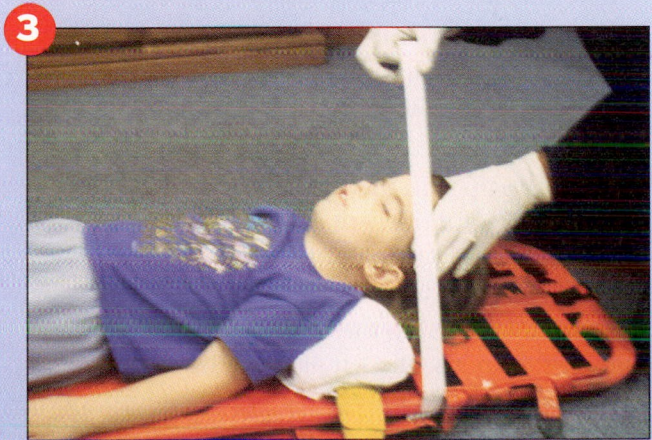

Place tape across the child's forehead to limit movement during transport.

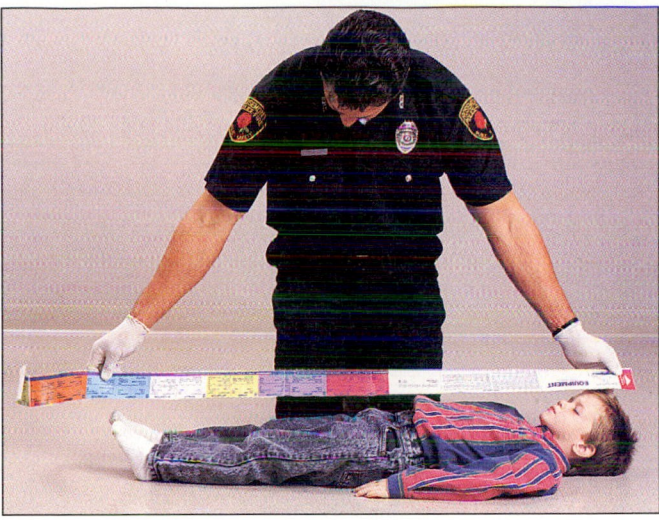

FIGURE 33-9 Use of a pediatric resuscitation tape measure is the best way to identify the appropriate size for pediatric airway equipment.

Oropharyngeal airway. An oropharyngeal airway is designed to keep the tongue from blocking the airway, and it makes suctioning the airway, if necessary, easier. An oropharyngeal airway should be used for pediatric patients who are unconscious and in possible respiratory failure. However, this adjunct should not be used in either conscious patients or those who have a decreased level of consciousness, as both will have a gag reflex. Patients with a gag reflex do not tolerate an oropharyngeal airway. In addition, this adjunct should not be used in children who may have ingested a caustic or petroleum-based product, as it may induce vomiting.

You should insert an oropharyngeal airway in a child in the following way (Figure 33-10):

1. **Determine the appropriately sized airway,** using the resuscitation tape to measure the patient.

2. **Place the airway next to the face** with the flange at the level of the central incisors and the bite block segment parallel to the hard palate. The tip of the airway should reach the angle of the jaw.

3. **Position the patient's airway.** If the emergency is medical, use the head-tilt/chin-lift maneuver, avoiding hyperextension; you may place a towel under the shoulders. If the patient has a traumatic injury, use the jaw-thrust maneuver, and provide in-line spinal stabilization.

4. **Open the patient's mouth** by applying pressure on the chin with your thumb.

5. **Insert the airway** by depressing the tongue with a tongue blade to the base of the tongue and inserting the airway directly over the tongue blade. If a tongue blade is not available, point the airway tip toward the roof of the mouth to depress the tongue, and

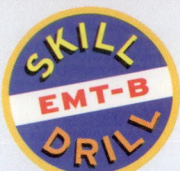

Inserting an Oropharyngeal Airway in a Child

Figure 33-10

1

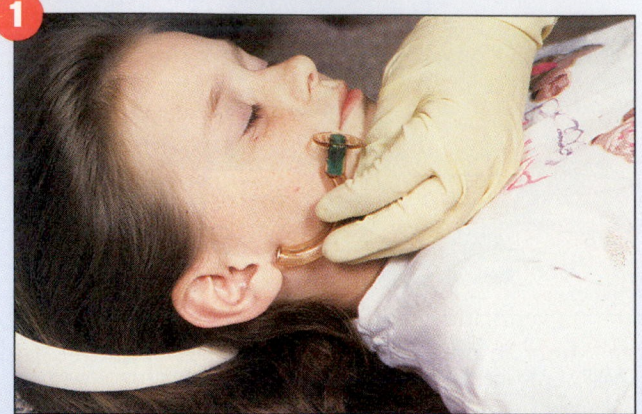

Determine the appropriately sized airway by measuring the airway from the corner of the patient's mouth to the earlobe.

2

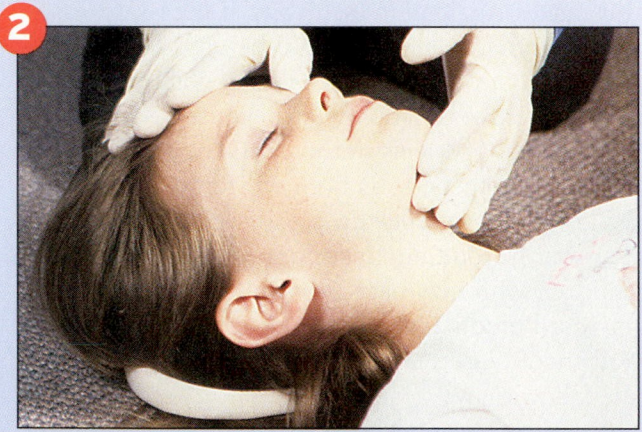

Position the patient's airway using either the head-tilt/chin-lift maneuver or the jaw-thrust maneuver.

3

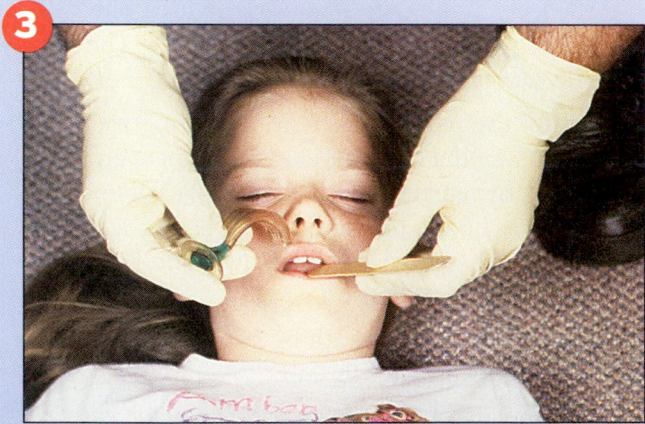

Open the patient's mouth using your thumb, and then insert the airway by depressing the tongue with a tongue blade to the base of the tongue. Insert the airway directly over the tongue blade.

then insert the airway until the flange rests against the lips. Gently rotate the airway 180° into position

6. **Reassess the airway** after insertion.

Take care to avoid injuring the hard palate as you insert the airway. Rough insertion can cause bleeding, which may aggravate airway problems and may even cause vomiting. Note also that if the patient's airway is too small, the tongue may be pushed back into the pharynx, obstructing the airway. If the airway is too large, it may obstruct the larynx.

Nasopharyngeal airway. A nasopharyngeal airway is also an adjunct and not a means of artificial ventilation. It is usually well tolerated and is not as likely as the oropharyngeal airway to cause vomiting. Unlike the oropharyngeal airway, the nasopharyngeal airway is used in conscious patients or in patients with altered levels of consciousness. In pediatric patients, it is typically used in association with possible respiratory failure. It is rarely used in infants younger than age 1 year.

A nasopharyngeal airway should not be used in patients with nasal obstruction or head trauma (possible basal skull fracture). Likewise, its use is contraindicated in patients with moderate to severe head trauma, as this adjunct could increase intracranial pressure in these patients.

You should insert a nasopharyngeal airway in a child in the following way (Figure 33-11):

1. **Determine the appropriately sized airway.** The external diameter of the airway should not be larger than the diameter of the external openings of the nose, called <u>nares</u>; and there should be no <u>blanching</u> (or turning white) of the nares after insertion.

2. **Place the airway** next to the patient's face to make sure the length is correct. The airway should extend from the tip of the nose to the tragus of the ear. The <u>tragus</u> is the small cartilaginous projection in front of the opening of the ear.

3. **Position the patient's airway,** using the techniques described for the oropharyngeal airway.

4. **Lubricate the airway** with a water-soluble lubricant.

5. **Insert the tip into the right nare** with the bevel pointing toward the <u>septum</u>, or center of the nose. Carefully move the tip forward until the flange rests against the outside of the nostril.

6. **If you are inserting the airway** on the left side, insert the tip into the left nare upside down, with the bevel pointing toward the septum. Move the airway forward slowly about 1″ until you feel a slight resistance, and then rotate the airway 180°

7. **Reassess the airway** after insertion.

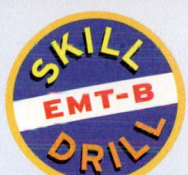

Inserting a Nasopharyngeal Airway in a Child

Figure 33-11

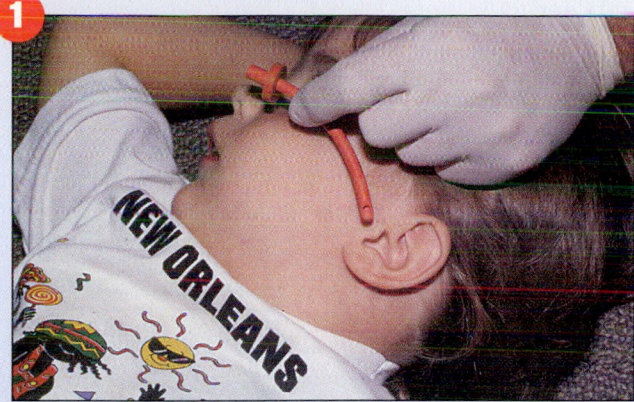

Place the airway next to the patient's face to make sure the length is correct. The airway should extend from the tip of the nose to the tragus. Then position the patient's airway.

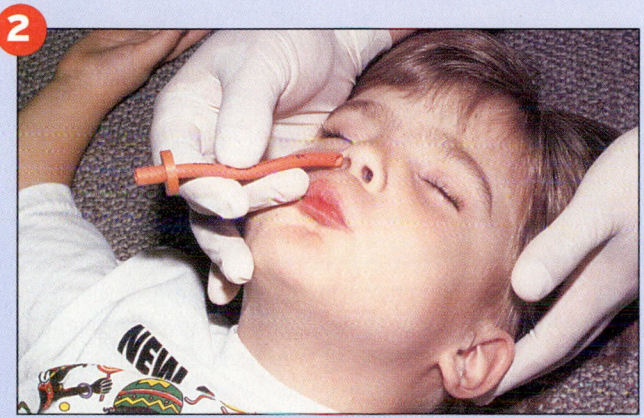

Lubricate the airway, and then insert the tip into the right nare with the bevel pointing toward the septum.

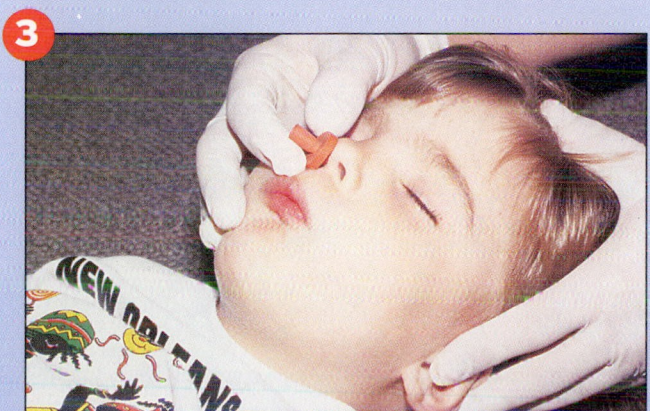

Move the tip forward until the flange rests against the outside of the nostril.

As with the oropharyngeal airway, there can be problems with the nasopharyngeal airway. An airway with a small diameter may easily become obstructed by mucus, blood, vomitus, or the soft tissues of the pharynx. If the airway is too long, it may stimulate the vagus nerve and slow the heart rate or enter the esophagus, causing gastric distention. Inserting the airway in responsive patients may cause a spasm of the larynx and result in vomiting. Nasopharyngeal airways should not be used in patients who have facial trauma, as the airway may tear soft tissues and cause bleeding into the airway.

Assisting Ventilation

After opening the airway, you should assess the patient's ventilation. Look, listen, and feel for breathing. Remember to observe chest rise in older children and abdominal rise in younger children and infants. Skin color indicates the amount of oxygen getting to the organs of the body. Patients who are pale, mottled, or blue may have inadequate levels of oxygen in their blood. All trauma patients should receive oxygen. If the patient has sustained trauma to the face, assisting ventilations may be difficult. Get the best seal with the mask you can to prevent inadequate oxygenation. Occasionally, mouth-to-mask ventilation may provide a better airway.

Oxygen Delivery Devices

In treating infants and children who require more than the usual 21% oxygen found in room air, you have several options, as follows:

- Nonrebreathing mask at 10 to 12 L/min provides up to 90% oxygen concentration.
- Blow-by technique at 6 L/min provides more than 21% oxygen concentration.
- Nasal cannula at 4 to 6 L/min provides 35% to 50% oxygen concentration.
- Simple face mask at 6 to10 L/min provides 30% to 60% oxygen concentration.
- BVM device (with oxygen reservoir) at 10 to 15 L/min provides 90% oxygen concentration.

Children need enough air to be delivered for adequate gas exchange in the lungs. Therefore, use of a nonrebreathing mask, a nasal cannula, or a simple face mask is indicated only for patients who have adequate respirations and/or tidal volumes. The **tidal volume** is the amount of air that is delivered to the lungs and airways. Children with respirations of less than 12 breaths/min or more than 60 breaths/min, an altered level of consciousness, and/or an inadequate tidal volume should receive assisted ventilations with a BVM device.

Blow-by oxygen is not an effective method for delivering oxygen. With this technique, an oxygen tube is held near the infant or child's nose and mouth. It is often used after childbirth to deliver a small amount of oxygen to the newborn. On rare occasions when other adjuncts cannot be used or the child will not tolerate any other adjunct, this technique may be necessary.

Nonrebreathing Mask

A nonrebreathing mask delivers 100% oxygen to the patient and allows the patient to exhale all carbon dioxide without rebreathing it (Figure 33-12).

1. **Select the appropriately sized** pediatric nonrebreathing mask. The mask should extend from the bridge of the nose to the cleft of the chin.
2. **Connect the tubing** to an oxygen source set at 10 to 12 L/min.

Blow-By Technique

The blow-by technique does not provide a high concentration of oxygen. However, if no other adjuncts are available, the blow-by technique is better than no oxygen.

1. **Place oxygen tubing** through a small hole in the bottom of a 6- to 8-oz paper or Styrofoam cup (Figure 33-13). A cup is a familiar object that is less likely than an oxygen mask to frighten young children. You may be able to use an oxygen mask with an older child if you make it a game. For example, have the child pretend that the mask belongs to a popular action hero.

2. **Connect tubing** to an oxygen source set at 6 L/min.
3. **Hold the cup** approximately 1" to 2" away from the child's nose and mouth.

Nasal Cannula

Some patients prefer this adjunct while others find it uncomfortable.

1. **Choose the appropriately sized** pediatric nasal cannula (Figure 33-14). The prongs should not fill the nares entirely. If the nares blanch, select a smaller cannula.
2. **Connect the tubing** to an oxygen source set at 4 to 6 L/min.

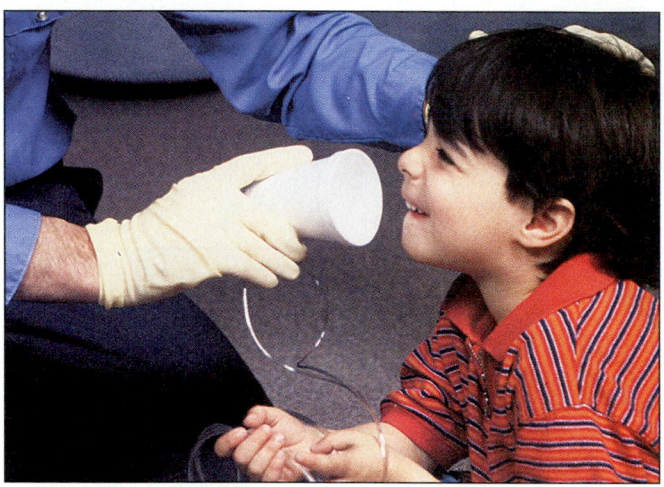

FIGURE 33-13 Blow-by techniques may be used, as oxygen masks frighten children. Make a small hole in a 6- to 8-oz paper or Styrofoam cup. Connect tubing to an oxygen source, and hold the cup about 2" from the child's face.

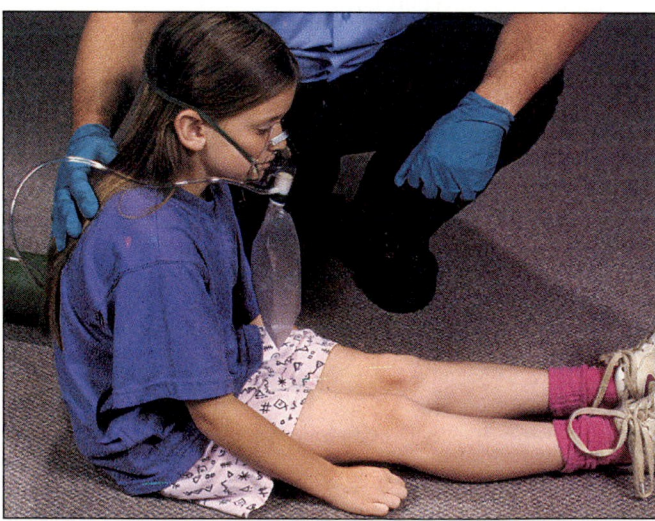

FIGURE 33-12 A pediatric nonrebreathing mask delivers 100% oxygen and allows the patient to exhale carbon dioxide without rebreathing it.

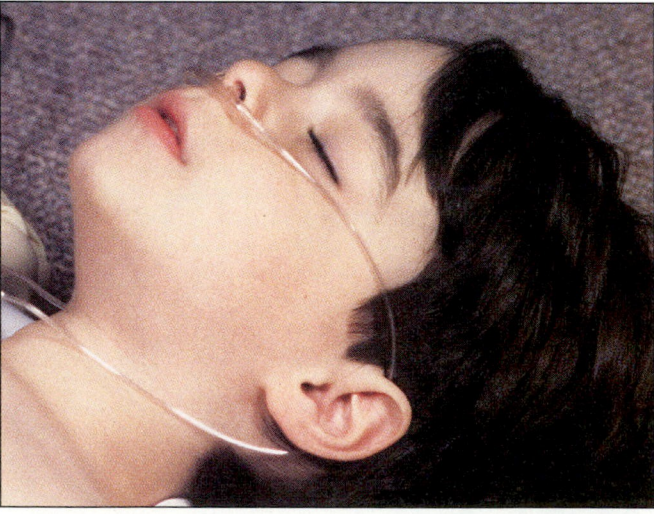

FIGURE 33-14 The prongs of a pediatric nasal cannula should not fill the nares entirely.

Simple Face Mask

Use of the appropriately sized mask is essential. A mask that is too small is uncomfortable while a mask that is too large will allow oxygen to leak into the environment. The face mask is tolerated best of all the adjuncts listed.

1. **Choose the appropriately sized** pediatric face mask (Figure 33-15). The mask should extend from the bridge of the nose to the cleft of the chin, between the lower lip and the bottom of the chin.

2. **Connect the tubing** to an oxygen source set at 6 to 10 L/min.

BVM Device

Assisting ventilations with a BVM device is indicated for patients who have respirations that are either too slow or too fast to provide an adequate volume of inhaled oxygen, who are unresponsive, or who do not respond in a purposeful way to painful stimuli.

Assist ventilation of an infant or child using a BVM device in the following way:

1. **Ensure that you have the appropriate** equipment in the right size. The mask should be the proper size so that it extends from the bridge of the nose to the cleft of the chin, avoiding compression of the eyes (Figure 33-16). The mask is transparent, so you can watch for cyanosis and vomiting. In addition, mask volume should be small to decrease dead space and avoid rebreathing; however, the bag should contain at least 450 mL of air. Use an infant bag, not a neonatal bag, for infants younger than age 1 year and a pediatric bag for children older than age 1 year. Older children and adolescents may need an adult bag. Make sure that there is no pop-off valve on the bag, or, if there is one, make sure that you can hold it shut as necessary to achieve chest rise.

2. **Maintain a good seal** with the mask on the face.

3. **Ventilate at the appropriate rate** and volume, using a slow, gentle squeeze, not a sharp, quick one. Stop squeezing and begin to release the bag as soon as the chest wall begins to rise, indicating that the lungs are filled to capacity. To keep from ventilating too rapidly, use the mnemonic "squeeze, release, release." Say "squeeze" as you squeeze the bag; when you see the chest start to rise, release pressure on the bag and say "release, release."

Errors in technique, including providing too much volume with each breath, squeezing the bag too sharply, or ventilating at too fast a rate, can result in gastric distention. An inadequate mask seal or improper head position can lead to hypoventilation or hypoxia.

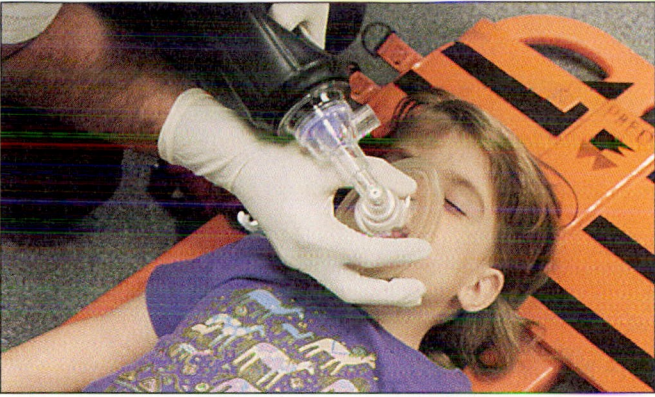

FIGURE 33-15 A pediatric face mask should extend from the bridge of the nose to the cleft of the chin, between the lower lip and the bottom of the chin.

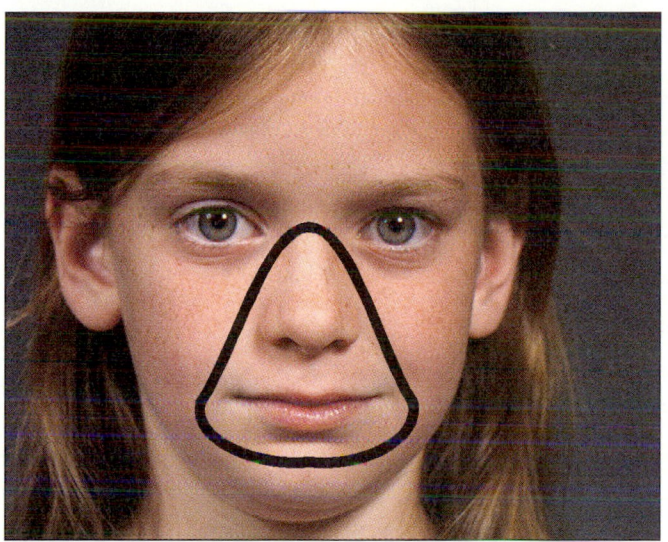

FIGURE 33-16 Proper mask size for BVM ventilation is critical. The mask should extend from the bridge of the nose to the cleft of the chin, avoiding compression of the eyes.

Even with the best technique in the world, the patient may regurgitate and aspirate the contents of his or her stomach, so stay alert.

One-rescuer BVM ventilation. You should perform one-rescuer BVM ventilation in the following way (Figure 33-17):

1. **Open the airway,** and insert the appropriate airway adjunct

2. **Hold the mask** on the patient's face with a one-handed head-tilt/chin-lift maneuver. With infants and toddlers, support the jaw with your third finger. Be careful not to compress the area under the chin, as you may push the tongue into the back of the mouth and block the airway. With older children, place your third, fourth, and fifth fingers on the ridge of the mandible to hold the jaw forward and to help maintain the proper head position.

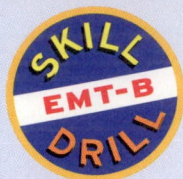

One-Person BVM Ventilation on a Child
Figure 33-17

1

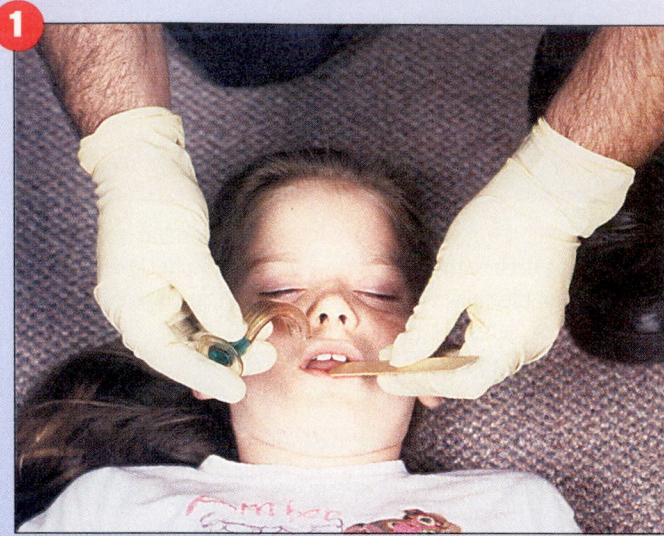

Open the airway, and insert the appropriate airway adjunct.

2

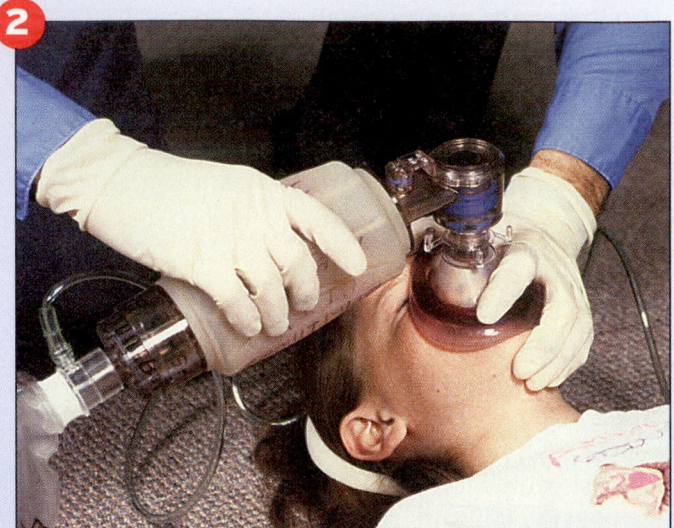

Hold the mask on the patient's face with a one-handed head-tilt/chin-lift maneuver.

3

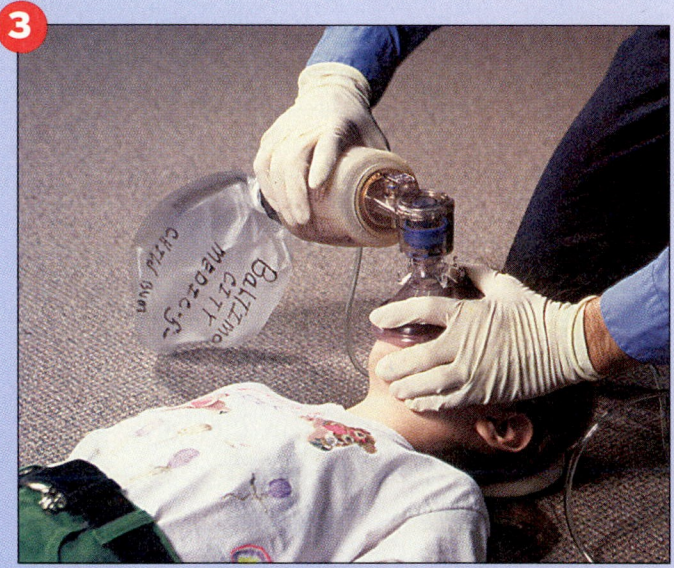

Squeeze the bag 20 times/minute for a child and 30 times/minute for an infant.

4

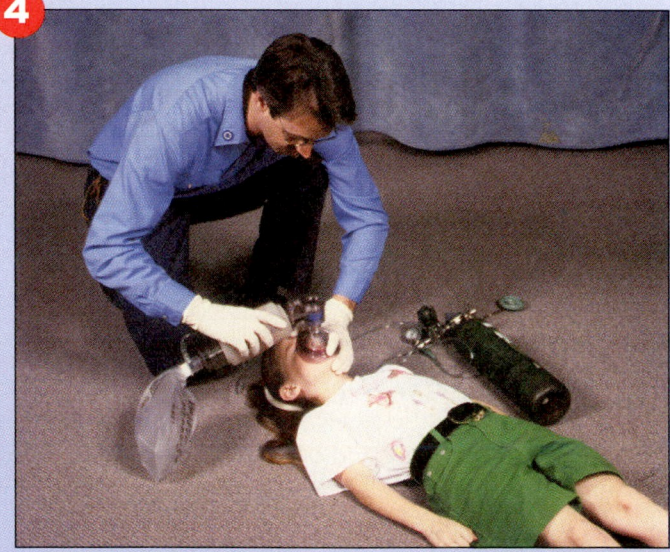

Assess effectiveness of ventilation by watching for adequate rise and fall of the chest.

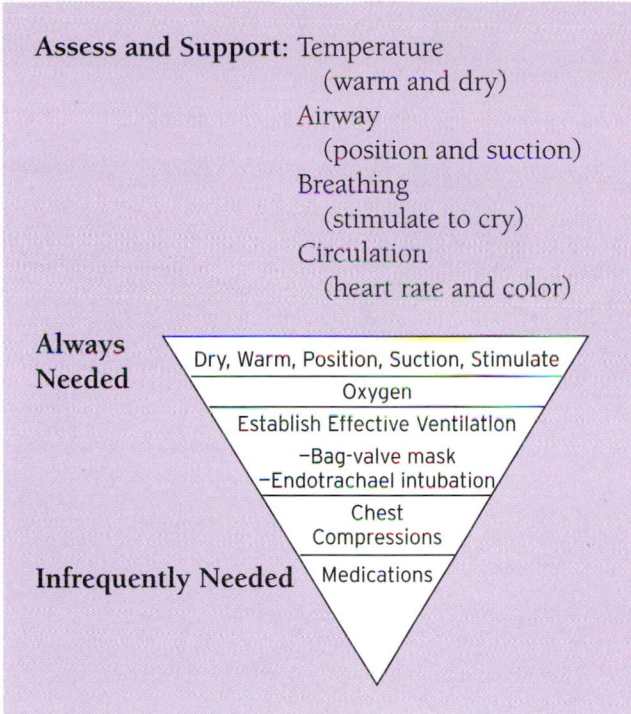

Assess and Support: Temperature
(warm and dry)
Airway
(position and suction)
Breathing
(stimulate to cry)
Circulation
(heart rate and color)

Always Needed

Dry, Warm, Position, Suction, Stimulate
Oxygen
Establish Effective Ventilation
–Bag-valve mask
–Endotrachael intubation
Chest Compressions
Medications

Infrequently Needed

FIGURE 33-18 The American Heart Association's resuscitation process for the newborn is designed to stimulate the newborn to breathe air and begin circulation of the blood through the lungs.

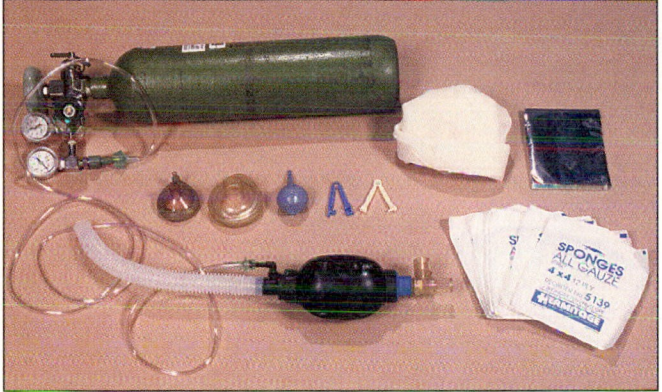

FIGURE 33-19 The proper equipment for neonatal resuscitation includes a bulb syringe, towels, an infant blanket, a BVM device, clear masks in two sizes, two umbilical clamps, sterile gauze, a stocking cap, and an oxygen source with tubing.

3. **Make sure the mask forms** an airtight seal on the face. Maintain the seal while checking that the airway is open.

4. **Squeeze the bag,** using the correct ventilation rate. For both infants and children, this is 20 breaths/min.

5. **Allow 1 to 1½ seconds per ventilation,** providing adequate time for exhalation. Use the "squeeze, release, release" mnemonic.

6. **Assess effectiveness of ventilation** by watching for adequate bilateral rise and fall of the chest. Also auscultate for bilateral breath sounds at the midaxillary line, third intercostal space.

Two-rescuer BVM ventilation. This procedure is exactly the same as one-rescuer ventilation except that it requires two rescuers, one to hold the mask to the patient's face and maintain the patient's head position, the other to ventilate the patient. This technique may be more effective in maintaining a tight seal.

Neonatal Resuscitation

At birth, most infants require only the resuscitation measures shown at the top of the American Heart Association's inverse pyramid, which are designed to stimulate the newborn to breathe air and begin circulation of blood through the lungs (Figure 33-18). These measures include positioning of the airway, drying, warming, suctioning, and tactile stimulation. Here are some tips to help you maximize the effects of the measures:

• Position the infant on his or her back with the head down and the neck slightly extended. Place a towel or blanket under the infant's shoulder to help maintain this position.

• Suction the mouth and nose using a bulb syringe or suction device with an 8 or 10 French catheter. Suction both sides of the back of the mouth, where secretions tend to collect, but avoid deep suctioning of the mouth and throat; this can cause the heart to slow down. It is always good practice to aim blow-by oxygen at the infant's mouth and nose during resuscitation.

• In addition to vigorously drying the infant's head, back, and body with dry towels, you may rub the infant's back and slap the soles of his or her feet.

In instances when a newborn is in distress, you should be properly equipped for resuscitation measures. All ambulances should have the following equipment and supplies for newborn resuscitation (Figure 33-19):

• A bulb syringe
• Clean dry towels
• An infant blanket
• A BVM device with a 450-mL reservoir
• Clear masks in both infant and premature infant sizes
• 2 umbilical clamps
• Sterile 4 x 4 gauze
• A stocking cap
• An oxygen source with tubing

Additional Resuscitation Efforts

Observe the infant for spontaneous respirations, skin color, and movement of the extremities. If the respiratory effort appears appropriate, evaluate the heart rate by palpating the pulse at the base of the umbilical cord or at the brachial artery. The heart rate is the most important measure in determining the need for further resuscitation (Table 33-3).

If chest compressions are required, give them at a rate of 120 beats/min using either the hand-encircling technique or the two-finger technique (Figure 33-20). Coordinate chest compressions with ventilations at a ratio of 5:1.

Any newborn who requires more than routine resuscitation requires transport, when possible, to a center with a level III neonatal intensive care unit. This type of unit is especially for newborns who require specialized care, including mechanical ventilation.

About 12% of deliveries are complicated by the presence of **meconium**, a dark green material in the amniotic fluid. Meconium can be thick or thin. If the newborn aspirates thick meconium, serious lung disease and sometimes death can occur. Therefore, if you see meconium in the amniotic fluid or meconium staining, you should continue vigorous suctioning of the infant after delivery.

Basic Life Support Review

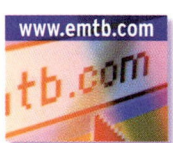 The reasons for cardiopulmonary arrest differ in children and adults. In adults, cardiac arrest is usually the result of an abnormal cardiac rhythm, which is itself caused by underlying cardiac disease. Because most children have healthy hearts, sudden cardiac arrest is rare. More commonly, children have cardiopulmonary arrest because of respiratory or circulatory failure from illness or injury. For this reason, the airway and breathing are the focus of pediatric basic life support (BLS) (Table 33-4).

Respiratory problems leading to cardiopulmonary arrest in children can have a number of different causes, including the following:

- Injury, both blunt and penetrating
- Infections of the respiratory tract or another organ system
- A foreign body in the airway
- Near drowning
- Electrocution
- Poisoning or drug overdose
- Sudden infant death syndrome (SIDS)

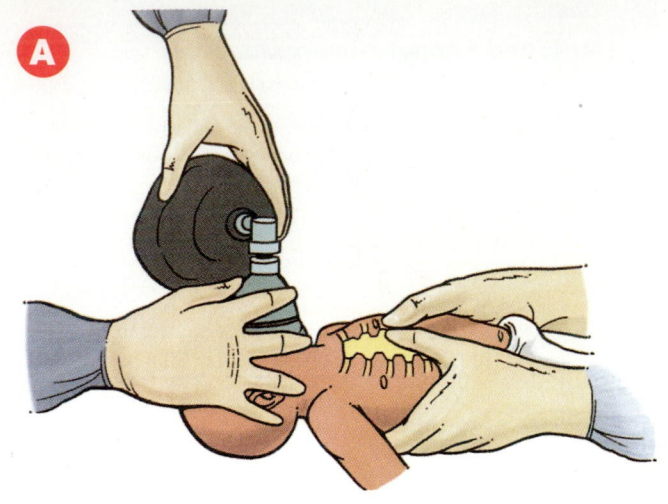

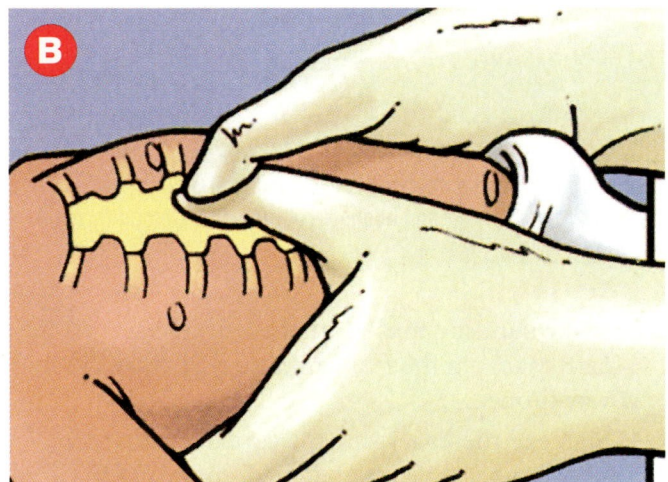

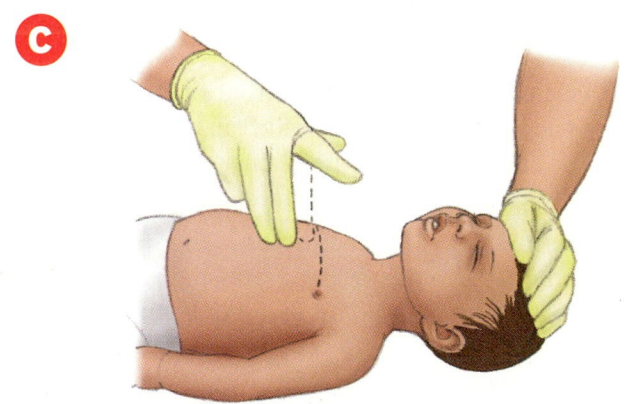

FIGURE 33-20 A: Chest compressions should be given with the hands encircling the infant and thumbs side by side. **B:** In very small infants, you may need to overlap the thumbs. **C:** In larger infants, you may use the two-finger technique, using the middle and ring fingers.

For purposes of pediatric BLS, infancy ends at 1 year of age, and childhood extends to 8 years. Although children older than age 8 years are still considered pediatric patients, they are treated with adult BLS methods. The goal, of course, is the same for all patients: To restore breathing and circulation of the blood.

Pediatric BLS can be divided into four steps, as follows:

1. Determining responsiveness
2. Airway
3. Breathing
4. Circulation

TABLE 33-3   Additional Neonatal Resuscitation Efforts

If the Heart Rate Is . . .	More Than 100 Beats/Min	60 to 100 Beats/Min	Fewer Than 80 and Not Rising
Do this:	Keep the infant warm.	Give blow-by oxygen.	Begin assisted ventilation with a BVM device and 100% oxygen.
	Transport the infant.	Stimulate the infant.	Reassess the infant every 15 to 30 seconds until heart rate and respirations are normal.
	Assess the infant continuously.	Keep the infant warm.	If the heart rate does not increase, begin chest compressions. Call for ALS backup.
		Continue to reassess the infant.	If the heart rate does not increase, medication and ALS may be necessary.

TABLE 33-4   Review of Pediatric BLS

Action	Infants Younger Than Age 1 Year	Children Between Age 1 and 8 Years
Airway	Head-tilt/chin-lift; jaw-thrust if spine injury is suspected	Head-tilt/chin-lift; jaw-thrust if spine injury is suspected
Breathing		
Initial	2 breaths at a rate of 1 to 1½ seconds/breath	2 breaths at a rate of 1 to 1½ seconds/breath
Subsequent	20 breaths/min	20 breaths/min
Circulation		
Pulse check	Brachial/femoral arteries	Carotid artery
Compression area	Lower half of sternum	Lower half of sternum
Compression width	2 or 3 fingers	Heel of hand
Compression depth	½" to 1"	1" to 1½"
Compression rate	At least 100/min	100/min
Ratio of Compressions to Ventilations	5:1 (pause for ventilation)	5:1 (pause for ventilation)
Foreign Body Obstruction	Back blows and chest thrusts	Abdominal thrusts

Table 33-4 has been adapted from "Summary of BLS Maneuvers in Infants and Children," *Basic Life Support for Healthcare Providers*, Dallas, American Heart Association, 1997, p. 6-10.

Determining Responsiveness

Never shake a child to determine whether he or she is responsive, especially if there is a possible neck or back injury. Instead, gently tap the child on the shoulder, and speak loudly (Figure 33-21). If a child is responsive but struggling to breathe, allow him or her to remain in whatever position is most comfortable.

If you find an unresponsive child while you are alone and not on duty, provide BLS for approximately 1 minute, and then stop to call the EMS system. Why not call right away, as you would with an adult? Because unlike an adult, an unconscious child may respond quickly to ventilation and oxygenation. Indeed, these actions may prevent the child from progressing to full cardiopulmonary arrest.

Airway

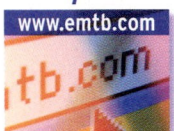

Because children often put toys and other objects, as well as food, in the mouth, foreign body obstruction of the upper airway is common. The steps for removing a foreign object are reviewed in chapter 34. You must make sure that the upper airway is open when dealing with pediatric respiratory emergencies or cardiopulmonary arrest. If the child is unconscious and lying in a supine position, the airway may become obstructed when the tongue and throat muscles relax and the tongue falls backward (Figure 33-22).

If the child is unconscious but breathing, place him or her on one side or the other in the recovery position, in which the upper leg is flexed and bent forward for stabilization and the head is positioned to allow drainage of saliva or vomitus (Figure 33-23). Do not use this position if you suspect a spinal injury unless you can secure the child to a backboard that can be tilted to the side. Do not attempt to open the airway at all if the child is conscious and breathing, but in a labored fashion. Instead, provide immediate transport to the nearest advanced life support facility.

There are two common techniques for manually opening the airway in a child who is neither conscious nor breathing: the head-tilt/chin-lift maneuver and the jaw-thrust maneuver (Figure 33-24). The latter is safer if there is a possibility of a neck injury.

Head-tilt/chin-lift maneuver. Perform this maneuver in a child in the following way:

1. **Place one hand on the child's forehead,** and tilt the head back gently, with the neck slightly extended.
2. **Place the fingers** (not the thumb) of your other hand under the child's chin, and lift the jaw upward and outward. Do not close the mouth or push under the chin; either move may obstruct rather than open the airway.
3. **If a foreign body** or vomitus is visible, remove it.

Jaw-thrust maneuver. Perform this maneuver in a child in the following way:

1. **Place two or three fingers** under each side of the angle of the lower jaw; lift the jaw upward and outward.
2. **If the jaw thrust alone** does not open the airway and cervical spine injury is not a consideration, tilt the head slightly. If cervical spine injury is suspected, use a second rescuer to immobilize the cervical spine.

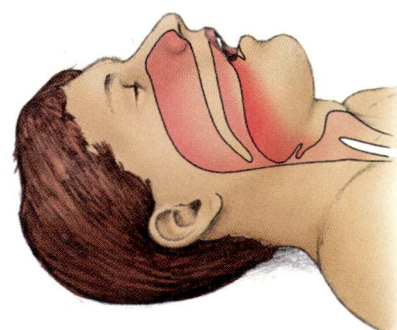

FIGURE 33-22 The airway may be obstructed when the tongue and throat muscles relax and the tongue falls back into the throat.

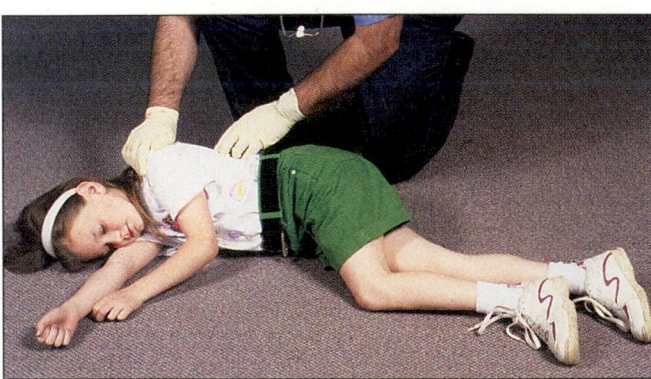

FIGURE 33-21 Never shake a child to determine responsiveness. Rather, gently tap the child on the shoulder, and speak loudly.

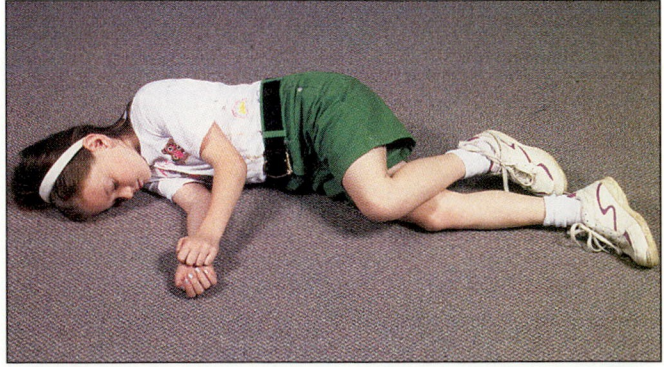

FIGURE 33-23 A child who is unconscious but breathing should be placed in the recovery position to allow saliva or vomitus to drain from the mouth.

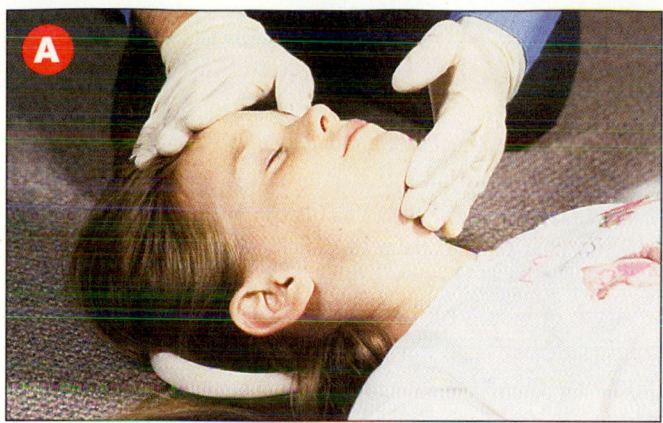

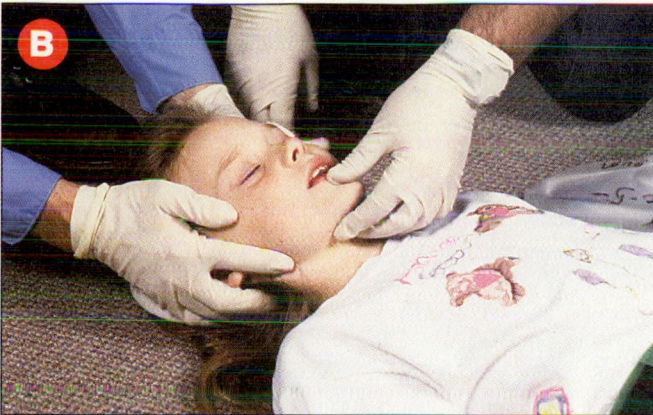

FIGURE 33-24 A: Use the head-tilt/chin-lift maneuver to open the airway in a child who has not sustained a traumatic injury.

B: Use the jaw-thrust maneuver to open the airway if there is a possibility that a traumatic injury has occurred.

Remember that the head of an infant or young child is disproportionately large in comparison to the chest and shoulders. As a result, when a child is lying flat on his or her back, especially on a backboard, the head will bend forward onto the upper chest. This can partially or completely obstruct the upper airway. To avoid this possibility, place a wedge of padding under the upper chest and shoulders.

Breathing

Once the airway is open, determine if the child is breathing spontaneously, using the Look, Listen, and Feel technique (Figure 33-25):

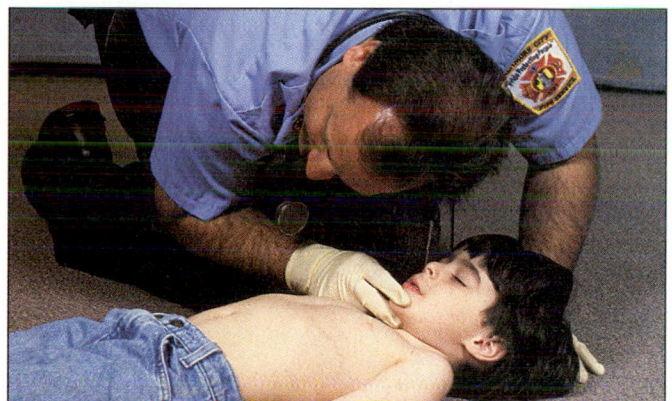

FIGURE 33-25 After you have opened the airway, use the look, listen, and feel technique to determine if the child is breathing spontaneously.

- **Look** for rise and fall of the chest or abdomen.
- **Listen** for exhalation of breath.
- **Feel** for exhaled air flow at the mouth.

If an infant or small child is breathing, provide immediate transport. Again, a child who is in respiratory distress should be allowed to stay in whatever position is most comfortable. Larger children who are unconscious and breathing with difficulty should be kept in the recovery position if possible.

If an infant or child is not breathing, provide rescue breathing while keeping the airway open. If you are using mouth-to-mouth resuscitation with an infant, place your mouth over the infant's mouth and nose to create a seal. If you are using a mask to assist ventilations in an infant, turning the mask upside down can sometimes create a better seal.

When two rescuers are available, use your thumb and index finger to apply pressure over the area just below the Adam's apple (the Sellick maneuver) (Figure 33-26). This will decrease the risk of gastric distention and aspiration of vomitus by pushing the larynx back to compress and close off the esophagus.

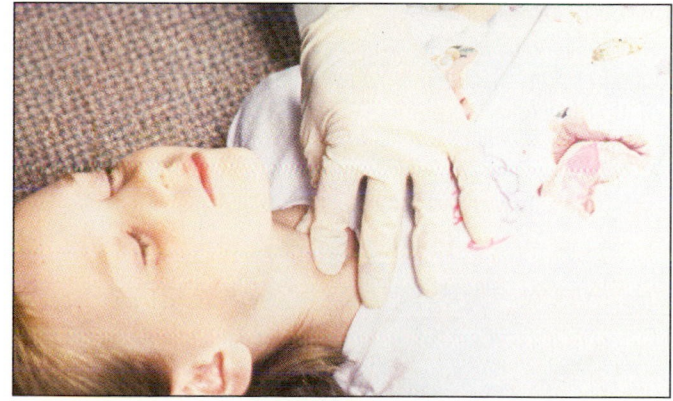

FIGURE 33-26 Perform the Sellick maneuver to decrease the risk of gastric distention and aspiration of vomitus

In a child with tracheostomy (breathing) tubes in the neck, place a mask, barrier device, or your mouth over the tracheotomy site. Then place your hand firmly over the child's mouth and nose to prevent the artificial breaths from leaking out of the upper airway.

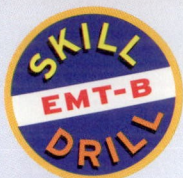

Performing Infant Chest Compressions

Figure 33-27

1

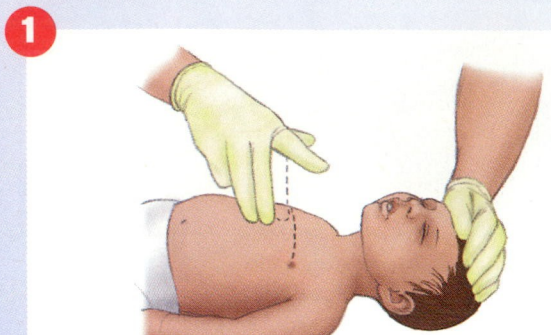

Place the infant on a firm surface, with one hand on the chest and the other maintaining the open airway. Draw an imaginary line between the nipples, and then place two fingers in the middle of the sternum one fingerwidth below the imaginary line.

2

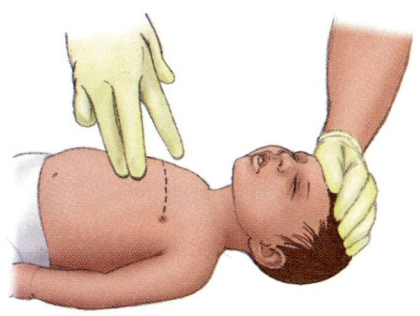

Compress the chest using the two-finger technique at a rate of 100 times/min.

3

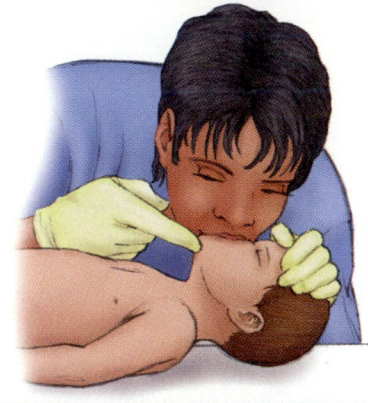

Coordinate rapid compressions and ventilations in a 5:1 ratio.

Circulation

Once you have opened the airway and provided two rescue breaths, you must determine the state of the child's circulation. Check for pulses in the carotid artery in older children and the brachial or femoral artery in young children and infants. Locate the carotid artery by placing one or two fingers over the groove between the Adam's apple and the neck muscles. Locate the brachial artery by placing two or three fingers on the inside of an infant's upper arm, between the elbow and the shoulder. The femoral artery can be felt in the crease between the upper leg and the groin. However, palpating the pulse in an infant or child is difficult; therefore, do not spend more than a few seconds trying. If an infant or child is not breathing, you can assume that there is no pulse.

For chest compressions to be effective, the patient should be placed on a firm, flat surface with the head at the same level as the body. If you need to carry an infant while providing CPR, your forearm and hand can serve as the flat surface. Follow these steps to perform infant chest compressions (Figure 33-27):

1. **Place the infant on a firm surface,** using one hand to keep the head in an open airway position. You can also use a pad or wedge under the shoulders and upper body to keep the head from tilting forward.

2. **Imagine a line drawn** between the nipples. Place two fingers in the middle of the sternum, about $1/2''$ below the level of the imaginary line.

3. **Using two fingers,** compress the sternum about one third to one half the depth of the chest; this is usually about $1/2''$ to $1''$. Compress the chest at a rate of 100 compressions per minute. With pauses for ventilation, you will actually compress the chest about 80 times a minute.

4. **After each compression,** allow the sternum to return briefly to its normal position. Allow equal time for compression and relaxation of the chest. Do not remove your fingers from the sternum, and avoid jerky movements.

5. **Coordinate rapid compressions** and ventilations in a 5:1 ratio, making sure the infant's chest rises with each ventilation. You will find this easier to do if you use your free hand to keep the head in the open airway position. If the chest does not rise, or rises only a little, use a chin lift to open the airway.

6. **Reassess the infant** for signs of spontaneous breathing or pulses after 1 minute and again after every few minutes.

SKILL EMT-B DRILL

Performing CPR in a Child
Figure 33-28

1

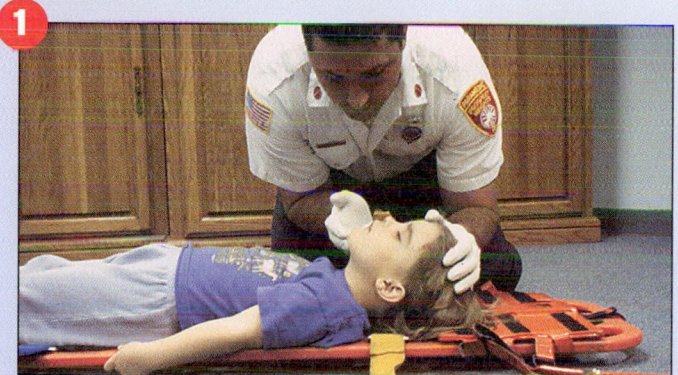

Place the child on a firm surface, and use one hand to maintain an open airway.

2

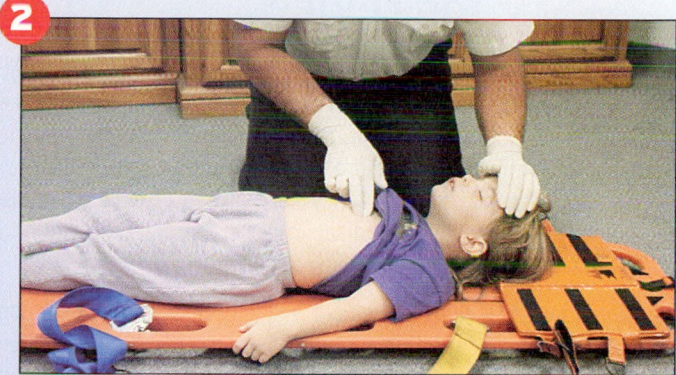

Locate the bottom of the sternum, and then place the heel of your hand over the lower half of the sternum.

3

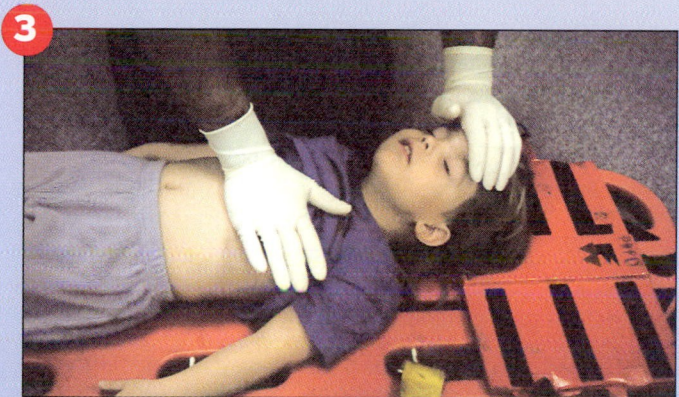

Compress the chest about one third to one half of its total depth at a rate of 100 times/min. Coordinate rapid compressions and ventilations in a 5:1 ratio.

4

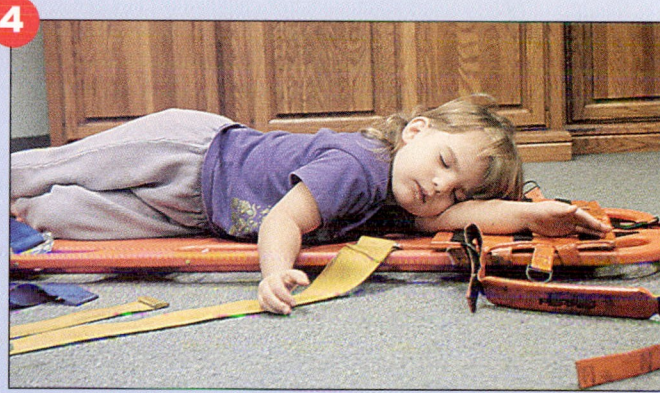

If the child resumes effective breathing, place him or her in the recovery position.

Follow these steps to perform CPR in children between ages 1 and 8 years (Figure 33-28).

1. **Place the child on a firm surface,** and use one hand to maintain the head in a tilted-back position.

2. **Using two fingers of the other hand,** locate the bottom of the sternum by tracing the lower margin of the rib cage to the notch where the ribs and sternum meet. Place the heel of your hand over the lower half of the sternum; this is the area between the meeting place of the ribs and sternum and an imaginary line drawn between the nipples. Avoid compression over the lower tip of the sternum, which is called the xiphoid process.

3. **Compress the chest** about one third to one half its total depth; this is usually 1 to 1½". Compress the chest at a rate of 100 compressions/min. With pauses for ventilation, the actual number of compressions will be about 80 per minute. Compression and relaxation should be about the same duration. Use smooth movements. Hold your fingers off the child's ribs, and keep the heel of your hand on the sternum.

4. **Coordinate rapid compressions** and ventilations in a 5:1 ratio, making sure the chest rises with each ventilation. At the end of every fifth compression, pause for 1 to 1½ seconds for artificial ventilation.

5. **Reassess the child** for signs of spontaneous breathing and pulses after about a minute and again every few minutes.

6. **If the child resumes effective breathing,** place him or her in the recovery position.

Remember, if the child is older than age 8 years or is equivalent to an adult in size, use the adult CPR sequence.

prep kit

ready for review

The airway in a child has a smaller diameter than the airway in an adult and is therefore more easily obstructed. Because the diaphragm is the principal muscle of respiration, gastric distention can create breathing difficulties. The three fundamentals of pediatric emergency care are to provide basic life support as needed, prevent disability by stabilizing the spine, and consult with an ALS unit when appropriate.

Always take vital signs in the field, and have pediatric resuscitation equipment ready at all times. To measure respirations in children younger than 3 years of age, count the rise and fall of the abdomen rather than of the chest. Feel for a pulse in the brachial or femoral artery in infants and small children and in the carotid artery in older children. Use a pediatric resuscitation tape measure to determine the appropriately sized equipment for children.

In treating possible respiratory failure in a child, always position the airway in a neutral position. Use an airway adjunct to maintain an open airway: an oropharyngeal airway in an unconscious patient (unless he or she has ingested a caustic or petroleum-based product) and a nasopharyngeal airway in a conscious patient (unless he or she is less than age 1 year and/or has sustained head trauma). Appropriate oxygen delivery devices include the blow-by technique at 6 L /min, a nasal cannula at 4 to 6 L/min, a simple face mask at 6 to 10 L/min, a nonrebreathing mask at 10 to 12 L/min, and a BVM device at 10 to 15 L/min.

Use a BVM device with a child whose breathing and tidal volume are inadequate and who has an altered level of consciousness. There are three keys to successful use of the BVM device in a child: (1) Have the appropriate equipment in the right size, (2) maintain a good face to mask seal, and (3) ventilate at the appropriate rate and volume: 20 breaths per minute for an infant or child, 30 for a neonate, 1 to $1\frac{1}{2}$ seconds per ventilation. Squeeze gently, and stop squeezing as the chest wall begins to rise; use the mnemonic "squeeze, release, release" to maintain a proper rhythm.

The heart rate is the most important measure in determining the need for extra resuscitation efforts in a normal newborn. If the heart rate is 80 to 100 beats/min, you should give blow-by oxygen and continue to reassess the infant. If the rate does not rise to more than 100 beats/min, begin assisted ventilations with a BVM device and 100% oxygen, and reassess the infant every 15 to 30 seconds. If the rate remains low, begin chest compressions, continue assisted ventilations, and call for ALS backup.

BLS for infants and children consists of determining responsiveness and assessing airway, breathing, and circulation. If the child is unconscious but breathing, place him or her in the recovery position unless you suspect a spinal injury. Use the head-tilt/chin-lift or jaw-thrust maneuver to open the airway in a child who is unconscious and not breathing. If a child is not breathing, provide rescue breathing while keeping the airway open. Breathe for an infant at a rate of 2 breaths/sec at first, then 20 breaths/min. Breathe for a child between ages 1 and 8 years at a rate of 2 breaths/sec at first, then 20 breaths/min. Do not spend more than a few seconds trying to feel a pulse in an infant or child; if he or she is not breathing, you can assume there is no pulse.

To provide CPR in an infant, compress the chest 100 times/min, pausing after every five compressions for ventilation; use two or three fingers, and compress the lower half of the sternum to a depth $\frac{1}{2}$ " to 1". In children, use the same rate and compressions to a depth of 1" to $1\frac{1}{2}$ " and the same 5:1 ratio of compressions to ventilations, but use the heel of your hand to compress the chest; avoid compressing the xiphoid process.

vital vocabulary

blanching Turning white.

meconium A dark green material in the amniotic fluid that can be a sign of serious lung disease.

nares The external openings of the nostrils.

occiput The back of the head.

pediatric resuscitation tape measure A tape that estimates an infant or child's weight on the basis of length and generates appropriate drug doses and equipment sizes on the tape.

pediatrics A separate medical practice devoted to the care of the young.

www.emtb.com

septum The center of the nose.

tidal volume The amount of air that is delivered to the lungs and airways.

tragus The small cartilaginous projection in front of the opening of the ear.

xiphoid process The lower tip of the sternum.

assessment in action

An 8-year-old boy, running for the door, slips and tumbles down the basement stairs. His mother calls 9-1-1, and you arrive to find the boy still lying on the concrete floor of the basement. He is scared and, through his crying, manages to tell you that everything hurts. You note multiple abrasions, several of which are still oozing blood. His mother states that she thinks he was unconscious briefly but that she is not certain. Assessment reveals that the boy's skin is warm and moist and that he has feeling and movement in all four extremities. You see a saucer-sized bruise over the right anterior chest area where he appears to have struck a support post as he went down the stairs. The boy reports that his chest "really hurts" when he breathes.

1. You should assess the patient's respiratory status:
   A. once during the initial assessment.
   B. only if the patient's skin color begins to change.
   C. on an ongoing basis throughout the call.
   D. en route, just before you arrive at the hospital.

2. You notice that the patient is beginning to look tired and is less responsive, conditions suggesting that he has:
   A. adult respiratory distress syndrome.
   B. missed his nap and should be put to bed.
   C. likely begun to have an allergic reaction.
   D. likely begun to experience ventilatory fatigue.

3. En route to the hospital, the boy begins to cry again. When you ask why he is crying, he states that "it hurts too bad to breathe." Of the following interventions, which is **NOT** appropriate at this time?
   A. Reassessing the patient's lung sounds
   B. Telling him to quit whining and tough it out
   C. Notifying the hospital about this information
   D. Increasing the oxygen flow

4. Ongoing assessment of this patient would **NOT** include which of the following steps?
   A. Reassessing the level of consciousness
   B. Reevaluating your patient care priorities
   C. Monitoring the overall quality of breathing
   D. Asking the patient's mother for proof of health insurance

5. Which of the following facts is likely to have the **LEAST** impact on your immediate care for this patient?
   A. The patient might have lost consciousness.
   B. The patient's chest hit a support post during the fall.
   C. The patient's father is at work and cannot come to the hospital.
   D. The patient fell down eight steps before hitting the basement floor.

prep kit **33**

points to ponder

Object. 1-5.4, 2-1.2, 2-1.9, 2-1.17, 3-2.9

Shortly after your partner begins rescue breathing on an infant, you notice that the infant has developed significant stomach distention. You point it out to your partner and assist in treating it. Within a few breaths, it occurs again, and your partner chooses to ignore it. The infant's skin color is not returning to normal, and the distention is getting worse.

• What may be causing this? How would you get your partner to treat the problem? Would you take the infant away from your partner? What would you do for the infant?

online outlook

There are many causes of respiratory distress and failure in children. Although you might not be able to identify the exact cause in every patient, you must be able to intervene appropriately to restore breathing in all of them. To learn more about upper airway problems in children, complete Exercise 33 at www.emtb.com.

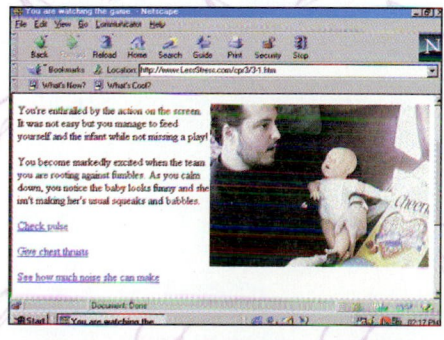

Pediatric Assessment and Medical Emergencies

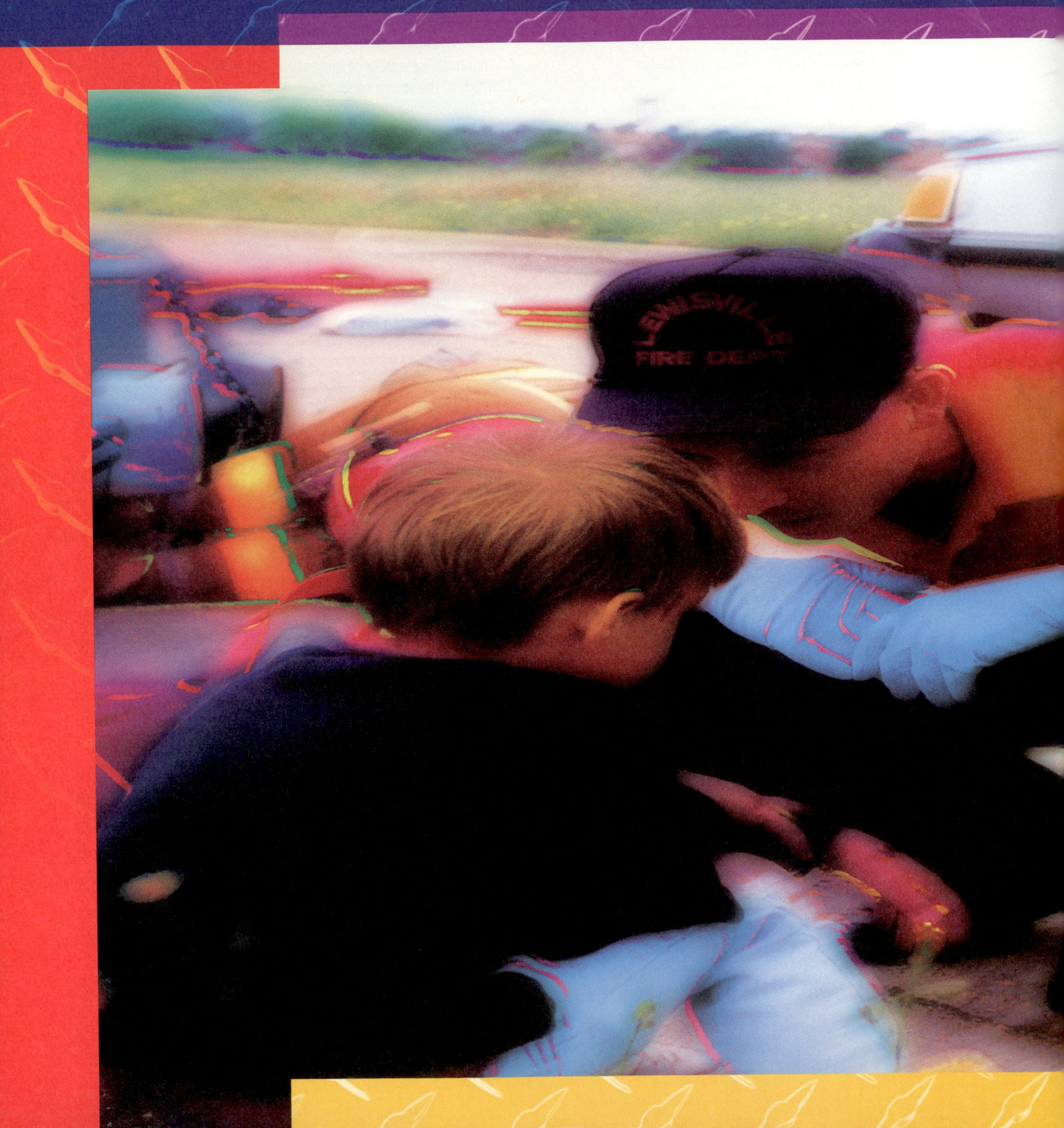

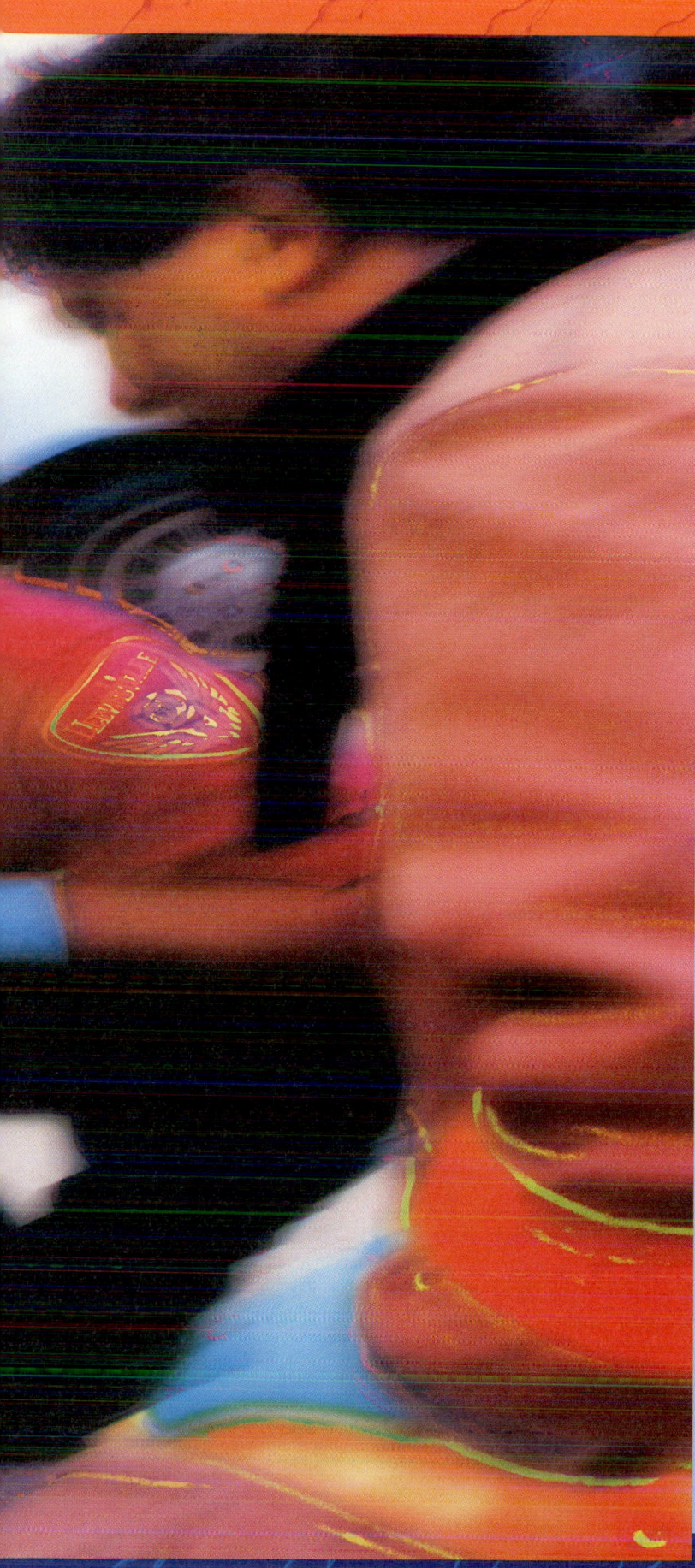

objectives

Cognitive

1. Identify the developmental considerations for the following age groups: infants, toddlers, preschool, school age, adolescent.

2. Describe differences in anatomy and physiology of the infant, child, and adult patient.

3. Differentiate the response of the ill or injured infant or child (age specific) from that of an adult.

4. Indicate various causes of respiratory emergencies.

5. Differentiate between respiratory distress and respiratory failure.

6. List the steps in the management of foreign body airway obstruction.

7. Summarize emergency medical care strategies for respiratory distress and respiratory failure.

8. Identify the signs and symptoms of shock (hypoperfusion) in the infant and child patient.

9. Describe the methods of determining end organ perfusion in the infant and child patient.

10. List the common causes of seizures in the infant and child patient.

11. Describe the management of seizures in the infant and child patient.

12. Recognize the need for EMT-Basic debriefing following a difficult infant or child transport.

Affective

13. Explain the rationale for having knowledge and skills appropriate for dealing with the infant and child patient.

14. Attend to the feelings of the family when dealing with an ill or injured infant or child.

15. Understand the provider's own response (emotional) to caring for infants or children.

Psychomotor

16. Demonstrate the techniques of foreign body airway obstruction removal in the infant.

17. Demonstrate the techniques of foreign body airway obstruction removal in the child.

18. Demonstrate the assessment of the infant and child.

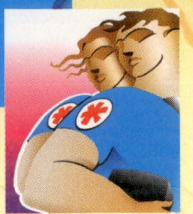

you are the emt

Squad 5, respond to 13422 Findley Avenue for "an unresponsive child." Also, please be advised that this is a duplex and you need to go to right, which is the B side.

A call involving an unresponsive child can be one of the most stressful, challenging, and difficult calls you will encounter. Over 1 million childhood poisonings occur each year alone and that just represents one possible cause for unresponsiveness in a child.

This chapter presents information on the most common pediatric emergencies that you will encounter as an EMT-B, and it will also help you to answer the following questions.

1. When it comes to emergencies, aren't pediatric patients just "little adults?"

2. Why do pediatric patients have more respiratory than cardiac problems?

Pediatric Assessment and Medical Emergencies

You will face some special challenges in caring for sick and injured children. Infants and children are not simply small adults. They come in a wide variety of sizes with anatomy and physiology that are different from those of adults. They cannot understand or use language as well as adults, if at all. In addition, caring for children usually means dealing with their caregivers at the same time. All these factors can complicate your job and, in many individuals, create extra anxiety.

However, once you learn how to approach children of different ages and what to expect while caring for them, you will find that they also offer some very special rewards. Not only are their innocence and openness appealing, but they often respond to treatment much more rapidly than adults do.

This chapter first describes the different developmental stages of childhood and provides some general advice on examining and coping with pain in children at each stage. The causes and management of airway obstruction from foreign objects are discussed next. Signs and symptoms of respiratory distress are then described, along with management techniques. The chapter then outlines the challenges of assessment and management of children with seizures, altered level of consciousness, poisoning, meningitis, shock, dehydration, and submersion injuries. Finally, an in-depth discussion of the troubling problem of sudden infant death syndrome (SIDS) and other circumstances of a child's death is presented. Some simple techniques for coping with the emotional stress surrounding the death of a child are presented in this section.

Growth and Development

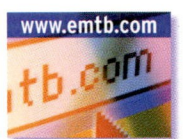

Adulthood begins at age 21. On this, the medical community has agreed. But when does childhood end? Many EMS systems use 18 years of age, others use 14, and still others use 12 or 16. Even though there are specific issues that are important to different age groups, there are also some general rules that apply when you care for children of any age (Table 34-1).

Between birth and adulthood, many physical and emotional changes occur in children. While each child is unique, the thoughts and behaviors of children as a whole are often grouped into stages: infancy, the toddler years, preschool age, school age, and adolescence. Children in each stage grapple with different developmental issues.

How you examine children and how you help them to cope with pain depend on several practical considerations, including the child's stability and mental status, the anticipated transport time, the availability of other personnel, and the protocols in your area. However, there are a number of simple techniques that will let you calm and comfort most children during emergency treatment and transport. Here are some suggestions about approaching and caring for the different age groups of childhood.

The Infant

Infancy is usually defined as the first year of life; the first month after birth is called the neonatal or newborn period. At first, infants respond mainly to physical stimuli such as light, warmth, cold, hunger, sound, and

TABLE 34-1 Helpful Tips in Caring for Infants and Children

1. **Try to remain calm and appear confident.** Children are used to having other people take charge. They are also easily frightened by noise, so speak with a soft voice whenever possible.

2. **Remember that you are caring for the whole family, not just the child.** Children are quick to pick up on their caregivers' anxiety. It may calm both parties if you can establish good rapport with the caregivers and allow them to help with the child's care. To avoid confusion, avoid using technical terms.

3. **Honesty is the best policy.** Telling a child or a caregiver that a procedure won't hurt (when you know that it will) or that it will be over quickly (when it won't) can boomerang: Once you lose their trust, any additional procedures that you attempt are more likely to meet with resistance.

4. **Tell both the caregivers and the child what is happening as often as you can.** Lack of information is very stressful for everyone; the

imagination can run wild in an effort to make sense of what is going on. In children, we call this frightening fantasies; in caregivers, we call it worst-case scenarios.

5. **Keep the family together as much as possible.** This is not always possible, but children and their caregivers generally feel safer when they are together. Parents can sometimes be encouraged to help by holding the child's hand, talking to the child, or telling a story

6. **Provide hope and reassurance to the caregivers and to the child.** Even when you are very concerned about the child's condition, be careful not to eliminate hope in patient and family. Children especially need reassurance, rewards, and praise during painful events. Remember that no one can be absolutely certain about the outcome. Children have an amazing ability to bounce back from what looks to be death's door.

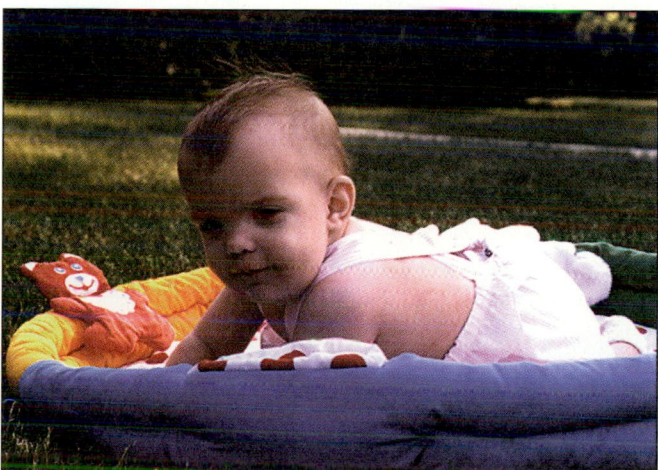

FIGURE 34-1 Infants are usually not afraid of strangers, but as they reach 6 months to 1 year, they may show signs that they prefer to be with their caregivers.

taste. Crying is one of their main avenues of expression during this period. After the first few months, however, they learn to coo, smile, roll over, and recognize their caregivers. Infants are usually not afraid of strangers, but they may show signs of preferring to be with their caregivers, particularly toward the end of the first year (Figure 34-1).

Begin your assessment by observing the infant from a distance, preferably in a caregiver's arms (Figure 34-2). Respirations, skin color, alertness, and level of activity provide a good overall picture of the infant's condition. Older infants, from 6 months to a year, may begin to cry when touched or picked up by a stranger, so let the caregiver continue to hold the baby as you start your examination. Warm your hands and the end of the stethoscope, then begin by listening to the chest and assessing the heart rate. Next examine the abdomen, then the head, and then the rest of the body.

Provide as much sensory comfort as you can: Keep the infant warm, and offer a pacifier if the caregiver allows it. Have a caregiver hold the infant, if possible, during procedures. Perform any painful procedure as quickly as you can.

The Toddler

After infancy, until about 3 years of age, a child is called a toddler. During this period, children begin to walk and to explore the environment. They are able to open doors, drawers, boxes, and bottles. Because of their fearlessness and increasing motor activity, injuries in this age group are more frequent.

Between birth and adulthood, many physical and emotional changes occur in children.

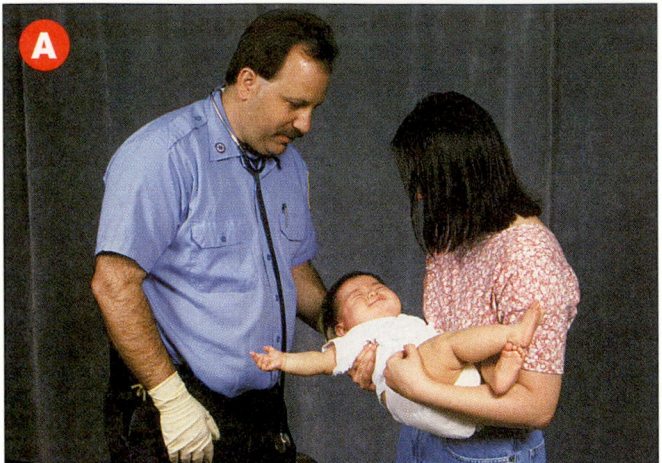

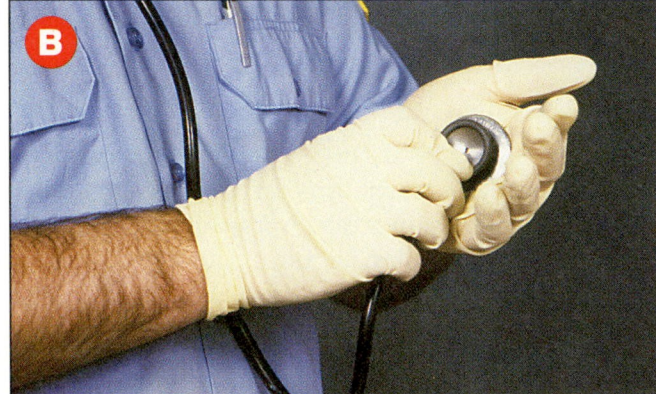

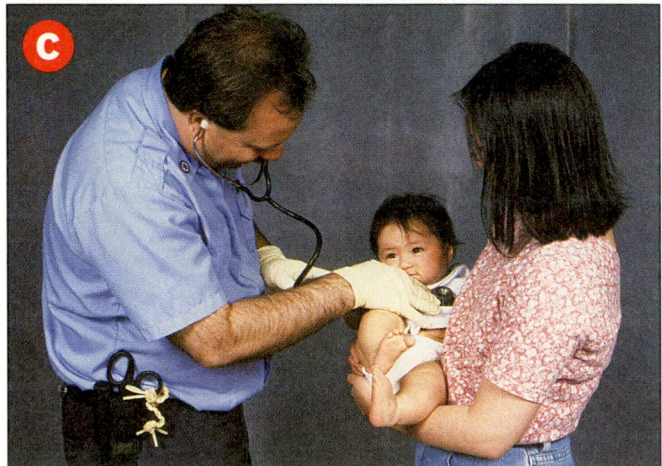

FIGURE 34-2 A: Begin assessing an infant from a distance, preferably in the caregiver's arms. **B:** Warm the end of the stethoscope with your hands. **C:** Listen to the chest and assess heart rate first.

Stranger anxiety may develop early in this period (Figure 34-3). Toddlers may resist separation from caregivers and be afraid to let others come near them. Because of their newly found independence, they may also be very unhappy about being restrained or held for procedures. Two-year-olds in particular have a well-deserved reputation for having their own ideas about almost everything, which is why these years are often called the "terrible twos."

Make as many observations as you can before touching the child: level of alertness, skin color, respirations. When appropriate, examine the child on the caregiver's lap, and use toys or puppets to distract him or her (Figure 34-4).

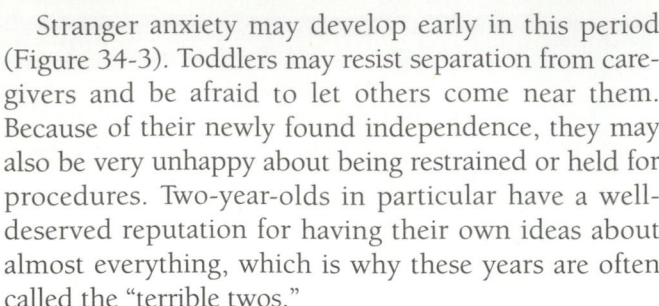

FIGURE 34-3 Because of their newly found independence, toddlers may be unhappy about being restrained or held for procedures.

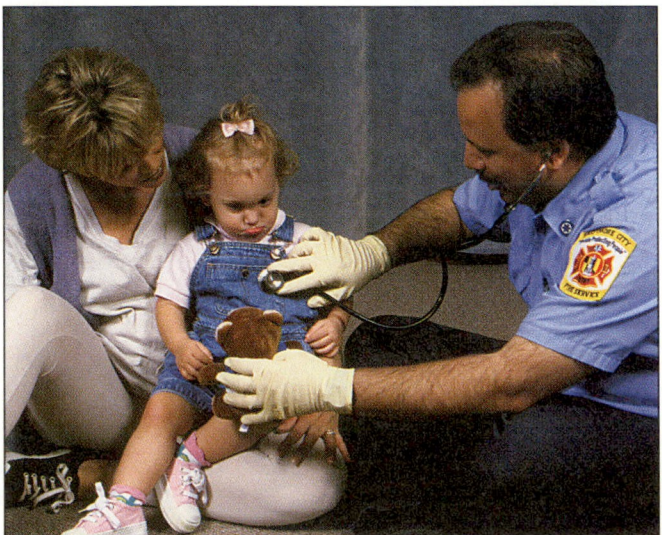

FIGURE 34-4 Leave a toddler on the caregiver's lap during your assessment, and use a toy to distract him or her.

Toddlers can be curious and adventuresome, so you may able to distract them. For example, you might allow the child to play with a tongue depressor. Restrain the child for as short a time as possible, and allow him or her to be comforted immediately after a painful procedure.

The Preschool-Age Child

Preschool-age children (age 3 to 6 years) are able to use simple language quite effectively and have lively imaginations (Figure 34-5). They can understand directions, be much more specific in describing their sensations, and identify painful areas when questioned. Much of their history must still be obtained from caregivers, however. Preschool-age children have a rich fantasy life, which can make them particularly fearful about pain and change involving their bodies. At this age, they often believe that their thoughts or wishes can cause injury or harm to themselves or to others.

Try to distract the child during the examination with simple conversation and questions, or use a toy, game, or puppet. Make the examination less threatening by allowing the child to handle some pieces of equipment, such as your stethoscope or a tongue blade (Figure 34-6). Do not use words that suggest invading the child's body, such as "shot," "cut," "poke," or "stick."

Tell the child what you are going to do immediately before you do it; this way, the child has no time to develop frightening fantasies. At this age, children are easily distracted with counting games, small toys, or conversation. Be sure to adjust the level of game to the developmental level of the child; health care providers often assume that preschool children understand more than they actually do. Use adhesive bandages to cover the site of an injection or other small wound, because the child might be worried about keeping his or her body together in one piece.

The School-Age Child

School-age children (age 6 to 12 years) usually are becoming more like adults. They can think in concrete terms, respond sensibly to direct questions, and help take care of themselves. Your assessment, therefore, is more like an adult assessment; talk to the child, not just the parent, in taking the medical history (Figure 34-7).

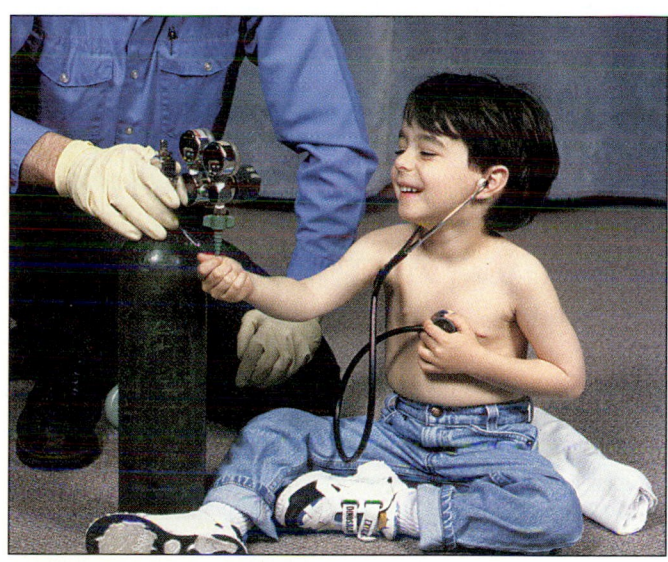

FIGURE 34-6 Make the exam less threatening by allowing the patient to handle some pieces of equipment.

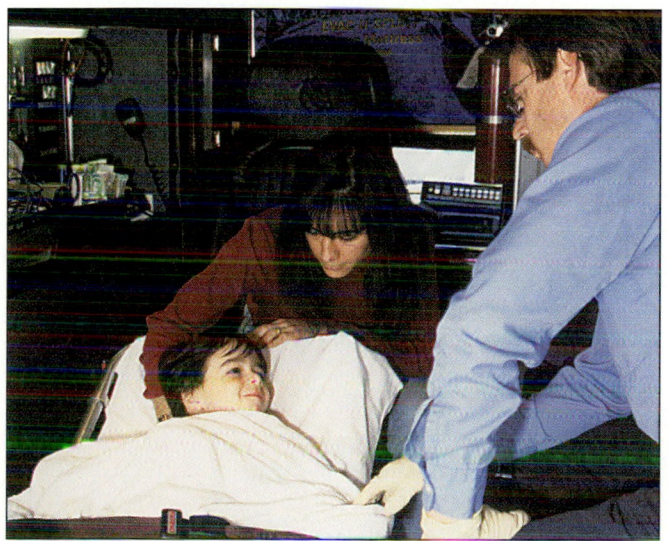

FIGURE 34-5 Preschool children have a vivid imagination, so much of the history must still be obtained from the caregiver.

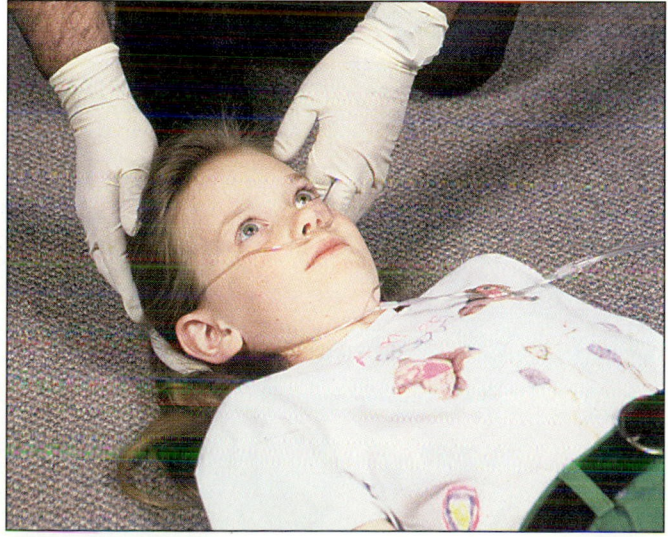

FIGURE 34-7 School-age children are more like adults in that they can answer your questions and can help to take care of themselves.

> Even though there are specific issues that are important to different age groups, there are also some general rules that apply when you care for children of any age.

The school-age child is usually familiar with the process of physical examination. Whenever possible, give the child choices: Would you like to sit up or lie down? Would you like to take off your clothes yourself? Encourage cooperation by allowing the child to listen to his or her own heartbeat through the stethoscope (Figure 34-8).

School-age children can understand the difference between emotional and physical pain; they have concerns about the meaning of pain. Give them simple explanations about what is causing their pain and what will be done about it (Figure 34-9). Games and conversation may distract them. Ask them to describe their favorite place, their pets, or their toys. Ask the caregiver's advice in choosing the right distraction. Rewarding the school-age child after a procedure can be very helpful in his or her recovery.

The Adolescent

Most adolescents (age 12 to 18 years) are able to think abstractly and can participate in decision making. They are very concerned about body image and how they appear to their peers and to others. They may have very strong feelings about being observed during procedures, even—or especially—by their caregivers.

Respect the adolescent's privacy at all times. Remember that adolescents can often understand very complex concepts and treatment options; you should provide them with information when they request it (Figure 34-10). You will find them more helpful and understanding of necessary procedures.

Adolescents have a clear understanding of the purpose and meaning of pain. Whenever possible, explain any necessary procedures well in advance. Assess their pain by facial and body expression as well as by asking questions; adolescents can be very stoic and may not request relief from pain even when they need it. To distract them, find out what they are interested in, such as sports, books, movies, or friends, and get them talking about this.

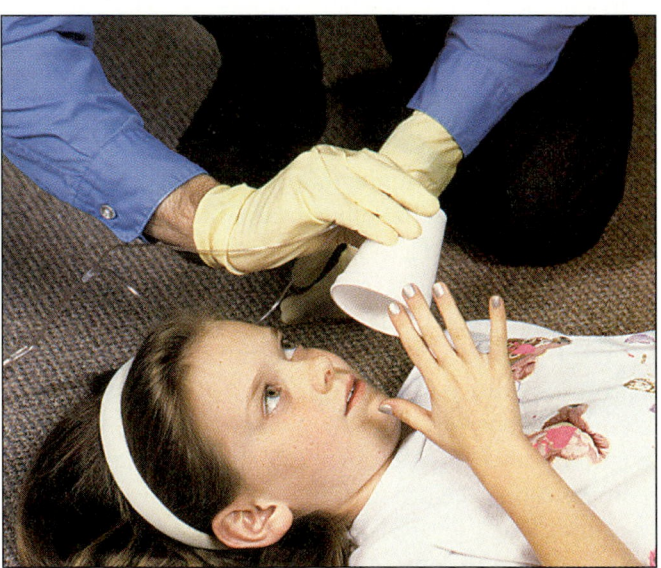

FIGURE 34-9 School-age children can understand simple explanations about their physical condition and the need for simple procedures.

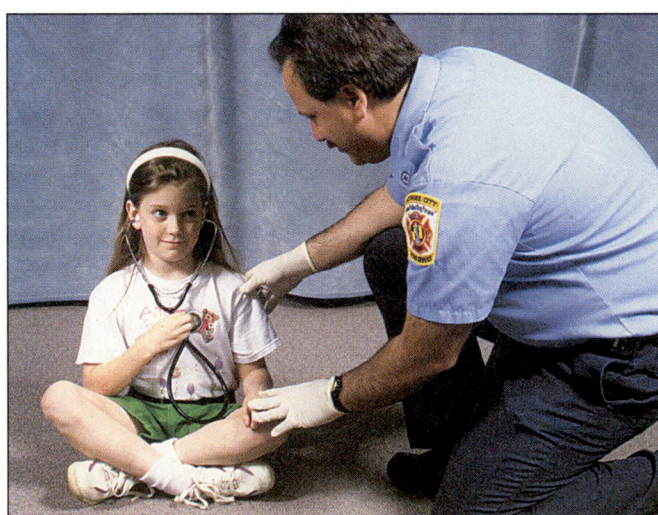

FIGURE 34-8 Encourage cooperation by allowing the child to listen to his or her own heartbeat through the stethoscope.

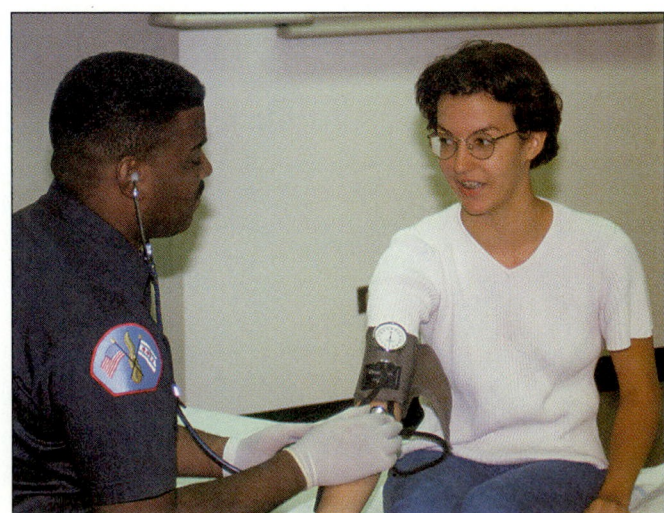

FIGURE 34-10 Respect the adolescent's privacy at all times; give the patient whatever information he or she requests.

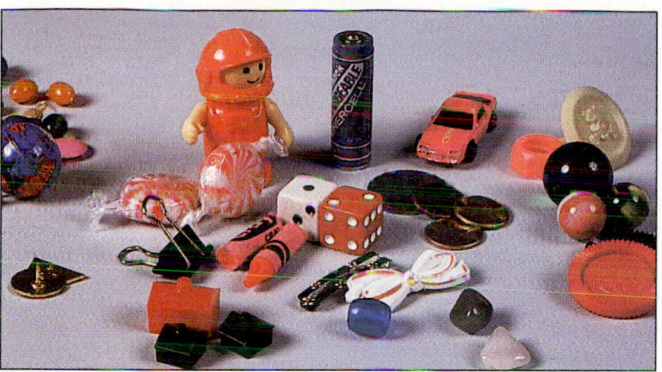

FIGURE 34-11 Any number of objects can obstruct a child's airway Some of the more common include batteries, coins, toys, buttons, and candy.

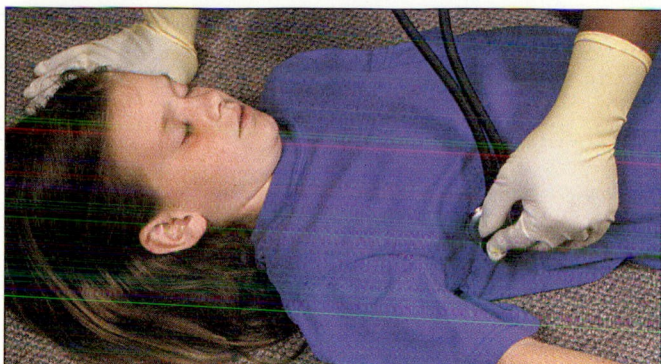

FIGURE 34-13 The best way to auscultate breath sounds in children is to listen on both sides of the chest at the level of the armpit.

Airway Obstruction

Children, especially those under age 5 years, can (and do) obstruct their airway with any object that they can fit into their mouth: hot dogs, balloons, grapes, coins (Figure 34-11). In cases of trauma, a child's teeth may have been dislodged into the airway. Blood, vomitus, or other secretions can also cause partial or complete obstruction.

Another source of airway obstructions is infections, including pneumonia, croup, and epiglottitis (Figure 34-12). **Croup** is an infection of the airway below the level of the vocal cords, usually caused by a virus. **Epiglottitis** is an infection of the soft tissue in the area above the vocal cords. Infection should be considered as a possible cause of airway obstruction if a child has congestion, fever, drooling, and cold symptoms. Such children must be taken immediately to the emergency department. Without special equipment and training, attempts to clear an airway that is blocked by infection can worsen the obstruction.

Signs and Symptoms

Obstruction by a foreign object may involve the upper or the lower airway. Signs and symptoms that are frequently associated with an upper airway obstruction include decreased or absent breath sounds and **stridor**, which is caused by swelling of the area surrounding the vocal cords. Stridor has been described as a high-pitched noise heard mainly on inspiration. In children with croup, it resembles the bark of a seal.

Signs and symptoms of a lower airway obstruction include **wheezing**, a whistling sound caused by air traveling through narrowed air passages within the bronchioles, and/or **rales**. Rales are caused by the flow of air through liquid, present in the air pouches and smaller airways in the lungs. They produce a crackling sound like that of blowing bubbles through a straw in a glass filled with liquid. The best way to auscultate breath sounds in a child is to listen on both sides of the chest at the level of the armpit (Figure 34-13).

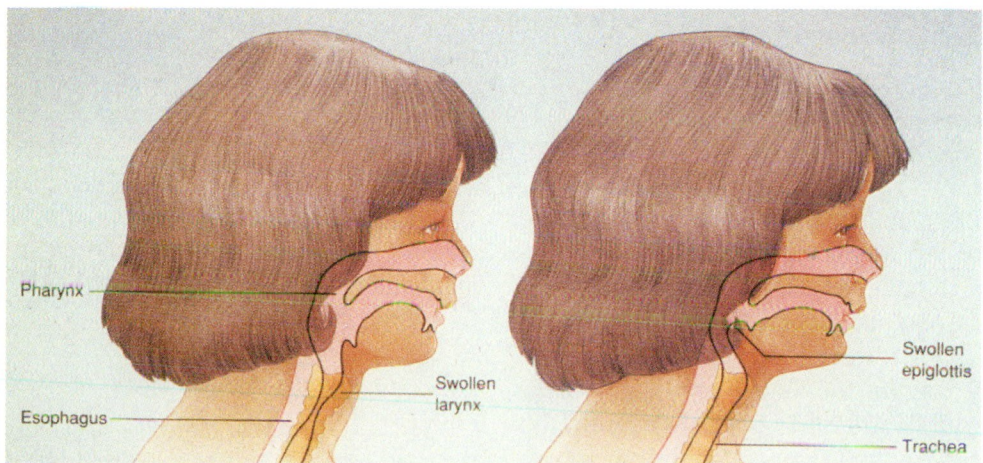

FIGURE 34-12 Croup and epiglottitis are infections that also cause airway obstruction in children.

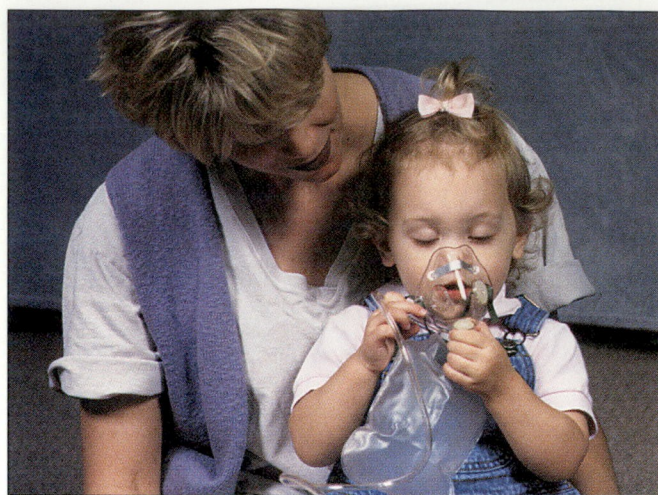

FIGURE 34-14 If a child has a partial airway obstruction, do not intervene except to give supplemental oxygen and allow the child to remain in whatever position is most comfortable.

Emergency Medical Care

Treatment of the child with an airway obstruction depends on whether or not the patient is unconscious and whether the obstruction is partial or complete.

If the child is conscious and you know for sure that there is a foreign body in the airway—that is, if someone actually saw the object go into the child's mouth—encourage the child to cough to clear the airway. If the obstruction is not complete, that is, if the material in the airway does not completely block the flow of air, the child may be able to breathe adequately on his or her own without any intervention. If the obstruction is only partial, do not intervene except to provide supplemental oxygen (Figure 34-14). Allow the child to remain in whatever position is most comfortable, and monitor his or her condition.

If you see signs of complete obstruction, however, you must attempt to clear the airway at once. The signs include the following:

- Ineffective cough (no sound)
- Inability to cry
- Increasing respiratory difficulty, with stridor
- Cyanosis
- Loss of consciousness

Management of airway obstruction in a child.

If there is reason to believe that an unconscious child has a foreign body obstruction, check the upper airway to see whether the obstructing object is visible. The best way to do this is to grasp the tongue and jaw between your finger and thumb and lift to open the mouth; this is called the tongue-jaw lift (Figure 34-15). If the object is visible, try to remove it using a finger sweep motion.

Never use finger sweeps in infants or children if you cannot see the object, as you may push it further into the airway.

Abdominal thrusts are recommended to relieve a complete airway obstruction in a child. These thrusts increase the pressure in the chest, creating an artificial cough that may force a foreign body from the airway.

The following steps are used to apply abdominal thrusts to the unconscious child who you suspect has a foreign body airway obstruction (Figure 34-16):

1. **Place the child** in a supine position on a firm, flat surface.

2. **Inspect the upper airway** using the tongue-jaw lift. If you see the foreign object, try to remove it.

3. **Attempt rescue breathing.** If the first try is unsuccessful, reposition the child's head and try again.

4. **If ventilation is still unsuccessful,** kneel beside or straddle the child's hips. Place the heel of one hand on the front of the child's abdomen just above the navel and well below the rib cage and sternum. Place your other hand on top of the first hand.

5. **Press both hands into the abdomen** in an upward motion, giving five distinct thrusts.

6. **Open the airway** using the tongue-jaw lift. If you see the foreign body, remove it.

7. **Attempt rescue breathing.** If the foreign body is not expelled on the first attempt, reposition the child's head and try again.

8. **If the airway remains obstructed,** repeat the abdominal thrusts.

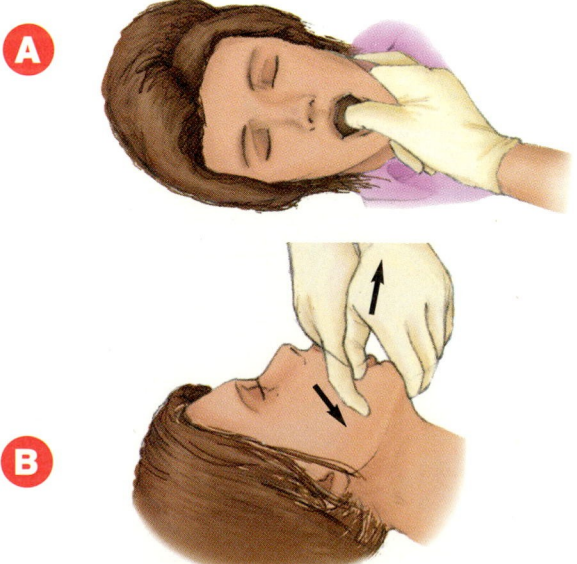

FIGURE 34-15 A: Use the tongue-jaw lift to open the mouth in an unconscious child. **B:** If the object is visible, try to remove it by using a finger sweep.

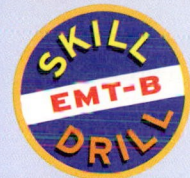

Removing Foreign Body Airway Obstruction in an Unconscious Child
Figure 34-16

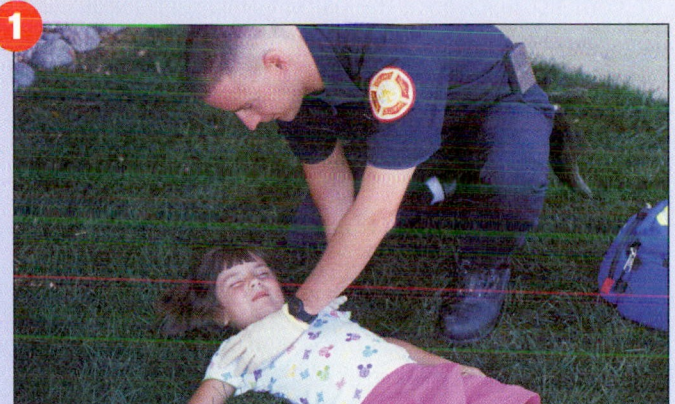

Place the child in a supine position on a firm, flat surface.

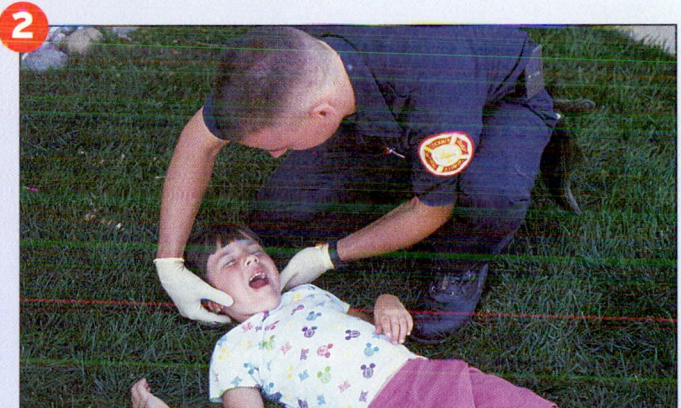

Inspect the airway. If you see a foreign object, try to remove it.

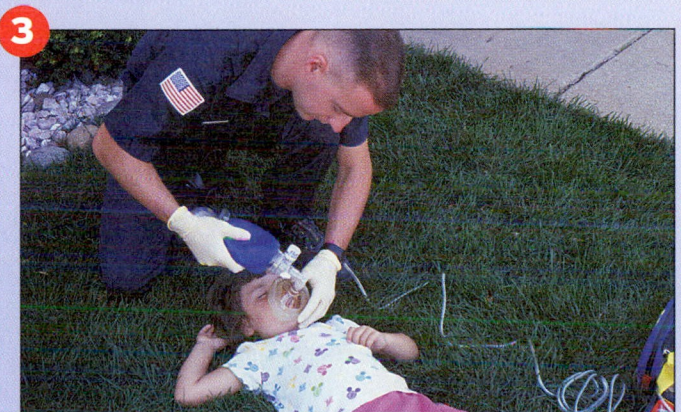

Attempt artificial ventilation.

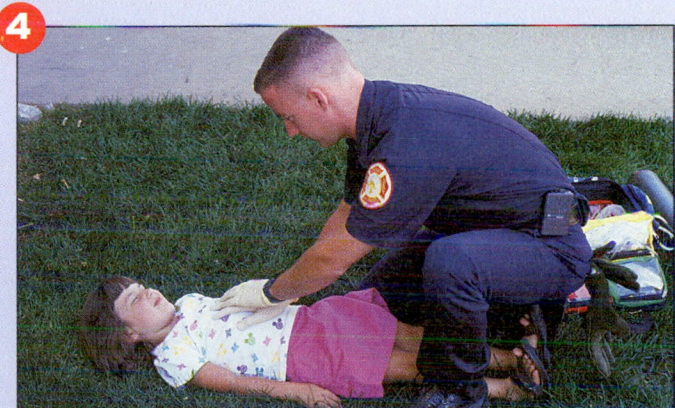

If ventilation is unsuccessful, kneel beside or straddle the child's hips. Place the heel of one hand on the front of the child's abdomen just above the navel. Place your other hand on top of the first hand. Press both hands into the abdomen in an upward motion, giving five distinct thrusts.

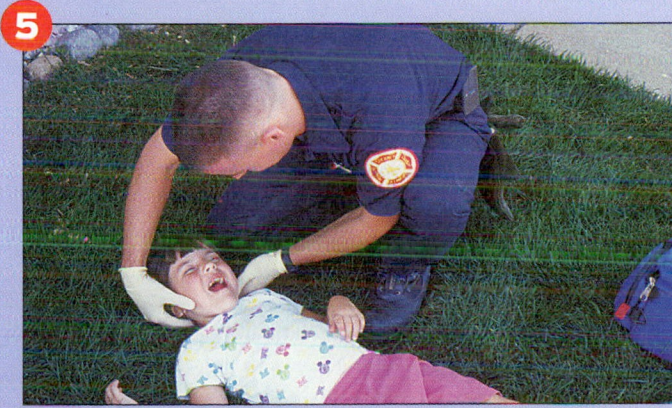

Open the airway again to try to see the object.

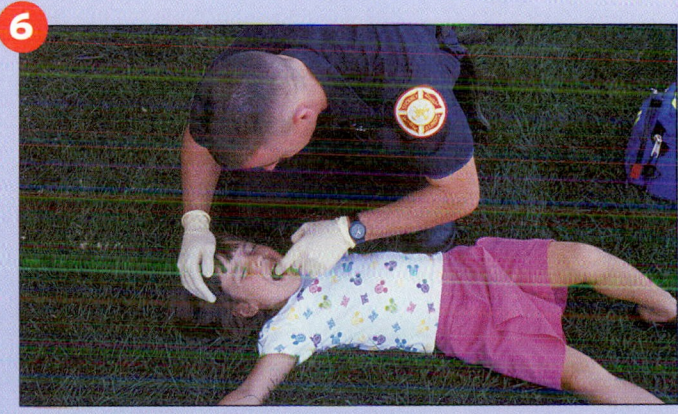

Remove the object only if you can see it.

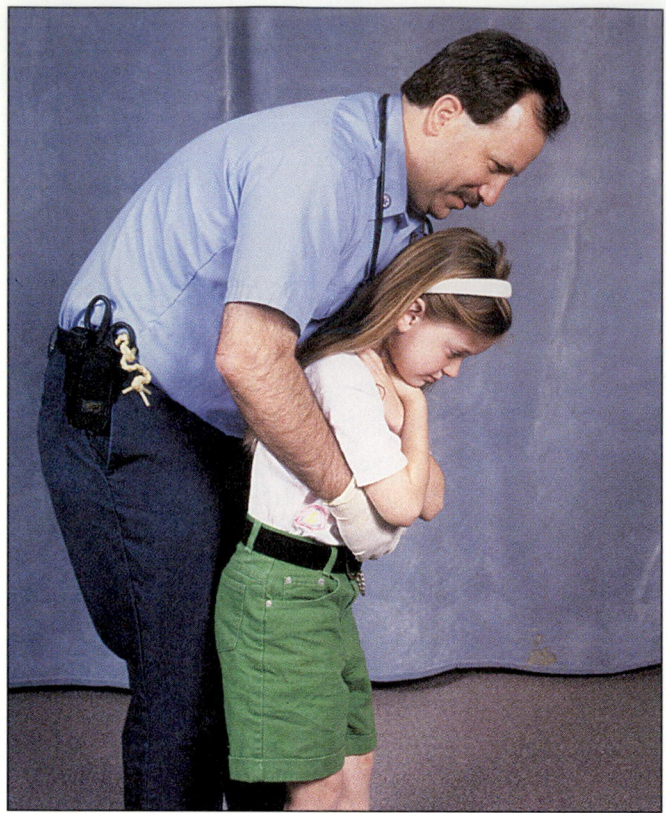

FIGURE 34-17 Stand behind the child, and circle his or her body with both arms. Place your fist just above the patient's navel and well below the lower tip of the sternum.

The following steps are used to remove a foreign body obstruction from a conscious child who is in a standing or sitting position (Figure 34-17):

1. **Stand behind the child,** and circle his or her body with both arms around the patient's chest. Place your fist just above the patient's navel and well below the lower tip of the sternum.

2. **Give the child five rapid,** distinct abdominal thrusts in an upward direction. Be careful to avoid applying force to the lower rib cage or sternum.

3. **Repeat this standing technique** until the child expels the foreign body or fully loses consciousness.

4. **If the child becomes unconscious,** inspect the airway using the tongue-jaw lift. If you see the foreign body, try to remove it.

5. **Attempt rescue breathing.** If the first attempt fails, reposition the head and try again.

6. **If the airway remains obstructed,** repeat the abdominal thrusts.

If you manage to clear the airway obstruction in an unconscious child but he or she remains without a pulse or spontaneous breathing, perform CPR, using the usual BLS sequence.

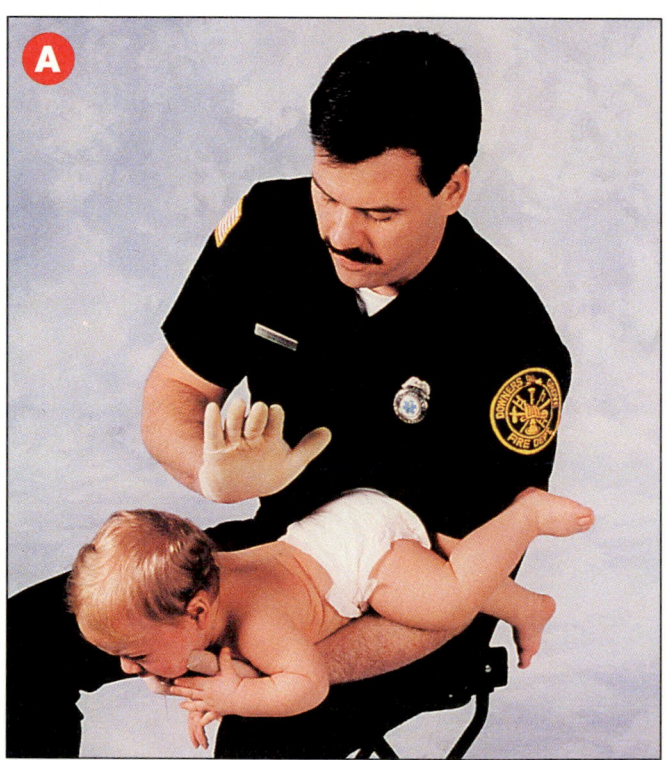
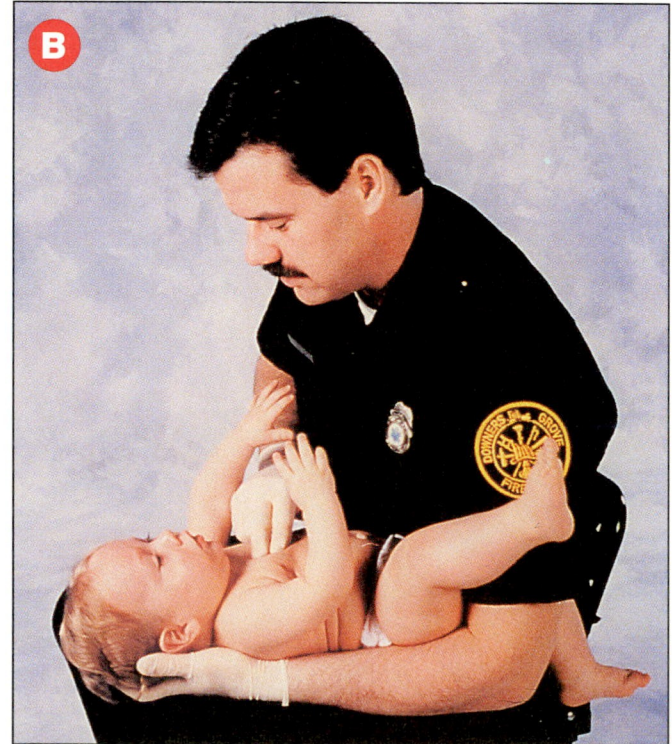

FIGURE 34-18 A: Hold the infant face down with the body resting on your forearm. Support the jaw and face with your hand, and keep the head lower than the rest of the body. Give the infant five back blows between the shoulder blades, using the heel of your hand. **B:** Give the infant five quick chest thrusts, using two fingers placed on the lower half of the sternum.

Management of airway obstruction in an infant. Abdominal thrusts are not recommended for infants because of the risk of injury to the immature organs of the abdomen. Instead, use back blows and chest thrusts to try to clear a complete airway obstruction in an infant, as follows (Figure 34-18):

1. **Hold the infant face down,** with the body resting on your forearm. Support the infant's jaw and face with your hand, and keep the head lower than the rest of the body.

2. **Deliver five back blows** between the shoulder blades, using the heel of your hand.

3. **Place your free hand** behind the infant's head and back, and bring the infant upright on your thigh, sandwiching the infant's body between your two hands and arms. The infant's head should remain below the level of the body.

4. **Give the infant five quick chest thrusts** in the same location and manner as chest compressions, using two fingers placed on the lower half of the sternum. For larger infants, or if you have small hands, you can perform this step by placing the infant in your lap and turning the infant's whole body as a unit between back blows and chest thrusts.

5. **Check the infant's airway.** If you can see the foreign body now, remove it. If not, repeat the cycle as often as necessary.

6. **If, after removal of the object,** the infant is still unconscious, perform CPR.

If the infant regains consciousness, keep him or her in the recovery position during transport.

Respiratory Emergencies

In the early stages of respiratory distress or failure, respirations may be too slow or too fast for the patient's age. This suggests that gases are not moving effectively into and out of the lungs. If, like most people, you find it hard to memorize normal vital sign ranges for infants and children, keep reference charts handy for this purpose. Respirations of greater than 60 breaths/min are a sign of a problem. In most cases, you should begin to assist ventilation immediately, even if the child appears to be breathing adequately. But remember, you are treating the child, not the numbers. A child breathing 60 times a minute who is playing happily does not need assisted ventilation; a child breathing 60 times a minute who is lying unconscious on the floor does.

Signs and Symptoms

In the early stages of respiratory distress, you may also note changes in the child's behavior, such as combativeness, restlessness, and anxiety. As the body attempts to maximize the amount of air going into the lungs, it works harder at breathing. Signs and symptoms of extra effort include the following:

- Nasal flaring, as the body tries to increase the size of the airway
- Grunting respirations, as the body attempts to keep the alveoli expanded at the end of expiration
- Accessory (intercostal) muscle use; remember that in children, the diaphragm is the major muscle of ventilation
- Retractions, or movements of the child's flexible rib cage

As the child progresses to possible respiratory failure, efforts to breathe decrease; the chest rises less with inspiration. A definite diagnosis of respiratory failure is made in the hospital. The body has used up its available energy stores and cannot continue to support the extra work of breathing under these conditions. At this point, cyanosis may develop. Be aware that not all children become cyanotic. You should be just as concerned about a child with pale skin as one with bluish skin.

Changes in behavior will also occur until the child demonstrates an altered level of consciousness. The patient may experience periods without respirations, a condition called **apnea**. As the lack of oxygen becomes more serious, the heart muscle itself becomes hypoxic and slows down. This leads to **bradycardia**, a condition in which the heart rate is less than 60 beats/min in children or less than 80 beats/min in infants. Bradycardia is almost always related to a lack of oxygen and is an ominous sign in pediatric patients. If the heart rate is fast, you need to investigate the cause. However, if the heart rate is slow or absent, you must intervene immediately. Without aggressive airway management, bradycardia may quickly progress to cardiopulmonary arrest.

Of course, respiratory failure does not always indicate airway obstruction. It may indicate trauma, problems with the nervous system, dehydration (often caused by vomiting and diarrhea), or metabolic disturbances.

> Respirations of greater than 60 breaths/min are a sign of a problem.

For example, a child with diabetes might have a blood glucose level that is too high or too low; or a child might have a pH imbalance, as can happen with some rare childhood diseases. Regardless of the cause, your first step is always to focus on ensuring adequate oxygenation and ventilation.

Never forget that a child can progress from respiratory distress to respiratory failure at any time. For this reason, you must reassess the child frequently.

Emergency Medical Care

A child or infant in respiratory distress or possible respiratory failure needs supplemental oxygen. Remember, anxiety, agitation, or crying may increase the effort or work of breathing, so use whichever method seems least upsetting to the child: mask, blow-by, or nasal cannula. You may need to get creative by distracting the child with games, a toy, or talking (Figure 34-19).

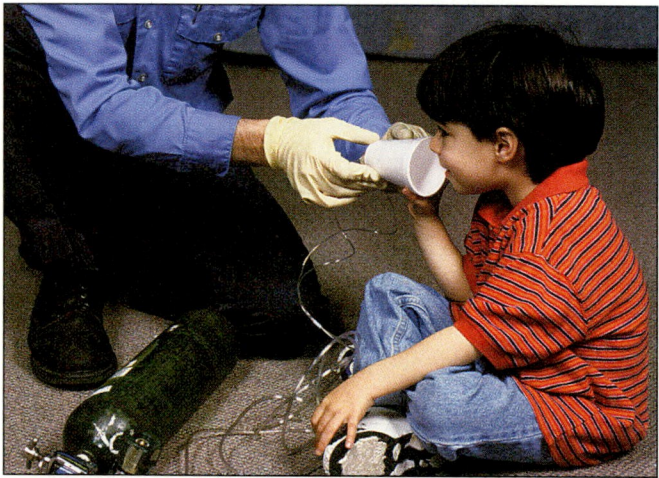

FIGURE 34-19 A child in respiratory distress needs supplemental oxygen; you should select whichever method seems least upsetting to the child.

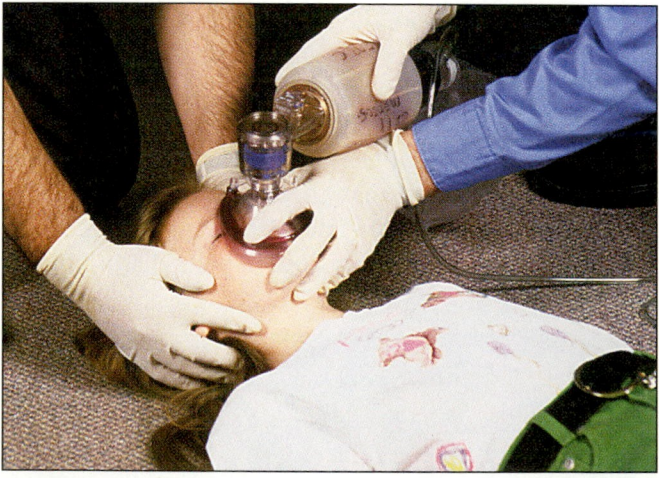

FIGURE 34-20 For an unconscious child, the best way to deliver oxygen is via a BVM device connected to high-flow oxygen.

Allow the child to remain in a comfortable position. For a small child, this may mean sitting on the caregiver's lap. Give nothing by mouth, in case the child's condition deteriorates suddenly.

If the patient has progressed to respiratory failure, you must begin assisted ventilation immediately and continue to provide supplemental oxygen. The best way to do this is with the BVM device connected to high-flow oxygen, *without* using an oral or nasopharyngeal airway (Figure 34-20). However, if the patient is unconscious, you should insert an oral airway. If a BVM device is not available, use mouth-to-mask rescue breathing; if you run into problems in ventilating the patient, you may need an airway adjunct. Make sure you have the proper equipment and are ventilating at the proper rate.

Reassess the patient at regular intervals, and be prepared to make appropriate adjustments if the patient's condition changes.

Seizures

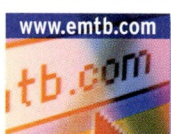

A seizure is the result of disorganized electrical activity in the brain. It can be very frightening to people around the patient. Therefore, it is important to reassure the family and to approach assessment and management in a calm, step-by-step manner.

Signs and Symptoms

Seizures in children may appear in several different ways, including shaking of the whole body or movement in just a single arm or leg. Seizures can also appear as lip smacking, eyes blinking, or staring off into space. The movements in a seizure are described as <u>tonic-clonic</u> if there is a rhythmic, back-and forth motion of an extremity and body stiffness. If the extremity is rigid and cannot be made to relax, the seizure is called <u>tonic</u>. <u>Myoclonic jerks</u> are short jerks of an extremity without the rhythmic back-and-forth motions that are found in tonic-clonic seizures. In a true seizure, movements cannot be stopped on command or by holding an extremity. The duration of movement varies from patient to patient.

There are several general categories of seizures. In the course of an epileptic episode, a patient may experience one or more of these types of seizures:

- **Generalized (grand mal) seizures** appear as back-and-forth motions of both upper and lower extremities. The patient is unresponsive to verbal commands or painful stimulation.

- **Partial seizures** may appear as movement in one limb, lip smacking, or eye deviation only (eyes turned to either side or up or down).

- **Absence (petit mal) seizures** appear as an unresponsiveness with or without any movement and may last seconds to minutes.

Altered mental status and the inability of others to stop a movement or range or movements in the affected limb are common to all seizures. Some patients may feel pins and needles, hear sounds, and see hallucinations. In all but absence seizures, there is a <u>postictal period</u> of extreme fatigue or unresponsiveness after the seizure for anywhere from a few minutes to several hours. During this time, the patient may appear sleepy and/or confused and is not able to interact appropriately.

A short period of seizure activity (under 30 minutes) is not in itself harmful to the patient. After 30 to 45 minutes, however, the brain may run low on energy stores, and continued activity can be harmful. <u>Status epilepticus</u> is the term that is used when a patient has had a continuous seizure or multiple seizures without a return to consciousness for 30 minutes.

Complications of seizure activity are due to injury from the seizure motion, airway obstruction, or poor breathing effort. Many patients injure themselves by hitting objects around them during a seizure. For this reason, you should take care to pad the stretcher and avoid placing hard objects, such as air tanks and monitors, near the patient.

Contrary to common belief, a person who is experiencing an epileptic seizure will not "swallow his or her tongue"; therefore, you should not try to force a spoon or other object into the mouth. This can cause dental and/or oral trauma, including bleeding and broken teeth, both of which pose a risk of airway obstruction. Remember that the tongue in a pediatric patient is proportionately larger than that in the adult and can become an obstruction if the patient is not positioned correctly. Other sources of obstruction during seizures include secretions or vomitus, and you should be ready to suction.

If you can identify the cause of the seizure, you will be better able to monitor the patient for any potential complications associated with the underlying problem (Table 34-2). In particular, be alert to the presence of medications, possible poisons, and indications of abuse or neglect.

Febrile Seizures

Febrile seizures are common in children between the ages of 6 months and 6 years. These seizures typically occur on the first day of a febrile illness, are characterized by generalized tonic-clonic seizure activity, and last less than 15 minutes with a short postictal phase or none at all. They may be a sign of a more serious problem, such

TABLE 34-2 Common Causes of Seizures
• Child abuse
• Electrolyte imbalance
• Fever
• Hypoglycemia (low blood glucose level)
• Idiopathic (no cause can be found)
• Infection
• Ingestion
• Lack of oxygen
• Medications
• Poisoning
• Previous seizure disorder
• Recreational drug use
• Trauma

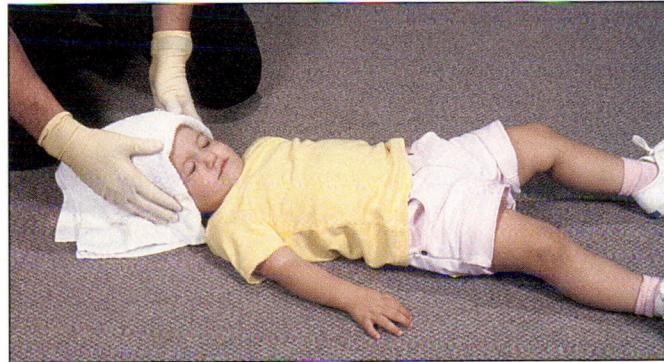

FIGURE 34-21 Following a febrile seizure, carefully assess the child's ABCD. Then begin cooling measures, and prepare the child for transport.

as meningitis. Obtain a history from the caregivers, as these children may have a history of a prior febrile seizure.

If you are called to care for a child who has had a febrile seizure, you often will find that the patient is awake, alert, and fully interactive when you arrive. Keep in mind that a persistent fever can lead to another seizure. Carefully assess ABCD, begin cooling measures, and provide prompt transport, as all children with febrile seizures need to be seen in the hospital setting (Figure 34-21).

Emergency Medical Care

Although medical management of seizures in the hospital setting may vary according to cause, your assessment and management of these patients remain essentially the same from patient to patient. First, ensure that the scene is safe for you and your partner and for the patient. Next, perform an initial assessment, focusing on ABCD. If possible, obtain a brief history from the caregivers about previous serious illnesses or seizures and current medication or trauma.

Securing and protecting the airway are your priority. To avoid obstruction from the tongue falling back into the airway, place a child who is having a seizure or who is postictal on his or her side (Figure 34-22). In the case of trauma, place the head in a neutral in-line position and ensure that the cervical spine is protected with spinal precautions. Be ready to use suction to prevent aspiration of stomach contents, blood, or vomitus. Do not place your fingers in the mouth of a patient who is having a seizure.

A patient who is actively seizing or who is postictal may not be breathing adequately. Assessing the rate and depth of respirations in this situation can be difficult but is essential. Patients may have shallow, rapid breathing or may have occasional deep respirations. Signs that a patient is not breathing adequately include the following:

- Very slow respirations
- Very shallow breaths
- Bluish tint to lips or pale lips
- Snoring respirations caused by the tongue blocking the airway

Deliver oxygen by mask, blow-by, or nasal cannula. If there are no signs of improvement, begin BVM ventilation with appropriately sized equipment.

Patients who are experiencing a seizure usually maintain adequate blood pressure and pulse rate unless the seizure is caused by an underlying circulatory or neurologic problem or trauma, including bleeding, heart

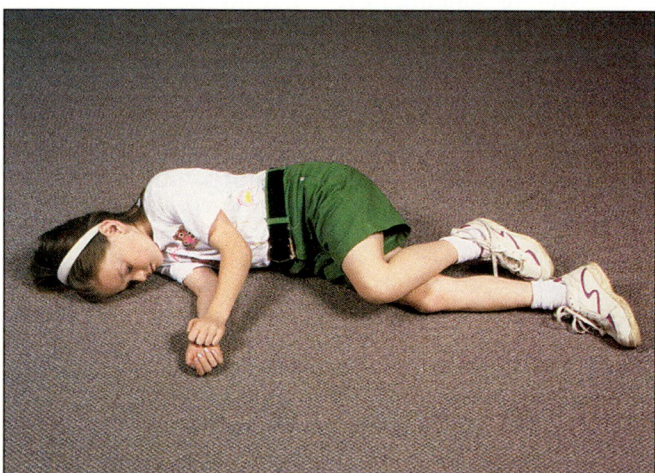

FIGURE 34-22 A child in the postictal state following a seizure should be placed on his or her side.

problems, brain injury, or multi-focal injury. Nevertheless, you must evaluate the pulse and blood pressure and *re-evaluate* them. Place the patient on a cardiac monitor if you are trained to do so and carry this equipment.

Once ABCD has been addressed, assessment and management should proceed as follows. If the patient is actively seizing, note the type of movement and position of the eyes, as this information may be very helpful for hospital staff in making a diagnosis. If there is a fever, begin cooling measures such as removing clothing and placing towels moistened with tepid water on the child. A child with febrile seizures can seize again if the temperature remains high. *Do not use alcohol or cold water to cool a patient.* Make sure the patient is protected from hitting the sides of the stretcher or nearby equipment. Bring any medications or possible poisons at the scene to the hospital with the patient. If patient is in status epilepticus, call for ALS backup, as medication is required to stop the seizures. In fact, you should always call for ALS backup when appropriate.

Altered Level of Consciousness

People who are aware of themselves and their surroundings are said to be *conscious*. Nonverbal infants may demonstrate consciousness by following a person's face or an object (tracking), by babbling and cooing, or by crying. Infants and children may exhibit an <u>altered level of consciousness</u> (also called altered mental status) in many ways, including lack of response to vocal commands and pain, combative behavior, confusion, thrashing about, drifting into and out of an alert state, or a change in the pitch and nature of their cry. Be aware of the many terms that are used to describe an altered level of consciousness, including coma, delirium, and stupor. However, you should avoid using all of these terms, as none are accurate.

Common causes of altered level of consciousness in a pediatric patient include the following:

- Head trauma
- Shock
- Meningitis
- Seizures
- Brain tumor
- Intracranial bleeding
- Metabolic disease such as diabetes
- Low blood glucose
- Severe dehydration
- Lack of oxygen to the brain
- Stroke

Your first step in caring for a patient with an altered level of consciousness is to assess ABCD and provide appropriate care as necessary. As you determine responsiveness, remember to use the AVPU scale. Then obtain a brief history from the patient's caregivers, focusing on the following points:

- Does the patient have any illnesses?
- Does the patient take any medications? When was the last dose?
- Did the patient ingest any substances (eg, poisons, drugs, or plant material)?
- Has the patient been ill?
- Has the patient had any behavior problems?

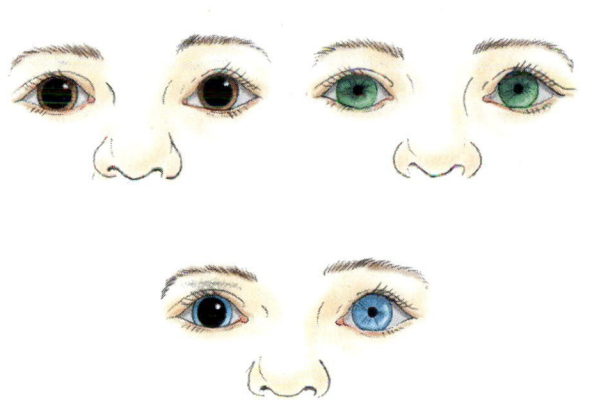

FIGURE 34-23 Observe a child's eyes for changes in pupillary size.

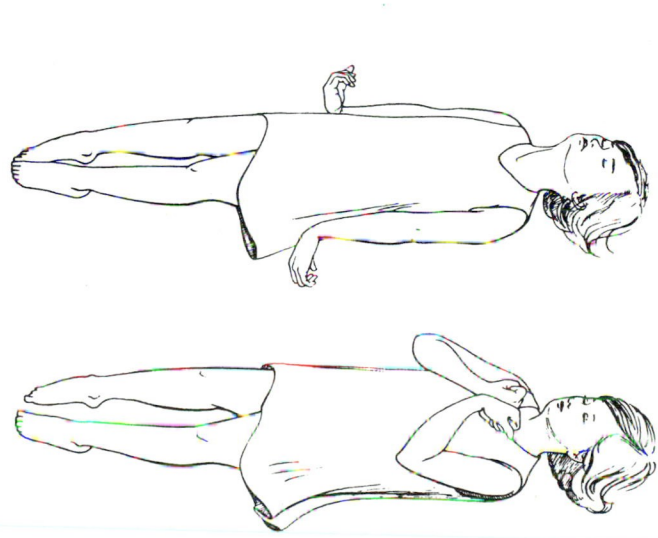

FIGURE 34-24 Observe a child for posturing.

Next, observe the child's pupils: Are they dilated or pinpoint? Do they react to a light by constricting (Figure 34-23)? Are the eyes turned to the right, left, up, or down? Is the child staring without moving his/her eyes? Is the child posturing (Figure 34-24)?

Once you have completed your initial assessment, immediately secure the airway. If respirations are inadequate, provide assisted ventilation with a BVM device. If you suspect trauma, log roll the child onto a backboard, and apply a cervical collar. If a collar is not available, tape the child's head to the backboard with towel rolls on both sides of the neck to prevent movement. Give supplemental oxygen by mask or nasal cannula.

If the child is actively seizing, follow the care described earlier in this chapter on seizures. Remember to call for ALS backup as necessary. No matter what the cause, you should support for the patient's vital functions and provide prompt transport.

Poisoning

Poisoning is common among children. It can occur by ingesting, inhaling, injecting, or absorbing a toxic substance (Figure 34-25). The signs and symptoms of poisoning vary widely, depending on the substance and the age and weight of the child (Table 34-3). The child may appear normal at first, even in serious cases, or he or she may be confused, sleepy, or unconscious.

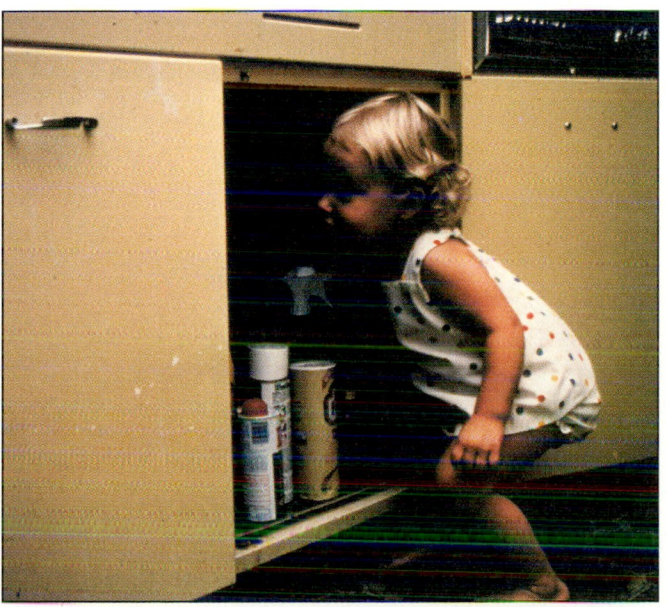

FIGURE 34-25 A curious child will try to taste or swallow almost any substance. A common victim of accidental ingestion of dangerous compounds is the unwatched toddler.

TABLE 34-3	Common Sources of Poisoning in Children

- Alcohol
- Aspirin and acetaminophen
- Household cleaning products such as bleach and furniture polish
- Houseplants
- Iron
- Prescription medications of family members
- Street drugs
- Vitamins

Infants may be poisoned as a result of being fed a harmful substance by a sibling or a caregiver or as a result of child abuse. Infants can be exposed to drugs and poisons left on floors and carpeting. They can also be exposed in a room or automobile in which harmful drugs, such as crack cocaine or PCP, are being smoked. Toddlers are curious and often ingest poisons when they find them in the home or garage. For example, some people store petroleum products in soda bottles. Toddlers may believe the substance to be soda. Adolescents are more likely to have ingested alcohol and street drugs while "partying" or in a suicide attempt.

After you have completed your initial assessment, you should ask the caregiver the following questions:

- What is the substance(s) involved?
- Approximately how much of the substance was ingested or involved in the exposure (eg, number of pills, amount of liquid)?
- What time did the incident occur?
- Are there any changes in behavior or level of consciousness?
- Was there any choking or coughing after the exposure? (These can be signs of airway involvement.)
- Are there any burns or changes in the color of the skin or mucous membranes?

Because a child's level of consciousness may be affected by the poison, your care will be guided by how awake and alert the child appears. For a child who is responsive, you must contact medical control *and your local poison control center* to report the situation. Focus on ABCD, keeping in mind that the child's condition may change over time. Assess the patient's level of consciousness, and support the vital functions as necessary, including giving supplemental oxygen. If the patient is combative and/or agitated, protect yourself from injury. *Do not administer activated charcoal or syrup of ipecac (if this is still used in your EMS system) unless directed to do so by medical control.* If the patient's condition becomes unstable, call for ALS backup. As you prepare the patient for transport, try to find the container that held the suspected poison, collect any vomitus from the child and place it in a plastic bag, and take both to the emergency department.

If the child is unresponsive, make sure that you focus immediately on ABCD, and be prepared to provide artificial ventilation if necessary. Give supplemental oxygen, and then call medical control to report the situation. Provide transport to the emergency department, ruling out trauma and keeping in mind that the child's condition could change at any time.

Fever

Fever is a common reason parents call 9-1-1. Simply defined, fever is an increase in body temperature, usually in response to an infection. Body temperatures of 100.4°F (38°C) or higher are considered to be abnormal. Fevers have many causes and are rarely life-threatening events. However, you should not underestimate the potential seriousness of fevers, such as those that occur in conjunction with a rash. You should try to determine whether the fever is a sign of serious illness, such as meningitis. Common causes of a high temperature in a child include the following:

- Infection, such as pneumonia, meningitis, or urinary tract infection
- Neoplasm (cancer)
- Drug ingestion
- Collagen vascular disease, including arthritis and systemic lupus erythematosus
- High environmental temperature

Note that there are other conditions in which the body temperature increases that are not a fever. Hyperthermia differs from fever in that it is an increase in body temperature caused by an inability of the body to cool itself. Hyperthermia is typically seen in warm environments, such as a closed car on a hot day.

Emergency medical care of a child with a fever begins with an initial assessment of ABCD, caring for immediate life threats as needed. Be sure to wear personal protective equipment, especially if meningitis is a possibility. Look carefully at the child to obtain a general impression: Does the child look sick? Then report your findings to medical control. Assess the patient's level of consciousness, and obtain vital signs. Evaluate the child for signs and symptoms of shock. If the child feels very warm, remove any covering so that the skin is exposed. Begin cooling measures en route, preferably by placing wet towels over the child's body and head. The towels should be room temperature, not cold; do not use ice.

Meningitis

Meningitis is an inflammation of the tissue, called the meninges, that covers the spinal cord and brain. It is caused by an infection by bacteria, viruses, fungi, or parasites. If left untreated, meningitis can lead to permanent brain damage and death. Being able to recognize a patient who may have meningitis is an important skill for the EMT-B.

Meningitis can occur in both children and adults, but some individuals are at greater risk than others, as follows:

- Males
- Newborn infants
- The elderly
- People whose immune systems have been weakened by AIDS or cancer
- People who have any past history of brain, spinal cord, or back surgery
- Children who have had head trauma
- Children with shunts, pins, or other foreign bodies within their brain or spinal cord

At especially high risk are children with a ventriculoperitoneal (VP) shunt. Usually, such children have tubing that can be seen and felt just under the scalp.

The signs and symptoms of meningitis vary, depending on the age of the patient. Fever and altered level of consciousness are common in patients of all ages. Changes in level of consciousness can range from a mild or severe headache to confusion, lethargy, and/or an inability to understand commands or interact appropriately. The child may also experience a seizure, which as described earlier may be a first sign of meningitis. Assess the level of consciousness using the AVPU scale. Infants younger than 2 to 3 months can have apnea, cyanosis, fever, or hypothermia.

In describing children with meningitis, physicians often use the term "meningeal irritation" or "meningeal signs" to describe pain that accompanies movement. Bending the neck forward or back increases the tension within the spinal canal and stretches the meninges, causing a great deal of pain. This results in the characteristic stiff neck of children with meningitis, who will often refuse to move their neck, lift their legs, or curl into a "C" position, even if coached to do so. One sign of meningitis in an infant is increasing irritability, especially when being handled. Another sign is a bulging fontanel.

One form of meningitis deserves special attention. **Neisseria meningitides** is a bacterium that causes a rapid onset of meningitis symptoms, often leading to shock and death. Children with *N. meningitides* typically have small, pinpoint, cherry-red spots or a larger purple/black rash. This rash may be on part of the face or body. These children are at serious risk of sepsis, shock, and death.

All patients with possible meningitis should be considered highly contagious and infectious. Therefore, you should use BSI techniques whenever you suspect meningitis and follow up with the hospital to learn the patient's final diagnosis. If you have been exposed to saliva and respiratory secretions from a child with *N. meningitides*, you should receive antibiotics to protect yourself and others from the bacteria. This is particularly true if you managed the patient's airway. If you were not in close contact with the patient or his or her respiratory secretions, you do not need treatment.

In taking the history of a child with meningitis, pay particular attention to the following details:

- Onset of illness, including any upper respiratory symptoms such as runny nose, cough, or other cold symptoms
- Presence and duration of fever
- Level of activity
- Change in behavior in older children, irritability in younger children

Emergency medical care of a patient who is believed to have meningitis should begin with an initial assessment of ABCD and immediate care of life threats. Some patients may experience episodes of cyanosis and/or apnea. If the patient is old enough to follow commands and respond, either verbally or nonverbally, determine responsiveness by asking, " What is your name?," "How old are you?," and "Hold up two fingers." Remember that you should be wearing appropriate protective equipment before you start caring for the child.

After you have secured the airway, give supplemental oxygen by mask or nasal cannula, as tolerated. You should be prepared to manage the airway with a BVM device if necessary. Assess the patient's vital signs, keep him or her warm, and watch for signs and symptoms of shock. If the patient's vital signs are unstable, call for ALS backup.

If possible, place the patient on a cardiac monitor if you are trained to do so and have the proper equipment. Continue to reassess vital signs during transport, and ensure that the patient is kept warm and monitored for signs of shock. If transport times are short, do not waste time in the field. You can perform assessment and any necessary procedures en route. Make sure that you either decontaminate or dispose of equipment that is used to care for the patient.

Shock

Shock is a condition that develops when the circulatory system is unable to deliver a sufficient amount of blood to the organs of the body. This results in organ failure and eventually cardiopulmonary arrest. In children, shock is rarely due to a primary cardiac event, such as a heart attack. Shock may be due to many things; the most common causes include the following:

- Traumatic injury with blood loss (especially abdominal)
- Dehydration from diarrhea and vomiting
- Severe infection
- Neurologic injury such as severe head trauma
- A severe allergic reaction to an insect bite or allergy (anaphylaxis)
- Diseases of the heart
- A collapsed lung (pneumothorax)
- Blood or fluid around the heart (cardiac tamponade or pericarditis)

Infants and children have less blood circulating in their bodies than adults do, so the loss of even a small volume of fluid or blood may lead to shock. Pediatric patients also respond differently than adults to fluid loss. They may respond by increasing their heart rate so that it is 160 to 220 beats/min; they may also breathe quickly and/or appear pale or blue. You must be able to recognize the signs of shock in infants and children.

Begin by assessing ABCD, intervening immediately as required; do not wait until you have completed a detailed assessment to take action. Children in shock often have increased respirations but do not demonstrate a fall in blood pressure until shock is severe.

In assessing circulation, you should pay particular attention to the following:

- **Pulse.** Assess both the rate and the quality of the pulse. A weak, "thready" pulse is a sign that there is a problem. The appropriate rate depends on the age; anything over 160 beats/min suggests shock (Table 34-4).
- **Skin signs.** Assess the temperature and moisture on the hands and feet. How does this compare with the temperature of the skin on the trunk of the body? Is the skin dry and warm, or cold and clammy?
- **Capillary refill.** Squeeze a finger or toe for several seconds until the skin blanches, then release it. The time it takes for the blood to return to the area is the capillary refill time. Does the fingertip return to its normal color within 2 seconds, or is it delayed?
- **Color.** Assess the patient's skin color. Is it pink, pale, ashen, or blue?

Changes in pulse rate, color, skin signs, and capillary refill are all important clues suggesting shock.

Blood pressure is the most difficult vital sign to take in pediatric patients. The cuff must be the proper size: two thirds the length of the upper arm. Cuffs that are too large will give pressures that are lower than actual; cuffs that are too small will give pressures that are higher than actual. The value for normal blood pressure is also age-specific. Remember that blood pressure may be normal; this is called *compensated* shock. If the blood pressure is low, this is a sign of *decompensated* shock, a serious condition that requires care an ALS team can provide.

Part of your assessment should also include talking with the caregivers to determine when the signs and

Age	**Respirations (breaths/min)**	**Pulse (beats/min)**	**Systolic Blood Pressure (mm Hg)**
Newborn	30–60	100–160	50–70
1–6 weeks	30–60	100–160	70–95
6 months	25–40	90–120	80–100
1 year	20–30	90–120	80–100
3 years	20–30	80–120	80–110
6 years	18–25	70–110	80–110

TABLE 34-4 Vital Signs by Age

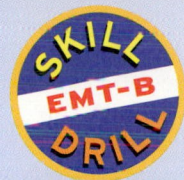

Caring for a Child in Shock
Figure 34-26

1

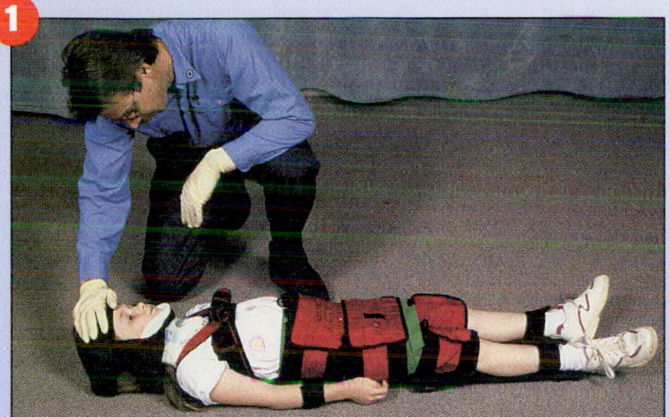

Immobilize the entire spine if you suspect trauma.

2

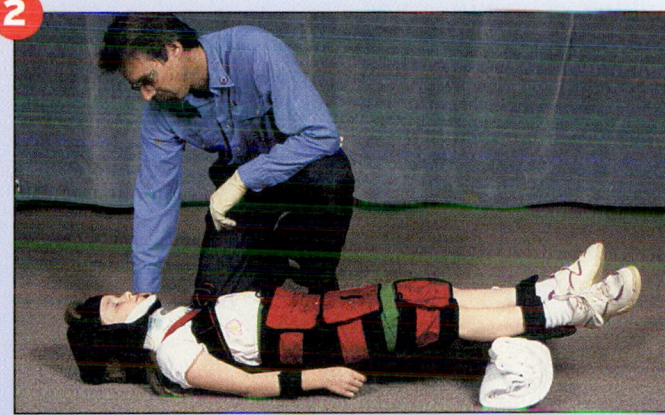

Position the patient with the head lower than the feet by elevating the feet with blankets.

3

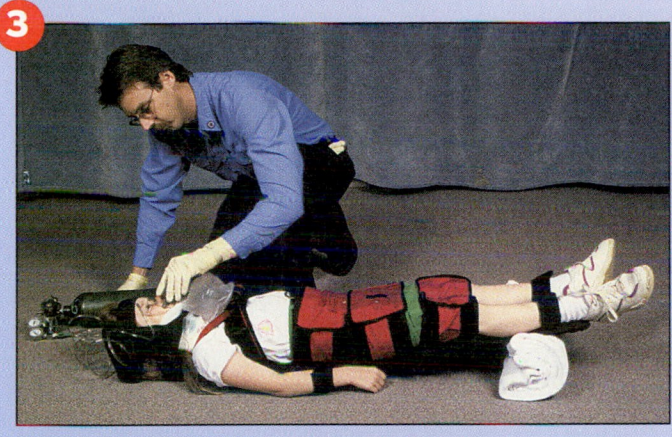

Ensure that the airway is open, and give supplemental oxygen.

4

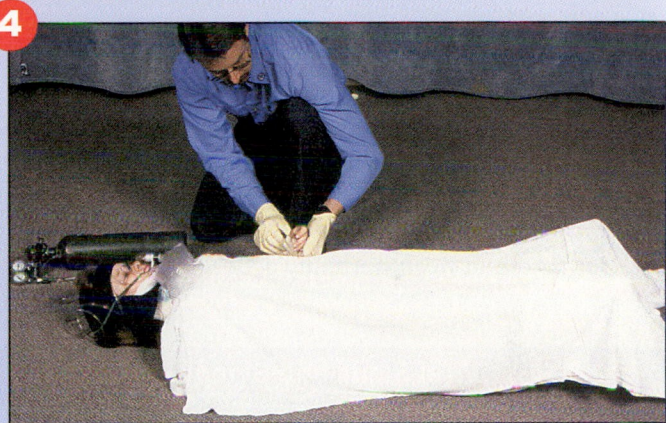

Keep the patient warm by covering him or her with blankets.

symptoms first appeared and whether any of the following has occurred:

- Decrease in urine output (with infants, are there fewer than 6 to 10 wet diapers?)
- Absence of tears, even when the child is crying
- Changes in level of consciousness and behavior

Shock is a serious condition; therefore, you should limit your care to the following interventions (Figure 34-26):

1. **Immobilize the entire spine** if you suspect trauma.
2. **Position the patient** with the head lower than the feet by elevating the feet with blankets.
3. **Ensure that the airway is open,** and give supplemental oxygen by mask or nasal cannula as tolerated.
4. **Be prepared to provide artificial ventilation** if necessary.
5. **Control bleeding** if present.
6. **Keep the patient warm** with blankets and by raising the rescue vehicle temperature.
7. **Provide immediate transport** to the nearest appropriate facility.
8. **Continue monitoring vital signs** en route to the hospital.
9. **Contact ALS backup** as needed.
10. **Whenever possible, allow a caregiver** to accompany the child.

Limit your management to these simple interventions. Time should not be wasted in field procedures. Immediate transport is of utmost importance.

Dehydration

Dehydration occurs when fluid losses are greater than fluid intake. The most common cause of dehydration in children is vomiting and diarrhea. If left untreated, dehydration can lead to shock and eventual death. Infants and children are at greater risk than adults for dehydration because their fluid reserves are smaller than those in adults. Life-threatening dehydration can overcome an infant in a matter of hours. Again, your ability to recognize a child with this condition is a critical part of your job.

Caregivers have important information that can help in treatment decisions. Be sure to ask the following questions about the child's history:

- If the child has vomiting and diarrhea, how long has he or she had these symptoms?

- How many wet diapers did the child have throughout the day (6 to 10 is normal)?

- What type of fluid has the caregiver been giving the child? Attempting to rehydrate the child with certain homemade solutions, tap water, or other fluids can lead to dangerous salt imbalances.

- What was the child's weight before the symptoms started?

- Has the child been normally active?

Dehydration can be described as mild, moderate, or severe. The severity of the dehydration can be gauged by looking at several clues (Table 34-5). For example, an infant with mild dehydration may have dry lips and gums, decreased saliva, and fewer wet diapers throughout the day (Figure 34-27). As the dehydration grows more severe, the lips and gums may become very dry, the eyes may look sunken, and the infant may be sleepy and/or irritable, refusing bottles. The skin may be loose and have no elasticity (tenting); this is called poor skin turgor.

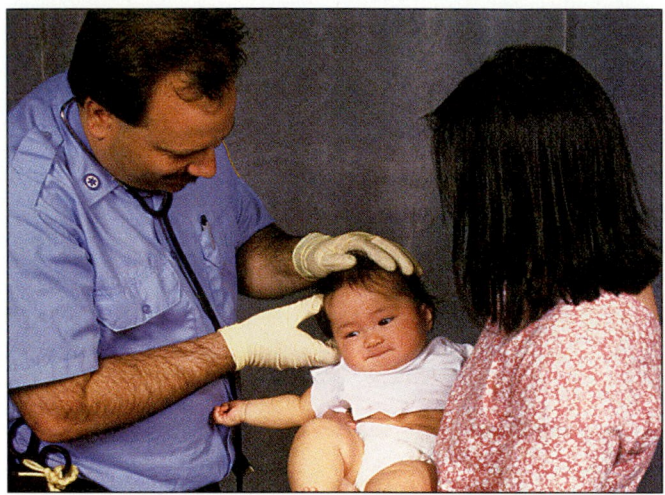

FIGURE 34-27 An infant with mild dehydration may have dry lips and gums, decreased saliva and fewer wet diapers throughout the day.

TABLE 34-5	Vital Signs and Symptoms of Dehydration		
	Mild	**Moderate**	**Severe**
Pulse	Normal	Increased	Increased; 160+ is sign of impending shock.
Level of Activity	Normal or slowed	Slowed	Variable, weak to unresponsive
Urine Output	Decreased	Decreased	No output
Skin	Normal	Cool, mottled; poor turgor	Cool, clammy; poor turgor; delayed capillary refill time
Mouth	Saliva may have drooling, bubbles	Dry mucous membranes	Dry mucous membranes
Eyes	Normal	Tears	Sunken eyes
Anterior Fontanel	Normal to sunken	Sunken	Very sunken
Level of Consciousness	Normal	Depressed	Decreased; lethargic
Blood Pressure	Normal	Normal	Elevated when shock sets in

Young children can compensate for fluid losses by decreasing blood flow to the extremities and directing it to vital organs such as the brain and heart. Their vital signs will reflect this. The heart rate of the dehydrated infant or child will generally be increased. A heart rate equal to or greater than 160 beats/min is a sign of a impending shock. Children who are moderately to severely dehydrated may have mottled, cool, clammy skin and delayed capillary refill. Respirations will usually be increased. Be aware that blood pressure may remain normal until the child is in shock.

Emergency medical care should include careful attention assessing ABCD, obtaining baseline vital signs, and reporting the degree of dehydration. You should begin fluid management, including giving fluids by mouth. However, if the dehydration is severe, ALS backup may be necessary so that IV access can be obtained and rehydration can begin.

All children with signs and symptoms of moderate to severe dehydration should be transported to the emergency department. However, if your transport time will be long, ALS backup will be necessary to administer IV fluids.

Submersion Injury

Submersion injuries include near drowning (the person survives) and drowning (the person dies). In submersion situations, you must always take steps to ensure your own safety when retrieving the patient from the water.

Drowning is the second most common cause of unintentional death among children in the United States; children under age 5 years are at particular risk. At this age, children often fall into swimming pools and lakes, but many drown in bathtubs and even buckets. Older adolescents, who account for the most drownings after toddlers, drown when swimming or boating; alcohol is frequently a factor.

The principal injury from submersion is lack of oxygen. Even a few minutes (or less) without oxygen affect the heart, lungs, and brain, causing life-threatening problems such as cardiac arrest, respiratory difficulty, and coma. Submersion in icy water can rob the body of heat, causing hypothermia. While a very few, very cold victims of submersion hypothermia have survived long periods in cardiac arrest in icy water, most people in this situation die. Diving into the water, of course, increases the risk of neck and spinal cord injuries.

Assessment and reassessment of ABCD are critical in submersion injuries. First assess breathing and pulse, because the patient may be in cardiac or respiratory arrest. Immediately check breathing effort, skin color, and capillary refill in addition to vital signs. Always immobilize the cervical spine of patients who were diving. Lung injuries may progress, causing breathing difficulty over time, so be sure to reassess the patient frequently during transport.

The usual basic and advanced life support measures should be used to ensure that the patient is getting adequate oxygen. If he or she is not breathing, provide artificial ventilation with a BVM device. Many patients who are unresponsive and not breathing respond to BLS, start breathing on their own, and wake up at the scene. If the patient is in cardiac arrest, perform CPR. Patients who are breathing on their own but show any signs of breathing difficulty or who are unconscious need oxygen. An unconscious patient who does not improve with oxygen or a patient with pink, frothy sputum at the nose or mouth requires intubation by ALS providers or in the emergency department.

If you cannot effectively ventilate the patient, consider the possibility of a foreign body airway obstruction; water alone does not obstruct the airway. If you can see the object, be sure to use removal techniques that are appropriate to the patient's age.

If it is within your scope of practice, consider using a nasogastric tube to protect the airway in unresponsive patients, as they will usually vomit. Always have a suction device ready in case of vomiting or water in the airway. Call for an ALS team if transport times are long and the patient needs advanced airway management or drugs.

Remove wet clothing so that the patient does not get colder. Keep the patient warm and monitor vital functions during transport.

A child may appear completely normal after being submersed in a liquid and then develop problems minutes or hours later. This is called *secondary drowning*; it is due to the lungs being filled with fluid from within the lung (pulmonary edema). This is why all children who have had a submersion injury require transport to the emergency department.

> In submersion situations, you must always take steps to ensure your own safety when retrieving the patient from the water.

Sudden Infant Death Syndrome

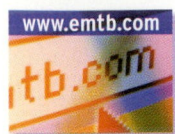 The death of an infant or a young child is called **Sudden Infant Death Syndrome (SIDS)** when, after a complete autopsy, the cause of death remains unexplained. SIDS is the leading cause of death in infants younger than age 1 year; most cases occur in infants younger than age 6 months.

Although it is impossible to predict SIDS, there are several known risk factors:

- Mother younger than 20 years old
- Mother smoked during pregnancy
- Lower socioeconomic status
- Low birth weight
- Infant sleeping in the prone position

Deaths due to SIDS can occur at any time of the day; however, these children are often discovered in the morning when the parents go in to check on the infant. If you are the first provider at the scene of suspected SIDS, you will face three tasks: assessment and management of the patient, communication and support of the family, and assessment of the scene.

Assessment and Management

SIDS is a diagnosis of exclusion. All other potential causes must first be ruled out, a process that may take physicians quite a while. An infant who has been a victim of SIDS will be pale or blue, not breathing, and unresponsive. Other causes for such a condition include the following:

- Overwhelming infection
- Child abuse
- Airway obstruction from a foreign object or as a result of infection
- Meningitis
- Accidental or intentional poisoning
- Hypoglycemia (low blood glucose)
- Congenital metabolic defects

Regardless of the cause, assessment and management of the infant remain the same. Remember that what you find in assessing the infant and the scene may provide important diagnostic information.

Begin with an assessment of ABCD, and provide interventions as necessary. Depending on how much time has passed since the child was discovered, he or she may show signs of postmortem changes. These include stiffening of the body, called **rigor mortis**, and **dependent lividity**, which is the pooling of blood in the lower parts of body or those that are in contact with the floor.

If the child shows such signs, call medical control. In some EMS systems, a victim of SIDS may be declared dead on the scene. Deciding whether to start CPR on a child who shows clear signs of rigor mortis or dependent lividity can be very difficult. Family members may consider anything less as withholding critical care. In this situation, the best course of action may be to initiate CPR and transport the patient and the family to the nearest emergency department, where the family can receive more extensive support. If there is no evidence of postmortem changes, begin CPR immediately.

As you assess the infant, pay special attention to any marks or bruises on the child *before* performing any procedures, including CPR. Also note any intervention such as CPR that was done by the parents before you arrived.

Communication and Support of the Family

The death of a child is a very stressful event for a family; it also tends to evoke strong emotional responses among health care providers, including EMS personnel. Part of your job at this point is to allow the family to express their grief in ways that may differ from your own cultural, religious, and personal practices. Provide support in whatever ways you can.

Many times family members will ask specific questions about the event: Why did this happen? How did this happen? Let them know that their concerns will be addressed but that answers are not immediately available. Always use the infant's name in speaking to family members. If possible, allow the family to spend time with the infant and to ride in the ambulance to the hospital.

Scene Assessment

Carefully inspect the environment, noting the condition of the scene where the caregivers found the infant. Your assessment of the scene should concentrate on the following:

- Signs of illness, including medications, humidifiers, thermometers, and so on
- The general condition of the house (Note any signs of poor hygiene.)
- Family interaction. Do not allow yourself to be judgmental about family interactions at this time. Do note and report any behavior that is clearly not within the acceptable range, such as physical and verbal abuse.
- The site where the infant was discovered. Note all items in the infant's crib or bed, including pillows, stuffed animals, toys, and small objects.

The death of a child is difficult for everyone involved: parents, relatives and friends, and health care professionals. You should arrange for a proper debriefing after your involvement with the case comes to a close. This can take the form of a session with a trained counselor or a group discussion with your colleagues or the entire health care team.

Apparent Life-Threatening Event

Infants who are not breathing and are cyanotic and unresponsive when found by their families sometimes resume breathing and color with stimulation. These children have had what is called an **apparent life-threatening event (ALTE)**, sometimes called "near-miss SIDS" in the past. In addition to cyanosis and apnea, a classic ALTE is characterized by a distinct change in muscle tone (limpness) and choking or gagging. After the event, a child may appear healthy and show no signs of illness or distress. Nevertheless, you must complete a careful assessment and provide immediate transport to the emergency department.

Pay strict attention to management of the airway. Assess the infant's history and, if possible, the environment. Allow caregivers to ride in the ambulance. If asked, explain that you cannot say what caused the event, that this is something that doctors will have to determine at the hospital.

Death of a Child

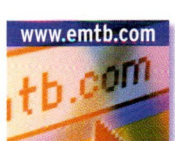
www.emtb.com

As with SIDS, the death of a child from any cause poses special challenges for EMS personnel. In addition to any medical treatment the child may require, you must be prepared to offer the family a high level of support and understanding as they begin the grieving process (Table 34-6). First, the family may want you to initiate resuscitation efforts, which may or may not conflict with your EMS protocols. If the child is clearly deceased and, under protocol, can be declared dead in the field, but the family is so distraught that they insist that resuscitation efforts be made, initiate CPR and transport the child.

The extent of your interaction with the family will depend, to some degree, on the number of providers available at the scene. Always introduce yourself to the child's caregivers, and ask about the child's date of birth and medical history. If and when the decision is made to start or stop resuscitation efforts, inform the family immediately. Find a place for family members from which they can watch resuscitation without being in the way.

TABLE 34-6	How You Can Help the Family of a Deceased Child

When Arriving on Site:

- Introduce yourself quickly.
- Obtain a brief history.
- When possible, one provider should stay with the family.

If Resuscitation is Attempted:

- Give brief, frequent updates and explanations.
- Allow family members to stay within viewing distance if they wish.
- Allow family members to accompany child to hospital when possible.

If No Resuscitation is Performed:

- Sit down with the family.
- Inform the family immediately.
- Explain why no resuscitation will be attempted.
- Offer to arrange for religious support, including baptism or last rites.

Beginning the Grieving Process:

- Learn and use the child's name.
- Allow family to express emotions; be nonjudgmental.
- Give brief explanations and answers.
- Mention the possibility of organ donation.
- Explain to the family that the cause of death is still unknown.
- Allow time for questions.

DO:

- Tell the family how sorry you are.
- Tell the family whom they can call if they have questions later.
- Give *written* instructions and referrals.

DON'T:

- Say, "I know how you feel."
- Say, "You have other children" or "You can have other children."
- Attempt to answer the question "Why did this happen?"
- Try to tell family that they will be feeling better in time.

Do not, in any case, speculate on the cause of the child's death. The family will want to see the child and should be asked whether they want to hold the child and say good-bye. Parents may be experiencing strong feelings of denial.

The following interventions are helpful in caring for the family at this time:

- Learn and use the child's name rather than the impersonal "your child."

- Speak to family members at eye level, maintaining good eye contact with them.

- Use the word "dead" or "died" when informing the family of the child's death; euphemisms such as "passed away" or "gone" are not effective.

- Acknowledge the family's feelings ("I know this is devastating for you"), but never say "I know how you feel," even if you have experienced a similar event; the statement will anger many people.

- Offer to call other family members or clergy if the family wishes.

- Keep any instructions short, simple, and basic. Emotional distress may limit their ability to process information.

- Ask each adult family member individually whether he or she wants to hold the child.

- Wrap the dead child in a blanket, as you would if he or she were alive, and stay with the family while they hold the child. Ask them not to remove tubes or other equipment that was used in an attempted resuscitation.

Remember that each individual and each culture expresses grief in a different way, some more visibly than others. Some will require intervention; others will not. Most caregivers feel directly or indirectly responsible for the death of a child and may express this immediately; this does not mean that they actually are responsible. Sometimes, it is helpful to address the issue of guilt by saying, "Many caregivers feel responsible for their child's death. Are you feeling that?" Parents often have questions that you should be prepared to answer (Table 34-7). Although you should keep the possibility of abuse or neglect in mind, you role is not that of investigator. Any further inquiry is the responsibility of law enforcement.

Some EMS systems arrange for home visits after the death of a child so that EMS providers and family members can come to some sort of closure together. This also gives the family an opportunity to ask any remaining questions about the event. However, you need special training for such visits.

Again, coping with the death of a child can be very stressful for health care professionals. You may find yourself with unexpected feelings of pain and loss. It is helpful to take some time before going back on the job to work through your feelings and to talk about the event with your EMS colleagues. Be alert for signs of posttraumatic stress in yourself and others: nightmares, restlessness, difficulty sleeping, lack of appetite, a constant need for food, and the like. Consider the need for professional help if these signs or symptoms continue. All EMS programs should have Critical Incident Stress Management protocols and debriefing teams available for traumatic incidents.

Although you may experience the death of a child as a failure, your skill at coping with this kind of emotional event can be a great comfort to the family, helping them to accept their loss and begin the long process of grieving.

TABLE 34-7 Common Questions Following Death of a Child	
Question	**Appropriate Response**
Was there pain?	This often can be answered by a simple "No." If you are uncertain, you may give an indirect answer such as "We really don't know what patients feel in these circumstances."
What did he/she die of?	Do not answer this question; you would probably be guessing at this point.
Why did this happen?	Do not attempt to answer this question either, as the answer depends on one's own individual philosophy, or religion. "I wish I had an answer for you" is usually the most appropriate response.
What happens now?	This question usually concerns the next few minutes or the next hour. If you know, you should give the family a general idea of what will happen. For example, if there is no history of illness, you can say that "the coroner (or medical examiner) will be examining [the child's name], and then he (or she) will be taken to the mortuary."

prep kit

ready for review

There are five development stages in childhood: infancy, the toddler years, preschool age, school age, and adolescence. Each requires a slightly different approach to assessment and pain management. General rules for dealing with children of all ages include appearing confident, being honest, and keeping caregivers together with the patient as much as possible.

Children younger than age 5 years often obstruct their upper and lower airway with a variety of foreign objects. If the child is conscious, encourage him or her to cough to clear the airway. If the child is unconscious, you should first use the tongue-jaw lift and finger sweeps to try to remove an object that you see. In treating an unconscious child with complete airway obstruction, use abdominal thrusts (in a series of five), alternating with attempts at artificial breathing; in infants, substitute back blows and chest thrusts. In a conscious child who is sitting or standing, apply abdominal thrusts from behind.

A child who is in early respiratory distress may be breathing too slow or too fast. Rates greater than 60 breaths/min are a sign of a problem requiring assisted ventilation in most cases. Look for signs of extra effort to breathe, including nasal flaring and grunting respirations; these may give way to cyanosis. You must intervene immediately if bradycardia develops in a child in respiratory distress. Use the least upsetting method to administer supplemental oxygen, adding assisted ventilations if these become necessary; use a BVM device without an artificial airway.

Seizures in children may appear as a shaking of the whole body (generalized), a movement in a single arm or leg or eye (partial), or a momentary unresponsiveness (absence seizure). Complications of seizures are due to injury from seizure motion, airway obstruction, or poor breathing effort. Do not put anything into the mouth of a seizing child. Do position the child so that the tongue is not an obstruction, and be prepared to suction secretions or vomitus. Febrile seizures, occurring on the first day of a fever, may be a sign of a more serious problem such as meningitis. Begin cooling measures, and transport the patient to the hospital.

Other childhood conditions that require immediate transport include altered level of consciousness, which you may assess using the AVPU scale; severe dehydration; and poisoning. The best way to cool a child with fever is with wet towels that are at room temperature, not cold. Children with meningitis will have fever, altered level of consciousness, and irritability, along with neck pain. All patients with possible meningitis should be considered highly contagious and infectious. *Neisseria meningitides*, characterized by tiny red spots or a large purple rash, is a fast-moving, dangerous form of meningitis. If you have been exposed to respiratory secretions from a child with this form of the disease, you should take antibiotics.

Infants and children can go into shock after the loss of even a small volume of fluid or blood, which may be caused by an injury, dehydration, severe infection or allergic reaction, heart disease, or a collapsed lung. Children who are in shock often have increased respirations but normal blood pressure until the condition is severe. Changes in skin color and capillary refill are important signs of shock.

The most common cause of dehydration in children is vomiting and diarrhea. Life-threatening diarrhea can develop in an infant in hours. You can determine whether a child's dehydration is mild, moderate, or severe by assessing the child's urine output, level of activity, mental status, skin tone, and pulse. For severe dehydration, ALS backup is necessary so that IV fluids can be given.

If you cannot effectively ventilate a victim of submersion, consider the possibility of a foreign body airway obstruction, as water alone does not obstruct the airway. Use a nasogastric tube to protect the airway in unresponsive patients who have been submersed.

A victim of sudden infant death syndrome (SIDS) will be pale or blue, not breathing, and unresponsive. He or she may show signs of postmortem changes, including rigor mortis and dependent lividity; if so, call medical control to report the situation. If family members insist, you should initiate CPR and transport infant and family to the emergency department, where the family can receive more extensive support. If the child does not have any evidence of postmortem changes, begin CPR immediately. Carefully inspect the environment where a SIDS victim was found, looking for signs of illness, abusive family interactions, and objects in the child's crib. Provide support for the family in whatever way you can. Allow them to spend time with the child and ride in the ambulance to the hospital.

Any death of a child is stressful for family members and for health care providers. In dealing with the family, acknowledge their feelings, keep any instructions short and simple, use the child's name, and maintain eye contact. Be prepared to respond to philosophical as well as medical questions, in most cases by indicating concern and understanding; do not be specific about the cause of death. Be alert for signs of posttraumatic stress in yourself and others after dealing with the death of a child. It can help to talk about the event and your feelings with your EMS colleagues.

prep kit

vital vocabulary

www.emtb.com

altered level of consciousnes A mental state in which infants and children may be unresponsive, combative, or confused, may thrash about, or may drift into and out of an alert state. Also called altered mental status.

apnea A period of not breathing.

apparent life-threatening event (ALTE) An event that causes unresponsiveness, cyanosis, and apnea in an infant, who then resumes breathing with stimulation.

bradycardia A heart rate of less than 60 beats/min in children or less than 80 beats/min in infants.

croup Infection of the airway below the level of the vocal cords, usually caused by a virus.

dehydration A state in which fluid losses are greater than fluid intake into the body, leading to shock and death if untreated.

dependent lividity Pooling of the blood in the lower parts of the body after death.

epiglottitis An infection of the soft tissue in the area above the vocal cords.

meningitis Inflammation of the meninges that covers the spinal cord and the brain.

myoclonic jerks Short jerks of an extremity during a seizure.

neisseria meningitides A form of bacterial meningitis characterized by rapid onset of symptoms, often leading to shock and death.

postictal period The period immediately following a seizure, characterized by extreme tiredness or listlessness.

rales A crackling breath sound caused by the flow of air through liquid in the lungs; a sign of lower airway obstruction.

rigor mortis Stiffening of the body after death.

shock A condition that develops when the circulatory system is not able to deliver sufficient blood to body organs, resulting in organ failure and eventual death if untreated.

status epilepticus The term used to describe a continuous seizure or multiple seizures without a return to consciousness for 30 minutes.

stridor A high-pitched breath sound heard mainly on inspiration that is a sign of upper airway obstruction.

Sudden Infant Death Syndrome (SIDS) Death of an infant or young child that remains unexplained after a complete autopsy.

tonic seizure A seizure in which there is a rigid extremity.

tonic-clonic seizure A seizure that features rhythmic back-and-forth motion of an extremity and body stiffness.

wheezing A whistling breath sound caused by air traveling through narrowed air passages within the bronchioles; a sign of lower airway obstruction.

assessment in action

The bank thermometer flashes an even 100° as it welcomes you back to the night shift. To make matters worse, your partner tells you that the air conditioning in the unit has not been working right for the last two shifts. Just then you are dispatched to an apartment for a child with "breathing difficulty."

You arrive to find an 8-year-old girl sitting at the kitchen table, in a slightly hunched-forward position. Her mother explains that this is the first time they have had to use the inhaler since the girl was diagnosed with asthma. They tried the inhaler twice with minimal results and were reluctant to try it again. The family doctor did not return a page, and they decided to call 9-1-1. The mother also states that the girl has had the flu for the past 2 days, including a low-grade temperature.

1. Which of the following signs should be used to determine whether this child is sick or well during your initial assessment?
   A. Blood pressure
   B. Capillary refill
   C. Pupil size
   D. Overall appearance

2. Which of the following signs does **NOT** suggest respiratory distress in this patient?
   A. Nasal flaring
   B. Audible wheezing
   C. Use of neck muscles for breathing
   D. Respirations of 24/min

3. The patient has a temperature of 101°F. Therefore, in addition to caring for her asthma, you must also monitor her for signs of:
   A. seizures.
   B. depression.
   C. shin splints.
   D. hip swelling.

4. En route, the mother whispers to you that she has never seen the child "this quiet." Which of the following is most likely responsible for the altered mental status in this patient?
   A. Hypoxia
   B. Angina pectoris
   C. Memory lapse
   D. Hereditary factors

5. En route, the patient looks at you with a scared expression and says, "It's getting harder to breathe!" You hear audible wheezing (without your stethoscope). Which of the following interventions would **NOT** be appropriate?
   A. Trying to calm the patient down
   B. Administering high-flow oxygen
   C. Providing a breathing treatment
   D. Having her breathe into a paper bag

points to ponder

Object. 1-1.1, 1-1.2, 2-1.2, 6-1.3, 6-1.5, 6-1.7, 6-1.19

You respond to a home in the middle of the night for a "child who can't breathe." When you arrive, you find a three-year-old child who is coughing and has noisy inhalations. The child has good skin color but feels warm to the touch. You attach a pulse oximeter and find that the child is well oxygenated. The parent explains that the child has had a cold but that the coughing is worse tonight. You question whether the child needs medical care at all and are confident that the child does not need to be transported in an ambulance.

- Would you refuse to transport the child? What would you tell the parent? What is your liability if you tell the parent that an ambulance is not needed?

online outlook

You will face some special challenges in caring for sick and injured children. Infants and children are not simply small adults; they come in a wide variety of sizes with anatomy and physiology that are different from those of adults. To learn more about pediatric medical emergencies, complete Exercise 34 at www.emtb.com.

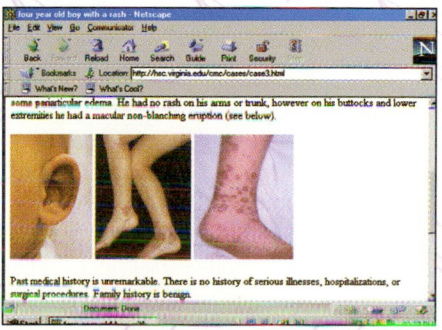

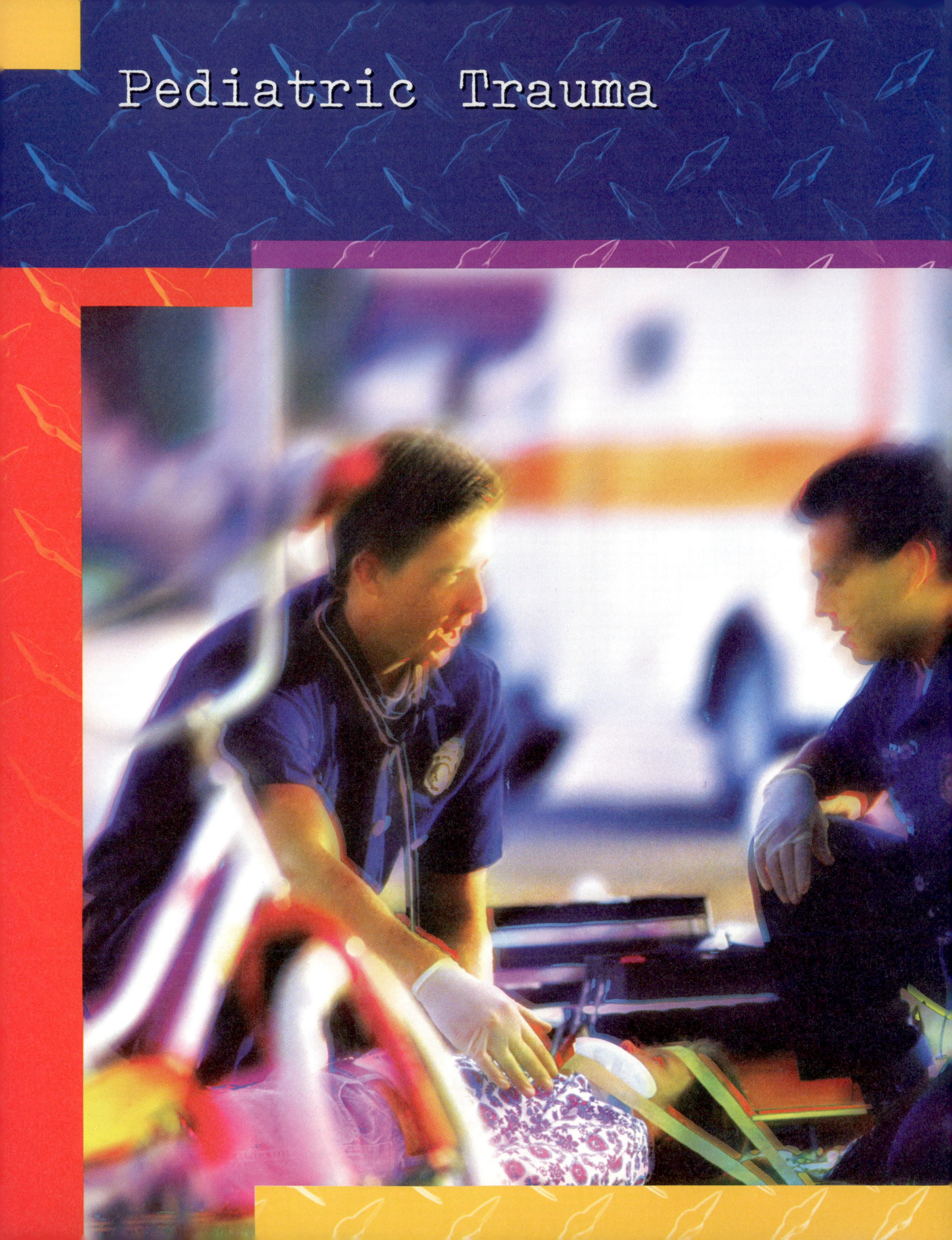

Pediatric Trauma

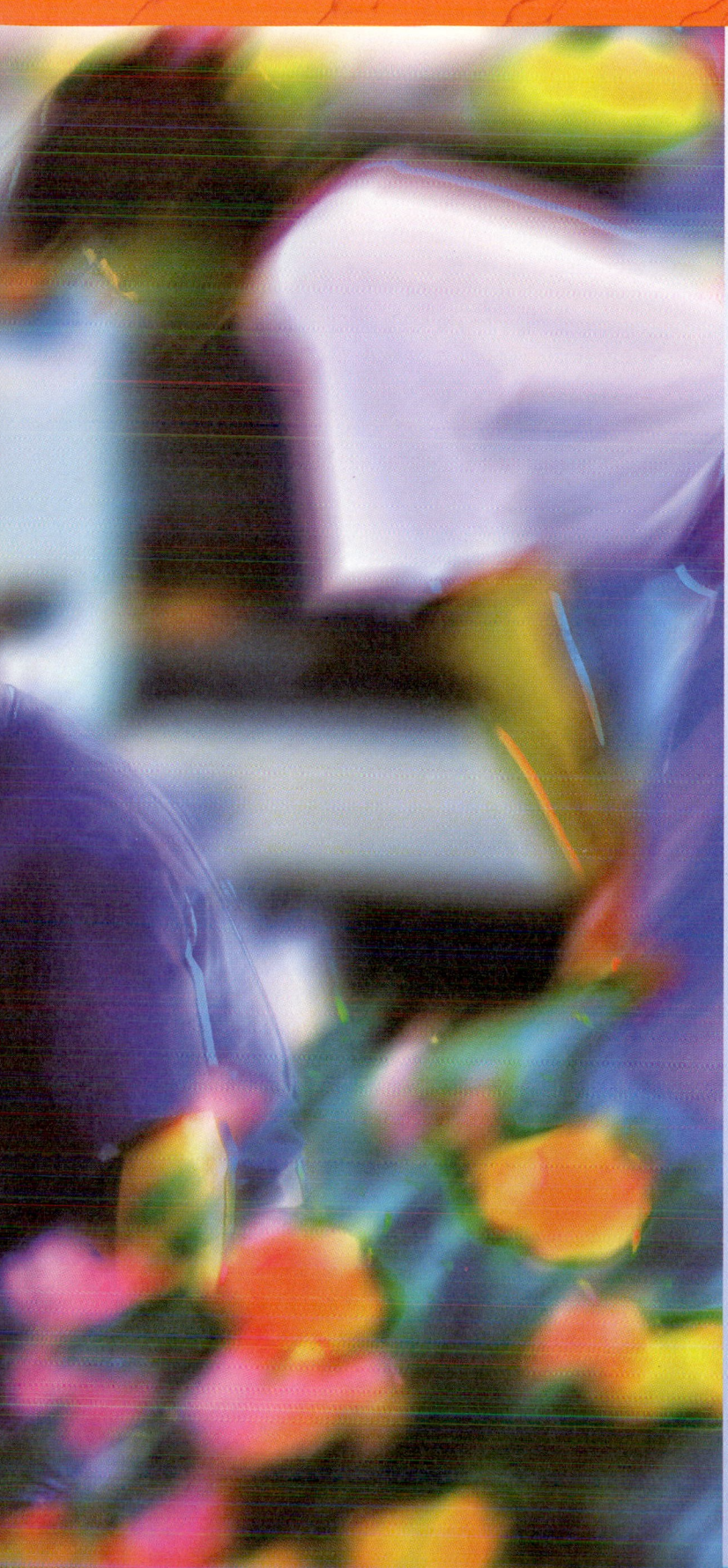

objectives

Cognitive

1. Describe differences in anatomy and physiology of the infant, child, and adult patient.

2. Differentiate between the injury patterns in adults, infants, and children.

3. Discuss the field management of the infant and child trauma patient.

4. Summarize the indicators of possible child abuse and neglect.

5. Describe the medicolegal responsibilities in suspected child abuse.

6. Recognize the need for EMT-Basic debriefing following a difficult infant or child transport.

Affective

7. Explain the rationale for having knowledge and skills appropriate for dealing with the infant and child patient.

8. Attend to the feelings of the family when dealing with an ill or injured infant or child.

9. Understand the provider's own response (emotional) to caring for infants or children.

Psychomotor

None

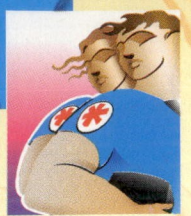

you are the emt

Squad 10 . . . You need to respond out in the county, at the corner of County A14 and Humbolt for "a child thrown from a horse."

The scene is about 20 minutes from your current location. You consider contacting the helicopter service to be on standby in case the child needs transport to a pediatric trauma center. Should you wait to make the decision until you are at the scene, or should you request the helicopter now? This chapter will introduce the unique and challenging world of pediatric trauma, as well as help you to answer the following questions:

1. What physical characteristics make children high-risk trauma patients?

2. Are pediatric patients the same as adult patients, only smaller?

Pediatric Trauma

Trauma is the number one killer of children in the United States. More children die of trauma-related injuries in 1 year than of all other causes combined. As an EMT-B, you will frequently treat injured children; therefore, you must have a thorough understanding of how trauma affects them. The quality of care in the first few minutes after a child has been injured can have an enormous impact on that child's chances for complete recovery.

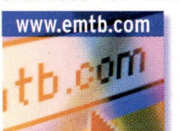

Treatment of traumatic injuries in children starts with understanding these injuries as completely as possible. The types of injuries differ, depending on the age of the child. Infants and toddlers are most commonly hurt as a result of falls or abuse. Older children and adolescents are usually injured as a result of mishaps involving automobiles. According to information collected by the National Pediatric Trauma Registry (NPTR) over the last 10 years, the automobile is the most significant threat to the well-being of the child. Approximately 41% of all injuries that the NPTR recorded in this time period were related to vehicular mishaps, including those involving bicycles. Other common causes of traumatic injury and death include falls, gunshot wounds, blunt injuries, and sports activities. Another extremely serious and troublesome cause of injury is child abuse.

Anatomic Differences

By now, you know that children are not simply small adults; they differ in many ways other than size. Children have less circulating blood than adults, so children cannot tolerate as much blood loss without going into shock. Children also lose body heat more easily than adults do because children have a larger body surface area in relation to body mass. A child's bones have not finished growing; they are more flexible and elastic than those in an adult's skeleton. Fat is distributed in a child in a somewhat different way than in an adult, so vital organs in the abdomen and the chest of a child are less well insulated. Therefore, a child may experience significant injuries to internal organs but have little or no evidence of external trauma. This is especially true of chest injuries. Because a child's ribs are softer and more flexible than those of an adult, they may compress the underlying lungs and heart, causing life-threatening conditions without obvious external damage (Figure 35-1).

Given these anatomic differences, you must be able to recognize severe injuries in children, as well as to identify potentially life-threatening injuries so that you can provide prompt emergency medical care. As with all patients, your focus is on ABCD:

- Evaluate responsiveness.
- Ensure that the child has an open airway and is breathing.
- If necessary, assist ventilation and give supplemental oxygen.

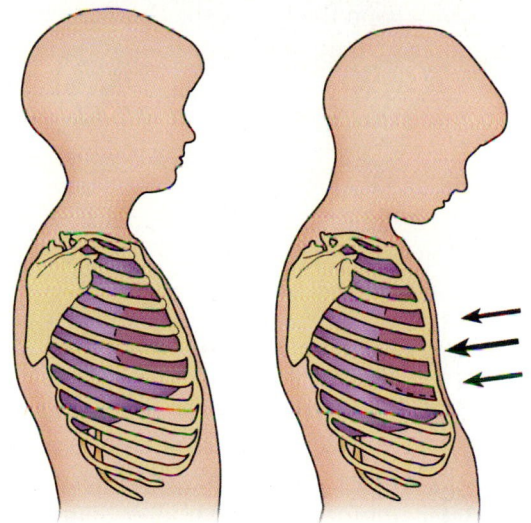

FIGURE 35-1 A child's ribs are softer and more flexible than an adult's. As a result, they may compress the lungs and heart, causing serious injury with no obvious external damage.

- Assess circulation by obtaining a pulse (brachial, carotid, femoral) and blood pressure, evaluating for external bleeding, and assessing skin color, temperature, and capillary refill.

Injury Patterns

Although you are not responsible for diagnosing injuries in children, your ability to recognize and report serious injuries will provide critical information to hospital staff. For this reason, it is important for you to understand the special physical and psychologic characteristics of children and what makes them more likely to have certain kinds of injuries. Situations that are unique to children also make them more susceptible to injury, such as their need to ride in child safety seats, their involvement in specific mishaps with motor vehicles, and their participation in organized sports.

Physical Differences

Children are smaller than adults; therefore, when they are hurt in the same type of accident as an adult, the location of their injuries may differ from those in an adult. For example, the bumper of a car will strike an adult in the lower leg, whereas that same bumper will strike a child in the pelvis. In a sudden deceleration accident, an adult might injure a ligament in the knee; in that same accident, a child might injure the bones in the leg.

Children's bones and soft tissues are less well developed than those of adults; therefore, the force of an injury affects these structures somewhat differently than it does in an adult. Because a child's head is proportionately larger than an adult's, it exerts greater stress on the neck structures during a deceleration injury. Because of these anatomic differences, you should always carefully assess for head and neck injuries in children.

Psychologic Differences

Children are also less mature psychologically than adults; therefore, they are often injured because they lack common sense. For example, children are more likely than adults to cross the street without looking for oncoming traffic. As a result, children are more likely than adults to be struck by cars. Children and adolescents are also more likely to sustain injuries from diving into shallow water because they forget to check the depth of the water before they dive. In such situations, you should always assume that the child has serious head and neck injuries. Other common injuries include wrist injuries from in-line roller skating and ankle fractures from bicycle accidents. Note that these examples do not apply to all children or all adults. In fact, some children have more common sense than some adults. However, you should be aware of these injury patterns when you are called to respond to pediatric emergencies.

Child Safety Seats

Children are often injured or killed in motor vehicle crashes. Those who are not restrained in child safety seats are at greater risk for head, neck, and spinal injuries. Although child safety seats are effective in decreasing the severity of injuries, children may still sustain abdominal and lower spinal injuries as the result of trauma caused by the restraints themselves. Head, neck, and spinal injuries are less common in restrained passengers but are certainly possible. Therefore, you should always immobilize the patient's cervical spine (Figure 35-2).

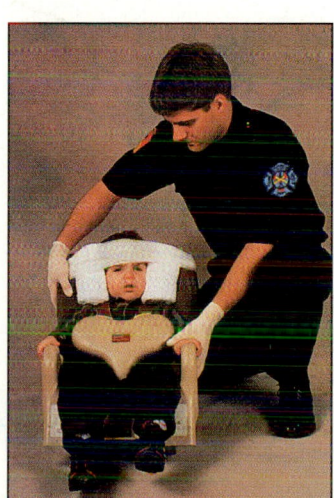

FIGURE 35-2
Even though head, neck, and spinal injuries are less common in children who are restrained, they are still possible. Therefore, you should always immobilize the patient's cervical spine.

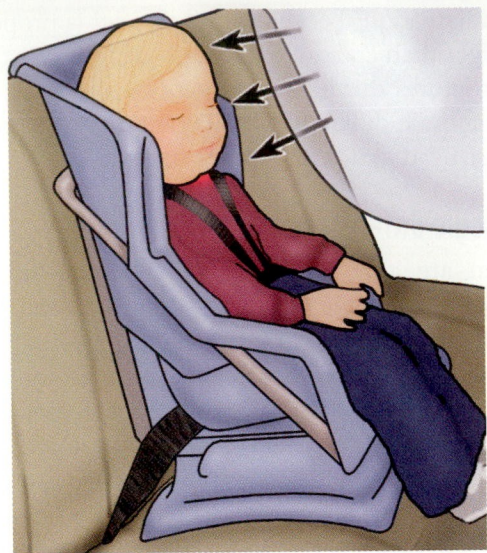

FIGURE 35-3 Children riding in a child safety seat in the front passenger seat of a car may be injured or killed by the force of a deploying airbag.

Young children, especially those who have been restrained in a child safety seat, may be injured or killed by airbags if they are riding in the front passenger seat of a car (Figure 35-3). This occurs because the child safety seat positions the child too close to the airbag. When the airbag deploys, the child may sustain a devastating spinal or head injury. For this reason, child safety seats should never be placed in the front seat of a vehicle that is equipped with passenger airbags.

Automobile Collisions

Children at play or riding a bicycle can dart out in front of motor vehicles without looking. In such a situation, the driver may have very little time to slow down or stop to prevent hitting the child. The area of greatest injury varies, depending on the size of the child and the height of the bumper at the time of impact. When vehicles slow down at the moment of impact, the bumper dips slightly, causing the point of impact with the child to be lowered. The exact area that is struck depends on the child's height and the final position of the bumper at the time of impact. Children who are injured in these situations often sustain high-energy injuries to the head, spine, abdomen, pelvis, or legs (Figure 35-4).

Sports Activities

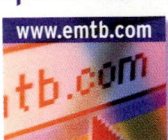

Children, especially those who are older or adolescent, are often injured in organized sports activities. Head and neck injuries can occur after high-speed collisions in contact sports such as football, wrestling, ice hockey, field hockey, soccer, or lacrosse. Remember to immobilize the cervical spine when caring for children with sports-related injuries. You should be familiar with your local protocols related to helmet removal, and/or follow the guidelines presented in Chapter 32.

Injuries to Specific Body Systems

Head Injuries

Head injuries are common in children. This is due, in part, to the fact that the size of a child's head, in relation to the body, is larger than that of an adult. The signs and symptoms of head injury in a child are similar to those in an adult, but there are some important differences. Nausea and vomiting are common signs and symptoms of head injury in children; however, it is easy to mistake these for an abdominal problem. You should suspect a

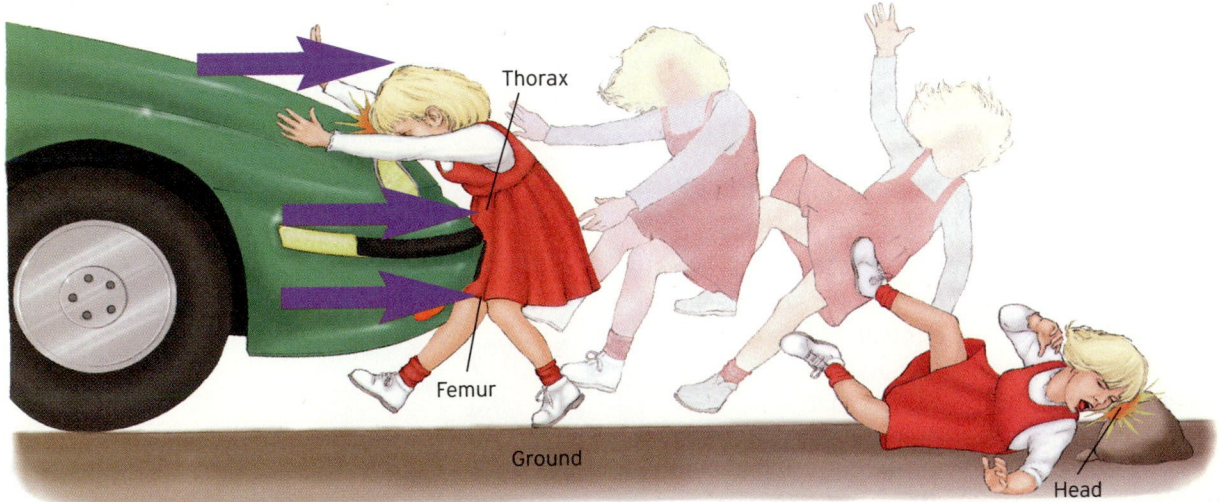

FIGURE 35-4 The exact area that is struck depends on the child's height relative to the position of the bumper at the time of impact.

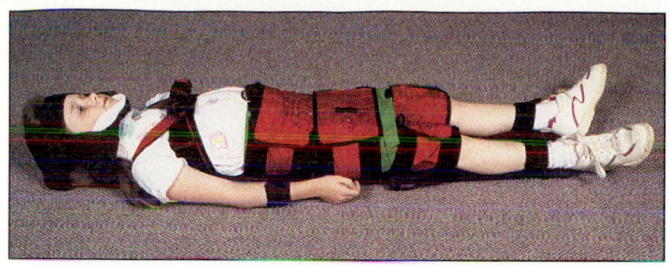

FIGURE 35-5 Avoid using sandbags to immobilize the head of a child.

serious head injury in any child who has nausea and vomiting after a traumatic event.

Your single most important step in caring for a child with a head injury is to ensure that the airway is open. Whenever you suspect trauma, you should immobilize the cervical spine and use the modified jaw-thrust maneuver to open the airway, as the child's tongue may have relaxed back into the throat, blocking the airway. As you immobilize the child onto a backboard, avoid using sandbags to immobilize the head (Figure 35-5). If the child begins to vomit and the board has to be turned

to the side, the weight of the bags on the head could cause additional injury.

All children with head injuries should be monitored for signs and symptoms of shock, including a weak, rapid pulse; cold, clammy skin; decreased capillary refill (an early sign); confusion; and decreased systolic blood pressure (a late sign). If a child has any one or any combination of these signs and symptoms, there is also a strong possibility of associated chest or abdominal injuries. Even in the absence of signs and symptoms of shock, or with only very few signs and symptoms, you should remain cautious about the possibility of internal injuries.

Children can lose a greater proportion of their blood volume than adults can before signs or symptoms of shock develop. What makes this situation dangerous is that infants and children have less blood circulating in their bodies than adults do, so the loss of even a small volume of fluid or blood may lead to shock (Figure 35-6).

Respiratory arrest can also occur as a result of head injuries in children. You should be prepared to assist ventilations or provide rescue breaths in any child who has evidence of severe head injury, if it becomes necessary.

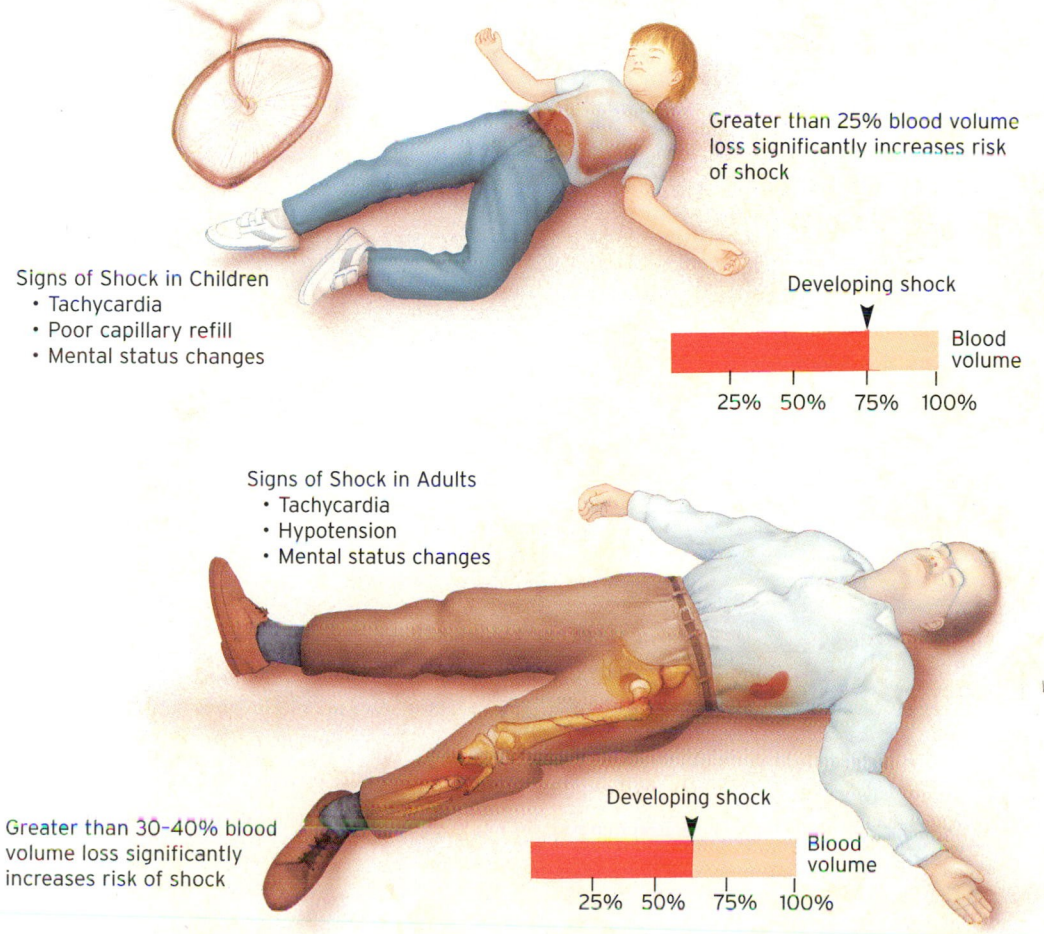

Greater than 25% blood volume loss significantly increases risk of shock

Signs of Shock in Children
• Tachycardia
• Poor capillary refill
• Mental status changes

Developing shock

Blood volume

25% 50% 75% 100%

Signs of Shock in Adults
• Tachycardia
• Hypotension
• Mental status changes

Developing shock

Blood volume

Greater than 30–40% blood volume loss significantly increases risk of shock

25% 50% 75% 100%

FIGURE 35-6 Children can lose a greater proportion of their blood volume than adults can before signs or symptoms of shock develop.

Abdominal injuries are more common in children than in adults.

Chest Injuries

Chest injuries in children are usually the result of blunt trauma rather than penetrating objects. Remember that children have very soft, flexible ribs that can be compressed a great deal without breaking. Keep this in mind as you assess a child who has sustained high-energy blunt trauma to the chest. Even though there may be no external sign of injury, such as broken ribs, there may be significant injuries within the chest.

Abdominal Injuries

Abdominal injuries are more common in children than in adults. Remember, though, that children can compensate for significant blood loss better than adults without signs or symptoms of shock developing. They can also have a serious injury without early external evidence of a problem. You should always suspect hidden internal injuries in children after a high-energy trauma injury. Abdominal injuries should also be considered if a child clearly has signs and symptoms of shock but no substantial evidence of external bleeding.

One of the problems associated with abdominal injuries in children is the presence of air in the stomach. Children, especially those who have had a traumatic injury, tend to swallow air. Air in the stomach can cause distention and interfere with your assessment. Air can also accumulate in the stomach with artificial ventilation, making it less effective. This is one of the reasons to use the modified jaw-thrust maneuver to position the airway, as it prevents air from accumulating in the stomach.

Injuries of the Extremities

Children have immature bones with active growth centers. Growth of long bones occurs from the ends at specialized growth plates. These growth plates are potential weak spots in the bone and are often injured as a result of trauma. In general, children's bones bend more easily than adults' bones. As a result, incomplete or greenstick fractures can occur.

Extremity injuries in children are generally managed in the same manner as those in adults. Painful deformed limbs with evidence of broken bones should be splinted. Specialized splinting equipment, such as a traction splint for fractures of the femur, should be used only if it fits the child. *You should not attempt to use adult immobilization devices on a child unless the child is large enough.*

Other Considerations

Pneumatic Antishock Garments

A pneumatic antishock garment (PASG) is rarely used in treating children. One situation in which you would use a PASG is when the child has obvious lower extremity trauma, particularly to both legs; pelvic instability; and clear signs and symptoms of severe shock. However, one problem with the use of this device for children is that it rarely fits. The PASG should be used on children only if it fits properly. Techniques such as placing the child in one leg of the garment are absolutely contraindicated and should *never* be used. The abdominal compartment of the garment should **never** be inflated on children because excessive pressure on the abdomen will cause pressure on the diaphragm and compromise breathing.

Burns

Children can be burned in a variety of ways. The most common involve exposure to hot substances such as scalding water in a bathtub or hot items on a stove or exposure to caustic substances such as cleaning solvents or paint thinners (Figure 35-7). You should suspect possible internal injuries from chemical ingestion when you see a child who has burns, particularly around the face and mouth.

One common problem following burn injuries in children is infection. Burned skin cannot resist infection

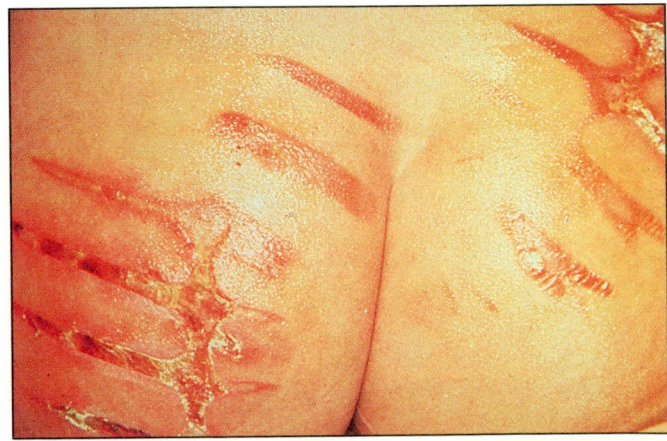

FIGURE 35-7 The most common burns in children involve exposure to hot surfaces. This child's buttocks was placed against a hot heating grate.

as effectively as normal skin can. For this reason, sterile techniques should be used in handling the skin of children with acute burns.

As when you are caring for adults, you should first remove all clothing from the burned skin as part of a complete exposure of the patient. Leaving charred clothing in place prevents you from clearly assessing the patient. In addition, the clothing may still be hot and continue to burn the underlying skin if it is not removed. After chemical burns, it is particularly important to remove the clothing rapidly, since chemical materials that are retained within the clothing may also cause damage to the underlying skin. After the skin has been exposed, you should place dry sterile dressings on the skin as soon as possible to decrease the risk of infection.

You must learn your local protocols regarding the immediate referral of children to burn centers. Table 35-1 provides some general guidelines to follow in assessing a child who has been burned.

These guidelines may help you to determine which children should be treated primarily at specialized burn centers. Also note that you should consider the possibility of child abuse in any burn situation. Make sure you report any information about your suspicions to hospital staff.

Emergency Medical Care

Emergency medical care of a child who has experienced a traumatic injury immediately focuses on ABCD, as with all patients.

Airway

You should be alert for airway problems in all children who have sustained traumatic injuries. Children who are awake, alert, and talking generally have open airways; however, unconscious children, even those who are initially breathing on their own with signs of an open airway, are at risk for airway obstruction. The airway can become blocked if the child's tongue relaxes back into the throat. Therefore, you should use the modified jaw-thrust maneuver when necessary in unconscious children to keep the airway open. One advantage of this maneuver is that it minimizes the risk of damage to the cervical spine because it keeps the head in a neutral position.

Because nausea and vomiting are common in children with traumatic head injuries, you must be prepared for it. Keep suctioning equipment readily available so that you can suction the mouth and oropharynx as necessary to

TABLE 35-1	Severity of Burns in Children
Severity of Burn	**Body Area Involved**
Minor	Partial-thickness burns involving less than 10% of the body surface
Moderate	Partial-thickness burns involving 10% to 20% of the body surface
Critical	Any full-thickness burn
	Any partial-thickness burn involving more than 20% of the body surface
	Any burn involving the hands, feet, face, airway, or genitalia

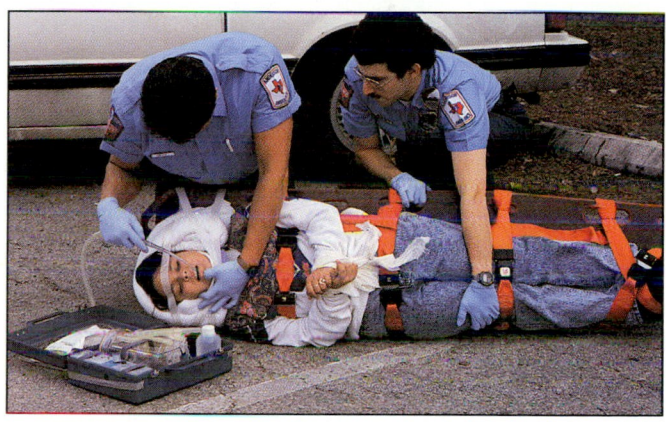

FIGURE 35-8 Turn the backboard to the side and suction the mouth when an immobilized child vomits.

keep the airway open. Be prepared to turn a backboard to one side if the child vomits (Figure 35-8). *Remember that you should not use sandbags to stabilize the cervical spine in children.* If you must turn the backboard to allow for vomiting, the weight of the sandbags may cause additional head injury when the backboard and patient are turned.

Breathing

You should give supplemental oxygen to all children with possible head, chest, or abdominal injuries or any evidence of shock, to correct for any hypoxia. Children who are breathing on their own should be given high-concentration oxygen via a nonrebreathing mask. Care should be taken to ensure that the mask fits

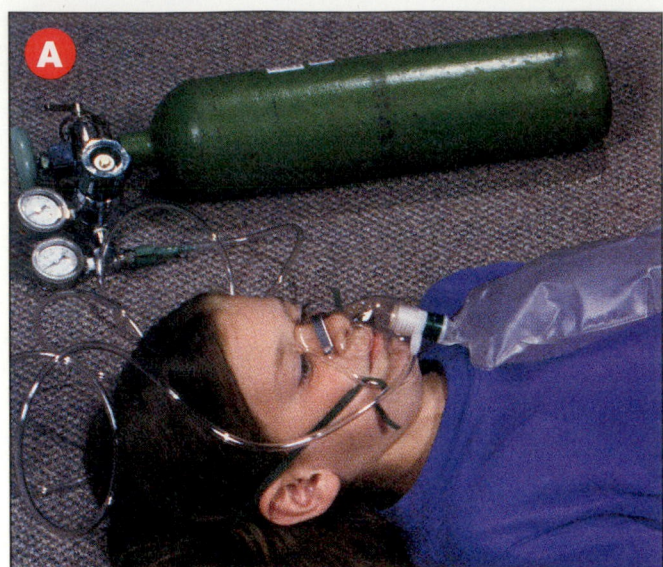

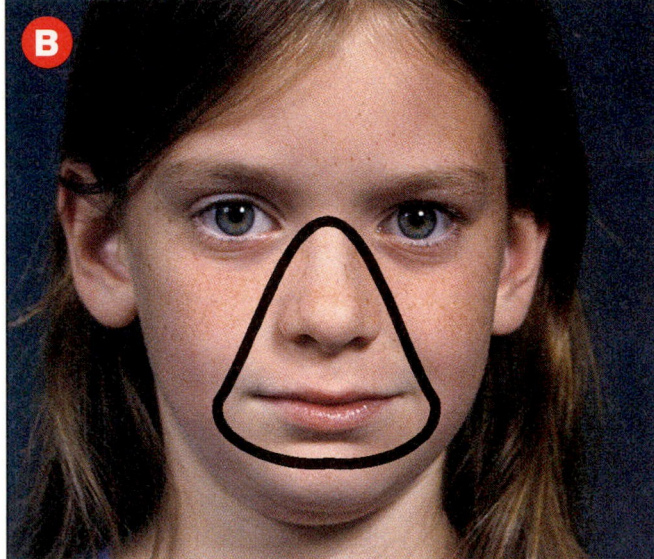

FIGURE 35-9 A: Use a properly fitting nonrebreathing mask to deliver supplemental oxygen. **B:** Area covered on a child's face with a properly fitting mask.

the child properly; adult masks used on children typically leak, making oxygen administration less effective (Figure 35-9).

You should be prepared to assist with ventilation in children who are in respiratory distress. For children who have had traumatic injuries, use a BVM device at a rate of about 20 breaths/min, or one breath every 3 seconds.

Immobilization

Immobilization is necessary for all children who have possible head or spinal injuries after a traumatic event. As with all patients who have unstable or potentially unstable injuries, immediate transport is indicated. The identification of the nearest appropriate facility depends on local protocols and the capabilities of local hospitals. In some areas of the country, you may be directed to take the patient directly to a pediatric trauma center or to arrange for air transport to a pediatric trauma center. In other areas of the country, children are evaluated primarily at local hospitals and are then transferred to a pediatric trauma center. You should be familiar with the local guidelines and protocols regarding transport issues.

Child Abuse

The term **child abuse** means any improper or excessive action that injures or otherwise harms a child or infant; it includes physical abuse, sexual abuse, neglect, and emotional abuse. The intentional injury of a child, whether physical or emotional, is not rare in our society. More than 2 million cases of child abuse are reported to child protection agencies annually. Many of these children suffer life-threatening injuries, and some die. If suspected child abuse is not reported, the child is likely to be abused again and again, perhaps suffering permanent injuries or even dying. Therefore, you must be aware of the signs of child abuse and neglect and of your responsibility to report *suspected* abuse to law enforcement or child protection agencies.

Signs of Abuse

As an EMT-B, you will be called to a home because of a reported injury to a child. If you suspect that physical or sexual abuse is involved, you should ask yourself the following questions:

- Is the method of injury reported by the parent or caregiver consistent with the child's injuries?

- Is the injury typical for the developmental level of the child?

- Does the child have multiple injuries at different stages of healing?

- Is the child clean and an appropriate weight for his or her age?

- Does the child have any unusual marks or bruises that may have been caused by cigarettes, grids, or branding injuries?

- Does the child have several types of injuries, such as burns, fractures, and bruises?

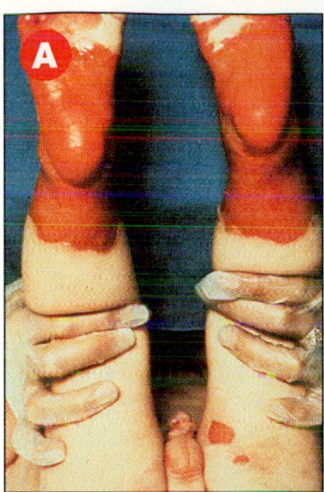 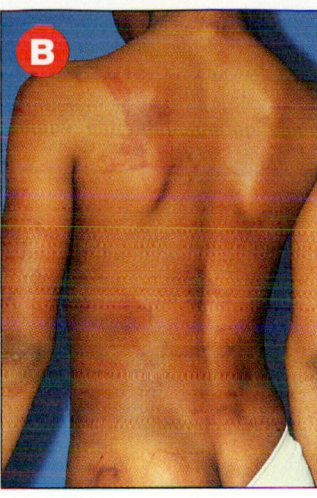

FIGURE 35-10 Signs of child abuse. **A:** Scald. **B:** Multiple injuries at different stages of healing.

- Does the child have any burns on the hands or feet that involve a glove distribution?
- Is there unexplained decreased level of consciousness?
- Is there a good relationship between the child and the caregiver?
- Is there any rectal or vaginal bleeding?
- Is the caregiver behaving appropriately (concerned about the child's well-being)?
- Is the caregiver drunk or abusing drugs?
- Is the home dirty?

As you assess the child, look for and pay particular attention to the following signs (Figure 35-10).

Bruises. Observe the color and location of any bruises. New bruises are pink or red. Over time, bruises turn blue, then green, then yellow-brown and faded. Note the location. Bruises to the back, buttocks, or face are suspicious and are usually inflicted by a person.

Burns. Burns to the penis, testicles, vagina, or buttocks are usually inflicted by someone else, as are burns that encircle a hand or foot to look like a glove. You should suspect abuse if the child has cigarette burns or grid burns.

Fractures. Fractures of the humerus or femur do not normally occur without major trauma, such as a fall from a high place or a motor vehicle crash. Falls from bed are not usually associated with fractures.

Shaken Baby Syndrome. Infants may sustain life-threatening head trauma by being shaken or struck on the head, a life-threatening condition called <u>Shaken</u> <u>Baby Syndrome</u>. With this condition, there is bleeding within the head and damage to the cervical spine as a result of intentional, forceful shaking. The infant will be found unconscious, often without evidence of external trauma. The call for help may be for an infant who has stopped breathing or is unresponsive to the caregiver. The infant may appear to be in cardiopulmonary arrest, but what has likely occurred is that the shaking tore blood vessels in the brain, resulting in bleeding around the brain. The pressure from the blood results in a coma.

Neglect. Children who are neglected are often dirty or too thin or appear developmentally delayed because of lack of stimulation. You may observe such children when you are making calls for unrelated problems. Report all cases of suspicious neglect.

Symptoms and Other Indicators of Abuse

An abused child may appear withdrawn, fearful, or hostile. You should be particularly concerned if the child refuses to discuss how an injury occurred. Occasionally, the parent or caregiver will reveal a history of several "accidents." Be alert for conflicting stories or a marked lack of concern from the parents or caregiver. Remember, the abuser may be a parent, caregiver, relative, or friend of the family. Sometimes the abuser is an acquaintance of a single parent.

Emergency Medical Care

Your priority is to care for ABCD, as in all other instances. Care for all wounds, splint fractures, and keep the infant or child warm and comfortable. Provide transport in all instances in which you suspect abuse has occurred. You are not there to solve the problem or to accuse a parent or caregiver. In fact, you need their cooperation, as you cannot transport a child without consent from the parent or guardian. Sometimes, you can persuade a parent to allow transport if you say that the child may need special X-rays or tests. If the parent still refuses and you are concerned about the child's well-being, consult law enforcement.

EMT-Bs in all states *must* report all cases of suspected abuse, even if the emergency department fails to do so. Most states have special forms for reporting. Supervisors are generally forbidden to interfere with the reporting of suspected abuse, even if they disagree with the assessment. You do not have to prove that there has been abuse. Law enforcement and child protection agencies are mandated to investigate all reported cases.

Sexual Abuse

Children of any age and either gender can be victims of sexual abuse. Most victims of rape are older than age 10 years, although younger children may be victims as well. This type of sexual abuse is often the result of long-standing abuse by relatives.

Your assessment of a child who has been sexually abused should be limited to determining the type of dressing any injuries require. Sometimes, a sexually abused child is also beaten. Therefore, you should treat any bruises or fractures as well. Do not examine the genitalia of a young child unless there is evidence of bleeding, or there is an injury that must be treated.

In addition, if you suspect that a child is a victim of sexual abuse, do not allow the child to wash, urinate, or defecate before a physician completes an exam. Although this step is difficult, it is important to preserve evidence. If the molested child is a girl, ensure that a female EMT or police officer remains with the child unless finding one will delay transport.

You must maintain professional composure the entire time you are assessing and caring for a sexually abused child. Assume a concerned, caring approach, and shield the child from onlookers and curious passersby. Obtain as much information as possible from the child and any witnesses. The child may be hysterical or unwilling to say anything at all, especially if the abuser is a relative or family friend. You are in the best position to obtain the most accurate firsthand information about the incident. Therefore, you should record any information carefully and completely on the run report.

Transport all children who are victims of sexual assault. Sexual abuse of a child is a crime. Make sure that you cooperate with law enforcement officials in their investigations.

Infants and Children with Special Needs

The approach to health care in our society continues to focus on decreasing lengths of hospitalization. Also, the technology that is used in the care of children with special needs at home continues to improve. As a result of these two factors, the number of infants and children with chronic diseases who are living at home or in other out-of-hospital environments continues to grow. You should be familiar with some of the special needs created by these chronic diseases or conditions, particularly as they relate to the potential need for emergency medical care.

Some examples of infants and children with special needs include the following:

- Children who were born prematurely and have associated lung disease problems
- Small children or infants with congenital heart disease
- Children with neurologic disease (occasionally caused by hypoxemia at the time of birth, as with cerebral palsy)
- Children with chronic disease or with functions that have been altered since birth

Occasionally, these children live at home but are dependent on artificial ventilators or other devices to maintain life. You assess and care for these children the same as for all other patients. Your focus on ABCD remains the priority.

Tracheostomy Tubes

Children who are dependent on home artificial ventilators or those who have chronic pulmonary medical conditions may breathe through a tracheostomy tube. A **tracheostomy tube** is a tube in the neck that passes directly into the major airways. Sometimes, the tube becomes obstructed by mucous plugs or foreign bodies; there may be bleeding or air leaking around the tube; and sometimes the tube becomes loose or dislodged. Occasionally, the opening around the tube may become infected. Your care of a patient with a tracheostomy tube includes maintaining an open airway, suctioning the tube if necessary to clear a mucous plug, maintaining the patient in a position of comfort, and providing transport to the hospital.

Artificial Ventilators

Children on home artificial ventilators need artificial ventilation during transport. Artificial ventilation is provided through the tracheostomy tube. To do this, remove the mask from a BVM device, and directly attach the bag and valve to the tracheostomy tube; this will allow you to ventilate through the tracheostomy tube. Remember that the patient's caregivers will know how the ventilator works and will be of great help to you in attaching the BVM device to the tube in preparation for transport.

Central IV Lines

Children with chronic medical conditions such as gastrointestinal disturbances that require prolonged IV feeding or those with infections that require prolonged IV antibiotics will have indwelling IV catheters placed near the heart for long-term use. Problems associated with these devices may include broken lines, infections around the lines, clotted lines, and bleeding around the line or from the tubing attached to the line. If bleeding occurs, you should apply direct pressure and provide transport to the hospital.

Gastrostomy Tubes

Gastrostomy tubes are tubes placed through the wall of the abdomen directly into the stomach for feeding in children who cannot be fed by mouth. Breathing problems in these children may be complicated by aspiration of the tube contents into the lungs. You should always have suction readily available to clear any materials from the mouth and to prevent airway problems. Patients with gastrostomy tubes who have difficulty breathing should be transported either sitting or lying on the right side with the head elevated to prevent the contents of the stomach from passing into the lungs. Give supplemental oxygen if the patient has any difficulty in breathing. Children with diabetes who receive insulin and tube feedings may become hypoglycemic quickly if tube feedings are discontinued. Be alert for altered mental status.

Shunts

Some children with chronic neurologic conditions may have shunts in place. Shunts are tubes that extend from the brain to the abdomen to drain excess cerebrospinal fluid that may accumulate near the brain. These children are prone to changes in mental status and respiratory arrest. Emergency medical care includes airway management and artificial ventilation during transport. During assessment, you will likely feel a device on the side of the head beneath the skin. This device is a fluid reservoir, and the presence of this device should alert you to the possibility that the child has an underlying shunt. Should the shunt become dysfunctional, the child could be predisposed to respiratory arrest.

Family Matters

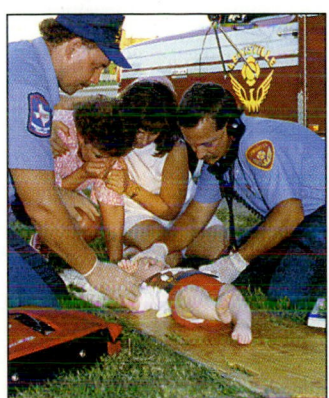

It is important to remember that when children are injured, especially those with chronic illnesses, you have not just one patient to treat but several (Figure 35-11). Family members, especially the primary caregiver, often need help or support when medical emergencies or problems

FIGURE 35-11 Remember that you are caring for at least two patients: the infant and the parent or caregiver.

develop. A calm parent usually helps to contribute to a calm child. An agitated parent usually means that the child will act the same way. Make sure that you are calm, efficient, professional, and sensitive as you deal with children and their families.

Transporting Infants and Children

Before you transport a sick or injured child, you should be aware of special transport considerations for infants and children. Infants and small children are very susceptible to temperature changes. They lose body heat rapidly and must always be transported wrapped in blankets. Very young and sick children are also extremely susceptible to infection. Therefore, you should avoid breathing or coughing directly on a small or sick child. Isolate an infant or child from bacterial contamination, particularly from your own nose, mouth, and hands.

Newborns should be transported in special incubators. If an incubator is not available, wrap the newborn in blankets. Be sure to keep the newborn's face uncovered, and make sure the ambulance is warm. Many large medical centers maintain specially equipped vehicles for transporting infants and small children. You should know the location and availability of these vehicles.

EMS Response to Pediatric Emergencies

After care and transport of a sick or injured child, you may experience a wide range of powerful emotions. These emotions result from the call itself or from your previous experience (or inexperience) in caring for infants and children. You may feel anxious if you have not had much experience in dealing with infants and children. You may also think of your own children or the children of a loved one.

As a result, you must be prepared to care for children. Practice with children and pediatric equipment is necessary. As you know, children are not simply small adults. However, many of the skills and principles you use to care for adults can be applied to children. You must simply remember that there are differences in anatomy and emotions.

After difficult incidents involving children, debriefing is helpful in working through the stress and trauma. It is also a means to help you in the future if you are faced with similar situations. The ability to seek help after difficult episodes is a sign of maturity and confidence.

prep kit

ready for review

For several reasons, you face special challenges when you are called on to care for children who have traumatic injuries. Children are not only smaller than adults and more vulnerable; they are also anatomically, physiologically, and psychologically different from adults in some important ways. You must understand these differences to provide the best possible care for children who have been injured. You should remember that children's bones are more flexible and bend more with injury and that the ends of the long bones, where growth occurs, are weaker and may be injured more easily. Children's heads are proportionately larger and are more likely to be injured in automobile mishaps. Children's internal organs are not as insulated by fat and may be injured more severely, and children have less circulating blood, so that, although children exhibit the signs of shock more slowly, they go into shock faster. Children are not always as cautious as adults and tend to have more accidental poisoning, diving, and bicycle injuries. You should also remember that infants and small children cannot communicate the source or cause of their injuries, and children of any age and background are at risk for child abuse and neglect.

There is rarely anything more satisfying than helping or saving the life of an injured child, but injured children who are unconscious or in pain can be difficult. Therefore, you must always be prepared emotionally to care for children who have been injured and seek counseling or debriefing if necessary after caring for a traumatically injured child.

vital vocabulary www.emtb.com

child abuse   Any improper or excessive action that injures or otherwise harms a child or infant.

gastrostomy tube   A feeding tube placed directly through the wall of the abdomen; used in patients who cannot ingest liquids or solids.

Shaken Baby Syndrome   Bleeding within the head and damage to the cervical spine of an infant who has been intentionally and forcibly shaken; a form of child abuse.

shunt   A tube that diverts excess cerebrospinal fluid from the brain to the abdomen.

tracheostomy tube   A tube inserted into the trachea in children who cannot breathe on their own.

points to ponder

Object.1-3.11, 1-3.12

You respond to a home to find an unconscious infant in a crib. The infant has irregular breathing and a weak, rapid pulse. There is a large red skin discoloration just in front of the infant's ear. The person who met you at the door told you that the baby fell out of the crib and hit its head, but the person in the bedroom says that the baby fell down the stairs. The baby does not appear old enough to have done either on its own. You suspect child abuse.

- Would you report this? If so, when and to whom? What would you ask the people who are with the child? How much time would you spend on the scene gathering information? Would you allow the adults to ride in the ambulance to the hospital?

online outlook

The treatment priorities in children who sustain serious trauma are similar to those in adults—the stabilization of the child and management of life-threatening injuries. To learn more about the diagnosis and treatment of pediatric trauma, complete Exercise 35 at www.emtb.com.

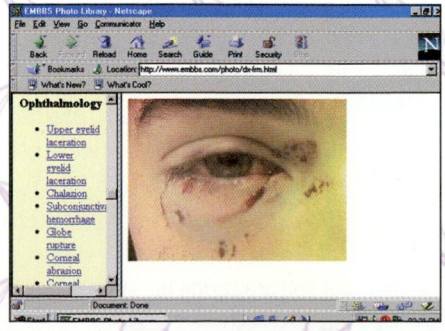

assessment **in action**

It's a hot, sunny Memorial Day, and the city parks are full of families out enjoying the holiday. Despite the big crowds, the day has been quiet so far. Your pager goes off, and you are dispatched to Hanson Park for "a child hit by a car."

You arrive to find a 3-year-old girl clinging to her mother. She is clearly frightened, and you can see that she has been crying, though she is quiet now. Her mother states that the girl chased a toy into the street, right into the path of the car, which knocked the child down with a glancing blow. She states that she is certain that her daughter did not lose consciousness. You see about 20′ of skid marks from where the child was struck. The patient has only minor abrasions, but you are concerned that her respirations are more than 40 breaths/min and that she cries in pain when you palpate her right side over the rib cage.

1. If you were to try to take the patient away from her mother, you should anticipate that the child will most likely:

   A. start screaming and crying almost immediately.

   B. laugh and play with your stethoscope and blood pressure cuff.

   C. be thrilled as long as you promise that you will not hurt her.

   D. cooperate with you as long as you smile and speak in a pleasant voice.

2. Which of the following statements about taking a pediatric blood pressure is true?

   A. Blood pressure readings can be obtained in children only at the hospital.

   B. A blood pressure measurement is required only if the patient is unconscious.

   C. You can only estimate blood pressure levels on a 3-year-old.

   D. You should use a pediatric blood pressure cuff to obtain an accurate measurement.

3. Your assessment and care of the patient's respiration problem would **NOT** include:

   A. evaluating and recording the skin color and moisture.

   B. carefully monitoring the patient's level of physical activity.

   C. monitoring for the onset of the use of accessory muscles during breathing.

   D. administer a breathing treatment if respirations exceed 18 breaths/min.

4. Which of the following statements about a child's respiratory system is **FALSE**?

   A. A child's airway is easily blocked with excess secretions.

   B. A child's smaller airways become blocked very easily.

   C. Compared to their large mandible, a child's tongue is very small.

   D. The airways throughout the pediatric respiratory system are small.

5. The patient's respirations increase to a point in which you begin assisting ventilations with a BVM device. At what rate should you squeeze the bag?

   A. Fewer than 6 to 8 times a minute

   B. No more than 10 times a minute

   C. Between 15 and 20 times a minute

   D. At least 60 times a minute

prep kit

35

Operations

Alasdair K.T. Conn, MD

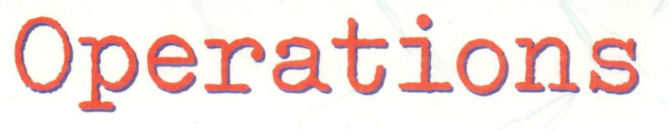

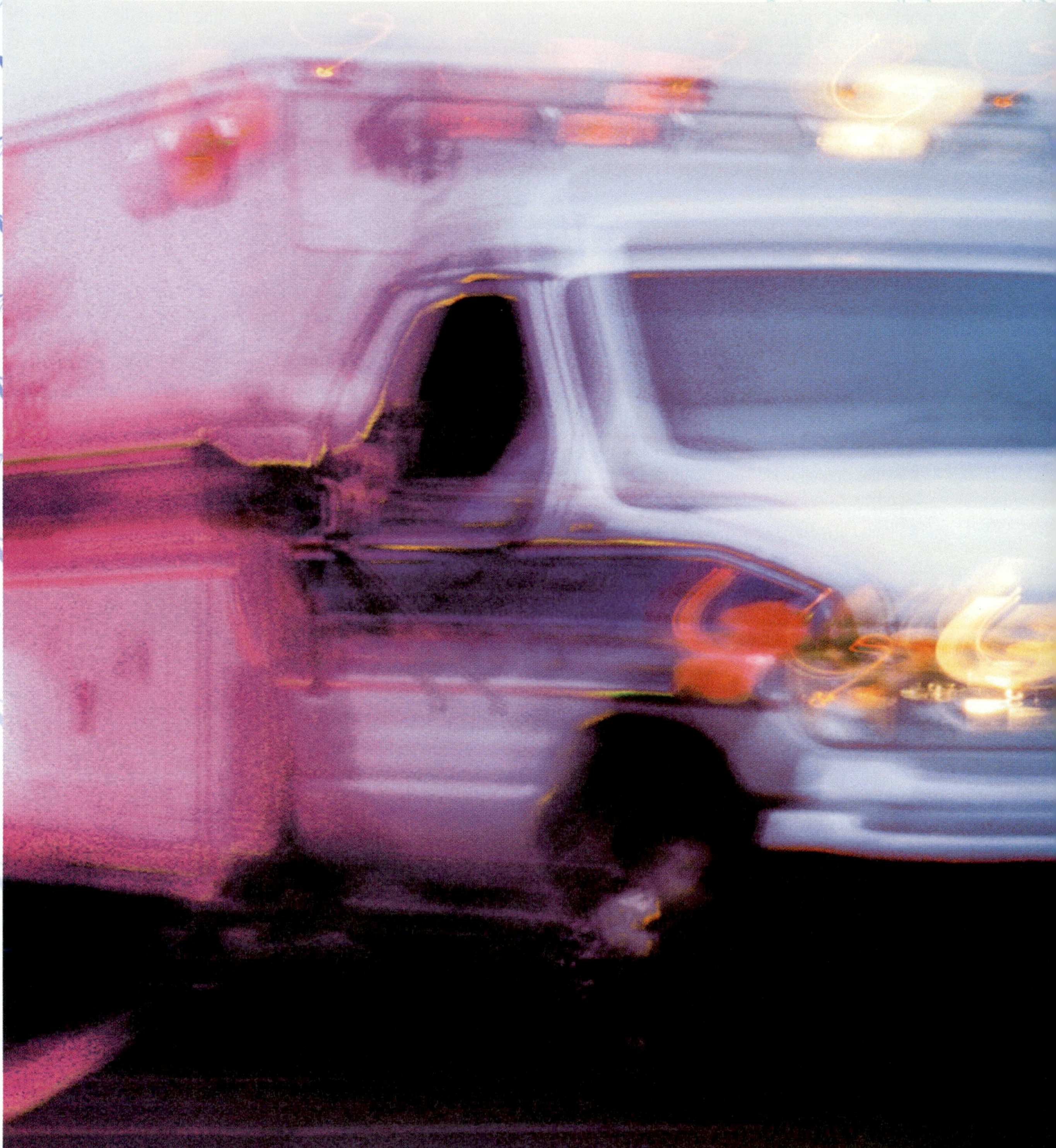

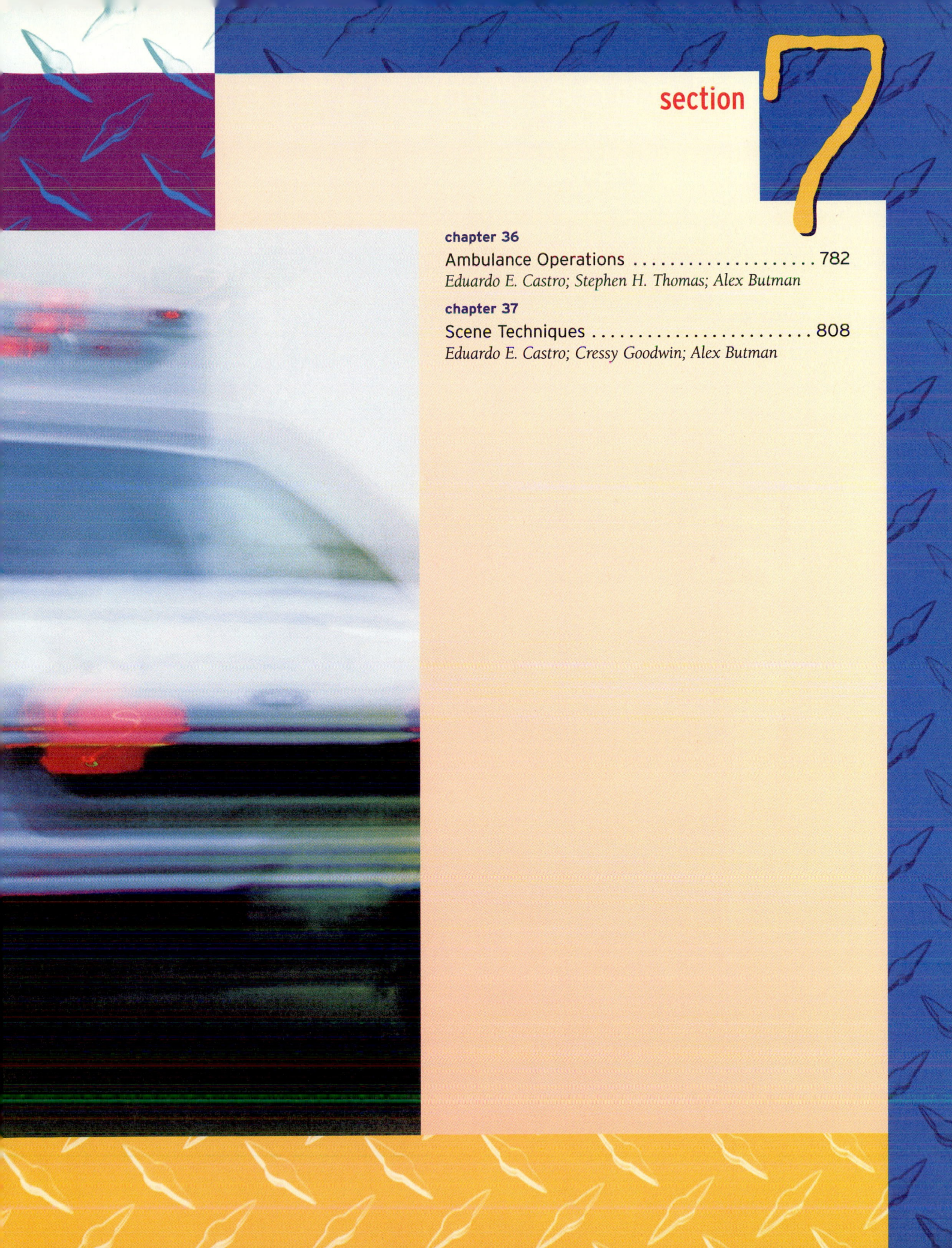

Ambulance Operations

objectives

Cognitive

1. Discuss the medical and nonmedical equipment needed to respond to a call.

2. List the phases of an ambulance call.

3. Describe the general provisions of state laws relating to the operation of the ambulance and privileges in any or all of the following categories:
   - speed
   - warning lights
   - sirens
   - right-of-way
   - parking
   - turning.

4. List contributing factors to unsafe driving conditions.

5. Describe the considerations that should be given to:
   - request for escorts
   - following an escort vehicle
   - intersections.

6. Discuss "Due Regard for Safety of All Others" while operating an emergency vehicle.

7. State what information is essential in order to respond to a call.

8. Discuss various situations that may affect response to a call.

9. Differentiate between the various methods of moving a patient to the unit based upon injury or illness.

10. Apply the components of the essential patient information in a written report.

11. Discuss the elements that dictate the use of lights and siren to the scene and to the hospital.*

12. Summarize the importance of preparing the unit for the next response.

13. Identify what is essential for completion of a call.

14. Distinguish among the terms cleaning, disinfection, high-level disinfection, and sterilization.

15. Describe how to clean or disinfect items following patient care.

Affective

16. Explain the rationale for appropriate reporting of patient information.

17. Explain the rationale for having the unit prepared to respond.

18. Explain the effects lights and siren have on emergency vehicle operator and other drivers.*

Psychomotor

None

* These are non-curriculum objectives.

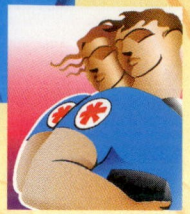

you are the emt

Emergency vehicles respond every hour to calls for help all across America. These portable emergency departments deliver care to patients in need, usually within minutes of their call to 9-1-1.

The ambulance is a virtual supply room that holds the tools of your trade. The public counts on you to respond quickly and for your equipment to work when it is needed. This chapter will help to familiarize you with the ambulance, as well as help you to answer the following questions:

1. What should you expect cars to do when you roll up behind them with your lights and sirens on?

2. Should lights and sirens be used on all ambulance runs?

Ambulance Operations

Many patients have said that the most frightening part of being suddenly ill or injured is the ambulance ride to the hospital. Already anxious, a patient may be made more so by a fast, bumpy ride with siren blaring. Sometimes, such a ride is truly lifesaving. However, in most cases, excessive speed is unnecessary and dangerous. What is necessary is that the patient be safely transported to a hospital in the shortest practical time. This takes common sense and defensive driving techniques. Speed is no substitute for these qualities.

This chapter focuses on the techniques and judgment that you will need to learn to drive an ambulance or ambulance service vehicle. It begins with a look at ambulance design, then discusses emergency vehicle control and operation, both important factors in safe driving. The chapter also discusses how to equip and maintain an ambulance, parking considerations, the effects of weather on driving, and common hazards that are encountered in driving an ambulance. Finally, it describes how to work safely with air ambulances.

> What is necessary is that the patient be safely transported to a hospital in the shortest practical time.

Emergency Vehicle Design

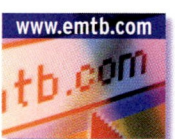

An **ambulance** is a vehicle that is used for treating and transporting patients who need emergency medical care from the scene to the hospital. The first motor-powered ambulance was introduced in 1906. For many decades after that, a hearse was the vehicle that was most often used as an ambulance, because it was the only vehicle with room enough for a person to lie down. Few supplies were carried on board, and there was little space for attendants.

The hearse-ambulance has gone the way of its horse-drawn predecessor. Ambulances today are designed according to strict government regulations based on national standards. The standards themselves are based in large part on suggestions from the ambulance industry, including EMS personnel. One of the most significant developments in ambulance design has been the enlargement of the patient compartment. Another development is the use of **ambulance service vehicles**, which respond initially to the scene with personnel and equipment to treat the sick and injured until an ambulance can arrive.

As defined by the National Academy of Sciences-National Research Council, the modern ambulance is a vehicle for emergency medical care that has the following features:

- A driver's compartment
- A patient compartment that can accommodate two EMTs and two patients on **litters**

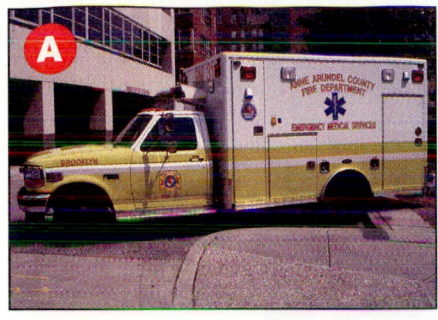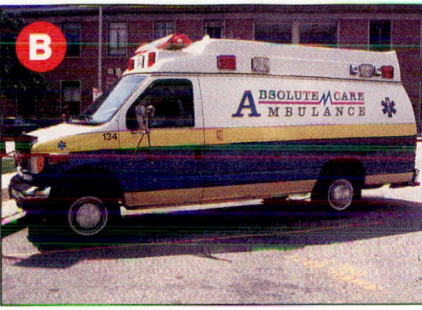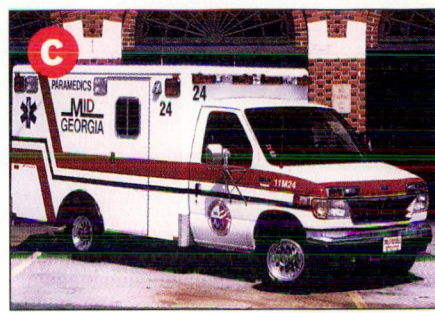

FIGURE 36-1 A: The conventional, truck cab-chassis has a modular ambulance body that can be transferred to a newer chassis (Type I). **B:** The standard van ambulance has a forward-control integral cab body (Type II). **C:** The specialty van ambulance has a forward-control integral cab body (Type III).

(a type of stretcher for moving or carrying patients), positioned so that at least one of the patients can receive CPR during transit

- Equipment and supplies to provide emergency medical care at the scene and during transport, to safeguard personnel and patients from hazardous conditions, and to carry out light extrication procedures

- Two-way radio communication so that ambulance personnel can speak with the dispatcher, the hospital, public safety authorities, and medical control

- Design and construction that ensure maximum safety and comfort

Each state establishes its own standards for licensing or certifying ambulances; however, most use the federal specifications (KKK-A-1822C, 1990) that cover the following three types of basic ambulance designs (Figure 36-1 and Table 36-1).

www.emtb.com

The six-pointed Star of Life® emblem identifies ambulances that meet federal specifications as licensed or certified ambulances. It should be affixed to the sides, rear, and roof of the ambulance. Local regulatory authorities determine what emblems may be displayed on the side of a prehospital care ambulance, but there is no regulation regarding emblems for inter-hospital transport ambulances, which may carry emblems that resemble the Star of Life® or a red cross.

Figures 36-2 and 36-3 illustrate the required features of a licensed or certified ambulance.

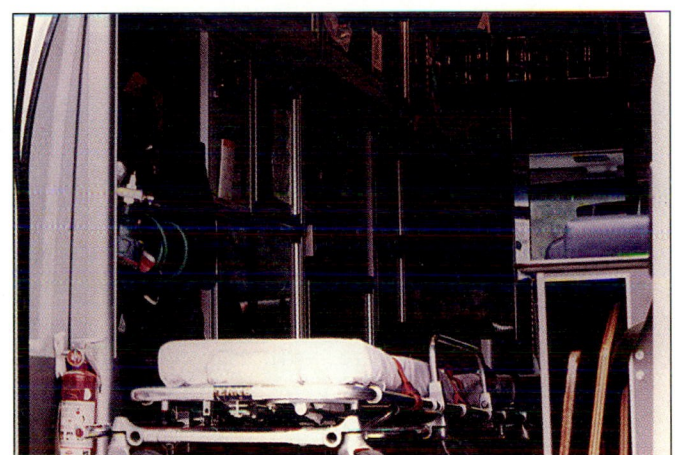

FIGURE 36-2 Parts of the ambulance.

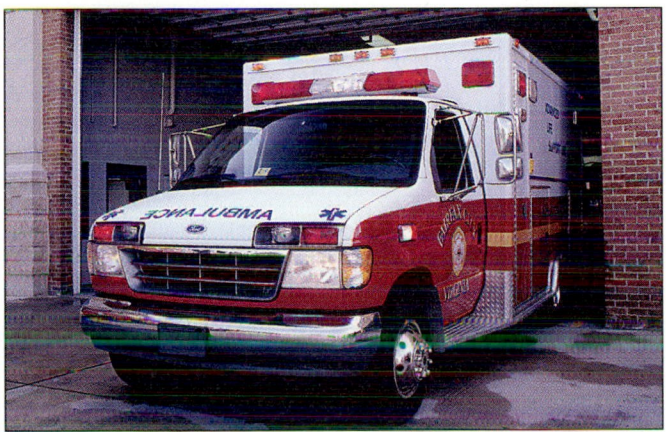

FIGURE 36-3 Warning lights and public address systems are necessary.

TABLE 36-1	Basic Ambulance Designs
Type I:	Conventional, truck cab-chassis with modular ambulance body that can be transferred to a newer chassis as needed
Type II:	Standard van, forward-control integral cab-body ambulance
Type III:	Specialty van, forward-control integral cab-body ambulance

Phases of an Ambulance Call

An ambulance call has nine phases: preparation, dispatch, en route, arrival at scene, transfer to ambulance, en route to receiving facility (transport), at receiving facility (delivery), en route to station, and postrun, as shown in Table 36-2.

The Preparation Phase

Making sure that equipment and supplies are in their proper place and ready for use is an important part of preparing for the call. Items that are missing or that do not work are of no use to you or the patient. As a general rule of thumb, the more complex a piece of equipment is, and the harder it is to learn to use, the more likely it is to malfunction during an emergency. Many EMS items have never been rigorously tested under field conditions and could turn out to be expensive mistakes. For this reason, you should never order a new piece of equipment without consulting with the medical director.

Equipment and supplies should be durable and, to the extent possible, standardized. This makes it easy to quickly exchange equipment with other ambulances or with the emergency department, thus saving time during patient transfer.

Store equipment and supplies in the ambulance according to how urgently and how often they are used (Figure 36-4). Give priority to items that are needed to care for life-threatening conditions. These include equipment for airway care, artificial ventilation, and oxygen delivery. Place these items within easy reach, at the head of the primary litter. Place items for cardiac care, control of external bleeding, and monitoring blood pressure at the side of the litter.

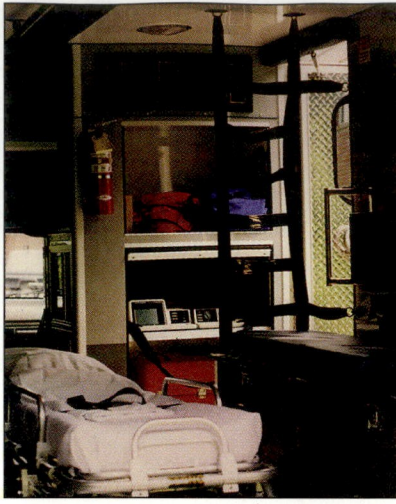

FIGURE 36-4
Store equipment and supplies in the ambulance according to how urgently and how often they are used.

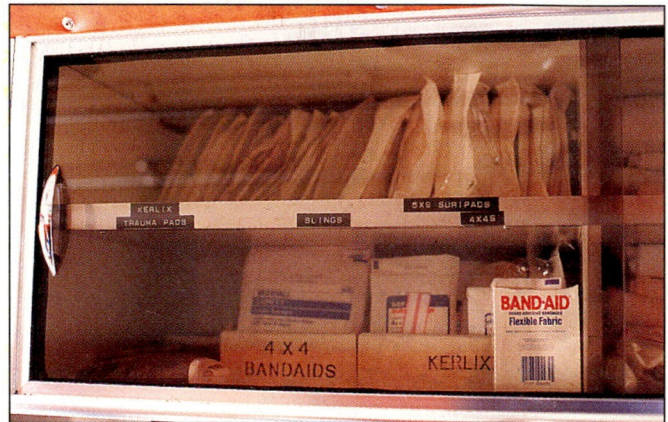

FIGURE 36-5 Containers should be placed in cabinets and drawers with transparent fronts for quick identification.

Storage cabinets and kits should open easily. They should also close securely so that they do not fly open while the ambulance is in motion. Cabinet and drawer fronts should be transparent so that you can quickly identify their contents; if they are not, be sure to label each container (Figure 36-5).

Medical equipment. As an EMT-B, you have access to a large variety of medical equipment and supplies, far more than can be described here. Certain items must be available on the ambulance at all times.

Basic supplies. Table 36-3 lists the basic supplies that should be carried on all ambulances.

Airway management. Airway management equipment that should be carried on all ambulances includes the following:

- Oropharyngeal airways for adults, children, and infants

- Nasopharyngeal airways for adults and children

- Two sets of equipment for advanced airway procedures if your service is authorized by state

TABLE 36-2 Phases of an Ambulance Call
• Preparation for the call
• Dispatch
• En route
• Arrival at scene
• Transferring the patient to the ambulance
• En route to the receiving facility (transport)
• At the receiving facility (delivery)
• En route to the station
• Postrun

TABLE 36-3   Basic Supplies

- At least 2 pillows and pillowcases
- Sterile sheets (at least 2 spare sheets)
- 4 blankets
- 4 towels
- 6 disposable emesis bags or basins
- 2 boxes of disposable tissue
- 1 bedpan (optional)
- 2 urinals (one male, one female; optional)
- 3 thermometers (one oral, one rectal, one hypothermia)
- 3 blood pressure cuffs (pediatric, adult, large adult)
- 1 stethoscope
- 1 pair of trauma shears
- 1 package of disposable drinking cups
- 1 unbreakable container of water
- 1 package of wet wipes
- 4 chemical cold packs
- 4 L of sterile irrigation fluid
- 2 restraining devices
- 1 package of plastic bags for waste or severed parts
- Latex disposable gloves (various sizes)
- 1 sharps container (minimum)
- 1 set of hearing protectors
- 2 infection control kits (goggles, masks, waterproof gowns)

regulation and the medical director to perform these: one in the ambulance and one in the jump kit that you carry to the patient

Ventilation devices. It is important that two portable artificial ventilation devices that operate independently of an oxygen supply are carried on the ambulance: one for use in the ambulance and one for use outside the ambulance or as a spare. These devices include pocket masks and bag valve mask (BVM) devices. In addition, BVM devices capable of oxygen enrichment that, when attached to an oxygen supply with the oxygen reservoir in place, are able to supply almost 100% oxygen, should also be carried on the ambulance. The nonrebreathing valve on the mask must allow patients to inhale oxygen during both artificial ventilation and spontaneous respirations. Devices should be either disposable or easy to clean and **decontaminate**, which means removal of radiation, chemical, or other hazardous material.

Masks for these devices come in a variety of sizes, from infant to adult, and are necessary materials to carry on the ambulance. The masks should be transparent so that you can monitor the patient's respirations, notice any color changes in the patient, and detect vomiting. Adult- and pediatric-size BVMs should be used with the appropriately sized mask to deliver the proper volume of oxygen-enriched air to the patient. In some regions, barrier devices for ventilation may be carried on the ambulance, depending on the preference of the medical director. Oxygen-powered devices are also available to provide ventilation to a patient.

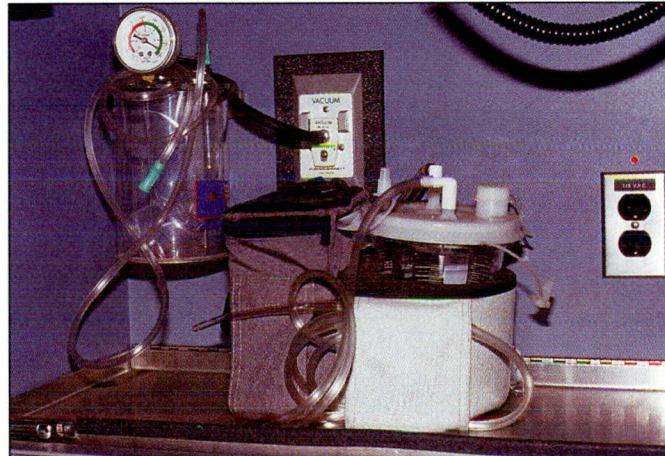

FIGURE 36-6 The ambulance should carry both a mounted suctioning unit and a portable unit.

Suctioning unit. The ambulance should carry both portable and installed suctioning units (Figure 36-6). These units must be powerful enough to provide an airflow of 30 L/min at the end of the tube and a vacuum of 300 mm Hg when the tube is clamped. The suctioning force must be adjustable for use on infants and children. The units should include large-bore, nonkinking suction tubing with a semirigid pharyngeal tip, with additional semirigid tips available.

The installed unit should include a suction yoke, an unbreakable collection bottle, water for rinsing the suction tips, and suction tubing, all easily accessible when you are sitting at the head of the litter. The tubing must reach the patient's airway, regardless of the patient's position. All components of the suctioning unit must be disposable or made of material that is easily cleaned and decontaminated.

Oxygen delivery. The ambulance should carry at least two oxygen supply units: one portable and one installed. The portable unit should be located near a door or in the jump kit, for easy use outside the ambulance. It should have a capacity of 300 L of oxygen and be equipped with a yoke, pressure gauge, flowmeter, oxygen supply tubing, nonrebreathing mask, and nasal cannula. This unit must be able to deliver oxygen at a variable rate between 2 and 15 L/min. At least one extra portable 300-L cylinder should be kept on the ambulance. Many services equip the backup cylinder with its own yoke, gauge, regulator, and tubing so that it can be used for a second patient.

The installed oxygen unit should have a capacity of 3,000 L of oxygen (Figure 36-7). It should also be equipped with visible flowmeters that are capable of delivering 2 to 15 L/min that are accessible when you are at the head of the litter. Position this unit so that the oxygen supply tubing will reach a patient who is lying on the stretcher or on the squad bench. Oxygen masks, with and without bags, should be semiopen, transparent, and disposable, in sizes for adults, children, and infants.

Ambulance services that often transport patients on runs lasting longer than 1 hour should consider using a disposable, single-use humidifier for the installed oxygen system. On runs of less than 1 hour, humidification may increase a patient's risk of infection unless the equipment is rigorously maintained.

CPR equipment. A <u>CPR board</u> provides a firm surface under the patient's torso so that you can give effective chest compressions (Figure 36-8). It also establishes an appropriate degree of head tilt. If you do not have a special CPR board, you can place a long or short backboard under the patient on the litter. Use a tightly rolled sheet or towel to raise the patient's shoulders 3″ to 4″; this will

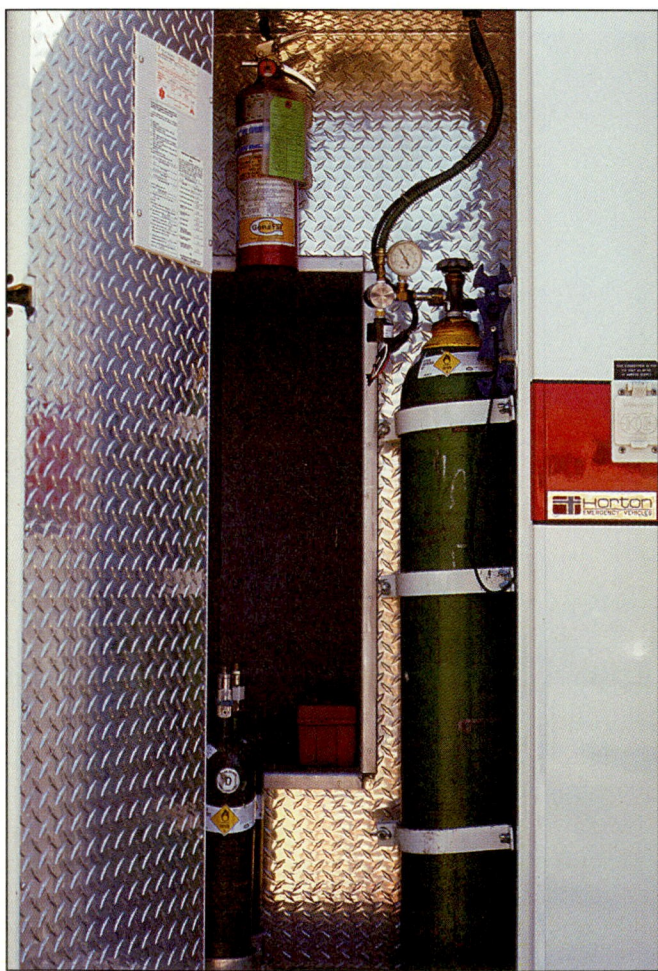

FIGURE 36-7 An oxygen unit with a capacity of 3,000 L of oxygen should be installed on the ambulance.

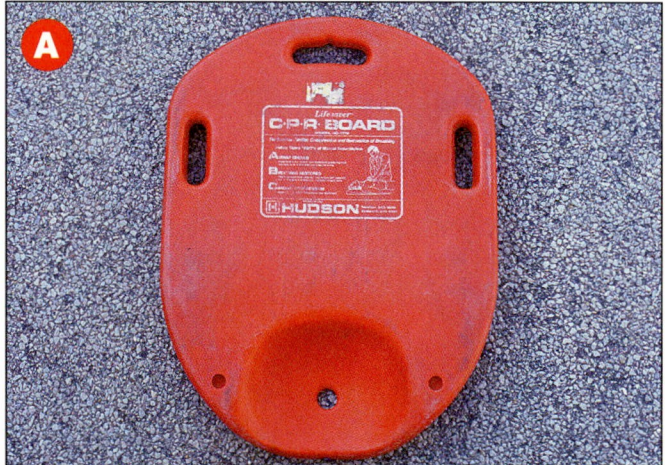

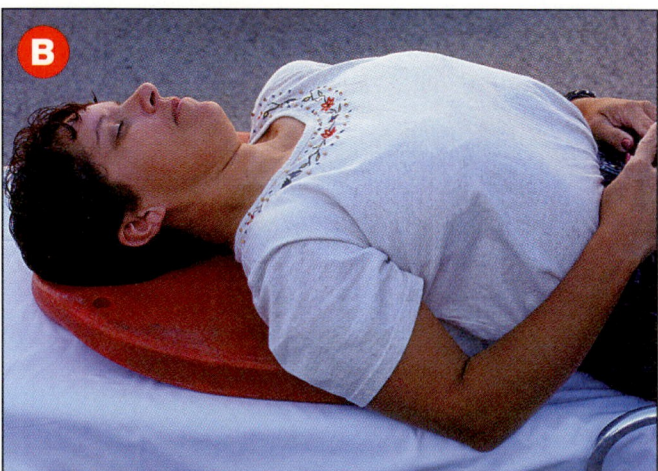

FIGURE 36-8 A: A CPR board should be carried on the ambulance. **B:** A patient on a CPR board has the appropriate degree of head tilt for effective artificial ventilation.

TABLE 36-4 Basic Wound Care Supplies

- Sterile sheets
- Large safety pins
- Adhesive tape in several widths
- Self-adhering, soft roller bandages, 4" x 5 yd
- Self-adhering, soft roller bandages, 2" by 5 yd
- Sterile dressings, gauze, 4" x 4"
- Sterile dressings, ABD or laparotomy pads, usually 6" x 9" or 8" x 10"
- Sterile universal trauma dressings, usually 10" x 36", folded into 9" x 10" packages
- Sterile, occlusive, nonadherent dressings (aluminum foil sterilized in original package)
- An assortment of Band-Aids®

TABLE 36-5 Splinting Supplies

- 1 adult-size traction splint
- 1 child-size traction splint
- A variety of arm and leg splints, such as inflatable, vacuum, cardboard, plastic, foam wire-ladder, or padded board. The number and type of splints should be determined by state regulations and your medical director.
- A variety of triangular bandages and roller bandages
- A short backboard device
- A long backboard
- Cervical collars in an adjustable size or a variety of sizes
- 1 adult-size pneumatic antishock garment (PASG)

TABLE 36-6 Emergency OB Pack

- 1 pair of surgical scissors
- 3 hemostats or special cord clamps
- Umbilical tape or sterilized cord
- Small rubber bulb syringe
- 5 towels
- 12 2" x 10" gauze sponges
- 3 or 4 pairs of sterile gloves
- Sanitary napkins
- A plastic bag
- 1 baby blanket

also keep the patient's head in a position of maximum backward tilt and keep the shoulders and chest in a straight position. Caution: Do not use this roll to hyperextend the neck if you suspect a spinal injury.

Mechanical devices that operate on compressed gas and deliver chest compressions and ventilations are also available.

Basic wound care supplies. Table 36-4 lists the basic supplies for dressing open wounds that should be included on the ambulance.

Splinting supplies. Supplies for splinting fractures and dislocations that should be carried on all ambulances are listed in Table 36-5 (Figure 36-9).

Childbirth supplies. You must carry a sterile emergency obstetric delivery (OB) pack that includes the supplies listed in Table 36-6 (Figure 36-10).

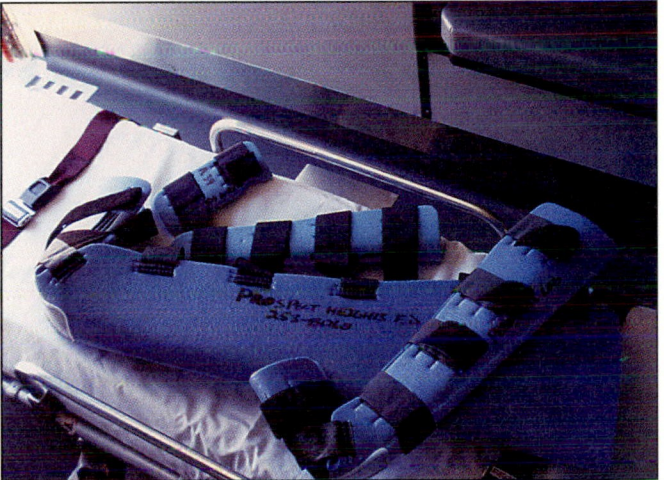

FIGURE 36-9 Supplies for splinting fractures and dislocations should be carried on the ambulance.

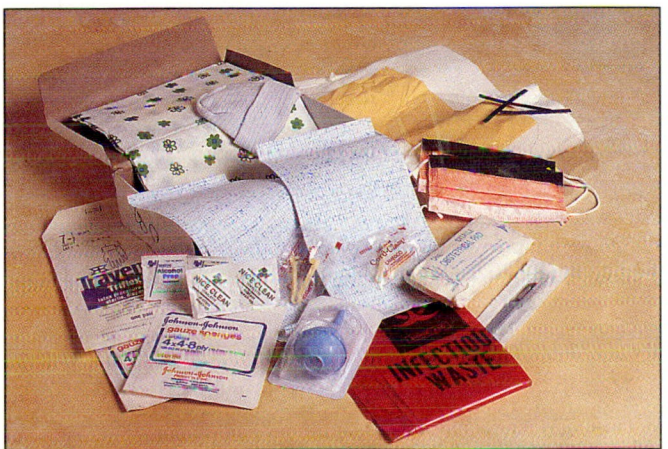

FIGURE 36-10 A sterile emergency obstetric delivery pack must be carried on the ambulance.

Medications. It is important that the ambulance carry the items listed in Table 36-7. Be certain that you have the telephone number and radio frequency of medical control or the local poison control center with you on the ambulance. The back of your clipboard is a good place to keep this information.

Automated external defibrillator. Semiautomated defibrillation equipment, as permitted by regulation and the local medical director, should always be carried on the ambulance (Figure 36-11).

The jump kit. The ambulance must be equipped with a portable, durable, and waterproof <u>jump kit</u> that you can carry to the patient (Figure 36-12). Think of the jump kit as the "5-minute kit," containing anything you might need in the first 5 minutes with the patient except for the semiautomated external defibrillator and possibly the oxygen bottle and portable suctioning unit.

It should also contain the phone number of medical control or the local poison control center, depending on your medical protocols. The jump kit must be easy to open and secure. Table 36-8 lists the items that are typically contained in a jump kit.

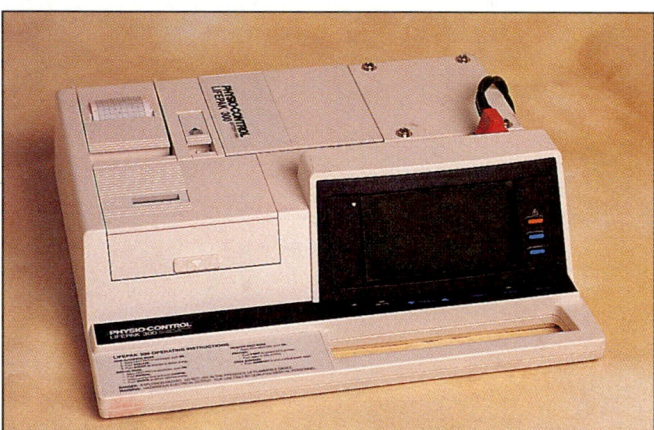

FIGURE 36-11 Every ambulance should carry an automated external defibrillator.

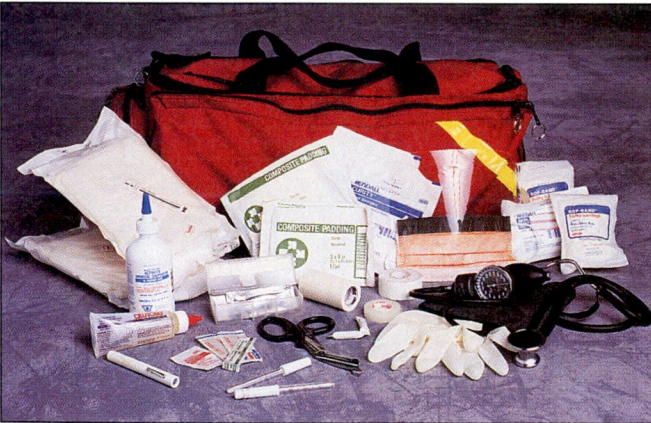

FIGURE 36-12 A portable jump kit contains anything you may need during the first 5 minutes with the patient except for the semi-automated external defibrillator and possibly the oxygen cylinder and portable suctioning unit.

TABLE 36-7	Medications Carried on the Ambulance

- Activated charcoal in premeasured doses
- Drinkable water and cups
- Tubes of oral glucose or other fluid or substance approved by local protocol
- Oxygen, as described above
- Supplies for irrigating the skin and eyes
- A snake bite kit or other regional equipment, depending on the area and local protocol

TABLE 36-8	Items Carried in a Jump Kit

- Latex gloves
- Triangular bandages
- Trauma shears
- Adhesive tape in various widths
- Universal trauma dressings
- Self-adhering soft roller bandages, 4" x 5 yd and 2" x 5 yd
- Oropharyngeal airways in adult, child, and infant sizes*
- BVM device with masks for adults, children, and infants*
- Blood pressure cuff
- Stethoscope
- Penlight
- Sterile gauze dressings, 4" x 4"
- Sterile dressings (ABD or laparotomy pads), 6" x 9" or 8" x 10"
- Thermometer
- Adhesive strips
- Oral glucose
- Activated charcoal

* These might be carried in a separate airway kit, along with the portable oxygen cylinder.

Patient transfer equipment. Each ambulance should carry the following patient transfer equipment:

- A primary wheeled ambulance stretcher

- A folding litter

- A collapsible chair device or stair chair for use in narrow spaces

The collapsible and folding litters may be combined in one unit. Litters must be easy to move, store, clean, and disinfect. The folding litter should keep the patient elevated above the floor when in the flat, extended position (Figure 36-13). The wheeled stretcher (or litter) should be adjustable in height. When it is secured in the lowest position, the top should be 11" to 15" above the floor of the ambulance (Figure 36-14). You should be able to tilt the head of the litter upward to at least a 60° semisitting position and tilt the entire litter into 10° to 15° of Trendelenburg's position (head down) for airway care and treatment of shock. Litters must be at least 76" long and 23" wide and must be provided with fasteners to secure them firmly to the floor or side of the ambulance during transport. Litter restraints should be capable of holding the litter in place in case the vehicle rolls over. Make sure there are at least two restraining devices for the patient.

Moving the patient to the ambulance can be done in different ways, depending on the injury or illness. Some patients can walk easily to the ambulance, which is sometimes easier and safer than trying to use a stretcher. For patients with spinal injuries, using a backboard or other immobilizing device, such as a Kendrick Extrication Device®, is usually best. For some patients with medical problems, especially patients with respiratory problems, transport with the patient sitting upright may allow the patient the most comfort and safety.

Personnel. Every ambulance must be staffed with at least one EMT-B in the patient compartment whenever a patient is being transported; two EMTs are strongly recommended. Some services may operate with a non-EMT driver and a single EMT-B in the patient compartment.

To do the job effectively, the EMT team will need the following equipment.

- Personal safety equipment
- Equipment for work areas
- Preplanning/navigation guides
- Extrication equipment

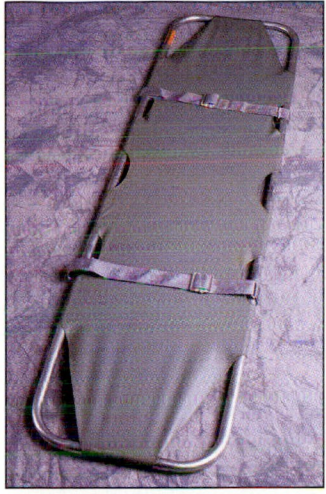

FIGURE 36-13 A folding litter is one of the three types of patient transfer equipment that should be carried on the ambulance.

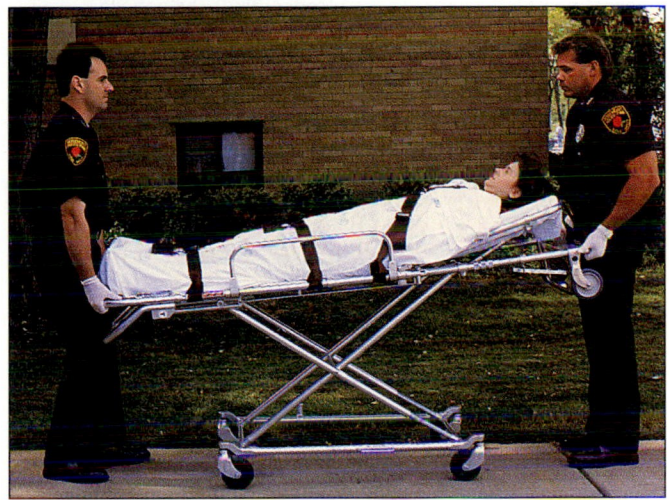

FIGURE 36-14 The wheeled ambulance stretcher should be adjustable in height.

Personal safety equipment. You should always carry personal protective equipment that allows you to work safely in a limited variety of hazardous or contaminated situations. These situations include the edges of a structural fire or explosion, vehicle extrication, and in crowds. The equipment should protect you from exposure to blood and other potentially infectious body fluids. Note that you will not be equipped to face all HazMat and other exposure situations that you may encounter; this is the job of specially trained HazMat technicians and response teams. Your equipment might include the following:

- Face shields

- Gowns, shoe covers, caps

- Turnout gear

- Helmets with face shields or safety goggles

- Safety shoes or boots

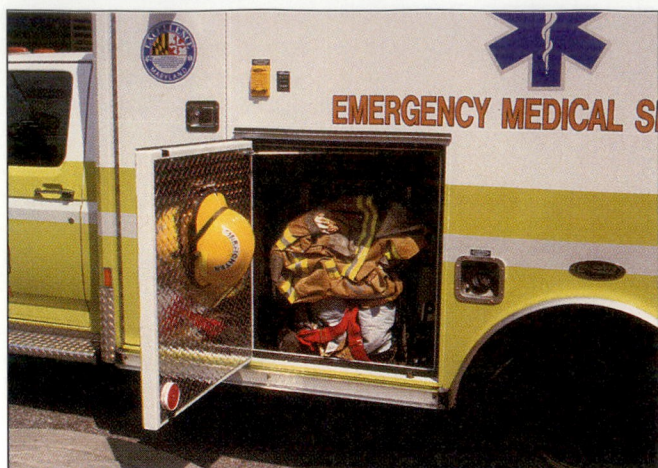

FIGURE 36-15 The ambulance should have a weatherproof compartment that can be reached from outside the patient compartment. It should hold equipment for safeguarding patients and EMTs, controlling traffic, and illuminating work areas.

Equipment for work areas. A weatherproof compartment that you can reach from outside the patient compartment should hold equipment for safeguarding patients and EMTs, controlling traffic and bystanders, and illuminating work areas (Figure 36-15). The following items are recommended:

- Warning devices that flash intermittently or have reflectors (road flares are not acceptable because they can pose an additional hazard, such as ignition of flammable liquids or gases)
- Two high-intensity halogen 20,000 candle flashlights of the recharging battery-powered, stand-up type
- Fire extinguisher, type BC, dry powder, size 5 lb minimum
- Hard hats or helmets with face shields or safety goggles
- Two portable floodlights

Preplanning and navigation. Make sure you have detailed street and area maps in the driver's compartment of the ambulance, along with directions to key locations, such as local hospitals. Become familiar with the roads and traffic patterns in your town or city so that you can plan alternative routes to common destinations. Pay particular attention to ways around frequently opened bridges, congested traffic, or blocked railroad crossings. Often, switching to an alternative route will save more time than driving faster. Also become familiar with special facilities and locations within your operating area, such as other medical facilities, arenas and stadiums, and chemical or research facilities that might pose unusual problems.

Extrication equipment. A weatherproof compartment outside the patient compartment should contain equipment that is needed for simple, light extrication, even if an extrication and rescue unit is readily available. Table 36-9 lists the items that should be included in the compartment.

If rescue and extrication services are not readily available, additional equipment may be needed.

Daily inspections. Being fully prepared means that you and your team must inspect both the ambulance and equipment daily to ensure that everything is in proper working order. The ambulance inspection should include the following:

✓ Fuel levels
✓ Oil levels
✓ Transmission fluid levels
✓ Engine cooling system and fluid levels
✓ Batteries
✓ Brake fluid
✓ Engine belts
✓ Wheels and tires, including the spare, if there is one. Check inflation pressure and look for signs of unusual or uneven wear.
✓ All interior and exterior lights
✓ Windshield wipers and fluid
✓ Horn
✓ Siren
✓ Air conditioners and heaters
✓ Ventilating system
✓ Doors. Make sure they open, close, latch, and lock properly.
✓ Communication systems, vehicle and portable
✓ All windows and mirrors. Check for cleanliness and position.

Check all medical equipment and supplies at least daily, including all the oxygen supplies, the jump kit, splints, dressings and bandages, backboards and other immobilization equipment, and emergency OB kit. Is the equipment functioning properly? Are the supplies clean? Are there enough of them? All battery-operated equipment, including the defibrillator, should be operated and checked each day. Rotate the batteries according to an established schedule.

TABLE 36-9 Extrication Equipment

- 12" wrench, adjustable, open-end
- 12" screwdriver, standard square bar
- 8" screwdriver, Phillips head #2
- Hacksaw with 12" carbide wire blades
- Vise-grip pliers, 10"
- 5-lb hammer with 15" handle
- Fire ax, butt, 24" handle
- Wrecking bar with 24" handle. This may be in a combination tool with a hammer and ax.
- 51" crowbar, pinch point
- Bolt cutter with 1" to 1¼" jaw opening
- Folding shovel, pointed blade
- Tin snips, double action, 8" minimum
- Gauntlets, reinforced, leather covering past midforearm; one pair per crew member
- Rescue blanket
- Ropes, 5,400-lb tensile strength in 50' lengths in protective bags
- Mastic knife (able to cut seat belt webbing)
- Spring-load center punch
- Pruning saw
- Heavy duty 2" x 4" and 4" x 4" shoring (cribbing) blocks, various lengths

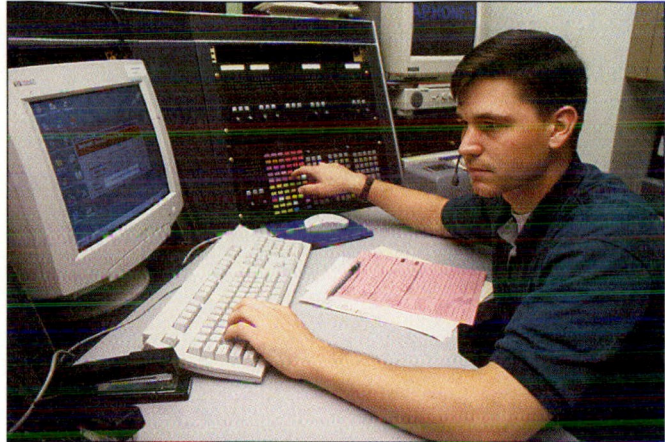

FIGURE 36-16 Dispatch must be easy to reach and always available.

Safety precautions. A final part of the preparation phase is reviewing safety precautions. These precautions, which include standard traffic safety rules and regulations, should be followed on every call. Check to make sure that safety devices, such as seat belts, are in proper working order.

The Dispatch Phase

Dispatch must be easy to access and in service 24 hours a day (Figure 36-16). It may be operated by the local EMS or by a shared service that also covers law enforcement and the fire department. The dispatch center might serve only one jurisdiction, such as a single city or town, or it might be an area or regional center serving several communities or an entire county. In either case, it should be staffed by trained personnel who are familiar with the agencies they are dispatching and the geography of the service area. For every emergency request, the dispatcher should gather and record the following minimum information:

- The nature of the call
- The name, present location, and call-back telephone number of the caller
- The location of the patient(s)
- The number of patients and some idea of the severity of their conditions
- Any other special problems or pertinent information about hazards or weather conditions

Many areas implement emergency medical dispatching, which allows the caller to receive instructions for patient care before the ambulance arrives.

En Route to the Scene

As you and your partner prepare to respond to the scene, make sure you fasten your seat belts and shoulder harnesses before you move the ambulance. At this point, you should inform dispatch that your unit is responding and confirm the nature and location of the call. This is also an excellent time to ask for any other available information about the location. For example, you might learn that the patient is on the third floor or that the best door to use is around the side of the house.

While en route, the team should prepare to assess and care for the patient. Review dispatch information about the nature of the call and the location of the patient. Assign specific initial duties and scene management tasks to each team member, and decide what type of equipment to take initially. Depending on your operation procedures, you may also decide which stretcher to bring to the patient.

Driver characteristics. In many ways, the en route or response phase of the call is the most dangerous for you. Collisions between automobiles and emergency vehicles

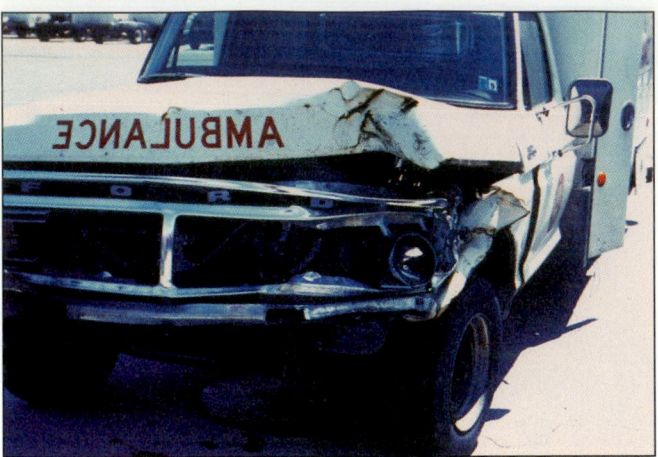

FIGURE 36-17 The en route or response phase may be the most dangerous part of the call.

cause most job-related injuries among EMS personnel (Figure 36-17). Therefore, drivers should be screened carefully. Not everyone who drives an automobile is qualified to drive an emergency vehicle. In some states, you must successfully complete an approved emergency vehicle operations course before you are allowed to drive the ambulance on emergency calls. In any state, diligence and caution are important characteristics, as are a positive attitude about your ability and tolerance of other drivers.

One basic requirement is physical fitness. Many accidents occur as a result of physical impairment of the driver. You should not be driving if you are taking medications that may cause drowsiness or slow your reaction times. These include cold remedies, analgesics, or tranquilizers. And, of course, you should never drive or provide medical care after drinking alcohol.

Another requirement is emotional fitness. Emotions should not be taken lightly. Personality often changes once an individual gets behind a steering wheel. Emotional stability is closely related to the ability to operate under stress. In addition to knowing exactly what to do, you must be able to do it under trying conditions.

The proper attitude is very important for an ambulance driver. Being able to drive to your destination without interruption and to move into the opposite lane are valuable, time-saving privileges that must never be abused. Do not ever get behind the wheel thinking that you can do whatever you like.

In addition to training and experience, the good judgment and knowledge that you need to drive an ambulance require practice. Remember, even the best drivers can benefit from practice. You can practice anytime, any place, in any vehicle.

Safe driving practices. Safe driving is a very important part of the emergency care of sick and injured patients.

The first rule of safe driving in an emergency vehicle is that speed does not save lives; good care does. The second rule is that the driver and all passengers must wear seat belts and shoulder restraints at all times. These are the most important items of safety equipment on every ambulance. Other EMTs should wear restraints en route to the scene and whenever they are not performing direct patient care.

Learn how your vehicle accelerates, corners, sways, and stops. For example, disc booster brakes make braking more efficient but increase sway. You must know exactly how your particular vehicle will respond to steering, braking, and accelerating under various conditions.

Getting a feel for the proper brake pressure comes with experience and practice. Each vehicle has a different braking action. For example, the brakes on types I and III vehicles have a heavier feel than the brakes on a type II vehicle. Braking on a diesel-powered unit will be different from braking on an identically equipped gasoline-powered unit. Certain heavy vehicles use air brakes, which have yet another feel. Get to know each vehicle you drive, and be sure you understand its braking characteristics and the best downshifting techniques.

The EMT driver often assumes that motorists and pedestrians will do the right thing when an emergency vehicle is in the vicinity. This is a mistake. Motorists may indeed pull over to the nearest curb and stop or drive as close to the curb as possible, but you cannot take this behavior for granted. At any time, a motorist might stop suddenly in front of the ambulance, causing a serious accident.

When you are driving an ambulance on a multi-lane highway, you should usually stay in the extreme left-hand (fast) lane. This allows other motorists to move over to the right when they see or hear you approach.

Most important, you must always drive defensively. Never rely on what another motorist will do unless you get a clear visual signal. Even then, you must be prepared to take defensive action in the case of a misunderstanding, panic, or careless driving on the part of the other driver.

The problem of excessive speed. Only in extreme life-and-death emergencies is speed an important factor. In most instances, if you properly assess and stabilize the patient at the scene, speed during transport is unnecessary and undesirable. No matter what the situation, you should never travel at a speed that is unsafe for the given road conditions.

Studies have shown conclusively that excessive speeds are unnecessary and, in most cases, do not add to patient survivability. More often, using excessive speed while driving to and from the scene has resulted in accidents in which the EMT, patient, and occupants of other vehicles are killed.

The following five factors contribute to the use of excessive speed:

1. **Lack of expertise** on the part of the dispatcher, resulting in calls being given an inappropriately high priority. Dispatching requires a trained, experienced EMT or emergency medical dispatcher. Only someone with training and a working knowledge of emergency calls can determine the urgency of a call, especially when the caller is excited and distraught. Untrained dispatchers cannot make such decisions properly.

2. **Inadequate equipment in the ambulance.** If you do not have the equipment and supplies that are necessary to stabilize the patient, you may have little choice but to speed to the hospital.

3. **Inadequate training of the EMT.** Without adequate training and confidence in your ability to care for the patient, you may tend to act like a chauffeur rather than an EMT.

4. **Inadequate driving ability.** This is the most important factor. If you do not understand the added risks that go with high-speed driving and the principles of safe ambulance operation, you might tend to choose speed over safety.

5. **Siren syndrome.** The siren may have a psychological effect on the driver, who may not recognize that he or she is driving faster and faster.

Emergency vehicle control. As the driver of an ambulance, you have only two ways to control the vehicle: by changing its direction or changing its speed. Either maneuver requires a continuous rolling contact between the surface of the tires and the surface of the road. Two factors are involved in this contact. The first is the <u>coefficient of friction</u>, which is a measure of the tire's grip on the road; <u>friction</u> is the resistance to motion of one body against another. The second factor is the <u>footprints</u> of the tires, which is the area of contact between the tire and surface of the road. On the typical ambulance, the footprint is about 8″ long and as wide as the tire.

The coefficient of friction may vary widely on different parts of the same road, depending on the condition of the surface, the age of the road, and the weather. It also varies according to the tire's tread design and wear. As a driver, you must constantly evaluate the road sur-

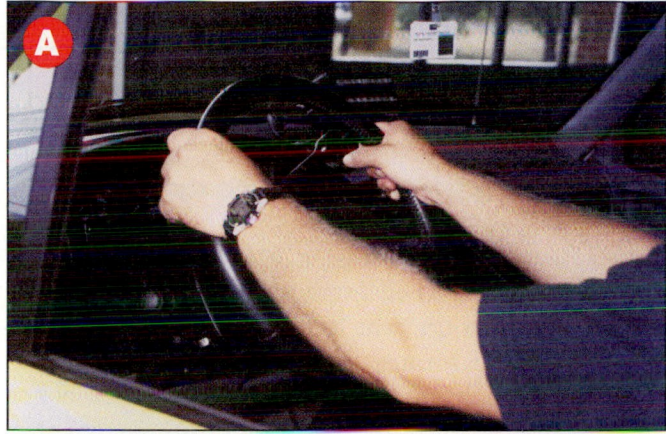

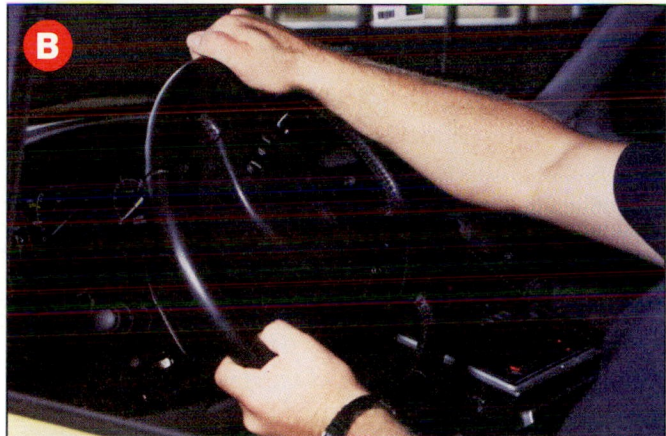

FIGURE 36-18 A: Hold the steering wheel with your hands at the nine o'clock and three o'clock positions so that you can turn the wheel without removing either hand. **B:** Turn the wheel by pulling with one hand and sliding the other. Make sure that both hands remain parallel.

face: At a given speed, how much frictional force can the tires apply before the ambulance becomes unstable? This is especially important in cornering, in which additional centrifugal force is acting on the vehicle.

Steering techniques. Steering technique includes the way you hold the steering wheel, the way it moves, and the timing of the movements. Hold the wheel with your hands at the nine o'clock and three o'clock positions. This allows you to turn the wheel without removing either hand; one hand pulls while the other slides so that they remain parallel (Figure 36-18). Your hands should not pass the twelve o'clock or six o'clock positions, because they will cross and become tangled; instead, let the hand that was pulling start to slide, and use the opposite hand to pull.

Timing of steering wheel movements relates to the speed of the vehicle. All vehicles lag somewhat when responding to steering input. The faster the speed, the greater the lag.

Chassis set. The <u>chassis</u> is the vehicle frame of the ambulance. <u>Chassis set</u> is the transfer of weight (center of mass) to different points on the chassis. Basically, the weight of a vehicle is concentrated over one of three points on the chassis: the front wheels, the rear wheels, or the center between the front and rear wheels. The transfer of weight from one point to another is caused by <u>acceleration</u>, or increasing speed, or <u>deceleration</u>, or slowing down. When a vehicle accelerates, the weight is transferred to the rear; the front wheels lose some traction, which means that you lose some ability to steer. The ambulance will have a tendency to travel in a straight line. With braking, the opposite weight shift occurs; this is why the rear end of the vehicle tends to slide to the outside of a curve when cornering.

Vehicle size and distance judgment. Vehicle length and width are critical factors in maneuvering, driving, and parking an emergency vehicle. They are especially important with types I and III vehicles, which are wider than they look from behind the steering wheel. To brake and pass effectively, you must know the width and length of your vehicle. Crashes often occur when the vehicle is backing up. Always use someone outside the ambulance as a ground guide when you are backing up, to avoid any surprises. Vehicle size and weight will greatly influence braking and stopping distances. Good peripheral vision and depth perception will help you to judge distances, but they are no substitute for intensive training, experience, and frequent evaluation of the vehicle.

Road positioning and cornering. Road position means the position of the vehicle on the roadway relative to the inside or outside edge of the paved surface. To corner efficiently, you must know the vehicle's present position and its projected path. The aim is to take the corner at the speed that will put you in the proper road position as you exit the curve. The process works in the following way: The apex of the turn through a curve is the point at which the vehicle is closest to the inside edge of the curve. If you reach the apex early in the curve, the vehicle will be forced toward the outside of the roadway as it exits the curve. If you reach the apex late in the curve, the vehicle will tend to stay on the inside of the roadway; this helps you to keep the vehicle in the proper lane (Figure 36-19).

Controlled acceleration. Controlled acceleration is the use of acceleration to control the vehicle; it is done by applying foot pressure on the accelerator pedal. Acceleration is most efficient when the vehicle is traveling in a straight line, because the force of linear acceleration is equally distributed to the rear wheels. If

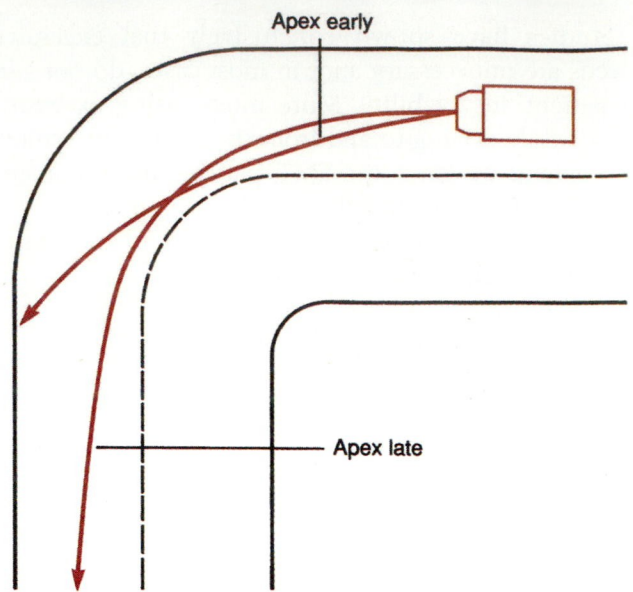

FIGURE 36-19 To keep the ambulance in the proper lane on a curve, you must know the vehicle's present position and projected path and take the corner at the correct speed.

you accelerate in a curve or during a turn, however, you force the vehicle to the outside of the curve. If acceleration in this direction becomes excessive, the vehicle may drift out of control and become unstable.

Controlled braking. Controlled braking is the use of the brakes to control the vehicle. Brakes not only control the movement of the vehicle, causing it to slow or stop; they also help to control its direction. Braking while the vehicle is traveling in a straight line is the safest, most efficient method. Braking in a turn causes a loss of efficiency. You might not notice this at low speed, but it becomes more apparent at higher speeds. Applying the brakes while cornering is not an effective way to slow the vehicle and may actually cause a skid or spin. Instead, maintain your speed by simultaneously easing off brake pressure and increasing accelerator pressure. Getting the feel for the proper brake pressure comes with experience and practice driving your assigned vehicle.

Weather and road conditions. You should be constantly alert to changing weather, road, and driving conditions (Figure 36-20). Whether going to or coming from an emergency, you must modify your speed according to road conditions. Take warnings of ice or hazardous conditions seriously, and be prepared to take an alternative route, if necessary. During a major disaster, all public safety and emergency services should be coordinated. If you run into unexpected traffic congestion, notify the dispatcher so that other emergency vehicles can select alternative routes.

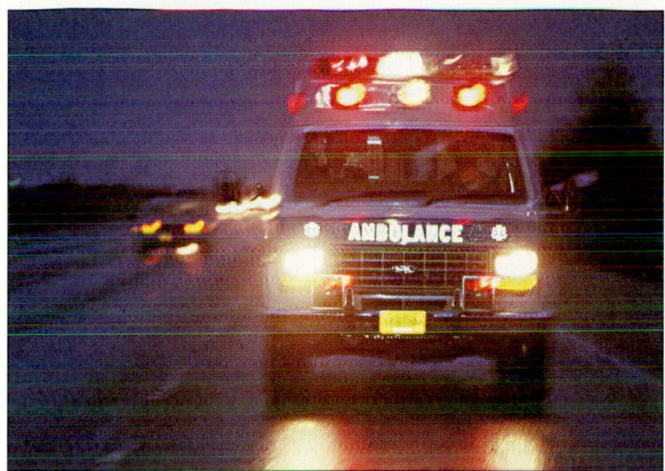

FIGURE 36-20 Modify your speed according to changing weather, road, and driving conditions.

Even the most careful drivers will occasionally run into unexpected situations that may require special driving skills. However, if you drive at a speed that is appropriate for the weather and road conditions, you will minimize these situations. For example, it is safer if you decrease speed in weather situations involving hard rain, snow, or ice.

Hydroplaning. On a wet road, a tire usually displaces the water on the road surface and stays in direct contact with the road. However, at speeds greater than 30 mph, the tire may be lifted off the road as water "piles up" under it; the vehicle feels as if it were floating. This is known as <u>hydroplaning</u>. At higher speeds on wet roadways, the front wheels may actually be riding on a sheet of water, robbing the driver of control of the vehicle. If hydroplaning occurs, you should gradually slow down without jamming on the brakes. Shimmying the steering wheel may also help to cut through the water and allow the tires to regain road surface, but this technique requires a great deal of practice.

Water on the roadway. Wet brakes will slow the vehicle and pull it to one side or the other. If at all possible, avoid driving through large pools of water; often, you cannot tell how deep they are. If you must drive through standing water, make sure to slow down and turn on the windshield wipers. After driving out of the pool, lightly tap the brakes several times until they are dry. If the vehicle is equipped with anti-lock brakes, apply a steady, light pressure to dry the brakes.

Decreased visibility. In areas where there is fog, smog, snow, or heavy rain, common sense tells you to slow down after warning cars behind you. At night, use only low headlight beams for maximum visibility without

reflection. You should always use headlights during the day to increase your visibility to other drivers. Also, watch carefully for stopped or slow-moving cars.

Ice and slippery surfaces. A light mist on an oily, dusty road can be just as slippery as a patch of ice. Good all-weather tires and an appropriate speed will reduce traction problems significantly. If you are in an area that often has snowy or icy conditions, consider using studded snow tires, if they are permitted by law. You should be especially careful on bridges and overpasses when temperatures are close to freezing. These road surfaces will freeze much faster than surrounding road surfaces, because they lack the warming effect of the ground underneath.

Laws and regulations. Regulations regarding vehicle operations vary from state to state and from city to city, but some things are the same everywhere. Drivers of emergency vehicles have certain limited privileges in every state. However, these privileges do not lessen drivers' liability in an accident. In fact, in most cases, the driver is presumed to be guilty if a collision occurs while the ambulance is operating with warning lights and siren. Motor vehicle accidents are the single largest source of lawsuits against EMS personnel and services.

While on a valid emergency call, emergency vehicles typically are exempt from usual vehicle operations. If you are on an emergency call and are using your warning lights and siren, you may be allowed to do the following:

- Park or stand in an otherwise illegal location
- Proceed through a red traffic light or stop sign
- Drive faster than the posted speed limit
- Drive against the flow of traffic on a one-way street, or make a turn that is normally illegal
- Travel left of center to make an otherwise illegal pass

Remember that these exemptions vary by state and local jurisdiction. Therefore, you should check your local statutes for regulations in your area.

An emergency vehicle is almost never allowed to pass a school bus that has stopped to load or unload children and is displaying its flashing red lights or extended "stop arm." If you approach a school bus that has its lights flashing, you should stop before reaching the bus and wait for the driver to make sure the children are safe, close the bus door, and turn off the warning lights. Only then may you carefully proceed past the stopped school bus.

Use of warning lights and siren. Three basic principles govern the use of warning lights and siren on an ambulance:

1. The unit must be on a true emergency call to the best of your knowledge.

2. Both audible and visual warning devices must be used simultaneously.

3. The unit must be operated with due regard for the safety of all others, on and off the roadway.

The siren is probably the most overused piece of equipment on an ambulance. In general, the siren does not help you as you drive, nor does it really help other motorists. Motorists who are driving at the speed limit with the windows up, the radio on, and the air conditioner or heater set on high cannot hear the siren until the ambulance is very close. If the radio is particularly loud, they may not hear the siren at all.

If you do have to use the siren, be sure to warn the patient before you turn it on. Be especially mindful not to increase the speed of the ambulance just because the siren is in use. Always travel at a speed that will allow you to stop safely at all times, especially if other drivers do not give you the right-of-way. And never assume that warning lights and sirens will allow you to drive through a congested area without stopping or slowing down.

Some ambulance headlights are equipped with a high-beam flasher unit. These are the most visible, effective warning devices for clearing traffic in front of the vehicle.

Right-of-way privileges. A right-of-way privilege is just that: a privilege. State motor vehicle statutes or codes often grant an emergency vehicle, such as an ambulance, the right to disregard the rules of the road when responding to an emergency. However, in doing so, the operator of an emergency vehicle must not endanger people or property under any circumstances.

Consider this case: an ambulance is approaching an intersection that is controlled by a four-way stop sign. The ambulance, with lights and audible warning device functioning, proceeds through the intersection without slowing or stopping and crashes into a car coming from its right. Did the operator of the ambulance act appropriately by going through the intersection in this manner?

Right-of-way privileges for ambulances vary from state to state. Some states allow you to proceed through a red light or stop sign after you stop and make sure it is safe to go on. Other states allow you to proceed through a controlled intersection "with due regard," using flashing lights and siren. This means that you may proceed only if you consider the safety of all people who are using the highway. If you fail to use due regard, your service might be sued. If you are found to be at fault, you may personally have to pay punitive damages or face both civil and criminal sanctions.

Get to know your local right-of-way privileges. Exercise them only when it is absolutely necessary for the patient's well-being. The use of lights and audible warning devices is a matter of state and local practice and protocol.

Use of escorts. Using a police escort is an extremely dangerous practice. When other motorists hear a siren and see a police car passing, they might assume that the police car is the only emergency vehicle and not see the ambulance. The only time an escort is justified is when you are in unfamiliar territory and truly need a guide more than an escort. In such cases, neither vehicle should use any warning lights or sirens. If you are being guided by a police car, make sure that you follow it at a safe distance.

Intersection hazards. Intersection accidents are the most common and usually the most serious type of collision in which ambulances are involved. Always be alert and careful when approaching an intersection. If you are on an urgent call and cannot wait for traffic lights to change, you should still come to a momentary stop at the light; look around for other motorists and pedestrians before proceeding into the intersection.

Motorists who "time the traffic lights" present a serious hazard. You may arrive at an intersection while the light is green. At the same time, a motorist who is timing the lights on the cross street arrives at the intersection. The motorist has a red light but knows that it is about to turn green and is expecting to go through. The stage is now set for a serious accident.

Another common intersection hazard occurs when the driver of one emergency vehicle follows another emergency vehicle through an intersection without assessing the situation carefully. A motorist who has yielded the right-of-way to the first vehicle may proceed into the intersection without expecting a second vehicle. You should exercise extreme caution in these situations. To signal motorists that a second unit is approaching, use a siren tone that is different from that of the first vehicle.

TABLE 36-10 Guidelines for Safe Ambulance Driving

Keep in mind the following guidelines whenever you are en route to a call:

1. Select the shortest and least congested route to the scene at the time of the dispatch.

2. Avoid routes with heavy traffic congestion; know alternative routes to each hospital during rush hours.

3. Avoid one-way streets; they may become clogged. Do not go against the flow of traffic on a one-way street.

4. Watch carefully for bystanders as you approach the scene. Curiosity seekers rarely move out of the way.

5. Park the ambulance in a safe place once you arrive at the scene. If you park facing into traffic, turn off your headlights so that they do not blind oncoming cars unless they are needed to illuminate the scene. If the vehicle is blocking part of the road, keep your warning lights on to alert oncoming motorists; otherwise, turn them off.

6. Drive within the speed limit while transporting patients, except in the rare extreme emergency.

7. Go with the flow of the traffic.

8. Use the siren as little as possible en route.

9. Always drive defensively.

10. Always maintain a safe following distance. Use the "4-second rule": Stay at least 4 seconds behind another vehicle in the same lane.

11. Try to maintain an open space in the lane next to you as an escape route in case the vehicle in front of you stops suddenly.

12. Use your siren if you turn on the emergency lights, except when you are on a freeway.

Guidelines for safe ambulance driving. Table 36-10 lists the guidelines to follow when you are en route to a call.

Arrival at the Scene

Once you reach the scene, you should inform dispatch that you have arrived and give a brief report of what you see. Also report any unexpected situations, such as the need for backup units, a heavy rescue unit, or a HazMat team (Figure 36-21). Do not enter the scene if there are any hazards to you. If there are dangerous hazards at the scene, the patient should be moved before you begin care. The patient may have to be moved by others if you are not appropriately equipped.

Immediately size up the scene by using the following guidelines:

- Look for safety hazards.
- Evaluate the need for additional units or other assistance.
- Determine the mechanism of injury in trauma patients or the nature of the illness on medical calls.

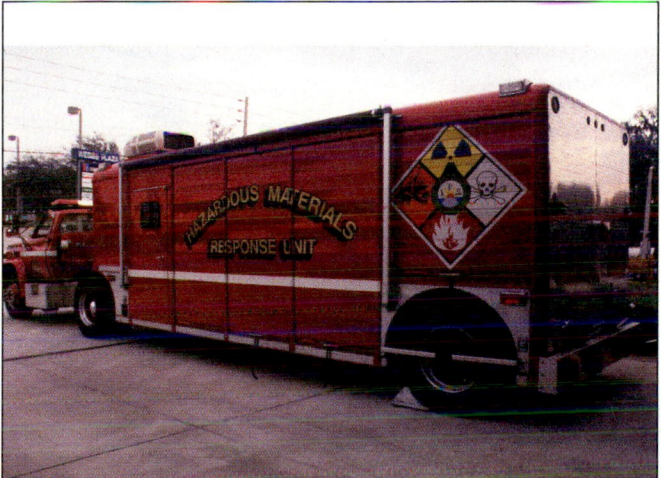

FIGURE 36-21 Once you arrive at the scene, you should report to dispatch and ask for backup, rescue, or HazMat units as needed.

- Evaluate the need to stabilize the spine.
- Make sure that you follow BSI techniques before touching the patient. The type of care that you expect to give will dictate what personal protective equipment you should wear.

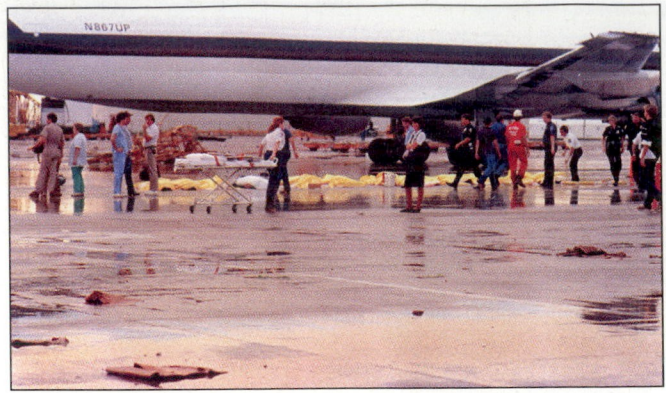

FIGURE 36-22 Quickly estimate the number of patients at a mass-casualty incident; then call dispatch for backup, and begin triage.

If you are at the scene of a mass-casualty incident, quickly estimate the number of patients (Figure 36-22). Inform dispatch that backup units are needed at the scene, then begin the triage process. Keep in mind that actions at the scene must be organized, and you must work rapidly and efficiently. Remember that your goal is to transport the patient to the hospital safely.

Safe parking. In assessing the situation, you must decide where to park the ambulance. Pick a position that will allow for efficient traffic control and flow around an accident scene. Do not park alongside the scene, as you may block the movement of other emergency vehicles. Instead, park about 100' past the scene on the same side of the road. It is best to park uphill and/or upwind of the scene if smoke or hazardous materials are present (Figure 36-23). If you must park on the back side of a hill or curve, leave your warning lights or devices on. Do the same when parking at night.

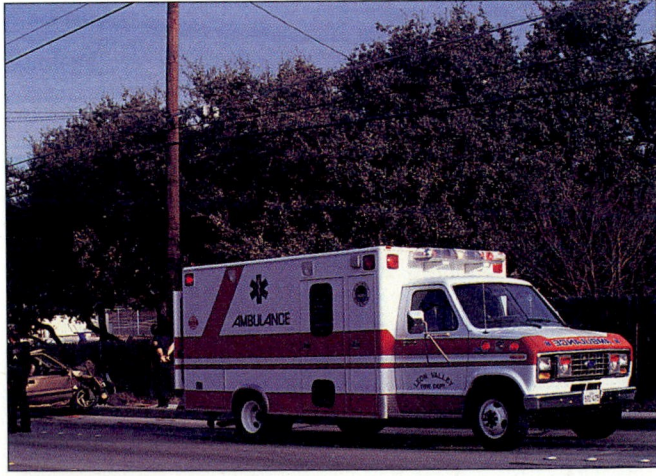

FIGURE 36-23 Park the ambulance about 100' past the scene on the same side of the road. Park uphill or upwind of the scene if hazardous materials are present.

Stay away from any structures that might collapse, fires, explosive hazards, or downed wires. Be sure to set the parking brake. If your vehicle is blocking part of the roadway, leave the emergency warning lights on. If your vehicle has them, leave only the flashing yellow lights on. Other drivers tend to drive toward emergency vehicles with flashing red or red and white lights. Within these safety guidelines, you should try to park your ambulance as close to the scene as possible to facilitate emergency medical care. If necessary, you can temporarily block traffic to unload equipment and to load patients quickly and safely. If you must do this, try to do it quickly so that traffic is not blocked any longer than is absolutely necessary. Also, park in a location that will not hamper your leaving the scene.

Traffic control. Your first responsibility at an accident scene is to care for the patients. Only when all the patients have been treated and the emergency situation is under control should you be concerned with restoring the flow of traffic. If the police are slow to arrive at the scene, you might then need to take action.

The purpose of traffic control is to ensure an orderly traffic flow and to prevent another accident. Under ordinary circumstances, traffic control is difficult. An accident or disaster scene presents serious additional problems. Passing motorists often "rubberneck," paying little attention to the roadway in front of them. Some curiosity seekers may park down the road and return on foot, creating still other hazards. As soon as possible, place appropriate warning devices, such as reflectors, on both sides of the accident. Remember, the main objectives in directing traffic are to warn other drivers, to prevent additional accidents, and to keep vehicles moving in an orderly fashion so that care of the injured is not interrupted.

The Transfer Phase

In almost every case, you will provide lifesaving care right where you find the patient, before moving the patient to the ambulance. You may then begin less critical measures, such as bandaging and splinting. Next, you must package the patient for transport, securing him or her to a device such as a backboard, a scoop litter, or the wheeled ambulance stretcher. Then move to the ambulance, and properly lift the patient into the patient compartment.

No matter how careful the driver may be, riding to the hospital while lying on one's back on a stretcher can be uncomfortable and even dangerous. So be sure to

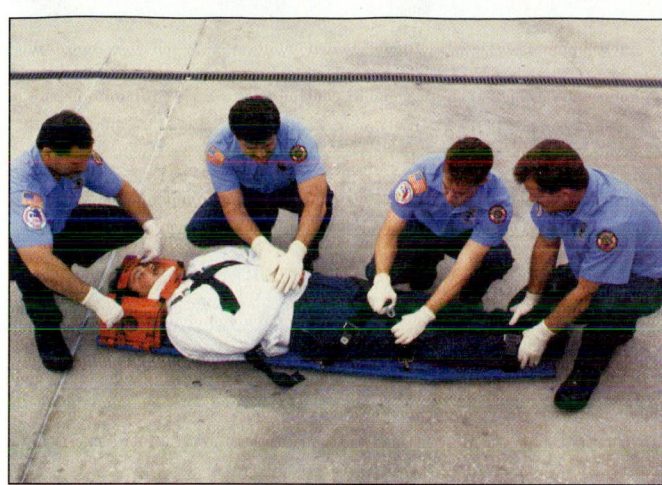

FIGURE 36-24 Be sure to secure the patient appropriately to protect the patient during transport.

secure the patient with at least three straps across the body (Figure 36-24). Use deceleration or stopping straps over the shoulders to prevent the patient from continuing to move forward in case the ambulance suddenly slows or stops.

The Transport Phase

Inform dispatch when you are ready to leave the scene with the patient. Report the number of patients you have and the name of the receiving hospital. Even though you have assessed and treated the patient at the scene, you should continue to monitor him or her en route. These ongoing assessments may uncover changes in the patient's vital signs and overall condition. Be sure to recheck the patient's vital signs en route. The frequency of checking vital signs depends on the situation, but checking them every 15 minutes for a stable patient and every 5 minutes for an unstable patient is a practice that many services use. In addition, it is important that you continually reassess the patient's clinical situation, and record and address new problems and the patient's responses to earlier treatment.

At this time, you should also contact the receiving hospital. Inform medical control about your patient(s) and the nature of the problem(s). Depending on the number of EMT-Bs on your team and how much care the patient needs, you might also want to begin working on your written report while en route.

Finally, and most importantly, do not abandon the patient emotionally. Do not become so involved in paperwork and ongoing assessments that you ignore the patient's fears. You are there to help the patient as a person, so use this time to reassure him or her. Some patients, such as the very young or elderly, may benefit from added attention during transport. Be aware of the differing levels of need of different patients.

The Delivery Phase

Inform dispatch as soon as you arrive at the hospital. Then follow these steps to transfer the patient to the receiving hospital:

1. Report your arrival to the triage nurse or other arrival personnel.
2. Physically transfer the patient from the stretcher to the bed directed for your patient.
3. Present a complete verbal report at the bedside to the nurse or physician who is taking over the patient's care.
4. Complete a detailed written report, and leave a copy with an appropriate staff member.

The written report should include a summary of the history of the patient's current illness or injury with pertinent positives and negatives, mechanism of injury, and findings on your arrival. In addition, you should list vital signs and briefly mention relevant past medical or surgical history, as well as information regarding medication and allergies. Also, be sure to include any treatment and its effect that occurred in the prehospital setting.

While at the hospital, you may be able to restock any items that were used during the run, such as oxygen masks or dressings and bandages (Figure 36-25). Remember, though, that your priority is transfer of the patient and patient information to the hospital staff. Restocking the ambulance comes second.

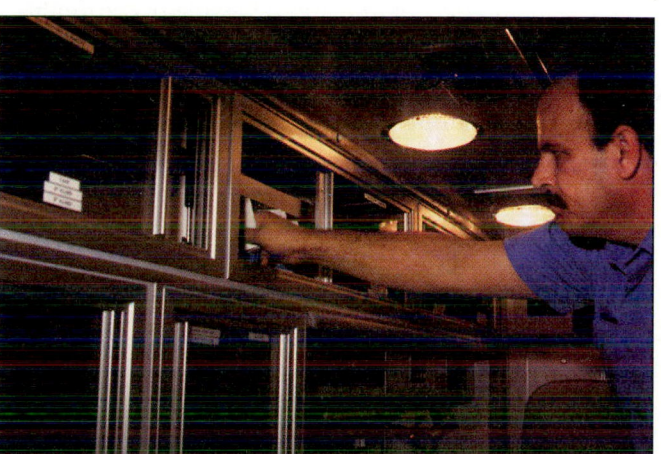

FIGURE 36-25 After transferring the patient and relating patient information to the hospital staff, you should restock any items that were used during the run.

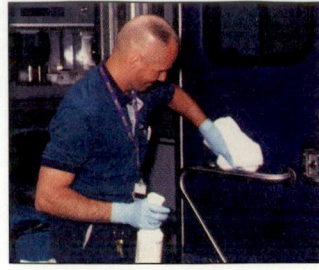

FIGURE 36-26 Be sure to clean and disinfect the ambulance and equipment at the station if you did not do so at the hospital.

En Route to the Station

Once you leave the hospital, inform dispatch whether or not you are in service and where you are going. As soon as you are back at the station, you should do the following:

- Clean and disinfect the ambulance and any equipment that was used, if you did not do so before leaving the hospital (Figure 36-26).

- Restock any supplies you did not get at the hospital.

The Postrun Phase

During the postrun phase, you should complete and file any additional written reports and again inform dispatch of your status, location, and availability.

You are also responsible for maintaining the ambulance so that it is safe and available on a moment's notice. This means routine inspections on a regular schedule. Use a written checklist to document needed repairs or replacement of equipment and supplies. In addition, you must ensure that the following steps are taken after each trip:

- Scrub blood, vomitus, and other substances from the floors, walls, and ceilings with soap and water.

- Clean and decontaminate the inside of the ambulance, according to state and local regulations. (You can use a 10% solution of bleach in water to clean the ambulance after any contamination.)

- Dispose of any contaminated waste in the manner prescribed by your agency.

- Clean the outside of the ambulance as needed.

- Replace or repair broken or damaged equipment without delay.

- Replace any other equipment or supplies that were used.

- Refuel the vehicle if the fuel tank is below required reserves. The oil level should be checked each time the vehicle is refueled.

It is important that you know the meanings of the terms "cleaning," "disinfection," "high-level disinfection," and "sterilization," as follows:

- **Cleaning**—The process of removing dirt, dust, blood, or other contaminants from a surface.

- **Disinfection**—The killing of pathogenic agents by directly applying a chemical made for that purpose to a surface.

- **High-level disinfection**—The killing of pathogenic agents by the use of potent means of disinfection.

- **Sterilization**—A process, such as the use of heat, that removes all microbial contamination.

Dispose of any contaminated materials that are not disinfected by placing them in the appropriate containers used for biohazard disposal.

Prescheduled preventive maintenance checks. The ambulance chassis and engine components are subjected to significantly greater stresses than the typical automobile or truck is. For this reason, the manufacturer's recommendations for periodic maintenance must be strictly followed, especially regarding lubrication, oil and filter changes, transmission and differential service, brakes, wheel alignment, wheel bearings, and steering components. Many services now use a Hobbs or engineer hour meter, which assesses hours of engine use, in addition to the odometer to help determine periodic maintenance requirements.

As is the case with emergency medical care report forms, local and individual differences will affect inspection routines. Your ambulance service should develop its own inspection forms for all three kinds of inspections so that nothing is overlooked. These forms should be filed for inspection and legal documentation and should be kept for at least 3 years.

> You are responsible for maintaining the ambulance so that it is safe and available on a moment's notice.

Air Ambulance Operations

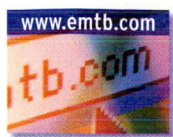

Air ambulances are used to evacuate medical patients, land at or near the accident scene, and transport patients to trauma facilities every day in many areas. You can expect to see the use of air ambulances increase in the future.

There are two basic types of air ambulances: fixed-wing and rotary-wing, otherwise known as helicopters (Figure 36-27). Fixed-wing aircraft generally are used for interhospital patient transfers over distances greater than 100 to 150 miles. For shorter distances, ground transport or rotary-wing aircraft are more efficient.

Specially trained medical flight crews accompany all air ambulance flights. Your role in fixed-wing aircraft transfers probably will be limited to providing ground transport for the patient and medical flight crew between the hospital and the airport.

Rotary-wing aircraft have become an important tool in providing emergency medical care. Trauma patient survival is directly related to the time that elapses between injury and definitive treatment. Most helicopters that are used for emergency medical operations fly well in excess of 100 mph in a straight line, without road or traffic hazards. The crew may include EMTs, paramedics, flight nurses, or physicians.

You should be familiar with the capabilities, protocols, and methods for accessing helicopters in your area. Helicopter services provide training for EMT-Bs in ground operations and safety.

Safety Precautions Around Helicopters

Helicopter safety is nothing more than good common sense, along with a constant awareness of the need for personal safety. The types of helicopters that are used for medical operations vary, but the dangers are the same. If you are familiar with the way helicopters work and follow the pilot's instructions, you will minimize these dangers. You should be sure to do nothing near the helicopter and go only where the pilot or crew directs you.

The most important rule is to keep a safe distance from the aircraft whenever it is on the ground and "hot," which means when the tail rotor is spinning. Stay away from the tail rotor; the tips of its blades move so rapidly that they are invisible. In fact, never approach the helicopter from the rear, even if it is not hot. If you must move from one side of the helicopter to another, go around the front. Never duck under the body, the tail boom, or the rear section of the helicopter; the pilot cannot see in these areas. The proper approach area is

> The types of helicopters that are used for medical operations vary, but the dangers are the same.

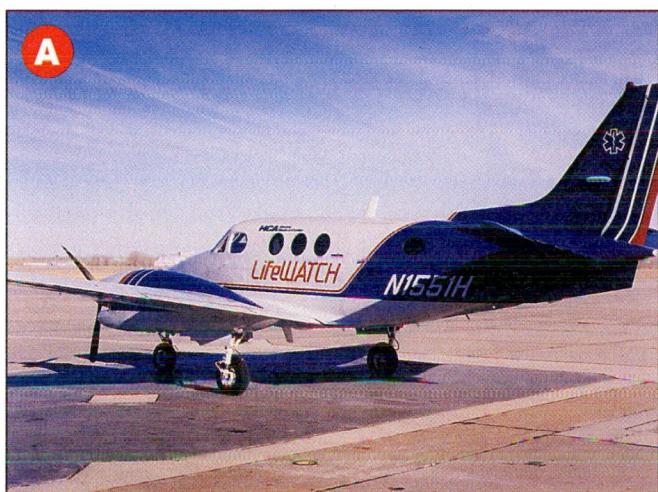

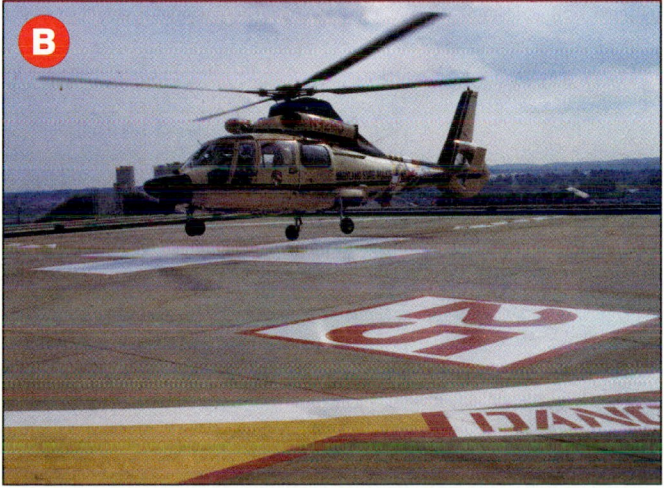

FIGURE 36-27 A: Fixed-wing aircraft are generally used to transfer patients from one hospital to another over distances greater than 100 to 150 miles. **B:** A rotary-wing aircraft, or helicopter, is used to help provide emergency medical care to patients who need to be transported quickly over shorter distances.

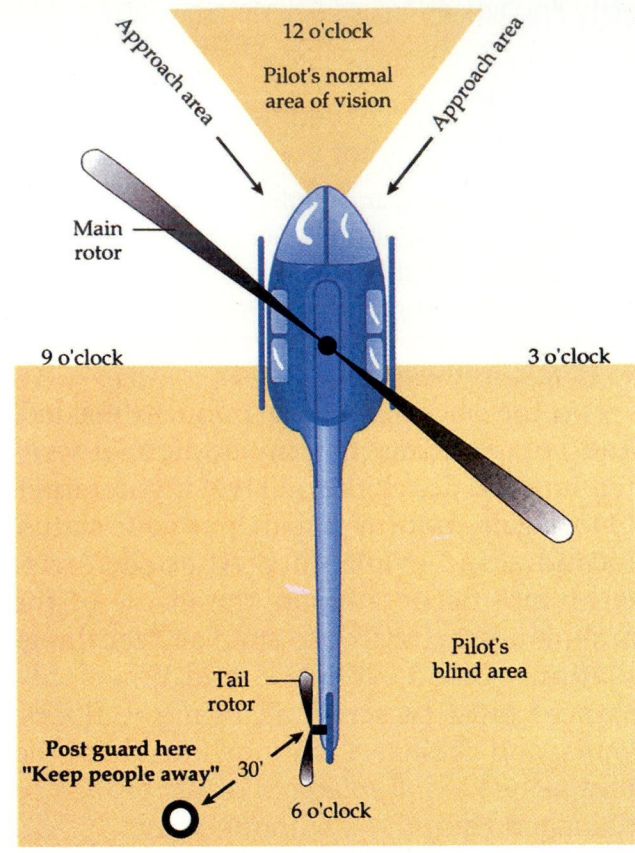

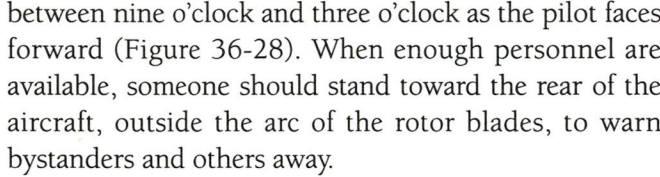

FIGURE 36-28 Approach a helicopter between the nine o'clock and three o'clock positions as the pilot faces forward.

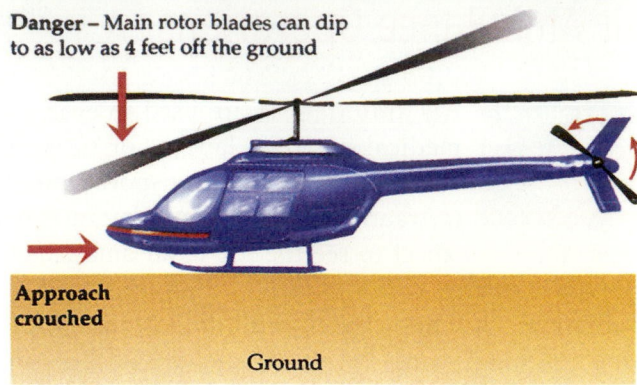

FIGURE 36-29 The main rotor blade of the helicopter is flexible and may dip as low as 4' off the ground.

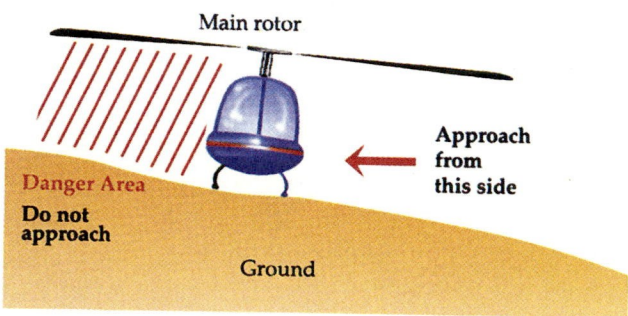

FIGURE 36-30 Approach a helicopter on a grade from the downhill side only.

between nine o'clock and three o'clock as the pilot faces forward (Figure 36-28). When enough personnel are available, someone should stand toward the rear of the aircraft, outside the arc of the rotor blades, to warn bystanders and others away.

Another area of concern is the height of the main rotor blade. It is flexible and may dip as low as 4' off the ground (Figure 36-29). When you approach the aircraft, walk in a crouched position. Wind gusts can alter the blade height without warning, so be sure to protect equipment as you carry it under the blades. Air turbulence created by the rotor blades can blow off hats and loose equipment. These, in turn, can become a danger to the aircraft and personnel in the area.

When accompanying a flight crew member, you must follow directions exactly. Never try to open any aircraft door or move equipment unless a crew member tells you to. When told to approach the aircraft, use extreme caution and pay constant attention to hazards.

Landing Sites

Although a helicopter can fly straight up and down, this is the most dangerous mode of operation. The safest and most effective way to land and take off is similar to that used by fixed-wing aircraft. Landing at a slight angle allows for safer operations. Takeoff combines a gradual lift and forward motion to travel up and out on a slight angle.

Clearing a landing site is another important role you can play. Look for loose debris, electric or telephone wires, poles, or any other hazards that might interfere with the safe operation of the helicopter. If you note any hazards, inform the pilot by radio or other signal. The pilot will usually "overfly," or survey the site, before final approach and landing to ensure that all potential dangers are identified. Depending on the time, temperature, winds, and the aircraft's weight, you might need to mark the proposed site with flags, lights, or other signaling devices. A clear landing zone that is at least 100' by 100' is recommended.

If the helicopter must land on a grade, extra caution is advised. The main rotor blade will be closer to the ground on the uphill side. In this situation, approach the aircraft from the downhill side only (Figure 36-30). Do not move the patient to the helicopter until the crew has signaled that they are ready to receive you. A flight crew member will direct and assist you in loading the patient.

Nighttime operations are considerably more hazardous than daytime operations because of the darkness. The pilot may fly over the area with the helicopter's lights on to spot obstacles and the shadows of overhead wires, which can be hard to see. Do not shine spotlights, flashlights, or any other lights in the air to help the pilot; they may temporarily blind the pilot. Instead, direct light beams toward the ground at the landing site. Even after the helicopter has landed, you should not aim lights anywhere near it. Of course, smoking, open lights or flames, and flares are prohibited within 50' of the aircraft at all times.

For further information on air ambulances, see the following publications:

- DOT publication HS805-703, *Air Ambulance Guidelines*, February 1981

- DOT publication HS806-841, *Proceedings: National MEDEVAC Helicopter Conference*

prep kit

ready for review

An ambulance is an emergency medical vehicle that contains a driver's compartment, a patient compartment, equipment and supplies to provide care at the scene and during transport, and two-way radio communication. It must be designed and constructed to ensure maximum safety and comfort. Ambulances should be white on the outside with an orange stripe, blue lettering, and reflectorized emblems. The Star of Life®, a six-pointed emblem that identifies ambulances that meet federal specifications, should be on the sides, rear, and roof of the ambulance.

The ambulance should be climate-controlled, insulated, and easy to clean. The patient compartment should be large enough to accommodate two litter patients, two EMTs, and all the necessary equipment and supplies to best take care of patients.

The 9 phases of an ambulance call are preparation for the call, dispatch, en route to the scene, arrival at the scene, transferring the patient to the ambulance, en route to the receiving facility, at the receiving facility, en route to the station, and postrun.

Specific supplies should be carried on the ambulance, including basic medical equipment, airway management equipment and ventilation devices, suctioning equipment, oxygen delivery equipment, CPR equipment, and basic wound care supplies. In addition, you must ensure that splinting supplies, childbirth supplies, and appropriate medications are on board. An automated external defibrillator, as permitted by medical control, should always be carried on the ambulance. A jump kit, patient transfer equipment, non-medical supplies, and initial extrication and rescue equipment are also needed.

The driver must be qualified to drive the ambulance; he or she must be physically and emotionally fit, with the proper attitude. The driver must know and follow safe driving practices.

In addition to ground ambulances, air ambulances in the form of fixed-wing aircraft or helicopters are used to evacuate patients, land at an accident scene, and transport patients to trauma facilities.

vital vocabulary

www.emtb.com

acceleration The process of increasing speed.

air ambulances Fixed-wing aircraft and helicopters that have been modified for medical care; used to evacuate and transport patients with life-threatening injuries to treatment facilities.

ambulance A specialized vehicle for transporting sick and injured patients.

ambulance service vehicle A specialized vehicle that is used to transport EMS equipment and personnel to scenes of medical emergencies.

chassis The vehicle frame.

chassis set The transfer of the center of mass of the ambulance to different points on the chassis.

cleaning The process of removing dirt, dust, blood, or other visible contaminants from a surface.

coefficient of friction A measure of the grip of the tire on the road surface.

CPR board A device that provides a firm surface under the patient's torso.

deceleration The process of slowing down.

decontaminate To remove or neutralize radiation, chemical, or other hazardous material from clothing, equipment, vehicles, and personnel.

disinfection The killing of pathogenic agents by direct application of chemicals.

footprint The area of contact between the ambulance tire and the road surface.

friction The resistance to motion of one body against another.

high-level disinfection The killing of pathogenic agents by using potent means of disinfection.

hydroplaning A condition in which the tires of a vehicle may be lifted off the road surface as water "piles up" under them.

jump kit A portable kit containing items that are used in the initial care of the patient.

litter A type of stretcher for moving or carrying patients.

Star of Life® The six-pointed star that identifies ambulances and other prehospital providers that meet federal specifications as licensed or certified ambulances.

sterilization A process, such as heating, that is used to remove microbial contamination.

assessment in action

All of your hard work has paid off. You have completed the EMT-B course, passed the state test, and have been certified. In addition, you have a new job as an EMT-B with a local private ambulance service. You put on your uniform and report to headquarters where you are introduced to your new partner. You shake hands, say your hellos, and head out to the bay to check out your rig and start your orientation.

1. Of the following, which issue with the ambulance is **LEAST** important to tell your supervisor about?
   A. Strange-sounding brakes
   B. Oil dripping under the engine
   C. A full tank of gas
   D. A screw stuck in the front tire

2. As you are checking the patient compartment, you find a small, dried puddle of blood under the stretcher. What should you do next?
   A. Wipe up the blood with a wet paper towel.
   B. Wait until the end of your shift to clean up the blood.
   C. Clean up the blood using appropriate BSI techniques.
   D. Leave the problem for the crew that left the ambulance dirty.

3. You notice that there are no cervical collars in the trauma bag. If you respond to a call without the required equipment on the ambulance, you could legally be charged with:
   A. slander.
   B. negligence.
   C. abandonment.
   D. malfeasance.

4. As you wait for your first call, you begin to review ambulance operations. According to state laws that govern ambulance operations, you are **NOT** allowed to:
   A. park in a no parking zone.
   B. endanger people's lives and property.
   C. go the wrong way down a one-way street.
   D. drive faster than the posted speed limit.

5. Which of the following statements about transporting a patient is **FALSE**?
   A. A patient who is in stable condition can ride alone in the patient compartment.
   B. Safety precautions should be observed for patients and providers alike whenever possible.
   C. All equipment that is not currently being used for patient care should be stowed.
   D. A patient on the cot should be strapped securely into place and the cot secured in place as well.

points to ponder

Object. 7-1.3, 7-1.4, 7-1.6

You have just been paired with a new partner, and after the first week, you are very uncomfortable with this person's driving. Your partner is not as bad when there is a patient on board, but when responding, protocols are not followed, and speed is excessive. When you mention it to your new partner, the response is that the partner has had only one accident in two years and is usually first on the scene. You are very uncomfortable with this situation.

- How would you deal with this situation? Would you report your partner? If so, when and to whom?

online outlook

Ambulance vehicles are classified as Type I, II, or III. To learn more about ambulance vehicle classifications, complete Exercise 36 at www.emtb.com.

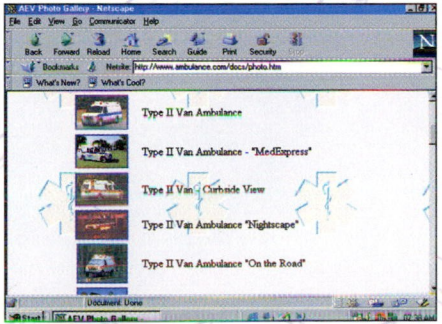

Scene Techniques

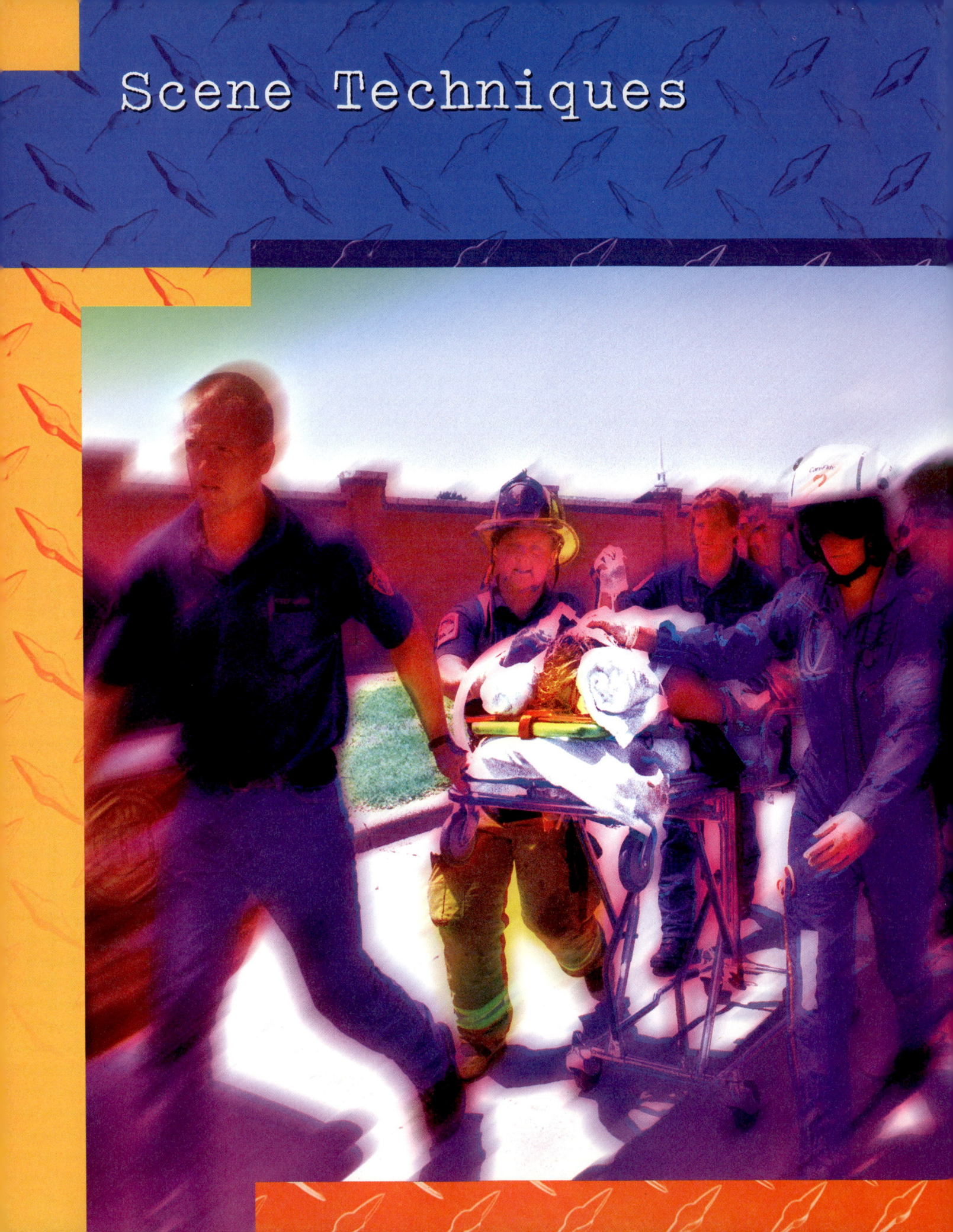

objectives

Cognitive

1. Describe the purpose of extrication.

2. Discuss the role of the EMT-B in extrication.

3. Identify what equipment for personal safety is required for the EMT-B.

4. Define the fundamental components of extrication.

5. State the steps that should be taken to protect the patient during extrication.

6. Evaluate various methods of gaining access to the patient.

7. Distinguish between simple and complex access.

8. Explain the EMT-B's role during a call involving hazardous materials.

9. Describe what the EMT-B should do if there is reason to believe that there is a hazard at the scene.

10. Describe the actions that an EMT-B should take to ensure bystander safety.

11. State the role the EMT-B should perform until appropriately trained personnel arrive at the scene of a hazardous materials situation.

12. Break down the steps to approaching a hazardous situation.

13. Discuss the various environmental hazards that affect EMS.

14. Describe the criteria for a multiple-casualty situation.

15. Evaluate the role of the EMT-B in the multiple-casualty situation.

16. Summarize the components of basic triage.

17. Define the role of the EMT-B in a disaster operation.

18. Describe basic concepts of incident management.

19. Explain the methods for preventing contamination of self, equipment, and facilities.

20. Review the local mass-casualty incident plan.

Affective

21. Discuss the psychological impact of wanting to act but recognizing that a scene is not safe to enter.*

Psychomotor

22. Given a scenario of a mass-casualty incident, perform triage.

* This is a non-curriculum objective.

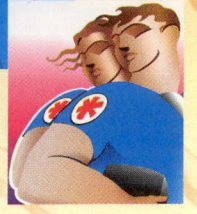

you are the emt

Unit 3, respond to the Belmont Loading Docks, Building 3, for a man with chest pain. You are en route for about 3 minutes when dispatch contacts you again to tell you that the Belmont Bridge is up and will be for at least 20 more minutes. You know you will need to reroute.

The prehospital environment is a dynamic, often uncontrolled place to work as an EMT-B. Getting to emergency scenes safely and in a timely fashion, managing bystanders effectively, and controlling or avoiding hazards represent just a few of the variables that come with EMS. This chapter will help you to better evaluate and manage emergency scenes effectively, and it will also help you to answer the following questions:

1. When the fire department, law enforcement, and a private ambulance are all on the same scene, who is in charge and what are they in charge of?

2. What exactly are the benefits of red lights and sirens?

Scene Techniques

As an EMT-B, you will usually not be responsible for rescue and extrication. Rescue involves many different processes and environments. It also requires training beyond the level of the EMT-B. In this chapter, you will learn basic concepts of extrication and situations involving hazardous materials and multiple casualty situations.

The chapter begins with a discussion of access: how to gain access to patients and how to keep patients and bystanders safe in the process. Your main concern is reaching the patient so that you can begin providing care. In most instances, once you have reached the patient, extrication will occur around you and the patient.

The next section describes your responsibilities at a hazardous materials incident. When you are responding to this type of incident, you cannot rush in to provide patient care. Rather, you must take time to accurately assess the scene by identifying the size of the hazard area, finding a safe location to which patients can be removed, and taking self-protective measures. *Safety is your prime consideration.* If a hazardous materials incident is not carefully handled, a lot of people, including rescue personnel, can become patients or casualties.

The final section of the chapter is a very basic introduction to incident management systems. The purpose of this section is to give you an idea of the larger structure that is at work during complex incidents. The role of the EMT-B within the system is explained, along with concepts such as triage and multiple-casualty incidents.

Fundamentals of Extrication

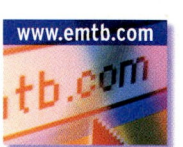

During all phases of rescue, your primary concern is safety, and your primary role is to provide emergency medical care and prevent further injury to the patient. You will provide care as extrication goes on around you unless this proves to be too dangerous for you or the patient. **Extrication** is the removal from entrapment or a dangerous situation or position. **Entrapment** means to be caught within a closed area with no way out. In the context of this chapter, extrication means removal of a patient from a wrecked automobile. However, the same principles and concepts apply to other situations.

You will need to coordinate your efforts with those of the rescue team. If you respect their job, they will respect yours. You should communicate with members of the rescue team throughout the extrication process. Start talking to the rescue team leader as soon as you arrive at the scene.

At any accident scene, four different basic functions must be addressed (Figure 37-1). When possible, responders work in clearly defined separate teams to ensure clear lines of responsibility and organization. Each team focuses on and is responsible for a different function:

- **Fire fighters** are responsible for putting out any fire, preventing additional ignition, ensuring that the scene is safe, and washing down any spilled fuel.

- **Law enforcement** is responsible for traffic control and direction, maintaining order at the scene, investigating the accident or crime scene, and establishing and maintaining lines so that bystanders are kept at a safe distance and out of the way of rescuers.

- **The rescue team** is responsible for properly securing and stabilizing the vehicle, providing safe entrance and **access** to patients (the ability to reach the patient), extricating any patients, ensuring that patients are properly protected during extrication or other rescue activities, and providing adequate room so that patients can be removed properly.

- **EMS personnel** are responsible for assessing and providing immediate medical care, triage and assigning priority to patients, providing additional assessment and care as needed once the patient has been removed, packaging the patient, and providing transport to the emergency department.

Good communication among team members and clear leadership are essential to safe, efficient provision of proper emergency care. Although your input at the scene is important, one member of your team must be clearly in charge. The team leader's assessment of the patient and the situation will dictate the way in which medical care, packaging, and transport will proceed. Customarily, the crew chief, who typically is clearly indicated on the shift schedule, is responsible for this role. If not, a team leader must be identified and agreed to before you arrive at the scene.

In some areas, there might not be enough personnel for two or multiple separate units. In these areas, you and your team may have two roles. However, one person still must be in charge of the overall rescue operation. If there is no identifiable leadership at the scene, the rescue effort and patient care will suffer. Leaders should be identified as part of a larger incident management system. They must be medically trained and qualified to judge the priorities of patient care, and they must also be experienced in extrication.

Scene Size-Up

You must always be prepared, mentally and physically, for any incident that requires rescue or extrication. *The most important part of this preparation is thinking about your safety and the safety of your team.* Safety begins with the proper mind-set and the proper protective equipment.

When you arrive, you should position the unit in a safe location that does not add a hazard to the scene. Before proceeding, make sure that the scene is properly marked and that either the road is closed or traffic flow is controlled safely around the scene (Figure 37-2). One of the important responsibilities of scene size-up is to determine what, if any, additional resources will be needed. These resources may include additional EMS units and personnel. If you are first on the scene, you may need to initiate a HazMat response or call in a utility crew.

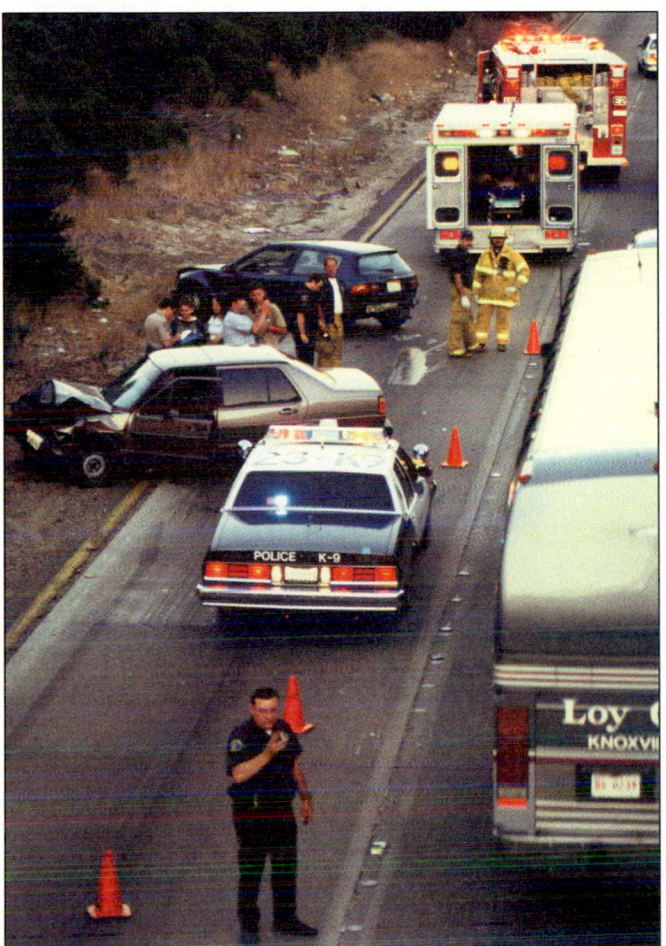

FIGURE 37-1 Every accident requires cooperation, as each responder has a specific role at the scene.

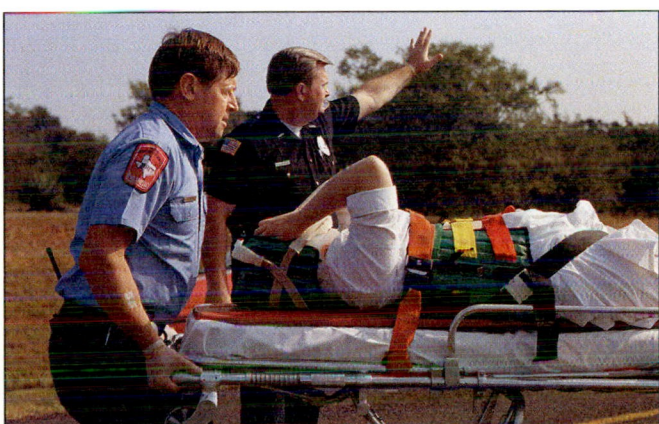

FIGURE 37-2 The scene of an accident should be marked properly, and traffic should be diverted so that responders have enough room to work.

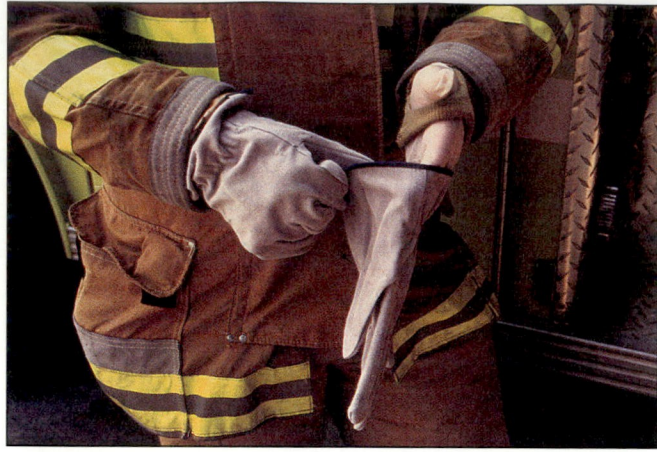

FIGURE 37-3 Proper protective equipment varies depending on the situation.

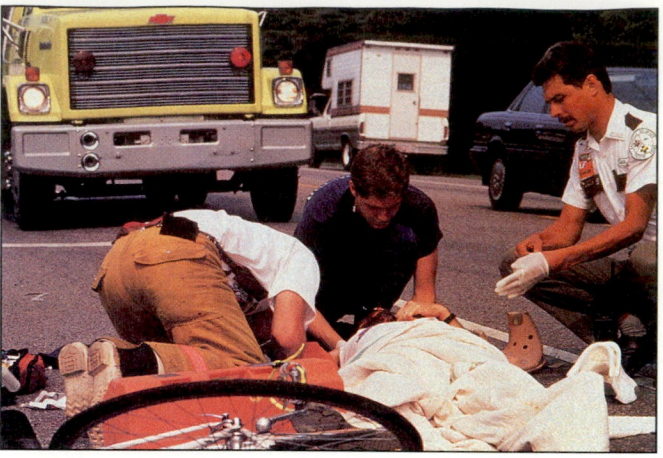

FIGURE 37-4 Always explain to the patient why you are there and what you are doing.

The equipment that you use and the gear that you wear will depend on the situation (Figure 37-3). However, the importance of wearing blood- and fluid-impermeable gloves at all times during patient contact cannot be emphasized enough. If you will be involved with extrication, you should wear a pair of leather gloves over your disposable gloves to protect you from injury in handling ropes, tools, broken glass, hot or cold objects, or sharp metal.

Remember, you should not access the patient or enter the vehicle until you are sure that the vehicle is stable and that any hazards have been identified and either properly controlled or eliminated.

Patient and Bystander Safety

While you are gaining access to the patient and during extrication, you must make sure that the patient remains safe. Always talk to the patient and describe what you are doing as you do it, even if you think the patient is unconscious (Figure 37-4). In many instances, you or another member of the team will provide immobilization of the cervical spine or other care during extrication. EMS personnel should wear proper protective gear while in the working area. Both personnel and the patient should be covered with a heavy, nonflammable blanket to protect against flying glass or other objects. A backboard may also be used as a protective shield (Figure 37-5). Try to keep heat, noise, and force to a minimum. Use only what is necessary to extricate the patient safely.

Bystanders and family members can be hazards themselves. If they are allowed to get too close, they are at risk of injury and may also interfere with the overall management of the incident. For these reasons, the rescue team will set up a danger zone that is off-limits to bystanders (Figure 37-6). A <u>**danger zone**</u> is an area

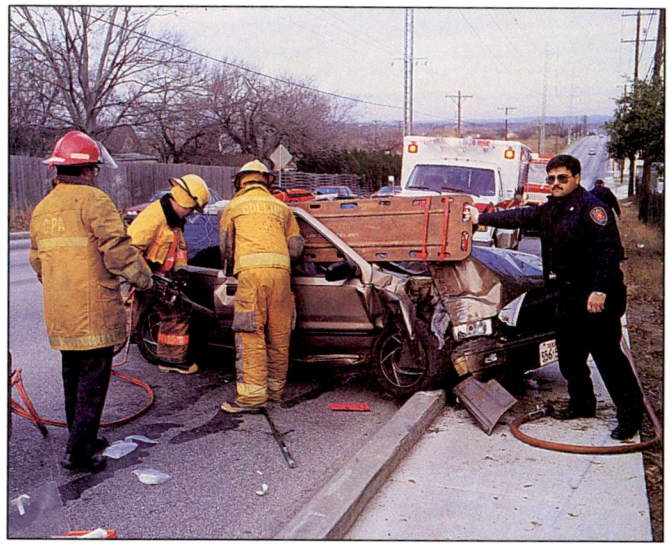

FIGURE 37-5 Use a spine board or blanket to protect the patient and any rescuers who are providing care.

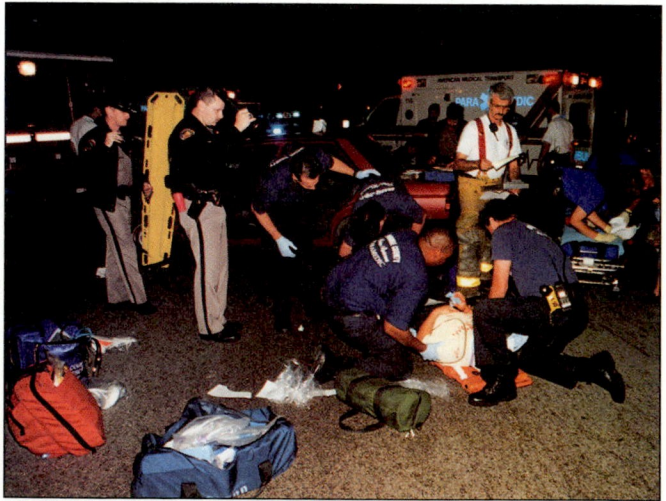

FIGURE 37-6 A danger zone should be established to prevent bystanders from entering the area around an incident.

where individuals can be exposed to toxic substances, lethal rays, or ignition or explosion of hazardous materials. You should help to set up and enforce this zone. If you arrive before the rescue team, you should coordinate crowd control with law enforcement officials.

Occasionally, a bystander may prove difficult to manage. This situation is especially challenging when the bystander claims to have medical credentials. Your EMS service should have a protocol for dealing with this situation. Many states provide physicians with wallet-sized copies of their medical license to use as identification (Figure 37-7). However, not all physicians have training in emergency medical care. If this situation occurs, inform medical control immediately. Communication between medical control and the physician at the scene may eliminate some of the problems. You may also assign such individuals duties that will allow them to become involved in a small way. This will reduce the risk of a possible confrontation.

Gaining Access to the Patient

The exact way you gain access to or reach the patient(s) depends on the situation. It is up to you to identify the safest, most efficient way to access the patient. Darkness, uneven terrain, tall grass, shrubbery, or wreckage may make patients hard to find (Figure 37-8). Multiple vehicles with multiple patients may be involved. If this is the case, you should locate and rapidly triage each patient to determine who needs urgent care. This step is important before you proceed with any treatment and patient packaging. Be sure to take these factors into account in your scene size-up. Remember that scene size-up is a continuing process, because the situation often changes. As a result, you may need to change your plans for gaining access and providing treatment.

To determine the exact location and position of the patient, you and your team should consider the following questions:

- Is the patient in a vehicle? In some other structure?
- Is the vehicle or structure severely damaged?
- What hazards exist that pose risk to the patient and rescuers?
- In what position is the vehicle? On what type of surface?

You must also take into account the patient's injuries and their severity. You may have to change your course of action as you learn more about the patient's condition. Do not try to access the patient until you are sure that the vehicle is stable and that hazards have been identified and eliminated. Hazards might include electrical or gas lines.

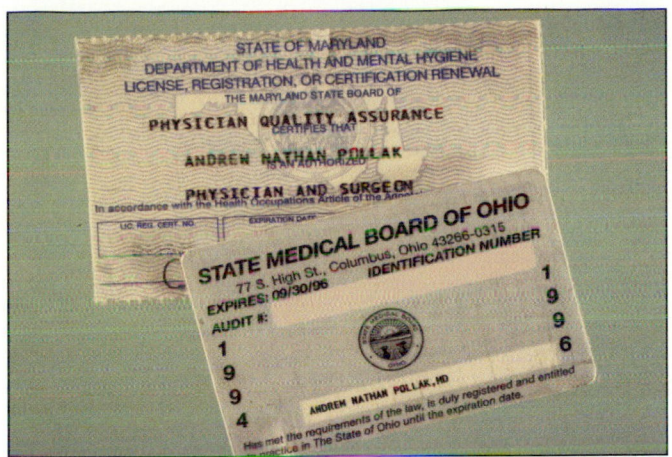

FIGURE 37-7 Many physicians carry a wallet-sized copy of their medical license.

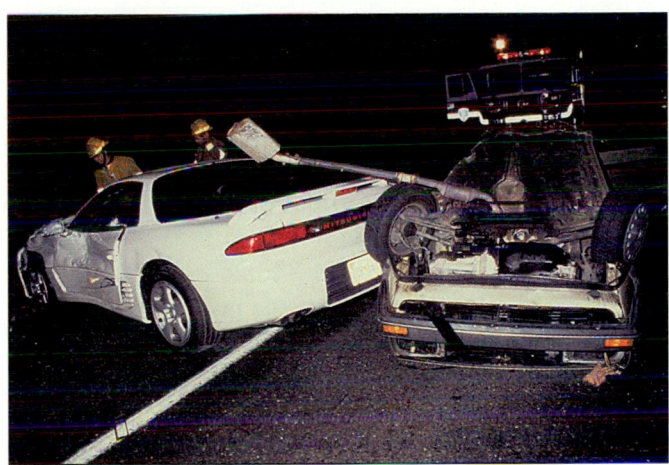

FIGURE 37-8 The exact way to gain access depends on many factors, including the terrain, the way in which the vehicle is situated, and the weather.

What if you have to remove a patient quickly because the environment is threatening or you need to perform CPR? CPR is not effective when the patient is in a sitting position or lying on the soft seat of a vehicle. In these instances, you and your team may have to use the Rapid Extrication technique to move a patient from a sitting position inside a vehicle to a supine position on a long backboard. A team of EMT-Bs who are experienced in using this technique should be able to remove a patient who is not entrapped rapidly and in the shortest time possible, keeping in mind the patient's condition and the team's safety. Use the Rapid Extrication technique only as a last resort.

Simple Access. Your first step is **simple access**, trying to get to the patient as quickly and simply as possible without using any tools or breaking any glass. Automobiles are built for easy entry and exit; however, it may be necessary to use tools or other forcible entry methods. Whenever possible, you should first try to

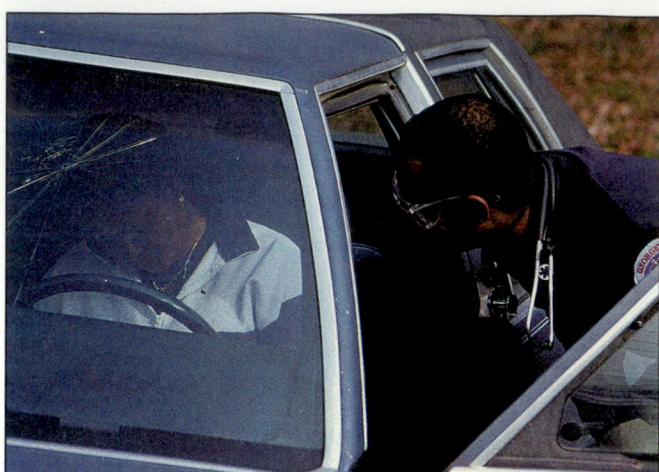

FIGURE 37-9 Get to the patient as quickly and simply as possible by opening the door without using tools or breaking any glass.

unlock the doors (or ask the patient to unlock them) or roll down the windows. Try to open every door using the door handles to gain access before breaking any windows or using other methods of forced entry (Figure 37-9). Enter through the doors when there is no danger to the patient. The rescue team should provide you with the entrance you need to access the patient.

Complex Access. <u>Complex access</u> requires the use of special tools and special training and includes breaking windows or other forcible entry. Most of these skills are too advanced for the 110-hour EMT-Basic course and are not covered in this text.

Entrapment and Extrication

Providing medical care to a patient who is trapped in a vehicle is principally the same as that for any other patient. Unless there is an immediate threat of fire, explosion, or other danger, once entrance and access to the patient have been provided, you should perform an initial assessment and stabilize the patient's vital functions before extrication begins, as follows:

1. Provide manual immobilization to protect the cervical spine, as needed.
2. Open the airway.
3. Assist or provide ventilation.
4. Control any significant external bleeding.
5. Treat any critical injuries.
6. Provide high-flow oxygen.

As a part of your assessment, determine how urgently the patient must be extricated, where you should be positioned to best protect the patient during extrication, and, once the patient has been freed, how you will best

> Your safety and that of the patient are paramount.

move the patient from within the vehicle onto the long backboard and onto the stretcher. Carefully examine the exposed area of the limb or other part of the patient that is trapped to determine the extent of injury and whether there is a possibility of hidden bleeding. If possible, you should also evaluate sensation in the trapped area so that you will know whether increased pain indicates that an object is pressing on the patient during extrication.

During this time, the rescue team is assessing exactly how the patient is trapped and determining the safest, easiest way to extricate him or her. Your input is essential so that the patient's injuries are considered as the rescue team plans a move that protects the patient from further harm. Once the plan has been devised and everyone understands what will be done, you should determine how best to protect the patient. Often, you or another EMT-B should be placed in the vehicle alongside the patient to monitor his or her condition and well-being as the vehicle is being forcibly cut, bent, or disassembled. Be sure to wear proper protective clothing.

Naturally, your safety and that of the patient are paramount during this process. Both you and the patient should be covered by a thick, fireresistant canvas or blanket for protection from broken glass, flying particles, tools, or other hazards during any cutting or forceful extrication maneuvers. Extrication is often extremely noisy, so you must be sure that you can communicate effectively with both the patient and the rescue team so that you can instantly let the rescuers know if it is necessary that they stop.

Once the patient has been freed, rapidly assess any previously unavailable parts, and recheck the patient's vital functions. Make sure that the spine is manually immobilized, and apply a cervical collar if this was not previously done. Reevaluate whether the patient needs to be immediately removed by using manual immobilization and the Rapid Extrication technique or whether the patient's condition and the scene allow for immobilization using an extrication vest or short backboard before he or she is moved further. In most cases, it is impractical and difficult to properly apply extremity splints within the vehicle. Extremity injuries can be rapidly supported and immobilized while the patient is being removed by securing an injured arm to the body and, if a leg is injured, securing one leg to the other.

This will be adequate until the patient is secured to the backboard or time allows for more detailed assessment and splinting of each injury.

Moving the patient in one fast, continuous step increases the risk of harm and confusion. To ensure that each EMT can be positioned so that he or she can lift and carry properly at all times, the patient should be moved in a series of smooth, slow, controlled steps, with stops designed between them to allow for the repositioning and adjustments that are needed. Plan the exact steps and pathway that you will follow in moving the patient from sitting in the vehicle to lying supine on the backboard and prepared ambulance cot. Choose a path that requires the least manipulation of the patient or equipment. Make sure that sufficient personnel are available. Once you are sure that everyone understands the steps and is ready, you can move the patient safely. Make sure that you move the patient as a unit, resisting the temptation to move the immobilization device instead. While moving the patient, continue to protect him or her from any hazards.

Once the backboard and patient have been placed on the cot, continue with any additional assessment and treatment that were deferred until the patient was out of the vehicle. If it is extremely cold or hot, raining, or snowing, you will want to load the cot and patient into the climate-controlled ambulance before continuing assessment and treatment. If the patient's condition requires that transport be initiated without further delay, you should provide only the additional care that is essential or necessary to package the patient. Leave the remaining steps to be performed while you are en route to the hospital.

Specialized Rescue Situations

Customarily, when on an ambulance call, you can drive the ambulance to within a short distance of the patient's location and, with either simple or complex access, reach and treat the patient. However, in some situations, the patient can be reached only by teams that are trained in making special technical rescues. Specialized skills of these teams include the following:

- Technical rope rescue (low- and high-angle rescue)
- Mountain, rock, and ice-climbing rescue
- Cross-field and trail rescue (park rangers)
- Water and small craft rescue
- White-water rescue
- Dive rescue (SCUBA)
- Cave rescue
- Mine rescue
- Confined space rescue
- Ski slope and cross-country or trail snow rescue (ski patrol)
- Lost person search and rescue (SAR)
- Tactical response and rescue (SWAT)

The EMT and Technical Rescue Situations. **Technical rescue situations** may contain hidden dangers, and special technical skills are needed for personnel to safely enter and move around. It is not safe to include any personnel who do not have the necessary special training and experience in such a rescue. A **technical rescue team** is made up of individuals from one or more departments in a region who are trained and on call for certain types of technical rescue. Many members of a technical rescue team are also trained as first responders or EMT-Bs so that they can provide the necessary immediate care when only they can safely reach the patient. Even when the technical rescue team includes a paramedic or physician, generally nothing but essential simple care is provided until the rescuers can bring the patient to the nearest point where a safe, stable setting exists.

If a technical rescue team is necessary but is not present when you arrive, you should immediately check with the incident commander to make sure that the team has been summoned and is en route to your location. The **incident commander** is the individual who has overall command of the scene in the field (Figure 37-10). If no incident commander is present, follow local guidelines.

When you arrive at a scene where a technical rescue is already in progress, you will usually be met by a member of the rescue team and directed or led to the actual rescue site. If the rescue scene is at some distance from the road, you may need to leave the ambulance on

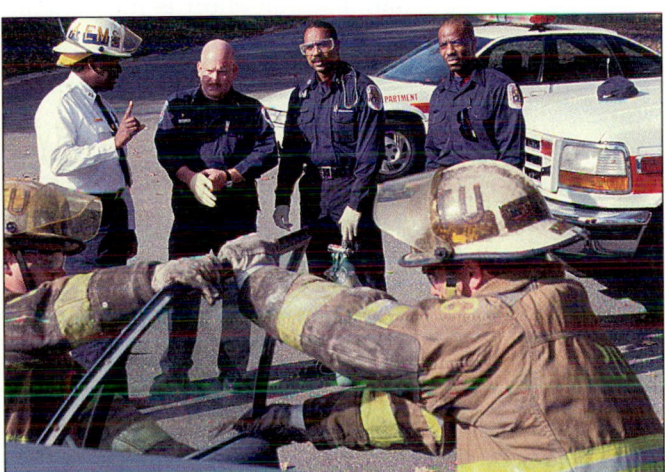

FIGURE 37-10 The incident commander is the individual who has overall command of the scene.

> Unless you have been instructed otherwise, only incident command should communicate any news or progress of the search to the family.

the road. The use of the ambulance cot is impractical in these situations; you should instead bring a long backboard and/or basket litter or similar rescue litter to carry the patient back to the waiting ambulance. Be sure that you take all of the carry-in kits and other equipment you may need to treat and immobilize the patient at the actual rescue base.

When you arrive at the rescue operation base, identify the stable location to which the rescue team will bring the patient, and set up your equipment there. As soon as the rescue team has brought the patient to this staging area, you should perform a rapid assessment and, after providing the treatment indicated, package the patient without delay. Although you and the other EMTs who responded with the ambulance will assume the primary responsibility for the patient's care at this point, it usually requires a cooperative effort by both the rescue and EMS teams to carry the patient to the waiting ambulance. Consider using an air medical helicopter if the patient will need to be carried and/or transported an extensive distance.

Lost Persons Search and Rescue. When someone is lost in the outdoors and a search effort is initiated, an ambulance is usually summoned to the search base. Each search team will be organized to include a member who is trained to either the first responder or EMT level, carrying the essential equipment to provide simple immediate care. Your role, and that of the other EMT-Bs who arrived with the ambulance, is to stand by at the search base until the lost person or people have been found.

As soon as you arrive at the scene and have been briefed on the situation, you should isolate and prepare the equipment you will need to carry in to the patient's location so that no time is lost once the patient has been found or a member of the search team becomes injured. The prepared carry-in equipment, including a long

backboard and other equipment you will need to immobilize the patient, should be left in the back of the ambulance so that it is protected from the weather. In addition, if the ambulance should need to be relocated, the equipment will not need to be reloaded or possibly be left behind. You will usually be given a walkie-talkie that is tuned to the search frequency so that you can monitor the progress of the search and communicate with and be contacted by those in charge of the search operation.

Sometimes, you may be asked to stay with relatives of the lost individual who are at the scene. Find out from relatives whether the lost person has any medical history that may need to be addressed, and pass this information on to those who are in charge of the search. Unless you have been instructed otherwise, only incident command should communicate any news or progress of the search to the family. For this reason, you must be sure that your walkie-talkie is set at a discreet volume.

Once the lost person has been found, you will be guided by search personnel to that location or a pre-arranged intersecting point where the patient will be carried to decrease the amount of time you need to reach the patient and begin treatment. You should be sure that the carry-in equipment is evenly distributed among personnel and that the pace is such that all can stay together easily. Sometimes, the time and effort that are needed to reach and carry out the patient can be decreased by relocating the ambulance or, if available, by using a four-wheel drive or all-terrain vehicle. As with other technical rescues, although the ambulance crew will assume the responsibility for patient care once they are at the patient's side, a cooperative effort of both the EMS and search team is necessary to safely carry the patient to the base and waiting ambulance.

Tactical Situations. If you are called to a scene where a tactical situation is taking place, such as an armed hostage situation, presence of a sniper, or exchange of shots, and the threat of violence remains, you should turn off the lights and sirens as you come close to the scene. In such situations, you should request direction from the incident commander or another appropriate authority in control of the scene. When you arrive at the outer perimeter barrier line that the police have established, you should ask a police officer to notify the incident commander of your arrival and for an officer to guide you to the shielded, safe staging area that has been selected for the ambulance and for care of the wounded and injured.

For your safety, you should exit the ambulance, stay low, and remain near the side of the vehicle unless you are directed to another place of safety. Do not turn on the vehicle's outside speakers, and turn down the volume of any walkie-talkies that you are carrying. No matter how tempting it is to look, be sure that you do not look around the corner of any building or around the sides or over the top of any structure that may be serving to shield you. If it is dark outside, turn off the headlights and all clearance lights, and do not display any other light that might be reflected and serve to highlight your general location.

As in other technical rescue situations, your role, and that of the other EMT-Bs, is to stand by at the staging area and treat and package injured patients after the SWAT team or other law enforcement officers have evacuated them to your shielded, safe location. When you are ready to transport a patient, you should ask a law enforcement officer to notify the incident commander. You should leave only after the incident commander has verified that it is safe for the ambulance to move. Be sure that you follow the specific route that is indicated by the incident commander or a law enforcement officer assigned to guide you. You should proceed slowly for a good distance from the incident perimeter before using your emergency lights and siren.

Structure Fires. In most areas, an ambulance is dispatched with the fire department truck to any structure fire, whether or not any injuries are reported. A fire in a house, apartment building, office, school, plant, warehouse, or other building is considered a **structure fire**. When responding to a major fire scene, you should determine whether, because of the fire, any special route will be necessary. Once you arrive at the scene, you should ask the incident commander where the ambulance should be parked. It is essential that the ambulance be parked far enough away from the fire to be safe from the fire itself or a collapsing building. You must also ensure that the ambulance will not block or hinder other arriving equipment or become locked in by other equipment or hose lines. However, you must also make sure that the ambulance will be close enough to be visible and that patients can be brought to it easily. The fire officer who is the incident commander will decide where this location should be.

Your next step is to determine whether there are any injured patients at the scene or whether you have been called to stand by. A number of ambulances may be dispatched to a major fire to ensure that one or more units will always remain immediately available at the scene if others leave to transport the injured.

As with other technical rescue situations, search and rescue in a burning building requires special training and equipment. Search and rescue is performed by teams of fire fighters wearing full turnout gear and self-contained breathing apparatus (SCBA), and carrying clearing tools and fully charged hose lines. These teams will bring patients out of the burning building to the area where the ambulance is standing by. Therefore, unless otherwise ordered, you should always stay with the ambulance. Do not wander off even after the fire is basically out, in case a firefighter becomes injured during further searches for pockets of fire or while the hoses and other equipment are being packed up. The ambulance should leave the scene only if transporting a patient or if the incident commander has dismissed it.

Sometimes, the scene at an accident or fire is further complicated by the presence of hazardous materials. A **hazardous material** is any substance that is toxic, poisonous, radioactive, flammable, or explosive and can cause injury or death with exposure. In addition to posing a threat to you and others at the immediate scene, hazardous materials may pose a threat to a much larger area and population. Whenever there is a possibility that a hazardous material is involved, you will have to follow a number of additional special procedures.

Introduction to Hazardous Materials

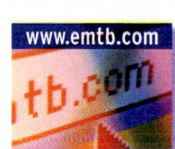

Your training has taught you that rapid response to the scene of an accident can save lives. You and your team can make quick decisions and act on them. Even so, sometimes you may be criticized for taking too much time at the scene of an accident. Such critics fail to appreciate a very important rule: When you arrive at the scene of a possible hazardous materials accident, you must first step back and assess the situation. This can be very stressful for you, particularly if you can see a patient. However, rushing in to such events can have catastrophic results. Because of the unique aspects of responding to and working at a HazMat incident, OSHA has set specific additional training requirements in 29CFR1910.120, which all individuals, including EMT-Bs, must meet before becoming involved in these situations. Because this text does not include the information to meet these requirements, you need to check with your agency for information about additional specific training.

Hazardous materials may be involved in any of the following situations (Figure 37-11):

- A truck or train accident in which a substance is leaking from a tank truck or railroad tank car

- A leak, accident, or fire at an industrial plant, refinery, or other complex where chemicals or explosives are produced, used, or stored

- A leak or rupture of an underground natural gas pipe

- Deterioration of underground fuel tanks and seepage of oil or gasoline into the surrounding ground

- Buildup of methane or other by-products of waste decomposition in sewers or sewage-processing plants

- A motor vehicle crash in which a gas tank has ruptured

Often, the presence of hazardous materials is easily recognized from warning signs, placards, or labels found in the following locations (Figure 37-12):

- On buildings or areas where hazardous materials are produced, used, or stored

- On trucks and railroad cars that carry any amount of hazardous material

- On barrels or boxes that contain hazardous material

Unfortunately, identifying materials still can be difficult. Little consistency is used on labels and placards. The laws and regulations that cover labeling of packages and transport vehicles can also be misleading. In most cases, the package or tank must contain a certain amount of a hazardous material before a placard is required. For example, because of the small quantities of hazardous materials that are involved, a truck carrying 99 lb of HazMat #1 and 99 lb of both HazMat #2 and HazMat #3 may not be required by law to display any labels or placards. The truck may show only a

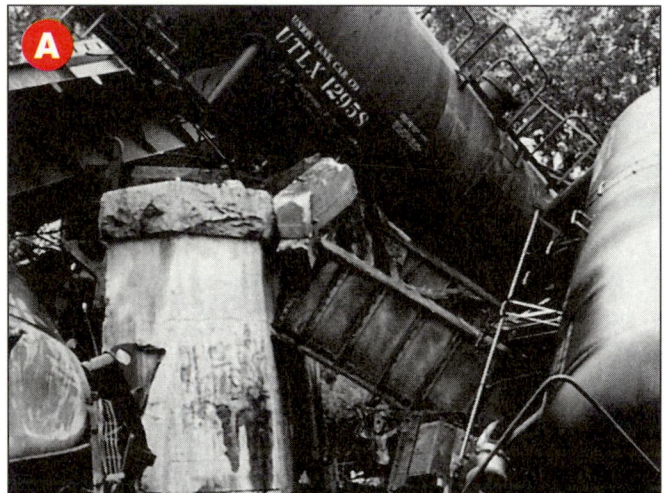

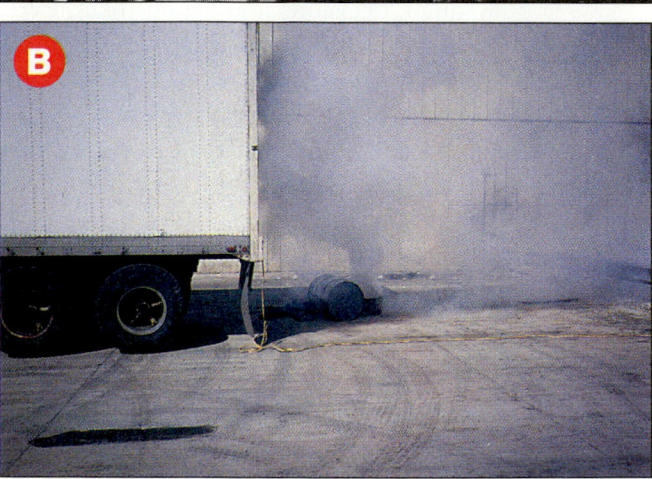

FIGURE 37-11 Hazardous materials incidents can occur in any community.

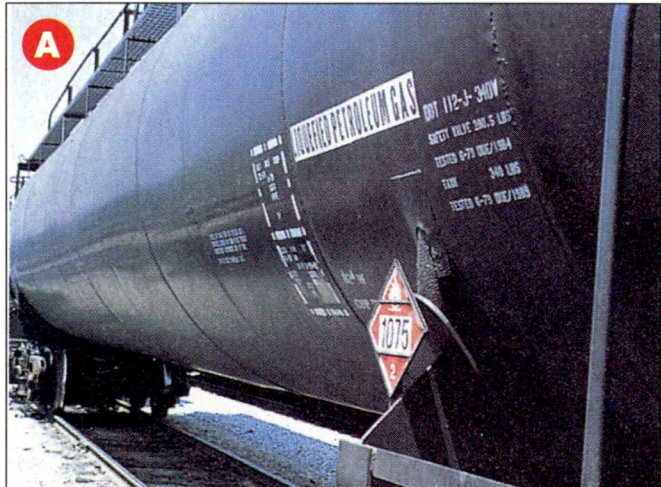

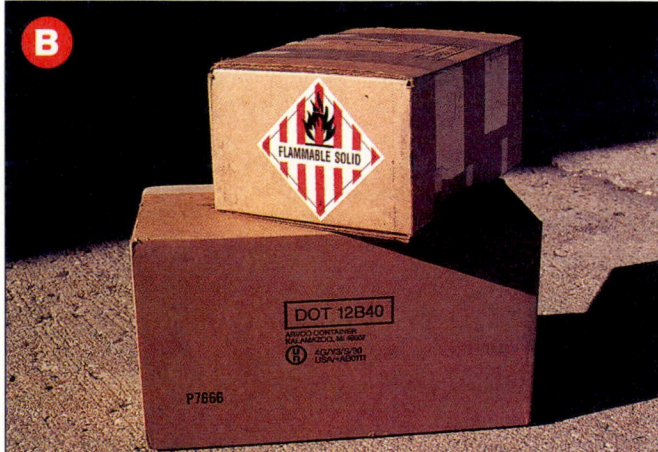

FIGURE 37-12 A: Warning placards are found on railroad cars that carry hazardous materials. **B:** Placards are also affixed to boxes that contain hazardous materials.

"Please Drive Carefully" placard. This placard implies that the truck carries no hazardous materials. An experienced HazMat technician knows that this is the most dangerous placard. However, other motorists are not aware that the truck is carrying a combination of hazardous materials. An accident involving this truck is a serious situation, but you would not know this if you relied on labels and placards.

Some substances are not hazardous; however, when mixed with another substance, they may become toxic or volatile. There may be no regulations against carrying such substances together on one truck or railroad car (or adjacent tank cars). No warnings are required.

However, the driver of a commercial truck and the conductor of a train must carry papers that identify what is being transported in their care. These papers may be your first clue that there is a possible HazMat problem; although, depending on the nature of the incident, the papers may not be available to you.

In the event of a leak or spill, the presence of a **hazardous materials incident** is often indicated by presence of the following:

- A visible cloud or strange-looking fumes resulting from the escaping substance
- A leak or spill from a tank, container, truck, or railroad car with or without hazardous material placards or labels
- An unusual, strong, noxious, acrid odor in the area

To indicate the presence of normally odorless toxic gases or fluids during a leak or spill, manufacturers may add a substance that produces a strong noxious odor. However, a large number of hazardous gases and fluids are *essentially odorless* (or do not have a distinctive unpleasant smell) even when a substantial leak or spill has occurred. In some incidents, a large number of people are exposed and may be injured or killed before the presence of a hazardous material incident is identified. If you approach a scene where more than one person has collapsed or is unconscious or in various degrees of acute distress, you should assume that there has been a hazardous material leak or spill and that it is unsafe to enter the area.

It is important for you to understand the potential danger of hazardous materials and know how to operate safely at a hazardous materials incident. If you do not follow the proper safety measures, you and many others could end up needlessly injured or dead. *Safety—of you and your team, the other responders, and the public—must be your most important concern.*

There will be times when the ambulance is the first to arrive at the scene. If, as you approach, any signs suggest that a hazardous material incident has occurred, you should stop at a safe distance; after rapidly sizing up the scene, call for a HazMat team. If you do not recognize the danger until you are too close, immediately leave the danger zone. Once you have reached a safe place, try to rapidly assess the situation and provide as much information as possible when calling for the HazMat team, including your specific location, the size and shape of the containers of the hazardous material, and what you have observed and been told has occurred. Do not reenter the scene. Do not leave the area until you have been cleared by the HazMat team, or you may worsen the situation by spreading hazardous material.

Identifying Hazardous Materials

Until the HazMat team arrives to determine the hazard zone, you should be aware of the safety perimeters that are necessary for hazardous materials that are toxic (poisons) and those in which the danger is of fire or explosion. When toxic gas, fumes, or airborne droplets or particles are involved, the safe area is upwind and at least 100′ from the site of any visible cloud or other discharge; in a hilly area, you should be uphill as well as upwind. Remember, wind direction can change quickly. A piece of narrow roller bandage, approximately 2′ long, tied to the top of your antenna will serve as a wind direction guide. Be sure to check the wind direction periodically, and relocate if a change in wind direction dictates.

If you can see and read the placard or other warning sign, note its color, wording, any symbols that it contains, and, if included, the four-digit number that appears on it or on any orange panel near it (Figure 37-13). This number, which may be preceded by the letters UN or NA, identifies the specific hazardous material. The name of the material may also be displayed

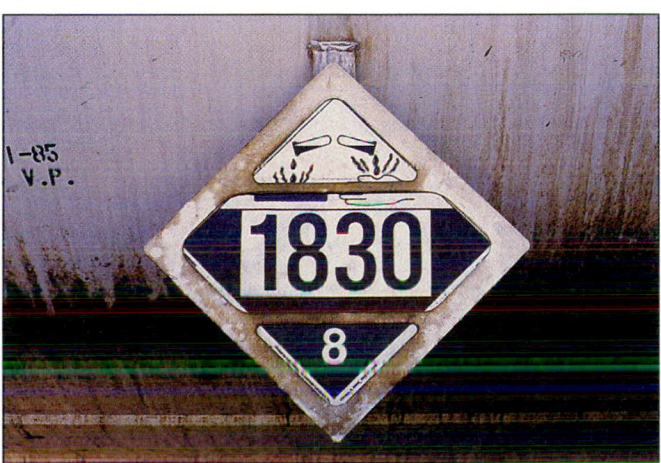

FIGURE 37-13 The four-digit number that appears on the warning placard identifies the specific hazardous material.

classification of hazardous materials

The NFPA 704 standard classifies hazardous materials according to health hazard or toxicity levels, fire hazard, and reactive hazard. Toxicity protection levels are also classified according to the level of protection provided. Even chemicals that are in the same category, on the basis of their chemical makeup, form, and concentration, will have different levels of hazard. The degree of health, fire, reactive hazard, and type of protection needed to operate safely near these substances must be known.

Toxicity Level. Toxicity levels are measures of the risk that a substance poses to someone who comes into contact with it. There are five toxicity levels: 0, 1, 2, 3, and 4 (Table 37-1). The higher the number, the greater the toxicity, as follows:

- **Level 0** includes materials that would cause little, if any, health hazard if you came into contact with them.

- **Level 1** includes material that would cause irritation on contact but only mild residual injury, even without treatment.

- **Level 2** includes materials that could cause temporary damage or residual injury unless prompt medical treatment is provided. Both Levels 1 and 2 are considered to be slightly hazardous but require use of SCBA if you are going to come into contact with them.

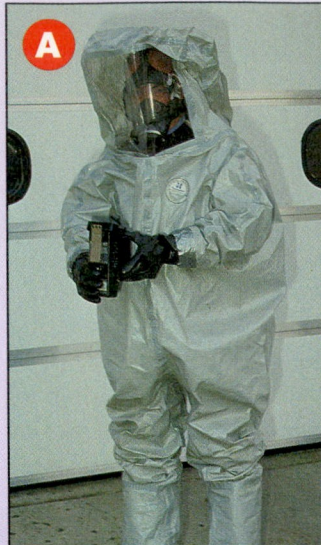
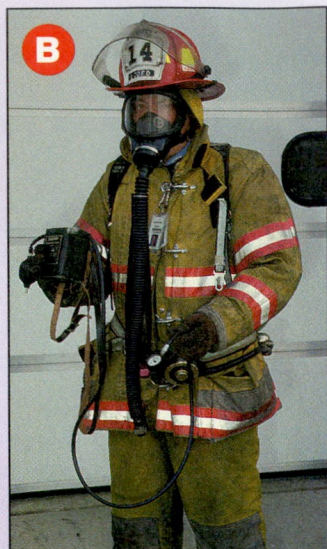
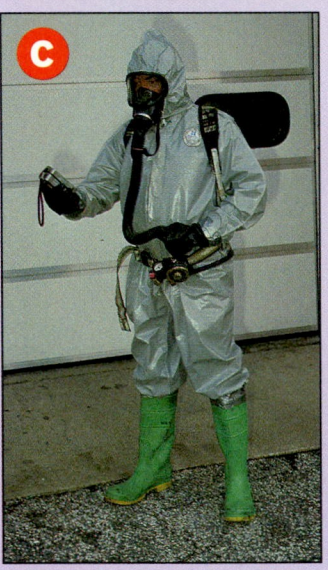
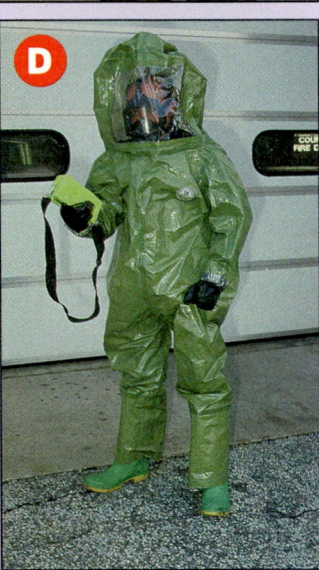

FIGURE 37-14 Four levels of protection.
A: Level A protection. **B, C, D:** Examples of Level B protection.

TABLE 37-1	Toxicity Levels of Hazardous Materials	
Level	**Health Hazard**	**Protection Needed**
0	Little to no hazard	None
1	Slightly hazardous	SCBA only
2	Slightly hazardous	SCBA only
3	Extremely hazardous	Full protection, with no exposed skin
4	Minimal exposure causes death	Special HazMat gear

- **Level 3** includes materials that are extremely hazardous to health. Contact with these materials requires full protective gear so that none of your skin surface is exposed.

- **Level 4** includes materials that are so hazardous that minimal contact will cause death. For Level 4 substances, you need specialized gear that is designed for protection against that particular hazard.

Protection Level. Protection levels indicate the amount and type of protective gear that you need to prevent injury from a particular substance. The four recognized protection levels, A, B, C, and D, are as follows (Figure 37-14):

- **Level A,** the most hazardous, requires fully encapsulated, chemical-resistant protective clothing that provides full body protection, as well as SCBA and special, sealed equipment.

- **Level B** requires nonencapsulated protective clothing, or clothing that is designed to protect against a particular hazard. Usually, this clothing is made of material that will let only limited amounts of moisture and vapor pass through (nonpermeable). Level B also requires breathing devices that contain their own air supply, such as SCBA, and eye protection.

- **Level C,** like Level B, requires the use of nonpermeable clothing and eye protection. In addition, face masks that filter all inhaled outside air must be used.

- **Level D** requires a work uniform, such as coveralls, that affords minimal protection.

All levels of protection require the use of gloves. Two pairs of rubber gloves are needed for protection in case one pair must be removed because of heavy contamination.

along with the number. The same number and name can also be found on the shipping papers and packaging of the material. If you are unable to read the placard or labels, *do not* move closer and risk exposure. The HazMat team will have binoculars that allow team members to read the placards or labels from a safe distance. If you are able to read the placard with the naked eye, you are too close and should move farther away. Figure 37-15 shows a chart illustrating the hazardous materials warning placards, and Figure 37-16 shows a chart illustrating the warning labels. You should study and be familiar with these warning materials.

You must also be sure to keep bystanders away. Often, well-meaning individuals try to help. However, unless they are trained for these types of incidents, they should be moved from the area.

Once you have called for the HazMat Team, you should focus your efforts on activities that will ensure the safety and survival of the greatest number of people. Use the ambulance's outside public address system to alert individuals who are near the scene and direct them to move to a location where they will be sufficiently far from and out of the line of danger. With the aid of others on your team, try to set up a perimeter to stop traffic and individuals from entering the danger zone.

The HazMat team is equipped to identify the specific substance that is involved and, using a number of complex factors, determine the size, direction or shape, and perimeter of the danger zone. The type, toxicity or concentration, and quantity of the hazardous material that is involved will help the team to determine the location of and safe distance from the danger zone. Determination of the danger zone will also be affected by the amount of wind and other weather factors.

When a material is hazardous because of its flammability or potential for explosion rather than its toxicity, you will need to be at an even greater distance and behind a windowless wall or other strong barrier that will shield you and others from heat, the blast force, and flying debris.

Once fire fighters and the HazMat team have arrived at a small incident, they will determine which specific hazardous material is involved and will mark the perimeter of the danger or hazard zone with warning tape. At a large incident, they may broadcast the zone's limits. Only individuals who are trained in HazMat and wearing the proper level of protective gear should enter the hazard zone. As an EMT-B, you do not have this role. Your job is to stand by at a designated treatment area outside of the hazard zone and provide treatment when HazMat team members bring patients to you.

Patients' skin and clothing may contain hazardous material, so a decontamination area should be set up

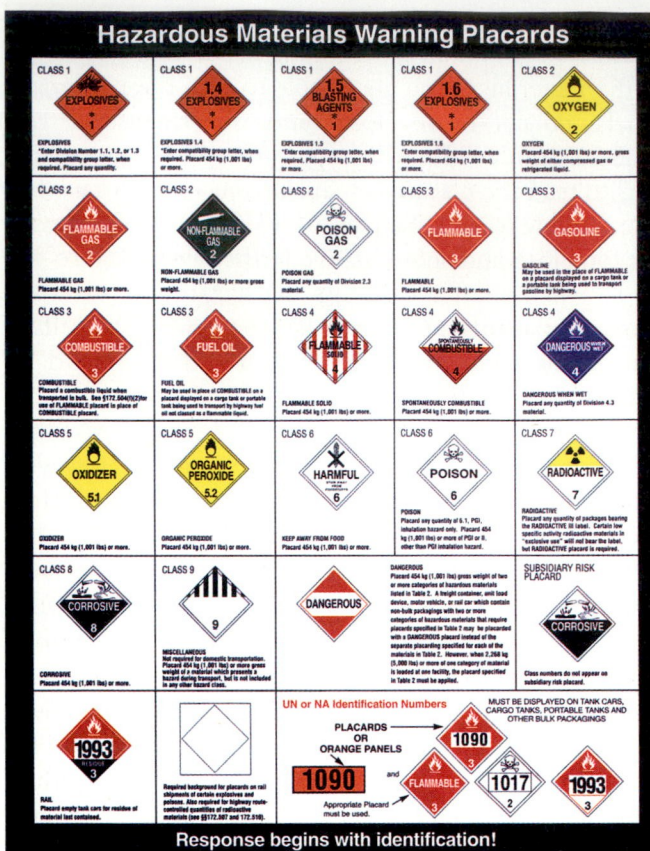

FIGURE 37-15 Hazardous materials warning placards.

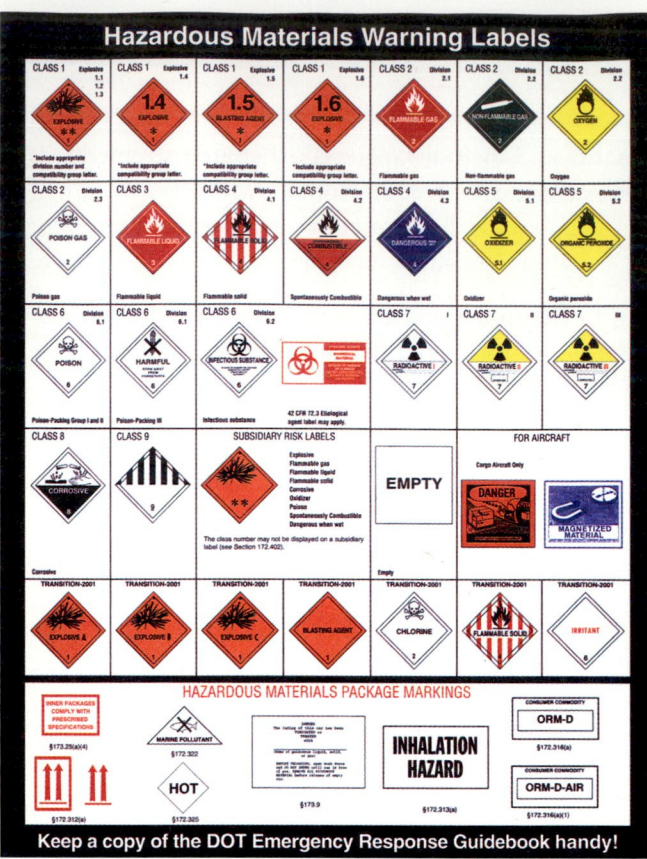

FIGURE 37-16 Hazardous materials warning labels.

between the hazard zone and the treatment area. The decontamination area is the designated area where contaminants are removed before an individual can go to another area. Decontamination is the process of removing or neutralizing and properly disposing of hazardous materials from equipment, patients, and rescue personnel. The decontamination area must include special containers for contaminated clothing and special bags to isolate each patient's personal effects safely until they can be decontaminated at a later time. The area will also contain a number of special facilities to thoroughly wash and rinse patients and backboards. The water that is used must be captured and delivered into special sealable containers.

Anyone who leaves the hazard zone must pass through the decontamination area. Fire fighters' and HazMat team members' outer protective gear is rinsed and washed in the decontamination area before it is removed (Figure 37-17). To prevent needless contact and communication of splash or residues, different personnel are used in the decontamination and treatment areas. You should not move into the decontamination area unless you are properly trained and equipped. You should wait for the patients to be brought to you.

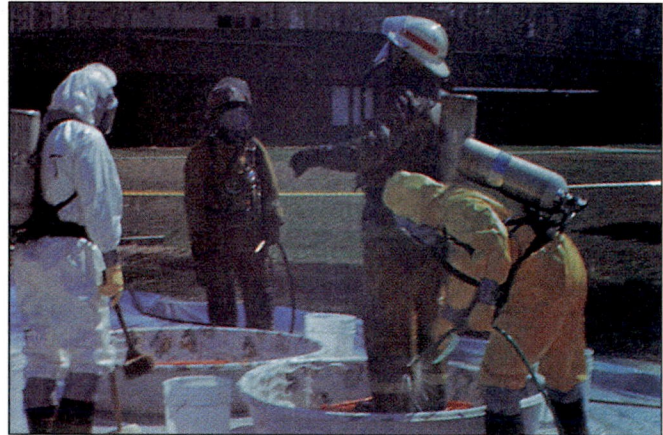

FIGURE 37-17 The decontamination zone is where firefighters and HazMat team members' outer protective gear is rinsed and washed before removal.

Caring for Patients at a Hazardous Materials Incident

Most HazMat team members are trained to the first responder or EMT-B level. Because of the dangers, time constraints, and inhibiting bulky protective gear, it is practical only to provide the simplest assessment and essential care in both the hazard zone and the decontamination area. In addition, to avoid entrapment and communication of contaminants, no bandages or splints are applied, except pressure dressings that are needed to control bleeding, until the "clean" patient has been moved to the treatment area. Therefore, the EMT-Bs providing care in the treatment area should assess and treat the patient in the same way as they would a patient who has not been previously assessed or treated.

Your care of patients at a HazMat incident must address the following two issues:

- Any trauma that has resulted from other related mechanisms, such as vehicle collision, fire, or explosion
- The injury and harm that have resulted from exposure to the toxic hazardous substance

You should treat the patient's injuries in the same way that you would treat any injury. There are very few specific antidotes or treatments for exposure to most hazardous materials. Different people may respond differently to contact with the same hazardous material. Therefore, your treatment for the patient's exposure to the toxic substance should focus mainly on supportive care and initiating transport to the hospital with a minimum of additional delay.

Most serious injuries and deaths from hazardous materials result from airway and breathing problems. Therefore, you should be sure to maintain the airway and, if the patient appears to be in distress, give oxygen at 10 to 15 L/min with a nonrebreathing mask. Monitor the patient's breathing at all times. If you see signs that would indicate that respiratory distress is increasing, you may need to provide assisted ventilation with a BVM device and high-flow oxygen.

If special antidotes or other special treatments need to be initiated in the field, they will be ordered by the medical control and relayed to the officer who is in charge of EMS operations at the scene. If special treatment includes medications, IVs, or other advanced care, paramedics or other advanced personnel will be sent to work with you at the treatment area.

Special care. In some cases, before the decontamination area has been completely set up, the HazMat Team will find one or two patients who need immediate treatment and transport without further delay if they are to survive. Even after the decontamination area is set up and functioning, some patients may have such respiratory distress or another urgent critical condition that the time necessary for full decontamination may prove fatal. If additional delay for proper decontamination appears to be life threatening in nontoxic exposure situations, it may be necessary to simply cut away all of the patient's

> Most serious injuries and death from hazardous materials result from airway and breathing problems.

clothing and do a rapid rinse to remove the majority of the contaminating matter before transport.

If you are treating and transporting a patient who has not been fully and properly decontaminated, you will need to increase the amount of protective clothing you wear, including the use of SCBA. At the least, this should include two pairs of gloves, goggles or a face shield, a protective coat, respiratory protection, and a disposable fluid-impervious apron or similar outfit. Many HazMat teams carry easy-to-use disposable fluid-impervious light protective suits for such a purpose. Remember, however, that transporting a contaminated patient merely increases the size of the event. The decision to transport even a patient with critical injuries rests with the incident commander, who bases his or her decision on recommendations made by the HazMat team.

To make decontaminating the ambulance afterwards easier, tape the cabinet doors shut. Any equipment kits, monitors, and other items that will not be used en route should be removed from the patient compartment and placed in the front of the ambulance or in outside compartments. Before loading the patient, you should turn on the power vent ceiling fan and patient compartment air-conditioning unit fan. Unless the weather is too severe, the windows in the driver's area and sliding side windows in the patient compartment should also be partially opened to prevent creating a "closed box" in the patient compartment and to ensure that the ambulance is properly ventilated for the patient's and EMT's safety.

When you leave the scene, inform the hospital that you are transporting a critically injured patient who has not been fully decontaminated at the scene. This will allow the hospital to prepare to receive the patient. Many emergency departments have a room with a separate outside entrance and decontamination facilities for such an event. You may be asked to reroute to a facility with these capabilities if the receiving hospital is not so equipped. Be sure that one EMT-B enters the emergency department and, after giving hospital staff the report and advising them again of the incomplete decontamination, obtains directions before the patient is unloaded and brought in. If there are enough ambulances at a hazardous materials scene, one may be isolated and used only to transport such patients. Remember, the ambulance needs to be decontaminated before transporting decontaminated patients.

Resources

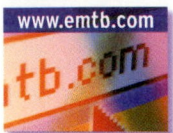

Every ambulance, as well as the dispatch center, should have a copy of *1996 North American Emergency Response Guidebook* (NAERG96), prepared by Transport Canada, the US Department of Transportation, and the Secretariat of Communications and Transportation of Mexico (Figure 37-18). This publication lists most hazardous materials. For each one, it describes the proper initial emergency action to control the scene and provide emergency medical care. Some state and local government agencies may also have information about hazardous materials that are commonly found in their areas. Be sure to keep these publications up to date and close at hand.

Another valuable resource is the **Chemical Transportation Emergency Center (CHEMTREC)**, located in Washington, D.C. CHEMTREC was established by the Chemical Manufacturers Association to assist emergency personnel in identifying and handling hazardous materials transport incidents. The center operates 24 hours a day, 7 days a week. Its toll-free number is 1-800-424-9300 from anywhere within the United States or Canada.

CHEMTREC provides information, warnings, and guidance for proper emergency management and treatment. However, it cannot identify an unknown substance. You must provide CHEMTREC with the correct DOT identification number, the chemical name, or the product name of the material.

If you are interested in learning more about hazardous materials incidents and rescue requirements, you can look to the following:

- National Fire Protection Association (NFPA) standard #479
- OSHA standard #1910.120
- Federal Emergency Management Agency (FEMA) guidelines for coping with hazardous materials incidents
- EPA protective clothing

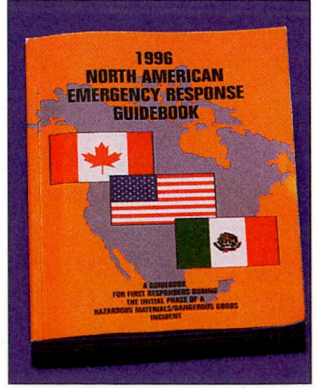

FIGURE 37-18
The *1996 North American Emergency Response Guidebook.*

Incident Management Systems

In recent years, a number of leadership and command systems have been developed to improve the on-scene management of emergency situations. Law enforcement, fire, and EMS systems have come up with similar programs to help control, direct, and coordinate emergency responders and resources. These programs are called **incident management systems (IMS)**, or incident command systems (ICS).

Components of an Incident Management System

At a large fire, a hazardous materials incident, or a mass-casualty incident, fire, rescue, HazMat, police, and EMS units from many different areas will all be involved in some way. To ensure clear lines of responsibility and authority, a preestablished system that identifies who is in charge and who reports to whom is necessary. Even on a call with only one patient and no need for any other services, the implementation of an incident management system is required to identify the roles and responsibilities of each crew member, particularly if the event begins to escalate.

Major incidents often require another level of management, known as *unified command*. With unified command, the incident commander is joined at the **command post**, the designated field command center, by an officer who is in charge of all fire operations, one who is in charge of all rescue or HazMat operations, one who is in charge of all EMS operations, and one who is in charge of all law enforcement operations at the incident. This group, under the direction of the incident commander, directs the overall operations at the scene. Because all officers are stationed at the command post, they can be easily found and can collectively advise the incident commander of changes and problems that are communicated to them. The incident commander can also involve them in making the necessary decisions and in rapidly conveying orders to those under their command. In addition to unified command, this system ensures that the actions of each different type of responder are properly coordinated. Often, representatives of the mayor (or prevailing civil authority) and specialized support personnel will be added at the command post as an incident escalates.

How these systems work together depends on the nature of the event. For example, with a major airplane crash, the leading agency is typically the fire department. In this situation, EMS is usually one aspect of the overall fire incident command system. Within their own system, EMS personnel establish and carry out their tasks. However, ultimate control of the incident will rest with the fire commander. Other situations, such as widespread injuries at a rock concert, are primarily civil events. Law enforcement would take the lead, establishing an incident management plan. Fire and EMS would follow the law enforcement commander's decision. EMS is seldom the lead agency.

At one time or another, your unit will probably be the first to respond to an incident that will involve more than one EMS unit or one or more non-EMS agencies. In this situation, the senior EMT should establish command and inform the dispatcher by saying, for example, "Dispatch, this is Squad 71, establishing 'Route 43' command." From that point on, all communications from the dispatcher to the scene will be directed to "Route 43 Command." If you arrive after command has been established, advise the dispatcher that you are on scene and "reporting to command." Then find the command post, and report for assignment.

When the activities at the scene are very spread out or are distinguished by specific geographic areas, a **sector commander** may be added to aid in the command and coordination of the activities in each assigned area. As at any accident scene, each team of fire, rescue, EMS and police personnel is led by an officer or crew chief who is a hands-on member of that team.

These systems will vary from place to place, and different terms may be used. You should become familiar with the specific terms and chain of command that are used in your area.

Structure of an Incident Management System

Incident management systems vary from town to town and from jurisdiction to jurisdiction. You may hear terms such as "sectors," "divisions," "task forces," or "platoons" used to mean much the same thing. In addition to learning your system's plan thoroughly, you must also be familiar with the terms and concepts that your local law enforcement and fire incident command systems use. You will be working closely with them.

As an example of how responsibilities may be assigned at a major EMS incident, consider the following typical assignments:

- **Extrication sector.** This is for disentangling and removing patients from the scene and moving them to the triage sector.
- **Triage sector. Triage** is the process of establishing treatment and transportation priorities according to the severity of injury and medical need. The triage sector is a sorting point, at which patients are directed to specific areas of the treatment sector, according to their assigned priority.

- **Treatment sector.** This is where thorough assessments are made and prioritized and on-scene treatment is begun while transport is being arranged.
- **Transportation sector.** This is where ambulances and crews are organized to transport patients from the treatment sector to area hospitals.
- **Staging sector.** This is a holding area for arriving ambulances and crews until they can be assigned a particular task.
- **Supply sector.** This is an area in which to assemble extra equipment and supplies, such as blankets, oxygen bottles, bandages, and backboards, for dispersal to other sectors as needed.
- **Mobile command center.** This is typically a vehicle or building at the scene where the EMS commander establishes an "office." From here, the commander oversees the activities of the various sectors and coordinates them with the activities of other agency commanders.

When you respond to this sort of incident, you will be assigned to a sector and a sector officer. Report at once to your sector officer for assignment. When you have finished your assigned task, report back to that same sector officer for another assignment. If your sector's duties are complete, you will be assigned to the staging area for reassignment to another sector.

The success of any incident management system depends on all personnel performing their assigned tasks and working within the system. For example, suppose an EMS team that is assigned to extrication decides instead to transport patients from the scene. This team thus bypasses the triage, treatment, and transport sectors. Discipline and coordination give way to chaos. Always remember that the cost of "doing your own thing" may include the loss of lives.

Multiple-Casualty Situations

A **multiple-casualty situation (MCS)** is any call involving more than one patient. A mass-casualty incident (MCI) is an event that places such a demand on available equipment or personnel resources that the system is stretched to its limit or beyond. Airplane crashes or earthquakes are the obvious examples. However, the truth is that MCSs and MCIs are far more common than these disasters and are usually much smaller in scope.

Ask yourself the following questions:

- How many seriously injured patients can you care for effectively and transport in your ambulance? One? Two?

- What happens when you have three patients to deal with?

- What do you do when two cars, each carrying four individuals, crash head-on at high speed?

Obviously, you and your team cannot treat and transport all those patients at the same time. Within the context of your team and unit, you have just encountered a multiple-casualty situation. It might not be an earthquake, but you will remember and talk about it for months.

When multiple-casualty situations occur, the local EMS resources may be increased by the use of additional ambulances and EMTs from around the immediate region (Figure 37-19). Operating procedures differ from those that are normally followed.

Not all multiple casualty situations require these changes. In many urban or densely populated suburban areas, accidents with fewer than 25 patients, called **limited victim incidents (LVI)**, are not uncommon. They may require additional leadership and some decrease in the patient radio reports; however, they are handled by the local on-duty units in generally the normal manner. This is achieved by focusing most of the available units at this scene, dividing the patient load among the crews, and equally distributing the patients to the various emergency departments that are in the area. But, when the number of patients is significantly higher (even in areas with abundant resources), a different system must be used to meet the urgent needs of patients so that increased deterioration and deaths do not result.

At any call involving more than one patient, you cannot just start at the nearest patient, assessing and treating each patient in turn. A more rapid method, such as triage, must be used to focus on the patients who have the greatest need.

Results of studies of past major incidents indicate that, regardless of the incident's mechanism (eg, plane crash, train derailment or collision, building collapse), patients generally experience the same injuries and conditions that are often seen at motor vehicle crashes.

Triage

An essential feature of multiple-casualty situations is triage, which is a French word that means "sorting." You have already learned that triage is a technique of establishing treatment and transport priorities in situations with more than one patient. Triage allows you to quickly assess all patients and sort them into categories on the basis of the severity and survivability of their injuries (Figure 37-20).

Usually, the most highly trained medical person at the scene directs triage. If you are the first EMT-B at the

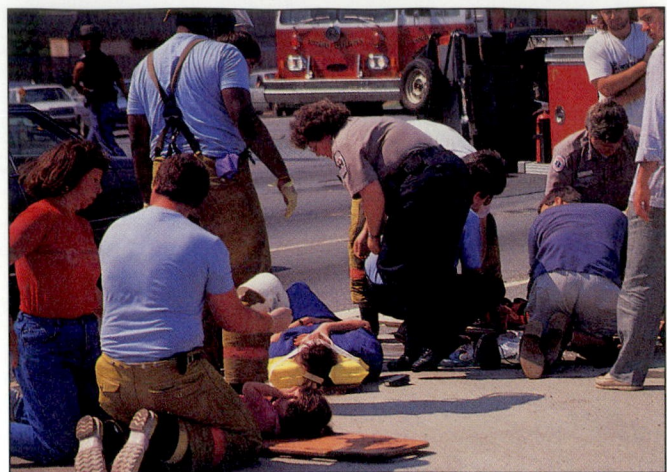

FIGURE 37-19 Multiple-casualty incidents require additional ambulances and EMS providers from the immediate region.

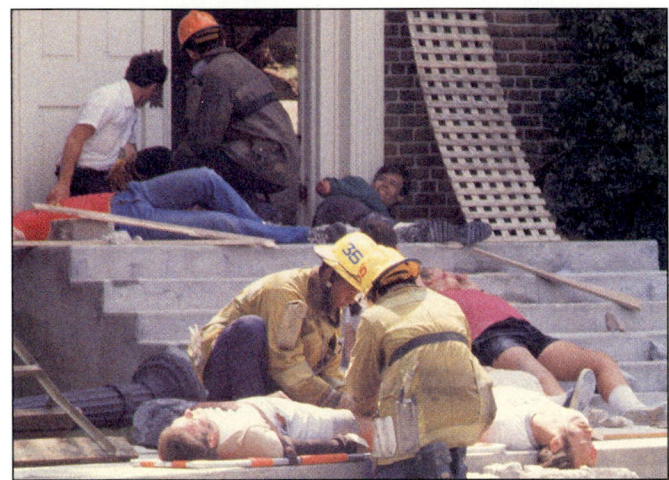

FIGURE 37-20 Triage is an essential component of a multiple-casualty incident.

scene, you should begin triage after you contact dispatch for additional resources. Remember that if you assume the initial duties of **triage officer**, you should not become involved in patient care. You are responsible for triaging patients in accordance with your protocols.

Precisely how and where triage will be carried out will vary depending on the event and your local protocol. It is difficult for one or two EMTs to wade through a field of patients. Whenever possible, it is better to establish one central triage clearinghouse. All patients are then brought to this clearinghouse on their way to the treatment areas. In major incidents, separate triage areas may have to be established to accommodate the size and geography of the area.

Triage priorities. Patients are sorted into four triage levels or groups. Each level may be identified by a certain color or number (Table 37-2). Treatment areas, too, are usually identified by colored flags or markers (Figure

TABLE 37-2 Triage Priorities	
Triage Category	**Typical Injuries**
Highest Priority (Red) Patients who need immediate care and transport. Treat these patients first, and transport as soon as possible.	• Airway and breathing difficulties • Uncontrolled or severe bleeding • Decreased level of consciousness • Severe medical problems • Shock (hypoperfusion) • Severe burns
Second Priority (Yellow) Patients whose treatment and transportation can be temporarily delayed	• Burns without airway problems • Major or multiple bone or joint injuries • Back injuries with or without spinal cord damage
Low Priority (Green) Patients whose treatment and transportation can be delayed until last	• Minor fractures • Minor soft-tissue injuries
Lowest Priority (Black) Patients who are already dead or have little chance for survival. If resources are limited, treat salvageable patients before these patients.	• Obvious death • Obviously non-survivable injury, such as major open brain trauma • Full cardiac arrest

37-21). The highest priority for treatment is given to patients whose injuries are critical but probably survivable with prompt intervention. Available personnel and equipment should be assigned to these patients first. Patients whose injuries are not an immediate threat to their airway, breathing, or circulation should be placed in lower priority categories. Low priority is given to patients with very minor injuries or those who are not physically injured. Individuals who are obviously dead or whose injuries are so catastrophic that certain death is very near are given lowest priority.

It might seem cruel to assign a low priority to those who are obviously dead or unlikely to survive their injuries. However, you must focus on patients who can benefit from your care. This is especially true if you have limited resources. The cardinal rule of triage is to do the greatest good for the greatest number. In a multiple-casualty situation, the criteria for triage include the consideration of both urgency and potential for survival.

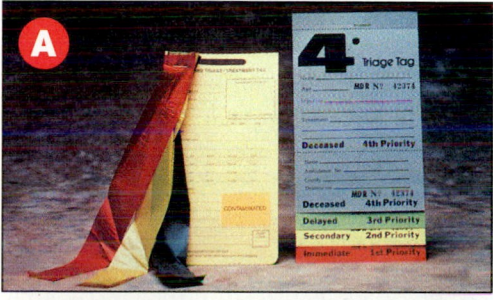

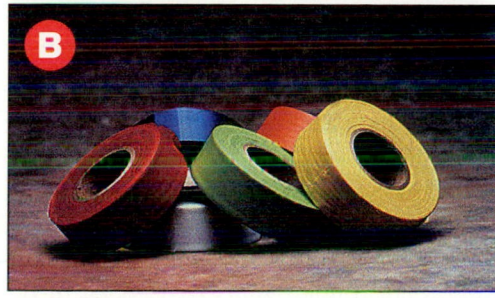

FIGURE 37-21 A: Triage tags. **B:** Triage tape.

Table 37-3 shows the important components of an incident management system in a multiple-casualty situation.

Triage procedures. Triage is a dynamic, ongoing process. Once the triage officer assigns a triage priority, the patient is taken to the appropriate treatment area. There, other EMS personnel will begin treatment and conduct a more thorough assessment. They will then reevaluate the patient's condition routinely on the basis of the following considerations:

- Is the patient improving? Can he or she be moved to a lower level of care?

- Is the patient becoming worse? Does he or she need more immediate transport?

A patient may be assigned a high priority (red) because of severe bleeding. However, once the bleeding is controlled, the patient's triage priority may change. Changing the patient's assigned category is the responsibility of the treatment sector officer. This officer is also responsible for communicating with the transportation sector officer to arrange transport for patients to the hospital.

The incident commander should determine exactly where patients should be triaged according to the situation and his or her judgment. Usually, a single **triage center** is essential to the orderly evaluation and evacuation of patients. Before moving patients to the triage center, you should provide initial treatment and stabilization. The triage officer should be either a highly experienced EMT-B, a paramedic, or an emergency physician (or trauma surgeon) with prior training specifically for this task. The triage officer must perform a rapid assessment, no more than 30 seconds long, and decide in which of the triage categories the patient belongs. Although the triage officer must do this on the basis of a rapid and somewhat subjective impression, the judgment of the triage officer is *not* to be questioned.

The priority that is assigned to each patient at this time reflects solely the patient's condition and is not relative to the condition of others. This initial triage puts patients into smaller, workable groups. Once the patient has been triaged, he or she is placed in the clearly identified area in the **treatment center** that is designated for that patient's priority level.

At the treatment center, other EMS personnel will perform a more thorough assessment and provide the treatment that is needed to stabilize the patient. Efforts at the treatment center will be focused initially on red-tagged patients, followed by yellow-tagged patients. The **treatment officer**, who should be an emergency physician or other physician trained and experienced in the stabilization of trauma patients, directs the EMTs and

---

TABLE 37-3 Key Components at a Multiple-Casualty Incident

- Incident commander, command post, and incident management system

- On-site communications system

- Adequate supply of long backboards, straps, or ties

- Extrication/retrieval group

- Triage officer and designated triage center

- Staffed patient collection and treatment area

- Supply location adjacent to the treatment area

- Transportation officer, transport area, and transport crew

- Staging area to hold resources until they are needed

- Fire and law enforcement personnel

- Secure perimeter

---

what would you do?

You are at the scene of a car accident in which three individuals have been injured. One patient is an alert 19-year-old woman with a profusely bleeding open fracture of the femur. The second patient is a conscious and distressed 68-year-old man with a sucking wound of the chest. The third patient is a 30-year-old man who is unconscious with massive head and chest injuries. His breathing is rapid, shallow, and irregular.

You can treat only one patient at a time. If you start treatment by resuscitating the 30-year-old patient, you will be treating him for a long time. Probably, he will die anyway. In addition, one or both of the other two patients will die. However, if you first occlude the sucking chest wound in the 68-year-old patient and then stop the bleeding in the 19-year-old patient with a pressure dressing, both, or at least one, of these patients will survive. If you treat the 30-year-old patient last, he will probably die, but you will have done the greatest good for the greatest number. The principle of triage is to treat the patient with survivable injuries first.

other personnel who are providing assessment and treatment. If a physician is not available, the role of the treatment officer should be filled by a senior paramedic or EMT.

On the basis of the assessment of patients in the same triage category, the treatment officer should determine which two patients should be transported next. These patients should then be moved to the area closest to the transport area, a designated area at one end of the treatment area where patients are loaded into ambulances and transported to the hospital.

The **transport officer** is the individual who is in charge of the transport area, news in the area, and all other activities pertaining to transport of patients to nearby hospitals. Under the direction of the transport officer, a third group of EMTs will load patients into the ambulances and care for them while transporting them to their assigned hospital. The treatment officer then recommends which two patients should be transported next, and the transport officer directs the EMTs to load them into one of the waiting ambulances and instructs the driver as to which hospital these patients should be taken. Fire fighters or law enforcement officers may be assigned to assist in loading or driving if there is a shortage of EMTs. However, because he or she is familiar with the location and operation of equipment and supplies in the ambulance, one of the EMTs who came with each ambulance should be assigned to care for the patients while en route to the hospital.

A rotation system is used to properly distribute patients to each hospital on the basis of hospital capacity and capabilities. The transport officer is responsible for sending the ambulance to the next hospital in turn. This rotation must occasionally be altered to allow specific patients to be taken to the most appropriate facility, such as a pediatric center, or because a hospital has notified the field that it needs to be skipped for one rotation.

Normally, no more than two patients are placed in the same ambulance. However, with severe weather, a patient who has been tagged green may be seated in an ambulance next to the driver to move the patient to a comfortable, safe indoor holding area at the hospital.

As the patients are loaded into the ambulance, the transport officer logs their MCS number, their overall condition, and the hospital to which they will be taken. As the ambulance leaves the scene, the transport officer radios the receiving hospital and briefly describes the patients and unit transporting them and the time they left the scene. To minimize radio traffic during such incidents, personnel on individual ambulances do not usually use their radios except to obtain advice from medical control or to notify the transport officer that they are leaving the hospital and returning to the field.

After giving a verbal report to hospital staff and transferring the patient, the ambulance returns to the staging area without further delay, helping to keep a continuous flow of ambulances moving between the MCS site and the hospital. Equipment that is collected at the hospital or additional supplies that are needed in the field are brought to the staging area in the next returning ambulance.

If the transport officer needs additional ambulances, he or she radios the EMS chief at the command center, who then summons them from the staging area. If none is available at the staging area, the EMS chief notifies the dispatcher to obtain them elsewhere. Given sufficient time from the onset of the incident, a lack of ambulances does not commonly occur.

After all the first-priority (red-tagged) patients have been transported, the second-priority (yellow-tagged) patients are transported, followed by the third-priority (green-tagged) patients. After all patients have been transported, several units stay at the incident site to protect the other responders who will remain. Often, ambulances will still be needed to transfer patients from the facility to which they were initially brought for stabilization to another, more appropriate facility.

Treatment and triage continue until all patients have been treated and transported. The transport officer should try to make transport decisions and allocate patients among local medical facilities on the basis of the number of patients, the severity of their injuries, and the available transportation resources. This minimizes overload on any one facility. These record-keeping and allocation duties may be delegated, but the ultimate responsibility belongs to the transport officer. If the incident is large in scale, this officer may designate a communications operator. A communications operator controls and directs radio traffic between the hospitals and the transport point.

Additional triage operations and roles. In the event of a fire at a multiple-casualty situation, the fire fighters' first responsibility is to contain and extinguish it. As fire fighters become available, they are assigned to other tasks. Some will join the police in marking and securing a perimeter to exclude spectators and others who do not have a role in the disaster functions. In some cases, spectators are enlisted to help secure this line or to help carry patients on backboards.

In "closed" incidents, such as a train wreck, patients must be removed from a cramped, unsafe environment before they can be assessed and triaged. In "open" incidents, such as a fire in a shopping mall, patients will be in widely separated groups spread around the outside of the building and must be collected for effective triage to be performed. The role of the <u>extrication/retrieval group</u> is to rapidly eyeball each patient and using a long spine board bring any patients in need of urgent care to the triage officer. The extrication/retrieval group will periodically also lead or bring patients who appear to have no urgent need for treatment to the triage center.

After the MCS has ended, all personnel who were involved should be debriefed and evaluated to determine whether they need counseling. Records are collected at this time. Multiple-casualty situations require regional preplanning and agreement, in addition to periodic simulation drills in which the fire, rescue, EMS, and police units in the region are alerted and a large number of mock victims are triaged and treated from the onset of the incident to receipt and re-triage at the hospital

special triage situations

Patients who have been contaminated by radiation or other hazardous materials and are covered with radiation particles or other hazardous materials are placed in a separate category of triage. This is the highest category of all. Contaminated patients must be moved away from all other patients. They must not be allowed to contaminate other patients, EMS personnel, ambulances, or hospitals.

Certain large urban areas that offer regionalized care use another concept of triage. Single patients with specific medical problems, such as burns, trauma, cardiac, or neonatal, are triaged to specialized regional centers for treatment. Making the decision to transport a patient to a special treatment center is difficult. The decision is based on many factors, including (but not limited to) the following:

- The specific illness or injury

- The severity of the illness or injury

- The availability of local resources at the time of the event

- Local rules and protocols

These decisions are often made only after on-line communication with medical control.

If there are special treatment centers in your area, you must know the specific triage protocols that apply. Also note that in the event of an MCS, these protocols might not be used. For example, a school bus accident in which all 30 or 40 patients are children can overwhelm a pediatric hospital. Similarly, 10 burn patients from a petroleum plant fire could immobilize a burn center. In these cases, good triage and communication with medical control are essential in providing each patient with the best available treatment.

Most urban areas have regional trauma care centers. Severe, life-threatening injuries should be treated in facilities that are prepared to deal immediately and completely with the problem. Ideally, severely injured patients should be identified in the field and sent to a designated Level One Trauma Center.

It is not enough to know the triage techniques that your EMS system uses to identify patients for transport to specialized treatment facilities. As with the other skills you are learning, you must practice these techniques as well. Your EMS system should conduct disaster drills yearly, preferably with the participation of local hospitals and other public safety and rescue units. Disaster plans must be developed and practiced in advance of need. The mass confusion of a disaster site is no time to experiment with organization.

prep kit

ready for review

During all phases of rescue, your primary concern is safety, and your primary role is to provide emergency medical care and prevent further injury to the patient. When there are not enough personnel for both an EMS team and a rescue team, you and your team may have to act as rescuers as well. Safety during rescue or extrication begins with the proper mind-set and the proper protective equipment. During size-up, you should identify the safest, most efficient way to access the patient. Try to get to the patient as simply and quickly as possible without using any tools or breaking any glass. Make sure that you and the patient are protected with a fireproof blanket. Unless there is immediate danger, perform an initial assessment of a patient while he or she is still in the vehicle. Immobilize the cervical spine before moving the patient from the vehicle. If you see that a special rescue team is needed, inform the dispatcher.

At a hazardous materials incident, safety—of you and your team, the patient, and the public—is your most important concern. If you arrive first, assess the situation, taking care to protect yourself, and then call for a trained HazMat team. The most important step in such an incident is to identify the substances involved. Do not enter the hazard zone; your job is to provide supportive care once the patient can be safely moved out of the area. Hazardous materials are classified according to five toxicity levels. Four protection levels are indicated for the amount and type of protective gear you need. Levels indicate the amount and type of protective gear that you need to prevent injury from a particular substance. The Chemical Transportation Emergency Center (CHEMTREC) is open around the clock to help you identify and handle hazardous materials transport incidents.

Incident management systems allow for coordination of police, fire, and EMS activities in an emergency situation. In major incidents, there is usually a unified command, with a single command post where decisions are made by agency leaders. If your unit arrives first at an incident that will involve more than one unit or agency, the senior EMT-B should establish command. Otherwise, you should report to the command post for assignment. You may be assigned to one of the following sectors: extrication, triage, treatment, transportation, staging, or supply.

In a multiple-casualty situation, the most highly trained medical person on the scene directs triage. This means assigning treatment and transport priorities according to the severity and survivability of patients' injuries. There are four triage levels, each with a separate treatment area. Highest priority is given to patients whose injuries are critical but probably survivable with prompt resuscitation. The cardinal rule of triage is to do the greatest good for the greatest number. Treatment and triage continue until all patients have been transported. In urban areas with special treatment centers, special protocols are used to triage patients with specific injuries to the appropriate centers. Communication with medical control is essential for good triage.

37

prep kit

prep kit

vital vocabulary

www.emtb.com

access The ability to gain entry to an enclosed area and reach a patient.

Chemical Transportation Emergency Center (CHEMTREC) An agency that assists emergency personnel in identifying and handling hazardous materials transport incidents.

command post The designated field command center where the incident commander and deputies are located.

complex access Complicated entry that requires special tools and training and includes breaking windows or using other force.

danger zone An area where individuals can be exposed to toxic substances, lethal rays, or ignition or explosion of hazardous materials.

decontamination The process of removing or neutralizing and properly disposing of hazardous materials from equipment, patients, and rescue personnel.

decontamination area The designated area in a hazardous materials incident where all patients and rescuers must be decontaminated before going to another area.

entrapment To be caught as in a trap within a vehicle, room, or container with no way out or to have a limb or other body part trapped.

extrication Removal of a patient from entrapment or a dangerous situation or position, such as removal from a wrecked vehicle, industrial accident, or building collapse.

extrication/retrieval group Personnel who are assigned to extricate and/or collect patients at a multiple-casualty situation and bring them to the triage center.

hazardous material Any substance that is toxic, poisonous, radioactive, flammable, or explosive and causes injury or death with exposure.

hazardous materials incident An accident in which a hazardous material is no longer properly contained and isolated.

incident commander The individual who has overall command of the scene in the field.

incident management systems (IMS) Organizational systems to help control, direct, and coordinate emergency responders and resources.

limited victim incident (LVI) A multiple-patient situation involving fewer than 25 patients.

multiple-casualty situation (MCS) An event that stretches the system to its limit in terms of available equipment or personnel; also called a mass-casualty incident (MCI).

protection level A measure of the amount and type of protective equipment that an individual needs to avoid injury during contact with a hazardous material.

sector commander The individual, working under the incident commander, who is delegated to oversee and coordinate a sector's activity.

simple access Access that is easily achieved without the use of tools or force.

structure fire A fire in a house, apartment building, office, school, plant, warehouse, or other building.

tactical situation A hostage, robbery, or other situation in which armed conflict is threatened or shots have been fired and the threat of violence remains.

technical rescue situation A rescue that requires special technical skills and equipment in one of many specialized rescue areas, such as technical rope rescue, cave rescue, and dive rescue.

technical rescue team A group of individuals from one or more departments in a region that is trained and on call for certain types of technical rescue.

toxicity level A measure of the risk that a hazardous material poses to the health of an individual who comes into contact with it.

transport area The area at one end of the treatment area in a multiple-casualty situation where patients are loaded into ambulances and transported to the receiving hospitals.

transport officer The individual in charge of the transport sector in a multiple-casualty situation, including the area, crews, and any activities related to the transport of patients to receiving hospitals.

treatment center Location in a mass-casualty situation where patients are brought after being triaged and assigned a priority, and where they are reassessed, treated, and monitored until it is their turn to be transported to the hospital.

treatment officer The individual, usually a physician, who is in charge of and directs EMS personnel at the treatment center in a multiple-casualty situation.

triage The process of establishing treatment and transportation priorities according to the severity of injury and medical need.

triage center Designated area in a multiple-casualty situation where the triage officer is located and patients are initially triaged before being taken to the treatment center.

triage officer The individual who is in charge of rapidly assessing and deciding into which triage category patients should be placed in a multiple-casualty situation.

prep kit

37

assessment in action

A pair of young men are involved in a house explosion where they allegedly were manufacturing illegal drugs. The explosion blows out part of the back and side walls, causing part of the roof to collapse. By the time you arrive, the fire department has put out the fire and has located the remains of one of the men. Within minutes, the HazMat team is carrying the other man on a long backboard out to the decontamination tank.

1. What is your priority when you arrive at the scene?
   A. Request that dispatch contact the news media.
   B. Extricate any survivors that you can find in the rubble.
   C. Start unloading all the gear from the ambulance.
   D. Ensure that the scene is safe for you and your partner.

2. Which of the following actions is **NOT** a generally accepted response to a potential HazMat situation?
   A. Park upwind, a safe distance away, if smoke or fire is visible.
   B. Allow bystanders to enter the scene if they accept responsibility for their safety.
   C. Avoid contact with any potentially hazardous materials.
   D. Do not approach the scene until you know it has been secured.

3. If you suspect that you have been dispatched to a potentially hazardous materials scene, when should you request the HazMat team?
   A. As soon as you are made aware or suspect that hazardous materials are involved
   B. After you have worked at the scene for about thirty minutes, then you can evaluate how personnel on scene are doing
   C. After you have entered the scene and done initial triage
   D. Never, as EMS does not request HazMat, law enforcement does

4. A crowd of unruly bystanders has gathered and begins yelling, "Get in there with them other guys and help out!" Before you enter the house, you should first:
   A. put on your coat, if you have one, and then some latex gloves.
   B. ask some of the bystanders to go in and look around.
   C. take a few deep breaths of oxygen off the on-board system.
   D. wait until the HazMat team gives you permission to come in.

5. The HazMat team brings out the sole survivor and removes all his clothes before turning him over to you. What should you do with the clothes?
   A. Leave them alone, and let the HazMat team dispose of them.
   B. Pick them up and place them in the side compartment on the unit.
   C. Get a shovel off the rescue truck and cover the clothes with dirt.
   D. Ask someone with a fireplace at home to take them home and burn them.

prep kit 37

points to ponder

Object. 1-2.10, 3-8.7, 7-3.2, 7-3.4

You arrive at the scene of an auto accident to find two vehicles, each with only a driver inside. One vehicle is a delivery van that is on its side with the driver halfway through the windshield. A placard on the van indicates that it is carrying radioactive materials. The driver is bleeding severely from a wound on the head and an open fracture of the left forearm. The driver is also unresponsive. The driver of the other car is responsive and has a bump on the forehead but is not bleeding anywhere and believes that she can walk. You can determine all of this because you initially approached close to the scene. Your partner yells to the conscious patient to walk to where your vehicle is parked and backs away from the scene to a safe location. Your partner then says, "Let's not tell anyone how close we were."

- How would you deal with this situation? What would be the likelihood that you or your vehicle was exposed? How serious are the radioactive materials that would be carried around in a delivery van?

online outlook

Incident management systems allow for coordination of police, fire, and EMS activities in an emergency situation. In major incidents, there is usually a unified command, with a single command post where decisions are made by agency leaders. To learn more about major incident management, complete Exercise 37 at www.emtb.com.

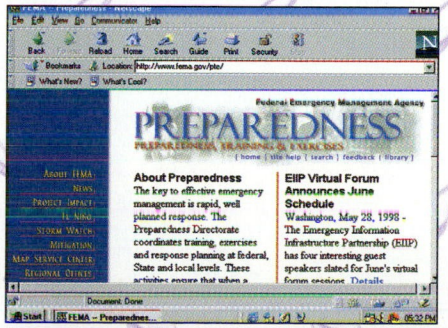

Enrichment

Twink Dalton, RN, MS

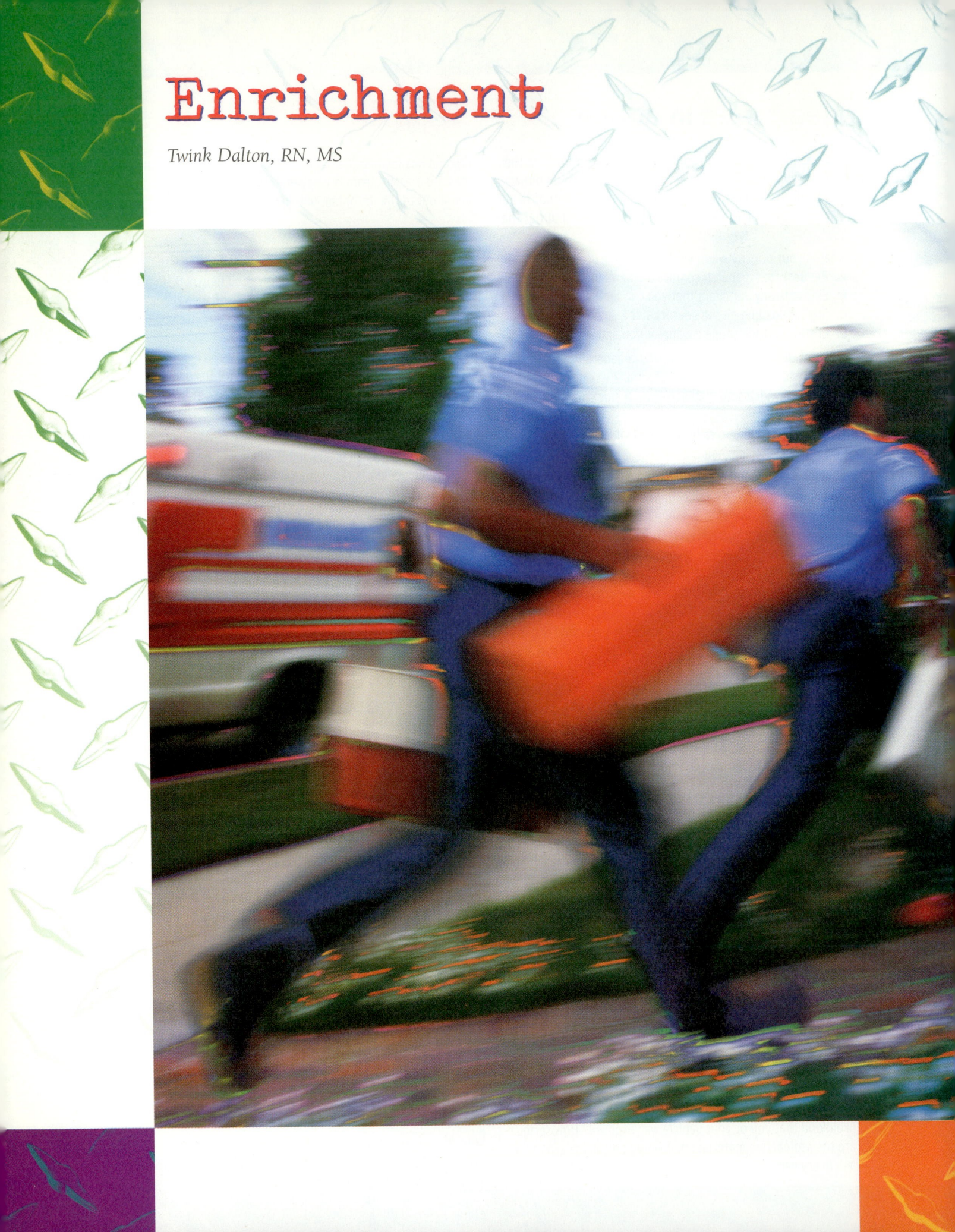

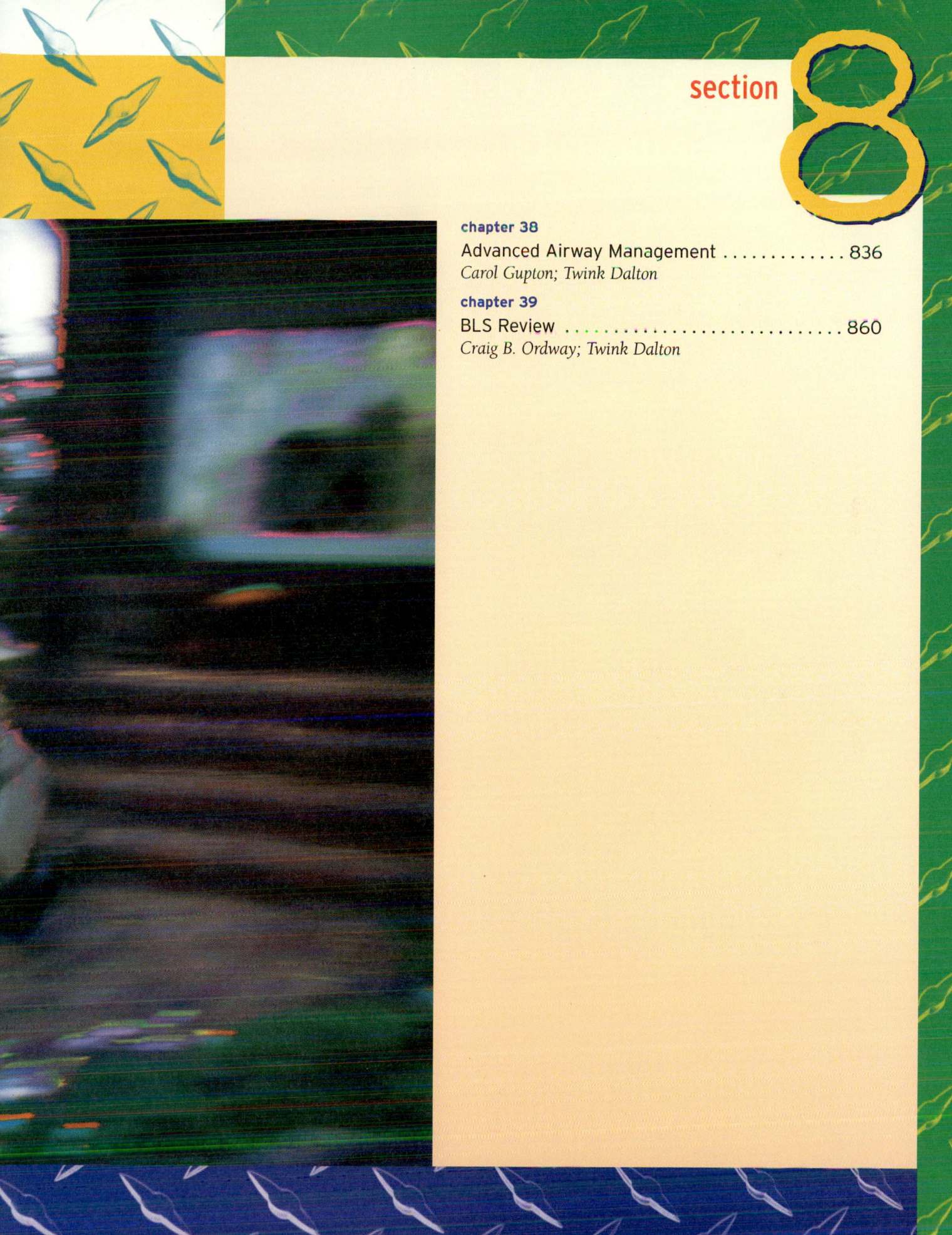

section 8

Advanced Airway Management

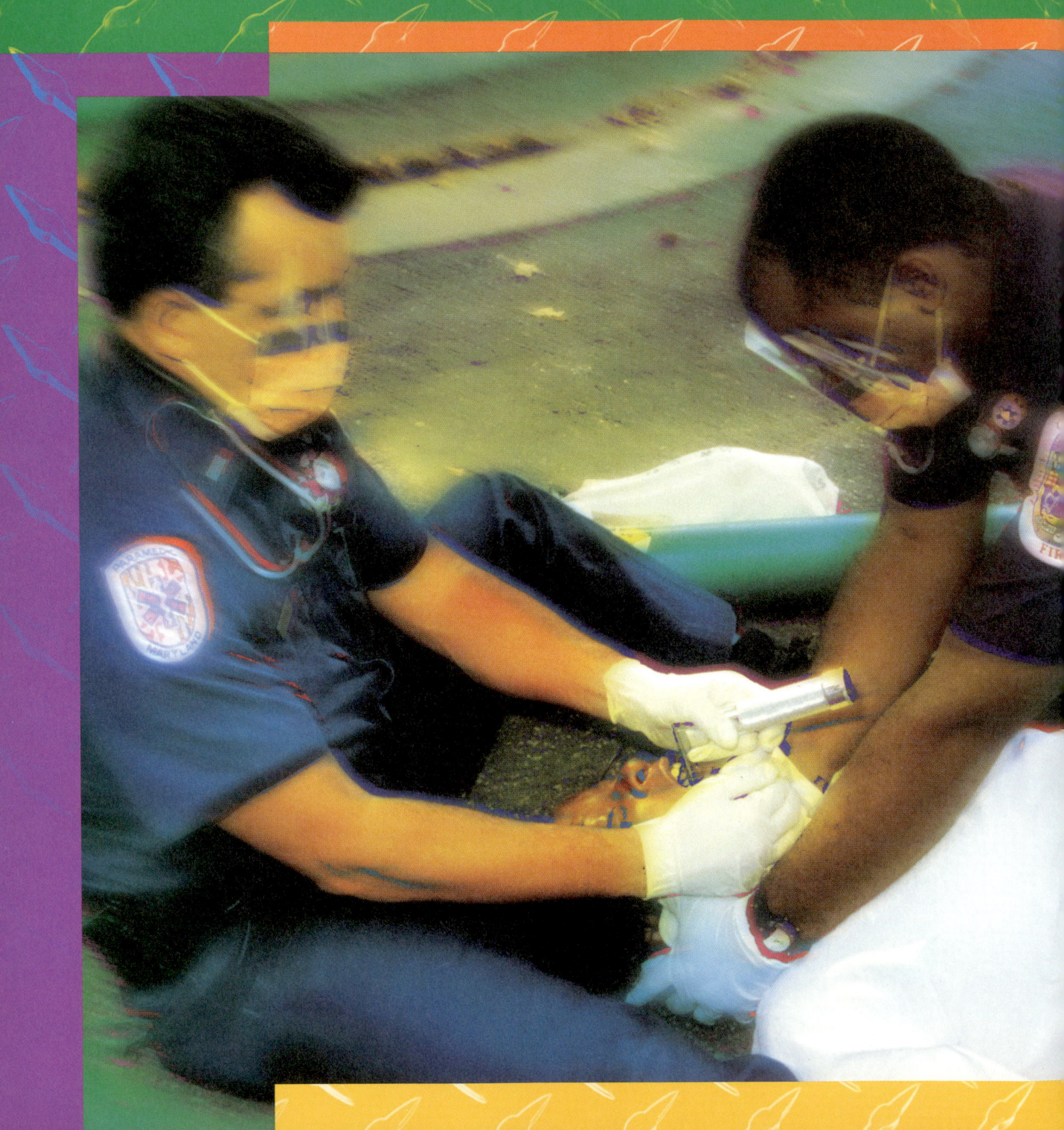

objectives

Cognitive

1. Identify and describe the airway anatomy in the adult.

2. Explain the pathophysiology of airway compromise.

3. Describe the proper use of airway adjuncts.

4. Review the use of oxygen therapy in airway management.

5. Describe the indications, contraindications, and technique for insertion of nasogastric tubes.

6. Describe how to perform the Sellick maneuver (cricoid pressure).

7. Describe the indications for advanced airway management.

8. List the equipment required for orotracheal intubation.

9. Describe the proper use of the curved blade for orotracheal intubation.

10. Describe the proper use of the straight blade for orotracheal intubation.

11. State the reasons for and proper use of the stylet in orotracheal intubation.

12. Describe the methods of choosing the appropriate size endotracheal tube in an adult patient.

13. State the formula for sizing an infant or child endotracheal tube.

14. List complications associated with advanced airway management.

15. Describe the skill of orotracheal intubation in the adult patient.

16. Describe the skill of orotracheal intubation in the infant and child patient.

17. Describe the skill of confirming endotracheal tube placement in the adult, infant, and child patient.

18. State the consequences of and the need to recognize unintentional esophageal intubation.

19. Describe the skill of securing the endotracheal tube in the adult, infant, and child patient.

Affective

20. Recognize and respect the feelings of the patient and family during advanced airway procedures.

21. Explain the value of performing advanced airway procedures.

22. Defend the need for the EMT-B to perform advanced airway procedures.

23. Explain the rationale for the use of a stylet.

24. Explain the rationale for having a suction unit immediately available during intubation attempts.

25. Explain the rationale for confirming breath sounds.

26. Explain the rationale for securing the endotracheal tube.

Psychomotor

27. Demonstrate how to perform the Sellick maneuver (cricoid pressure).

28. Demonstrate the skill of orotracheal intubation in the adult patient.

29. Demonstrate the skill of orotracheal intubation in the infant and child patient.

30. Demonstrate the skill of confirming endotracheal tube placement in the adult patient.

31. Demonstrate the skill of confirming endotracheal tube placement in the infant and child patient.

32. Demonstrate the skill of securing the endotracheal tube in the adult patient.

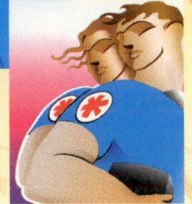

you are the emt

Squad 16, respond to the main pool at Smithee High School for a "diving accident and possible drowning." You snap on the lights and sirens and proceed to the high school.

This situation represents one of the most difficult in all of EMS: an almost certain spine or spinal cord injury, coupled with the airway complications of drowning. This chapter will provide you with the knowledge and skills to make good choices and provide quality care when you are confronted with a call like this. It will also help you to answer the following questions

1. How does intubating a child differ from intubating an adult?
2. In the situation above, does airway care take priority over care of the spine? Is it vice versa?

Advanced Airway Management

The single most important manipulative skill you will use as an EMT-B is establishing and maintaining a patient's airway. While the obviously broken leg or amputated finger may be eye-catching, the blocked airway must be cleared immediately, or the patient will die. As long as the gag reflex is present, most patients can clear their own airways. Therefore, in managing the conscious patient, you may need only to provide oxygen and monitor the patient closely for any changes. Semiconscious patients may require an oropharyngeal or nasopharyngeal airway and suctioning. However, patients who are unresponsive and not breathing on their own will fare better with advanced airway techniques. The purpose of advanced airway management is to protect and improve ventilation in such patients by using a tube to create a direct channel to the trachea. Endotracheal intubation, or simply intubation, is a difficult skill to master and requires additional training for the EMT-B.

The chapter begins with a brief review of the anatomy and physiology of the respiratory system, followed by a look at gastric tubes, which are used primarily to relieve gastric distention. Endotracheal intubation, including proper equipment and technique, is discussed in detail. For reference, the chapter concludes with a section on the use of multi-lumen airway adjuncts, which are easier to use than endotracheal tubes.

Anatomy and Physiology of the Airway

As you learned earlier, the respiratory system consists of all the structures in the body that are used for breathing (Figure 38-1). The upper airway begins with the nose, mouth, and throat (pharynx). The lower airway includes the larynx (vocal cords), trachea, bronchi, and lungs. The epiglottis is a leaf-shaped structure located at the glottic opening (or top of the trachea) that prevents food and liquid from entering the lower airway during swallowing. The bronchi and other air passages branch off from the trachea, extending into each lung, subdividing into bronchioles (smaller passages) down to the alveoli, where the exchange of gases occurs.

The mechanical process of breathing occurs through the use of the diaphragm and intercostal muscles. The diaphragm is a thin, dome-shaped muscle that separates the thoracic cavity from the abdominal cavity. The diaphragm and intercostal muscles contract during the active phase of breathing (inhalation), increasing the size of the chest cavity. Contraction of the diaphragm pulls the chest cavity down; contraction of the intercostal muscles pulls the rib cage up and out. The increased size of the chest cavity allows air to flow into the lungs. During the passive phase of breathing (exhalation), air flows out of the lungs. The diaphragm and intercostal muscles relax, and the size of the chest cavity decreases. The diaphragm moves up, and the ribs move down.

The respiratory system delivers oxygen to the body and removes carbon dioxide, a process that takes place on two levels: the alveolar/capillary exchange and the capillary/cellular exchange (Figure 38-2).

The alveolar/capillary exchange works in the following way:

1. **Air breathed in during inspiration** travels through the airways to the alveoli.

2. **As this oxygen-containing air** enters the alveoli, oxygen-poor blood is circulated through the capillaries around each alveoli.

3. **Oxygen in the alveoli** crosses over into the bloodstream. Carbon dioxide in the blood from the capillaries crosses over into the alveoli, creating a shift of oxygen and carbon dioxide.

The capillary/cellular exchange occurs throughout the body's cells. Cells give up carbon dioxide into the capillaries, and capillaries give up oxygen to the cells.

> **After 4 to 6 minutes without oxygen, cells in the brain and nervous system may die.**

Each living cell in the body requires a regular supply of oxygen; some cells, such as those in the heart, brain, and nervous system, need a constant supply of oxygen to survive. Cells in the heart will be damaged if the oxygen supply is interrupted for more than a few minutes. After 4 to 6 minutes without oxygen, cells in the brain and nervous system may die. Dead brain cells can never be replaced. Brain damage and other permanent changes in the body result from damage caused by a lack of oxygen.

Other cells in the body that are not as dependent on a constant oxygen supply can tolerate short periods without oxygen and still survive.

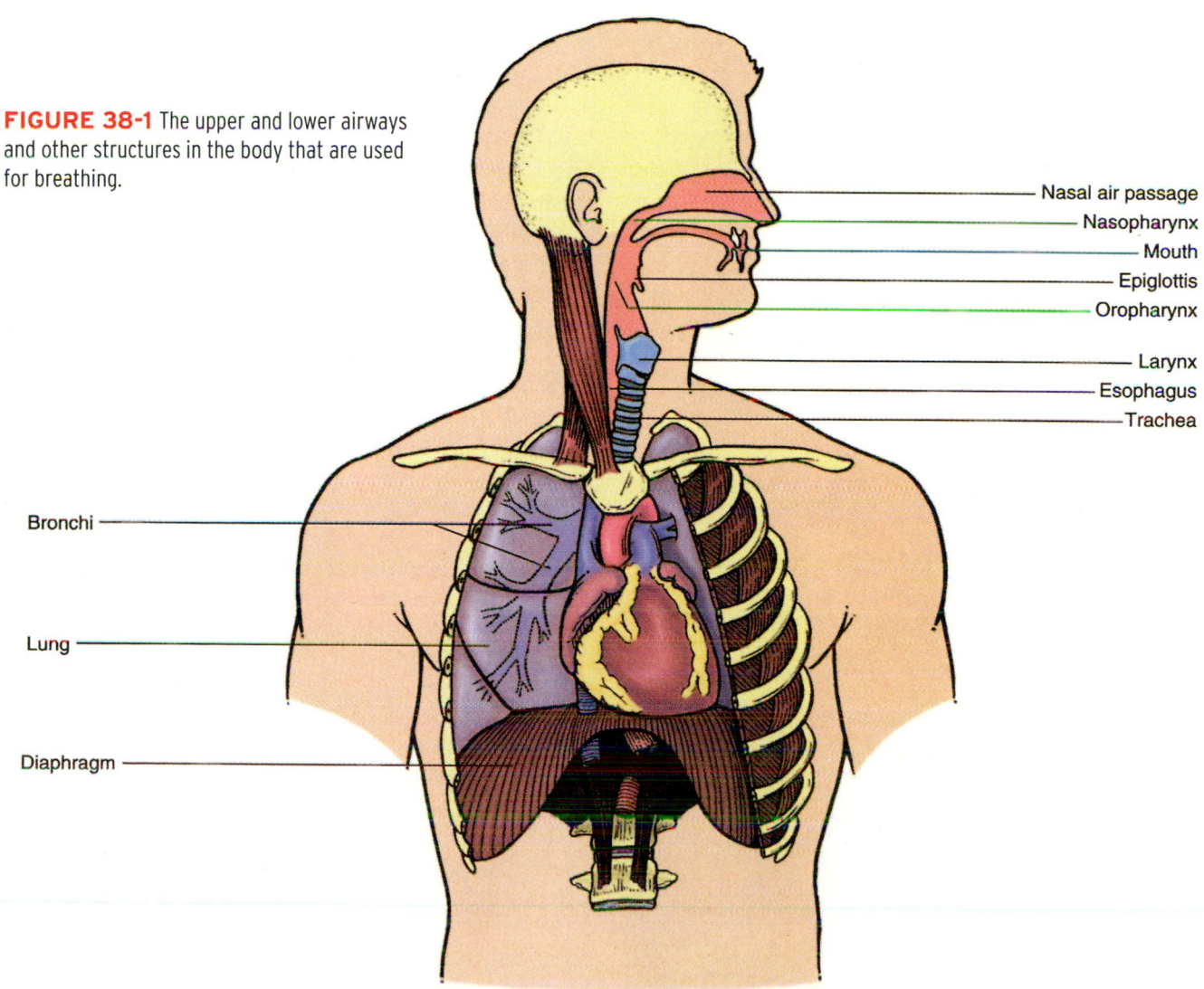

FIGURE 38-1 The upper and lower airways and other structures in the body that are used for breathing.

Nasal air passage
Nasopharynx
Mouth
Epiglottis
Oropharynx
Larynx
Esophagus
Trachea
Bronchi
Lung
Diaphragm

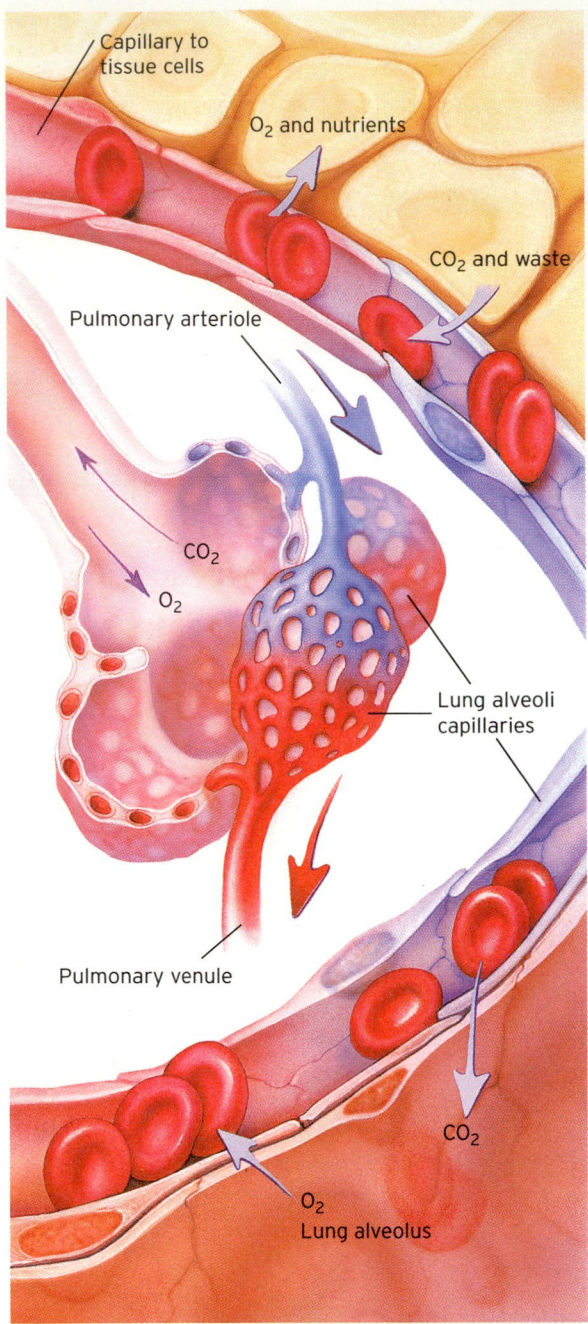

Capillary to
tissue cells

O_2 and nutrients

CO_2 and waste

Pulmonary arteriole

CO_2

O_2

Lung alveoli
capillaries

Pulmonary venule

CO_2

O_2
Lung alveolus

FIGURE 38-2 The exchange of oxygen and carbon dioxide occurs at the cellular level, where cells give up carbon dioxide into the capillaries and the capillaries give up oxygen to the cells.

> The capillary/cellular exchange occurs throughout the body's cells. Cells give up carbon dioxide into the capillaries, and capillaries give up oxygen to the cells.

Basic Airway Management

You should always assess the airway first in an injured or ill patient. This rule applies to both the basic and advanced levels of airway management. Advanced airway techniques are begun only after proper basic airway management has been completed.

As you have already learned, the first step in airway management is opening a patient's airway. You should use the head-tilt/chin lift maneuver in the patient with no spinal injury and the jaw-thrust maneuver in a patient you suspect has a spinal injury. After you have opened the airway, you should assess the airway and evaluate the need for suctioning to remove foreign bodies, liquid, or blood from the patient's mouth.

After the airway has been cleared, you need to determine whether the patient needs an airway adjunct. The basic airway adjuncts that are already available to you are oropharyngeal and nasopharyngeal airways. The more advanced airway adjuncts that may be available to you, with approval of your medical director, will be discussed in this chapter.

Gastric Tubes

Patients who have gastric distention or are vomiting are especially challenging to manage. You must use basic suctioning techniques to prevent aspiration in a patient who is vomiting. Patients with gastric distention are prone to vomiting; therefore, you should consider using a gastric tube in these patients.

A **gastric tube** is an advanced airway adjunct that provides a channel directly into a patient's stomach, allowing you to remove gas, blood, and toxins or to insert medications and nutrition. In the field, you will use a gastric tube primarily to decompress the stomach of a patient with gastric distention, a problem that is most common in children but is also seen in adults.

There are two types of gastric tubes: nasogastric tubes, which are inserted through the nose, and orogastric tubes, which are inserted through the mouth. A nasogastric tube is contraindicated in a patient with major facial, head, or spinal trauma. In these patients, an orogastric tube is safer. A nasogastric tube can cause nasal trauma with bleeding, or it can accidentally be passed into the trachea, interfering with the airway and ventilation. In a patient with a basal skull fracture, a nasogastric tube can accidentally be passed into the brain.

Inserting a gastric tube can activate a patient's gag reflex, causing vomiting and aspiration. Clearly, inserting a gastric tube is a delicate task that must be done strictly according to local EMS protocol and medical

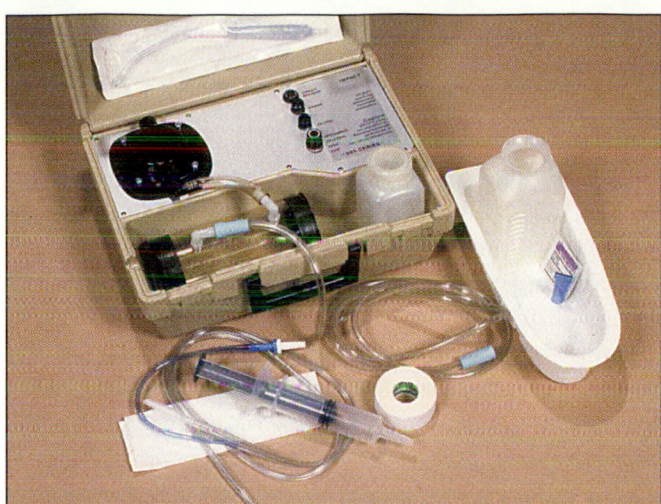

FIGURE 38-3 Equipment for gastric intubation includes gastric tubes, a catheter-tipped 20-mL syringe, water-soluble lubricant, an emesis container, tape, a stethoscope, and a suctioning unit.

direction. Special care is called for if the patient has head, spinal, or major facial trauma. Be sure to follow local protocol.

You will need the following equipment for gastric intubation (Figure 38-3):

- Proper-sized tubes
  —newborn/infant, 8 French
  —toddler/preschool, 10 French
  —school-age child, 12 French
  —adolescent, 14 to 16 French
- Catheter-tipped 20-mL syringe
- Water-soluble lubricant
- Emesis container
- Tape
- Stethoscope
- Suctioning unit and catheters

Once you have prepared and assembled the proper equipment, use the following procedure to insert a nasogastric tube:

1. **Measure the tube from the tip of the nose,** around the ear, to the epigastric area below the xiphoid process. (If you are using an orogastric tube, measure from the teeth to the angle of the jaw and down to the epigastric area.) Mark the measured length on the tube with a piece of tape, or note the number on the tube.

2. **Lubricate the distal end** of the tube with a water-soluble lubricant.

3. **Place the patient** in the proper position. If you do not suspect a spinal injury, place the patient supine, with the head turned to the left side.

4. **Pass the tube** along the nasal floor (or, for an orogastric tube, over the tongue to the back of the throat) until you reach the tape marker.

5. **Confirm proper tube placement** by aspirating stomach contents with the syringe or injecting 20 mL of air into the tube and listening for gurgling over the stomach with the stethoscope.

6. **Aspirate air and stomach contents** with the syringe, once placement is confirmed, to decompress the stomach, or attach to on-board suction. Follow local protocols concerning the type of suction to use (intermittent or continuous).

7. **Secure the tube** in place with tape.

The Sellick Maneuver

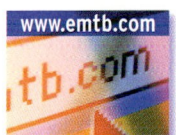

Intubating an unresponsive patient who has no cough and/or gag reflex may cause vomiting and aspiration, which can ultimately damage tissues and block the lower airway passages. A procedure called the Sellick maneuver, which was originally developed for intubating patients during surgery, can be helpful in avoiding these complications in the field (Figure 38-4). To perform this maneuver, apply posterior pressure on

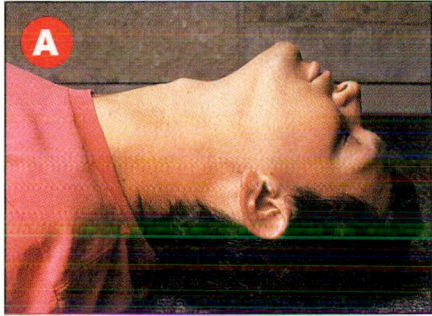
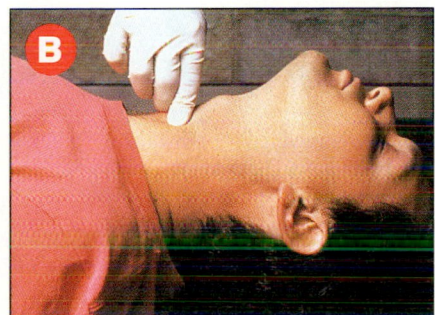
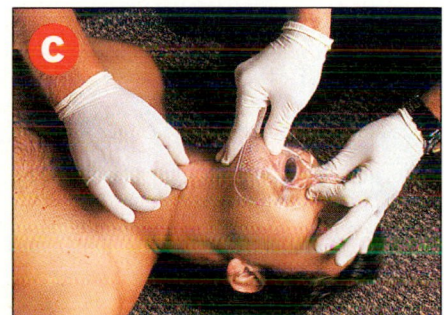

FIGURE 38-4 Performing the Sellick maneuver. **A:** Visualize the cricoid cartilage just below the thyroid cartilage. **B:** Palpate the location of the cricoid cartilage using the index finger. **C:** Place your thumb and index finger on either side of the midline of the cricoid cartilage, then apply firm pressure.

the cricoid cartilage to compress and shut off the esophagus behind it.

The cricoid cartilage, located just below the thyroid cartilage (Adam's apple), is a rigid, ring-shaped structure that completely encircles the larynx at the top of the trachea. It can be hard to locate in infants, children, and small adults. The depression between the thyroid cartilage and the cricoid cartilage is called the cricothyroid membrane. (In certain cases, ALS providers will insert an emergency airway though this membrane.) The esophagus is much softer than the trachea and does not have rings of cartilage to hold it open. It is normally closed, opening only as we eat or drink. By applying pressure on the cricoid cartilage, you can squeeze the esophagus shut and thus prevent solids and fluids from leaving the esophagus and eventually being aspirated into the larynx and trachea.

To perform this maneuver, place a thumb and index finger on either side of the midline of the cricoid cartilage. Apply firm but not excessive pressure; too much pressure could collapse the larynx. Maintain this pressure until the patient is intubated.

The Sellick maneuver should be performed by a third EMT-B and might not be possible if you and your partner are alone. When performing this maneuver, be sure to correctly identify anatomic landmarks to avoid damaging other structures.

Endotracheal Intubation

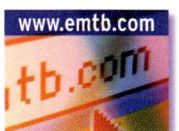
www.emtb.com

Endotracheal intubation is the insertion of a tube into the trachea to maintain the airway. This can be done through the mouth (called **orotracheal intubation**) or through the nose (called **nasotracheal intubation**). In either case, the tube passes directly through the larynx between the vocal cords and then into the trachea.

Endotracheal intubation on patients who are conscious or drifting into and out of consciousness is extremely difficult. As an EMT-B, you will be intubating only patients who are unresponsive with no gag reflex, or in cardiac arrest. However, you should not immediately intubate a patient who is unresponsive or in cardiac arrest. First, you must try to open the airway with the appropriate BLS maneuver, clear the airway, and ventilate the patient with a BVM or oxygen-powered breathing device. When BLS maneuvers fail to open the airway, you should then consider endotracheal intubation based on your local medical protocols.

The remainder of this section will focus on orotracheal, rather than nasotracheal, intubation.

Orotracheal Intubation

Orotracheal intubation is the most effective way to control a patient's airway and has many advantages over other airway management techniques (Table 38-1). It is indicated for patients who cannot protect their own airways as a result of unconsciousness or cardiac arrest (Figure 38-5). It is also used for patients who need prolonged artificial ventilation, are unresponsive to painful stimuli, or have no gag reflex or ability to cough. *Remember that defibrillation is the priority for patients in cardiac arrest from ventricular fibrillation.* Intubation is done only after defibrillation and during the 1 minute time lapse for CPR.

Equipment

Endotracheal intubation requires all your attention. You should not be searching for forgotten or misplaced equipment as you work. Therefore, you should assemble all the equipment that you will need before starting the procedure, while the patient is being hyperventilated (Figure 38-6). As in all patient care situations, be sure to follow

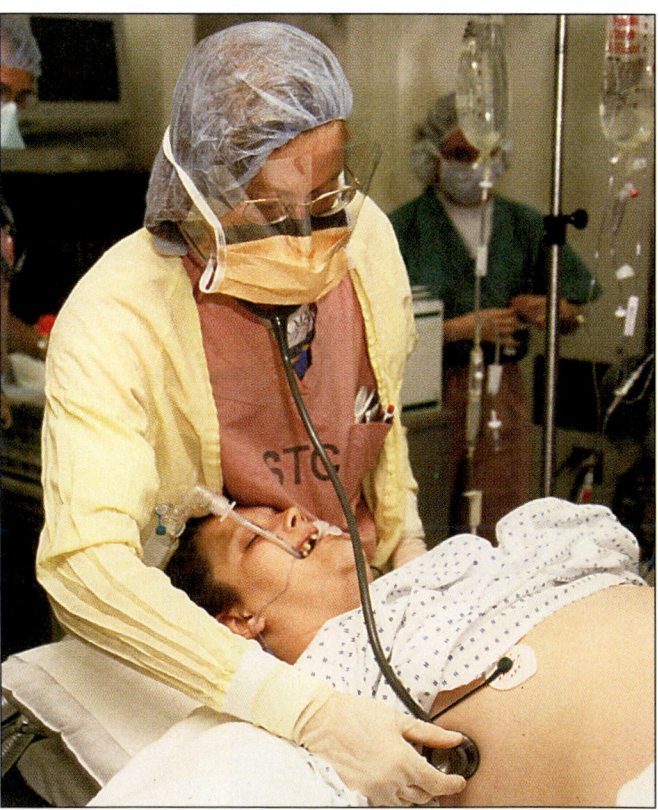

FIGURE 38-5 Endotracheal intubation is indicated for patients who are unconscious and cannot protect their own airways. *(This patient is in a hospital setting. This is an example of a completed procedure.)*

TABLE 38-1 Advantages of Orotracheal Intubation	
• Completely controls and protects the airway • Delivers better minute volume without the difficulty of maintaining an adequate mask seal, as is needed with a BVM device. (The minute volume is the volume of air cycled through the alveoli in 1 minute.) • If prolonged ventilation is required, it may be left in place for a long time. • Prevents gastric distention, which means less regurgitation of stomach contents and greater opportunity for good tidal volume	• Minimizes the risk of aspiration of stomach contents into the respiratory system because a balloon seals off the trachea • Allows for direct access to the trachea for suctioning • Allows for the delivery of high volumes of oxygen at higher than normal pressures • Provides a route for administration of certain medications

BSI techniques. You will be working in close proximity to the patient's airway, so the minimum BSI materials include gloves, eye protection, and a mask.

You will need the following equipment for endotracheal intubation:

- BSI materials
- Proper-sized endotracheal tube (ETT)
- Laryngoscope handle and blade
- Stylet
- 10-mL syringe
- Oxygen, with BVM device or oxygen-powered breathing device, for ventilation before and after intubation
- A suctioning unit with rigid and soft-tip catheters
- Magill forceps
- Towels for raising the patient's head and/or shoulders
- A stethoscope

- Water-soluble lubricant for tubes and scopes
- Tape or a commercial securing device

You must check your equipment daily to ensure that it is all available and to be certain that it is properly assembled and working, especially before you try to intubate a patient.

Laryngoscope. The purpose of a <u>**laryngoscope**</u> is to sweep the tongue out of the way and align the airway so that you can see the vocal cords and pass the ETT through them (Figure 38-7). The handle of the laryngoscope contains two C or D cell batteries to provide power to the light and has a locking bar to connect the handle to the blade; the blade is detachable from the

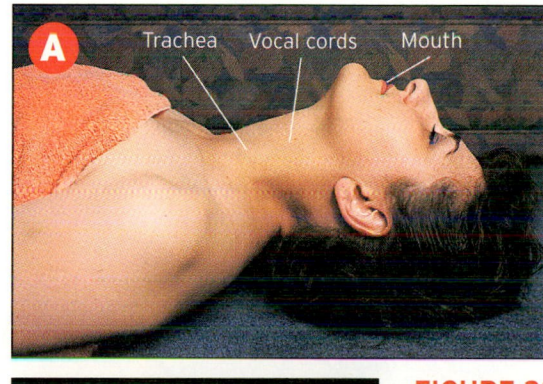

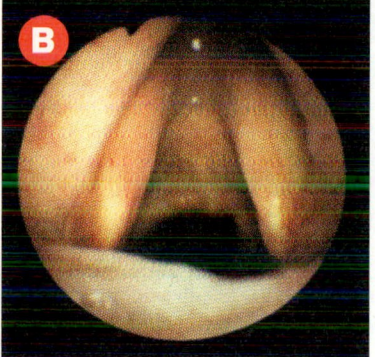

FIGURE 38-7
A: You must see the vocal cords to pass an ETT through them. The vocal cords are located in the upper airway at the entrance to the larynx. **B:** A view of the vocal cords.

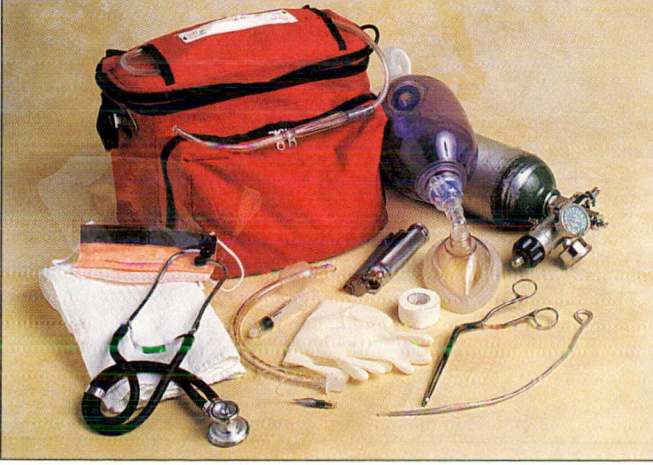

FIGURE 38-6 Assemble all necessary equipment before you begin intubation.

handle. Blades are either curved or straight and range in size from 0 to 4 (Figure 38-8). The two blade designs function differently to align the structures so that you can visualize the vocal cords. The straight blade is inserted past the epiglottis; the curved blade is inserted just in front of it (Figure 38-9). More precisely, the curved blade is inserted into the <u>vallecula</u> (the space between the base of the tongue and the epiglottis), allowing you to see the glottic opening and vocal cords.

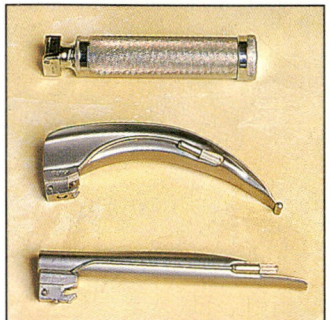

FIGURE 38-8
Laryngoscope blades are curved or straight and come in different sizes.

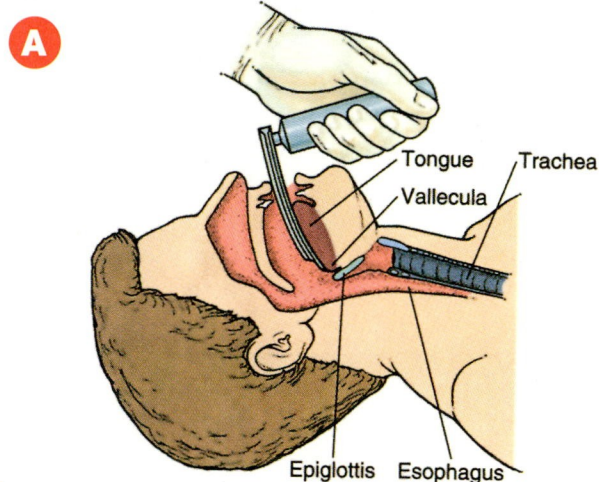

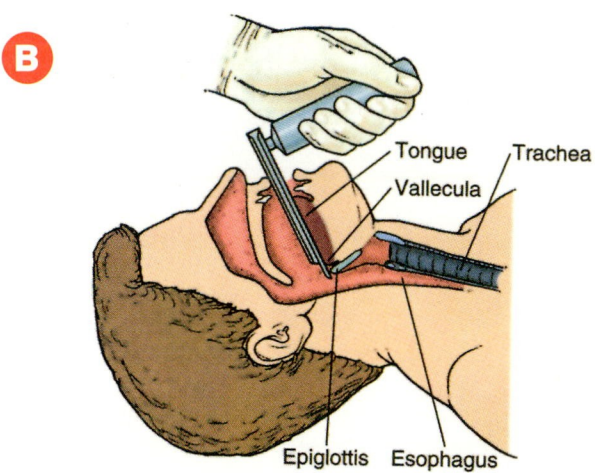

FIGURE 38-9 A: Insert a curved blade just in front of the epiglottis into the vallecula. **B:** Insert a straight blade past the epiglottis.

Because its broader base and flange provide better displacement of the tongue, a curved blade is preferred for use in older children. A straight blade, which actually lifts the epiglottis out of the way to allow for visualization of the glottic opening and vocal cords, is preferred for use in infants. You should practice intubation with both curved and straight blades so that you will feel comfortable using both techniques in a real patient situation.

A notch on the blade locks onto the locking bar of the handle. Because adequate lighting is essential for you to visualize the epiglottis and vocal cords, the light source is near the tip of the blade. You can activate the light by lifting the blade away from the handle until it locks at a right angle (Figure 38-10). The light should be bright white. However, the bulb will not come on if the blade is not attached properly, the bulb is burned out or loose, or the batteries in the handle are dead. Always carry extra batteries for the handle and extra light bulbs in assorted sizes for each blade.

Endotracheal tubes. Endotracheal tubes come in many sizes; the size is specified by the measurement of the inside diameter of the tube. Sizes range from 2.5 mm to 9 mm. The length of the ETT is marked on the outside of the tube in centimeters. The usual length of a tube for an adult is 33 cm. The following are general guidelines to use when you are intubating an average-sized adult patient (Figure 38-11):

- The centimeter markings on the outside of the tube will usually indicate that it is 15 cm to the vocal cords, 20 to 21 cm to the sternal notch, and 25 cm to the carina.

- You can mark the length placement of the ETT by looking at where the tube lines up with the teeth on an intubated patient. This tube-to-teeth mark is usually at around 22 cm.

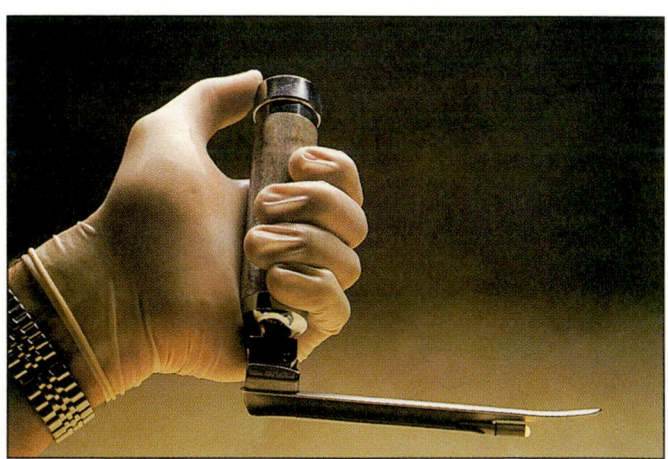

FIGURE 38-10 Once the blade is locked in place at 90° angle, the light will turn on.

The proper-sized tube for adult male patients ranges from 7.5 to 8.5 mm; for adult female patients, it ranges from 6.5 to 8.0 mm (Figure 38-12). For most efficient use of the tube, use the largest-diameter ETT you can. A good rule of thumb is to always have a 7.5-mm ETT on hand; this size tube will fit most male or female adult patients. However, you should carry a complete selection of tube sizes in the unit to ensure that no matter what size you choose, you have one tube smaller and one tube larger, in case you need it.

Tube components include a standard 15-mm adapter, which attaches to either the BVM device or the oxygen-powered breathing device. Make sure that the adapter is securely pushed into the tube so that it does not pull off when you ventilate the patient. The tube has a pilot balloon attached to it to indicate how well the balloon cuff at the end of the ETT is inflated. The cuff at the end of the tube holds about 10 mL of air. The small hole at the distal end of the tube across from the bevel end, called a Murphy eye, helps to prevent tube obstruction (Figure 38-13).

For children, it is best to have a chart or tape device to help you with sizing the ETT (Figure 38-14). Generally, for newborns and small infants, the proper tube size ranges from 3.0 to 3.5 mm; for infants up to 1 year, it is 4.0 mm. You may also follow a formula for sizing tubes in children. You can calculate tube size in children by adding 16 to the child's age and then dividing by 4. Another method is to select a tube that roughly equals the size of the diameter of the patient's

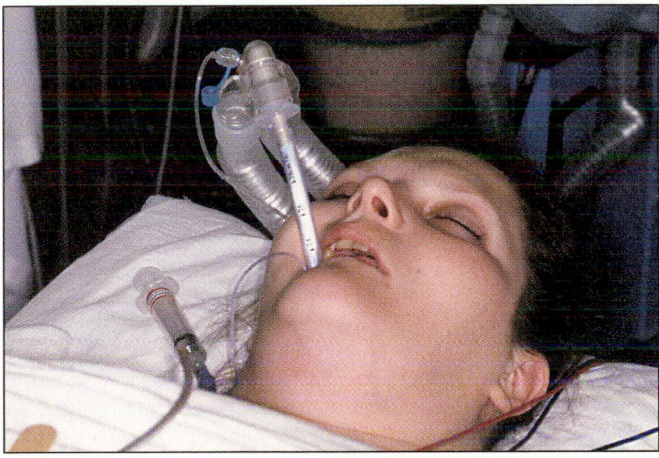

FIGURE 38-11 Prior to securing the tube, note the mark on the ETT. The ETT typically lines up with the teeth on an intubated patient around the 22 cm mark. (On this patient the mark is between 23 and 24 cm.)

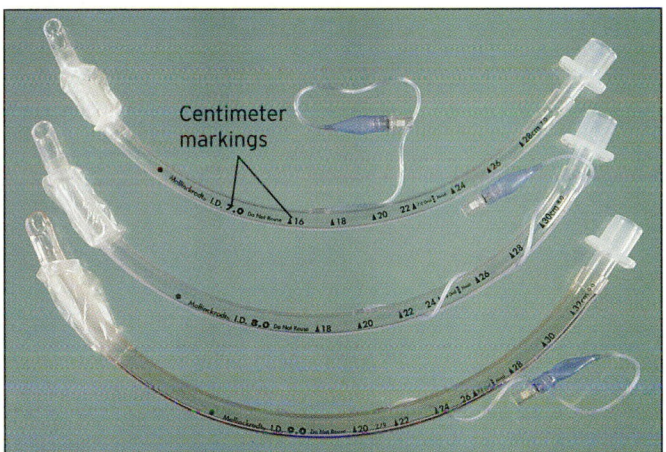

FIGURE 38-12 Endotracheal tubes that are used on adults generally range in size from 6.5 to 8.5 mm. Note the centimeter markings.

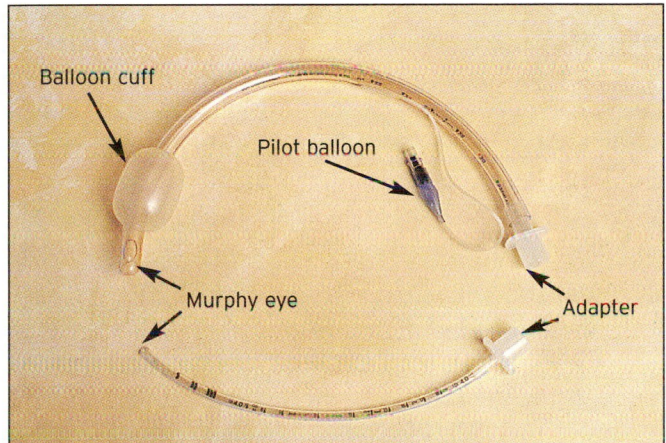

FIGURE 38-13 The components of the adult endotracheal tube include a 15-mm adapter that attaches to a ventilating device, a pilot balloon, the tube, a balloon cuff (shown inflated), and the Murphy eye. The pediatric tube shown at the bottom includes an adapter and a Murphy eye at the uncuffed distal end of the tube.

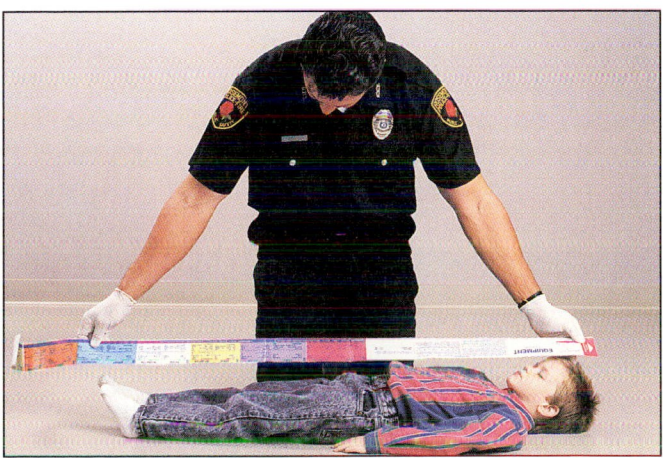

FIGURE 38-14 A chart or tape device is best for estimating the size of an ETT for children.

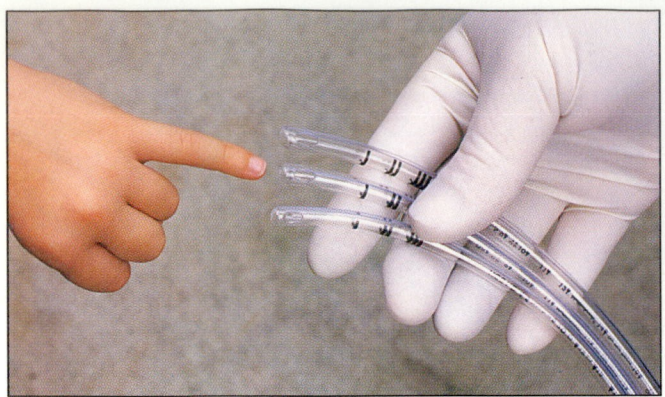

FIGURE 38-15 Another method of sizing endotracheal tubes in children is to select a tube that roughly equals the size of the diameter of the patient's little finger across the nailbed.

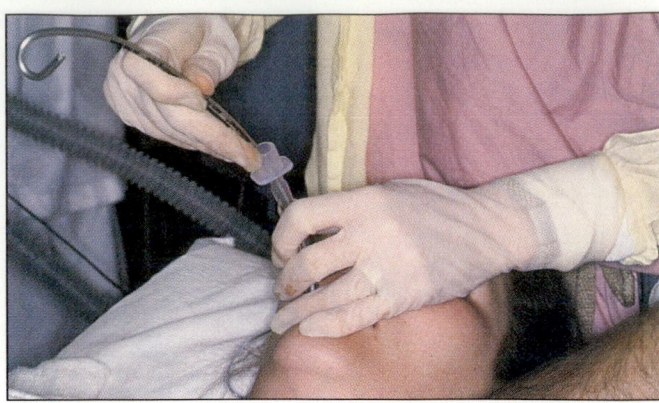

FIGURE 38-16 A wire stylet adds rigidity and shape to the tube and must be removed.

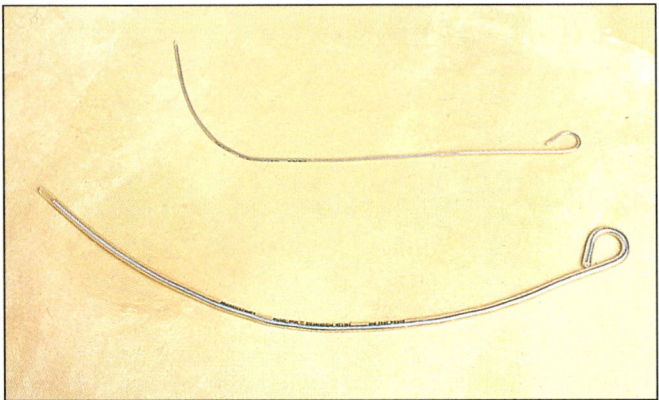

FIGURE 38-17 Bend the tip of the stylet into a hockey stick shape for a pediatric patient, as shown at the top. Bend the stylet to form a gentle curve for an adult patient, as shown at the bottom.

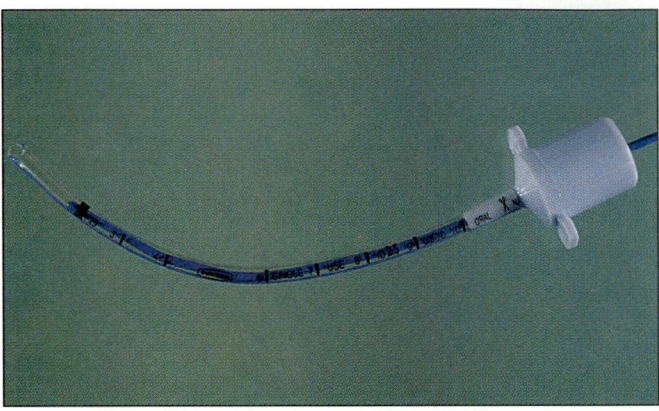

FIGURE 38-18 Do not insert the stylet past the Murphy eye, as it could damage airway tissues. Keep the stylet ¹/₄" from the cuff in the adult tube and 1" from the end of the pediatric tube.

little finger across the nailbed (Figure 38-15). No matter what size you decide to use, you should also have one tube larger and one tube smaller available, in case you need it.

With children older than age 8 years and with adults, you will use cuffed tubes. However, in younger children, the circular narrowing of the trachea at the level of the cricoid cartilage functions as a cuff. Therefore, uncuffed tubes are used in children younger than 8 years. Always watch the tube pass through the vocal cords in a child (as well as in an adult) to make sure that the tip of the ETT is in the proper position.

Stylet. A plastic-coated wire called a <u>stylet</u> may be inserted into the ETT to add rigidity and shape to the tube (Figure 38-16). You should bend the tip of the stylet to form a gentle curve in adults. Because an infant's or child's airway is more angular and less aligned than an adult's, you should bend the tip of the stylet into a hockey stick shape for use in an infant or child (Figure 38-17). You should also apply a little water-

soluble lubricant to the tube to make it easier to insert and to the end of the stylet to make it easier to remove once the tube is in place. Do not insert the stylet past the Murphy eye, as it could puncture or lacerate delicate airway tissues (Figure 38-18). A good rule of thumb is to keep the stylet ¹/₄" from the cuff, or proximal end in adults and 1" from the end of the tube in infants and children. Before you attempt intubation, you should always confirm that the stylet is not sticking out past the end of the ETT.

Syringe. You will use the 10-mL syringe to test for air leaks in the ETT before intubation. You will use it again after the ETT is in place to inflate the cuff and provide a seal inside the trachea to prevent aspiration and help to secure the ETT. Note that this step is done only in ETTs with cuffs; therefore, you will not perform this step with the uncuffed tubes that are used on infants and children.

Take the following steps to properly use the syringe (Figure 38-19):

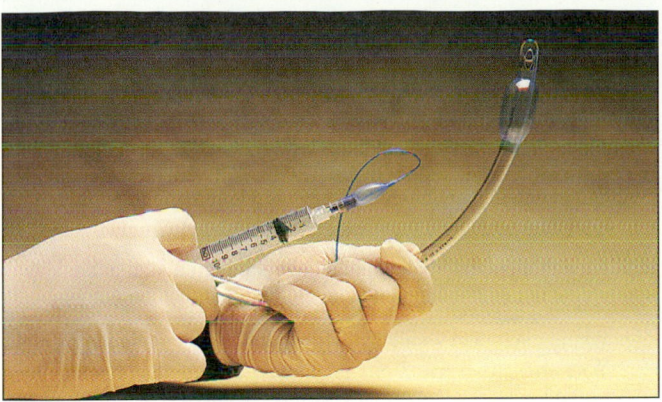

FIGURE 38-19 Inflate the cuff with 5 to 10 mL of air to check for air leaks.

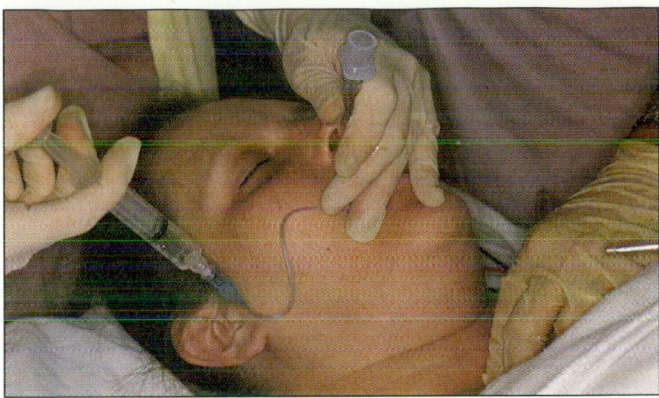

FIGURE 38-20 Inflate the cuff with 5 to 10 mL of air, and then remove the syringe from the pilot balloon to prevent air from leaking out back into the syringe.

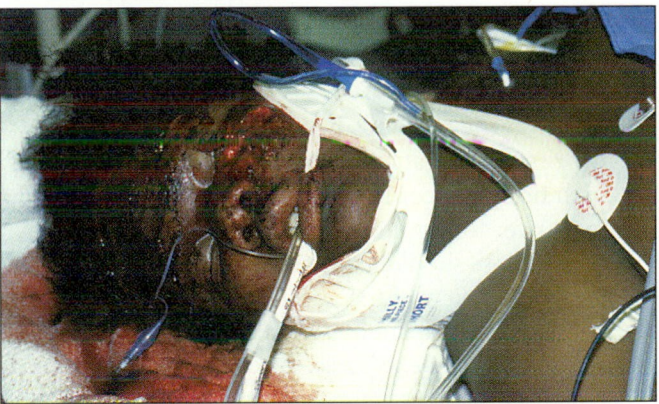

FIGURE 38-21 You must secure the ETT in place with either tape or a commercial device. Note that the cervical collar alone does not ensure spinal immobilization.

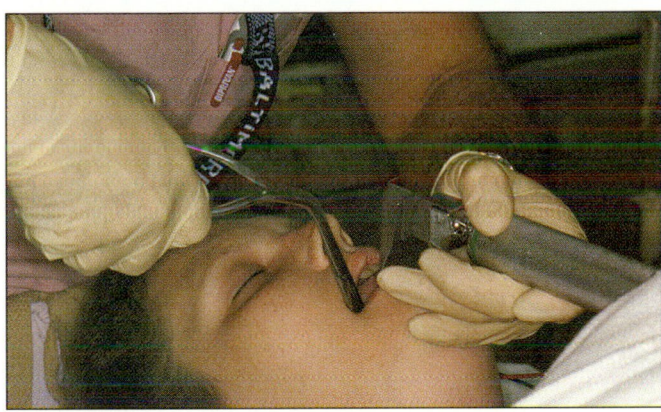

FIGURE 38-22 Magill forceps can be used to help guide the tube.

1. **As you are assembling** and checking your equipment before intubation, pull back on the plunger of the syringe to the 10-mL mark to fill the syringe with the amount of air that is needed to inflate the cuff.

2. **Attach the syringe** to the pilot balloon, and test the cuff by inflating it with 5 to 10 mL of air.

3. **Deflate the cuff** after you have confirmed that there are no air leaks.

4. **With the syringe still attached,** remove the air from the cuff by pulling back on the plunger to the 10-mL mark. Be sure that the syringe remains attached to the pilot balloon with the plunger pulled back to the 10-mL mark.

After the ETT has been properly inserted in the patient, you will inflate the cuff with 5 to 10 mL of air and then remove the syringe from the pilot balloon to prevent air from leaking out back into the syringe (Figure 38-20).

Other equipment. You must also have a securing device available, in the form of either tape or a commercial device (Figure 38-21). Be sure that medical control has approved the commercial device you are using or the technique you use when securing the ETT with tape. Medical control may also advise you to use an oral airway or similar device as a bite block in the intubated patient.

In addition, you will need the following equipment for airway and ventilation assistance:

- Oxygen

- A suctioning unit

- A ventilation device (either a BVM device or an oxygen-powered breathing device)

- Magill forceps (can be used to help guide the tube) (Figure 38-22)

- Towels for raising the patient's head or shoulders if necessary

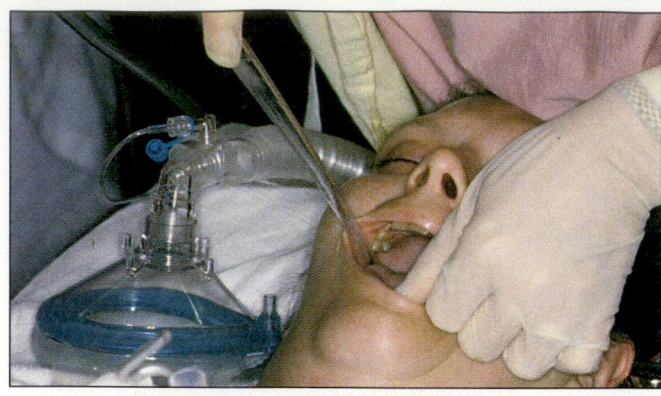

FIGURE 38-23 Suction any fluid or particles from the mouth before any attempt to intubate.

You will use the BVM device to ventilate the patient before you first try to intubate and then to ventilate the intubated patient. The suctioning unit should be readily available to clear any fluid or particles from the mouth (Figure 38-23). Use a rigid, large-bore suction catheter to clear the mouth before intubation. Once the patient is intubated, you might need to use a French catheter to suction any fluids from inside the ETT.

The Intubation Procedure

You may intubate only if authorized to do so by off-line or on-line medical control, according to your local medical protocols. Once you and medical control have made the decision to intubate, you must act quickly, carefully, and efficiently. Be sure to follow BSI techniques, including gloves, eye protection, and a mask. You should not use more than 30 seconds in an attempt to properly position the ETT. The 30-second time limit begins when you stop ventilation and insert the laryngoscope blade into the patient's mouth; it ends when the ETT has been properly placed. If you are not successful in placing the ETT, stop, withdraw the tube, hyperventilate the patient, and try again according to your local protocols.

Intubation is a multiple-person task, especially in a situation involving cardiac arrest and use of an AED. The following tasks should be divided among the EMT-Bs who are present:

- First EMT-B applies and uses the AED.
- Second EMT-B ventilates the patient with a BVM device with 100% oxygen at a rate of one ventilation every 5 seconds.
- Third EMT-B provides CPR.
- Fourth EMT-B prepares and intubates the patient.

You should note that defibrillation with an AED remains the highest priority. Intubating a patient who is in cardiac arrest should occur only after the necessary defibrillations and CPR have been performed for 1 minute. Consult with medical control regarding protocol on the sequence of these events.

The steps of the intubation procedure are as follows (Figure 38-24):

1. **Open the patient's airway** with a BLS maneuver, and clear the airway of any foreign material.

2. **Insert an oropharyngeal airway** and ventilate the patient with a BVM device at the appropriate rate, which will vary depending on the age of the patient. You should hyperventilate the patient at a rate of at least 24 breaths/min before attempting intubation.

3. **As your partner ventilates** the patient, you should quickly assemble and test your equipment. Verify that the bulb on the laryngoscope is working, make sure the ETT cuff has no leaks, and select the proper-sized tube. If you are using a stylet, insert it in the ETT. Lubricate the tube and stylet as needed.

4. **Position the patient's head** and neck to allow for the best visualization of the vocal cords. In a patient with no spinal cord injury, use the head-tilt/chin-lift maneuver to align the structures. Place towels under the patient's shoulders, if necessary, to raise the head for a better view of the vocal cords.

   Intubating a patient with a possible spinal cord injury is not an easy task. If you must intubate a patient whom you suspect has a spinal cord injury, you should make sure that your partner maintains manual in-line stabilization of the head and neck in the neutral position with a cervical collar in place while you attempt the intubation. You might need to lie on your stomach or straddle the patient's head while leaning back to adequately visualize the vocal cords.

5. **Confirm that the patient** has been properly hyperventilated. Remove the oral airway if it is in place.

6. **Grasp the laryngoscope** handle in your left hand. Make sure the blade is locked into place and the bulb is illuminated. Open the patient's mouth with the gloved fingers of your right hand. Gently place the blade in the right side of the patient's mouth, then move it toward the center of the mouth, gently pushing the tongue to the left. The tongue must be displaced for you to visualize the vocal cords. Visualize the epiglottis. Advance a curved blade along the base of the tongue until its tip rests at the vallecula; advance a straight blade along the base of the tongue until you see it catch the epiglottis. Lift the laryngoscope away from the posterior pharynx so that you can see the vocal cords. The lifting force is directed straight up, parallel to the long axis of the laryngoscope handle, not back toward the

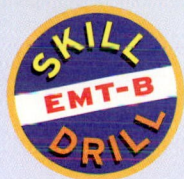

Performing Orotracheal Intubation
Figure 38-24

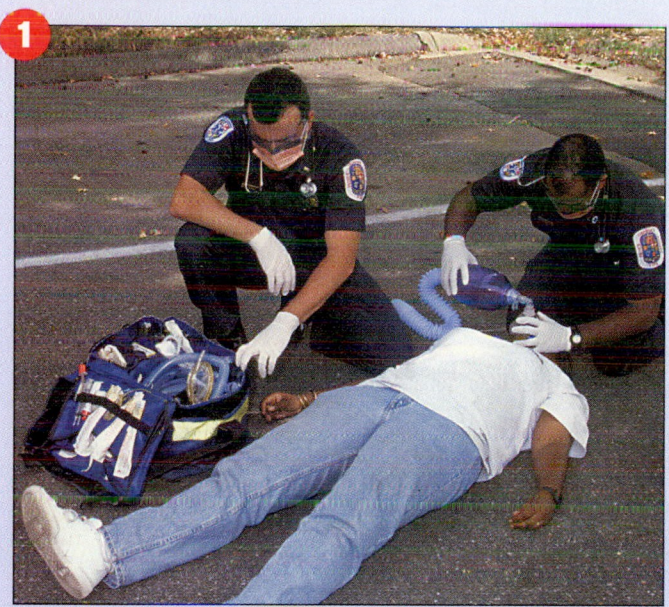

Ensure that the patient's airway is open, and ventilate with a BVM device. Hyperventilate the patient at a rate of 24 breaths/min.

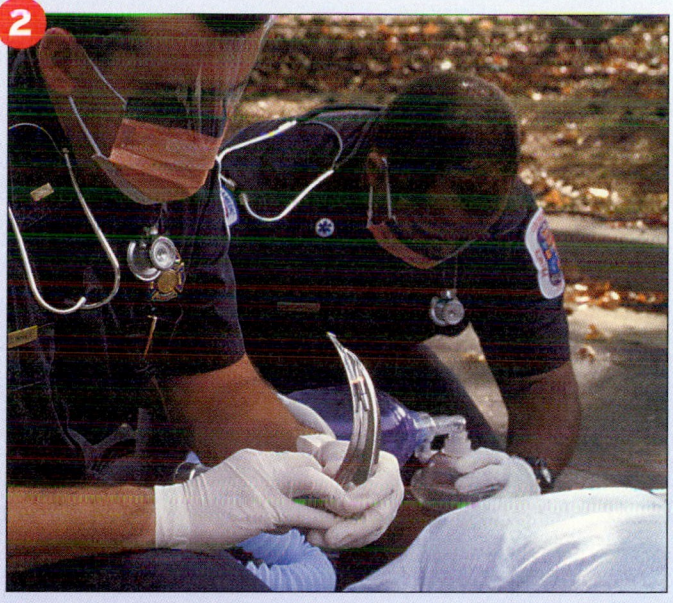

Continue to ventilate the patient as your partner tests the intubation equipment.

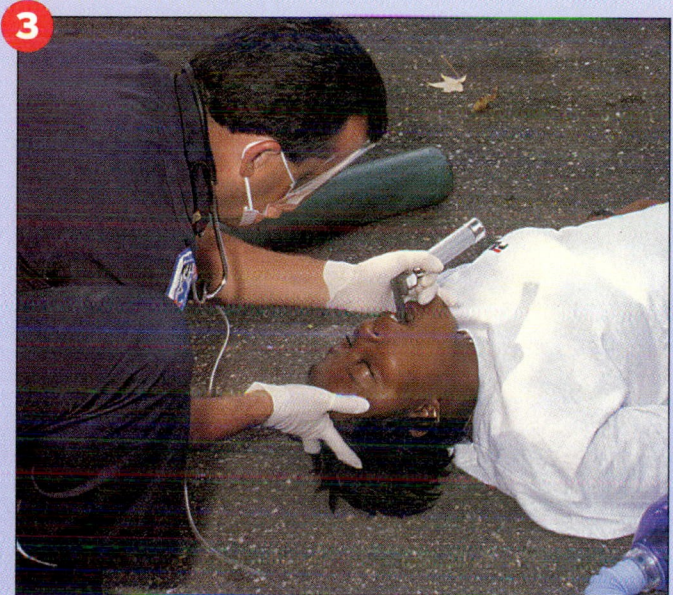

Position the nontrauma patient using the head-tilt/chin-lift maneuver, and insert the laryngoscope, pushing the tongue to the left.

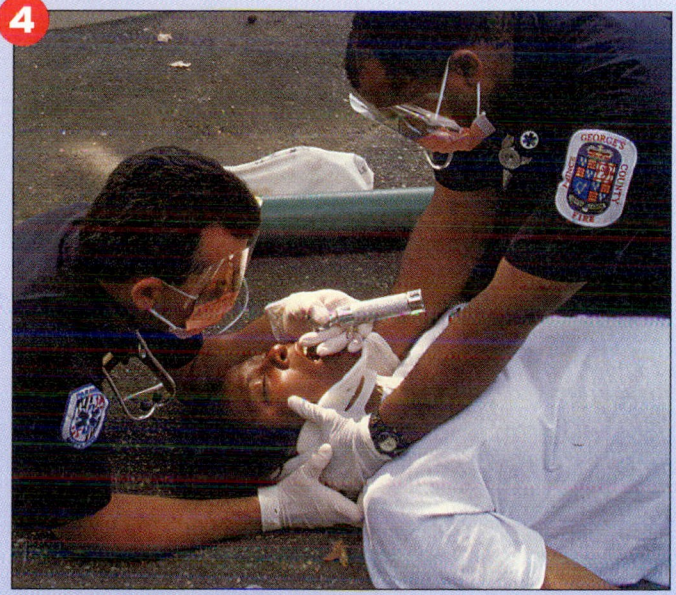

With a trauma patient, you must maintain the cervical spine in a neutral, in-line position as your partner lies down on his or her stomach to visualize the vocal cords.

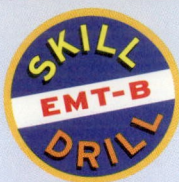

Performing Orotracheal Intubation–cont'd.
Figure 38-24

5

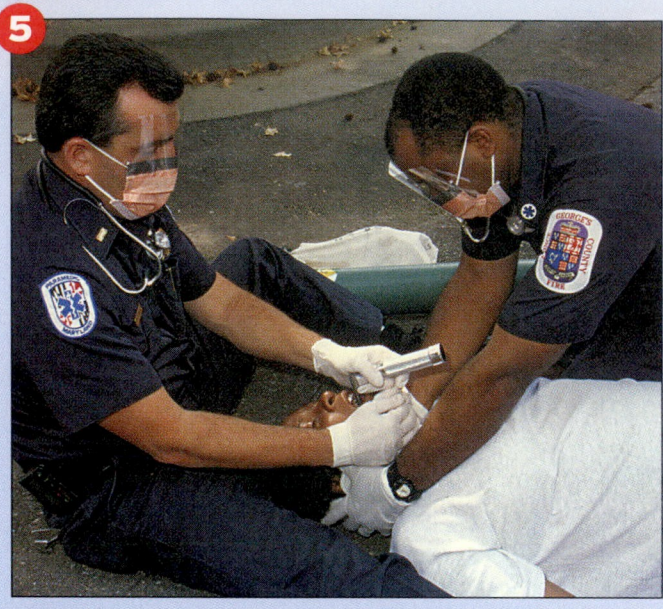

You may also visualize the vocal cords in a trauma patient by maintaining the cervical spine in a neutral position as your partner straddles the patient's head and leans back.

6

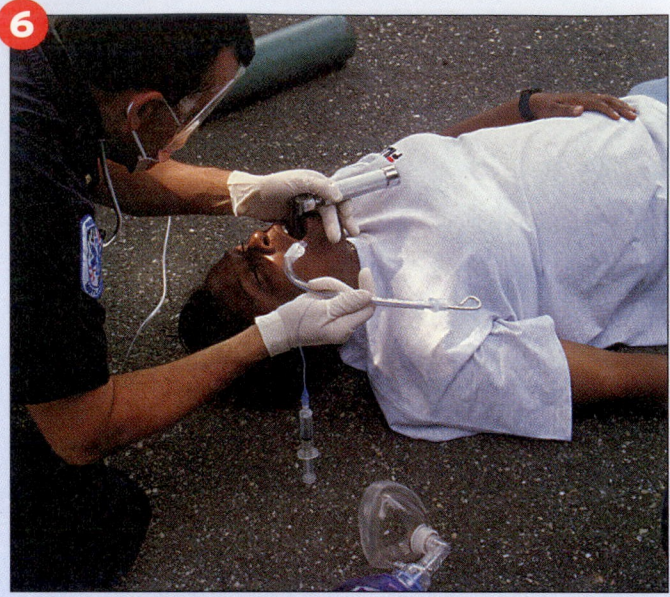

Lift the laryngoscope away from the posterior pharynx so that you can see the vocal cords. Insert the ETT from the right side of the patient's mouth.

7

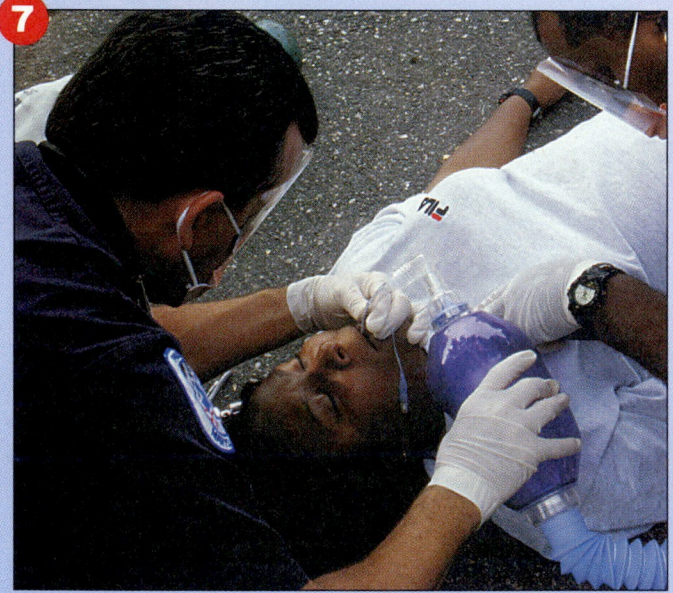

Confirm placement of the ETT by listening with a stethoscope over both lungs and the stomach as your partner ventilates the patient through the tube.

8

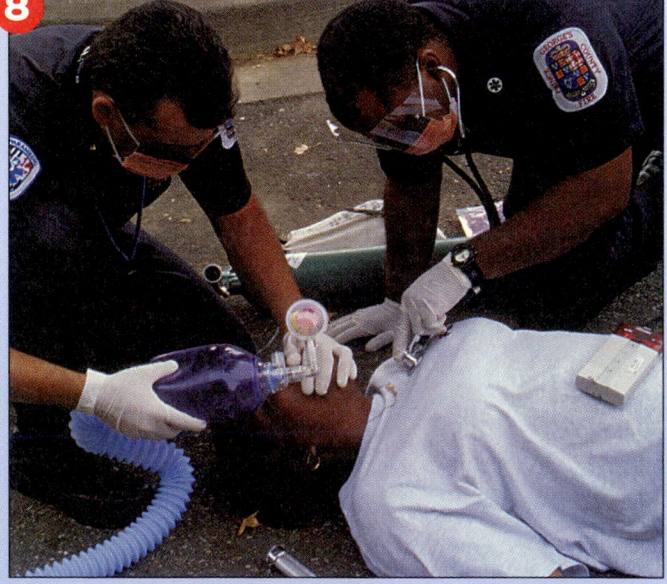

Confirm placement with readings from an end tidal carbon dioxide detector.

patient's head. It should feel as if you are picking up the patient's head by the jaw. To avoid breaking the patient's teeth or lacerating the lips, never use the blade as a lever or fulcrum against the upper teeth. Do not lose sight of the vocal cords at any time after you have visualized them. Proper placement of the ETT depends on your visualization of the ETT as it is placed through the vocal cords.

7. **If another EMT-B is available,** have him or her perform the Sellick maneuver to improve visualization of the vocal cords and prevent vomiting and aspiration. Maintain pressure on the cricoid cartilage until the ETT cuff is inflated.

8. **Insert the ETT** with your right hand, keeping the vocal cords and the tip of the tube in sight at all times. Do not advance the ETT down the center of the laryngoscope blade, or your view of the vocal cords will be obstructed.

   Advance the tube from the right side of the patient's mouth. Watch the uninflated cuff on the tube as it passes through the vocal cords, then advance the ETT until the cuff is just past the vocal cords. Note and document the centimeter markings on the outside of the ETT at the level of the teeth.

   Once the tube has been inserted through the vocal cords into the trachea, gently remove the laryngoscope and stylet, if a stylet was used. Inflate the soft balloon cuff on the end of the tube with 5 to 10 mL of air. This will seal the trachea and anchor the tube so that air can be blown directly into the lungs. Gently squeeze the pilot balloon cuff to verify the amount of air you should use. The pilot balloon should be full but easily compressed between your fingers. Detach the syringe so that the air in the cuff will not empty back into it. Continue to hold the tube in place at all times until it is secured, by either tape or a special commercial device. You or your partner (whoever is not holding the ETT in place) should begin ventilating the patient with a BVM device.

9. **Confirm placement of the ETT.** Listen with a stethoscope over both lungs and the stomach as you ventilate the patient through the tube. You should be able to hear equal breath sounds over both right and left lung fields. Also listen at the sternal notch in children. You should see both sides of the chest rise and fall with each ventilation. This is especially important in children, as breath sounds in children may be misleading. You may hear them even if the tube is in the esophagus. You should not be able to hear breath sounds in the stomach.

   Proper confirmation of ETT placement is essential for care of the patient. If you do not actually visualize the ETT passing through the vocal cords, you may place the ETT in the esophagus rather than in the trachea, which can prove fatal for the patient. The actual visualization of the ETT as it passes through the vocal cords is the best way to confirm proper placement.

   A previously unresponsive patient may become combative after being intubated. This is an indication that the ETT has been properly placed and the patient is now receiving high concentrations of oxygen through the ETT. Local medical control may decide whether an ETT can be pulled after being correctly placed. Usually, if a resuscitated patient can obey commands, the pilot balloon is deflated and the tube is removed.

   For further confirmation of proper placement, medical control may direct you to use an end tidal carbon dioxide detector. The **end tidal carbon dioxide detector** is a disposable plastic indicator with chemically treated paper that changes from purple to yellow in the presence of carbon dioxide. Of course, patients who are in full respiratory and cardiac arrest will not produce respiratory carbon dioxide, and the color indicator will not change until the patient is ventilated. As the patient is being ventilated, oxygen and carbon dioxide cross the alveolar membrane. Carbon dioxide coming out of the ETT will change the color of the indicator. If the ETT is in the stomach, ventilation will not create carbon dioxide, so there will be no change in color. Therefore, placement can be confirmed. The carbon dioxide detector should not be used as a substitute for seeing the tube go through the vocal cords, hearing good bilateral breath sounds, and seeing the patient's chest rise and fall with each ventilation. Consult your medical director for more information about this device. The pulse oximeter is not a useful device to confirm tube placement.

10. **Once you have verified** that the tube is properly placed, secure the ETT in place with the device and technique that have been approved by your medical director.

11. **Keep in mind that,** even when placed properly, the ETT will move if it is not secured. For this reason, you must never let go of the ETT until it is secured. Even then, you must continuously check the tube to make sure it is secure and in the correct place. Continue to artificially ventilate the patient at an age-appropriate rate. Also, again remember to note the distance the tube has been inserted. Be sure to reassess breath sounds each time you move the patient.

Complications

Endotracheal intubation is a difficult skill to master. If intubation takes longer than 30 seconds, the resulting delay in oxygenation may lead to brain damage. Obviously, you will need a great deal of expert instruction and practice to master this skill. Among the possible complications of endotracheal intubation are the following, as summarized in Table 38-2.

Intubating the right mainstem bronchus. This is the most common error that is made during intubation. If you push or accidentally slip the tube in too far, the ETT will pass into the right mainstem bronchus. In this position, it will ventilate the right lung only. Therefore, you will hear breath sounds on the right side only. The best way to correct this problem is to deflate the cuff and pull the ETT back about 1″. Listen again for bilateral breath sounds. Make sure you do not completely remove the ETT.

Intubating the esophagus. This often occurs when you insert the ETT without first seeing the vocal cords and, as a result, the ETT is inserted into the esophagus rather than the trachea. The result is rapid inflation of the patient's stomach rather than ventilation of the lungs; if the situation is not corrected, the patient will die. To avoid this, carefully watch the ETT as it passes through the vocal cords. Next, check breath sounds over the left and right apices and bases of the lungs. Watch for the rise and fall of the chest. If there is any doubt, pull out the ETT, hyperventilate the patient for 2 to 3 minutes, and then try to intubate the patient again. Some EMS systems allow a maximum of two attempts at intubation. Be sure that you follow the protocol established by your medical director. If you are still unsuccessful after two attempts at intubation, insert an oral airway, ventilate the patient with a BVM device, and provide transport to the hospital.

Aggravating a spinal injury. Whenever there is concern about a spinal injury, you must intubate without moving the patient's neck from the neutral, in-line position. This makes it difficult to lift the lower jaw and tongue enough to see the vocal cords; indeed, this can be done only by two EMT-Bs working together.

Taking too long to intubate. Do not take any longer than 30 seconds trying to intubate, or the patient will become more hypoxic. Your partner or another member of the team should actually time the intubation. If you cannot complete the procedure within 30 seconds, you should ventilate the patient again with a BVM device at 100% oxygen for 2 to 3 minutes before trying again. Ask a third EMT-B to perform the Sellick maneuver so that you can better see the vocal cords. If after two tries, the tube cannot be passed, try another airway technique, or ask another qualified rescuer to try. If the patient is difficult to intubate, you should not waste time in the field. Use another airway adjunct, and provide immediate transport, assisting ventilations as needed.

Patient vomiting. A patient who is not totally unresponsive may begin to gag or try to remove the tube. Gagging may cause the patient to vomit and aspirate stomach contents. To avoid this, always check for a gag reflex before intubation, using a tongue blade, the laryngoscope blade, or an oral airway. Patients who tolerate an oral airway do not have an intact gag reflex and may need intubation. Be aware that checking for a gag reflex can make the patient vomit. You should always have a suctioning unit ready. Trying to insert an ETT through the vocal cords can also cause the cords to spasm. This is called **laryngospasm**. If this occurs, stop intubating,

---

TABLE 38-2	Benefits and Complications of Endotracheal Intubation

Benefits	Complications
Provides complete protection of airway	Intubating the right mainstem bronchus
Can be left in for long periods of time	Intubating the esophagus
Delivers better oxygen concentration than a BVM device	Aggravating a spinal injury
Prevents gastric distention and aspiration	Vomiting and/or removing the tube
Allows for deep suctioning of the trachea	Causing soft-tissue trauma
Allows for administration of certain medications	Mechanical failure
	Patient intolerance

> You may intubate only if authorized to do so by off-line or on-line medical direction, according to your local medical protocols.

and try to ventilate the patient with a BVM device or oxygen-powered breathing device.

Soft-tissue trauma. The laryngoscope and the tip of the ETT can injure the lips, teeth, tongue, gums, and other airway structures. Used as a lever, the laryngoscope blade can easily break teeth, while a tube pushed blindly through the vocal cords can lacerate the oropharynx. Careful attention to your technique will minimize the risk of these complications.

Mechanical failure. You may hear or feel air coming from the oropharynx when ventilating the patient. In an adult, this means that the cuff does not have enough air in it or that it has been torn and is leaking. If this occurs, you must get more air into the cuff (check the pilot balloon), or you must replace the tube. In a child, an air leak means that the uncuffed tube is too small or the child is large enough to need a cuffed tube.

Patient intolerant of ETT. Because of the reversal of hypoxia from direct oxygenation, a patient may regain a gag reflex or regain consciousness and try to remove the ETT. Before extubating the patient in these circumstances, you should determine that the patient can obey commands. If he or she can, ensure that the suctioning unit is nearby and turned on. Then deflate the cuff, and carefully withdraw the ETT as the patient inhales.

Sometimes, you may have to ask the patient to cough. Provide immediate suctioning if the patient vomits, then reassess the airway and administer supplemental oxygen. Always consult medical control before removing the ETT.

Decrease in heart rate. Be sure to carefully and continuously monitor the patient's vital signs, particularly the heart rate. In children, it is particularly important to check heart rate and skin color. With endotracheal intubation, the heart rate may decrease when the airway has been stimulated. Also be sure to evaluate the lung sounds and chest wall motion any time you move the patient. It is easy to dislodge the ETT while moving the patient. Always check placement after the patient has been moved in any way.

Multi-Lumen Airways

In addition to endotracheal intubation, other advanced airway devices are available to the EMT-B. These devices are called multi-lumen airways, and depending on local protocol and your medical director, you may be trained in the use of these airways. The benefits and complications associated with use of the multi-lumen airway are shown in Table 38-3.

The multi-lumen airways, which are inserted with no direct visualization of the vocal cords, have been designed to provide lung ventilation when placed in either the trachea or the esophagus, making them much easier to insert than an ETT. Two of these adjuncts are described here: the Esophageal Tracheal Combitube (ETC), and the Pharyngeotracheal Lumen Airway (PtL). Remember that you must be trained and authorized to use these devices.

TABLE 38-3 Benefits and Complications of Multi-Lumen Airways	
Benefits	**Complications**
Ease of proper placement	Loses effectiveness (cuff malfunction)
No mask seal necessary	Requires deeply comatose patient
Requires minimal skill and practice to maintain	Requires constant balloon observation
Easily used in spinal injury patients	Cannot be used on patients smaller than 5' tall
May be inserted blindly	Requires great care in listening for breath sounds
Protects the airway from upper airway secretions	Large balloon is easily broken and tends to push the PtL out of the mouth when inflated
Stays in place well (ETC)	
Sturdy balloon (ETC)	

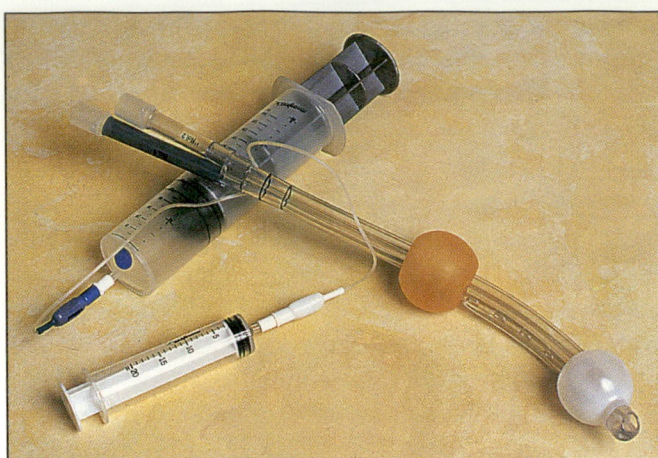

FIGURE 38-25 The ETC consists of a double lumen tube and two balloon cuffs. The blue lumen is the primary ventilation port, and the clear lumen is the ventilation port if the tube is placed in the trachea.

Esophageal Tracheal Combitube

The ETC consists of a double lumen tube and two balloon cuffs (Figure 38-25). The blue lumen (No. 1) is the primary ventilation port when the tube is inserted in the esophagus. The clear lumen (No. 2) is the ventilation port if the tube is placed in the trachea. The clear cuff at the tip of the tube (distal cuff) seals off the esophagus

or the trachea; the larger, flesh-colored cuff near the midway point seals off the oropharynx and naso-pharynx. A blue pilot balloon and a white pilot balloon correspond to the flesh-colored and distal cuffs. Two syringes are also included in the kit. The ETC is a single-use item and must be discarded after use. It should not be cleaned and reused.

The ETC is inserted blindly (Figure 38-26). If the tube happens to go into the trachea, ventilations are provided directly into the trachea. If the tube goes into the esophagus, as occurs most often, ventilations can still be provided to the patient. You do not need to maintain a constant face mask seal with either place-ment. Instead, the ETC forms an inflated cuff seal in the oropharynx, so you can ventilate the trachea via a tube, rather than a mask. This ease of ventilation is an advan-tage of the ETC.

Contraindications. You should not attempt to insert an ETC in the following individuals:

- Conscious or semiconscious patients with a gag reflex
- Children younger than age 16 years
- Adults shorter than 5′ tall
- Patients who have ingested a caustic substance
- Patients who have a known esophageal disease

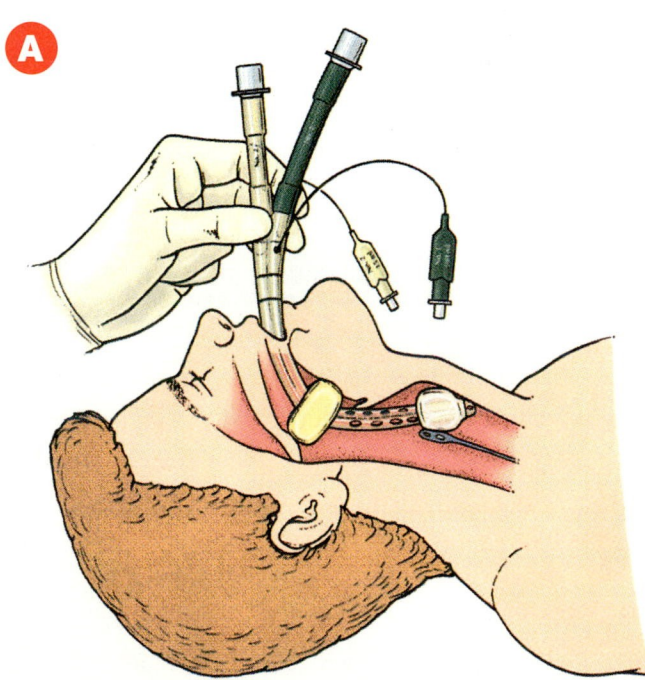

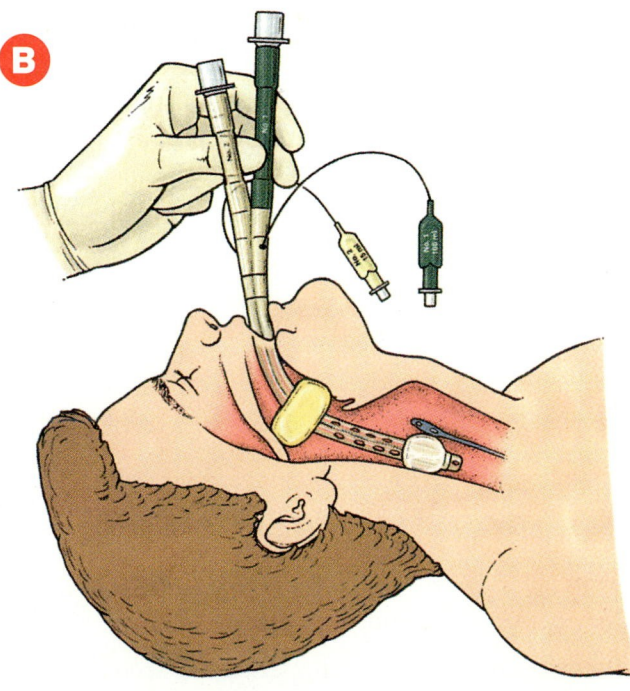

FIGURE 38-26 A: If the ETC is inserted into the trachea, it functions as an ETT with ventilations provided directly into the trachea.
B: If the ETC is inserted into the esophagus, ventilations can still be provided to the patient.

Inserting the ETC. As with endotracheal intubation, you must act quickly and carefully once you have received permission from medical control to use the ETC. Remember to follow BSI techniques, including gloves, eye protection, and a mask, any time you may be exposed to blood or other body fluids.

The steps for insertion of the ETC are as follows:

1. **Assemble and check** the proper equipment, including the following:
   —BSI materials
   —ETC kit with syringes
   —Water-soluble lubricant
   —Suctioning unit with suction catheters
   —BVM device or flow-restricted oxygen-powered breathing device

2. **Apply a water-soluble lubricant** to the ETC.

3. **Position the patient.** Open the patient's mouth and clear it of any foreign objects, including vomitus, dentures, and blood clots. Remove the oral airway if one has been inserted. Open the airway of a patient who has no possible spinal injury by hyperextending the patient's head and neck. Note that with an unconscious patient who may have a spinal injury, you must maintain the neck in a neutral, in-line position during insertion of the ETC.

4. **Hyperventilate the patient** with 100% oxygen using either a BVM device or oxygen-powered breathing device.

5. **Lift the lower jaw and tongue** away from the posterior pharynx by inserting your thumb deep into the patient's mouth and grasping the tongue and lower jaw between your thumb and index finger.

6. **Gently guide the ETC** along the base of the tongue and into the airway. Hold the ETC so that it curves in the same direction as the natural curvature of the pharynx. Insert the tip into the mouth, and advance it carefully along the tongue. Do not use force. If you meet resistance, pull back and redirect the ETC. When the ETC is at the proper depth, the teeth will be between the heavy black lines.

7. **Inflate the blue pilot balloon** (and flesh-colored cuff) with the predrawn 100-mL blue-tipped syringe. Once the cuff is inflated and the pilot balloon is tense, immediately inflate the white pilot balloon (and the distal cuff) with the smaller, predrawn 15-mL syringe. The ETC may move forward a bit, but this is normal.

8. **Ventilate the patient** through the blue (No. 1) tube, using a BVM or an oxygen-powered breathing device.

9. **Confirm the placement** of the tube. If the chest rises and falls and you hear breath sounds, the ETC is in the esophagus. When this is the case, continue to ventilate through the blue (No. 1) tube. If the chest does not rise and fall, and you do not hear breath sounds, the ETC is in the trachea. In this case, put the BVM device or the oxygen-powered ventilation device on the shorter, clear tube, and ventilate the patient through it. Again, listen for breath sounds in all lung fields and in both axillae. Also listen over the stomach to verify that proper placement has occurred.

10. **Continuously monitor the patient.** Watch for balloon cuff leaks by carefully squeezing the pilot balloon. Use the syringes to keep the balloon cuffs properly inflated. Balloon cuffs may be torn by broken teeth, dentures, and bones. Therefore, you must use special care with this device, especially in the event of facial trauma.

Removing the ETC. Removal of the ETC airway is fairly simple. If the patient will no longer tolerate the ETC, you should remove it. Remember that the patient will likely vomit when the ETC is removed, so you must have a suctioning unit readily available. Be sure to turn the patient on his or her side to keep the airway clear of vomitus. When you are ready, simply deflate both balloon cuffs, and gently remove the tube.

Remember to follow BSI techniques, including gloves, eye protection, and a mask, any time you may be exposed to blood or other body fluids.

Pharyngeotracheal Lumen Airway

The PtL consists of two tubes, two balloon cuffs, a bite block, and a neck-retaining strap (Figure 38-27). The long, clear (No. 3) tube contains a stylet and a low-pressure balloon cuff near its tip. The stylet is left in as a plug if the tube is placed in the esophagus but is removed if the tube ends up in the trachea. In either case, the balloon cuff prevents gastric contents from entering the lungs when the cuff is inflated.

The No. 3 tube passes through the larger-diameter green (No. 2) tube. The No. 2 tube has a large balloon cuff designed to seal the oropharynx. This allows ventilation gas to pass through it into the trachea (if the No. 3 tube is placed in the esophagus) but also prevents blood and debris from entering the airway from above. The balloon cuff in the No. 2 tube functions as the mask seal. The No. 1 tube is connected to these balloon cuffs to assist with inflation of these important airway seals.

As with the ETC, this device is designed to be inserted blindly into the oropharynx and esophagus, but you must be trained and authorized to use it (Figure 38-28). If the tube happens to go into the trachea when blindly inserted, it acts like an endotracheal tube. If the long tube goes into the esophagus, you can still provide adequate ventilations to the patient. However, with the PtL, you need not maintain a constant face mask seal. The PtL forms an inflated cuff seal in the oropharynx, and the trachea may be ventilated via a tube rather than a mask.

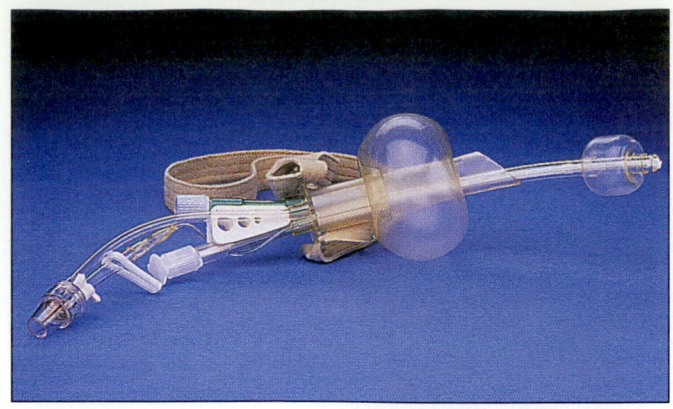

FIGURE 38-27 The PtL consists of two tubes, two balloon cuffs, a bite block, and a neck-retaining strap.

Contraindications. You should not attempt to use the PtL in the following individuals:

- Conscious or semiconscious patients with a gag reflex
- Children younger than age 14 years
- Adults shorter than 5' tall
- Patients who have ingested a caustic substance
- Patients who have a known esophageal disease

Inserting the PtL. Once you have confirmed with medical control your decision to insert a PtL, you must act quickly and carefully. Remember to follow BSI techniques, including gloves, eye protection, and a mask, any time you may be exposed to blood or other body fluids. Take the following steps to insert the PtL:

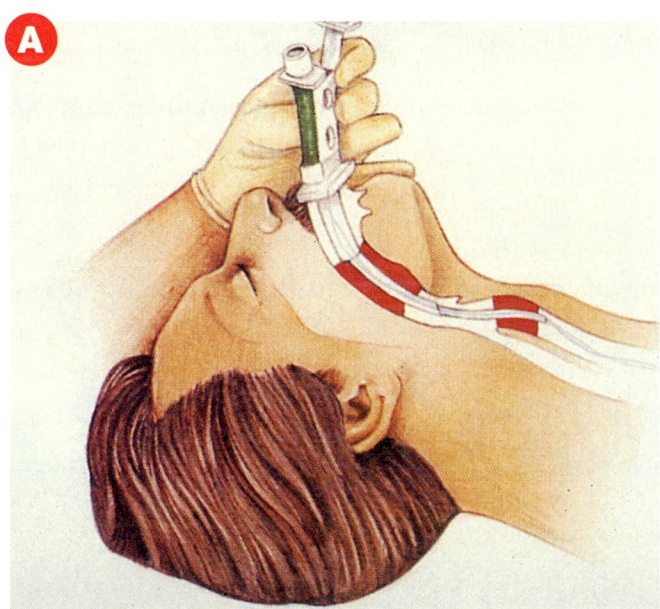

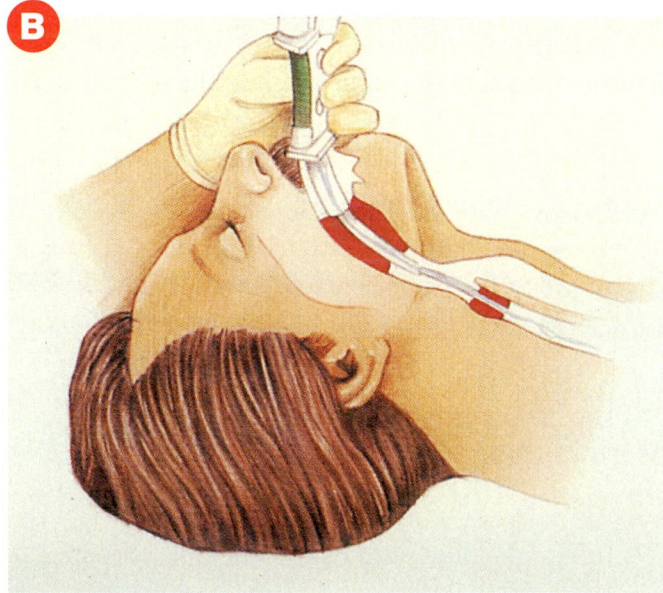

FIGURE 38-28 The PtL is inserted blindly into the oropharynx. **A:** If the PtL is inserted into the trachea, it functions as an ETT with ventilations provided directly into the trachea. **B:** If the PtL is inserted into the esophagus, ventilations can still be provided to the patient.

1. **Assemble and check** the proper equipment, including the following:
   —BSI materials
   —PtL
   —Water-soluble lubricant
   —Suctioning unit with suction catheters
   —BVM device or oxygen-powered ventilation device

2. **Lubricate the tube** on the PtL with a water-soluble lubricant.

3. **Position the patient.** Open the patient's mouth and clear it of any foreign objects, such as vomitus, dentures, and blood clots. Remove the oral airway if one has been inserted. If the patient has no spinal injury, open the airway by hyperextending the head and neck. With a trauma patient, maintain the neck in a neutral in-line position during insertion of the PtL.

4. **Hyperventilate the patient** with 100% oxygen with the BVM device or oxygen-powered ventilation device.

5. **Lift the lower jaw and tongue** away from the posterior pharynx by inserting your thumb deep into the patient's mouth and grasping the tongue and lower jaw between your thumb and index finger.

6. **Hold the PtL** so that it curves in the same direction as the natural curvature of the pharynx. Gently guide the PtL along the base of the tongue and into the airway until the teeth are against the teeth strap. If resistance is met, pull back and redirect the PtL. When the PtL is at the proper depth, place the neck strap over the patient's head and tighten.

7. **Inflate the balloon cuffs** with the No. 1 tube. Be sure to close the white cap.

8. **Ventilate the patient** through the short, green No. 2 tube, and then check the patient's chest for equal breath sounds.

9. **If you see the chest rise** and hear equal breath sounds, the No. 3 tube is in the esophagus, and you should ventilate the patient with the No. 2 tube. If the chest does not rise and fall and you do not hear equal breath sounds, the No. 3 tube is likely in the trachea. In this case, you should remove the stylet from the No. 3 tube and ventilate the patient using the No. 3 tube.

10. **Verify that the patient** is receiving adequate ventilation by listening to the lungs on both sides of the chest anteriorly, in both axillae, and over the stomach as you ventilate the patient with a BVM or oxygen-powered ventilation device.

11. **Continuously monitor the patient.** Watch for balloon cuff leaks, and use inlet tube No. 1 to keep the balloon cuffs properly inflated. Jagged, broken teeth, dentures, and bones can easily tear balloon cuffs, so you must use special care if the patient has facial trauma.

Removing the PtL. Removing the PtL is a simple procedure. You should remove the PtL if the patient will no longer tolerate it. The patient will likely vomit when the PtL is removed, so you must keep a suctioning unit readily available. Turn the patient to one side to help keep the airway clear of vomitus. When you are ready to remove the PtL, simply deflate the balloon cuffs and gently remove the tube.

prep kit

ready for review

Gastric tubes provide a channel directly into a patient's stomach, allowing you to remove gas, blood, and toxins or to administer medications and nutrition. In the field, gastric tubes are mostly used to decompress the stomach of a patient with gastric distention.

There are two types of gastric tubes: nasogastric tubes and orogastric tubes. An orogastric tube, which is inserted through the mouth, is safer and easier to use. A nasogastric tube, which is inserted through the nose, can cause nasal trauma with bleeding and, in patients with a basal skull fracture, can be accidentally passed into the brain. Either type of tube can be accidentally passed into the trachea. Insertion of a gastric tube is a delicate task that must be done strictly according to local EMS protocol, with special care being taken for a patient who has head, spinal, or major facial trauma.

Endotracheal intubation, the insertion of a tube into the trachea to maintain a patient's airway, can be done through the mouth (orotracheal intubation) or through the nose (nasotracheal intubation). You will intubate only patients who are unconscious, unresponsive, or in cardiac arrest.

Orotracheal intubation controls and protects the airway and may be employed long-term if necessary. It also allows for direct access to the trachea for suctioning and the delivery of high volumes of oxygen at higher than normal pressures.

Some of the equipment that is needed for endotracheal intubation includes the correctly sized endotracheal tube (ETT); a laryngoscope, stylet, and syringe; oxygen with a BVM device or oxygen-powered breathing device; a suctioning unit; and Magill forceps.

Complications of endotracheal intubation include intubating the mainstem bronchus, intubating the esophagus, aggravating a spinal injury, taking too long to intubate, causing soft-tissue trauma, and mechanical failure. The patient may also vomit and/or try to remove the tube.

A patient who has undergone endotracheal intubation must be monitored continuously to evaluate the heart rate and lung sounds. In addition, movement of the patient can cause the ETT to become dislodged.

Multi-lumen airways, such as the Esophageal Tracheal Combitube (ETC) and the Pharyngeotracheal Lumen Airway (PtL), are inserted blindly and are easier to insert than an ETT. However, you must be trained and authorized to use these devices.

vital vocabulary

www.emtb.com

cricoid cartilage A rigid, ring-shaped structure that completely encircles the larynx at the top of the trachea.

end tidal carbon dioxide detector A plastic disposable indicator that signals, by color change, that the ETT is in the proper place.

endotracheal intubation A method of intubation in which an endotracheal tube (ETT) is placed through a patient's mouth, directly through the larynx between the vocal cords, and into the trachea, to open and maintain an airway.

gastric tube An advanced airway adjunct that provides a channel directly into a patient's stomach, allowing you to remove gas, blood, and toxins or insert medications and nutrition.

laryngoscope An instrument that is used to give a direct view of the patient's vocal cords during endotracheal intubation.

laryngospasm Vocal cord spasm.

nasotracheal intubation The placement of a tube through the nose into the trachea.

orotracheal intubation The placement of a tube through the mouth into the trachea.

Sellick maneuver A technique that is used with intubation in which pressure is applied on the cricoid cartilage to prevent gastric distention and allow better visualization of vocal cords.

stylet A plastic-coated wire that gives added rigidity and shape to the endotracheal tube.

vallecula The space between the base of the tongue and the epiglottis.

assessment in action

It's Friday night. You and your partner have already been on 6 calls, and you are not even halfway through the shift. "Rescue 9, PD requests your presence at the Parkside Motor Inn for a possible overdose."

The 3-minute run across town goes without incident, and you arrive at a seedy motel. The trail of police officers points to the patient, and as you walk into the room, one of the officers states, "I think he just quit breathing." You kneel to assess the patient, and one of the man's friends asks, "He ain't doin' that breathing thing is he, man?" You confirm to your partner that the patient is in respiratory arrest, but still has a weak but regular pulse.

1. The patient's friend continues to ask you the same question over and over as you try to initiate care, despite your firm request that he leave. At this point, you should:
   A. take the man aside and provide a few minutes of counseling.
   B. push him as hard as possible and tell him to stand back.
   C. ask a law enforcement official to handle the matter.
   D. try to involve him during resuscitation.

2. Whenever possible, why is it important to hyperventilate a patient before you attempt inserting the endotracheal tube?
   A. It is required by federal law.
   B. It prevents accidental intubation of the esophagus.
   C. It provides additional oxygen for the brain and heart.
   D. It makes passing the tube through the glottic opening much easier.

3. Your first attempt took about 20 seconds, and you were still unable to visualize the vocal cords. Your most appropriate step at this time would be to:
   A. immediately attempt to revisualize the vocal cords for up to another 45 seconds.
   B. withdraw the laryngoscope and ventilate the patient for 2 minutes.
   C. log roll the patient onto his side and deliver five back blows.
   D. deliver five quick abdominal thrusts and then recheck the airway.

4. You realize that the patient's trachea is extremely anterior, and you are concerned about the increasing possibility of vomiting. What procedure helps prevent vomiting while at the same time improving visualization?
   A. Heimlich maneuver
   B. Gallop procedure
   C. Sellick maneuver
   D. Marriott procedure

5. Once you have inserted the ETT, you need to confirm placement by listening with the stethoscope over:
   A. either the right or left lung.
   B. one lung and then the stomach.
   C. both lungs only.
   D. both lungs and the epigastrium.

prep kit 38

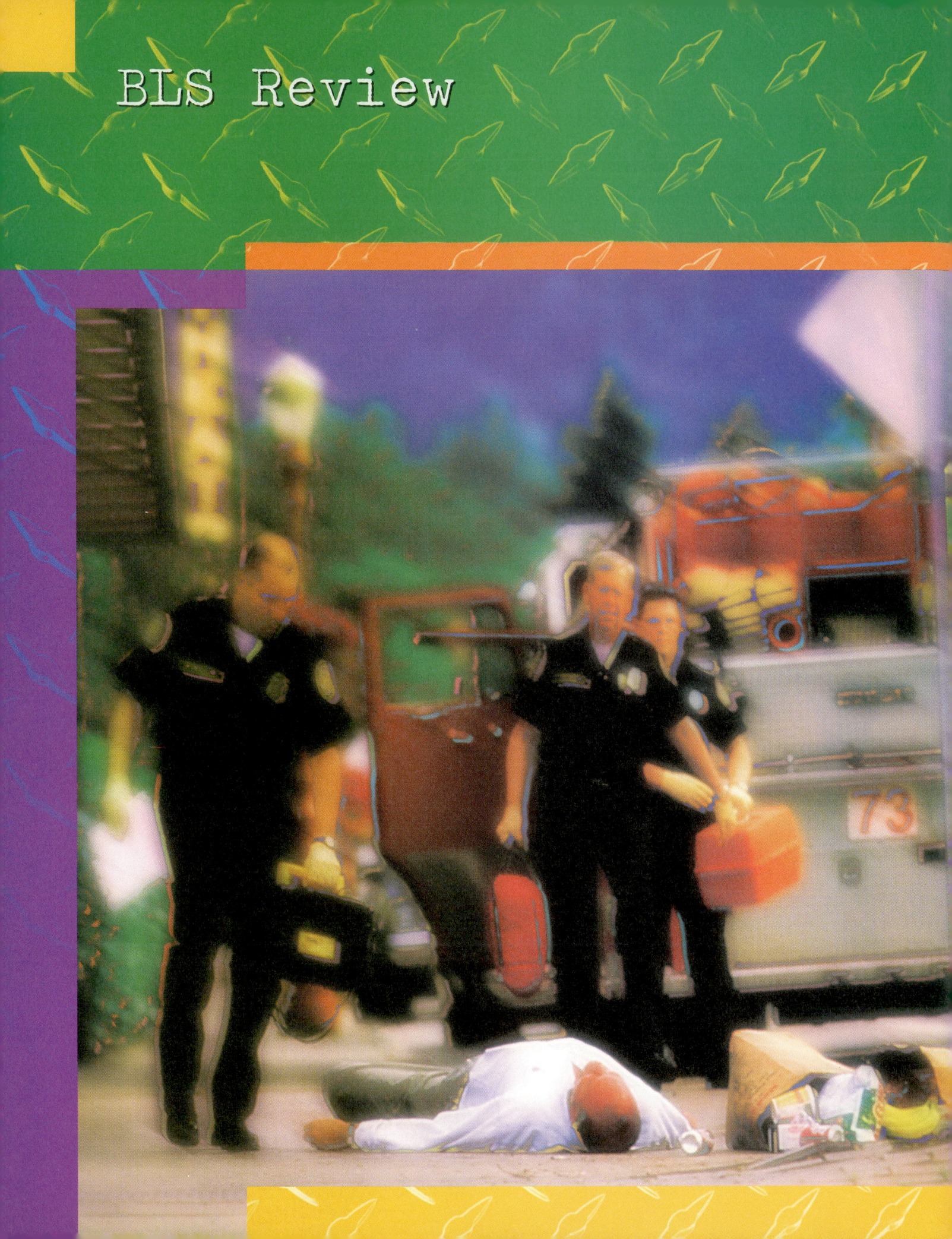

BLS Review

objectives*

Cognitive

1. Identify the need for basic life support, including the urgency surrounding its rapid application.

2. List the EMT-B's responsibilities in beginning and terminating CPR.

3. Describe the proper way to position an adult patient to receive basic life support.

4. Describe the proper way to position an infant and child to receive basic life support.

5. Describe the three techniques for opening the airway in infants, children, and adults.

6. List the steps in providing artificial ventilation in infants, children, and adults.

7. Describe how gastric distention occurs.

8. Define the recovery position.

9. Describe infectious disease issues related to rescue breathing.

10. List the steps in providing chest compressions in an adult.

11. List the steps in providing chest compressions in an infant and child.

12. List the steps in providing one-rescuer CPR in an infant, child, and adult.

13. List the steps in providing two-rescuer CPR in an infant, child, and adult.

14. Distinguish foreign body obstruction from other conditions that cause respiratory failure.

15. Distinguish a complete airway obstruction from a partial airway obstruction.

16. Describe the steps in removing a foreign body obstruction in an infant, child, and adult.

Affective

17. Recognize and respect the feelings of the patient and family during basic life support.

18. Explain the urgency surrounding the rapid initiation of basic life support measures.

19. Explain the EMT-B's responsibilities in starting and terminating CPR.

20. Explain the rationale for removing a foreign body obstruction.

Psychomotor

21. Demonstrate how to position the patient to open the airway.

22. Demonstrate how to perform the head-tilt/chin-lift maneuver in infants, children, and adults.

23. Demonstrate how to perform the jaw-thrust and modified jaw-thrust maneuvers in infants, children, and adults.

24. Demonstrate how to place a patient in the recovery position.

25. Demonstrate how to perform chest compressions in an adult.

26. Demonstrate how to perform chest compressions in an infant and child.

27. Demonstrate how to perform one-rescuer CPR in an infant, child, and adult.

28. Demonstrate how to perform two-rescuer CPR in an infant, child, and adult.

29. Demonstrate how to remove a foreign body obstruction in an infant, child, and adult

* These are non-curriculum objectives.

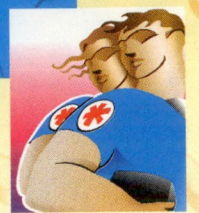

you are the emt

Squad 14, respond to East Gate Mall at the main entrance for a man down. Be advised that security called this in and CPR is in progress.

With over a million cardiac-related deaths annually in the United States, scenarios like this occur every day. Despite almost 50 years of advances in emergency cardiac care, heart attacks are often fatal, however, recent advances with AED technology may dramatically impact survival rates.

This chapter will review the principles and practices of basic life support, and will also help you to answer the following questions:

1. With more ALS services becoming available, how does BLS fit in to emergency cardiac care? Does it fit in at all?
2. What link in the chain of survival is the most important when caring for a patient who has had a sudden cardiac arrest?

BLS Review

The principles of basic life support were first introduced in 1960, but the specific techniques are reviewed and revised every 5 to 6 years. The updated guidelines are published in the *Journal of the American Medical Association*. The most recent revision occurred as a result of the 1992 Conference on Cardiopulmonary Resuscitation and Emergency Cardiac Care. The guidelines in this appendix follow those proposed at the 1992 conference and later adopted by the American Heart Association. Note that the 1994 EMT-Basic National Standard Curriculum requires basic life support (BLS) as a prerequisite to the EMT-Basic course; it is presented here as a review.

This chapter begins with a definition and general discussion of BLS. The next sections describe methods for opening and maintaining an airway, providing artificial ventilation to a person who is not breathing, providing artificial circulation to a person with no pulse, and removing a foreign body airway obstruction. Each of these sections is followed by a review of the changes in technique that are necessary to treat infants and children. The chapter concludes with a discussion of the methods of preventing the transmission of infectious diseases during cardiopulmonary resuscitation (CPR).

Airway   **Breathing**   **Circulation**

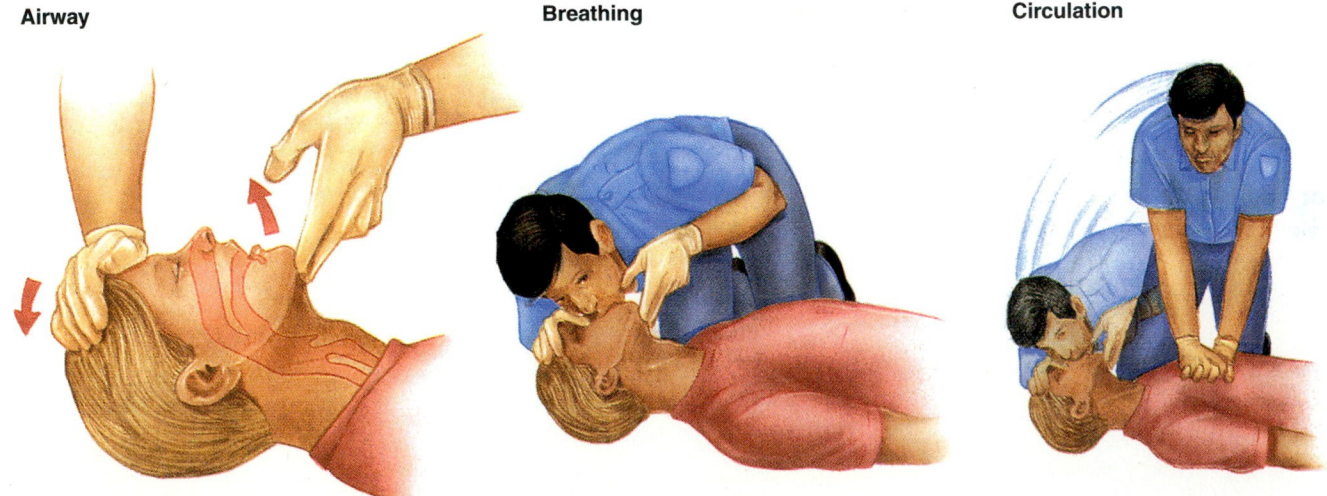

FIGURE 39-1 The ABCs of basic life support are Airway, Breathing, and Circulation.

Elements of Basic Life Support

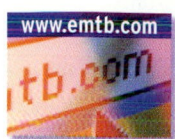

Basic life support is noninvasive emergency lifesaving care that is used to treat airway obstruction, respiratory arrest, or cardiac arrest. This care focuses on what is often termed ABCD: airway (obstruction), breathing (respiratory arrest), circulation (cardiac arrest or severe bleeding), and disability (level of consciousness) (Figure 39-1). BLS follows a specific sequence for adults and for infants and children (Table 39-1). Ideally, only seconds should pass between the time you recognize that a patient needs BLS and the start of treatment. Remember, brain cells die every second that oxygen does not reach the brain. Permanent brain damage may occur if the brain is without oxygen for 4 to 6 minutes. After 6 minutes without oxygen, some brain damage is almost certain (Figure 39-2).

If a patient is not breathing well or at all, you may simply need to open the airway. Very often, this will help the patient to breathe normally again. However, if the patient has no pulse, you must combine artifi-cial ventilation with artificial circulation. If breathing stops before the heart stops, the patient will have enough oxygen in the lungs to stay alive for several minutes. But when a patient goes into cardiac arrest first, the heart and brain stop receiving oxygen right away.

Cardiopulmonary resuscitation (CPR) is a series of steps that are used to establish artificial ventilation and circulation in a patient who is not breathing and has no pulse. These include artificial ventilation, opening the

TIME IS CRITICAL!

0 to 1 minute: Cardiac irritability

0 to 4 minutes: Brain damage not likely

4 to 6 minutes: Brain damage possible

6 to 10 minutes:
Brain damage very likely

Above 10 minutes:
Irreversible brain
damage

FIGURE 39-2 Time is critical for patients who are not breathing. If the brain is deprived of oxygen for 4 to 6 minutes, brain damage is likely to occur.

TABLE 39-1	Review of Pediatric BLS	
Action	**Infants younger than age 1 year**	**Children age 1 to 8 years**
Airway	Head tilt/chin lift; jaw thrust if spinal injury is suspected	Head tilt/chin lift; jaw thrust if spinal injury is suspected
Breathing		
Initial	2 breaths at a rate of 1 to 1½ seconds/breath	2 breaths at a rate of 1 to 1½ seconds/breath
Subsequent	20 breaths/min	20 breaths/min
Circulation		
Pulse check	Brachial/femoral arteries	Carotid artery
Compression area	Lower half of sternum	Lower half of sternum
Compression width	2 or 3 fingers	Heel of hand
Compression depth	½" to 1"	1" to 1 ½"
Compression rate	100/min	100/min
Ratio of Compressions to Ventilations	5:1 (pause for ventilation)	5:1 (pause for ventilation)
Foreign-Body Obstruction	Back blows and chest thrusts	Abdominal thrusts

Chart patterned after: "Summary of BLS Maneuvers in Infants and Children," *Basic Life Support for Healthcare Providers*, Dallas, American Heart Association, 1994, pp. 6-14.

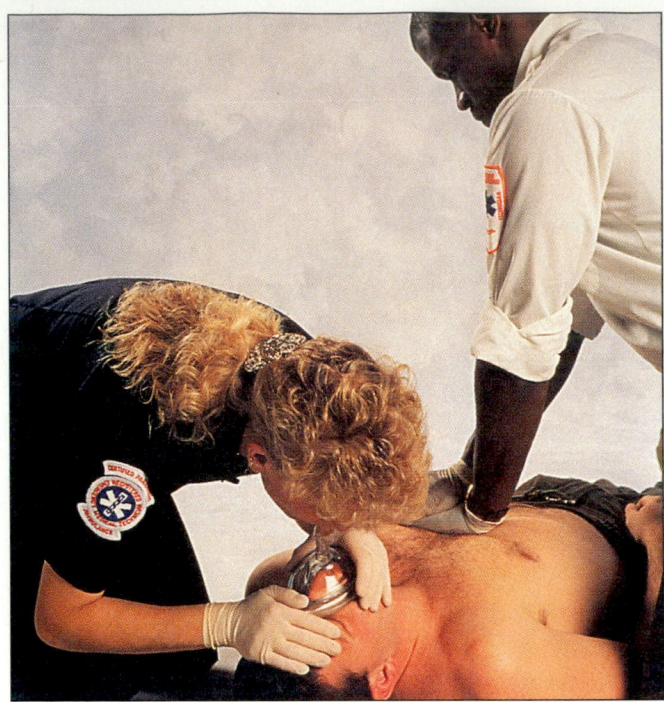

FIGURE 39-3 You must quickly identify patients in distress so that BLS measures can begin immediately.

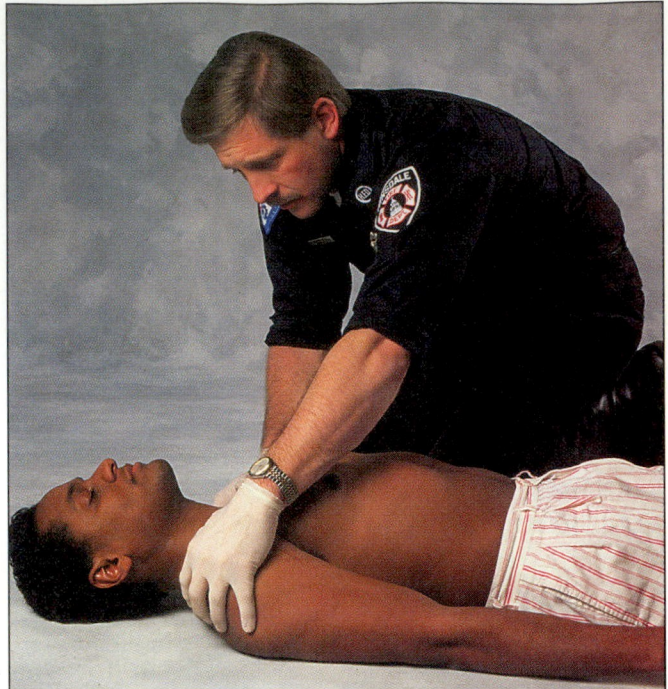

FIGURE 39-4 Assess airway, breathing, and circulation in an unconscious patient by first attempting to rouse the patient.

airway and restoring breathing by mouth-to-mouth or mouth-to-nose ventilation and by the use of mechanical devices, and artificial circulation, providing blood circulation to the body by external chest compressions. For CPR to be effective, you must be able to easily identify a patient who is in respiratory and/or cardiac arrest and begin treatment with BLS measures immediately (Figure 39-3).

BLS can be given by one or two EMT-Bs, by first responders, or by alert and well-trained bystanders. It does not require any equipment; however, you should use a barrier device to perform rescue breathing. Rescue breathing delivers exhaled gas from you to the patient. This gas contains 16% oxygen, which is more than enough to maintain the patient's life. Once you determine that the patient needs BLS, you should begin rescue breathing immediately, along with efforts to support the circulation and correct cardiac problems.

BLS differs from **advanced life support (ALS)**, which involves advanced lifesaving procedures, such as cardiac monitoring, starting IV fluids, giving medications, and using advanced airway adjuncts. However, when done correctly, BLS can maintain life for a short time until ALS measures can be started. In some instances, such as choking, near drowning, or lightning injuries, early BLS measures may be all that a patient needs to be resuscitated. Of course, these patients also require transport to the hospital for evaluation.

BLS measures are only as effective as the person who

is performing them. Your skills will be very good immediately after training. However, as time goes on, your skills will deteriorate unless you practice them regularly.

Assessing the Need for BLS

Because of the urgent need to start CPR in a pulseless patient who is not breathing, you must complete an initial assessment as soon as possible, evaluating the patient's airway, breathing, circulation, and level of consciousness. The first step is determining unresponsiveness (Figure 39-4). A patient who is alert and oriented does not need CPR; a person who is not conscious may or may not. You may also suspect the presence of a cervical spine injury. If so, you must protect the spinal cord from further injury as you perform CPR. If there is even a remote possibility of this type of injury, you should begin taking appropriate precautions during the initial assessment.

The basic principles of BLS are the same for infants, children, and adults. For the purposes of BLS, anyone younger than age 1 year is considered an infant. A child is between ages 1 and 8 years. For children older than age 8 years, you can usually use the same techniques that you use for adults. However, these are guidelines, not rules. Children vary in size. Some small children may best be treated as infants, some larger children as adults. There are two basic differences in providing CPR for infants, children, and adults. The first is that the

> The most important element for successful CPR is immediate opening of the airway.

emergencies in which infants and children require CPR have different underlying causes. The second is that anatomically, the airways of infants and children are smaller than those of adults.

Although cardiac arrest in adults usually occurs before respiratory arrest, the reverse is true in infants and children. In most cases, full cardiac arrest in children younger than age 9 years results from respiratory arrest. If untreated, respiratory arrest will quickly lead to cardiac arrest and death. Respiratory arrest in infants and children has a variety of causes, including aspiration of foreign bodies into the airway, such as parts of hot dogs, peanuts, candy, or small toys; airway infections, such as croup and epiglottitis; near-drowning accidents or electrocution; and sudden infant death syndrome (SIDS).

When to Start and Stop BLS

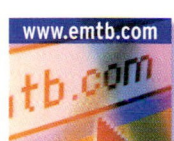

As an EMT-B, it is your responsibility to start CPR in virtually all patients who are in cardiac arrest. There are only two general exceptions to the rule.

First, you should not start CPR if the patient has obvious signs of irreversible or biological death. These are called "dead on arrival" (DOA) criteria. Signs of irreversible or biological death include clinical death, absence of a pulse, and absence of breathing, along with any one of the following:

- Rigor mortis, or stiffening of the body after death
- Dependent lividity (livor mortis), a discoloration of the skin due to pooling of blood (Figure 39-5)
- Putrefaction or decomposition of the body
- Evidence of non-survivable injury, such as decapitation.

Rigor mortis and dependent lividity develop after a patient has been dead for a long period of time.

Second, you should not start CPR if the patient and his or her physician have previously agreed upon DNR (do not resuscitate) or no-CPR orders (Figure 39-6). This may apply only to situations in which the patient is known to be in the terminal stage of an incurable dis-

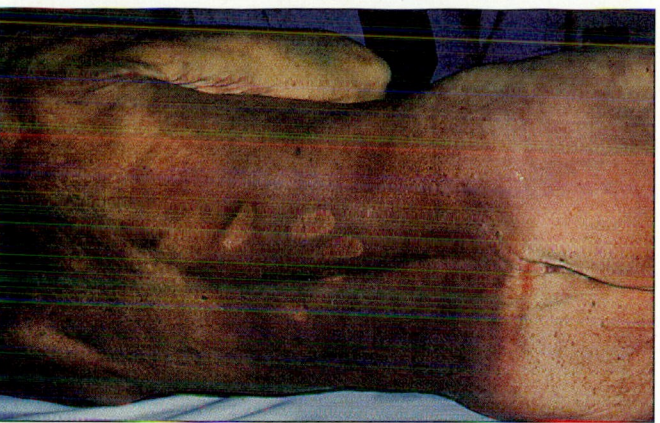

FIGURE 39-5 Dependent lividity is an obvious sign of death, caused by blood settling to the lower parts of the body. The lividity in this figure is seen as purple discoloration of the back, except in areas that are in firm contact with the ground (scapula and buttock).

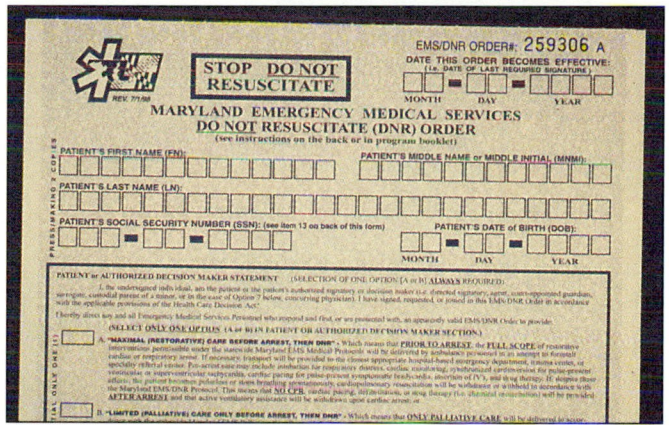

FIGURE 39-6 You should not start CPR if the patient and his or her physician have previously agreed upon DNR or no-CPR orders. Learn your local protocols for treating terminally ill patients.

ease. In this situation, CPR serves only to prolong the patient's dying. However, this can be a complicated issue. Advance directives, such as living wills, may express the patient's wishes, but these documents are not binding for all healthcare providers, especially outside of a hospital or nursing home. The safest course is to assume that an emergency exists and begin CPR under the rule of implied consent. Learn your local protocols and the standards in your system for treating terminally ill patients. Some EMS systems have computer notes on patients who are preregistered with the system. These notes usually specify the amount and extent of treatment that are desired.

In all other instances, you should begin CPR on anyone who is in cardiac arrest. It is usually impossible to know how long the patient has been without oxygen to the brain and vital organs. Factors such as air temperature and the basic health of the patient's tissues and organs can affect the ability to survive. Therefore, most

caring for kids

Opening the airway in an infant or child is done by using the same techniques as are used for an adult. However, because a child's neck is so flexible, the head-tilt maneuver should be modified so that as you tilt the head back, you are moving it only into the neutral position or a slightly extended position (Figure 39-7). You may also use the jaw-thrust maneuver without a head tilt. In fact, this is the best method to use if you suspect a spinal injury in a child. If a second rescuer is present, he or she should immobilize the child's cervical spine.

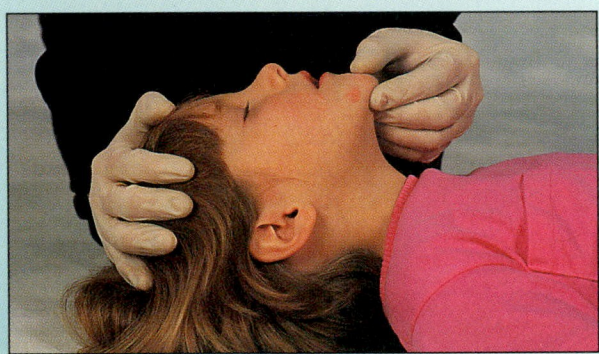

FIGURE 39-7 The head-tilt/chin-lift maneuver on a child is slightly modified in that as you tilt the head back, you move it only into the neutral position or a slightly extended position.

legal advisers recommend that, when in doubt, you should always give too much care rather than too little. You should always start CPR if any doubt exists.

You are not responsible for making the decision to stop CPR. Once you begin CPR in the field, you must continue until one of the following events occurs:

- **S** The patient **starts** breathing and has a pulse.
- **T** The patient is **transferred** to another person who is trained in BLS, ALS-trained personnel, or another emergency medical responder.
- **O** You are **out** of strength or too tired to continue.
- **P** A **physician** who is present assumes responsibility for the patient.

"Out of strength" does not mean merely weary; rather, it means no longer physically able to perform CPR. In short, CPR should always be continued until the patient's care is transferred to a physician or higher medical authority in the field. In some cases, your medical director or a designated medical control physician may order you to stop CPR on the basis of the patient's condition.

Every EMS system should have clear standing orders or protocols that provide guidelines for starting and stopping CPR. Your medical director and your system's legal adviser should agree on these protocols, which should be closely administered and reviewed by your medical director.

Positioning the Patient

The next step in providing CPR is to position the patient to ensure that the airway is open. For CPR to be effective, the patient must be lying supine on a firm surface, with enough clear space around the patient for two rescuers to perform CPR. If the patient is crumpled up or lying facedown, you will need to reposition him or her. The few seconds that you spend to properly position the patient will greatly improve the delivery and effectiveness of CPR.

Follow these steps to reposition an unconscious adult patient for airway management (Figure 39-8):

1. **Kneel beside the patient.** You and your partner must be far enough away so that, when rolled toward you, the patient does not come to rest in your lap.

2. First EMT-B: **Place your hands** behind the patient's back, head, and neck to protect the cervical spine. Second EMT-B: Place your hands on the distant shoulder and the hip.

3. Second EMT-B: **Turn the patient toward you** by pulling on the distant shoulder and the hip. First EMT-B: Control the head and neck so that they move as a unit with the rest of the torso. This single motion will allow the head, neck, and back to stay in the same vertical plane and will minimize aggravation of any spinal injury.

4. First EMT-B: **Place the patient in a supine position,** with the legs straight and both arms at the sides.

If possible, log roll the patient onto a long backboard as you are positioning him or her for CPR. This device will provide support during transport and emergency department care. Once the patient is properly positioned, you can easily assess airway, breathing, circulation, and disability and start CPR if necessary.

Opening the Airway in Adults

The most important element for successful CPR is immediate opening of the airway. Without an open airway, artificial ventilation will not be effective. There are

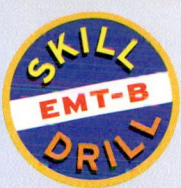

Positioning the Patient
Figure 39-8

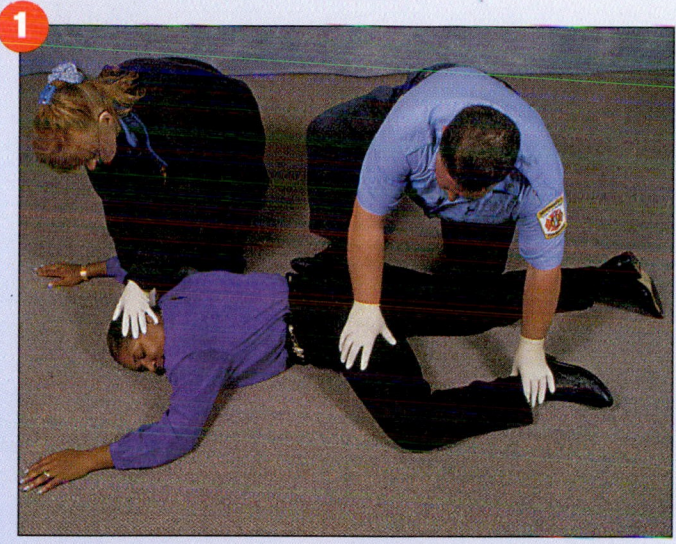

Kneel beside the patient. Place your hands behind the patient's back, head, and neck to protect the cervical spine as your partner places his or her hands on the distant shoulder and hip.

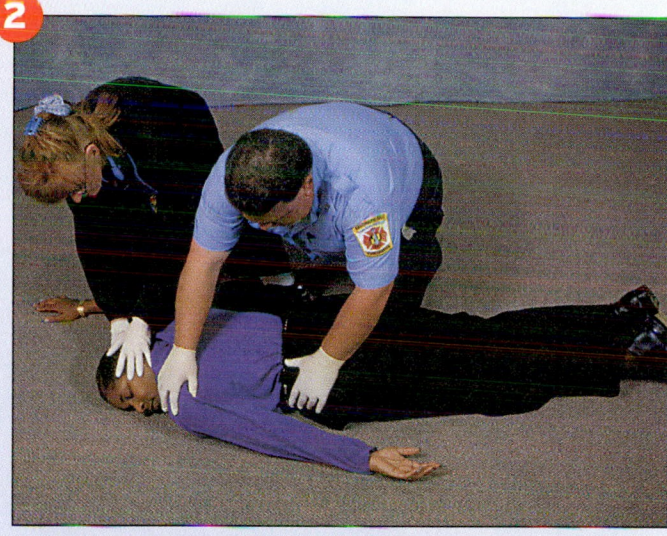

Continue to protect the cervical spine as your partner begins to turn the patient by pulling on the distant shoulder and hip.

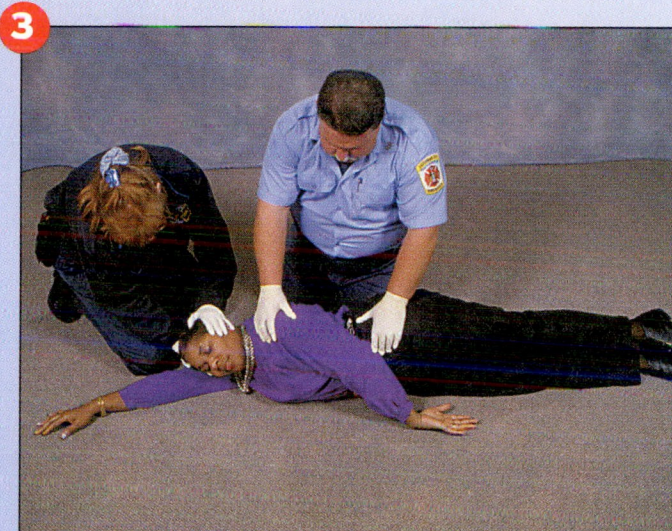

Control the head and neck so that they move as a unit with the rest of the torso as your partner continues to turn the patient.

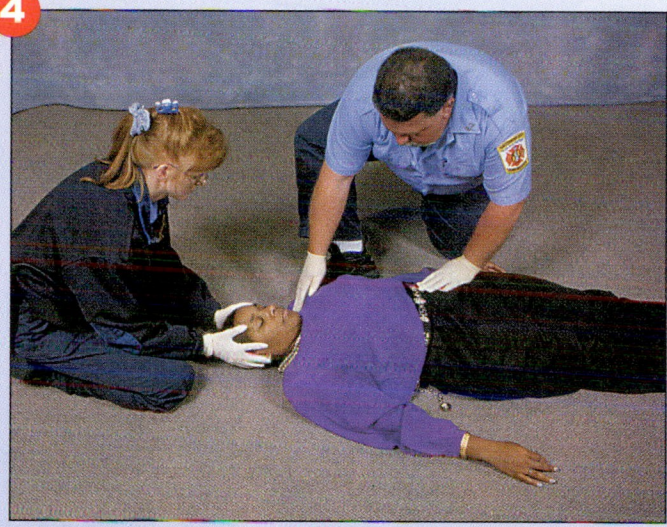

Ensure that the patient is in a supine position, with the legs and arms straight and at the sides.

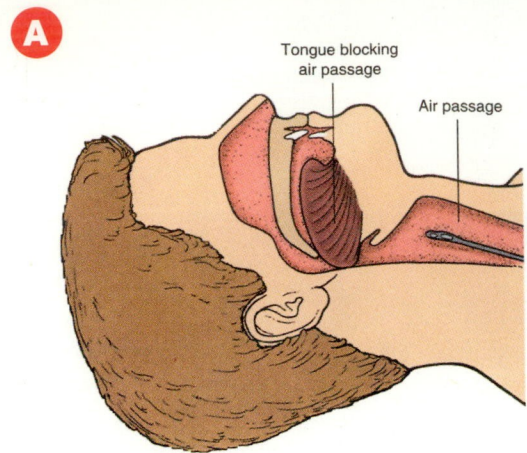

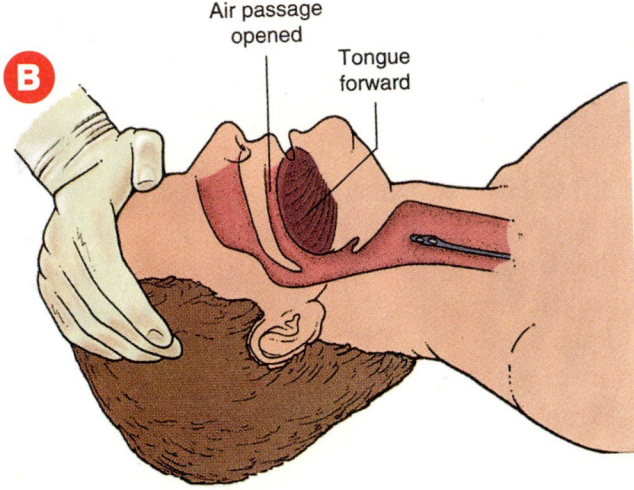

FIGURE 39-9 A: Relaxation of the tongue back into the throat causes airway obstruction. **B:** The head-tilt/chin-lift maneuver combines two movements to open the airway.

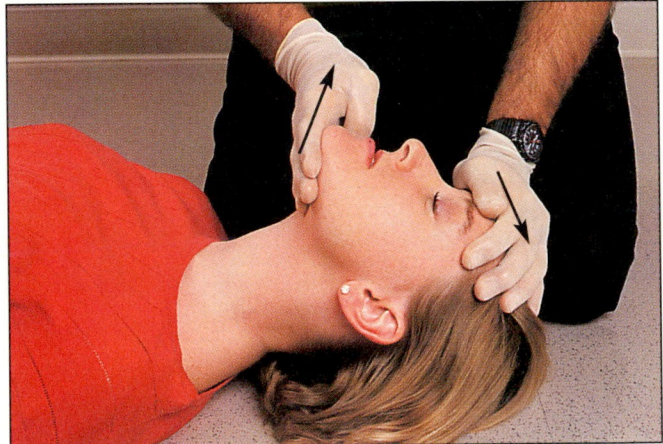

FIGURE 39-10 To perform the head-tilt/chin-lift maneuver, place one hand on the patient's forehead, and apply firm backward pressure with your palm to tilt the head back. Next, place the tips of the fingers of your other hand under the lower jaw near the bony part of the chin. Lift the chin forward, bringing the entire lower jaw with it, helping to tilt the head back.

three techniques for opening the airway in adults: the head-tilt/chin-lift maneuver, the jaw-thrust maneuver, and the modified jaw-thrust maneuver.

Head-Tilt/Chin-Lift Maneuver

Opening the airway to relieve an obstruction caused by relaxation of the tongue can often be accomplished quickly and easily with the <u>head-tilt/chin-lift maneuver</u> (Figure 39-9). In patients who have not sustained trauma, this simple maneuver is sometimes all that is required for the patient to resume breathing. If the patient has any foreign material or vomitus in the mouth, you should quickly remove it. Wipe out any liquid materials from the mouth with a piece of cloth held by your index and middle fingers; use your hooked index finger to remove any solid material. You should perform the head-tilt/chin-lift maneuver in an adult in the following way (Figure 39-10):

1. **Make sure the patient is supine.** Kneel close beside the patient.

2. **Place one hand on the patient's forehead**, and apply firm backward pressure with your palm to tilt the patient's head back. This extension of the neck will move the tongue forward, away from the back of the throat, and will clear the airway, if the tongue is blocking it.

3. **Place the tips of the fingers** of your other hand under the lower jaw near the bony part of the chin. Do not compress the soft tissue under the chin, as this would block the airway.

4. **Lift the chin forward,** bringing the entire lower jaw with it, helping to tilt the head back. Do not use your thumb to lift the chin. Lift so that the teeth are nearly brought together, but avoid closing the mouth completely.

The chin lift has the added advantage of holding loose dentures in place, making obstruction by the lips less likely. Performing ventilation is much easier when dentures are in place. However, dentures that do not stay in place should be removed. Partial dentures (plates) may come loose as a result of an accident or as you are providing care, so check these periodically.

Jaw-Thrust Maneuver and Modified Jaw-Thrust Maneuver

The head-tilt/chin-lift maneuver is effective for opening the airway in most patients. However, in cases of suspected spinal injury, a jaw thrust may be needed.

The <u>jaw-thrust maneuver</u> is a technique in which you place your fingers behind the angles of the patient's lower jaw and then forcefully move the jaw forward. When no spinal injury is suspected, you may tilt the head back slightly to further open the airway without significantly extending the cervical spine. If the patient's mouth remains closed, you can use your thumbs to pull the patient's lower lip down, to allow breathing through both the nose and mouth.

You should perform the jaw-thrust maneuver in an adult in the following way (Figure 39-11):

1. **Kneel above the patient's head.** Place your index or middle finger behind the angle of the patient's lower jaw on both sides, and forcefully move the jaw forward and tilt the head backward.

2. **Use your thumbs to pull the patient's** lower jaw down to allow breathing through the mouth as well as the nose.

If you suspect that the patient has a spinal injury, you can modify the jaw-thrust maneuver to keep the head in a neutral position as you move the jaw forward and open the mouth (Figure 39-12). Only a truly unconscious patient will tolerate the modified jaw-thrust maneuver. Note that you can easily apply a face mask with both hands doing the jaw thrust while at the same time you seal the mask around the mouth. The nose may also be sealed with your thumbs in the modified jaw-thrust maneuver. To perform the modified jaw-thrust maneuver, maintain the head in neutral alignment and use your index and long fingers to thrust the jaw forward.

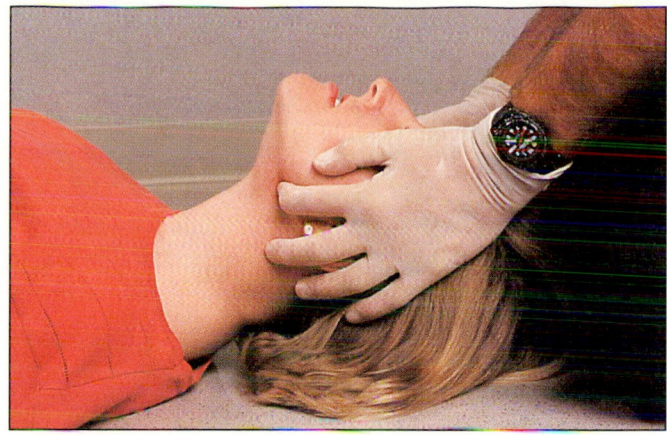

FIGURE 39-11 To perform the jaw-thrust maneuver, place your index or middle finger behind the angle of the lower jaw on both sides. Forcefully move the jaw forward, and tilt the head back.

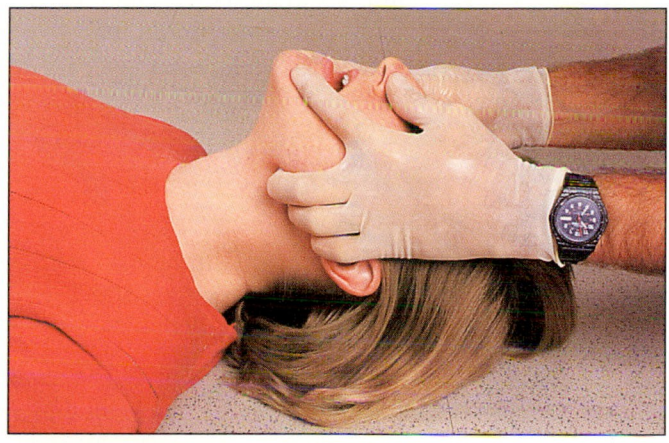

FIGURE 39-12 To perform the modified jaw-thrust maneuver, maintain the head in neutral alignment and use your index and long fingers to thrust the jaw forward while the thumbs compress the nose.

Artificial Ventilation in Adults

Once you open the airway, the patient may start to breathe on his or her own. To assess this, place your ear about 1″ above the patient's nose and mouth; listen carefully for sounds of breathing. Turn your head so that you can watch for movement of the patient's chest and abdomen (Figure 39-13). This is called the look, listen, and feel technique. You know that the patient is breathing if you see the chest and abdomen rise and fall and, more important, if you feel and hear air move during exhalation. With airway obstruction, there may be no movement of air, even though the chest and abdomen rise and fall as the patient tries to breathe. You may also have difficulty seeing movement of the chest and abdomen if the patient is fully clothed. Finally, you may see very little or no chest movement at all in some patients, particularly those with chronic

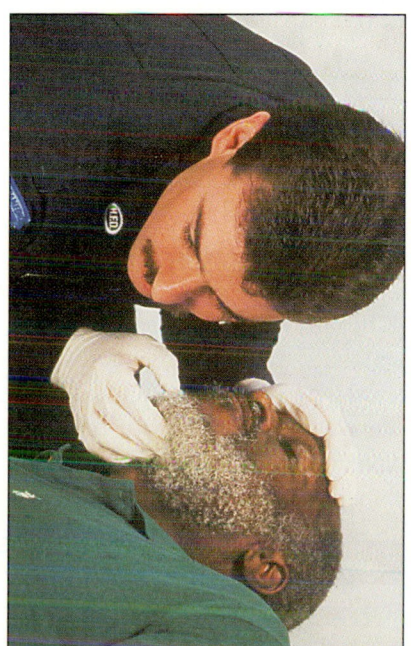

FIGURE 39-13
The look, listen, and feel technique is used to watch for movement of the chest and abdomen as the patient breathes. More important are feeling and hearing air move during exhalation.

lung disease. Therefore, if you do not feel any air movement as you look, listen, and feel, you must begin artificial ventilation. This evaluation should take no more than 5 seconds.

A lack of oxygen, combined with too much carbon dioxide in the blood, is lethal. To correct this condition, you must provide slow, deliberate inhalations that last $1^1/_2$ to 2 seconds. This gentle, slow method of ventilating the patient prevents air being forced into the stomach.

Ventilation

Ventilations are now done routinely with a barrier device, such as a mask. These feature a plastic barrier that covers the patient's mouth and nose and a one-way valve to prevent backflow of secretions and gases (Figure 39-14). Such devices provide good infection control as well. Providing ventilations without a barrier device is appropriate only in extreme conditions.

You should perform artificial ventilation with a simple barrier device in an adult in the following way (Figure 39-15):

1. **Open the airway** with the head-tilt/chin-lift maneuver (nontrauma patient).

2. **Press on the forehead** to maintain the backward tilt of the head. Pinch the patient's nostrils together with your thumb and index finger.

3. **Depress the lower lip** with the thumb of the hand that is lifting the chin. This will help to keep the patient's mouth open.

4. **Open the patient's mouth widely,** and place the barrier device over the patient's mouth and nose.

5. **Take a deep breath,** then make a tight seal with your mouth around the barrier device. Give two slow rescue breaths, each lasting $1^1/_2$ to 2 seconds, followed by 10 to 12 breaths/min.

6. **Remove your mouth,** and allow the patient to exhale passively. Turn your head slightly to watch for movement of the patient's chest.

If you use the jaw-thrust maneuver to open the airway, you must move to the patient's side to provide ventilations. Keep the patient's mouth open with both thumbs, and seal the nose by placing your cheek against the patient's nostrils (Figure 39-16). Note that this maneuver is very difficult; practice with a manikin will help you gain familiarity with this technique.

Stoma Ventilations

Patients who have undergone surgical removal of the larynx often have a permanent tracheal stoma at the midline in the neck or at the front base of the neck.

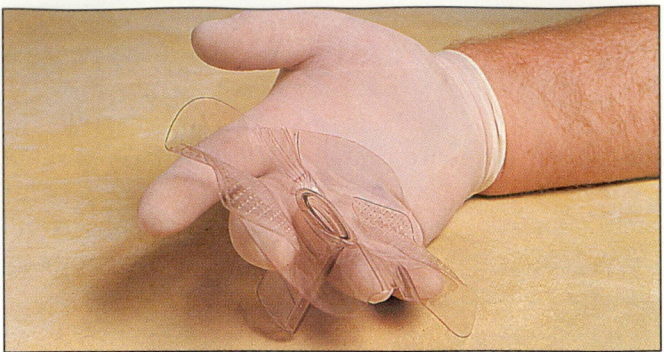

FIGURE 39-14 A barrier device is used in performing ventilation, as it prevents backflow of saliva, blood, and vomitus.

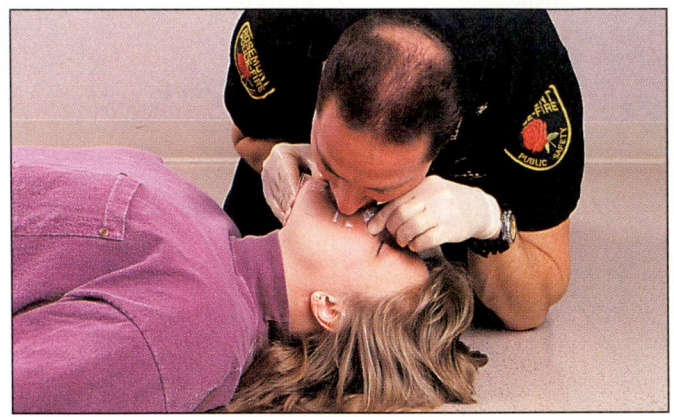

FIGURE 39-15 To perform ventilations, ensure that you make a tight seal with your mouth around the barrier device, and then give two slow gentle breaths, each lasting $1^1/_2$ to 2 seconds.

A stoma is an opening that connects the trachea directly to the skin (Figure 39-17). Because it is at the midline, the stoma is the only opening that will move air into the patient's lungs; you should ignore any other openings. Patients with a stoma should be ventilated with a BVM device, as described in Chapter 7.

Gastric Distention

Artificial ventilation often results in the stomach becoming filled with air, a condition called **gastric distention**. Although it most commonly happens in children, it also happens in adults. Gastric distention is most likely to occur if you blow too hard as you ventilate, if you give breaths too rapidly, or if the patient's airway is obstructed. Therefore, it is important for you to give slow, gentle breaths. Such breaths are also more effective in ventilating the lungs. Serious inflation of the stomach is dangerous, as it can cause the patient to vomit during CPR. It can also reduce lung volume by elevating the diaphragm.

If massive gastric distention interferes with adequate ventilation, you should contact medical control.

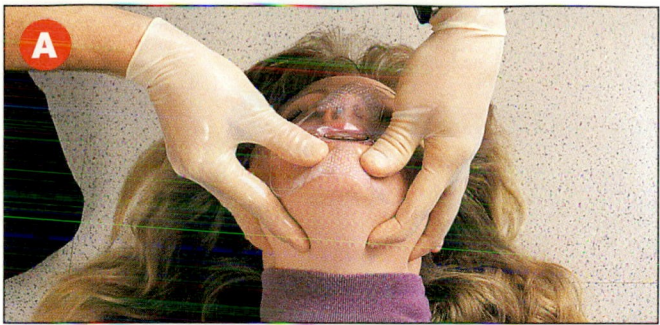

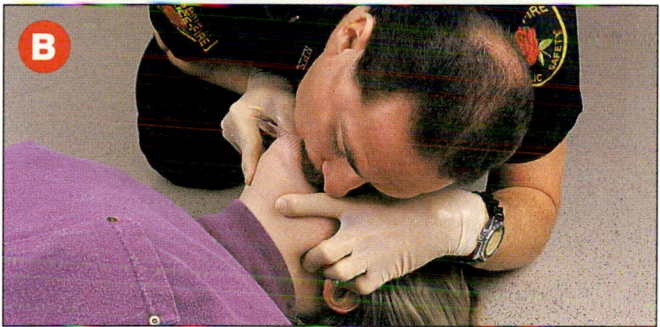

FIGURE 39-16 A: If you use the jaw-thrust maneuver to open the airway, keep the patient's mouth open with both thumbs as you move from above the patient's head to the side. **B:** Seal the nose by placing your cheek against the patient's nostrils.

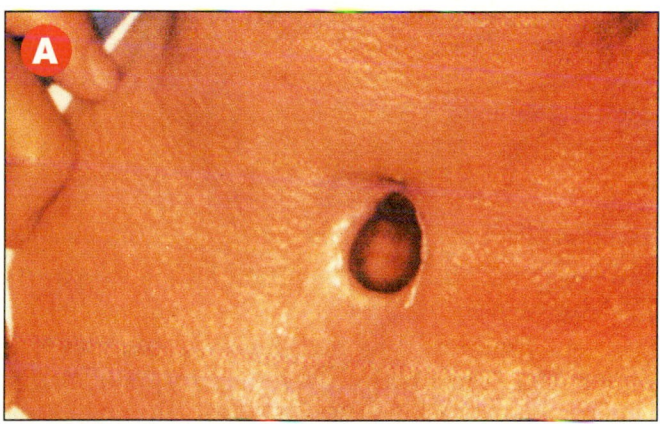

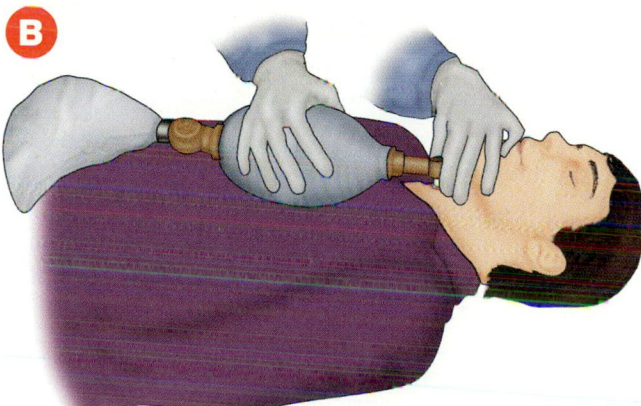

FIGURE 39-17 A: A stoma is an opening that connects the trachea directly to the skin. **B:** Use a BVM device to ventilate a patient with a stoma.

caring for kids

Children who are in respiratory distress are usually struggling to breathe. As a result, they usually position themselves in a way that keeps the airway open enough for air to move. Let them stay in that position as long as their partially obstructed airway does not become a complete airway obstruction. If you and your partner arrive at the scene and find that an infant or child is not breathing or has cyanosis, one of you should begin one-rescuer CPR while the other calls for additional help.

For infants, the preferred technique of artificial ventilation is mouth-to-nose-and-mouth ventilation. With this technique, a seal must be made over the mouth and the nose. Various pocket masks or other barrier devices are recommended for this technique. If the patient is a large child (age 1 to 8 years) for whom a tight seal cannot be made over both mouth and nose, you should perform mouth-to-mouth ventilation as you would for an adult.

Once you have made an airtight seal over the mouth, give two gentle breaths lasting 1 to 1½ seconds. These initial breaths will help you to assess for airway obstruction as well as expand the lungs. Because the lungs of infants and children are much smaller than those of adults, you do not need to blow in a great amount of air. Limit the amount of air to that needed to cause the chest to rise.

Remember, too, that a child's airway is smaller than that of an adult. Therefore, there is greater resistance to airflow. As a result, you will need to use a bit more ventilatory pressure to inflate the lungs. You know you are giving the correct amount of air volume as soon as you see the chest rise. Infants and children should be ventilated once every 3 seconds or 20 times per minute.

If air enters freely with your initial breaths and the chest rises, the airway is clear. You should then check the pulse. If air does not enter freely, you should check the airway for obstruction. Reposition the patient to open the airway, and give another two breaths. If air still does not enter freely, you must then clear the airway.

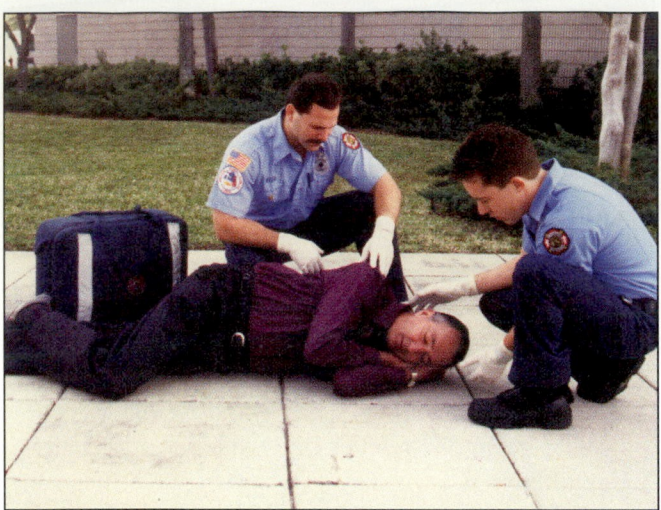

FIGURE 39-18 The recovery position is used to maintain an open airway in a patient with a decreased level of consciousness who has not had traumatic injuries. It allows vomitus, blood, and any other secretions to drain from the mouth.

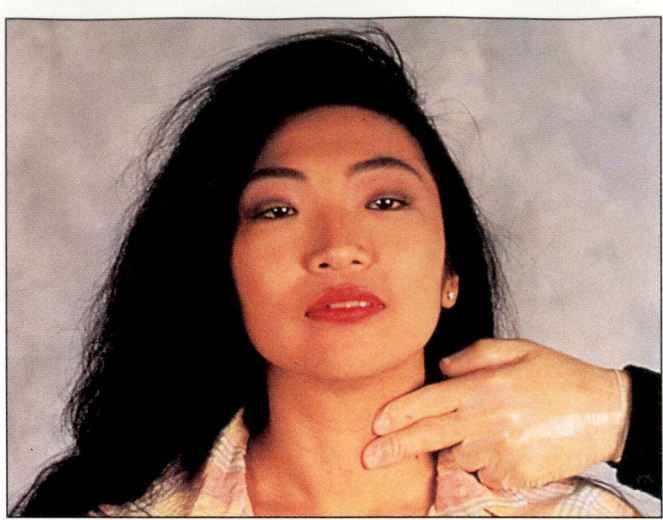

FIGURE 39-19 Feel for the carotid artery by locating the larynx, then sliding two fingers toward one side. You can feel the pulse in the groove between the larynx and the sternocleido-mastoid muscle.

Check the airway again and reposition the patient, watch for rise and fall of the chest, and avoid giving forceful breaths. You should continue to provide slow rescue breaths without trying to expel the stomach contents. Any attempt to do so with manual pressure over the upper part of the abdomen is likely to result in vomiting.

Recovery Position

The <u>**recovery position**</u> is used once a patient begins breathing on his or her own after artificial ventilation. This position helps to maintain a clear airway in a patient with a decreased level of consciousness who has not had traumatic injuries and is breathing on his or her own (Figure 39-18). It also allows vomitus to drain from the mouth. Roll the patient onto his or her side so that the head, shoulders, and torso move as a unit, without twisting. Then place the patient's hands under his or her cheek. Never place a patient who has a suspected head or spinal injury in the recovery position as maintenence of spinal alignment in this position is difficult and spinal cord injury could result.

Artificial Circulation in Adults

Once you have arrived at the scene and determined that the patient is unresponsive and not breathing, you must position the patient and begin artificial ventilation. After you begin rescue breathing, you must assess the patient's circulation. Cardiac arrest is determined by the absence of a palpable pulse in the carotid artery. Feel for

the carotid artery by locating the larynx at the front of the neck and then sliding two fingers toward one side. The pulse is felt in the groove between the larynx and the sternocleidomastoid muscle, with the pulp of the index and long fingers held side by side (Figure 39-19). Light pressure is sufficient to palpate the pulse. Excessive pressure must not be applied because it can obstruct the carotid circulation, dislodge blood clots, or produce marked reflex slowing of heart rate.

External Chest Compression

You can provide artificial circulation by applying rhythmic pressure and relaxation to the lower half of the sternum. The heart is located slightly to the left of the middle of the chest between the sternum and the spine (Figure 39-20). The blood that circulates through the lungs by chest compressions is likely to receive adequate oxygen to maintain life when accompanied by artificial ventilation. However, keep in mind that, at its best, external chest compression provides only 25% to 33% of the blood that is normally pumped by the heart, so it is very important to do it properly.

The patient must be placed on a firm, flat surface, in a supine position. The head should be not be elevated at a level above the heart, as this will further reduce blood flow to the brain. The surface can be the ground, the floor, or a backboard on a stretcher. You cannot perform chest compressions adequately on a bed; therefore, a patient who is in bed should be moved to the floor or have a board placed under the back. Remember, too, that external chest compressions must always be accompanied by artificial ventilation.

Proper hand position. Correct hand position is established by sliding the index and long fingers of the hand near the patient's feet along the edge of the rib cage until they reach the xiphoid notch in the center of the chest (Figure 39-21). Push your long finger as high as possible into the notch, and then lay your index finger on the lower portion of the sternum with the two fingers touching. The heel of your other hand is then placed on the lower half of the sternum so that it touches the index finger of the first hand. Then remove your first hand from the notch in the center of the rib cage, and apply it over and parallel to the hand that is resting on the patient's lower sternum. Only the heel of one hand should be in contact with the lower half of the sternum. Take great care not to place your hand either on the xiphoid process, which extends down over the upper abdomen and liver, or beside the sternum onto the ribs or costal cartilage. Your technique may be improved or made more comfortable if you interlock the fingers of your lower hand with the fingers of your upper hand; either way, your fingers should be kept off the patient's chest.

Proper compression technique. You must pay considerable attention to your technique when performing compressions because, even when it is well done, it carries some risk. Complications include fractured ribs, a lacerated liver, or a fractured sternum. Although these injuries cannot be entirely avoided, you can minimize the chance that they will occur if you use good, smooth technique and proper hand placement.

Proper compressions begin by locking your elbows, with your arms straight, and positioning your shoulders directly over your hand so that the thrust of each compression is straight down on the sternum. Depress the sternum 1½" to 2" in an adult, using a rocking motion and rising gently upward. This motion allows pressure to be delivered vertically down from your shoulders. Vertical downward pressure produces a compression that must be followed immediately by an equal period of relaxation. The ratio of time devoted to compression versus relaxation should be 1:1.

The actual motions must be smooth, rhythmic, and uninterrupted. Short, jabbing compressions are not effective in producing artificial blood flow. Do not remove the heel of your hand from the patient's chest during relaxation, but make sure that you completely release pressure on the sternum so that it can return to its normal resting position between compressions (Figure 39-22).

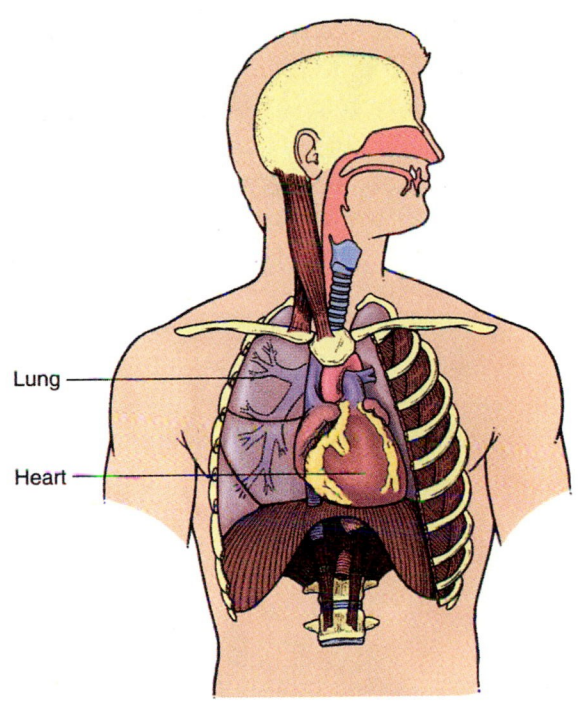

FIGURE 39-20 The heart lies slightly to the left of the middle of the chest between the sternum and the spine.

FIGURE 39-22 A: Compression and relaxation should be rhythmic and of equal duration. Do not remove the heel of the hand from the sternum. **B:** Pressure on the sternum must be released so that it can return to its normal resting position between compressions.

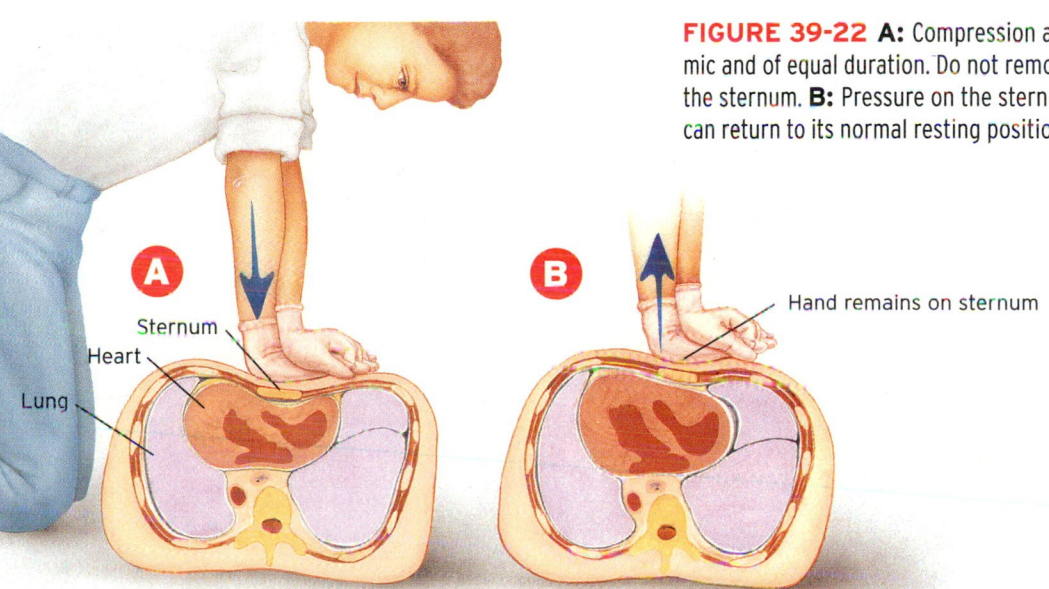

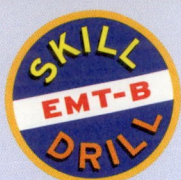

Performing Chest Compressions
Figure 39-21

1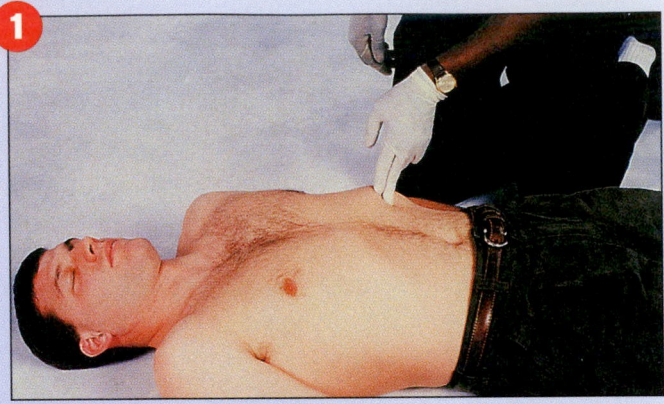

Slide your index and long fingers nearest the patient's feet along the center of the patient's rib cage to the notch in the center of the chest.

2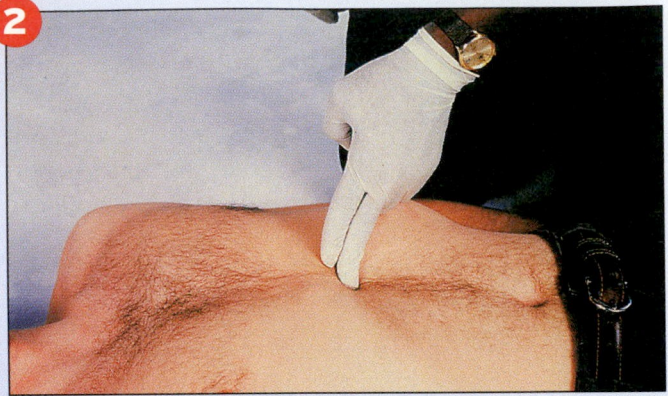

Push the long finger high into the notch, and lay the index finger on the lower portion of the sternum.

3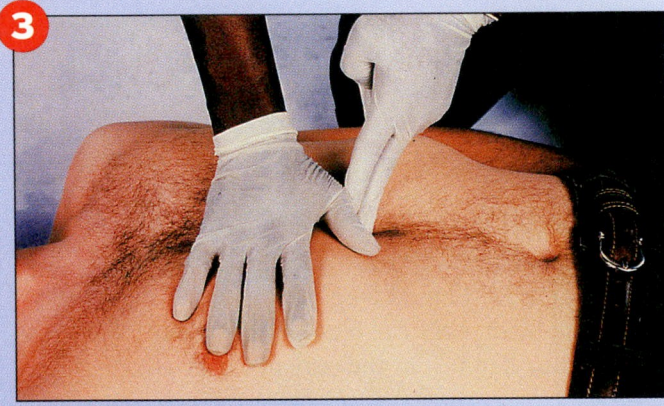

Place the heel of the second hand on the lower half of the sternum, touching the index finger of your first hand.

4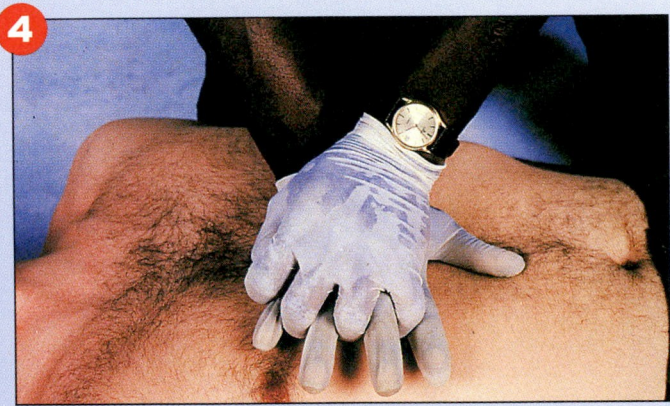

Remove your first hand from the notch, and place it over and parallel to the hand on the sternum.

5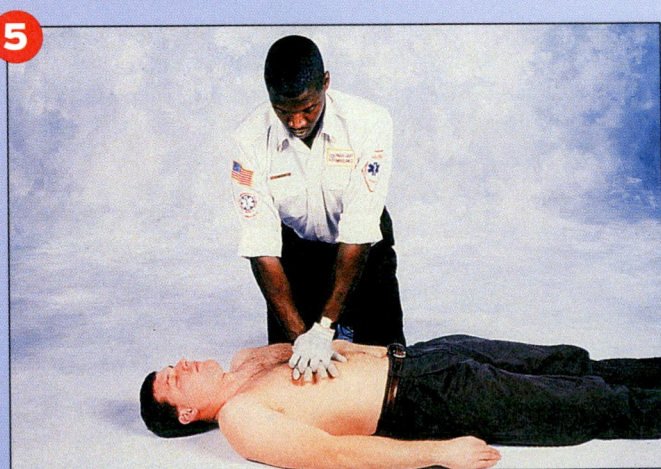

With your arms straight, lock your elbows, and position your shoulders directly over your hands. Depress the sternum 1$\frac{1}{2}$" to 2", using a rocking motion and rising gently upward.

One-Rescuer Adult CPR

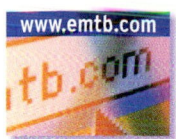

When you are doing CPR alone, you must give both artificial ventilations and chest compressions in a ratio of compressions to ventilations of 15:2 (Figure 39-23 on page 876):

1. **Perform the initial assessment** to determine the need for CPR, and then call for additional help.

2. **Position the patient** properly to open the airway.

3. **Determine breathlessness,** and then give artificial ventilations. If the patient is unconscious but breathing, place him or her in the recovery position, and maintain the open airway.

4. **Determine pulselessness,** and then begin artificial circulation.

5. **Place your hands** in the proper position for delivering external chest compression, as described above.

6. **Give 15 compressions** at a rate of 80 to 100/min for an adult. Each set of 15 compressions should take about 10 seconds. Using a rocking motion, apply pressure vertically from your shoulders down through both arms to depress the sternum $1^1/_2''$ to $2''$ in the adult, then rise up gently. Count the compressions aloud.

7. **Open the airway,** and then give two full ventilations, each lasting $1^1/_2$ to 2 seconds. The second ventilation will be completely exhaled by the effects of the next chest compression.

8. **Locate the proper position,** and begin another cycle of chest compressions.

9. **Perform four cycles** of compressions and ventilations.

10. **After four cycles** of compressions and ventilations, check for the return of a spontaneous carotid pulse. If there is no change, resume CPR. If the patient has a pulse, then check for breathing. If the patient has a pulse and has resumed breathing, closely monitor the patient. If the patient is still not breathing but has a pulse, resume rescue breathing at a rate of 10 to 12 breaths/min.

Two-Rescuer Adult CPR

You and your team should be able to perform both one-rescuer and two-rescuer CPR with ease. Two-rescuer CPR is always the first choice, since it is both less tiring for rescuers and more effective. Once one-rescuer CPR is in progress, a second rescuer can be added very easily. He or she should enter the procedure after a cycle of 15 compressions and 2 ventilations. You should use airway adjuncts, such as mouth-to-mask ventilations, whenever possible (Figure 39-24 on page 877):

1. **First EMT-B:** Position yourself at the patient's head, maintain an open airway, and assess the carotid pulse.

2. **Second EMT-B** (simultaneously): Position yourself at the patient's side so that you can deliver chest compressions.

3. **Second EMT-B:** Begin chest compressions, as described above, at a compression to ventilation ratio of 5:1. As in one-rescuer CPR, compressions should be given at a rate of 80 to 100/min.

4. **First EMT-B:** After 1 minute of CPR (and every 5 minutes thereafter), check the patient's pulse to determine whether the carotid pulse has returned. Because chest compressions produce a pulse, you must check for the pulse after a ventilation. Continue to check for a pulse every few minutes.

Switching Positions

The best time to switch positions is during the pulse checks. However, you can switch positions any time one of you needs to change by following the same sequence of steps: The EMT-B who has been performing chest compressions checks for a spontaneous carotid pulse following the final ventilation by the other EMT-B, who then moves to the chest and establishes his or her hand position on the sternum. Compressions start with the command, "No pulse. Continue CPR." You and your partner should be on opposite sides of the patient so that you can easily switch positions when necessary, as follows:

1. **First EMT-B:** Move into position to begin chest compressions after giving a breath.

2. **Second EMT-B:** Give the fifth compression, then move to the patient's head.

3. **Second EMT-B:** Check the carotid pulse for 3 to 5 seconds. If the patient has no pulse, say "No pulse. Continue CPR."

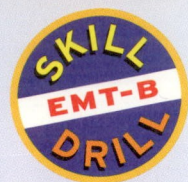

Performing One-Rescuer Adult CPR
Figure 39-23

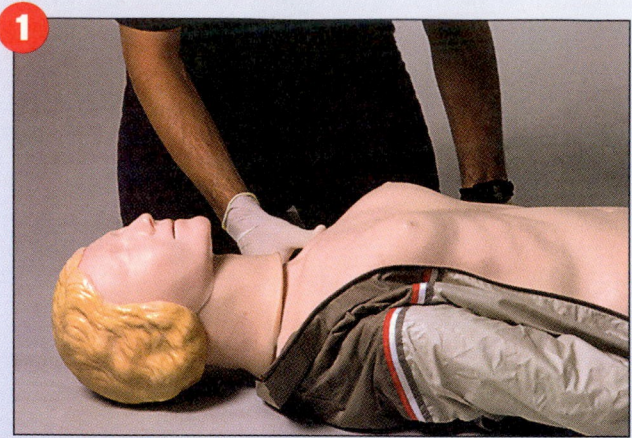

Establish the need for CPR by determining responsiveness.

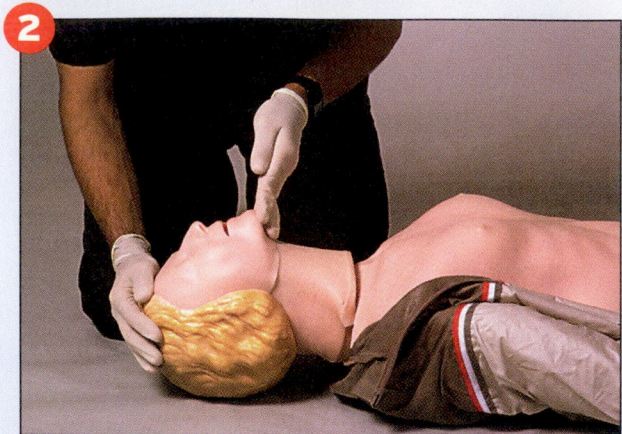

Position the patient to open the airway.

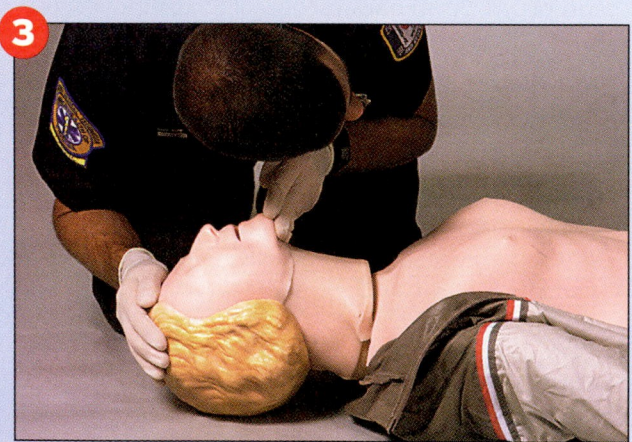

Check for breathing by using the look, listen, and feel technique.

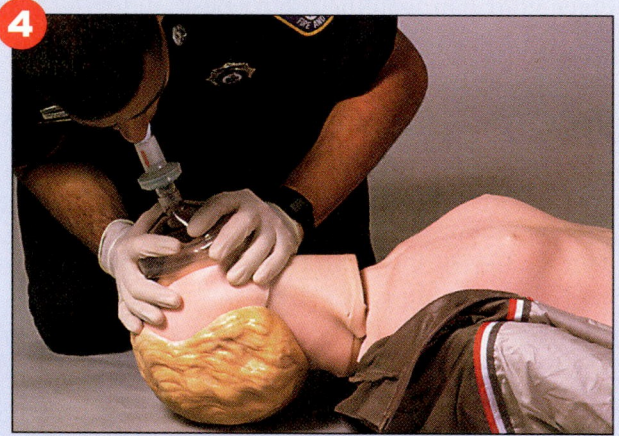

Begin rescue breathing by delivering two breaths, for 1½ to 2 seconds each.

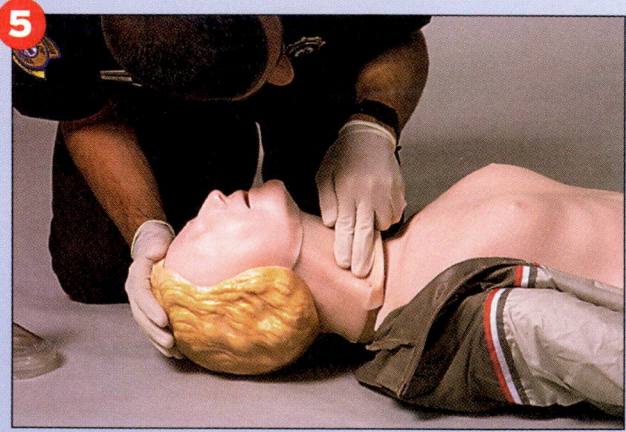

Determine pulselessness by checking the carotid pulse.

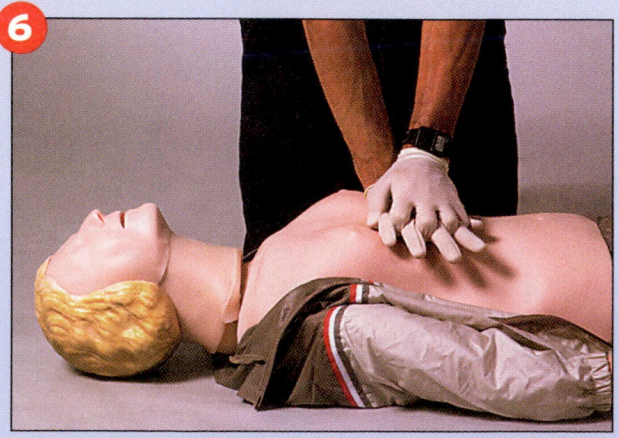

Perform chest compressions at a rate of 80 to 100/min at a ratio of 15 compressions to 2 ventilations.

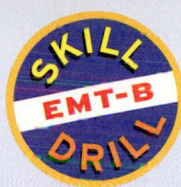

Performing Two-Rescuer Adult CPR
Figure 39-24

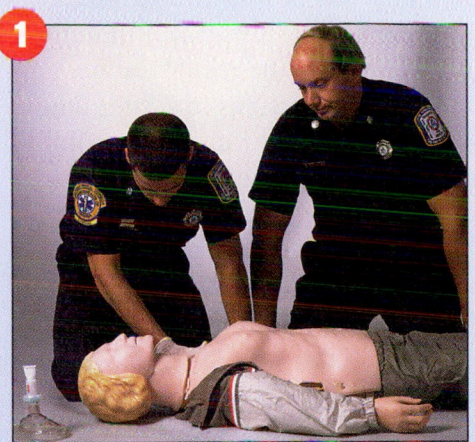

Establish the need for CPR by determining responsiveness as your partner moves to the patient's side to be ready to deliver chest compressions.

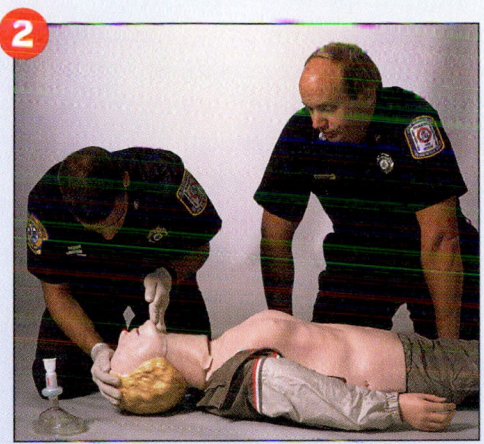

Position the patient to open the airway.

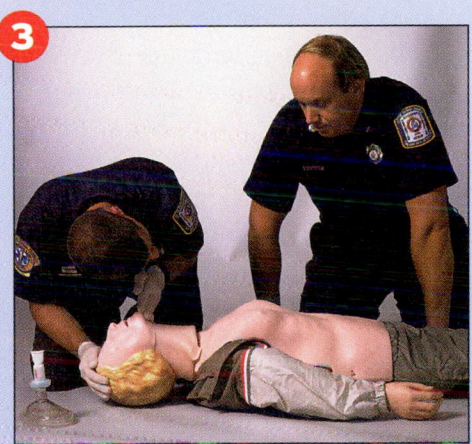

Check for breathing by using the look, listen, and feel technique.

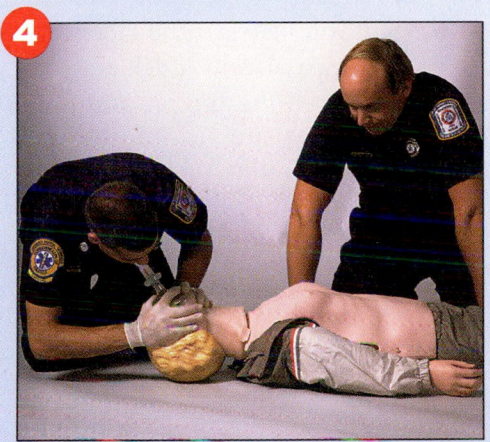

Begin rescue breathing by delivering two breaths, for 1½ to 2 seconds each.

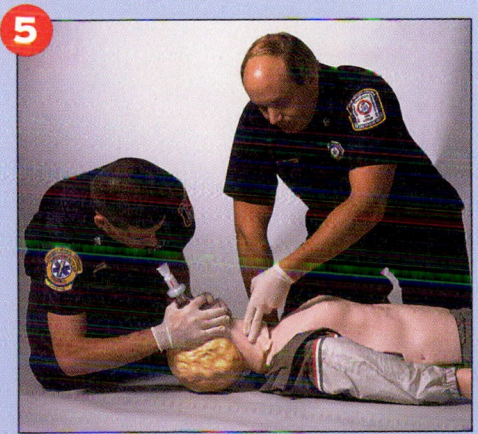

Determine pulselessness by checking the carotid pulse.

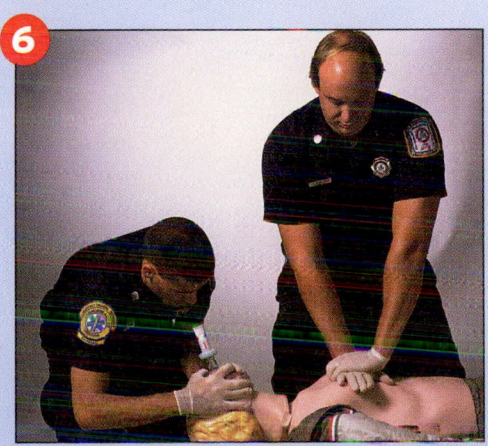

Perform chest compressions at a rate of 80 to 100/min at a ratio of 5 compressions to 1 ventilation.

caring for kids

In most instances, cardiac arrest in infants and children follows respiratory arrest, triggered by hypoxia and ischemia of the heart. Children consume oxygen two to three times as rapidly as adults. Therefore, you must first focus on opening the airway and providing artificial ventilation. Often, this will be enough to get the patient breathing again.

Once the airway is open and you have delivered two artificial ventilations, you need to assess circulation. As with an adult, you should first check for a palpable pulse in a large central artery. Absence of a palpable pulse in a major artery means that you must begin external chest compressions. You can usually palpate the carotid pulse in children older than age 1 year, but it is difficult in infants, who have short and often fat necks. Therefore, in infants, palpate the brachial artery, which is located on the inner side of the arm, midway between the elbow and shoulder. Place your thumb on the outer surface of the arm between the elbow and shoulder. Then place the tips of your index and long fingers on the medial side of the biceps, and press lightly toward the bone (Figure 39-25).

External chest compression. Most BLS techniques are the same for infants, small children, larger children, and adults. As with an adult, an infant or child must be lying on a hard surface for the best results. For an infant, the hard surface can be your hand or forearm, with your palm supporting the infant's back. In this way, the infant's shoulders are elevated, and the head is slightly tilted back in a position that will keep the airway open. However, you must ensure that the infant's head is not higher than the rest of the body. The technique for chest compressions in infants and children differs because of a number of anatomic differences, including the position of the heart, the size of the chest, and the fragile organs of a child. The liver is relatively large, immediately under the right side of the diaphragm, and very fragile, especially in infants. The spleen, on the left, is much smaller and much more fragile in children than in adults. These organs are easily injured if you are not careful in performing chest compressions, so be sure that your hand position is correct before you begin.

Proper hand position. As the chest grows, the proportion of space occupied by the heart decreases, but the heart in the infant or child is located at about the same level as that in adults. Imagine a line drawn between the nipples, over the sternum. The proper area for compression is one fingerbreadth below this line on the sternum. If you place your index finger just below this line, your adjacent middle and ring fingers will be at the proper point for compression (Figure 39-26). Finger position is important, as you must take care to avoid compressing the xiphoid process.

Proper compression technique. The chest of an infant or child is both smaller and more pliable than that of an adult. Therefore, you should not use both hands to compress the chest. In an infant, two or three fingers are enough. With your fingers on the lower sternum, compress the sternum $1/2$" to 1" at a rate of 100/min. When combined with ventilations, the compression rate averages around 80/min. After each compression, release pressure from the sternum without removing your fingers from the patient's chest. Use smooth, rhythmic motions to deliver compressions, as with adult CPR.

For a child older than age 1 year, the way in which you deliver chest compressions differs somewhat. You might need to use more force with a child than with an infant, compressing the sternum 1" to $1\frac{1}{2}$" at a rate of 100/min with the heel of one hand. Your other hand should be used to maintain the child's

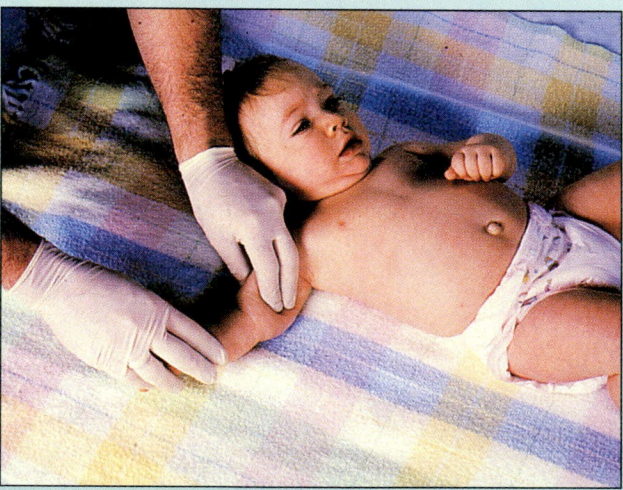

FIGURE 39-25 To assess circulation in an infant, you should palpate the brachial artery, which is located on the inner side of the arm, midway between the elbow and shoulder.

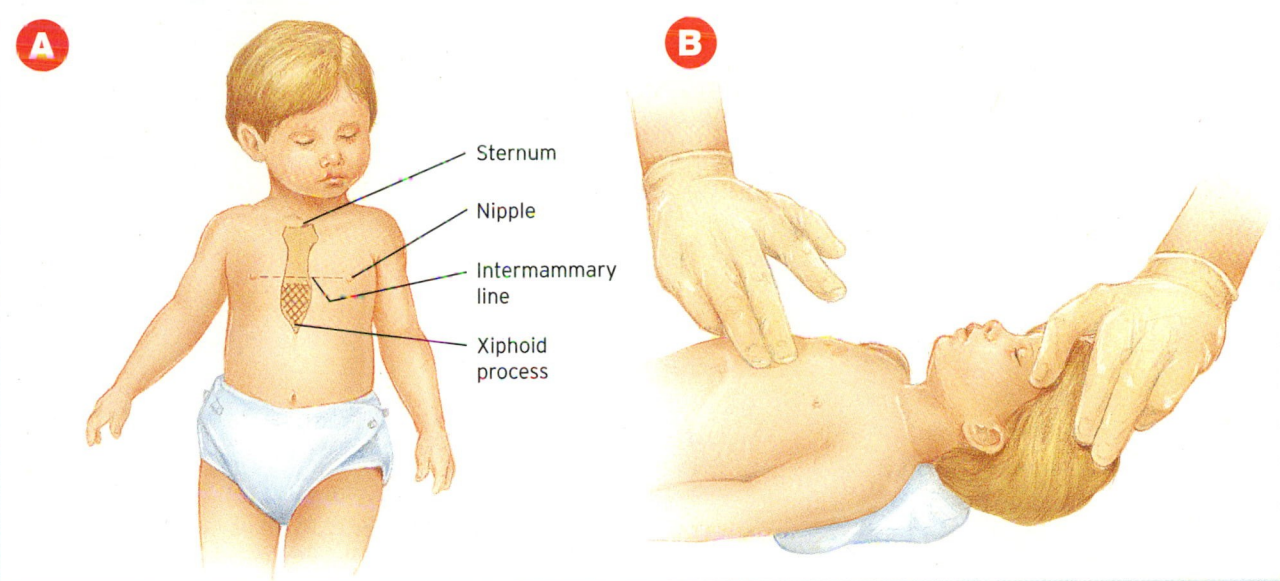

FIGURE 39-26 **A:** The proper location for chest compressions in an infant is in the midline, one fingerbreadth below an imaginary line drawn between the nipples at the sternum. **B:** With your middle and ring fingers, compress the sternum ¹/₂" to 1" at a rate of 100/min.

head position so that you can provide artificial ventilation without repositioning the head (Figure 39-27). Compressions should be delivered in a smooth, rhythmic manner in which the chest returns to its resting position after each compression, leaving your hand on the patient's chest. Note that large children or those older than age 8 years should be given chest compressions as an adult.

As with an adult, external chest compressions on a child or infant must be coordinated with ventilations. The rate of compression to ventilation for infants and children is 5:1 for both one-rescuer and two-rescuer CPR. This means that you should open the airway and ventilate the patient once after each set of five compressions. One ventilation should take 1 to 1¹/₂ seconds.

Make sure that the hand closest to the head remains on the infant's forehead during chest compressions. Your other hand may remain on the chest as you give artificial ventilations. If the chest does not rise, remove the hand that is on the patient's chest, and reposition the airway using the head-tilt/chin-lift maneuver. Then return the compression hand to the chest. In this instance, you do not need to physically relocate the exact position on the sternum. You can find the correct position visually to save time.

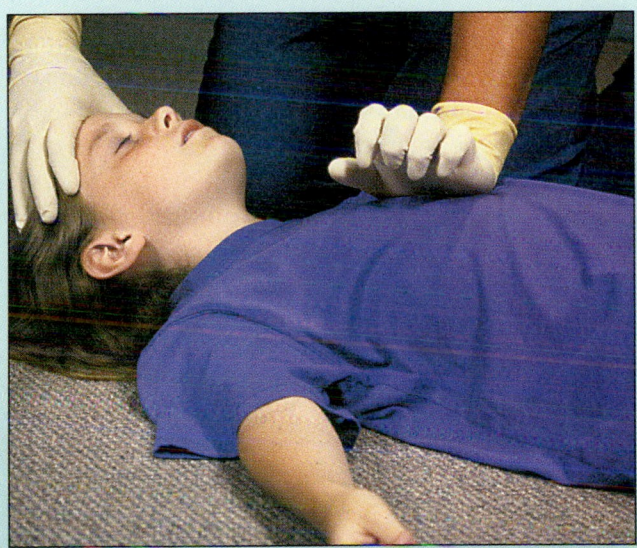

FIGURE 39-27 When performing chest compressions on a child, use the heel of one hand to compress the sternum 1" to 1¹/₂" at a rate of 100/min. The other hand should remain on the child's head to maintain the open airway.

Interrupting CPR

CPR is an important holding action that provides minimal circulation and ventilation until the patient can receive definitive care in the form of defibrillation or further care at the hospital. No matter how well it is performed, however, CPR is rarely enough to save a patient's life. If ALS is not available at the scene, you must provide immediate transport, continuing two-rescuer CPR on the way.

Try not to interrupt CPR for more than 5 seconds, except when it is absolutely necessary. For example, if you have to move a patient up or down stairs, you should continue CPR until you arrive at the head or foot of the stairs, interrupt CPR at an agreed-upon signal, and move quickly to the next level where you can resume CPR. Do not move the patient until all transport arrangements are made so that your interruptions of CPR can be kept to a minimum.

Foreign Body Airway Obstruction in Adults

Airway obstruction may be caused by many things, including relaxation of the throat muscles in an unconscious patient, vomited or regurgitated stomach contents, a blood clot, bone fragments or damaged tissue after an injury, dentures, or foreign bodies in the airway.

Loose dentures, large pieces of vomited food, mucus, or blood clots in the mouth should be swept forward and out with your gloved index finger. Use suctioning to maintain a clear airway. Occasionally, a large foreign body will be aspirated and block the upper airway.

Recognizing Foreign Body Obstruction

Sudden airway obstruction by a foreign body in an adult usually occurs during a meal. In a child, it usually occurs during mealtime or at play. Children commonly choke on peanuts, large bits of hot dog, or small toys. If the foreign body is not removed quickly, the lungs will use up their oxygen supply; unconsciousness and death will follow. Your treatment will be based on the cause of the obstruction. Therefore, you must learn to tell the difference between obstructions caused by a foreign body and those due to respiratory failure or arrest, such as fainting, stroke, or heart problems.

Conscious patients. Sudden airway obstruction is usually easy to recognize in someone who is eating or has just finished eating. The person is suddenly unable

FIGURE 39-28
Hands at the throat represent the universal sign to indicate choking.

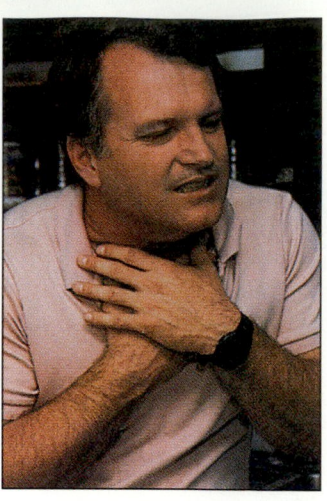

to speak or cough, grasps his or her throat, turns cyanotic, and makes exaggerated efforts to breathe. Either air is not moving into and out of the airway or the air movement is so slight that it is not detectable. At first, the patient will be conscious and able to clearly indicate the nature of the problem. Ask the patient, "Are you choking?" The patient will usually answer by nodding yes. Alternatively, he or she may use the universal sign to indicate airway blockage (Figure 39-28).

Unconscious patients. When you discover an unconscious patient, your first step is to determine whether he or she is breathing and has a pulse. The unconsciousness may be due to airway obstruction, cardiac arrest, or a number of other problems. Only after ruling out cardiac arrest can you concentrate on possible airway obstructions.

You should suspect an airway obstruction if the standard maneuvers to open the airway and ventilate the lungs are not effective. If you feel resistance to blowing into the patient's lungs or pressure builds up in your mouth, the patient probably has some type of obstruction.

Removing a Foreign Body Obstruction

Two manual maneuvers are recommended for removing a foreign body airway obstruction: the abdominal-thrust maneuver (the Heimlich maneuver) and finger sweeps and manual removal of the object.

Abdominal-thrust maneuver. The <u>abdominal-thrust maneuver</u>, also called the Heimlich maneuver, is the preferred way to dislodge and force food or other material from the throat of a choking victim. Residual air, which is always present in the lungs, is compressed upward and used to expel the object. You should give abdominal thrusts in sets of five until the foreign body is dislodged.

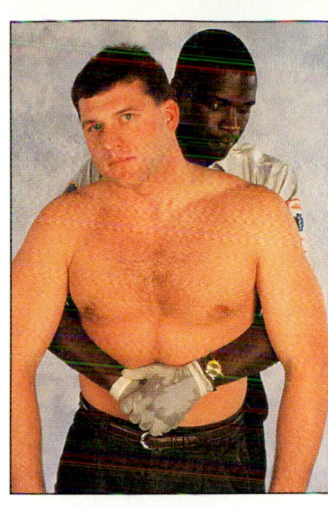

FIGURE 39-29 The abdominal-thrust maneuver. Stand behind the patient, and wrap your arms around his or her waist. Press your fists into the patient's abdomen in a series of five quick inward and upward thrusts.

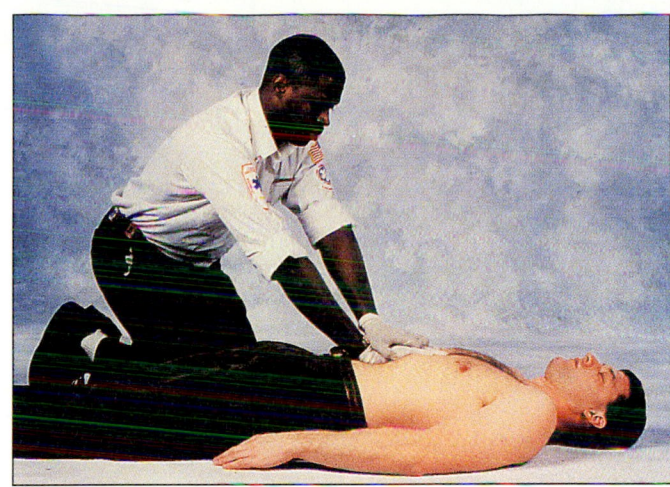

FIGURE 39-30 The abdominal-thrust maneuver with the patient in a supine position. Straddle the hips or legs. Place the heel of one hand against the patient's abdomen and the other hand on top of the first. Press your hands into the patient's abdomen in a series of five quick inward and upward thrusts.

With the patient sitting or standing, follow these steps (Figure 39-29):

1. **Stand behind the patient,** and wrap your arms around his or her waist.

2. **Make a fist with one hand;** grasp the fist with the other hand. Place the thumb side of the fist against the patient's abdomen, just above the umbilicus and well below the xiphoid.

3. **Press your fist into the patient's abdomen** with a quick inward and upward thrust.

4. **Repeat the thrusts in sets of five** until the object is expelled from the airway or the patient becomes unconscious.

For the patient who is crumpled up or lying flat, modify the technique as follows (Figure 39-30):

1. **Place the patient** in a supine position.

2. **Straddle the patient's** hips or legs.

3. **Place the heel of one hand** against the patient's abdomen above the umbilicus and well below the xiphoid process. Then place your other hand on top of the first.

4. **Press the hand** into the patient's abdomen with quick inward and upward thrusts, and repeat five times

Chest thrusts. You can perform the abdominal-thrust maneuver safely on all adults and children. However, you should use chest thrusts for women in advanced stages of pregnancy, patients who are very obese, and children younger than age 1 year.

To perform chest thrusts when the patient is standing or sitting, use the following technique (Figure 39-31):

1. **Stand behind the patient** with your arms directly under the patient's armpits, and wrap your arms around the patient's chest.

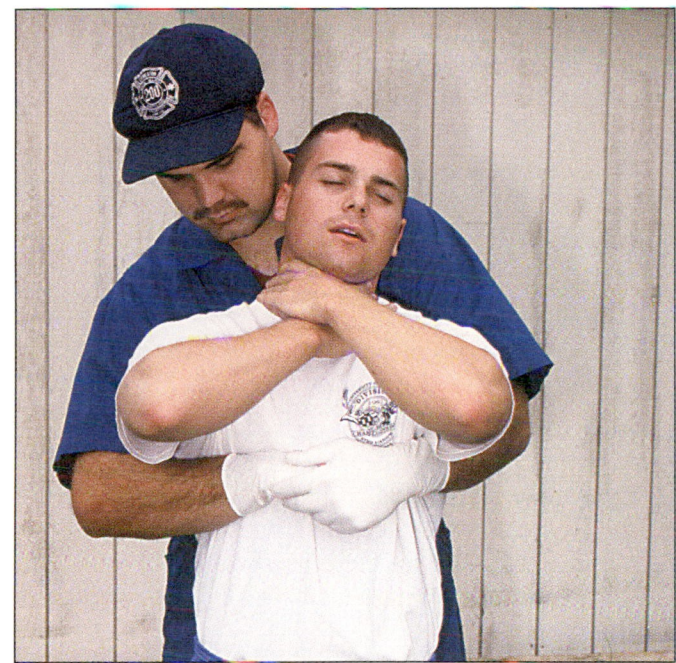

FIGURE 39-31 Chest thrusts. Stand behind the patient, and wrap your arms under the armpits and around the patient's chest. Press your fists into the patient's chest with backwards thrusts until the object is expelled or the patient becomes unconscious.

2. **Make a fist with one hand;** grasp the fist with the other hand. Place the thumb side of the fist against the patient's sternum, avoiding the xiphoid process and the edges of the rib cage.

3. **Press your fist into the patient's chest** with backward thrusts until the object is expelled or the patient becomes unconscious.

If the patient is lying down, modify the technique as follows (Figure 39-32):

1. **Place the patient** in a supine position.
2. **Kneel** next to the patient.
3. **Use the same hand position** as that for chest compressions.
4. **Deliver slow, deliberate chest thrusts** to expel the object.

Manual Removal of Foreign Objects

Use of finger sweeps should be limited to unconscious patients. If you can see a foreign object in the patient's mouth, you should remove it carefully with your gloved fingers. This may be necessary if the abdominal-thrust maneuver dislodges but does not expel the foreign body.

Use the following technique to manually remove the foreign material (Figure 39-33):

1. **Place the patient** in a supine position.
2. **Open the patient's mouth** by grasping the tongue and the lower jaw between your thumb and fingers and lifting them forward (tongue-jaw lift). This pulls the tongue away from the back of the throat and from the foreign body that may be lodged there.
3. **Use the index finger** of your opposite hand as a hook to sweep down inside the patient's cheek to the base of the tongue.
4. **Dislodge any impacted foreign body** up into the mouth.
5. **When the foreign body** comes up within reach, grasp and carefully remove it.

Make sure that you do not push the dislodged foreign body farther back into the airway. Since this is very easy to do in infants and small children, blind finger sweeps are not recommended for these patients. Instead, look first, and then reach for the object with your index finger and thumb only after you see it. If you don't see anything, don't reach.

Partial Airway Obstruction

Some patients may have only a partial airway obstruction. They are able to exchange some air but still have signs of respiratory distress. Breathing is noisy, and the patient may be coughing. *Your main concern is to prevent a partial airway obstruction from becoming a complete airway obstruction.* The abdominal-thrust maneuver is generally not effective in these situations. Manual removal is dangerous because you could force the object farther down the airway, causing a complete obstruction.

Therefore, for a patient with a partial airway obstruction, you should first encourage the patient to cough. Do not interfere with the patient's attempts to expel the foreign body; rather, simply stay with and monitor

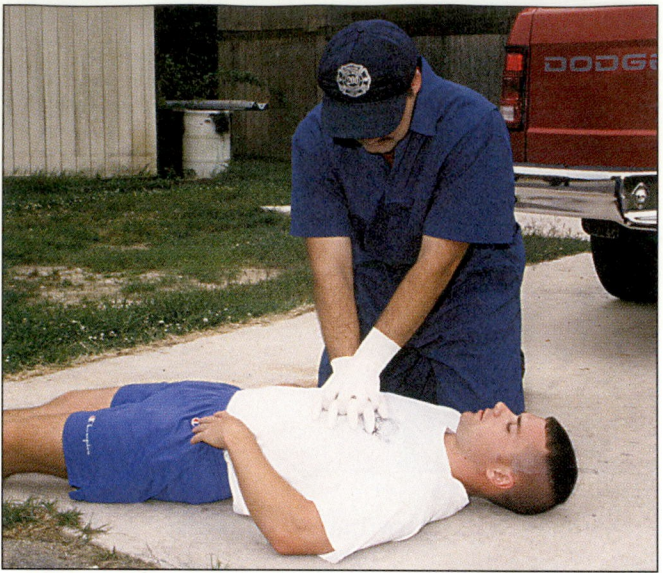

FIGURE 39-32 Chest thrusts with the patient in a supine position. Kneel next to the patient. Place your hands as you would to deliver chest compressions. Deliver slow chest thrusts until the object is expelled.

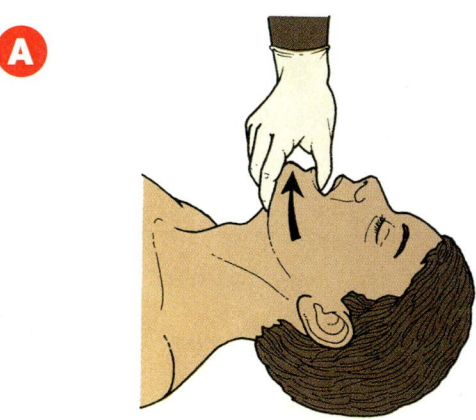

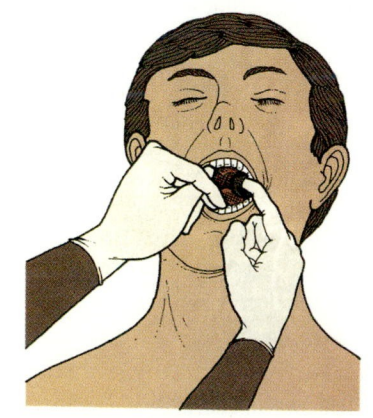

FIGURE 39-33 A: To manually remove a foreign object in an unconscious patient, use the tongue-jaw lift to open the mouth and to help see the object. **B:** Hook the index finger of your opposite hand to sweep down inside the cheek to the base of the tongue.

the patient. Give 100% oxygen to the patient using a nonrebreathing mask, and provide prompt transport. A partial airway obstruction with poor exchange (ie, ineffective cough, high-pitched inspiratory sound, increased respiratory difficulty, and cyanosis) should be treated as a complete airway obstruction.

Foreign Body Obstruction in Infants and Children

Airway obstruction is a common problem in infants and children, usually caused by a foreign body or an infection, such as croup or epiglottitis, resulting in swelling and narrowing of the airway. You should try to identify the cause of the obstruction as soon as possible. In patients who have signs and symptoms of an airway infection, you should not waste time trying to dislodge a foreign body. The child needs immediate transport to the emergency department.

A previously healthy child who is eating, playing with small toys, or crawling about the house and who suddenly has difficulty breathing has probably aspirated a foreign body. As in adults, foreign bodies may cause a partial or complete airway obstruction. With a partial airway obstruction, air exchange can be either good or poor.

With good air exchange, the patient can cough forcefully, although there may be wheezing between coughs. As long as the patient can breathe, cough, or talk, you should not interfere with his or her own attempts to expel the foreign body. In fact, you should encourage the child to continue coughing and breathing. You should attempt to remove the obstruction only if the cough becomes ineffective; if the patient has stridor, increased respiratory difficulty, or cyanosis; or if the patient loses consciousness. You should give this patient oxygen and provide transport, evaluating him or her often, as good air exchange may progress to poor air exchange.

Give patients with partial airway obstruction oxygen. If the oxygen does not convert poor air exchange into good air exchange, you must treat the patient as if he or she had a complete airway obstruction.

Removing a Foreign Body Airway Obstruction

For a child who is sitting or standing, use the following technique (Figure 39-34):

1. **Stand behind the patient.** Place your arms under the patient's armpits, and wrap your arms around the patient's chest.
2. **Make a fist with one hand**; grasp the fist with the other hand. Place the thumb side of your fist against the patient's abdomen, just above the umbilicus and well below the xiphoid process.

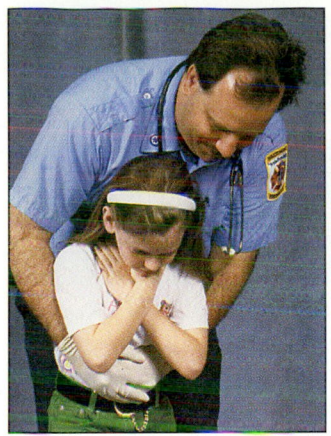

FIGURE 39-34
Stand behind the patient, place your arms under the armpits, and wrap your arms around the patient's chest. Press your fists into the patient's abdomen in a series of five quick, upward thrusts.

3. **Press your fist into the patient's abdomen** with a set of five quick upward thrusts.
4. **Repeat the thrusts in sets of five** until the object is expelled or the patient loses consciousness.

For a child who is lying down or unconscious, modify the technique, as follows (Figure 39-35):

1. **Place the patient** in a supine position.
2. **Kneel beside the patient,** or straddle the patient's hips.
3. **Place the heel of one hand** against the patient's abdomen above the umbilicus and well below the xiphoid process. Then place your other hand on top of the first.
4. **Press the hand into the patient's abdomen** with quick inward and upward thrusts, and repeat five times.
5. **Open the airway,** and attempt rescue breathing. If the obstruction is not cleared, repeat abdominal thrusts.

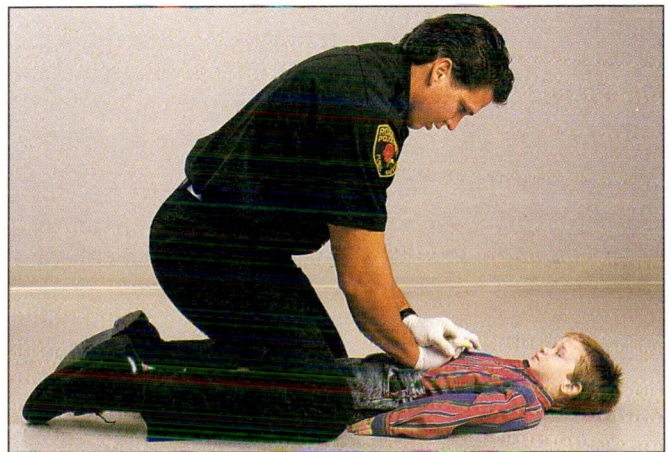

FIGURE 39-35 Place the patient in a supine position, and kneel beside the patient or straddle the patient's hips. Place the heel of one hand against the patient's abdomen, with the other hand on top of the first. Press your hands into the patient's abdomen in a series of five quick upward thrusts.

> Airway obstruction
> is a common problem
> in infants and children.

If the foreign body is not expelled, open the child's mouth. If you see the foreign body, perform the tongue-jaw lift, and then use a finger sweep to remove it. Do not use blind finger sweeps on infants and children, as you may force foreign objects farther into the airway. In rare instances, when you cannot remove the foreign body, perform mouth-to-mask ventilation en route to the hospital.

The abdominal-thrust maneuver might injure the liver or other abdominal organs in an infant. Therefore, use the following technique to remove a foreign body in an infant (Figure 39-36):

1. **Place one hand on the infant's back** and neck and the other on his or her chest, jaws, and face, holding the jaw firmly to support the head at a level lower than the trunk. This sandwiches the infant between your hands and arms. Your forearm should rest on your thigh to support the infant.

2. **Deliver five quick back blows** between the shoulder blades, using the heel of your hand.

3. **Next, turn the infant face up**, making sure that you support the head and neck. Hold the infant in a supine position on your thigh, with the head slightly lower than the trunk.

4. **Give five quick chest thrusts** on the sternum in the same fashion as for CPR, except at a slightly slower rate. If the infant is large or your hands are small, you might need to place the infant on your lap to deliver the chest thrusts.

5. If the infant is unconscious, you should **perform the tongue-jaw lift** to open the mouth. Remove the object manually if you can see it.

If the infant does not start breathing after these maneuvers, try to open the airway again, and give artificial ventilation. If the chest does not rise, reposition the head, and attempt ventilation again. If the chest still does not rise, continue giving back blows followed by chest thrusts until the obstruction is cleared or you reach the hospital.

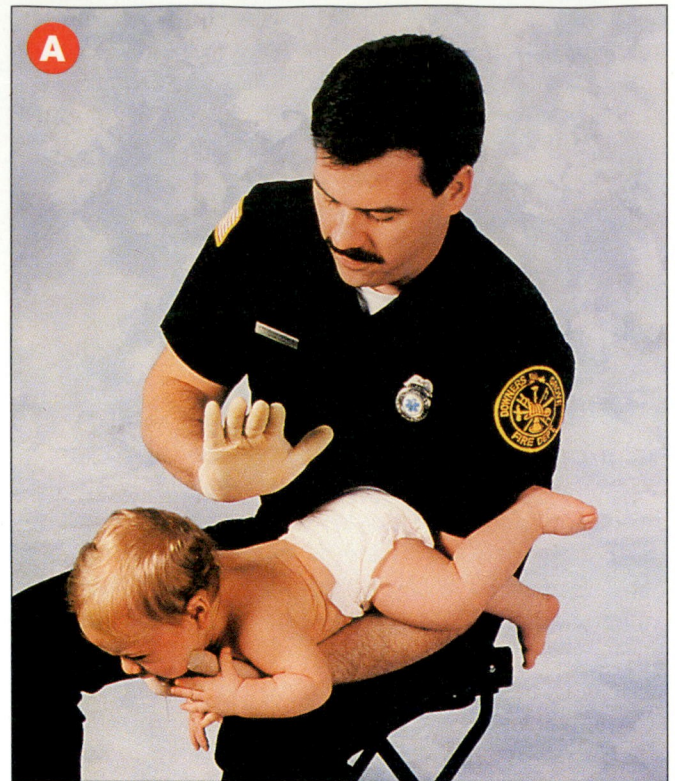

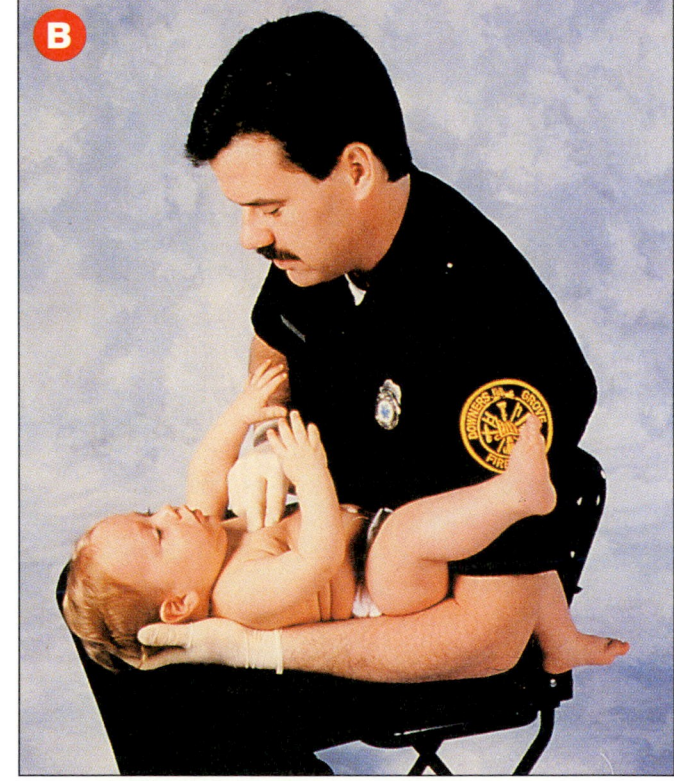

FIGURE 39-36 A: Deliver five quick back blows between the shoulder blades, using the heel of your hand. **B:** Give five quick chest thrusts on the sternum at a slightly slower rate than you would give for CPR.

Infectious Disease and the EMT-B

Transmission of infectious disease such as HBV, HIV, or herpes simplex can occur both during CPR training and while performing CPR in the field. There is also a risk of aerosol transmission of airborne diseases, such as tuberculosis and meningitis.

Although there has never been a documented case of anyone catching a bacterial, fungal, or viral disease from a manikin, these tools must be strictly maintained according to the manufacturer's instructions. Students and instructors with known active infectious disease should postpone CPR training until their treatment is complete.

Because there is no opportunity to disinfect the manikin during two-rescuer CPR training, the second student should simply simulate ventilation. In addition, individual protective face shields should be changed after use by a single student. Finally, students and instructors in CPR should always practice good hygiene by washing their hands and avoiding eating in class.

The probability that you will become infected with HIV or HBV while administering CPR is minimal. In theory, at least, the risk is greater for transmission of herpes simplex or *Neisseria meningitis*. The use of plastic nose covers with filtered openings or one-way valves may offer some degree of protection.

The emergence of multi-drug-resistant tuberculosis also poses a threat to the EMT-B, although transmission of tuberculosis usually involves close physical contact over long periods of time. If you know that you have been exposed to tuberculosis, you should be evaluated by a physician using the standard tests for this disease.

ready **for review**

Basic life support (BLS) is a series of emergency lifesaving procedures that are carried out in order to treat respiratory arrest, cardiac arrest, or both. Commonly known as cardiopulmonary resuscitation (CPR), it is a method of providing artificial ventilation and circulation. CPR depends for its effectiveness on prompt recognition of respiratory and/or cardiac arrest and the immediate start of treatment. You are expected to be able to recognize cardiac or respiratory arrest without difficulty and quickly to institute proper basic life support measures.

BLS can be given by one or two EMT-Bs, by first responders, or by alert and well-trained bystanders. It does not require any equipment; however, a barrier device should be used to perform rescue breathing.

The basic principles of BLS are the same for infants, children, and adults. For the purposes of BLS, anyone younger than age 1 year is considered an infant. A child is between ages 1 and 8 years. For children older than age 8 years, you should use the same techniques as you use for adults.

Several methods exist for opening the airway and providing artificial ventilation. Each has specific applications for conscious or unconscious patients, with or without head or spinal injury. The head-tilt/chin-lift maneuver is effective for opening the airway of most patients. However, for patients who have suspected spinal injury, the jaw-thrust or modified jaw-thrust maneuver is indicated. Artificial ventilation is done routinely with a barrier device, such as a mask, in order to provide infection control. Sometimes, artificial ventilation results in too much air forced into the stomach. The resulting condition is called gastric distention. A patient with gastric distention may vomit during CPR. If this condition develops, you should continue to provide slow rescue breaths without trying to expel the stomach contents.

If a patient begins breathing again following artificial ventilation, you should place the patient in the recovery position. This position helps to maintain a clear airway in a patient with a decreased level of consciousness who has not had traumatic injuries and is breathing on his or her own.

After you begin artificial ventilation, you must assess the patient's circulation. If the patient has no pulse, you must provide artificial circulation by applying rhythmic pressure and relaxation to the lower half of the sternum. Remember that the patient must be on a firm, flat surface for chest compressions to be effective. Proper hand position and proper compression technique are necessary for artificial circulation to be effective.

CPR can be done with one or two rescuers. Two-rescuer CPR is always the first choice. When a rescuer is doing adult CPR alone, the ratio of compressions to ventilations is 15:2. With two-rescuer adult CPR, the ratio of compressions to ventilations is 5:1. In infants and children, the ratio of compressions to ventilations is 5:1 for both one-rescuer and two-rescuer CPR. Remember that you should try not to interrupt CPR for more than 5 seconds, except when it is absolutely necessary.

Similarly, specific techniques must be used for removing foreign bodies that obstruct the airway. Obstruction may be caused by many things, including relaxation of the throat muscles in an unconscious patient, vomited or regurgitated stomach contents, a blood clot, bone fragments or damaged tissue after an injury, dentures, or foreign bodies in the airway. Recognition of the obstruction and prompt initiation of interventions are critical.

Two manual maneuvers are recommended for removing a foreign body airway obstruction: the abdominal-thrust maneuver (Heimlich maneuver) and finger sweeps and manual removal of the object. In infants and children, the cause of airway obstruction may be infectious. Therefore, you should try to identify the cause of an obstruction as soon as possible. Infants and children with these infections need immediate transport to the hospital.

vital **vocabulary**

abdominal-thrust maneuver The preferred method to dislodge and force food or other material from the throat of a choking victim. Also called the Heimlich maneuver.

advanced life support (ALS) Advanced lifesaving procedures, such as cardiac monitoring, starting IV fluids, giving medications, and using advanced airway adjuncts.

basic life support (BLS) Noninvasive emergency lifesaving care that is used to treat airway obstruction, respiratory arrest, or cardiac arrest.

cardiopulmonary resuscitation (CPR) A series of steps that are used to establish artificial ventilation and circulation in a patient who is not breathing and has no pulse.

www.emtb.com

gastric distention A condition in which air fills the stomach as a result of high volume and pressure during artificial ventilation

head-tilt/chin-lift maneuver A technique to open the airway that combines tilting back the forehead and lifting the chin.

jaw-thrust maneuver A technique to open the airway in which your fingers are placed behind the angles of the patient's lower jaw and then the jaw is moved forcefully forward.

recovery position A position that helps to maintain a clear airway in a patient with a decreased level of consciousness who has not had traumatic injuries and is breathing on his or her own.

assessment in action

You and your partner have been on the scene at the Friendship Village Nursing Home for about 5 minutes, assessing a 78-year-old woman who has "been feeling weak all morning." She is sitting partially upright in bed, is alert and oriented times three, but looks as though she does not feel very well. In addition, her skin appears dusky, is cool, and slightly moist. Her medical history includes heart problems and diabetes, with the recent addition of osteoporosis. Your partner is just wrapping the blood pressure cuff around her arm when the patient suddenly grabs her chest and slumps forward. A quick assessment confirms that the patient is in cardiac arrest.

1. Before initiating CPR, you should first:
   A. radio medical control for orders.
   B. run to the nurses station to check for a DNR.
   C. remove the patient's dentures and night shirt.
   D. move the patient out of her bed and down to the floor.

2. Your partner heads out to the unit for the AED as you begin CPR. What is the proper ratio of compressions to ventilations for one-rescuer adult CPR?
   A. 1 to 5
   B. 2 to 15
   C. 5 to 1
   D. 15 to 2

3. After approximately 1 minute of CPR (or four cycles of compressions and ventilations), you should:
   A. double the rate of compressions for the next 3 minutes.
   B. stop CPR and reassess the patient's pulse and respirations.
   C. deliver five quick abdominal thrusts and recheck the airway.
   D. provide rescue breathing for 60 seconds, and then reassess the patient.

4. When your partner arrives with the AED, you should now:
   A. perform CPR for 3 more minutes, and then apply the AED.
   B. perform a second complete assessment before you apply the AED.
   C. immediately apply the AED and start the analysis sequence.
   D. apply the AED, but leave the power off unless CPR is not successful.

5. Once the AED is in place and completes its initial analysis of the patient, the voice prompt says, "No shock advised." Your next step is to:
   A. stop CPR and provide immediate transport to the hospital.
   B. turn off the AED and perform CPR until the ALS unit arrives.
   C. stop CPR and wait for the ALS unit to arrive to assume control.
   D. reassess the patient's airway, breathing, and circulation.

prep kit

39

Appendix A

National Registry Skill Sheets

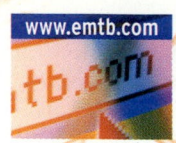

The following skill sheets are supplied by the National Registry of Emergency Technicians (NREMT). You will want to find out more about the NREMT and the state licensure process.

AIRWAY, OXYGEN AND VENTILATION SKILLS
UPPER AIRWAY ADJUNCTS AND SUCTION

Start Time: _____
Stop Time: _____   Date: _____
Candidate's Name: _____
Evaluator's Name: _____

OROPHARYNGEAL AIRWAY

	Points Possible	Points Awarded
Takes, or verbalizes, body substance isolation precautions	1	
Selects appropriately sized airway	1	
Measures airway	1	
Inserts airway without pushing the tongue posteriorly	1	
Note: The examiner must advise the candidate that the patient is gagging and becoming conscious		
Removes the oropharyngeal airway	1	

SUCTION

Note: The examiner must advise the candidate to suction the patient's airway

	Points Possible	Points Awarded
Turns on/prepares suction device	1	
Assures presence of mechanical suction	1	
Inserts the suction tip without suction	1	
Applies suction to the oropharynx/nasopharynx	1	

NASOPHARYNGEAL AIRWAY

Note: The examiner must advise the candidate to insert a nasopharyngeal airway

	Points Possible	Points Awarded
Selects appropriately sized airway	1	
Measures airway	1	
Verbalizes lubrication of the nasal airway	1	
Fully inserts the airway with the bevel facing toward the septum	1	
Total:	**13**	

Critical Criteria

_____ Did not take, or verbalize, body substance isolation precautions

_____ Did not obtain a patent airway with the oropharyngeal airway

_____ Did not obtain a patent airway with the nasopharyngeal airway

_____ Did not demonstrate an acceptable suction technique

_____ Inserted any adjunct in a manner dangerous to the patient

---

BLEEDING CONTROL/SHOCK MANAGEMENT

Start Time: _____
Stop Time: _____   Date: _____
Candidate's Name: _____
Evaluator's Name: _____

	Points Possible	Points Awarded
Takes, or verbalizes, body substance isolation precautions	1	
Applies direct pressure to the wound	1	
Elevates the extremity	1	
Note: The examiner must now inform the candidate that the wound continues to bleed.		
Applies an additional dressing to the wound	1	
Note: The examiner must now inform the candidate that the wound still continues to bleed. The second dressing does not control the bleeding.		
Locates and applies pressure to appropriate arterial pressure point	1	
Note: The examiner must now inform the candidate that the bleeding is controlled		
Bandages the wound	1	
Note: The examiner must now inform the candidate the patient is now showing signs and symptoms indicative of hypoperfusion		
Properly positions the patient	1	
Applies high concentration oxygen	1	
Initiates steps to prevent heat loss from the patient	1	
Indicates the need for immediate transportation	1	
Total:	**10**	

Critical Criteria

_____ Did not take, or verbalize, body substance isolation precautions

_____ Did not apply high concentration of oxygen

_____ Applied a tourniquet before attempting other methods of bleeding control

_____ Did not control hemorrhage in a timely manner

_____ Did not indicate a need for immediate transportation

BAG-VALVE-MASK
APNEIC PATIENT

Start Time: _____   Date: _____

Stop Time: _____

Candidate's Name: _____

Evaluator's Name: _____

	Points Possible	Points Awarded
Takes, or verbalizes, body substance isolation precautions	1	
Voices opening the airway	1	
Voices inserting an airway adjunct	1	
Selects appropriately sized mask	1	
Creates a proper mask-to-face seal	1	
Ventilates patient at no less than 800 ml volume *(The examiner must witness for at least 30 seconds)*	1	
Connects reservoir and oxygen	1	
Adjusts liter flow to 15 liters/minute or greater	1	
The examiner indicates arrival of a second EMT. The second EMT is instructed to ventilate the patient while the candidate controls the mask and the airway		
Voices re-opening the airway	1	
Creates a proper mask-to-face seal	1	
Instructs assistant to resume ventilation at proper volume per breath *(The examiner must witness for at least 30 seconds)*	1	
Total:	**11**	

Critical Criteria

_____ Did not take, or verbalize, body substance isolation precautions

_____ Did not immediately ventilate the patient

_____ Interrupted ventilations for more than 20 seconds

_____ Did not provide high concentration of oxygen

_____ Did not provide, or direct assistant to provide, proper volume/breath *(more than two (2) ventilations per minute are below 800 ml)*

_____ Did not allow adequate exhalation

Cardiac Arrest Management/AED

Start Time: _____   Date: _____

Stop Time: _____

Candidate's Name: _____

Evaluator's Name: _____

	Points Possible	Points Awarded
ASSESSMENT		
Takes, or verbalizes, body substance isolation precautions	1	
Briefly questions the rescuer about arrest events	1	
Directs rescuer to stop CPR	1	
Verifies absence of spontaneous pulse (skill station examiner states "no pulse")	1	
Directs resumption of CPR	1	
Turns on defibrillator power	1	
Attaches automated defibrillator to the patient	1	
Directs rescuer to stop CPR and ensures all individuals are clear of the patient	1	
Initiates analysis of the rhythm	1	
Delivers shock (up to three successive shocks)	1	
Verifies absence of spontaneous pulse (skill station examiner states "no pulse")	1	
TRANSITION		
Directs resumption of CPR	1	
Gathers additional information about arrest event	1	
Confirms effectiveness of CPR (ventilation and compressions)	1	
INTEGRATION		
Verbalizes or directs insertion of a simple airway adjunct (oral/nasal airway)	1	
Ventilates, or directs ventilation of, the patient	1	
Assures high concentration of oxygen is delivered to the patient	1	
Assures CPR continues without unnecessary/prolonged interruption	1	
Re-evaluates patient/CPR in approximately one minute	1	
Repeats defibrillator sequence	1	
TRANSPORTATION		
Verbalizes transportation of patient	1	
Total:	**21**	

Critical Criteria

_____ Did not take, or verbalize, body substance isolation precautions

_____ Did not evaluate the need for immediate use of the AED

_____ Did not direct initiation/resumption of ventilation/compressions at appropriate times.

_____ Did not assure all individuals were clear of patient before delivering each shock

_____ Did not operate the AED properly (inability to deliver shock)

_____ Prevented the defibrillator from delivering indicated stacked shocks

VENTILATORY MANAGEMENT
DUAL LUMEN DEVICE INSERTION FOLLOWING
AN UNSUCCESSFUL ENDOTRACHEAL INTUBATION ATTEMPT

Start Time: _____

Stop Time: _____   Date: _____

Candidate's Name: _____

Evaluator's Name: _____

	Points Possible	Points Awarded
Continues body substance isolation precautions	1	
Confirms the patient is being properly ventilated with high percentage oxygen	1	
Directs the assistant to hyper-oxygenate the patient	1	
Checks/prepares the airway device	1	
Lubricates the distal tip of the device *(may be verbalized)*	1	
Note: The examiner should remove the OPA and move out of the way when the candidate is prepared to insert the device		
Positions the patient's head properly	1	
Performs a tongue-jaw lift	1	
USES ☐ COMBITUBE ☐ USES THE PTL		
Inserts device in the mid-line and to the depth so that the printed ring is at the level of the teeth	Inserts the device in the mid-line until the bite block flange is at the level of the teeth	1	
Inflates the pharyngeal cuff with the proper volume and removes the syringe	Secures the strap	1	
Inflates the distal cuff with the proper volume and removes the syringe	Blows into tube #1 to adequately inflate both cuffs	1	
Attaches/directs attachment of BVM to the first (esophageal placement) lumen and ventilates		1	
Confirms placement and ventilation through the correct lumen by observing chest rise, auscultation over the epigastrium and bilaterally over each lung		1	
Note: The examiner states, "You do not see rise and fall of the chest and hear sounds only over the epigastrium."			
Attaches/directs attachment of BVM to the second (endotracheal placement) lumen and ventilates		1	
Confirms placement and ventilation through the correct lumen by observing chest rise, auscultation over the epigastrium and bilaterally over each lung		1	
Note: The examiner states, "You see rise and fall of the chest, there are no sounds over the epigastrium and breath sounds are equal over each lung."			
Secures device or confirms that the device remains properly secured		1	
Total:	**15**	

Critical Criteria

____ Did not take or verbalize body substance isolation precautions

____ Did not initiate ventilations within 30 seconds

____ Interrupted ventilations for more than 30 seconds at any time

____ Did not hyper-oxygenate the patient prior to placement of the dual lumen airway device

____ Did not provide adequate volume per breath (maximum 2 errors/minute permissible)

____ Did not ventilate the patient at a rate of at least 10 breaths per minute

____ Did not insert the dual lumen airway device at a proper depth or at the proper place within 3 attempts

____ Did not inflate both cuffs properly

____ **Combitube** - Did not remove the syringe immediately following the inflation of each cuff

____ **PTL** - Did not secure the strap prior to cuff inflation

____ Did not confirm, by observing chest rise and auscultation over the epigastrium and bilaterally over each lung, that the proper lumen of the device was being used to ventilate the patient

____ Inserted any adjunct in a manner that was dangerous to the patient

---

VENTILATORY MANAGEMENT
ESOPHAGEAL OBTURATOR AIRWAY INSERTION FOLLOWING
AN UNSUCCESSFUL ENDOTRACHEAL INTUBATION ATTEMPT

Start Time: _____

Stop Time: _____   Date: _____

Candidate's Name: _____

Evaluator's Name: _____

	Points Possible	Points Awarded
Continues body substance isolation precautions	1	
Confirms the patient is being ventilated high percentage oxygen	1	
Directs the assistant to hyper-oxygenate the patient	1	
Identifies/selects the proper equipment for insertion of EOA	1	
Assembles the EOA	1	
Tests the cuff for leaks	1	
Inflates the mask	1	
Lubricates the tube *(may be verbalized)*	1	
Note: The examiner should remove the OPA and move out of the way when the candidate is prepared to insert the device		
Positions the head properly with the neck in the neutral or slightly flexed position	1	
Grasps and elevates the patient's tongue and mandible	1	
Inserts the tube in the same direction as the curvature of the pharynx	1	
Advances the tube until the mask is sealed against the patient's face	1	
Ventilates the patient while maintaining a tight mask-to-face seal	1	
Directs confirmation of placement of EOA by observing for chest rise and auscultation over the epigastrium and bilaterally over each lung	1	
Note: The examiner must acknowledge adequate chest rise, bilateral breath sounds and absent sounds over the epigastrium		
Inflates the cuff to the proper pressure	1	
Disconnects the syringe from the inlet port	1	
Continues ventilation of the patient	1	
Total:	**17**	

Critical Criteria

____ Did not take or verbalize body substance isolation precautions

____ Did not initiate ventilations within 30 seconds

____ Interrupted ventilations for more than 30 seconds at any time

____ Did not direct hyper-oxygenation of the patient prior to placement of the EOA

____ Did not successfully place the EOA within 3 attempts

____ Did not ventilate at a rate of at least 10 breaths per minute

____ Did not provide adequate volume per breath (maximum 2 errors/minute permissible)

____ Did not assure proper tube placement by auscultation bilaterally and over the epigastrium

____ Did not remove the syringe after inflating the cuff

____ Did not successfully ventilate the patient

____ Did not provide high flow oxygen (15 liters per minute or greater)

____ Inserted any adjunct in a manner that was dangerous to the patient

IMMOBILIZATION SKILLS
JOINT INJURY

Start Time: _____

Stop Time: _____   Date: _____

Candidate's Name: _____

Evaluator's Name: _____

	Points Possible	Points Awarded
Takes, or verbalizes, body substance isolation precautions	1	
Directs application of manual stabilization of the shoulder injury	1	
Assesses motor, sensory and circulatory function in the injured extremity	1	
Note: The examiner acknowledges "motor, sensory and circulatory function are present and normal."		
Selects the proper splinting material	1	
Immobilizes the site of the injury	1	
Immobilizes the bone above the injured joint	1	
Immobilizes the bone below the injured joint	1	
Reassesses motor, sensory and circulatory function in the injured extremity	1	
Note: The examiner acknowledges "motor, sensory and circulatory function are present and normal."		
Total:	8	

Critical Criteria

_____ Did not support the joint so that the joint did not bear distal weight

_____ Did not immobilize the bone above and below the injured site

_____ Did not reassess motor, sensory and circulatory function in the injured extremity before and after splinting

---

SPINAL IMMOBILIZATION
SUPINE PATIENT

Start Time: _____

Stop Time: _____   Date: _____

Candidate's Name: _____

Evaluator's Name: _____

	Points Possible	Points Awarded
Takes, or verbalizes, body substance isolation precautions	1	
Directs assistant to place/maintain head in the neutral in-line position	1	
Directs assistant to maintain manual immobilization of the head	1	
Reassesses motor, sensory and circulatory function in each extremity	1	
Applies appropriately sized extrication collar	1	
Positions the immobilization device appropriately	1	
Directs movement of the patient onto the device without compromising the integrity of the spine	1	
Applies padding to voids between the torso and the board as necessary	1	
Immobilizes the patient's torso to the device	1	
Evaluates and pads behind the patient's head as necessary	1	
Immobilizes the patient's head to the device	1	
Secures the patient's legs to the device	1	
Secures the patient's arms to the device	1	
Reassesses motor, sensory and circulatory function in each extremity	1	
Total:	14	

Critical Criteria

_____ Did not immediately direct, or take, manual immobilization of the head

_____ Released, or ordered release of, manual immobilization before it was maintained mechanicall

_____ Patient manipulated, or moved excessively, causing potential spinal compromise

_____ Patient moves excessively up, down, left or right on the patient's torso

_____ Head immobilization allows for excessive movement

_____ Upon completion of immobilization, head is not in the neutral position

_____ Did not assess motor, sensory and circulatory function in each extremity after immobilization to the device

_____ Immobilized head to the board before securing the torso

IMMOBILIZATION SKILLS
LONG BONE INJURY

Start Time: _____
Stop Time: _____   Date: _____

Candidate's Name: _____

Evaluator's Name: _____

	Points Possible	Points Awarded
Takes, or verbalizes, body substance isolation precautions	1	
Directs application of manual stabilization of the injury	1	
Assesses motor, sensory and circulatory function in the injured extremity	1	
Note: The examiner acknowledges "motor, sensory and circulatory function are present and normal"		
Measures the splint	1	
Applies the splint	1	
Immobilizes the joint above the injury site	1	
Immobilizes the joint below the injury site	1	
Secures the entire injured extremity	1	
Immobilizes the hand/foot in the position of function	1	
Reassesses motor, sensory and circulatory function in the injured extremity	1	
Note: The examiner acknowledges "motor, sensory and circulatory function are present and normal"		
Total:	**10**	

Critical Criteria

_____ Grossly moves the injured extremity

_____ Did not immobilize the joint above and the joint below the injury site

_____ Did not reassess motor, sensory and circulatory function in the injured extremity before and after splinting

---

Patient Assessment/Management - Medical

Start Time: _____
Stop Time: _____   Date: _____

Candidate's Name: _____

Evaluator's Name: _____

	Points Possible	Points Awarded
Takes, or verbalizes, body substance isolation precautions	1	
SCENE SIZE-UP		
Determines the scene is safe	1	
Determines the mechanism of injury/nature of illness	1	
Determines the number of patients	1	
Requests additional help if necessary	1	
Considers stabilization of spine	1	
INITIAL ASSESSMENT		
Verbalizes general impression of the patient	1	
Determines responsiveness/level of consciousness	1	
Determines chief complaint/apparent life threats	1	
Assesses airway and breathing	Assessment	1
	Initiates appropriate oxygen therapy	1
	Assures adequate ventilation	1
Assesses circulation	Assesses/controls major bleeding	1
	Assesses pulse	1
	Assesses skin (color, temperature and condition)	1
Identifies priority patients/makes transport decision	1	

FOCUSED HISTORY AND PHYSICAL EXAMINATION/RAPID ASSESSMENT

Signs and symptoms (Assess history of present illness)

Respiratory	Cardiac	Altered Mental Status	Allergic Reaction	Poisoning/ Overdose	Environmental Emergency	Obstetrics	Behavioral		
*Onset?	*Onset?	*Description of the episode.	*History of allergies?	*Substance?	*Source?	*Are you pregnant?	*How do you feel?	1	
*Provokes?	*Provokes?	*Onset?	*What were you exposed to?	*When did you ingest/become exposed?	*Environment?	*How long have you been pregnant?	*Determine suicidal tendencies.	1	
*Quality?	*Quality?	*Duration?	*How were you exposed?	*How much did you ingest?	*Duration?	*Pain or contractions?	*Is the patient a threat to self or others?	1	
*Radiates?	*Radiates?	*Associated Symptoms?	*Effects?	*Over what time period?	*Loss of consciousness?	*Bleeding or discharge?	*Is there a medical problem?	1	
*Severity?	*Severity?	*Evidence of Trauma?	*Progression?	*Interventions?	*Effects – general or local?	*Do you feel the need to push?	*Interventions?	1	
*Time?	*Time?	*Interventions?	*Interventions?	*Estimated weight?		*Last menstrual period?		1	
*Interventions?	*Interventions?	*Seizures?							
		*Fever?							

Allergies	1	
Medications	1	
Past pertinent history	1	
Last oral intake	1	
Event leading to present illness (rule out trauma)	1	
Performs focused physical examination (assesses affected body part/system or, if indicated, completes rapid assessment)	1	
Vitals (obtains baseline vital signs)	1	
Interventions (obtains medical direction or verbalizes standing order for medication interventions and verbalizes proper additional intervention/treatment)	1	
Transport (re-evaluates the transport decision)	1	
Verbalizes the consideration for completing a detailed physical examination	1	
ONGOING ASSESSMENT (verbalized)		
Repeats initial assessment	1	
Repeats vital signs	1	
Repeats focused assessment regarding patient complaint or injuries	1	
Total:	**30**	

Critical Criteria

_____ Did not take, or verbalize, body substance isolation precautions when necessary
_____ Did not determine scene safety
_____ Did not obtain medical direction or verbalize standing orders for medical interventions
_____ Did not provide high-concentration of oxygen
_____ Did not find or manage problems associated with airway, breathing, hemorrhage or shock (hypoperfusion)
_____ Did not differentiate patient's need for transportation versus continued assessment at the scene
_____ Did detailed or focused history/physical examination before assessing the airway, breathing and circulation
_____ Did not ask questions about the present illness
_____ Administered a dangerous or inappropriate intervention

OXYGEN ADMINISTRATION

Start Time: _____   Stop Time: _____   Date: _____

Candidate's Name: _____

Evaluator's Name: _____

	Points Possible	Points Awarded
Takes, or verbalizes, body substance isolation precautions	1	
Assembles the regulator to the tank	1	
Opens the tank	1	
Checks for leaks	1	
Checks tank pressure	1	
Attaches non-rebreather mask to oxygen	1	
Prefills reservoir	1	
Adjusts liter flow to 12 liters per minute or greater	1	
Applies and adjusts the mask to the patient's face	1	
Note: The examiner must advise the candidate that the patient is not tolerating the non-rebreather mask. The medical director has ordered you to apply a nasal cannula to the patient.		
Attaches nasal cannula to oxygen	1	
Adjusts liter flow to six (6) liters per minute or less	1	
Applies nasal cannula to the patient	1	
Note: The examiner must advise the candidate to discontinue oxygen therapy		
Removes the nasal cannula from the patient	1	
Shuts off the regulator	1	
Relieves the pressure within the regulator	1	
Total:	**15**	

Critical Criteria

_____ Did not take, or verbalize, body substance isolation precautions

_____ Did not assemble the tank and regulator without leaks

_____ Did not prefill the reservoir bag

_____ Did not adjust the device to the correct liter flow for the non-rebreather mask (12 liters per minute or greater)

_____ Did not adjust the device to the correct liter flow for the nasal cannula (6 liters per minute or less)

MOUTH TO MASK WITH SUPPLEMENTAL OXYGEN

Start Time: _____   Date: _____

Stop Time: _____

Candidate's Name: _____

Evaluator's Name: _____

	Points Possible	Points Awarded
Takes, or verbalizes, body substance isolation precautions	1	
Connects one-way valve to mask	1	
Opens patient's airway or confirms patient's airway is open (manually or with adjunct)	1	
Establishes and maintains a proper mask to face seal	1	
Ventilates the patient at the proper volume and rate (800–1200 ml per breath/10-20 breaths per minute)	1	
Connects the mask to high concentration of oxygen	1	
Adjusts flow rate to at least 15 liters per minute	1	
Continues ventilation of the patient at the proper volume and rate (800–1200 ml per breath/10-20 breaths per minute)	1	
Note: The examiner must witness ventilations for at least 30 seconds		
Total:	**8**	

Critical Criteria

_____ Did not take, or verbalize, body substance isolation precautions

_____ Did not adjust liter flow to at least 15 liters per minute

_____ Did not provide proper volume per breath (more than 2 ventilations per minute were below 800 ml)

_____ Did not ventilate the patient at a rate a 10-20 breaths per minute

_____ Did not allow for complete exhalation

SPINAL IMMOBILIZATION
SEATED PATIENT

Start Time: _____

Stop Time: _____   Date: _____

Candidate's Name: _____

Evaluator's Name: _____

	Points Possible	Points Awarded
Takes, or verbalizes, body substance isolation precautions	1	
Directs assistant to place/maintain head in the neutral in-line position	1	
Directs assistant to maintain manual immobilization of the head	1	
Reassesses motor, sensory and circulatory function in each extremity	1	
Applies appropriately sized extrication collar	1	
Positions the immobilization device behind the patient	1	
Secures the device to the patient's torso	1	
Evaluates torso fixation and adjusts as necessary	1	
Evaluates and pads behind the patient's head as necessary	1	
Secures the patient's head to the device	1	
Verbalizes moving the patient to a long board	1	
Reassesses motor, sensory and circulatory function in each extremity	1	
Total:	**12**	

Critical Criteria

____ Did not immediately direct, or take, manual immobilization of the head

____ Released, or ordered release of, manual immobilization before it was maintained mechanicall

____ Patient manipulated, or moved excessively, causing potential spinal compromise

____ Device moved excessively up, down, left or right on the patient's torso

____ Head immobilization allows for excessive movement

____ Torso fixation inhibits chest rise, resulting in respiratory compromise

____ Upon completion of immobilization, head is not in the neutral position

____ Did not assess motor, sensory and circulatory function in each extremity after voicing immobilization to the long board

____ Immobilized head to the board before securing the torso

VENTILATORY MANAGEMENT
ENDOTRACHEAL INTUBATION

Start Time: _____

Stop Time: _____

Candidate's Name: _____

Date: _____

Evaluator's Name: _____

*Note: If a candidate elects to initially ventilate the patient with a BVM attached to a reservoir and oxygen, full credit must be awarded for steps denoted by "***" provided the first ventilation is delivered within the initial 30 seconds*

	Points Possible	Points Awarded
Takes of verbalizes body substance isolation precautions	1	
Opens the airway manually	1	
Elevates the patient's tongue and inserts a simple airway adjunct (oropharyngeal/nasopharyngeal airway)	1	
Note: The examiner must now inform the candidate "no gag reflex is present and the patient accepts the airway adjunct."		
** Ventilates the patient immediately using a BVM device unattached to oxygen	1	
** Hyperventilates the patient with room air	1	
Note: The examiner must now inform the candidate that ventilation is being properly performed without difficulty		
Attaches the oxygen reservoir to the BVM	1	
Attaches the BVM to high flow oxygen (15 liter per minute)	1	
Ventilates the patient at the proper volume and rate (800-1200 ml/breath and 10-20 breaths/minute)	1	
Note: After 30 seconds, the examiner must auscultate the patient's chest and inform the candidate that breath sounds are present and equal bilaterally and medical direction has ordered endotracheal intubation. The examiner must now take over ventilation of the patient.		
Directs assistant to hyper-oxygenate the patient	1	
Identifies/selects the proper equipment for endotracheal intubation	1	
Checks equipment { Checks for cuff leaks	1	
{ Checks laryngoscope operation and bulb tightness	1	
Note: The examiner must remove the OPA and move out of the way when the candidate is prepared to intubate the patient.		
Positions the patient's head properly	1	
Inserts the laryngoscope blade into the patient's mouth while displacing the patient's tongue laterally	1	
Elevates the patient's mandible with the laryngoscope	1	
Introduces the endotracheal tube and advances the tube to the proper depth	1	
Inflates the cuff to the proper pressure	1	
Disconnects the syringe from the cuff inlet port	1	
Directs assistant to ventilate the patient	1	
Confirms proper placement of the endotracheal tube by auscultation bilaterally and over the epigastrium	1	
Note: The examiner must ask, "If you had proper placement, what would you expect to hear?"		
Secures the endotracheal tube (may be verbalized)	1	
Total:	**21**	

Critical Criteria

____ Did not take or verbalize body substance isolation precautions when necessary

____ Did not initiate ventilation within 30 seconds after applying gloves or interrupts ventilations (for greater than 30 seconds at any time

____ Did not voice or provide high oxygen concentrations (15 liter/minute or greater)

____ Did not ventilate the patient at a rate of at least 10 breaths per minute

____ Did not provide adequate volume per breath (maximum of 2 errors per minute permissible)

____ Did not hyper-oxygenate the patient prior to intubation

____ Did not successfully intubate the patient within 3 attempts

____ Used the patient's teeth as a fulcrum

____ Did not assure proper tube placement by auscultation bilaterally over each lung and over the epigastrium

____ The stylette (if used) extended beyond the end of the endotracheal tube

____ Inserted any adjunct in a manner that was dangerous to the patient

____ Did not immediately disconnect the syringe from the inlet port after inflating the cuff

IMMOBILIZATION SKILLS
TRACTION SPLINTING

Start Time: _____

Stop Time: _____ Date: _____

Candidate's Name: _____

Evaluator's Name: _____

	Points Possible	Points Awarded
Takes, or verbalizes, body substance isolation precautions	1	
Directs application of manual stabilization of the injured leg	1	
Directs the application of manual traction	1	
Assesses motor, sensory and circulatory function in the injured extremity	1	
Note: The examiner acknowledges "motor, sensory and circulatory function are present and normal"		
Prepares/adjusts splint to the proper length	1	
Positions the splint next to the injured leg	1	
Applies the proximal securing device (e.g... ischial strap)	1	
Applies the distal securing device (e.g...ankle hitch)	1	
Applies mechanical traction	1	
Positions/secures the support straps	1	
Re-evaluates the proximal/distal securing devices	1	
Reassesses motor, sensory and circulatory function in the injured extremity	1	
Note: The examiner acknowledges "motor, sensory and circulatory function are present and normal"		
Note: The examiner must ask the candidate how he/she would prepare the patient for transportation		
Verbalizes securing the torso to the long board to immobilize the hip	1	
Verbalizes securing the splint to the long board to prevent movement of the splint	1	
Total:	**14**	

Critical Criteria

____ Loss of traction at any point after it was applied

____ Did not reassess motor, sensory and circulatory function in the injured extremity before and after splinting

____ The foot was excessively rotated or extended after splint was applied

____ Did not secure the ischial strap before taking traction

____ Final Immobilization failed to support the femur or prevent rotation of the injured leg

____ Secured the leg to the splint before applying mechanical traction

Note: If the Sagar splint or the Kendricks Traction Device is used without elevating the patient's leg, application of manual traction is not necessary. The candidate should be awarded one (1) point as if manual traction were applied.

Note: If the leg is elevated at all, manual traction must be applied before elevating the leg. The ankle hitch may be applied before elevating the leg and used to provide manual traction.

Patient Assessment/Management – Trauma

Start Time: _____

Stop Time: _____ Date: _____

Candidate's Name: _____

Evaluator's Name: _____

	Points Possible	Points Awarded
Takes, or verbalizes, body substance isolation precautions	1	
SCENE SIZE-UP		
Determines the scene is safe	1	
Determines the mechanism of injury	1	
Determines the number of patients	1	
Requests additional help if necessary	1	
Considers stabilization of spine	1	
INITIAL ASSESSMENT		
Verbalizes general impression of the patient	1	
Determines responsiveness/level of consciousness	1	
Determines chief complaint/apparent life threats	1	
Assesses airway and breathing — Assessment	1	
— Initiates appropriate oxygen therapy	1	
— Assures adequate ventilation	1	
— Injury management	1	
Assesses circulation — Assesses/controls major bleeding	1	
— Assesses pulse	1	
— Assesses skin (color, temperature and condition)	1	
Identifies priority patients/makes transport decision	1	
FOCUSED HISTORY AND PHYSICAL EXAMINATION/RAPID TRAUMA ASSESSMENT		
Selects appropriate assessment *(focused or rapid assessment)*	1	
Obtains, or directs assistance to obtain, baseline vital signs	1	
Obtains S.A.M.P.L.E. history	1	
DETAILED PHYSICAL EXAMINATION		
Assesses the head — Inspects and palpates the scalp and ears	1	
— Assesses the eyes	1	
— Assesses the facial areas including oral and nasal areas	1	
Assesses the neck — Inspects and palpates the neck	1	
— Assesses for JVD	1	
— Assesses for tracheal deviation	1	
Assesses the chest — Inspects	1	
— Palpates	1	
— Auscultates	1	
Assesses the abdomen/pelvis — Assesses the abdomen	1	
— Assesses the pelvis	1	
— Verbalizes assessment of genitalia/perineum as needed	1	
Assesses the extremities — 1 point for each extremity includes inspection, palpation, and assessment of motor, sensory and circulatory function	4	
Assesses the posterior — Assesses thorax	1	
— Assesses lumbar	1	
Manages secondary injuries and wounds appropriately 1 point for appropriate management of the secondary injury/wound	1	
Verbalizes re-assessment of the vital signs	1	
Total:	**40**	

Critical Criteria

____ Did not take, or verbalize, body substance isolation precautions

____ Did not determine scene safety

____ Did not assess for spinal protection

____ Did not provide for spinal protection when indicated

____ Did not provide high concentration of oxygen

____ Did not find, or manage, problems associated with airway, breathing, hemorrhage or shock (hypoperfusion)

____ Did not differentiate patient's need for transportation versus continued assessment at the scene

____ Did other detailed physical examination before assessing the airway, breathing and circulation

____ Did not transport patient within (10) minute time limit

The National Registry of Emergency Medical Technicians

EMT-Basic Practical Examination

The purpose of this checklist is to help the examination coordinator establish a quality control process for the examination and to provide the testing agency with a means of helping to assure standardization of practical examinations. To achieve this, the examination coordinator, or designee, must personally oversee or observe the various components of the examination as presented in this checklist. As each control criterion is completed, a check should be placed in the space provided. If a check is not placed in the space provided, an explanation why that criterion was not met should be listed on the reverse side of this checklist. This checklist should be completed and signed by the examination coordinator before an examination is accepted for credit by the testing agency.

Examination Site: _____   Examination Date: _____

A. ORGANIZATION OF THE EXAMINATION
- ☐ Established a minimum of six (6) examination skill stations
- ☐ Scheduled the appropriate number of qualified skill station examiners
- ☐ Registered and identified candidates to assure eligibility to participate in the examination
- ☐ Reviewed qualification of skill station examiners prior to the examination

B. FACILITIES
- ☐ Skill stations had adequate room to conduct the examination without interference
- ☐ Equipment was in working order
- ☐ An adequate variety of equipment was provided

C. SKILL STATION EXAMINERS
- ☐ Read and understood their role in the examination process
- ☐ Remained objective in recording each candidate's performance
- ☐ Did not introduce extraneous elements into the skill station
- ☐ Read the "Instructions to the Practical Skills Candidate" to each individual tested
- ☐ Did not show preference toward any agency or individual for any reason

D. ORIENTATION OF CANDIDATES AND SKILL STATION EXAMINERS
- ☐ Read the standardized orientation script clearly and completely
- ☐ Allowed adequate time for candidates to ask questions concerning the examination
- ☐ Oriented programmed patients and EMT assistance as required

E. CANDIDATES
- ☐ Were instructed concerning the practical examination retest policy
- ☐ Were instructed concerning the process for filing an official complaint

F. SCORING THE PERFORMANCE
- ☐ Used proper criteria for determining the final grade of the candidate
- ☐ Recorded the overall grade on the Practical Examination Report Form

By virtue of my signature and completion of this checklist, I attest to the fact that this examination was organized and administered according to standards established by

_____
Signature Examination Coordinator

_____
Signature Medical Director

The National Registry of Emergency Medical Technicians

EMT-Basic Practical Examination Report Form

Examination Attempt	
Initial Attempt	
1st Retest	
2nd Retest	

Overall Score	
Pass	
Fail	
Retest	

Name _____ _____ _____
     Last Name   First Name   Middle Initial

Address _____ _____ _____ _____
        Street   City   State   Zip Code

Exam Site: _____   Date: _____

		Pass	Fail
Station #1	Patient Assessment/Management - Trauma	Pass	Fail
Station #2	Patient Assessment/Management - Medical	Pass	Fail
Station #3	Cardiac Arrest Management/AED	Pass	Fail
Station #4	Bag-Valve-Mask Apneic Patient	Pass	Fail
Station #5	Spinal Immobilization (Specify) Seated/Supine	Pass	Fail
Station #6	Random Skill Verification (Specify)	Pass	Fail

Examination Coordinator: _____
                                    Signature

Physician Medical Director: _____
                                    Signature

Candidates failing three (3) or less stations are eligible for a same day retest of the skills failed. Failing a same day retest will require the candidate to retest only those skills failed at a different site with a different examiner. Failure of the retest attempt at a different site and with a different examiner constitutes a complete failure of the practical examination. A candidate is allowed to test a single skill a maximum of three (3) times before he/she must retest the entire practical examination. Failing four (4) or more stations, constitutes a complete failure of the practical examination. Any complete failure of the practical examination will require the candidate to document remedial training over all skills before re-attempting all stations of the practical examination.

Remarks: _____

Appendix B

Registry Review

These review questions are designed to help you assess your knowledge of the principles of emergency medical care, as discussed in *Emergency Care and Transportation of the Sick and Injured, Seventh Edition*. The questions are not endorsed by the National Registry of Emergency Medical Technicians.

appendix b

1. Which of the following statements about a child's respiratory system is true?

   A. Children depend less heavily on the diaphragm for breathing.
   B. Infants younger than 1 month are able to breathe through the mouth.
   C. The larynx and cricoid cartilage are smaller and softer than that of an adult.
   D. The tongue takes up less space in a child's mouth than in an adult's mouth.

2. As an EMT-B, your first responsibility at the scene of a sudden illness or injury is:

   A. sorting patients based on the degree of illness or injury.
   B. maintaining the airway of an unconscious patient.
   C. your safety and the safety of others.
   D. removing trapped patients.

3. When trying to manage a disruptive patient, you should:

   A. turn your back on the patient to show that you are not a threat.
   B. attempt to disarm the patient yourself if the patient has a gun or knife.
   C. leave the patient alone for a few minutes to think about the situation.
   D. keep your eyes on the patient at all times and be alert for aggressive behavior.

4. The normal pulse rate for a child is approximately how many beats per minute?

   A. 60 to 100
   B. 80 to 100
   C. 100 to 120
   D. 100 plus the child's age

5. You are called to a restaurant where a woman who is at least 8 months pregnant is choking on a piece of meat. She is grasping her throat and coughing as she tries to breathe. What information about the patient is most important in determining whether she has a complete airway obstruction or a partial airway obstruction?

   A. She is grasping her throat.
   B. Audible coughing is noted.
   C. The foreign body is meat.
   D. The pregnancy is almost full term.

6. Orders communicated to the EMT-B in the form of standing orders, protocols, or SMOPs are known as:

   A. on-line medical direction.
   B. off-line medical direction.
   C. general medical orders.
   D. specific medical orders.

7. A conscious and alert woman who has severe abdominal pain refuses to go to the hospital. Her husband asks you to transport the patient regardless of her wishes. The most appropriate course of action would be to:

   A. respect the patient's wishes.
   B. transport the patient because her husband requests it.
   C. transport the patient because her condition warrants it.
   D. explain to the husband that transport is not needed because the patient's condition is not life threatening.

8. When assessing a patient's knee, you would NOT expect to find:

   A. swelling.
   B. bruising.
   C. paradoxical motion.
   D. loss of motor function.

9. To protect yourself from exposure to blood or other body fluids while in the field, you must wear:

   A. an oxygen mask.
   B. gloves and eye protection.
   C. full turnout gear and an SCBA.
   D. three protective layers of clothing.

10. The Critical Incident Stress Debriefing (CISD) program is designed to help:

    A. families deal with the sudden death of a loved one.
    B. law enforcement officials interview victims of a crime.
    C. law enforcement officials interview witnesses to a crime.
    D. emergency medical personnel cope with personal and group anxieties and stress.

appendix b

11. Chest compressions on a 3-year-old patient should be performed at a depth and rate of:

    A. $1/2''$ to $1''$, at a rate of 140/min.
    B. $1''$ to $1^1/2''$, at a rate of 100/min.
    C. $1''$ to $2''$, at a rate of 60 to 80/min.
    D. $3/4''$ to $2''$, at a rate of 100 to 120/min.

12. A local celebrity has severe injuries as a result of an automobile-truck accident. The highway is closed by law enforcement officials, but the media is allowed to cover the story. A reporter approaches you and asks the condition of the patient. You should:

    A. ignore the reporter.
    B. answer the reporter's questions as best you can.
    C. tell the reporter the patient will be fine to protect his privacy.
    D. explain that you cannot comment and that the reporter should contact the hospital.

13. Gastric distention during artificial ventilation is considered dangerous because it can:

    A. stimulate hyperventilation.
    B. result in bacterial pneumonia.
    C. cause the patient to vomit during CPR.
    D. increase lung volume by elevating the diaphragm.

14. The best way to estimate a patient's skin temperature is to use the:

    A. back of your hand.
    B. tips of your fingers.
    C. palm of your hand.
    D. index and middle fingers.

15. The state of the pupils is a rapid reflection of:

    A. circulation.
    B. blood pressure.
    C. retinal pressure.
    D. central nervous system injury or disease.

16. Which of the following is NOT an acceptable reason for you to stop CPR once you have started?

    A. The patient starts breathing and you feel a pulse.
    B. You are too fatigued and exhausted to continue any longer.
    C. A bystander tells you that the patient may have a living will.
    D. A physician at the scene assumes responsibility and tells you to stop.

17. In most instances, cardiac arrest in infants and children results from:

    A. electrocution.
    B. respiratory arrest.
    C. severe head trauma.
    D. severe hypothermia.

18. In which of the following situations has expressed consent been given?

    A. A 5-year-old child who says, "Make me better"
    B. An unconscious 26-year-old woman who has a bleeding head wound
    C. A 35-year-old man who has a slight concussion but holds his bleeding arm out for bandaging
    D. An 86-year-old man who stares blankly at his bleeding leg and says, "What happened to me?"

19. Which of the following signs is seen in respiratory depression?

    A. Rapid, shallow respirations
    B. Deep, labored, noisy respirations
    C. Strong airflow at the nose and mouth
    D. Little or no movement of the chest and abdomen

20. If an injured patient needs to be moved, but is not in immediate danger from fire or building collapse, you should first:

    A. determine the number of people you will need to help move the patient.
    B. remove the patient with the Rapid Extrication technique.
    C. check the patient's airway, breathing, and circulation.
    D. order the equipment you will need for extrication.

21. When you are dealing with an emotionally disturbed patient, the best legal situation is to:

    A. always transport the patient with restraints.
    B. try to obtain the patient's consent to medical treatment.
    C. have law enforcement restrain the patient with police-type handcuffs.
    D. allow the patient to refuse treatment when the patient presents a threat to self or others.

22. A woman in labor appears to have a part of the umbilical cord protruding from the vagina. You should first place the woman in Trendelenburg's position, and then carefully:

    A. push the cord back into the vagina and provide prompt transport.
    B. push the baby's head back into the vagina and provide prompt transport.
    C. moisten the cord with sterile saline solution and provide prompt transport.
    D. insert your gloved finger into the vagina and gently push the baby's head away from the umbilical cord.

23. The usual dosage of activated charcoal for a child is how many grams per kilogram of body weight?

    A. 1
    B. 2
    C. 3
    D. 5

24. An 8-year-old boy has a deep cut on his arm with severe bright red bleeding. You have tried to contact the parents, but they cannot be reached. Your next step would be to:

    A. phone the emergency department physician and ask for permission to proceed with treatment.
    B. take the boy to the emergency department but give no treatment.
    C. ask the police for permission to proceed with treatment.
    D. assume the parents would give consent for treatment.

25. A patient who is lying on the ground with his left leg bent out to the side appears to have a deformed knee. He is in extreme pain and states that he cannot move the leg. On assessment, you find that the patient has strong distal pulses. You should prepare the patient for transport by:

    A. wrapping the leg with a pillow.
    B. splinting the leg in the position in which it is found.
    C. straightening the leg and applying and inflating an air splint.
    D. straightening the leg and applying two standard rigid leg splints.

26. Normal systolic blood pressure in an adult male patient is approximately:

    A. 90 mm Hg plus the patient's age, up to 150 mm Hg.
    B. 95 mm Hg plus the patient's age, up to 150 mm Hg.
    C. 100 mm Hg plus the patient's age, up to 150 mm Hg.
    D. 105 mm Hg plus the patient's age, up to 150 mm Hg.

27. When evaluating respirations, you should observe and record the:

    A. rate, quality, and rhythm.
    B. rate and amount of oxygen exhaled.
    C. rate and amount of carbon dioxide exhaled.
    D. number of breaths in a 60-second period and multiply by 2.

28. What is the single most important measure, outside of wearing PPE, for controlling risk of exposure to communicable disease?

    A. Handwashing
    B. Taking antibiotics
    C. Disinfecting with alcohol
    D. Ensuring immunizations are up to date

29. Signs that a conscious patient is not breathing well include all of the following EXCEPT:

    A. cool, damp skin.
    B. pale or cyanotic skin.
    C. slowing of the heart rate.
    D. muscle retractions above the clavicles and between the ribs.

30. You are on the first ambulance to reach a multiple-casualty scene. As the most experienced EMT-B on the team, you serve as triage officer. You identify one critical patient and other less severely injured patients. When the next ambulance reaches the scene, you should:

    A. assign the critical patient to the second ambulance and accompany him or her on the transport.
    B. immediately transport the critical patient and transfer triage duties to the officer on the second ambulance.
    C. assign the critical patient to the second ambulance; once the critical patient is removed, you can eliminate the role of triage officer.
    D. assign the critical patient to the second ambulance, keep any extra personnel at the scene to help, and continue as triage officer.

31. What happens to the pressure inside the chest at the onset of inhalation?

   A. It increases.
   B. It decreases.
   C. It remains the same.
   D. It is always equal to atmospheric pressure.

32. A man is found sitting behind the steering wheel after an accident. He has a painful, deformed lower right leg and an open wound to his right forearm. Your care of him should include:

   A. giving him oxygen, then moving him to the ambulance and providing transport.
   B. moving him to the ambulance, then bandaging the wound and splinting the leg.
   C. applying a traction splint to the leg injury before moving him to the ambulance.
   D. performing an initial assessment and stabilizing his vital functions before extrication begins.

33. The normal respiratory rate for an infant is approximately how many breaths per minute?

   A. 6 to 12
   B. 12 to 20
   C. 15 to 30
   D. 25 to 50

34. Which of the following terms is described as an audible high-pitched breath sound that usually results from a blockage of the smaller air passages?

   A. Stridor
   B. Wheezing
   C. Exhalation
   D. Rales

35. Which of the following statements about using a bag-valve-mask (BVM) device is true?

   A. One-person BVM is more effective than two-person BVM.
   B. Two-person BVM is more effective than one-person BVM.
   C. You should try to deflate the bag simultaneously with the patient's expiratory effort.
   D. When using the BVM device with chest compressions, you should ventilate twice after every fifth compression.

36. A properly sized oropharyngeal airway should:

   A. be the same size as the little finger.
   B. reach from the nose to the forehead.
   C. reach from the lips to the epiglottis.
   D. reach from the earlobe to the corner of the mouth.

37. A man is found unconscious and slumped over the steering wheel after an automobile accident. He regains consciousness and is not able to feel pain in his legs and feet. This finding suggests that the:

   A. patient has a hematoma.
   B. spinal cord has been injured.
   C. cervical spine has been displaced.
   D. back has not been seriously injured.

38. Your patient is a 4-month-old infant who is awake but appears to be listless and has dry, tented skin. His mother states that he has had a 3-day history of diarrhea. Your treatment should include:

   A. giving two baby bottles of water.
   B. providing prompt transport.
   C. giving oxygen with a nonbreathing face mask at 4 L/min.
   D. helping the mother give the infant 2 tablespoons of an antidiarrheal medication.

39. How many seconds should your breaths last when you are using mouth-to-mouth breathing to ventilate a patient?

   A. $1\frac{1}{2}$ to 2
   B. 2 to $2\frac{1}{2}$
   C. $2\frac{1}{2}$ to 3
   D. 3 to $3\frac{1}{2}$

40. Artificial ventilation for a patient involved in a near-drowning accident should begin as soon as the patient is:

   A. positioned faceup.
   B. moved into the ambulance.
   C. pulled from the water and placed on a firm surface.
   D. pulled from the water and placed on a spine board.

41. You are assisting at an emergency home delivery, and the baby's head is delivered still covered by the membranes of the unruptured amniotic sac. What should you do next?

   A. Wait for the sac to break on its own, then clear the baby's nose and mouth.
   B. Leave the sac intact, monitor the baby's vital signs, and provide immediate transport.
   C. Immediately, but carefully, puncture the sac with your gloved fingers, a sterile clamp, or scissors, and clear the baby's nose and mouth.
   D. Wait until the delivery is complete, carefully puncture the sac with your gloved fingers, a sterile clamp, or scissors, and clear the baby's nose and mouth.

42. You are called to the home of a woman who has frostbite. Upon arrival, you find that she is in her warm house, but there is a snowstorm outside. The nearest hospital is one hour away. In this situation, treatment should consist of:

   A. rubbing the affected area with snow.
   B. rubbing the affected area with your warm hands.
   C. attempting active, rapid rewarming.
   D. immersing the affected area in a cold water bath.

43. An unconscious patient with possible spinal injuries seems to have trouble breathing. The patient's chest wall is moving only slightly, but the diaphragm is moving in and out with each breath. These findings suggest that the patient:

   A. needs CPR immediately.
   B. needs supplemental oxygen immediately, and possibly assisted ventilations.
   C. should be placed in Trendelenburg's position to increase blood flow to the heart.
   D. is breathing normally following trauma, but requires immediate transport.

44. Respiratory distress in a child is suggested by all of the following EXCEPT:

   A. screaming.
   B. nasal flaring.
   C. active exhalation.
   D. seesaw respirations.

45. Assessment of a patient with low blood glucose is most likely to reveal which of the following findings?

   A. Salivation, sweating, and diarrhea
   B. Nausea, vomiting, and abdominal pain
   C. Decreased mental status and convulsions
   D. Agitation, mood swings, and cardiac abnormalities

46. A suspected fractured elbow should be immobilized in the position in which it is found because movement may result in:

   A. further injury to the bone.
   B. damage to nerves and blood vessels.
   C. unnecessary increase in pain to the patient.
   D. a separation or dislocation of the elbow joint.

47. You are called to a construction site and find a construction worker buried to midchest in mud from a trench cave-in. Other workers are trying to dig him out. The patient is cyanotic, has a pulse of 128/min, and shallow respirations of 30/min. Given the patient's vital signs, which of the following supplemental oxygen devices would be most appropriate at this time?

   A. Nasal cannula
   B. Simple face mask
   C. Nonrebreathing mask
   D. Bag-valve-mask device

48. You are called to the home of a child who has been injured in a bicycle accident. Upon arrival, you find the child sitting on the porch of his house, about 25' from the accident site. He tells you he skidded on some sand and then fell off the bicycle. He remembers everything that happened and says that he only hurt his knee. You note an abrasion on the knee with a small amount of bleeding. Given the circumstances in this situation, your first concern when assessing the patient is to:

   A. splint the knee injury.
   B. check the capillary refill in the injured extremity.
   C. find and treat all injuries in the order you find them.
   D. focus on finding and treating the most life-threatening injuries.

49. A man is conscious and alert after an automobile accident in which he was the driver. He states that his fingers are tingling and that his shoulders hurt. Your assessment should include:

   A. gently feeling along the spine for any point tenderness.
   B. gently moving the patient's arms, legs, and shoulders to determine the severity of his pain.
   C. asking the patient to move his head from side to side to determine if he has neck pain.
   D. asking the patient to roll and shrug his shoulders in an attempt to determine the severity of his pain.

50. Which of the following is the method of choice for providing artificial ventilation?

   A. Mouth-to-mask ventilation
   B. One-person bag-valve-mask
   C. Two-person bag-valve-mask
   D. Oxygen-powered manually triggered breathing device

51. A teenage boy is successfully resuscitated at the scene after a near-drowning accident. Your next step in caring for the patient is to:

    A. take the patient home.
    B. provide transport to the hospital.
    C. provide transport to the patient's doctor.
    D. advise him to visit his own doctor as soon as possible.

52. When evaluating a patient who complains of a painful left leg, your detailed physical exam should include assessing:

    A. skin color, temperature, and moisture.
    B. distal pulse rate, sensation, and motor function.
    C. skin color, distal pulse rate, and skin temperature.
    D. deformity, proximal pulse rate, and ability to move.

53. Which of the following is considered a significant mechanism of injury for a child?

    A. A bicycle collision
    B. A fall from higher than 5'
    C. A slow-speed vehicle collision
    D. An abrasion injury of the abdomen

54. A woman appears to have fractures of the left leg and arm as a result of a head-on collision. The patient is conscious and states that her "stomach hurts." During your assessment, you notice a bloody discharge from the urethral area. You should prepare the patient for transport by immobilizing her on a:

    A. long spine board.
    B. long spine board with a PASG in place.
    C. stretcher, with her leg and arm supported with pillows.
    D. stretcher, with her leg in a traction splint and her arm in a sling.

55. The chance to save a patient experiencing cardiac arrest from VF is greater if:

    A. CPR is initiated within 10 minutes.
    B. oxygen and rapid transport are provided.
    C. rapid transport to the hospital is provided.
    D. defibrillation or CPR is initiated within 4 minutes.

56. Your primary responsibility in the initial management of a disruptive patient is to:

    A. make a specific diagnosis.
    B. lecture the patient about the dangers of substance abuse.
    C. take charge of the situation, but protect yourself if necessary.
    D. play along with the patient if he or she sees or hears things that are not real.

57. A man is found unconscious in his car with the window open. His face is severely swollen and he is barely breathing. A law enforcement officer at the scene tells you that he saw the man's car slow down and then park at the side of the road. You should first:

    A. search for an epinephrine kit in the car.
    B. give oxygen and perform an initial assessment.
    C. place cool compresses on his face and provide immediate transport.
    D. check the patient for an embedded insect stinger and then pull it out before providing transport.

58. The primary purpose of the scene size-up is to:

    A. verify if news media have arrived.
    B. ensure the well-being of the EMT-B.
    C. get names and addresses of witnesses.
    D. determine the patient's respiratory rate.

59. Any order from medical control should be:

    A. automatically questioned.
    B. followed immediately as stated.
    C. repeated back word for word and confirmed.
    D. discussed with your partner to ascertain its accuracy.

60. Which of the following statements about the prehospital care report is true?

    A. It is only valuable as a legal document.
    B. It cannot be used for patient billing information.
    C. It helps ensure efficient continuity of patient care.
    D. It is only for the prehospital care provider's information.

61. What is the most important first step when dealing with a patient having a heart attack?

    A. Starting an IV
    B. Initiating CPR
    C. Performing defibrillation
    D. Showing support and a caring attitude

62. Which of the following parts of the body deteriorates the fastest without constant perfusion?

   A. Heart
   B. Liver
   C. Kidneys
   D. Skeletal muscle

63. A patient has severe bleeding from a chest wound, and no dressing or bandage is available. The most appropriate action in this case would be to:

   A. use a pressure point.
   B. use your gloved hand to apply direct pressure.
   C. quickly try to find a bandage, clean cloth, or sanitary napkin.
   D. wash your bare hand with soap and then apply direct pressure.

64. Altered mental status that often accompanies diabetic emergencies is often mistaken for:

   A. a migraine.
   B. alcohol intoxication.
   C. a severed spinal cord.
   D. a swollen or deformed lower extremity.

65. A 5-year-old child requires full spinal immobilization after falling from a tree. As the child is log rolled onto the backboard, you should:

   A. place blanket rolls under the child's knees to prevent the legs from moving.
   B. place a small pillow under the child's head to prevent hyperextension of the neck.
   C. place a rolled towel under the child's neck to prevent hyperextension of the neck.
   D. place padding between the shoulders and the backboard to prevent hyperflexion of the neck.

66. When ventilating a patient with a bag-valve-mask device, you should squeeze the bag until:

   A. it is empty.
   B. the patient's chest rises.
   C. 100% oxygen is delivered.
   D. the patient has spontaneous respirations.

67. A mass-casualty plan should be activated when:

   A. there is more than one patient.
   B. there are as many patients as EMT-Bs.
   C. an incident occurs on a weekend or holiday.
   D. patient needs are greater than the available resources.

68. If use of an AED is indicated and the patient has a pacemaker, you should:

   A. not defibrillate the patient.
   B. place both pads near the pacemaker.
   C. avoid placing the pads over the pacemaker.
   D. place one pad over the pacemaker and the other on the left side of the back.

69. Treatment of a patient who is hyperventilating should include:

   A. reassuring the patient and providing prompt transport.
   B. having the patient breathe into a bag without providing transport.
   C. giving oxygen, having the patient breathe into a bag, and providing transport.
   D. having the patient breathe into a bag, giving reassurance, and providing transport.

70. Chest compressions on a 9-month-old patient should be performed at a depth and rate of:

   A. 1/4" to 1/2", at a rate of 140/min.
   B. 1/2" to 1", at a rate of 100/min.
   C. 1" to 1 1/2", at a rate of 80 to 100/min.
   D. 1 1/2" to 2", at a rate of 100 to 120/min.

71. You are called to care for a patient in respiratory distress. He is breathing noisily and coughing. You should consider that the patient is experiencing:

   A. gastric distention.
   B. a cyanotic episode.
   C. a partial airway obstruction.
   D. a complete airway obstruction.

72. The size of the nasopharyngeal airway is determined by measuring from the:

   A. lips to the angle of the jaw.
   B. chin to the angle of the jaw.
   C. tip of the nose to the earlobe.
   D. incisors to the base of the tongue.

73. For the purpose of administering CPR, patients classified as children are between the ages of:

   A. 1 and 3 years.
   B. 1 and 8 years.
   C. 2 and 12 years.
   D. 3 and 6 years.

74. The first question to ask yourself at the scene of a train or bus accident is:

   A. "How severe are the patients' injuries?"
   B. "How many patients are there?"
   C. "What caused the crash?"
   D. "Who will do the triage?"

appendix b

75. You have been called to the scene of an automobile accident. You should park the ambulance:

    A. alongside the accident site.
    B. 25' from the accident site on the same side of the street.
    C. 50' from the accident site on the opposite side of the street.
    D. 100' from the accident site on the same side of the street.

76. A man is found slumped over the steering wheel, unconscious and making "snoring" sounds, after an automobile accident. The patient's head is turned to the side, and his neck is flexed. The first steps in caring for this patient would be to secure the airway and then:

    A. rotate the head to correct the deformity.
    B. splint the head in the position you found it.
    C. hyperextend the neck to correct the deformity.
    D. attempt manual stabilization and move the head to a neutral, in-line position.

77. During the first stage of labor, you should usually:

    A. prepare for an emergency delivery at home.
    B. have time to transport the woman to the hospital.
    C. help the woman walk around between contractions.
    D. hold the woman's legs together to slow down delivery.

78. The best way to gain the confidence of and effectively communicate with a frightened patient is to:

    A. shout at the patient.
    B. use medical terminology.
    C. let the patient have some time alone.
    D. make and keep eye contact with the patient.

79. If a life-threatening condition, such as an airway obstruction, is found during assessment, you should:

    A. assess the patient's circulation next.
    B. note it and continue the assessment.
    C. give priority to emergency care of the ABCD.
    D. abandon the assessment and transport the patient immediately.

80. Pale skin generally suggests which of the following underlying problems?

    A. Heat cramps
    B. Poor oxygenation
    C. Liver abnormalities
    D. Inadequate circulation

81. The treatment of partial-thickness burns on the legs of a child should include:

    A. giving oxygen with a nasal cannula at 2 L/min.
    B. covering the burn with dry bandages and clean sheets.
    C. putting the child in ice water to stop the burning process.
    D. asking the caregiver for butter to cover the burn.

82. What are the two main purposes of the oropharyngeal airway?

    A. Prevents airway obstruction and eases suctioning
    B. Prevents airway injury and eases suctioning
    C. Prevents airway obstruction and tachycardia
    D. Prevents aspiration and airway obstruction

83. Which of the following is NOT considered a link in the Chain of Survival?

    A. BLS
    B. ACLS
    C. Rapid transport
    D. Early defibrillation

84. A splint is applied to a patient with a fractured elbow. Five minutes later, the radial pulse in the injured arm is very weak, and the patient states that he has no feeling in the arm. Because the nearest hospital is 30 minutes away, the appropriate course of action would be to:

    A. transport the patient immediately.
    B. position the splinted arm lower than the patient's body.
    C. position the splinted arm higher than the patient's body.
    D. contact medical control for a decision on realigning the limb.

85. Cardiac arrest in children is usually preceded by respiratory arrest, because children:

    A. have large, overdeveloped lungs.
    B. often have long-term, chronic diseases.
    C. consume oxygen two to three times faster than adults.
    D. do not consume much oxygen due to their slower heart rate.

86. Assessment of the patient's airway begins with:

    A. assisting ventilations.
    B. checking capillary perfusion.
    C. noting skin color and temperature.
    D. noting how well the patient responds to the question, "Are you okay?"

87. The use of oxygen in treatment of shock is considered to be:

    A. a routine part of treatment.
    B. of no particular benefit to the patient.
    C. a last resort measure if all other treatment fails.
    D. useful only if the patient has difficulty breathing.

88. As you open the airway of an elderly man who is not breathing, you do not feel, hear, or see any air exchange. You deliver two quick breaths, mouth-to-mask. The patient's chest does not rise, and your breaths meet no resistance, but the patient's stomach inflates with each breath. Your attempts at rescue breathing have not been effective most likely because the:

    A. patient has had a laryngectomy, and the breaths are exiting via the stoma.
    B. patient has an open pneumothorax, and the breaths are exiting via the wound.
    C. seal around the mask is inadequate, and the air is leaking out around the patient's cheeks.
    D. rescue breaths are too fast or too strong, and the air is being forced into the patient's stomach.

89. A 53-year-old man leaps from a third floor apartment window to escape a fire. The man tumbles in midair, but manages to land on his feet. The most appropriate course of action is to first:

    A. assess the patient thoroughly for third-degree burns.
    B. assess and treat the patient for possible lower extremity and spinal fractures.
    C. treat any serious cuts and burns, then transport the patient to the hospital.
    D. ask the patient to come over to the ambulance immediately so he can be examined.

90. If the patient is pulseless and the AED recommends no shock, you should next:

    A. restart CPR.
    B. shock anyway.
    C. provide immediate transport.
    D. provide transport and deliver three stacked shocks en route.

91. The first step in caring for a patient who has an airway obstruction without spinal injury is to:

    A. apply a cervical collar.
    B. activate the EMS system.
    C. perform CPR and give supplemental oxygen.
    D. open the mouth using the head-tilt/chin-lift maneuver.

92. A woman has frostbite in both feet after walking several miles in a frozen field. Her feet are white, hard, and cold to touch. Treatment at the scene should include:

    A. rubbing her feet gently with your own warm hands.
    B. trying to restore circulation by helping her walk around.
    C. removing her wet clothing and rubbing her feet briskly with a warm, wet cloth.
    D. removing her wet clothing and covering her feet with dry, sterile dressings.

93. A general impression of a patient is formed to determine:

    A. scene safety.
    B. treatment priority.
    C. transport speed.
    D. response speed.

94. You and your partner are called to the scene of a possible crime. Upon arrival, you find one dead patient and one seriously injured patient. Law enforcement is present. Your initial responsibilities include:

    A. protecting the scene and securing potential evidence.
    B. witnessing bystander statements and assisting law enforcement.
    C. protecting yourself and your partner and providing emergency medical care.
    D. assisting law enforcement with crowd control and providing emergency medical care.

95. You are called to the scene of an accident in which a car with a lone driver has hit a utility pole. Witnesses say that the accident just happened. The driver is not breathing, has no carotid pulse, and has widely dilated pupils. The driver is also being held in an upright position by the steering wheel. An extrication team has been called. To stabilize the patient's vital functions before extrication begins, your first step should be to:

    A. give high-flow oxygen.
    B. gently shake the patient to awaken him.
    C. establish and maintain an open airway.
    D. apply direct pressure to control bleeding.

96. A man trips and falls down a flight of stairs. Upon your arrival, he does not respond to your greeting or questions. The most appropriate initial course of action would be to treat the patient as if he has had a:

    A. spinal injury.
    B. diabetic emergency.
    C. fractured extremity.
    D. reaction to medication.

97. You suspect that a 17-year-old boy has dislocated his shoulder in a game of touch football. The patient is in extreme pain and shouts for you to "do something." Your first step in caring for the patient should be to:

    A. give him pain medication.
    B. give him supplemental oxygen.
    C. immobilize the shoulder in the position you found it.
    D. attempt to reduce the shoulder or "put it back in place."

98. When communicating with an elderly patient, you should:

    A. approach the patient slowly and calmly.
    B. avoid the patient and speak only to family members.
    C. step back to avoid making the patient uncomfortable.
    D. raise your voice to ensure that the patient can hear you.

99. Which of the following conditions can occur if an unconscious patient is given oral glucose?

    A. Shock
    B. Aspiration
    C. Hypotension
    D. Hyperglycemia

100. A man has an open, bleeding gash on his forehead after an automobile accident. To control the bleeding, you should apply:

    A. pressure to the carotid artery.
    B. pressure to the subclavian artery.
    C. a sterile dressing with a snug bandage.
    D. a sterile dressing with a loose bandage.

101. The first step in the management of a patient exhibiting disruptive behavior is to:

    A. call the police.
    B. assess the situation.
    C. give supplemental oxygen.
    D. notify the emergency department.

102. Which pulse should you palpate in an infant to assess the quality of the pulse?

    A. Radial
    B. Carotid
    C. Brachial
    D. Popliteal

103. A teenage girl states that she was stung on the arm and that she knows she is allergic to bee stings. You see a raised, white area on the arm at the site of the sting. To slow the spread of the toxin, you should place which of the following directly over the site?

    A. A cold pack
    B. A warm compress
    C. A constricting band
    D. A saline-moistened dressing

104. Premature ventricular contractions may occur when the heart:

    A. needs to beat faster.
    B. requires less oxygen.
    C. receives too much blood.
    D. does not receive enough oxygen.

105. The treatment of hypothermia in the field should include:

    A. preventing blood loss.
    B. massaging the patient's extremities.
    C. giving the patient hot coffee to drink.
    D. stabilizing the vital signs and preventing further heat loss.

106. You are at the scene of a hazardous materials incident and are outside of the hazard zone you have established. The HazMat team has not yet arrived. An unconscious patient is lying in the danger area, and the wind is blowing from behind you toward the scene and beyond. You should:

    A. stay upwind of the materials, but remain on site.
    B. evacuate the area and await the arrival of the HazMat team.
    C. enter the zone rapidly with the wind at your back, and quickly remove the patient.
    D. approach the patient and provide only lifesaving care until the HazMat team can arrive and decontaminate you both.

107. What is the most serious underlying problem that must be addressed during the initial assessment of a patient with a severe facial injury?

    A. Fracture of facial bones
    B. Injury to the lumbar spine
    C. Possible hypovolemic shock
    D. Partial or complete upper airway obstruction

108. Nitroglycerin helps a patient with chest pain by:

    A. causing coronary vasoconstriction.
    B. increasing the blood pressure.
    C. dilating the coronary arteries.
    D. relieving anxiety.

109. A 3-year-old child is found at the bottom of an ice-covered pond after being submerged for about 15 minutes. The patient is not breathing and has no palpable pulse. The most appropriate course of action would be to:

    A. pronounce the child dead.
    B. begin full resuscitation efforts.
    C. wrap the child in blankets and give back blows.
    D. give supplemental oxygen and begin rewarming.

110. How does the heart get more blood when it is working hard?

    A. The aorta constricts.
    B. The heart beats faster.
    C. The coronary arteries dilate.
    D. The pulmonary vascular resistance increases.

111. The first step in treating a patient with a head injury is to:

    A. control bleeding.
    B. immobilize the patient's head.
    C. establish and maintain an airway.
    D. check for and stabilize any cervical spine injuries.

112. You are ventilating a patient with a stoma and air is escaping from the mouth and nose. To prevent this, you should:

    A. use less pressure.
    B. suction the stoma.
    C. suction the breathing tube.
    D. seal the mouth and pinch the nostrils.

113. Assessment of a patient whose core temperature has dropped to 95°F (35°C) is most likely to reveal which of the following findings?

    A. Rigid muscles
    B. Rapid pulse rate
    C. Impaired judgment
    D. Decreased level of consciousness

114. Which of the following conditions is considered the most serious?

    A. Asystole
    B. Atrial fibrillation
    C. Ventricular fibrillation
    D. Ventricular tachycardia

115. Use of a police escort may be a dangerous practice in an intersection because:

    A. bystanders could gather to watch and cause traffic problems.
    B. too many emergency vehicles with sirens and lights could cause motorists to panic.
    C. trying to move two emergency vehicles through congested traffic is more difficult than one and may take much time.
    D. a motorist seeing the police car pass might assume it is the only emergency vehicle and could proceed, hitting the ambulance.

116. Your care of a premature baby should include:

    A. keeping the baby cool.
    B. removing the clamp on the umbilical cord.
    C. keeping the mouth and nose clear of mucus.
    D. directing a stream of oxygen directly into the baby's mouth.

117. A young boy with a severe soft-tissue injury to the leg has rather extensive bleeding, which has frightened him. The best way to control the bleeding in this situation is to apply:

    A. a conventional tourniquet.
    B. pressure to the femoral artery.
    C. direct pressure with a dry, sterile dressing.
    D. a blood pressure cuff to act as a tourniquet.

118. The proper way to perform chest compressions on an infant is with:

    A. two fingers placed on the xiphoid process.
    B. two fingers placed on the lower half of the sternum.
    C. the heel of one hand placed at midsternum.
    D. the heel of one hand placed on the lower sternum.

119. A woman who is having her third baby tells you she must move her bowels. The most appropriate step would be to:

    A. provide prompt transport because there is still plenty of time before the delivery.
    B. ask her if she is about to deliver, and if she says no, provide prompt transport.
    C. provide immediate transport because it is always safer to deliver at the hospital.
    D. prepare to deliver the baby at the scene, because delivery is about to occur.

120. When obtaining a history from a diabetic patient, you should ask which of the following questions in addition to the SAMPLE history?

    A. "Are you allergic to insulin?"
    B. "What kind of insulin do you take?"
    C. "Have you taken your insulin today?"
    D. "How long have you been a diabetic?"

121. A small car crashes into a utility pole, resulting in two power lines falling over the car. A woman is lying partially out of the car with one leg on the ground. After the fire department removes her from the car, you begin cardiac monitoring and confirm that she is in ventricular fibrillation. You should immediately:

    A. begin CPR.
    B. defibrillate the patient.
    C. give high-flow oxygen.
    D. perform a focused history and physical exam.

122. If you discover an error as you are writing the patient report, you should:

    A. erase the error and rewrite the correct information.
    B. draw the error to the attention of your supervisor, but do not change the form.
    C. draw a line through the error, initial it, and write the correct information next to the error.
    D. cover the incorrect information with correction fluid, initial it, and write the correct information in the corrected area.

123. What is the proper ratio of compressions to ventilations for two-rescuer adult CPR?

    A. 1:5
    B. 2:15
    C. 5:1
    D. 15:2

124. When evaluating a patient who complains of chest pain, you should find out when the pain began, what caused it, what it feels like, if it is radiating and to where, how severe it is, and whether the:

    A. pain causes nausea.
    B. pain is constant or intermittent.
    C. patient is under the influence of alcohol.
    D. patient was able to call for the ambulance.

125. Which of the following patients would be the highest priority in a triage situation?

    A. A 24-year-old man with a deformed lumbar spine and paralyzed legs
    B. A 26-year-old woman with multiple lacerations, no pulse, and no respirations
    C. A 32-year-old woman with bilateral deformed femurs and no signs of shock
    D. A 35-year-old man who is unconscious and has a significant head laceration

126. What is the most common cause of airway obstruction in an unconscious 27-year-old patient?

    A. Vomitus
    B. The tongue
    C. Blood clots
    D. Aspirated food

127. You have responded to the scene of an accident where a bystander who claims to have medical credentials becomes difficult to manage. You should:

    A. inform medical control immediately.
    B. inform law enforcement immediately.
    C. flatly tell the bystander to leave or he may be arrested.
    D. let the bystander take over patient care as he has higher medical credentials.

128. You should NOT assist with nitroglycerin if the patient:

    A. is older than 80 years.
    B. took a pill 5 minutes earlier.
    C. has a heart rate over 100 beats per minute.
    D. has a systolic blood pressure of less than 100 mm Hg.

129. A traffic light turns red as the ambulance on an emergency call is approaching an intersection. There are no vehicles in front of the ambulance. You should:

   A. sound the siren, maintain speed, and proceed.
   B. bypass the traffic light by turning into a side street.
   C. stop, sound the siren if necessary, and proceed when safe.
   D. turn off the lights and siren and wait for the light to change.

130. A patient who has just had a severe asthma attack is now very sleepy. This may indicate that the patient:

   A. may stop breathing.
   B. does not need transport.
   C. has recovered from the attack.
   D. is probably having a drug reaction.

131. The principal goal in treatment of heat-related emergencies is to:

   A. provide rapid transport.
   B. make the patient comfortable.
   C. replace lost fluids with salt water.
   D. reduce the patient's body temperature.

132. You are called to a scene where a 5-year-old child has ingested a poison. The child is awake and responsive. You should first:

   A. consult medical control.
   B. give the child syrup of ipecac.
   C. give the child activated charcoal.
   D. give the child an injection of epinephrine.

133. You should assist with delivery of the baby's head by:

   A. placing one hand at the top of the head and the other in back.
   B. maintaining finger pressure against the center of the baby's skull.
   C. placing the palm of your hand firmly against the back of the baby's skull.
   D. placing the flats of your fingers on the bony part of the skull and exerting very gentle pressure on it.

134. Shivering in the presence of hypothermia indicates that the:

   A. muscular system is damaged.
   B. nerve endings are damaged, causing loss of muscle control.
   C. body is trying to generate more heat through muscular activity.
   D. circulatory system is impaired, and the body cannot maintain its temperature.

135. The driver in a one-car crash has no apparent injuries, but is acting unruly. A half-full whiskey bottle is lying on the passenger seat. The appropriate course of action would be to:

   A. assume that the driver is drunk.
   B. ask bystanders to help you restrain the driver.
   C. let law enforcement officials handle the matter.
   D. assess the situation to determine why the driver is acting unruly.

136. You are called to an apartment where two men have been fighting and one has been stabbed. You should:

   A. put on body armor before entering the apartment.
   B. enter the apartment and attempt to grab the knife from the man.
   C. enter the apartment and begin treating the patient who was stabbed.
   D. remain outside, evaluate the potential for violence, and call for help from law enforcement.

137. What is the proper ratio of compressions to ventilations for one-rescuer adult CPR?

   A. 1:5
   B. 2:15
   C. 5:1
   D. 15:2

138. Initial treatment of a man who is disoriented, stuporous, and drifting in and out of consciousness as a result of swallowing 30 sleeping pills should include:

   A. checking his breath odor for alcohol.
   B. contacting medical control immediately.
   C. diluting the poison while waiting for instructions from poison control.
   D. covering the patient with a blanket and then turning him on his side while waiting for him to vomit.

139. A woman who is having her first child is having contractions 2 minutes apart. You should:

    A. prepare to deliver the baby at the scene.
    B. examine for crowning before deciding whether to transport.
    C. provide slow transport while monitoring the woman's vital signs.
    D. place the woman in Trendelenburg's position and provide immediate transport.

140. Which of the following conditions may develop as a result of severe hypothermia?

    A. Jaundice
    B. Cardiac arrhythmia
    C. Congestive heart failure
    D. Cerebrovascular accident

141. Which of the following signs strongly suggests early stages of shock in a child?

    A. Delayed capillary refill time
    B. Systolic blood pressure of less than 50 mm Hg
    C. Diastolic blood pressure of less than 50 mm Hg
    D. A combined blood pressure of less than 100 mm Hg

142. Which of the following is NOT an important consideration when caring for a patient believed to have ingested or been exposed to a poison?

    A. Type of substance
    B. Time of ingestion/exposure
    C. Amount of substance ingested
    D. What kind of food was eaten last

143. A man is cut above the ankle by a lawn mower blade. If the bleeding cannot be controlled with direct pressure, you should apply pressure on which of the following arteries?

    A. Dorsalis pedis
    B. Subclavian
    C. Temporal
    D. Femoral

144. When caring for a patient with a suspected extremity fracture, you should:

    A. move the limb across the body to provide support.
    B. move the limb to determine the severity of the fracture.
    C. splint the part first, then control bleeding in open fractures.
    D. splint the part in the position you find it, whenever possible.

145. A newborn is not breathing on its own shortly after delivery. The 1-minute Apgar score is 4. The first step in caring for this newborn is to:

    A. begin CPR.
    B. resuction the nose and mouth.
    C. stimulate the newborn with gentle shaking.
    D. give assisted ventilations with a BVM device.

146. Signs of internal bleeding include:

    A. increased pulse rate and warm skin.
    B. increased pulse rate and clammy skin.
    C. reduced pulse rate and dilated pupils.
    D. reduced pulse rate and a soft abdomen.

147. To help a patient in shock maintain adequate blood flow and oxygen supply to the heart and brain, you should:

    A. tilt the entire body up at the head.
    B. elevate the lower extremities 6″ to 12″.
    C. elevate the upper part of the body 6″ to 12″.
    D. elevate the lower extremities and trunk of the body.

148. After applying both a dressing and a bandage to a laceration below the elbow, you should check for signs of impaired circulation in the patient's:

    A. neck.
    B. elbow.
    C. fingers.
    D. shoulder.

149. A 17-year-old boy is found unconscious, floating facedown in a swimming pool. You and your partner should first:

    A. roll him over as a unit and then place him on a backboard.
    B. roll him over as a unit, extend his neck to open the airway, and then prepare to float a backboard under him.
    C. place him on a backboard in a facedown position, then remove him from the pool.
    D. stabilize his neck and back with your hands while you and your partner roll him over as a unit and then establish an open airway.

150. What is the absolute minimum information that you should obtain from the dispatcher while you are en route to the scene of an emergency?

    A. Whether or not the scene is safe
    B. The number of patients and their locations
    B. The nature of the call and the number of patients
    B. The nature and location of the call

Answers

1. **C.** A child's nose and mouth are much smaller than that of an adult. The larynx, cricoid cartilage, and trachea are smaller and softer as well. This makes the mechanics of breathing much more delicate.

2. **C.** Your first responsibility at the scene is your own safety and the safety of others.

3. **D.** When trying to manage a disruptive patient, you should keep your eyes on the patient at all times and be alert for aggressive behavior.

4. **B.** The normal pulse rate for a child is approximately 80 to 100 beats per minute.

5. **B.** In this case, audible coughing is a good sign. With a partial obstruction, the patient is able to exchange some air, but breathing is noisy and the patient may be coughing. Your main concern is to prevent a partial airway obstruction from becoming a complete airway obstruction.

6. **B.** Off-line medical direction is delivered to the EMT-B by protocol, standing orders, or standard medical operating procedures (SMOPs).

7. **A.** A competent patient has the right to refuse treatment. The EMT-B should explain to the patient why transportation to the hospital for treatment is advisable. However, the EMT-B in this case must respect the patient's wishes if she refuses treatment. In any case of patient refusal, the EMT-B should follow local protocols.

8. **C.** You would not expect to find paradoxical motion with an extremity injury. Paradoxical motion is chest movement in the opposite direction of the normal rise and fall of breathing.

9. **B.** Gloves and eye protection are the minimum standard for all patient care if there is any possibility for exposure to blood or body fluids. These are part of the body substance isolation techniques you should follow whenever exposure to blood or other body fluids is possible.

10. **D.** The purpose of Critical Incident Stress Debriefing (CISD) is to help emergency medical personnel relieve personal and group anxieties and stress. These debriefings should not be dismissed as trivial or nonessential.

11. **B.** For child CPR, the chest should be compressed 1" to 1 1/2", at a rate of at least 100/min.

12. **D.** Confidential information cannot be disclosed without permission from the patient or a court order. The EMT-B should not comment on the condition of any patient, except to report to the hospital or to turn the patient over to equally or better trained health care professionals.

13. **C.** Serious gastric distension is dangerous, as it causes the patient to vomit during CPR. It can also reduce lung volume by elevating the diaphragm.

14. **A.** The best way to estimate skin temperature is to place the back of your hand on the patient's skin.

15. **D.** The state of the pupils, especially any progressive change, is a rapid reflection of central nervous system injury or disease.

16. **C.** If you begin CPR in the field, you must continue unless one of the following occurs: the patient starts breathing and has a pulse; the patient is transferred to a higher medical authority; you are out of strength or too fatigued to continue; or a physician present assumes responsibility for the patient.

17. **B.** With infants and children, full cardiac arrest results from respiratory arrest. If uncorrected, respiratory arrest will lead to cardiac arrest and death.

18. **C.** Expressed consent occurs when the patient expressly authorizes you to provide care or transport to the hospital. Expressed consent may take the form of words, a nod of agreement, or other expressions of approval.

19. **D.** With respiratory depression or arrest, there is little or no movement of the chest and abdomen. There is also little or no airflow felt or heard at the nose and mouth.

20. **C.** The only time your attention should be directed away from initial assessment of the patient is when the patient's life or your life is in immediate danger.

21. **B.** When dealing with emotionally disturbed patients, the best legal situation is to try to obtain the patient's consent to medical treatment. This may be difficult, since these patients often resist treatment or try to threaten you. If the patient presents a threat to self or others, you can legally care for, and even restrain, the patient against his or her will.

22. **D.** When presented with a prolapsed umbilical cord, you should place the woman in Trendelenburg's position, carefully insert your gloved finger into the vagina, and then gently push the baby's head away from the umbilical cord.

23. **A.** The usual dosage for a child is 1 g of activated charcoal per kilogram of body weight, to a maximum of 12.5 to 25 g.

24. **D.** You should assume that the parents would give consent for treatment.

25. **B.** A patient with a dislocated knee will be in extreme pain. If the patient has strong distal pulses in the injured leg, splint the knee in the position in which you found it.

26. **C.** Normal systolic blood pressure in an adult male patient is 100 mm Hg plus the patient's age, up to 150 mm Hg.

27. **A.** Rate, quality, and rhythm should all be assessed when evaluating respirations.

28. **A.** Most infectious diseases are spread by surface contact; therefore, handwashing remains a most effective way to prevent the spread of disease.

29. **C.** The heart rate will be elevated in respiratory distress in a conscious patient. All the other signs are seen in respiratory distress.

30. **D.** As triage officer, you must remain at the scene to coordinate prioritized patient care. The triage officer should not become involved in patient care. An incident commander, transport officer, and others will be identified, as needed, depending on the scope of the problem. Leaving the scene, even with a critical patient, defeats the concept of continuity of care and breaks down the command process.

31. **B.** Air pressure within the thorax decreases at the onset of inhalation. Air then moves from the outside into the trachea and fills the lungs.

32. **D.** Except in cases where an emergency rapid extrication is warranted by the patient's condition or safety concerns at the scene, appropriate patient care should be provided before removing the patient from the vehicle. In this case, performing the initial assessment and stabilizing the vital functions should be done before extrication.

33. **D.** The normal respiratory rate for an infant is approximately 25 to 50 breaths per minute.

34. **B.** Wheezing is described as an audible, high-pitched breath sound usually resulting from a blockage of the smaller air passages.

35. **B.** Two-person BVM is more effective than one-person BVM. It is very difficult for one EMT-B to maintain a proper seal between the mask and face with one hand while getting adequate air into the patient with the other hand.

36. **D.** The proper sized oropharyngeal airway is determined by measuring from the corner of the mouth to the earlobe.

37. **B.** In this situation, it is likely that the patient has sustained spinal injuries because the patient does not feel pain in the extremities.

38. **B.** Dehydration may cause shock in infants and children. Therefore, prompt transport is necessary.

39. **A.** When using mouth-to-mouth breathing to ventilate a patient, your breaths should last 11/2 to 2 seconds.

40. **A.** Artificial ventilation for a patient involved in a near-drowning accident should begin as soon as possible, even before you remove the patient from the water.

41. **C.** If the baby's head is still covered by the membranes of the amniotic sac after delivery, you must break the membranes immediately to prevent suffocation. You should then clear the baby's nose and mouth and complete the delivery.

42. **C.** For the situation where prompt hospital care is not available, you should attempt active, rapid rewarming.

43. **B.** An unconscious patient who is seen breathing with the diaphragm rather than with the chest muscles has likely sustained a severe spinal injury. When the diaphragm is unable to substitute for the chest muscles, the patient is likely to have respiratory difficulty. Therefore, you should give the patient supplemental oxygen at 100% and monitor breathing.

44. **A.** A child in respiratory distress will show all the signs listed except screaming. In order to scream, a child must be breathing well and have a respiratory reserve.

45. **C.** Decreased level of consciousness is the most common sign of low blood sugar. Seizures or convulsions may also occur at a later time.

46. **B.** A fractured elbow should be immobilized in the position in which it is found because movement may result in damage to nerves and blood vessels.

47. **C.** A nonrebreathing mask would be the most beneficial to this patient. Patients breathing fewer than 12 breaths per minute or more than 24 breaths per minute are not breathing adequately. Fast, shallow breathing does not allow for adequate exchange of air and carbon dioxide in the alveoli. The nonrebreathing mask is capable of providing up to 95% inspired oxygen.

48. **D.** Even though the patient's injuries appear only minor, your primary concern is to find and/or rule out any obvious or hidden life-threatening injuries. Only after you have completed this step can you direct your attention to less serious problems.

49. **A.** A patient who is conscious and complaining of shoulder pain and tingling in the extremities should be treated for possible spinal injuries. Your assessment should include gently feeling along the spine for any point tenderness. To prevent further injury, you should not ask the patient to move the head, neck, or extremities.

50. **A.** The four methods for providing artificial ventilation by an EMT-B, in order of preference, are mouth-to-mask ventilation, two-person bag-valve-mask, oxygen-powered manually triggered breathing device, and one-person bag-valve-mask.

51. **B.** You must provide transport of all patients involved in near-drowning accidents. Even if initial resuscitation in the field appears completely successful, the patient can still aspirate fluids. This may result in complications lasting days or weeks.

52. **B.** When assessing the extremities, you should look for injuries, swelling, deformities, and bleeding. When assessing the legs, you should also check the distal pulses, whether the patient can feel what you are doing, and the strength of each foot.

53. **A.** Falls greater than 10' for children, as well as bicycle collisions and medium-speed vehicle collisions, are considered significant mechanisms of injury.

54. **B.** The patient's abdominal pain and bloody discharge suggest a possible pelvic fracture. The appropriate course of action in this situation would be to immobilize the patient on a long spine board with a PASG in place under the patient.

55. **D.** The best results in resuscitating patients who have sudden cardiac death include rapid BLS (within 4 minutes) and ready availability of defibrillation.

56. **C.** Your primary responsibility in the initial management of a disruptive patient is to take charge of the situation and to be mindful of your personal safety.

57. **B.** If a patient seems to be having an allergic reaction, you should give oxygen as you complete the initial assessment. Next, obtain baseline vital signs and, if the patient is conscious, a SAMPLE history.

58. **B.** In addition to beginning the process of gathering important patient information, the scene size-up is also your first real opportunity to evaluate whether the environment is safe so that you can begin caring for the patient. If the scene is unsafe, this is the time to make it safe before entering.

59. **C.** Once you receive an order from medical control, you must repeat the order back word for word and then receive confirmation.

60. **C.** Prehospital care reports help to ensure efficient continuity of patient care. This report describes the nature of the patient's injuries or illness at the scene and the initial treatment you provide.

61. **D.** Providing support and reassurance to the patient will help reduce anxiety. This will also physically help the patient because fear can stimulate the heart and make matters worse.

62. **A.** The heart needs constant perfusion in order to function properly. Without adequate perfusion, it will deteriorate much more quickly than the liver, kidneys, or skeletal muscle. No part of the body can tolerate inadequate perfusion indefinitely.

63. **B.** Use your gloved hand to apply direct pressure. Do not waste valuable time washing or looking for a dressing of any kind.

64. **B.** Altered mental status associated with diabetes has often been mistaken for alcohol or drug intoxication.

appendix **b**

65. **D.** As you log roll a child onto an immobilization device, make sure you place padding under the child's shoulders to prevent hyperflexion of the neck.

66. **B.** After positioning the BVM device on the patient, you should hold the mask in place while your partner squeezes the bag with two hands until the patient's chest rises.

67. **D.** A mass-casualty or multiple-casualty plan should be invoked whenever patient needs are greater than available resources. Depending on the severity of the injuries, this may involve as few as two or three patients, or as many as nine or ten.

68. **C.** Defibrillator pads should not be placed over or near a pacemaker.

69. **A.** Reassurance remains the best way to treat hyperventilation. Breathing into a bag may be dangerous. Because there usually is a cause for the hyperventilation, the patient should be transported to the hospital for evaluation.

70. **B.** For infant CPR, the chest should be compressed $1/2$" to 1", at a rate of at least 100/min.

71. **C.** A patient with a partial airway obstruction will have some degree of respiratory distress, but will probably be able to cough and breathe noisily.

72. **C.** The proper sized nasopharyngeal airway is determined by measuring from the tip of the nose to the earlobe.

73. **B.** For the purposes of BLS, patients classified as children are between the ages of 1 and 8 years.

74. **B.** The first question to be answered at the scene of a multiple-casualty incident is, "How many patients are there?" Once that is determined, additional resources can be summoned immediately. Triage should be started by the most experienced EMT on the scene, and assessing the severity of injuries will be a function of the triage and treatment process. Determinations of what caused the crash are left to the proper investigating agencies.

75. **D.** When responding to an accident, the ambulance should be parked about 100' from the accident on the same side of the street.

76. **D.** The patient's "snoring" sounds indicate an airway problem. Therefore, you should secure the airway and then hold the head still, in a neutral, in-line position, until it can be fully immobilized.

77. **B.** If the woman is in the first stage of labor, you usually have enough time to transport her to the hospital.

78. **D.** The best way to communicate with a frightened patient is to make and keep eye contact in order to help the patient keep calm.

79. **C.** Priority is always given to emergency care of the ABCD. When a life-threatening problem is found, such as an airway obstruction, you should act immediately to clear it.

80. **D.** Pale skin indicates inadequate circulation. Poor oxygenation will usually cause cyanosis, liver problems produce a jaundiced skin color, and a flushed skin color is often seen with heat cramps.

81. **B.** A burn destroys the patient's protective skin layer and covering the skin with dry bandages and clean sheets helps minimize the risk of infection.

82. **A.** The oropharyngeal airway prevents obstruction of the airway, primarily from the tongue. It also makes it easier to suction the airway.

83. **C.** The links in the Chain of Survival include early activation of EMS, early BLS, early defibrillation, and early ACLS.

84. **D.** The appropriate course of action in this situation would be to contact medical control for a decision on realigning the limb.

85. **C.** Since children consume oxygen two to three times faster than adults, cardiac arrest is usually secondary to hypoxia and ischemia of the heart.

86. **D.** Assessment of the patient's airway begins with the evaluation of the patient's level of consciousness. Level of consciousness is assessed by the patient's response to the question, "Are you okay?"

87. **A.** Oxygen should be given to all patients in shock.

88. **D.** Blowing too fast or too vigorously can cause air to enter the esophagus and stomach rather than the trachea. This will cause inflation of the stomach (gastric distention) rather than the lungs.

89. **B.** In this situation, you should suspect impacted fractures of the lower extremities and possible fractures of the spine.

90. **A.** BLS should be performed on all pulseless patients. CPR is immediately indicated after the rhythm is analyzed as requiring no shock, as in asystole.

91. **D.** The first step in determining why an airway is obstructed is to open the patient's mouth using the head-tilt and chin-lift maneuver. You should always take care to protect the neck in a trauma situation, but remember that the priority is always the airway.

92. **D.** When treating a patient with frostbite, you should remove any wet clothing and cover the injured area with a dry cloth or dry, sterile dressings. Do not break any blisters, and do not apply heat or try to rewarm the area.

93. **B.** The general impression formed by the EMT-B determines the priority in treating the patient.

94. **C.** Your primary responsibility is always to protect yourself and to provide emergency medical care. When a crime is involved, it is important to make every effort to preserve the crime scene and protect any evidence while still providing appropriate prehospital care.

95. **C.** In this situation, although the patient appears to be dead, you must establish an open airway and attempt to ventilate so that you can begin effective CPR as soon as possible.

96. **A.** You should assume a spinal injury with any patient who is unresponsive. After checking the head and cervical spine for deformities, the cervical spine should then be immobilized.

97. **C.** A patient with a dislocated shoulder will be in extreme pain; therefore, immobilization is difficult. You should immobilize the shoulder in the position that is most comfortable for the patient. Never attempt to reduce or "put back in place" the shoulder.

98. **A.** Approach an elderly patient slowly and calmly. Allow plenty of time for the patient to respond to your questions.

99. **B.** When oral glucose is properly given, placing it between the cheek and gum of a conscious patient who is able to swallow and protect the airway, there are no side effects. However, if given to a patient who is unconscious or unable to swallow, aspiration can occur.

100. **C.** Bleeding from a wound should be treated with direct pressure from your gloved hand or with a pressure dressing. Once the bleeding has been controlled, you should firmly wrap a sterile roller bandage around the wound to maintain the pressure.

101. **B.** The first step in the management of a patient exhibiting disruptive behavior is to assess the situation.

102. **C.** The brachial pulse is the easiest to access and evaluate in an infant.

103. **A.** To slow the spread of the toxin from a bee sting, you should apply ice or cold packs to the injected site, but not directly on the skin.

104. **D.** Premature ventricular contractions may result if the heart does not receive enough oxygen.

105. **D.** Management of hypothermia in the field focuses on stabilizing the vital signs, preventing further heat loss, and providing prompt transport.

106. **A.** Stay upwind (and uphill, when applicable) of the hazardous material, but remain on site to protect others from entering the area. Await the arrival of properly trained and equipped HazMat technicians, and NEVER knowingly enter a hazard zone without the proper protection and training.

107. **D.** The most serious underlying problem associated with a facial injury is partial or complete upper airway obstruction.

108. **C.** Nitroglycerin causes dilation of the blood vessels in the heart and elsewhere. You should watch the blood pressure closely after giving nitroglycerin.

109. **B.** Never give up on resuscitating a drowning victim. Submersion in very cold water will produce hypothermia and lower the metabolic rate, which protects the vital organs from lack of oxygen. Once the child has been removed from the water, you should begin full resuscitation efforts.

110. **C.** When the heart is working hard, the coronary arteries dilate. Oxygen-rich blood from the aorta can then nourish the heart.

111. **C.** Establishing and maintaining an airway is the first step in treating a patient with a head injury.

112. **D.** A stoma is a permanent opening in the neck that connects the trachea directly to the skin. When ventilating a patient with a stoma, the air will leak out. To prevent this, you must seal the mouth and pinch the nostrils and then ventilate through the stoma. Release the patient's mouth and nostrils for exhalation.

113. **B.** Mild hypothermia occurs when the core temperature is between 90° and 95°F (32° and 35°C). The patient is usually alert and shivering. The pulse rate and respirations are usually rapid. The skin may appear red, but may eventually appear cyanotic.

114. **A.** Atrial fibrillation, ventricular tachycardia, and ventricular fibrillation all involve some activity of the heart muscle. Asystole does not. A heart that has no activity will probably not recover, despite BLS and ALS.

115. **D.** Use of a police escort may be dangerous in an intersection because a motorist hearing a siren and seeing the police car pass may assume that only one emergency vehicle is passing. The motorist may then proceed into the intersection and possibly hit the ambulance.

116. **C.** Your care of a premature baby should include keeping the mouth and nose clear of mucus.

117. **C.** The best way to control bleeding in an extremity injury to a child is to apply direct pressure with a dry, sterile dressing.

118. **B.** To perform chest compressions on an infant, place two fingers on the lower half of the sternum.

119. **D.** If a woman who has had a child tells you she feels as if she must move her bowels, you should prepare to deliver the baby at the scene. The baby's head is pressing on her rectum and delivery is about to occur.

120. **C.** When called to the scene of a diabetic emergency, you should ask the patient or his or her family if insulin had been taken that day, whether a meal had been missed, if the patient had vomited after a meal, and whether the patient had done any strenuous exercise.

121. **B.** The longer a patient remains in ventricular fibrillation, the less likely that he or she can be resuscitated successfully or without serious long-term neurologic problems. Since this patient is already in ventricular fibrillation, she has most likely been fibrillating for some time and will need to be shocked as soon as possible.

122. **C.** If you discover errors as you are writing a report, draw a single horizontal line through the error, initial it, and write the correct information next to it.

123. **C.** The proper ratio of compressions to ventilations for two-rescuer adult CPR is 5:1.

124. **B.** Pertinent information to gather when evaluating a patient experiencing pain follows the OPQRST mnemonic: Onset, Provoke, Quality, Radiation, Severity, and Time. Whether the pain is constant or intermittent falls into the time category.

125. **D.** Unconsciousness qualifies as a first priority condition, while back injuries and bone or joint injuries are second priority. The pulseless patient is dead, which is considered the lowest priority.

126. **B.** In an unconscious patient, the tongue and throat tissues relax causing the airway to be obstructed.

127. **A.** Each EMS service should have a protocol for dealing with bystanders who are physicians. Not all physicians are trained in emergency medical care. Medical control may be able to communicate with the physician and help eliminate some problems.

128. **D.** Do not give nitroglycerin to a patient with a systolic blood pressure of less than 100 mm Hg. Nitroglycerin may further lower the pressure.

129. **C.** When the ambulance approaches a red light at an intersection and there is no traffic in front of it, the driver should stop at the light, sound the siren, and proceed when certain that the intersection is clear.

130. **A.** A patient having a severe asthma episode could become exhausted. This may mean that the patient may soon stop breathing.

131. **D.** The principal goal in treatment of heat exposure is to reduce the patient's body temperature.

132. **A.** Consult medical control first when caring for an alert child who has ingested a poison. You should discuss with medical control the possibility of giving activated charcoal.

133. **D.** Assist with delivery of the baby's head by placing the flats of your fingers on the bony part of the skull as it emerges and then exert very gentle pressure. Avoid pressing your fingers into the baby's fontanels.

134. **C.** Shivering in the presence of hypothermia indicates that the body is trying to generate more heat through muscular activity.

135. **D.** The appropriate course of action in this situation would be to assess the scene to determine why the driver is being disruptive. Do not "write off" the unruly or abusive patient as "just another drunk."

136. **D.** Whenever you are in doubt about your safety, do not put yourself at risk. Never enter an unstable environment. As part of your scene size-up, evaluate the potential for violence. If it is a possibility, call for additional help. Rely on the advice of law enforcement.

137. **D.** The proper ratio of compressions to ventilations for one-rescuer adult CPR is 15:2.

138. **B.** It is critical to consult medical control before you treat any poisoning victim. If the ingested substance is an opiate, sedative, or barbiturate, expect CNS depression. You may need to provide aggressive ventilatory support and even CPR.

139. **B.** You should examine for crowning before deciding whether there is time to transport when a woman expecting her first child is having contractions 2 minutes apart.

140. **B.** One result of severe hypothermia, a core temperature of 80°F (27°C), is the possibility of cardiac arrhythmia.

141. **A.** Delayed capillary refill time in a peripheral extremity strongly suggests early stages of shock in a child.

142. **D.** When caring for a patient believed to have ingested or been exposed to a poison, determining what kind of food was eaten last is not an important consideration. Factors to consider are the type of substance, the time of ingestion/exposure, the amount of substance ingested, the amount of time exposed, and the weight of the patient.

143. **D.** Since the bleeding is above the ankle, you should use the femoral pressure point, which is proximal to the wound.

144. **D.** You should splint a suspected extremity fracture in the position in which you found it, whenever possible.

145. **B.** The first step in caring for an infant who is not breathing spontaneously after 30 seconds is to resuction the nose and mouth.

146. **B.** An increased pulse rate and clammy skin suggest possible internal bleeding.

147. **B.** Elevation of the lower extremities increases the amount of blood available to the chest and head.

148. **C.** Once the dressing and bandage are applied, check for signs of impaired circulation or loss of sensation in the patient's fingers.

149. **D.** The first step in caring for a patient who is found unconscious, floating facedown in a pool, is for you and your partner to stabilize the patient's neck and back with your hands. You should then roll him over as a unit and establish an airway while you are still in the water.

150. **D.** The minimum information that should be obtained from the dispatcher is the location of the scene and the general nature of the situation. The dispatcher cannot reliably advise you of the scene's safety until you arrive and can survey the area yourself.

appendix b

Glossary

abandonment   Unilateral termination of care by the EMT-B without the patient's consent and without making provision for transferring care to another medical professional with skills at the same level or higher.

abdomen   The second major body cavity that contains the major organs of digestion and excretion.

abdominal-thrust maneuver   The preferred method to dislodge and force food or other material from the throat of a choking victim. Also called the Heimlich maneuver.

abduction   Motion of a limb away from the midline.

abortion   Delivery of the fetus and placenta before 20 weeks; miscarriage.

abrasion   Loss or damage of the superficial layer of skin as a result of a body part rubbing or scraping across a rough or hard surface.

absence seizure   Seizure that may be characterized by a brief lapse of attention in which the patient may stare and does not respond. Also known as *petit mal seizure*.

absorption   The process by which medications travel through body tissues until they reach the bloodstream.

acceleration   The process of increasing speed.

access   The ability to gain entry to an enclosed area and reach a patient.

accessory muscles   The secondary muscles of respiration.

acetabulum   The depression in which the femoral head fits snugly.

acidosis   A pathologic condition resulting from the accumulation of acids in the body.

acromioclavicular (A/C) joint   A simple joint where the bony projections of the scapula and the clavicle meet at the top of the shoulder.

action   Effect of a drug on the body.

activated charcoal   Charcoal ground into a very fine powder that provides the greatest possible surface area for binding drugs that have been taken by mouth; it is carried on the EMS unit.

activities of daily living (ADL)   The basic activities a person usually accomplishes during a normal day, such as eating, dressing, and washing.

acute abdomen   A condition of sudden onset of pain within the abdomen, demanding immediate medical or surgical treatment.

acute myocardial infarction (AMI)   Heart attack; death of the heart muscle following obstruction of blood flow to it. Acute in this context means "new" or "happening right now."

Adam's apple   The firm prominence in the upper part of the larynx formed by the thyroid cartilage. It is more prominent in men than in women.

addiction   A state characterized by an overwhelming obsession or physical need to continue the use of a drug or agent.

adduction   Motion of a limb toward the midline.

adsorption   To bind to or stick to a surface

advance directive   Written documentation that specifies medical treatment for a competent patient should the patient become unable to make decisions; also called a living will.

advanced life support (ALS)   Advanced lifesaving procedures, such as cardiac monitoring, starting IV fluids, giving medications, and using advanced airway adjuncts, some of which are now being provided by the EMT-B.

agonal respirations   An irregular, gasping respiration, sometimes heard in dying patients.

air ambulances   Fixed-wing aircraft and helicopters that have been modified for medical care, used to evacuate and transport patients with life-threatening injuries to treatment facilities.

air embolism   The presence of air in the veins, which can lead to cardiac arrest if it enters the heart.

airway   The upper airway tract or the passage above the larynx, which includes the nose, mouth, and throat.

allergen   A substance that causes an allergic reaction.

allergic reaction   The body's immune response to an internal or surface agent.

altered level of consciousness   A mental state in which infants and children may be unresponsive, combative, confused, thrash about, or drift in and out of an alert state. Also called altered mental status.

altered mental status (AMS)   A change in the way a person thinks and behaves that signals disease in the central nervous system.

alveoli   The air sacs of the lungs in which the exchange of oxygen and carbon dioxide takes place.

ambient temperature   The temperature of the surrounding environment.

ambulance   A specialized vehicle for transporting sick and injured patients.

ambulance service vehicle   A specialized vehicle used to transport EMS equipment and personnel to scenes of medical emergencies.

American Standard System   A safety system for large oxygen cylinders, designed to prevent the accidental attachment of a regulator to a wrong cylinder.

Americans with Disabilities Act (ADA)   Comprehensive legislation that is designed to protect individuals with disabilities against discrimination.

amniotic sac   The fluid-filled, bag-like membrane in which the fetus develops.

anaphylactic shock   Severe shock caused by an allergic reaction.

anaphylaxis   An extreme, life-threatening systemic allergic reaction that may include shock and respiratory failure.

anatomic position   Position of reference with the patient standing, facing you, arms at the side, with the palms of the hands forward.

aneurysm   A swelling or enlargement of a part of an artery, resulting from weakening of the arterial wall.

angina pectoris   Transient (short-lived) chest discomfort caused by partial or temporary blockage of blood flow to the heart muscle.

angle of Louis   A ridge on the sternum that lies at the level where the second rib is attached to the sternum; provides a constant and reliable bony landmark on the anterior chest wall.

anorexia   Lack or loss of appetite for food.

anterior   A directional term meaning the front surface of the body, the side facing you.

anterior superior iliac spines   The hard bony prominences at the front on each side of the lower abdomen just below the plane of the umbilicus.

anterograde (posttraumatic) amnesia   Inability to remember events after an injury.

antidote   Substance used to neutralize or counteract a poison.

glossary

antivenin   A substance produced to counteract the effect of venom from an animal or insect.

aorta   The main artery, which receives blood from the left ventricle and delivers it to all the other arteries that carry blood to the tissues of the body.

aortic valve   A structure that lies between the left ventricle and the aorta. It keeps blood from flowing back into the left ventricle after the left ventricle ejects its blood into the aorta. It is one of four heart valves that ensure that blood flows in only one direction.

apex (plural: apices)   The tip or the topmost portion of a structure.

apgar score   A scoring system for assessing the status of a newborn that assigns a number value to each of five areas of activity.

aphasia   The inability to understand or produce speech.

apices   See apex.

apnea   Periods of not breathing.

apparent life-threatening event (ALTE)   An event causing unresponsiveness, cyanosis, and apnea in an infant, who then resumes breathing with stimulation.

appendix   A small tubular structure that is attatched to the lower border of the cecum in the lower right quadrant of the abdomen.

arrhythmia   An irregular or abnormal heart rhythm.

arterial rupture   Rupture of a cerebral artery that may contribute to interruption of cerebral blood flow.

arteriole   The smallest branch of an artery leading to the vast network of capillaries.

arteriosclerosis   A disease characterized by hardening and thickening of the arterial walls.

articular cartilage   A pearly layer of specialized cartilage covering the articular surface of bones in synovial joints.

assault   Unlawfully placing a patient in fear of bodily harm.

asthma   A disease of the lungs in which muscle spasm in the small air passageways and the production of large amounts of mucus result in airway obstruction.

asystole   Complete absence of heart electrical activity.

atherosclerosis   A disorder in which cholesterol and calcium build up inside the walls of blood vessels, forming plaque, which eventually leads to partial or complete blockage of blood flow. An atherosclerotic plaque can also become a site where blood clots can form, break off, and embolize elsewhere in the elsewhere in the circulation.

atrium   One of two (right and left) upper chambers of the heart. The right atrium receives blood from the vena cava and delivers it to the right ventricle, which, in turn, pumps blood into the blood vessels of the lungs. The left atrium receives blood from pulmonary veins and delivers it to the left

auscultation   A method of listening to sounds within an organ with a stethoscope.

autonomic (involuntary) nervous system   The part of the nervous system that regulates functions, such as digestion system and sweating, that are not controlled by conscious will.

AVPU scale   A method of assessing a patient's level of consciousness by determining whether a patient is awake and alert, responsive to verbal stimulus or pain, or unresponsive, used principally in the initial assessment; used primarily in the initial survey.

avulse   To pull or tear away.

avulsion   An injury in which soft tissue is either torn completely loose or is hanging as a flap.

backboard   A device used to provide support to patients suspected of having a hip, pelvic, spinal, or lower extremity injury. Also called a spine board, trauma board, or longboard.

bag-valve-mask (BVM) device   A device with face mask attached to a bag containing a reservoir and connected to oxygen; delivers more than 90% supplemental oxygen.

ball-and-socket joint   A joint that allows internal and external rotation as well as bending.

barrier device   A protective item, such as a pocket mask with a valve, that limits exposure to a patient's body fluids.

base station   Any radio hardware containing a transmitter and receiver that is located in a fixed place.

basic life support (BLS)   Noninvasive emergency lifesaving care that is used to treat airway obstruction, respiratory arrest, or cardiac arrest.

basket stretcher   A rigid stretcher commonly used in technical and water rescues that surrounds and supports the patient, yet allows water to drain through holes in the bottom. Also called a Stokes litter.

battery   Touching a patient or providing emergency care without consent.

behavior   How a person functions or acts.

behavioral crisis   The point at which a person's reactions to events interfere with activities of daily living; a behavioral crisis becomes a psychiatric emergency when it causes a major life interruption, such as attempted suicide.

biceps   Large muscle that covers the front of the humerus.

bilateral   A body part that appears on either side of the midline.

bile ducts   Ducts that convey bile between the liver and the intestine.

birth canal   The vagina and the lower part or neck of the uterus.

blanching   Turning white.

blood pressure (BP)   The pressure of circulating blood against the walls of the arteries.

bloody show   A plug of pink-tinged mucous discharged when the cervix begins to dilate.

blowout fracture   Fracture of the orbit or of the bones that support the floor of the orbit.

blunt trauma   A mechanism of injury in which force occurs over a broad area, and the skin is not usually broken.

body substance isolation (BSI)   An infection control concept and practice that assumes that all body fluids are potentially infectious.

brachial artery   The major vessel in the upper extremity that supplies blood to the arm.

bradycardia   Slow heart rate, less than 60 beats/min.

brain   Controlling organ of the body; center of consciousness; functions include perception, control of reactions to the environment, emotional responses, and judgement.

brain stem   Area of the brain between the spinal cord and cerebrum, surrounded by the cerebellum; controls functions necessary for life, such as respirations.

breath sounds   An indication of air movement in the lungs.

breath-holding syncope   Loss of consciousness caused by a decreased breathing stimulus.

breech presentation Presentation of an infant who comes out buttocks first.

bronchitis Irritation of the major lung passageways, either from infectious disease or irritants such as smoke.

burnout A condition of chronic fatigue and frustration that results from mounting stress over time.

burns Injury in which the soft tissue receives more energy than it can absorb without injury. Types of burns include thermal heat, frictional heat, toxic chemicals, electricity, or nuclear radiation.

calcaneus The heel bone.

capillary refill A test that evaluates the ability of the circulatory system to restore blood to the capillary system.

capillary vessels Fine end divisions of the arterial system that allow contact between cells of the body tissues and the plasma and the red blood cells.

carbon dioxide retention A condition characterized by a chronically high blood level of carbon dioxide in which the respiratory center no longer responds to high blood levels of carbon dioxide.

cardiac arrest A state in which the heart fails to generate an effective and detectible blood flow; pulses are not palpable in cardiac arrest, even if muscular and electrical activity continues in the heart.

cardiogenic shock A state in which not enough oxygen is delivered to the tissues of the body, caused by low output of blood from the heart. It can be a severe complication of a large acute myocardial infarction, as well as other conditions.

cardiopulmonary resuscitation (CPR) Noninvasive emergency lifesaving care that is used to treat airway obstruction, respiratory arrest, or cardiac arrest.

carotid artery The major artery that supplies blood to the head and brain.

carpometacarpal joint The joint between the wrist and the metacarpal bones; the thumb joint.

carrier An animal or person who may transmit an infectious disease but does not display any symptoms of it.

cataract Clouding of the lens of the eye or its surrounding transparent membrane.

catheter A hollow, cylindrical structure that drains or delivers fluids.

cavitation A phenomenon in which speed causes a bullet to generate pressure waves, which cause damage distant from the bullet's path.

cecum The first part of the large intestine, into which the ileum opens.

cellular telephone A low-power portable radio that communicates through an interconnected series of repeater stations called "cells."

central nervous system (CNS) The brain and spinal cord.

cerebellum One of the three major subdivisions of the brain, sometimes called the "little brain"; coordinates the various activities of the brain, particularly body movements.

cerebral edema Swelling of the brain.

cerebral embolism Obstruction of a cerebral artery caused by a clot that was formed elsewhere in the body and traveled to the brain.

cerebrovascular accident (CVA) The interruption of blood flow to the brain that results in the loss of brain function.

cerebrum The largest part of the three subdivisions of the brain, sometimes called the "gray matter"; it is made up of several lobes that control movement, hearing, balance, speech, visual perception, emotions, and personality.

certification A process in which a person, an institution, or program is evaluated and recognized as meeting certain predetermined standards to provide safe and ethical care.

cervical spine The portion of the spinal column consisting of the first seven vertebrae that lie in the neck.

cervix The neck of the uterus.

channel An assigned frequency or frequencies used to carry voice and/or data communications.

chassis Vehicle frame.

chassis set The transfer of the center of mass of the ambulance to different points on the chassis.

Chemical Transportation Emergency Center (CHEMTREC) Agency that assists emergency personnel in identifying and handling hazardous materials transport incidents.

chief complaint The reason a patient called for help. Also, the patient's response to general questions such as "What's wrong?" or "What happened?"

child abuse Any improper or excessive action that injures or otherwise harms a child or infant.

chronic obstructive pulmonary disease (COPD) A slow process of dilation and disruption of the airways and alveoli, caused by chronic bronchial obstruction.

ciphtheria An infectious disease in which a membrane lining the pharynx is formed that can severely obstruct passage of air into the larynx.

circulatory system Complex arrangement of connected tubes, including the arteries, arterioles, capillaries, venules, and veins. System moves blood, oxygen, nutrients, carbon dioxide, and cellular waste throughout the body.

clavicle The collarbone. It is medially to the sternum and laterally to the scapula.

cleaning The process of removing dirt, dust, blood, or other visible contaminants from a surface.

closed (blunt) chest injury Injury to the chest in which the skin is not broken, usually due to blunt trauma.

closed abdominal injury Any injury of the abdomen caused by a nonpenetrating instrument or force in which the skin remains intact. Also called blunt abdominal injury.

closed fracture Any fracture in which the skin is not broken.

closed head injury Injury usually associated with trauma in which the brain has been injured, but the skin has not been broken and there is no obvious bleeding.

closed injury Injury in which damage occurs beneath the skin or mucous membrane but the surface remains intact.

coagulation Formation of clots to plug openings in injured blood vessels and stop blood flow.

coccyx The last three or four vertebrae that form the tailbone.

coefficient of friction A measure of the "grip" of the tire on the road surface.

colic Acute cramping abdominal pain.

collagen A protein that is the chief component of connective tissue fibrils and bones.

command post The designated field command center where the incident commander and deputies are located.

common cold Usually associated with swollen nasal mucous membranes and the production of fluid from the sinuses and nose.

communicable disease Any disease that can be spread from person to person, or from animal to person.

compartment syndrome An elevation of pressure within the fibrous tissue that surrounds and supports muscles and neurovascular structures, characterized by extreme pain, hypesthesia (decreased pain sensation), pain on stretching of affected muscles, and decreased power; most frequently seen in fractures below the elbow or knee in children.

compensated shock The early stage of shock, while the body can still compensate for blood loss.

competent Able to make rational decisions about personal well-being.

complex access Complicated entry that requires special tools and training and includes breaking windows or other force.

conduction The loss of heat by direct contact (e.g., when a body part comes in contact with a colder object).

congestive heart failure (CHF) A disorder in which the heart loses part of its ability to effectively pump blood, usually as a result of damage to the heart muscle, and usually resulting in a back-up of fluid into the lungs.

conjunctiva The delicate membrane that lines the eyelids and covers the exposed surface of the eye.

conjunctivitis Inflammation of the conjunctiva.

connecting nerves Nerves that connect the sensory and motor nerves.

consent Granting permission to another to render care.

contagious An infectious disease that is capable of being transmitted from one person to another.

contamination The presence of infective organisms (or foreign bodies such as dirt, gravel, metal) on or in objects such as dressings, water, food, needles, wounds, or a patient's body.

continuous quality improvement (CQI) A system of internal and external reviews and audits of all aspects of an EMS.

contraindication Situations in which a drug should not be given because it would not help or may actually harm a patient.

contusion A bruise without a break in the skin.

convection The loss of body heat caused by air movement (e.g., breeze blowing across the body).

core temperature The temperature of the central part of the body (e.g., the heart, lungs, and vital organs).

cornea The transparent tissue layer in front of the pupil and iris of the eye.

coronary artery A blood vessel that carries blood and nutrients to the heart muscle.

costal arch A bridge of cartilage that connects the ends of the sixth through tenth ribs with the lower portion of the sternum.

costovertebral angle An angle that is formed by the junction of the spine and the tenth rib.

cover The tactical use of an impenetrable barrier to conceal and protect the presence of EMS personnel from projectiles (e.g., bullets, bottles, rocks).

CPR board A device that provides a firm surface under the patient's torso.

cranium The area of the head above the ears and eyes; the skull. The cranium contains the brain.

crepitus A grating or grinding sensation caused by fractured bone ends or joints rubbing together. Also air bubbles under the skin, giving the skin a crinkly feeling.

cricoid cartilage A rigid, ring-shaped structure that completely encircles the larynx at the top of the trachea.

cricothyroid membrane A thin sheet of fascia that connects the thyroid and cricoid cartilages that make up the larynx.

critical incident stress debriefing (CISD) A confidential group discussion of a highly traumatic incident that usually occurs within 24 to 72 hours of the incident.

critical incident stress management (CISM) A process that confronts the responses to critical incidents and defuses them, directing the emergency service personnel toward physical and emotional equilibrium.

croup An infectious disease of the upper respiratory system that may cause partial airway obstruction and is characterized by a barking cough; usually seen in children.

crowning The appearance of the infant's head at the vaginal opening during labor.

cyanosis A bluish, gray skin color caused by reduced levels of oxygen in the blood

cyspnea Shortness of breath or difficulty breathing.

danger zone An area where individuals can be exposed to toxic substances, lethal rays, or ignition or explosion of hazardous materials.

DCAP-BTLS A mnemonic for assessment in which each area of the body is evaluated for Deformities, Contusions, Abrasions, Punctures/Penetrations, Burns, Tenderness, Lacerations, and Swelling.

deceleration The slowing of an object.

decompensated shock The late stage of shock, when blood pressure is falling.

decompression sickness (the bends) A condition seen in divers in which gas, especially nitrogen, forms bubbles in blood vessels, obstructing them.

decontamination The process of removing and properly disposing of hazardous materials from equipment, patients, and rescue personnel.

decontamination area The designated area in a hazardous materials incident where all patients and rescuers must be decontaminated before going to another area.

dedicated line A special telephone line used for specific point-to-point communications. Also known as a "hot line."

deep Further inside the body and away from the skin.

defibrillate To shock a fibrillating (chaotically beating) heart with specialized electrical current in an attempt to restore a normal rhythmic beat.

dehydration A state in which fluid losses are greater than fluid intake into the body, leading to shock and death if untreated.

delirium A change in mental status marked by the inability to focus, think logically, and maintain attention.

delirium tremens (DTs) Clinical withdrawal syndrome seen in alcoholics who are deprived of ethyl alcohol; characterized by restlessness, fever, sweating, disorientation, agitation, and convulsions; in some cases, there is risk of death when untreated.

dementia The slow onset of progressive disorientation, shortened attention span, and loss of cognitive function.

dependent lividity Pooling of the blood in the lower parts of the body after death.

depression A persistent mood of sadness, despair, and discouragement; depression may be a symptom of many different mental and physical disorders, or it may be a disorder on its own.

dermis The inner layer of the skin containing hair follicles, sweat glands, nerve endings, and blood vessels.

designated officer The individual in the department charged with the responsibility of managing exposures and infection control issues.

detailed physical exam Part of the assessment process in which a detailed area-by-area exam is performed in patients whose problems cannot be readily identified, or when more specific information about problems identified in the focused history and physical exam is necessary.

diabetes mellitus A metabolic disorder in which the ability to metabolize carbohydrates (sugars) is impaired, usually because of a lack of insulin.

diabetic coma Unconsciousness caused by dehydration, very high blood glucose, and acidosis in diabetes.

diabetic ketoacidosis Form of acidosis in uncontrolled diabetes in which an accumulation of certain acids occurs when insulin is not available in the body.

diamond carry A carrying technique in which one EMT-B is located at the head end, one at the foot end, and one at each side of the patient; the two EMT-Bs at the sides each use one hand to support the stretcher so that all are able to face forward as they walk.

diaphragm A muscular that forms the undersurface of the thorax, separating the chest from the abdominal cavity. Contraction of the diaphragm (and the chest wall muscles) brings air into the lungs. Relaxation allows air to be expelled from the lungs.

diastole The dilation, or period of dilatation, of the heart, especially of the ventricles.

diastolic pressure The component of blood pressure in which pressure remains in the arteries during the relaxing phase of the heart's cycle when the left ventricle is at rest.

diffuse pain Pain that is not identified as specific to a single location.

diffusion A process in which molecules move from an area of higher concentration of molecules to an area of lower concentration.

digestion The processing of food that nourishes the individual cells of the body.

dilation Widening of a tubular structure such as a coronary artery.

diptheria An infectious disease in which a membrane lining the pharynx is formed that can severely obstruct passage of the air into the larynx.

direct contact Exposure or transmission of a communicable disease from one person to another, by physical touching.

direct ground lift A lifting technique used for patients who are found lying supine on the ground, with no suspected spinal injury.

disinfection The killing of pathogenic agents by direct application of chemicals.

dislocation Disruption of a joint in which ligaments are damaged and the bone ends are completely displaced.

displaced fracture Fracture in which fracture fragments are separated from one another and not in anatomic alignment.

distal Structures that are nearer to the free end of the extremity.

distracted The action of pulling the spine along its length.

diving reflex Slowing of the heart rate caused by sudden submersion in cold water.

DNR orders Written documentation giving permission to medical personnel not to attempt resuscitation in the event of cardiac arrest.

dorsal The posterior surface of the body, including the back of the hand.

dorsalis pedis artery Artery on the anterior surface of the foot between the first and second metatarsals.

dose The amount of medication given based on the size and age of the patient.

drowning Death from suffocation by submersion in water.

duplex The ability to transmit and receive simultaneously.

duty to act A medicolegal term relating to certain personnel who either by statute or function have a responsibility to provide care.

dysarthria The inability to pronounce speech clearly, often due to loss of the nerves or brain cells that control the small muscles in the larynx.

dyspnea Shortness of breath or difficulty breathing.

ecchymosis Bruising or discoloration associated with bleeding within or under the skin.

eclampsia Convulsions (seizures) resulting from severe hypertension in the pregnant woman.

ectopic pregnancy A pregnancy that develops outside the uterus, typically in a fallopian tube.

edema The presence of abnormally large amounts of fluid in the extracellular spaces of body tissues, causing swelling of the affected area.

elder abuse Any action on the part of an elderly individual's family member, caretaker, or other associated person that takes advantage of the elderly individual's person, property, or emotional state; also called granny battering or parent battering.

electrolytes Certain salts and other chemicals that are dissolved in body fluids and cells.

embolus A blood clot or other substance that has formed in a blood vessel or in the heart that breaks off and travels to another blood vessel, where it causes blockage.

emergency A serious situation, such as injury or illness, that arises suddenly, threatens the life or welfare of a person or group of people, and requires immediate intervention.

emergency medical care Immediate care or treatment; the EMT-B is often the first link in the chain of prehospital care.

emergency medical services (EMS) A multidisciplinary system that represents the combined efforts of several professionals and agencies to provide prehospital emergency care to the sick and injured.

emergency medical technician (EMT) An EMS professional who is trained and licensed by the state to provide emergency medical care in the field.

emergency move A move in which the patient is dragged or pulled from a dangerous scene before initial assessment and care are provided.

emesis Vomiting.

emphysema A disease of the lungs in which there is extreme dilation and eventual destruction of pulmonary alveoli with poor exchange of oxygen and carbon dioxide; it is one form of chronic obstructive pulmonary disease (COPD).

EMT-Basic An EMT who has training in basic emergency care skills, including automated defibrillation, use of a definitive airway adjunct, and assisting patients with certain medications.

EMT-Intermediate An EMT who has advanced training in specific aspects of advanced life support, such as intravenous therapy.

EMT-Paramedic   An EMT who has extensive training in advanced life support, including intravenous therapy, pharmacology, cardiac monitoring, and other advanced assessment and treatment skills.

end tidal carbon dioxide detector   A plastic disposable indicator that signals, by color change, that the ETT is in the proper place.

endocrine system   Complex message and control system that integrates many body functions, including the release of hormones.

endotracheal intubation   A method of intubation in which an endotracheal tube (ETT) is placed through a patient's mouth, directly through the larynx between the vocal cords, and into the trachea, to open and maintain an airway.

entrance wound   The area of the body where a penetrating trauma occurs. In gunshot wounds, this would be the area where the bullet entered.

entrapment   To be caught as in a trap within a vehicle, room, or container with no way out, or to have a limb or other body part trapped.

envenomation   The act of injecting venom.

epidermis   The outer layer of skin that acts as a watertight protective covering.

epidermis   The outer layer of skin, which is made up of cells that are sealed together to form a watertight protective covering for the body.

epiglottis   A thin, leaf-shaped valve that allows air to pass into the trachea but prevents food or liquid from entering.

epiglottitis   An infectious disease in which the epiglottis becomes inflamed and enlarged and may cause upper airway obstruction.

epinephrine   A substance produced by the body (adrenaline) and a drug produced by pharmaceutical companies to increase pulse and blood pressure; the drug of choice for an anaphylactic reaction.

epistaxis   Nosebleed.

esophagus   A collapsible tube about 10 inches long that extends from the pharynx to the stomach; contractions of the muscle in the wall of the esophagus propel food and liquids through it to the stomach.

eustachian tube   The internal auditory canal that connects the middle ear to the nasal cavity.

evaporation   Conversion of water from a liquid to a gas.

evisceration   The displacement of organs outside the body.

exhalation   Part of the breathing process in which the diaphragm and the intercostal muscles relax.

exit wound   The area of the body where a penetrating trauma exited. In gunshot wounds, this would be the area where the bullet exited.

exposure   A situation in which a person has had contact with blood, body fluids, tissues, or airborne particles in a manner that suggests that disease transmission may occur.

exposure control plan   Comprehensive plan that helps employees reduce their risk of exposure to or acquisition of communicable diseases.

expressed consent   A type of consent in which a patient gives express authorizes for provision of care or transport.

extend   To straighten.

external auditory canal   The ear canal.

extremity lift   A lifting technique used for patients who are supine or in a sitting position with no suspected extremity or spinal injuries.

extrication   Removal of a patient from entrapment or a dangerous situation or position, such as removal from a wrecked vehicle, industrial accident, or building collapse.

extrication/retrieval group   Personnel assigned to extricate and/or collect patients at a multiple-casualty situation and bring them to the triage center.

eyes forward position   Position in which head is gently lifted until the patient's eyes are looking straight ahead and the head and torso are in line.

fallopian tube   Long, slender tube that extends from the uterus to the region of the ovary on the same side, and through which the ovum passes from ovary to uterus.

fascia   A sheet or band of tough fibrous connective tissue. It lies deep under the skin and forms an outer layer for the muscles.

febrile seizures   Convulsions that result for sudden high fevers, particularly in children.

Federal Communications Commission (FCC)   Federal agency with jurisdiction over interstate and international telephone and telegraph services and satellite communications, all of which may involve EMS activity.

femoral artery   The principal artery of the thigh, a continuation of the external iliac artery. It supplies blood to the lower abdominal wall, external genitalia, and legs. It can be palpated in the groin area.

femoral head   The proximal end of the femur, articulating with the acetabulum.

femur   The thigh bone extending from the pelvis to the knee, responsible for formation of the hip; the longest and largest bone in the body.

fetal alcohol syndrome   A condition of infants born to alcoholic mothers characterized by physical and mental retardation and a variety of congenital abnormalities.

fetus   The developing, unborn infant inside the uterus.

fibrillation   Completely disorganized, ineffective twitching of the heart muscle.

fibula   The outer and smaller bone of the two bones of the leg.

first responder   The first trained individual, such as a police officer, fire fighter, or other rescuer, to arrive at the scene of an emergency to provide initial medical assistance.

flail chest   A condition in which three or more ribs are fractured in two or more places, or in association with a fracture of the sternum so that a segment of chest wall is effectively detached from the rest of the thoracic cage.

flex   To bend.

flexible stretcher   A stretcher that is a rigid carrying device when secured around a patient, but can be folded or rolled when not in use.

floating ribs   These are the eleventh and twelfth ribs because they do not attach to the sternum through the costal arch.

flutter valve   A one-way valve that allows air to leave the chest cavity but not return.

focal pain   Pain that is easily identified as specific to a single location.

focused history and physical exam   Part of the assessment process in which the patient's major complaints or any problems that are immediately evident are further and more specifically evaluated.

footprint   The area of contact between the ambulance tire and the road surface.

foramen magnum   A large opening at the base of the skull where the brain connects to the spinal cord.

forcible restraint   The process of confining an individual from any mental or physical action.

four-person log roll   Recommended procedure for moving a patient with a suspected spinal injury from the ground to a long spine board.

Fowler's position   The position where the patient is sitting up with the knees bent.

fracture   Any break in the continuity of a bone.

friction   The resistance to motion of one body against another.

frostbite   Damage to tissues as the result of exposure to cold; frozen body parts.

full-thickness burn   A burn that affects all skin layers and may affect the subcutaneous layers, muscle, bone, and internal organs, leaving the area dry, leathery, and white, dark brown, or charred; traditionally called a third-degree burn.

functional disorder   A disorder in which there is no known physiologic reason for the abnormal functioning of an organ or organ system.

gag reflex   A normal reflex mechanism that causes retching and is activated by touching the soft palate or the back of the throat.

gallbladder   A pear-shaped sac on the undersurface of the liver that collects bile from the liver and discharges it into the duodenum through the common bile duct.

gastric distention   A condition in which air fills the stomach as a result of high volume and pressure during artificial ventilation.

gastric tube   An advanced airway adjunct that provides a channel directly into a patient's stomach, allowing you to remove gas, blood, and toxins, or insert medications and nutrition.

gastrostomy tube   A feeding tube placed directly through the wall of the abdomen used in patients who cannot ingest liquids or solids.

gel   A semi-liquid substance administered orally through capsules or plastic tubes.

general impression   Overall initial impression formed to determine the priority for patient care. Based on the patient's surroundings, the mechanism of injury, or the patient's chief complaint.

generalized seizure   Seizure characterized by severe twitching of all the body's muscles that may last several minutes or more; also known as a grand mal seizure.

generic name   The original chemical name of a drug (in contrast to one of its "trade names").

genital system   The male and female reproductive systems.

Glasgow coma scale   A method of assessing a patient's level of consciousness by scoring the patient's response to eye opening, motor response, and verbal response; used primarily in the detailed and ongoing assessment.

glenoid fossa   The part of the scapula that joins with the humeral head to form the glenohumeral joint.

globe   The eyeball.

glucose   D-glucose or dextrose; one of the basic sugars; it is the primary fuel, along with oxygen, for cellular metabolism.

Golden Hour   The period of time during which treatment of a patient in shock or with traumatic injuries is most critical. This period of time is generally thought to be the first 60 minutes after injury.

Good Samaritan laws   Statutory provisions enacted by many states to protect citizens from civil and criminal liability for errors and omissions in giving good faith emergency medical care, unless there is wanton, gross, or willful negligence.

greater trochanter   A bony prominence on the proximal lateral side of the thigh, just below the hip joint.

guarding   Involuntary muscle contractions of the abdominal wall, an effort to protect the inflamed abdomen.

hair follicles   The small organs that produce hair.

hallucinogen   An agent that produces false perceptions in any one of the five senses.

hazardous material   Any substance that is toxic, poisonous, radioactive, flammable, or explosive, and causes injury or death with exposure.

hazardous materials incident   An accident in which a hazardous material is not longer properly contained and isolated.

head-tilt/chin-lift maneuver   A technique to open the airway that combines tilting back the forehead and lifting the chin.

heart   A hollow muscular organ that receives blood from the veins and propels it into the arteries.

heart rate (pulse)   The wave of pressure that is created by the heart contracting and forcing blood out the left ventricle and into the major arteries.

heat cramps   Painful muscle spasms usually associated with vigorous activity in a hot environment.

heat exhaustion   A form of heat injury in which the body loses significant amounts of fluid and electrolytes from heavy sweating, which results in dizziness, nausea, confusion, collapse, and severe weakness; also called heat prostration or heat collapse.

heatstroke   A life-threatening condition caused by exposure to excessive natural or artificial heat, marked by warm, dry skin, severely altered mental status, and often irreversible coma.

hematemesis   Vomiting blood.

hematoma   Blood collected within the body's tissues or in a body cavity, occasionally palpable as a discrete mass.

hematuria   The presence of blood in the urine.

hemiparesis   Weakness on one side of the body.

hemophilia   Congenital condition in which the patient lacks one or more of the blood's normal clotting factors.

hymoptysis   The spitting or coughing up of blood.

hemorrhage   Bleeding.

hemorrhagic stroke   One of the two main types of stroke; occurs as a result of bleeding inside the brain.

hemothorax   A collection of blood in the pleural cavity.

hepatitis   An infection of the liver, usually caused by a virus, that causes fever, loss of appetite, jaundice, fatigue, and altered liver function.

hernia   The protrusion of a loop of an organ or tissue through an abnormal body opening.

Hh   A substance produced by the body that is responsible for many of the symptoms of anaphylaxis.

high-level disinfection   The killing of pathogenic agents by using potent means of disinfection.

hinge joints   Joints that can bend and straighten but cannot rotate.

histamine   A substance produced by the body that is responsible for many of the symptoms of anaphylaxis.

HIV infection   Infection with the human immunodeficiency virus (HIV) that can progress to acquired immunodeficiency syndrome (AIDS).

hollow organs   Tubes through which materials pass, such as the stomach, small intestines, large intestines, ureters, and bladder.

glossary

glossary

hormone One of several chemical substances that regulate the activity of body organs and tissues; produced by a gland.

host The organism or individual attacked by the infecting agent; the host is infected by the agent.

humerus The supporting bone of the upper arm that joins with the scapula (glenoid) to form the shoulder joint and with the ulna and radius to form the elbow joint.

hydroplaning A condition in which the tires of a vehicle may be lifted off the road surface as water "piles up" under them.

hyperbaric chamber A chamber, usually a small room, pressurized to more than atmospheric pressure.

hyperglycemia Abnormally increased glucose level in the blood.

hypertension Blood pressure that is higher than the normal range.

hyperthermia A condition in which the internal body temperature rises to 101°F (38.3°C) or more.

hyperventilation A lowering of blood carbon dioxide levels, usually through rapid or deep breathing.

hyphema Bleeding into the anterior chamber of the eye, obscuring the iris.

hypnotic A sleep-inducing effect or agent.

hypoglycemia Condition characterized by an abnormally decreased glucose level in the blood.

hypotension Blood pressure that is lower than the normal range.

hypothermia A condition in which the internal body temperature falls below 95°F (35°C) after exposure to a cold environment.

hypovolemic shock Condition in which low blood volume, due to either massive internal or external bleeding or extensive loss of body water, results in inadequate perfusion.

hypoxia A dangerous condition in which the body tissues and cells do not have enough oxygen.

hypoxic drive A "backup system" to control respiration.

ieneric name The original chemical name of a drug (as opposed to one of its "trade names").

ileus Paralysis of the bowel, arising from any one of several causes.

iliac crest The rim of the pelvic bone.

ilium One of three bones that fuse to form the pelvic ring.

implied consent Type of consent in which a patient who is unable to give consent is given treatment under the legal assumption that he or she would want treatment.

incident commander The individual with overall command of the scene in the field.

incident management systems Organizational systems to help control, direct, and coordinate emergency responders and resources.

indication A therapeutic use for a specific medication.

indirect contact Exposure or transmission of disease from one person to another by contact with a contaminated object.

infarcted cells Cells in the brain that die as a result of loss of blood flow to the brain.

infarction Death of a body tissue, usually caused by interruption of its blood supply.

infection The abnormal invasion of a host or host tissue by organisms such as bacteria, viruses, or parasites, with or without signs or symptoms of disease.

infection control Procedures to reduce transmission of infection among patients and health care personnel.

infectious disease A disease that is caused by infection, as opposed to one caused by faulty genes, metabolic or hormonal disturbances, emotional trauma, or another cause.

inferior A directional term meaning below or "at the bottom;" the part of the body, or any body part nearer to the feet.

inferior vena cava One of the two largest veins in the body that carry blood from the lower extremities and the pelvic and the abdominal organs into the heart.

informed consent Permission for treatment given by a competent patient after the potential risks, benefits, and alternatives to treatment have been explained.

ingestion Swallowing; taking a substance by mouth.

inguinal ligament Tough, fibrous ligament that stretches between the lateral edge of the pubic symphysis and the anterior superior iliac spine.

inhalation Breathing into the lungs; a medication delivery route.

initial assessment Part of the assessment process that helps you to identify any immediate or potential life threats so that you can initiate live saving care.

insulin A hormone produced by the pancreas that enables sugar in the blood to enter the cells of the body; used in synthetic form to treat and control diabetes mellitus.

insulin shock Unconsciousness or altered mental status in a patient with diabetes caused by significant hypoglycemia; usually the result of excessive exercise and activity or failure to eat after a routine dose of insulin.

intervertebral disk A cushion that lies between the vertebrae.

intramuscular (IM) injection An injection into a muscle.

intraosseous (IO) Into the bone; a medication delivery route.

intravenous (IV) injection An injection directly into a vein.

involuntary activity Those actions we do not consciously control.

involuntary muscle Muscle that continues to contract, rhythmically, regardless of the conscious will of the individual.

iris The muscle and surrounding tissue behind the cornea that dilate and constrict the pupil, regulating the amount of light that enters the eye.

irreversible shock The final stage of shock, resulting in death.

ischemia A lack of oxygen that deprives tissues of necessary nutrients, resulting from partial or complete blockage of blood flow; ischemia implies that the problem is still potentially reversible and that permanent injury has not yet occurred.

ischemic cells Cells in the brain that receive enough blood after a cerebrovascular accident to stay alive, but not to function properly.

ischemic stroke One of the two main types of stroke; occurs when blood flow to a particular part of the brain is cut off by a blockage (e.g., a clot) inside a blood vessel.

ischium One of three bones that fuse to form the pelvic bones.

jaundice A yellow skin color seen in patients with liver disease or dysfunction.

jaw-thrust maneuver A technique to open the airway in which your fingers are placed behind the angles of the patient's lower jaw and then the jaw is moved forcefully forward.

joint (articulation) The place where two bones come in contact.

joint capsule The fibrous sac with synovial lining that encloses a joint.

jump kit A portable kit containing items used in the initial care of the patient.

kidneys Two retroperitoneal organs that excrete the end products of metabolism as urine regulate teh bodies salt and water content.

kinetic energy The energy of a moving object.

labored breathing A way in which to describe breathing that requires increased effort; characterized by grunting, stridor, and use of accessory muscles.

laceration A smooth or jagged open wound.

lacrimal glands The tear glands and ducts of the eyes

large intestine The portion of the digestive tune that extends from the ileocecal valve to the anus. It is made up of the cecum, colon, and rectum.

laryngoscope An instrument used to give a direct view of the patient's vocal cords during endotracheal intubation.

laryngospasm Vocal cord spasm.

larynx Voice box; a structure composed of thyroid cartilage on the top and cricoid cartilage on the bottom.

lateral Parts of the body that lie at some distance from the midline. Also called outer structures.

lens The transparent part of the eye, through which images are focused on the retina.

leukotrienes Chemical substances made by the body that contribute to anaphylaxis.

ligament A band of fibrous tissue that connects bones to bones. It supports and strengthens a joint.

limb presentation A delivery in which the presenting part of the infant is a single arm, leg, or foot.

limited victim incident A multiple patient situation involving fewer than 25 patients.

litter A type of stretcher for moving or carrying patients.

liver A large solid organ that lies in the right upper quadrant immediately below the diaphragm; it produces bile, stores sugar for immediate use by the body, and produces many substances that help regulate immune responses.

lumbar spine The lower part of the back; formed by the lowest five non-fused vertebrae.

lumbar vertebrae Vertebrae of the lumbar spine.

lumen The inside diameter of an artery or other hollow structure.

mandible The bone of the lower jaw.

manubrium The upper quarter of the sternum.

mastoid process Prominent bony mass at the base of the skull about 1" posterior to the external opening of the ear.

maxilla The bone that forms the upper jaw on either side of the face and contains the upper teeth, the orbit of the eye, the nasal cavity, and the palate.

maxillae The upper jawbones that assist in the formation of the orbit, the nasal cavity, and the palate, and lodges the upper teeth.

mechanism of injury The way in which traumatic injuries occur; the forces that act on the body to cause damage.

meconium A dark green material in the amniotic fluid which can be a sign of serious lung disease.

MED channels VHF and UHF channels designated by the FCC exclusively for EMS use.

medial Parts of the body that lie closer to the midline. Also called inner structures.

medical direction Physician instructions that are given directly by radio (on-line/direct) or indirectly by protocol/guidelines (off-line/indirect), as authorized by the medical director.

medical control The physician who authorizes or delegates the authority to perform medical care in the field.

medicolegal A term relating to medical jurisprudence (law) or forensic medicine.

memoptysis The spitting or coughing up of blood.

meninges Three distinct layers of tissue that surround and protect the brain and the spinal cord within the skull and the spinal canal.

meningitis Inflammation of the meninges that covers the spinal cord and the brain; usually caused by a virus or bacterium.

mental disorder An illness with psychological or behavioral symptoms and/or impairment in functioning, due to a social, psychological, genetic, physical, chemical or biologic disturbance.

metabolism The sum of all the physical and chemical processes of living organisms; the process by which energy is made available for the uses of the organism.

metered-dose inhaler (MDI) A miniature spray canister through which droplets or particles may be inhaled.

midaxillary line Imaginary vertical line drawn through the middle of the axilla (armpit), parallel to the midline.

midclavicular line Imaginary vertical line drawn through the middle portion of the clavicle and parallel to the midline.

midline Imaginary vertical line drawn from the middle of the forehead through the nose and the umbilicus (navel) to the floor.

motor nerves Nerves that carry information from the central nervous system to the muscles of the body.

mucous membranes The lining of body cavities and passages that are indirect contact with the outside environment.

mucus The opaque, sticky secretion of the mucous membranes that lubricates the body openings.

multigravida A woman who has previously given birth.

multiple-casualty situation (MCS) An event that stretches the system to its limit in terms of available equipment or personnel; also called a mass-casualty incident (MCI).

musculoskeletal system The bones and voluntary muscles of the body.

myocardial contusion A bruise of the heart muscle

myocardium The heart muscle.

myoclonic jerks Short jerks of an extremity during a seizure.

nares The external openings of the nostrils.

nasal cannula An oxygen delivery device in which oxygen flows through two small, tube-like prongs that fit into the patient's nostrils.

nasal flaring When nostrils flare out, indicating that there is an airway obstruction.

nasopharyngeal (nasal or trumpet) airway Airway adjunct inserted into the nostril of a conscious patient who is not able to maintain a natural airway.

nasopharynx The part of the pharynx that lies above the level of the soft palate.

nasotracheal intubation   The placement of a tube through the nose into the trachea.

near drowning   Survival, at least temporarily, after suffocation in water.

negligence   Failure to provide the same care that a person with similar training would provide. Also defined as a deviation from accepted standards of care.

neisseria meningitides   A form of bacterial meningitis characterized by rapid onset of symptoms, often leading to shock and death.

nervous system   System that controls virtually all activities of the body, both voluntary and involuntary activities.

neurogenic shock   Circulatory failure caused by paralysis of the nerves that control the size of the blood vesselsl. Seen in spinal cord injuries.

nitroglycerin   Medication that increases blood flow by relieving spasms or causing arteries to dilate; the EMT-B may be allowed to help the patient self-administer the medication.

nondisplaced fracture   A simple crack in the bone that has not caused the bone to move from its normal anatomic position; also called a hairline fracture.

nonrebreathing mask   A mask and reservoir bag system that is the preferred way to give oxygen in the prehospital setting; delivers up to 90% inspired oxygen.

nuchal cord   An umbilical cord that is wrapped around the infant's neck.

occiput   The most posterior portion of the skull.

occlusion   Blockage, usually of a tubular structure such as a blood vessel.

Occupational Safety and Health Administration (OSHA)   The federal regulatory compliance agency that develops, publishes, and enforces guidelines concerning safety in the workplace.

ongoing assessment   Part of the assessment process in which problems are reevaluated and responses to treatment assessed.

open abdominal injury   Any injury of the abdomen caused by a penetrating or piercing instrument or force in which the skin is lacerated or perforated and the cavity itself is opened to the atmosphere. Also called penetrating injury.

open chest injury   Injury to the chest in which the chest wall itself is penetrated by some object.

open fracture   Any break in the bone in which the overlying skin has been damaged.

open head injury   Injury to the head often caused by a penetrating object in which there may be bleeding and exposed brain tissue.

open injury   Injury in which there is a break in the surface of the skin or the mucous membrane, exposing deeper tissue to potential contamination.

opioids   Any drug or agent with actions similar to morphine.

OPQRST   The six pain questions: Onset, Provoke, Quality, Radiation, Severity, Time.

optic nerve   A cranial nerve that transmits visual sensations to the brain.

oral   By mouth; a medication delivery route.

oral glucose   A simple sugar that is readily absorbed by the bloodstream; it is carried on the EMS unit.

orbit   The eye socket.

organic brain syndrome   Temporary or permanent dysfunction of the brain, caused by a disturbance in the physical or physiologic functioning of brain tissue.

orientation   The mental status of a patient; the patient's memory of person (his or her name), place (the current location), time (the current year, month, and approximate date), and event (what happened).

oropharyngeal airway   Airway adjunct inserted into the mouth to keep the tongue from blocking the upper airway and to make suctioning the airway easier.

oropharynx   A tubular structure that extends vertically from the back of the mouth to the esophagus and trachea; the throat.

orotracheal intubation   The placement of a tube through the mouth into the trachea.

osteoporosis   A generalized bone disease common among post-menopausal women, in which there is a reduction in the amount of bone mass, leading to fractures after minimal trauma.

ovary   A female gland that produces sex hormones and ova (eggs).

over-the-counter (OTC) drugs   Drugs that may be purchased directly by a patient without a prescription.

oxygen   A gas that is needed by all cells in order to metabolize; the heart and brain, especially, cannot function without oxygen.

paging   The use of a radio signal and a voice or digital message that is transmitted to pagers ("beepers") or desktop monitor radios.

palmar   The front region of the hand.

palpate   Examination by touch.

pancreas   A flat, solid organ that lies below the liver and the stomach, it is a major source of digestive enzymes and produces the hormone insulin.

paradoxical motion   The motion of the portion of the chest wall that is detached in a flail chest; the motion is exactly the opposite of normal motion during breathing: in during inhalation, out during exhalation.

parietal regions   The region between the temporal and occiput regions of the cranium.

partial airway obstruction   Condition in which the patient is able to exchange air in the lungs, but has some degree of respiratory distress.

partial-thickness burn   A burn affecting the epidermis and some portion of the dermis but not the subcutaneous tissue, characterized by blisters and skin that is white to red, moist, and mottled; traditionally called a second-degree burn.

patella   The knee cap; a specialized bone that lies within the tendon of the quadriceps muscle.

pathogen   A microorganism that is capable of causing disease in a susceptible host.

pedal edema   Swelling of the feet and ankles caused by collection of fluid in the tissues.

pediatric resuscitation tape measure   A tape that estimates weight based upon length and generates appropriate drug doses and equipment sizes on the tape.

pediatrics   A separate medical practice devoted to the care of the young.

penetrating trauma   A mechanism of injury in which force occurs in a small point of contact between the skin and the object.

penetrating wound   An injury resulting from a sharp, pointed object.

per os   Through the mouth; a medication delivery route.

per rectum   Through the rectum; a medication delivery route.

perfusion   The circulation of blood within an organ or tissue in adequate amounts to meet the cells' current needs.

pericardial tamponade   Acute compression of the heart due to a buildup of blood or other fluid in the pericardial sac.

pericardium   The fibrous sac that surrounds the heart.

perineum   The area of skin between the vagina and the anus.

peripheral nervous system   The part of the nervous system that consists of 31 pairs of spinal nerves and 12 pairs of cranial nerves. These peripheral nerves may be sensory nerves, motor nerves, or connecting nerves.

peristalsis   The wavelike movement by which the ureters or other tubular organs propel their contents.

peritoneal cavity   The abdominal cavity.

peritoneum   The membrane lining the abdominal cavity (parietal peritoneum) and covering the abdominal organs (visceral peritoneum).

peritonitis   Inflammation of the peritoneum.

personal protective equipment (PPE)   Protective equipment required by OSHA to be made available to the EMT.

pharmacology   The study of the properties and effects of medications.

pin-indexing system   A system established for portable cylinders to ensure that a regulator is not connected to the wrong cylinder.

pinna   The external, visible part of the ear.

placenta   Body tissue attached to the inner lining of the wall of the uterus, connected to the fetus by the umbilical cord.

placenta abruptio   Premature separation of the placenta from the wall of the uterus.

placenta previa   A condition in which the placenta develops over and covers the cervix.

plantar   The bottom of the foot.

plasma   A sticky, yellow fluid that carries the blood cells and nutrients and transports cellular waste material to the organs of excretion.

platelets   Tiny, disk-shaped elements that are much smaller than the cells; they are essential in the initial formation of a blood clot, the mechanism that stops bleeding.

pleura   The serous membrane covering the lungs and lining the thoracic cavity, completely enclosing a potential space known as the pleural space.

pleural space   The potential space between the parietal pleura and the visceral pleura. It is described as "potential" because under normal conditions the lungs fill this space.

pleural effusion   A collection of fluid between the lung and chest wall that may compress the lung.

pleuritic chest pain   Sharp, stabbing pain in the chest that is worsened by a deep breath often caused by inflammation or irritation of the pleura.

pneumonia   An infectious disease of the lung that damages and destroys lung tissue.

pneumothorax   A partial or complete accumulation of air in the pleural space.

point tenderness   Tenderness sharply localized at the site of the injury found by gently palpating along the bone with the tip of one finger.

poison   A substance whose chemical action could damage structures or impair function when introduced into the body.

polydipsia   Excessive thirst persisting for long periods of time despite reasonable fluid intake; often the result of excessive urination; in patients with diabetes, the excessive urination is caused by the wasting of glucose in the urine when blood levels are high.

polyphagia   Excessive eating; in diabetes, the inability to use glucose properly can cause a sense of hunger.

polyuria   The passage of an unusually large volume of urine in a given period; in diabetes, this can result from wasting of glucose in the urine.

portable stretcher   A stretcher with a strong rectangular tubular metal frame and rigid fabric stretched across it.

position of function   A hand position in which the wrist is slightly dorsiflexed and all finger joints are moderately flexed.

posttraumatic stress disorder (PTSD)   A delayed stress reaction to a prior incident. This delayed reaction is the result of one or more unresolved issues concerning the incident that may have been alleviated with the use of critical incident stress management.

posterior   A directional term meaning the back surface of the body, the side away from you.

posterior tibial artery   Artery just posterior to the medial malleolus; supplies blood to the foot.

postictal period   The period immediately following a seizure, characterized by extreme tiredness or listlessness.

postictal state   Period following a seizure that lasts between 5 and 30 minutes, characterized by labored respirations and some degree of altered mental status.

potential energy   The product of mass, gravity, and height, which is converted into kinetic energy and results in injury, such as from a fall.

power grip   Technique in which the litter or backboard is gripped by inserting each hand under the handle with the palm facing up and the thumb extended, fully supporting the underside of the handle on the curved palm with the fingers and thumb.

power lift   Lifting technique in which the EMT-B's back is held upright with legs bent, and the patient is lifted when the EMT-B raises his or her upper body and arms and straightens his or her legs.

prescription drugs   Drugs distributed to patients only by pharmacists according to a physician's order.

presentation   The manner in which an infant is born; the part of the infant that appears first.

pressure point   Point where a blood vessel lies near a bone.

primary service area (PSA)   The area in which the EMS service is responsible for the provision of prehospital emergency care and transportation to the hospital.

primigravida   A woman who is having her first infant.

prolapse of the umbilical cord   A situation in which the umbilical cord comes out of the vagina before the infant.

prone position   The position in which the body is lying face down.

prostate gland   A small gland that surrounds the male urethra where it emerges from the urinary bladder; it secretes fluid that is part of the ejaculatory fluid.

protection level   A measure of the amount and type of protective equipment that an individual needs to avoid injury during contact with a hazardous material.

proximal   Structures that are closer to the trunk.

psychogenic   A symptom or illness that is caused by mental factors as opposed to physical ones.

psychogenic shock   Shock caused by a temporary reduction in blood supply to the brain. The common faint.

pubis   One of three bones that fuse to form the pelvic ring.

pulmonary artery   The major artery leading from the right ventricle of the heart to the lungs. It carries oxygen-poor blood.

pulmonary contusion   A bruise of the lung.

pulmonary edema   A build-up of fluid in the lungs, usually as a result of congestive heart failure.

pulmonary embolism   The condition in which a blood clot breaks off from a large vein and travels to the blood vessels of the lung, causing obstruction of blood flow.

pulmonary veins   One of the four veins that return oxygenated blood from the lungs to the left atrium of the heart.

pulse (heart rate)   The pressure wave that occurs as each heartbeat causes a surge in the blood circulating through the arteries; the rate at which the heart is contracting. The normal pulse rate in an adult is 60 to 80 beat/min; for a child, the normal rate is 80 to 100 beats/min.

pupil   The circular opening in the middle of the iris of the eye.

quadrants   The way to describe the sections of the abdominal cavity. Imagine two lines intersecting at the umbilicus dividing the abdomen into four equal areas.

quality control   The responsibility of the medical director to ensure that the appropriate medical care standards are met by EMT-Bs on each call.

rabid   An adjective describing an animal that is infected with rabies.

radial artery   The major artery in the lower arm and is palpable at the wrist on the thumb side.

radiation   A continuation of an area of pain or discomfort distal to the site of the origin of the pain; the direct loss of body heat to a colder air environment.

radius   The bone on the thumb side of the forearm, most important in wrist function.

rales   A crackling breath sound caused by the flow of air through liquid in the lungs; a sign of lower airway obstruction. Also called crackles.

Rapid Extrication Technique   A technique that was developed to move a patient from a sitting position inside a vehicle to supine on a backboard in less than 1 minute.

rapport   A trusting relationship that you build with your patient.

recovery position   A position that helps to maintain a clear airway in a patient with a decreased level of consciousness who has not had traumatic injuries and is breathing on his or her own.

rectum   The lowermost end of the large intestine.

red blood cells   Cells that carry oxygen to the body's tissues; also called erythrocytes.

reduce   Return of a dislocated joint or fractured bone to its normal position; set.

referred pain   Pain felt in an area of the body other than where the cause of pain is located.

renal pelvis   A cone-shaped collecting area that connects the ureter and the kidney.

repeater   A special base station radio that receives messages and signals on one frequency and then automatically retransmits them on a second frequency.

respiratory system   All the structures of the body that contribute to the process of breathing, consisting of the upper and lower airways.

responsiveness   The way in which a patient responds to external stimuli, including verbal stimuli (sound), tactile stimuli (touch), and painful stimuli.

retina   The light-sensitive area of the eye where images are projected; a layer of cells at the back of the eye that changes the light image into electrical impulses, which are carried by the optic nerve to the brain.

retinal detachment   A condition in which the retina is separated from its attachments at the back of the eye.

retractions   Movements in which the skin pulls in around the ribs during inspiration.

retrograde amnesia   The inability to remember events leading up to a head injury.

retroperitoneal   Behind the abdominal cavity.

retroperitoneal space   The space between the abdominal cavity and the posterior abdominal wall containing the kidneys, certain large vessels, and parts of the gastrointestinal tract.

rhonchi   Coarse breath sounds heard in patients with chronic mucus in the airways.

rigor mortis   Stiffening of the body after death.

Rule of Nines   A system that assigns percentages to sections of the body, allowing calculation of the amount of skin surface involved in the burn area.

sacrum   One of three bones (sacrum and two pelvic bones) that make up the pelvic ring.

salivary glands   Gland that produces saliva to keep the mouth and pharynx moist.

SAMPLE history   A key brief history of a patient's condition to determine Signs/symptoms, Allergies, Medications, Pertinent past history, Last oral intake, and Events leading to the illness/injury.

scalp   The thick skin covering the cranium and usually bearing hair.

scanner   A radio receiver that searches or "scans" across several frequencies until the message is completed. The process is then repeated.

scapula   The shoulder blade.

scene size-up   Part of the assessment process in which a quick assessment of the scene and the surroundings is made to provide as much information as possible about the safety of the scene.

sciatic nerve   The major nerve to the lower extremity.

sclera   The white portion of the eye; the tough outer coat of the eye that gives protection to the delicate, light-sensitive inner layer.

scoop stretcher   A stretcher that is designed to be split into two or four sections that can be fitted around a patient lying on the ground or other relatively flat surface. Also called a split litter.

sebaceous glands   Glands that produces an oily substance called sebum, which discharges along the shafts of the hairs.

sector commander   The individual, working under the incident commander, who is delegated to oversee and coordinate a sector's activity.

sedative   A substance that decreases activity and excitement.

seizure   Generalized, uncoordinated muscular activity associated with loss of consciousness; a convulsion.

self-contained underwater breathing apparatus (SCUBA)   A system that delivers air to the mouth and lungs at various atmospheric pressures, increasing with the depth of the dive.

Sellick maneuver   A technique used with intubation in which pressure is applied on the cricoid cartilage to prevent gastric distention and allow better visualization of vocal cords.

semen   Seminal fluid ejaculated from the penis containing sperm.

seminal vesicles Storage sacs for sperm and seminal fluid, which empty into the urethra at the prostate.

sensitization Developing a sensitivity to a substance that initially caused no allergic reaction.

sensory nerves Nerves that transmit sensory input, such as touch, taste, heat, cold, and pain, from the body to the central nervous system.

septic shock Shock caused by severe bacterial infection.

septum The center of the nose.

Shaken Baby Syndrome Bleeding within the head and damage to the cervical spine of an infant who has been intentionally and forcibly shaken; a form of child abuse.

shock A condition that develops when the circulatory system is not able to deliver sufficient blood to body organs, resulting in organ failure and eventual death if untreated ; also called hypoperfusion.

shock position The position that has the head and torso (truck) supine and the lower extremities elevated 8" to 12". This helps to increase blood flow to the brain; also referred to as the modified Trendelenburg's position.

shoulder girdle The proximal portion of the upper extremity, made up of the clavicle, the scapula, and the humerus.

shunt A tube that diverts excess cerebrospinal fluid from the brain to the abdomen.

side effects Any effects of a drug other than the desired ones.

sign An objective finding that can be seen, heard, felt, smelled, or measured.

simple access Access that is easily achieved without the use of tools or force.

simplex Single-frequency radio; transmissions can occur in either direction but not simultaneously in both; when one party transmits the other can only receive, and when one party is transmitting it is unable to receive.

skeletal muscle Striated muscle that is attached to bones and usually crosses at least one joint. It is also called voluntary muscle and striated muscle.

skeleton Framework that gives us our recognizable form. Also designed to allow motion of the body and protection of vital organs.

sling Any bandage or material that helps support the weight of an injured upper extremity.

small intestine The protion of the digestive tube between the stomach and the cecum, consisting of the duodenum, jejunum, and the ileum.

smooth muscle Nonstriated, involuntary muscle; it constitutes the bulk of the gastrointestinal tract and is present in nearly every organ to regulate automatic activity.

sniffing position An unusually upright position in which the patient's head and chin are thrust slightly forward; also called a tripod position.

solid organs Solid masses of tissue where much of the chemical work of the body takes place, e.g., the liver, spleen, pancreas, and kidneys.

solution A liquid mixture that cannot be separated by filtering or allowing the mixture to stand.

somatic (voluntary) nervous system The part of the nervous system that regulates our voluntary activities, such as walking, talking, and writing.

sphincters Circular muscles that encircle and, by contracting, constrict a duct, tube, or opening.

spinal cord An extension of the brain, composed of virtually all the nerves carrying messages between the brain and the rest of the body. It lies inside of and is protected by the spinal canal.

splint A flexible or rigid appliance used to protect and maintain the position of an injured extremity.

spontaneous pneumothorax When a weak area on the lung ruptures spontaneously, allowing air to leak into the pleural space.

spontaneous respirations Breathing in a patient that occurs with no assistance.

sprain Any joint injury with damage to supporting ligaments.

stair chair A lightweight folding device that is used to carry a conscious, seated patient up or down stairs.

standard of care Written, accepted levels of emergency care expected by reason of training and profession; written by legal or professional organizations so that patients are not exposed to unreasonable risk or harm.

standing orders Written documents, signed by the EMS system's medical director, that outline specific directions, permissions, and sometimes prohibitions regarding patient care; also called protocols.

Star of Life® The six-pointed star that identifies ambulances and other prehospital providers that meet federal specifications as licensed or certified ambulances.

status epilepticus The term used to describe a continuous seizure or multiple seizures without a return to consciousness for 30 minutes.

sterilization A process, such as heating, that is used to remove microbial contamination.

sternocleidomastoid muscles Muscles on either side of the neck that allow movement of the head.

sternum The breastbone.

stimulant Any agent that produces an excited state.

stoma Opening in the neck that connects the trachea directly to the skin.

strain Stretching or tearing of a muscle; also called a muscle pull.

strangulation Complete obstruction of blood circulation in a given organ as a result of compression or entrapment; a situation causing death of tissue.

striated muscle Muscle that has characteristic stripes, or striations, under the microscope; voluntary, skeletal muscle.

stridor A harsh, high-pitched inspiratory sound, such as the sound often hear in acute laryngeal (upper airway) obstruction.

stroke A loss of brain function in certain brain cells because they suddenly do not get enough oxygen. Usually caused by obstruction of the blood vessels in the brain that feed oxygen to those brain cells.

structure fire A fire in a house, apartment building, office, school, plant, warehouse, or other building.

stylet A plastic-coated wire that gives added rigidity and shape to the endotracheal tube.

subcutaneous (SC) injection An injection into the tissue between the skin and muscle.

subcutaneous emphysema The presence of air in soft tissues, causing a characteristic crackling sensation on palpation.

subcutaneous tissue Tissue, largely fat, that lies directly under the dermis and serves as an insulator of the body.

sublingual (SL) Under the tongue; a medication delivery route.

substance abuse The knowing misuse of any substance to produce some desired effect.

sucking chest wound An open or penetrating chest wall wound through which air passes during inspiration and expiration.

glossary

Sudden Infant Death Syndrome (SIDS)   Death of an infant or young child that remains unexplained after a complete autopsy.

superficial   Closer to or on the skin.

superficial burn   A burn affecting only the epidermis, characterized by skin that is red but not blistered or actually burned through; traditionally called a first-degree burn.

superior   A directional term meaning above or "on top;" the part of the body, or any body part nearer to the head.

superior vena cava   One of the two largest veins in the body that carries blood from the upper extremities, head, neck, and chest into the heart.

supine hypotensive syndrome   Low blood pressure resulting from compression by weight of the fetus on the inferior vena cava.

supine position   When the body is lying face up.

suspension   A mixture of ground particles that are distributed evenly throughout a liquid.

swathe   A bandage passing around the chest to secure an injured arm to the chest.

sweat glands   The glands that secrete sweat.

symphysis pubis   The firm cartilaginous joint between the two pubic bones.

symptom   A subjective finding that the patient feels, but can only be identified by the patient.

syncope   Fainting spell or transient loss of consciousness.

systole   The contraction, or period of contraction, of the heart, especially that of the ventricles.

systolic pressure   The component of blood pressure in which pressure is increased along an artery with each contraction of the ventricle.

tachycardia   Rapid heart rhythm, more than 100 beats/min.

tachypnea   Rapid respirations.

tactical situation   A hostage, robbery, or other situation in which armed conflict is threatened or shots have been fired, and the threat of violence remains.

tagus   The small cartilaginous projection in front of the opening of the ear.

technical rescue situation   A rescue that requires special technical skills and equipment in one of many specialized rescue areas, such as technical rope rescue, cave rescue, and dive rescue.

technical rescue team   A group of individuals from one or more departments in a region that is trained and on-call for certain types of technical rescue.

telemetry   A process in which electronic signals are converted into coded, audible signals. These signals can then be transmitted by radio or telephone to a receiver at the hospital with a decoder.

temporal regions   The lateral portions on each side of the cranium.

temporomandibular joint   The joint formed where the mandible and cranium meet, just in front of the ear.

tendon   A tough rope-like cord of fibrous tissue that attaches a skeletal muscle to a bone.

tension pneumothorax   An accumulation of air or gas in the pleural cavity that progressively increases and causes a rise in intrathoracic pressure.

testicle   A male genital gland that contains specialized cells that produce hormones and sperm.

thoracic cage   The chest or rib cage.

thoracic spine   The 12 vertebrae that lie between the cervical vertebrae and the lumbar vertebrae. One pair of ribs is attached to each of the thoracic vertebrae.

thorax   The cavity that contains the heart, lungs, esophagus, and the great vessels (the aorta and two venae cavae).

thrombosis   Clotting of the cerebral arteries that may result in the interruption of cerebral blood flow and subsequent stroke.

thyroid cartilage   A firm prominence of cartilage that forms the upper part of the larynx; the Adam's apple.

tibia   The larger of the two leg bones responsible for supporting the major weightbearing surface of the knee and the ankle; the shin bone.

tidal volume   The amount of air that is exchanged with each breath.

tolerance   The need for increasing amounts of a drug to obtain the same effect.

tonic seizure   A seizure in which there is a rigid extremity.

tonic-clonic seizure   A seizure that features rhythmic back-and-forth motion of an extremity and body stiffness.

tonsil tip   A large, somewhat rigid suction tip recommended for suctioning the pharynx.

topical medications   Lotions, creams, and ointments that are applied to the surface of the skin and affect only that area.

topographic anatomy   The superficial landmarks of the body that serve as guides to the structures that lie beneath them.

torso   The trunk without the head and limbs.

toxicity level   A measure of the risk that a hazardous material poses to the health of an individual who comes in contact with it.

toxin   A poison or harmful substance produced by bacteria, animals, or plants.

trachea   The windpipe; the main trunk for air passing to and from the lungs.

tracheostomy tube   A tube inserted into the trachea in children who cannot breathe on their own.

traction   The act of exerting a pulling force on a structure.

trade name   The brand name a manufacturer gives a drug.

tragus   Small rounded fleshy bulge that lies immediately anterior to the ear canal.

tral   By mouth; a medication delivery route.

transcutaneous   Through the skin; a medication delivery route.

transdermal medications   Medications designed to be absorbed through the skin.

transient ischemic attack (TIA)   A disorder of the brain in which brain cells temporarily stop working because of insufficient oxygen, causing stroke-like symptoms that resolve completely within 24 hours of onset.

transmission   The way in which an infectious agent is spread: contact, airborne, by vehicles, or by vectors.

transport area   The area at one end of the treatment area in a multiple-casualty situation where patients are loaded into ambulances and transported to the receiving hospitals.

transport officer   The individual in charge of the transport sector in a multiple-casualty situation, including the area, crews, and any activities related to the transport of patients to receiving hospitals.

treatment center   Location in a mass-casualty situation where patients are brought after being triaged and assigned a priority, and where they are reassessed, treated, and monitored until it is their turn to be transported to the hospital.

treatment officer   The individual, usually a physician, who is in charge of and directs EMS personnel at the treatment center in a multiple-casualty situation.

Trendelenburg's position   The position where the body is supine with the head lower than the feet.

triage   The process of establishing treatment and transportation priorities according to severity of injury and medical need.

triage center   Designated area in a multiple-casualty situation where the triage officer is located and patients are initially triaged before being taken to the treatment center.

triage officer   The individual who is in charge of rapidly assessing and deciding into which triage category patients should be placed in a multiple-casualty situation.

triceps   The muscle in the back of the upper arm.

tuberculosis (TB)   A chronic bacterial disease, caused by Mycobacterium tuberculosis, that usually affects the lungs, but can also affect other organs such as the brain or kidneys.

turbinates   Layers of bone within the nasal cavity.

two- to three-word dyspnea   A condition in which a patient can speak only two to three words at a time without taking a breath.

tympanic membrane   The eardrum, which lies between the external and middle ear.

type I diabetes   The type of diabetic disease that usually starts in childhood and requires insulin for proper treatment and control.

type II diabetes   The type of diabetic disease that usually starts in later life and often can be controlled through diet and oral medications.

UHF   Ultra High Frequency. Radio frequencies between 300 and 3,000 MHz.

ulna   The bone on the small finger side of the forearm, most important for elbow function.

ulnar artery   One of the major arteries of the arm; it can be palpated at the medial wrist at the base of the fifth finger.

umbilical cord   The conduit connecting mother to infant via the placenta; contains two arteries and one vein.

universal precautions   Protective measures that have traditionally been developed by the Centers for Disease Control and Prevention (CDC) for use when dealing with objects, blood, body fluids, or other potential exposure risks of communicable disease.

ureter   A small, hollow tube that carries urine from the kidneys to the bladder.

urethra   The membranous canal that conveys urine from the bladder to outside the body.

urinary bladder   A sac made of smooth muscle that collects and stores urine.

urinary system   The organs that control the discharge of certain waste materials filtered from the blood and excreted as urine.

urticaria   Small spots of generalized itching and/or burning that appear as multiple raised areas on the skin; hives.

uterus   The muscular organ where the fetus grows, responsible for contractions during labor; the womb.

vagina   A muscular distensible tube that connects the uterus with the vulva (the external female genitalia); also called the birth canal.

vallecula   The space between the base of the tongue and the epiglottis.

vasa deferentia   The Spermatic duct of the testicles; also called vas deferans.

vasodilation   Widening of a blood vessel.

ventilation   Exchange of air between the lungs and the air of the environment, either spontaneously by the patient or with assistance from an EMT-B.

ventral   The anterior surface of the body.

ventricle   One of two (right and left) lower chambers of the heart. As the main pumping chamber of the heart, the left ventricle receives blood from the left atrium (upper chamber) and delivers blood to the aorta which, in turn, delivers it to the rest of the body.

ventricular fibrillation   Disorganized, ineffective twitching of the ventricles, resulting in no blood flow and a state of cardiac arrest.

ventricular tachycardia   Rapid heart rhythm in which the electrical impulse begins in the ventricle (instead of the atrium), which may result in inadequate blood flow and eventually deteriorate into cardiac arrest.

VHF   Very High Frequency. Radio frequencies between 30 and 300 MHz. The VHF spectrum is further divided into "high" and "low" bands.

virulence   The strength or ability of a pathogen to produce disease.

vital signs   The key signs used to evaluate the patient's overall condition, including respirations, pulse, blood pressure, level of consciousness, and skin characteristics.

voluntary activity   Actions that we consciously perform, in which sensory input determines the specific muscular activity.

voluntary muscle   Muscle under direct voluntary control of the brain that can be contracted or relaxed at will; skeletal muscle.

vomitus   Vomited material.

wheal   A raised, swollen area on the skin resulting from an insect bite or allergic reaction.

wheeled ambulance stretcher   A specially designed stretcher that can be rolled along the ground. A collapsible undercarriage allows it to be loaded into the ambulance. Also called the cot or an ambulance cot.

wheeze   A high-pitched, whistling breath sound, characteristically heard on expiration in patients with asthma or COPD.

wheezing   A whistling breath sound caused by air traveling through narrowed air passages within the bronchioles and characteristically heard on expiration; a sign of lower airway obstruction.

white blood cells   They play a role in the body's immune defense mechanisms against infection.

xiphoid process   The narrow, cartilaginous lower tip of the sternum.

zygomas   The quadrangular bones of the cheek, articulating with the frontal bone, the maxillae, the zygomatic processes of the temporal bone, and the great wings of the sphenoid bone.

glossary

Index

index

Additional Credits

Chapter 1
1-1, 1-5 © Linda Gheen

Chapter 2
Opener © Skedco, Inc.
2-1 © James Shaffer, PhotoEdit; 2-2 © Hiroyuki Matsumoto, Tony Stone Images; 2-3 © Spencer Grant, Liaison International; 2-4 © Craig Jackson, In the Dark Photography; 2-7: Reproduced with permission of the USDA and DHHS; 2-21 © U.S. Department of Transportation

Chapter 3
Opener © Craig Jackson, In the Dark Photography
3-4, © Craig Jackson, In the Dark Photography; 3-5 © Kenneth Murray, Photo Researchers Inc.; 3-7 © Linda Gheen; 3-8 © Bill Brett, Boston Globe

Chapter 4
4-8: Rolin Graphics

Chapter 6
Opener © Lt. Luis Fernandez, Metro-Dade Fire Rescue

Section 3
Opener © Bo Saunders, The Stock Market

Chapter 8
Opener © Linda Gheen
8-4: Reproduced with permission of the Maryland Institute of Emergency Medical Services System (MIEMSS); 8-8, 8-9 © Linda Gheen

Chapter 9
9-14 © Lawrence Migdale, Photo Researchers, Inc.; 9-15 © Linda Gheen

Chapter 10
Opener © Bruce Ayers, Tony Stone Images
10-6 Courtesy of Hartwell Medical

Section 4
Opener © Bruce Ayers, Tony Stone Images

Chapter 12
Opener © Kevin Anderson, Tony Stone Images
12-12: Rolin Graphics

Chapter 13
Opener: Courtesy of Laerdal Medical Corp.
13-10: Rolin Graphics; 13-17: Courtesy of Physio-Control Corp.; 13-18: Reproduced courtesy of the American Heart Association;

Chapter 14
Opener © Craig Jackson, In the Dark Photography

Chapter 16
Opener © Yellow Dog Prod., The Image Bank

Chapter 17
Opener © Craig Jackson, In the Dark Photography

Chapter 18
18-6A © Andrea Randolph; 18-19A © Charles Seaborn, Tony Stone Images; 18-19B © Doug Perrine, Innerspace Visions; 18-19C © Kevin McConnell

Chapter 20
20-10: Studio Montage; 20-11: Rolin Graphics

Chapter 21
Opener © Yuri Dojc, The Image Bank

Chapter 22
Opener © Bert Vandermark
22-12: Reproduced with permission. *Textbook of Pediatric Advanced Life Support,* 1994. © Copyright American Heart Association; 22-15, 22-16, 22-17: Reproduced with permission from *Mayo Clinic Complete Book of Pregnancy and Baby's First Year.* New York, NY, William Morrow and Co., 1994, © Mayo Foundation for Education and Research.

Chapter 23
Opener © Lew Long, The Stock Market
23-3: Reproduced with permission of the Maryland Institute of Emergency Medical Services System (MIEMSS); 23-6C: Rolin Graphics; 23-7, 23-8, 23-12: Reproduced with permission of the Maryland Institute of Emergency Medical Services System (MIEMSS)

Chapter 24
24-8: Rolin Graphics

Chapter 25
Opener © Craig Jackson, In the Dark Photography.
25-6 © Andrea Randolph

Chapter 26
Opener © Marc Romanelli, The Image Bank
26-5B, 26-6B, 26-7B, 26-8B: Rolin Graphics

Chapter 27
Opener © 1996 Tim McCandless

Chapter 31
31-15, 31-16: Reproduced with permission of the Maryland Institute of Emergency Medical Services System (MIEMSS); 31-21 © Craig Jackson, In the Dark Photography

Chapter 32
32-7 Rolin Graphics; 32-15 Fred Schall, NREMT-B

Section 6
Opener © Richard Gaul, FPG International

Chapter 33
Opener © Bruce Ayers, Tony Stone Images
33-3 © Linda Gheen; 33-18: Reproduced with permission. *Textbook of Pediatric Advanced Life Support,* 1994. © Copyright American Heart Association
33-20C, 33-22, 33-27: Rolin Graphics

Chapter 34
Opener © Linda Gheen
34-15A, 34-23: Rolin Graphics; 34-24: Reprinted with permission. D. P. Henderson and J. S. Seidel (eds.). *Pediatric Neurologic Assessment* (Los Angeles: Pediatric Rural Emergency Services System Education Project, Robert Wood Johnson Foundation, 1989).

Chapter 35
Opener © Bruce Ayers, Tony Stone Images
35-4: Rolin Graphics; 35-11 © Linda Gheen

Chapter 36
Opener © Andy Sacks, Tony Stone Images
36-1C, 36-2, 36-3: Courtesy of American Emergency Vehicles, Jefferson, NC.; 36-20 © A. Nance, FPG International; 36-22 © Linda Gheen

Chapter 37
Opener © Linda Gheen
37-1 © Spencer Grant, The Picture Cube; 37-2 © Linda Gheen; 37-4 © Kenneth Murray, Photo Researchers, Inc; 37-6 © Craig Jackson, In the Dark Photography; 37-8: Reproduced with permission of the Maryland Institute of Emergency Medical Services System (MIEMSS); 37-15, 37-16 © U.S. Department of Transportation; 37-17: Reproduced with permission of the Maryland Institute of Emergency Medical Services System (MIEMSS); 37-18 © U.S. Department of Transportation; 37-19 © Jay Higgins, Unicorn Stock Photos

Section 8
Opener © Adam Smith, FPG International

Chapter 39
Opener: Courtesy of Physio-Control Corp.

Photographs also supplied by Elizabeth Sawyer, Susan Steinkamp, Martin H. Simon, the American Academy of Orthopaedic Surgeons and Jones and Bartlett Publishers.

AAOS

Emer
Care and Transporta

Prepare for class, exams, and the field

These materials, especially designed for you, use realistic scenarios and challenging exercises to reinforce what you have learned and to focus your study time where it is needed. They were made specifically for the Seventh Edition of the "Orange Book" and are ideal for EMT students preparing for initial certification or veterans studying for recertification.

Student Workbook

The Student Workbook makes your study time more effective. Use it's additional review questions—focusing on curriculum objectives, basic concepts, and principles—to test your knowledge and review the answers provided to gauge your progress.
ISBN: 0-7637-0804-6

Student Review Manual, 3e

The Student Review Manual contains multiple-choice questions and great scenario-based exercises keyed to the Seventh Edition of the "Orange Book." Put your classroom knowledge to the test in realistic situations. Available in print and on computer disc. The disc generates a customized plan, guiding you to specific pages in the Seventh Edition for areas needing further study.
Text — **ISBN: 0-7637-1026-1**
Disk — **ISBN: 0-7637-1043-1**
Text and Disk — **ISBN: 0-7637-1042-3**

The Student Review Manual is also available online at **www.emtb.com**, for easy, instant access.

EMT-B Field Guide

This handy, full-color, pocket-sized reference will provide easy access to the vital emergency information you need. It's a great resource for fast review of important step-by-step procedures, offering just the right amount of information to guide your actions and reactions in the field. It also includes a prescription medication reference, a spell-checker, and documentation tips.
ISBN: 0-7637-0880-1

Order today by calling
Jones and Bartlett Publishers toll-free:
1-800-71-ORANGE
and visit us at www.emtb.com

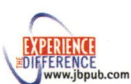